Oxford Textbook of

Advanced Heart Failure and Cardiac Transplantation

Oxford Textbook of
Advanced Heart Failure and Cardiac Transplantation

Edited by

Michael J. Domanski

Division of Cardiology, Peter Munk Center, University Health Network; the University of Toronto School of Medicine, Toronto, Canada; the Ichan School of Medicine at Mount Sinai, New York, NY, USA

Mandeep R. Mehra

Harvard Medical School; BWH Heart and Vascular Center, Brigham and Women's Hospital, Boston, MA, USA

Marc A. Pfeffer

Harvard Medical School; Cardiovascular Division, Brigham and Women's Hospital, Boston, MA, USA

OXFORD

UNIVERSITY PRESS

OXFORD
UNIVERSITY PRESS

Great Clarendon Street, Oxford, OX2 6DP,
United Kingdom

Oxford University Press is a department of the University of Oxford.
It furthers the University's objective of excellence in research, scholarship,
and education by publishing worldwide. Oxford is a registered trade mark of
Oxford University Press in the UK and in certain other countries

Impression: 3

Published in the United States of America by Oxford University Press
198 Madison Avenue, New York, NY 10016, United States of America

British Library Cataloguing in Publication Data
Data available

Library of Congress Control Number: 2015958813

ISBN 978–0–19–873487–1

Printed in Great Britain by
Bell & Bain Ltd., Glasgow

Foreword

During the last half century there have been extraordinary advances in the diagnosis and management of many forms of heart disease. A variety of drugs, devices, surgical and catheter-based interventions have resulted in dramatic reductions of morbidity and mortality of many cardiovascular disorders. For example, in the early 1960s, the one year mortality in patients with acute myocardial infarction who reached the hospital was about 50% and has been reduced to 10% since then. Surgical and catheter-based interventions have prolonged the lives of most patients with valvular and congenital heart disease. Hypertension can now be controlled with pharmacotherapy in the majority of patients. Patients at high risk of sudden cardiac death can be identified and this outcome can be prevented in many patients.

Concomitant with these spectacular advances, there has been a progressive and alarming increase in the prevalence of heart failure, which has become the most frequent diagnosis of hospital admission in Medicare patients. The development of heart failure has actually become the price of successful treatment of heart disease, and for many patients this price has been high indeed. How can this seeming paradox be explained? While the life of patients with most forms of heart disease has certainly been prolonged and its quality improved, with some exceptions the underlying condition is rarely cured. For example, while most patients with acute myocardial infarction now survive for years after the event, they often develop additional episodes of myocardial infarction which "chip away" at their remaining viable myocardium leading to left ventricular dysfunction and ultimately to heart failure. Similar scenarios play out in patients with hypertension, who might have died as a consequence of a hemorrhagic stroke in 1960, but who now develop heart failure later in life as a consequence of prolonged and progressive ventricular hypertrophy despite receiving antihypertensive drugs. While the development and more widespread use of implanted cardiac defibrillators has reduced sudden cardiac death, this treatment has increased the prevalence of patients who survive to develop failure of the myocardial pump. Co-morbidities such as diabetes mellitus, obesity, atrial fibrillation, chronic obstructive lung disease and severely reduced renal function, which are common in the elderly, increase the risk of heart failure in patients with the aforementioned underlying cardiac disorders.

Fortunately, there has been progress in the treatment of one form of heart failure—that which occurs in patients with reduced ejection fraction. However, while the prognosis in such patients has improved, this improvement is usually temporary, and after several years, the condition often progresses. Treatment of patients with heart failure and preserved ejection fraction as well as of patients with acute decompensated heart failure has improved relatively little in the last few decades. As a consequence, many patients with a history of heart failure enter a phase commonly known as advanced heart failure. This pre-morbid condition is the subject of this excellent book, edited by Michael Domanski, Marc Pfeffer, and Mandeep Mehra, three acknowledged leaders of this field. They have been joined by a team of expert co-authors and have produced a volume which reviews the fundamental pathobiology and pathophysiology of advanced heart failure, including right heart failure. It then goes on to describe and assess diagnostic procedures, pharmacologic and device management, and treatment with mechanical circulatory support and cardiac transplantation.

This well written, carefully edited book will be of great interest to clinicians faced with the challenge of caring for the growing number of patients with advanced heart failure. It will be of particular value to trainees who will join the ranks of specialists in advanced heart failure. It is this next generation who, in addition to providing care to these patients, will advance this importance branch of cardiology, and this book will help them on their journey.

Eugene Braunwald, M.D.
Boston, MA, USA

Contents

Contributors *ix*

Abbreviations *xi*

1 **Advanced heart failure in perspective** *1*
Marc A. Pfeffer, Michael J. Domanski, and Mandeep R. Mehra

2 **Cell biology of heart failure** *12*
Kenneth B. Margulies and J. Eduardo Rame

3 **Physiology and hemodynamic assessment of the failing heart: Current knowledge and unmet needs for advanced heart failure** *43*
J. Julia Shin, Mandeep R. Mehra, and Ileana L. Piña

4 **Transplantation immunology** *57*
James F. George

5 **Implantable devices for cardiovascular monitoring** *74*
Max J. Liebo and W. H. Wilson Tang

6 **Endomyocardial biopsy in the failing heart** *92*
Michael J. Domanski, Mark Halushka, and Sean P. Pinney

7 **Imaging in advanced heart failure** *102*
Mayank Kansal, Manish Bansal, Jagat Narula, and Partho P. Sengupta

8 **Pharmacologic management of advanced heart failure** *137*
Akshay S. Desai and Marc A. Pfeffer

9 **Arrhythmias in heart failure: The atrioventricular node and above** *153*
Steven Stevens, Kalyanam Shivkumar, and Noel G. Boyle

10 **Ventricular arrhythmias in heart failure** *165*
John D. Ferguson and John P. DiMarco

11 **Cardiac resynchronization** *179*
James P. Daubert, Brett Atwater, and Kevin Jackson

12 **Advanced heart failure in valvular heart disease** *202*
Blase A. Carabello

13 **High-risk heart failure surgery: Strategies for coronary artery bypass grafting and valve surgery in patients with reduced ejection fraction** *215*
Marzia Leacche, Garrick C. Stewart, and John G. Byrne

14 **Mechanical circulatory support: Patient selection, optimization, and in-patient management of the patient with a left ventricular assist device** *231*
Michael J. Domanski and Mandeep R. Mehra

15 **Mechanical circulatory support: Outpatient management** *248*
Mandeep R. Mehra and Michael J. Domanski

16 **Cardiac transplantation: Overview** *255*
Josef Stehlik MD, PhD and Joann Lindenfeld MD

17 **Immunosuppression strategies** *279*
Jon A. Kobashigawa

18 **Rejection surveillance: Types and treatment** *307*
Natasha Lipson Altman and Sean P. Pinney

19 **Complications after cardiac transplantation** *314*
Howard J. Eisen

20 **Right heart failure: Anatomy, physiology, and pathobiology** *329*
Thomas G. Di Salvo and Simon Maltais

21 **Right ventricular failure: Clinical features and management** *346*
Thomas G. Di Salvo and Simon Maltais

22 Pulmonary arterial hypertension *385*
Myung H. Park

23 End of life care in advanced heart failure *420*
Jessi Khangura and Sarah J. Goodlin

24 Future directions in advanced heart failure *427*
Michael J. Domanski, Mark A. Pfeffer, and Mandeep R. Mehra

Index *433*

Contributors

Natasha Lipson Altman University of Colorado Hospital, Aurora, CO, USA

Brett Atwater Duke University Medical Center, Durham, NC, USA

Manish Bansal Baptist Medical Center Jacksonville, Jacksonville, Florida, USA

Noel G. Boyle David Geffen School of Medicine at UCLA, Los Angeles, CA, USA

John G. Byrne Brigham and Women's Hospital, Boston, MA, USA

Blase A. Carabello Mount Sinai Beth Israel, NY, USA

James P. Daubert Duke University Medical Center, Durham, NC, USA

Akshay S. Desai Brigham and Women's Hospital, Boston, MA, USA

John P. DiMarco University of Virginia School of Medicine, Charlottesville, VA, USA

Thomas G. Di Salvo Vanderbilt Heart and Vascular Institute, Nashville, TN, USA

Michael J. Domanski Icahn School of Medicine and Mount Sinai School of Medicine, NY, USA and Peter Munk Cardiac Centre, University of Toronto, Canada

Howard J. Eisen Drexel University College of Medicine, Philadelphia, PA, USA

John D. Ferguson University of Virginia School of Medicine, Charlottesville, VA, USA

James F. George University of Alabama at Birmingham, Birmingham, AL, USA

Sarah J. Goodlin Oregon Health and Science University, Portland, OR, USA

Mark Halushka The John Hopkins Hospital, Baltimore, MD, USA

Kevin Jackson Duke University Medical Center, Durham, NC, USA

Mayank Kansal University of Illinois at Chicago, Chicago, IL, USA

Jessi Khangura Oregon Health and Science University, Portland, OR, USA

Jon A. Kobashigawa Cedars-Sinai Heart Institute, Los Angeles, CA, USA

Marzia Leacche Brigham and Women's Hospital, Boston, MA, USA

Max J. Liebo Stritch School of Medicine, Loyola University Chicago, Maywood, IL, USA

Joann Lindenfeld Vanderbilt University, Nashville, TN, USA

Simon Maltais Vanderbilt University Medical Center, Nashville, TN, USA

Kenneth B. Margulies Perelman School of Medicine at the University of Pennsylvania, Philadelphia, PA, USA

Mandeep R. Mehra Brigham and Women's Hospital, Boston, MA, USA

Jagat Narula Mount Sinai School of Medicine, New York

Myung H. Park University of Maryland Medical Center, Baltimore, MD, USA

Ileana L. Piña Montefiore Einstein Center for Heart and Vascular Care, NY, USA

Marc A. Pfeffer Brigham and Women's Hospital, Boston, MA, USA

Sean P. Pinney Mount Sinai School of Medicine, NY, USA

J. Eduardo Rame Perelman School of Medicine at the University of Pennsylvania, Philadelphia, PA, USA

Partho P. Sengupta Mount Sinai School of Medicine, NY, USA

J. Julia Shin Montefiore Medical Center, NY, USA

Kalyanam Shivkumar David Geffen School of Medicine at UCLA, Los Angeles, CA, USA

Josef Stehlik University of Utah School of Medicine, Salt Lake City, UT, USA

Steven Stevens David Geffen School of Medicine at UCLA, Los Angeles, CA, USA

Garrick C. Stewart Brigham and Women's Hospital, Boston, MA, USA

W.H. Wilson Tang Clever Clinic Lerner Research Institute, Cleveland, OH, USA

Abbreviations

ABIM	American Board of Internal Medicine
AC	adenylyl cyclase
AC	arrhythmogenic cardiomyopathy
ACC	American College of Cardiology
ACE	angiotensin converting enzyme
ACEI	angiotensin converting enzyme inhibitor
ACHD	adult congenital heart disease
ACLS	adult cardiac life support
ACR	acute cellular rejection
ACT	activated clotting time
ADCC	antibody-dependent cellular cytotoxicity
ADHF	acute decompensated heart failure
ADL	activities of daily living
AF	atrial fibrillation
AHA	American Heart Association
AHG	anti-human globulin
AMPK	AMP-sensitive kinase
AMR	antibody-mediated rejection
ANS	autonomic nervous system
APC	antigen presenting cells
AR	aortic regurgitation
ARB	angiotensin receptor blocker
ARVC	arrhythmogenic right ventricular cardiomyopathy
AS	aortic stenosis
ASD	atrial septal defect
ASE	American Society of Echocardiography
ASO	arterial switch operation
AT	atrial tachycardia
ATG	anti-thymocyte globulin
ATP	anti-tachycardia pacing
ATR	atrial tachycardia remodeling
AUC	area under the curve
AV	atrioventricular
AVA	aortic valve area
AVM	arteriovenous malformations
AVR	aortic valve replacement
AZA	azathioprine
BiVAD	biventricular assist device
BiVP	biventricular pacing
BMI	body mass index
BMV	balloon mitral valvotomy
BNP	brain natriuretic peptide
BR	breathing reserve
BTT	bridge to transplant
BUN	blood urea nitrogen
CABG	coronary artery bypass grafting
CAD	coronary artery disease
CARE	cholesterol and recurrent events
CARP	cardiac ankyrin repeat protein
CAV	cardiac allograft vasculopathy
cCTGA	congenitally corrected transposition of the great arteries
CDC	complement-dependent cytotoxicity
CHD	congenital heart disease
CHF	congestive heart failure
CI	cardiac index
CICR	calcium-induced calcium release
CIED	cardiovascular implantable electronic devices
CK	creatine kinase
CMR	cardiac magnetic resonance
CMV	cytomegalovirus
CNI	calcineurin inhibitor
CO	cardiac output
COPD	chronic obstructive pulmonary disease
CPAP	continuous positive airway pressure
CPET	cardiopulmonary exercise testing
CREB	CAMP response binding
CRT	cardiac resynchronization therapy
CS	coronary sinus
CSA	cyclosporine
CTD	connective tissue disease
CTEPH	chronic thromboembolic pulmonary hypertension
CTL	cytotoxic T lymphocyte
CTPH	chronic thromboembolic pulmonary hypertension
CTRD	cardiac transplant research database
CVP	central venous pressure
CXR	chest radiograph
DAMPS	damage-associated molecular patterns
DAVID	dual-chamber and vvi implantable defibrillator
DC	dendritic cell
DCD	donation after circulatory death
DENSE	displacement encoding with stimulated echoes
DSA	donor-specific antibodies
DSE	dobutamine stress-echocardiography

EBV	Epstein–Barr virus
ECG	electrocardiography
ECMO	extracorporeal membrane oxygenation
EDV	end-diastolic volume
EEPV	end-ejection pressure/volume
EF	ejection fraction
EGFR	epidermal growth factor receptor
ELISA	enzyme-linked immunosorbent assay
EMB	endomyocardial biopsy
EPR	external pressure reference
ER	endoplasmic reticulum
ERA	endothelial receptor antagonist
ESC	European Society of Cardiology
ESV	end-systolic volume
EVR	everolimus
FAC	fractional area change
FC	functional class
FDA	food and drug administration
FDG	fluorodeoxyglucose
FFA	free fatty acid
FHF	first heart field
FI	fluid index
FSV	forward stroke volume
FVC	forced vital capacity
GALT	gut-associated lymphoid tissue
GCM	giant cell myocarditis
GEP	gene expression profiling
GFR	glomerular filtration rate
GI	gastrointestinal
GLS	global longitudinal strain
GPCR	G-protein-coupled receptors
H&E	hematoxylin and eosin (strain)
HBV	hepatitis B virus
HCV	hepatitis C virus
HF	heart failure
HFpEF	heart failure with preserved ejection fraction
HFrEF	heart failure with reduced ejection fraction
HIT	heparin-induced thrombocytopenia
HLA	human leukocyte antigen
HMR	heart-to-mediastinum ratio
HPV	human papillomavirus
HRS	Heart Rhythm Society
HRV	heart rate variability
HTLV	human T-lymphotropic virus
IABP	intra-aortic balloon pump
ICD	implantable cardioverter defibrillator
ICU	intensive care unit
IDC	interdigitating dendritic cell
IHM	implantable hemodynamic monitors
INR	international normalized ratio
INTERMACS	Interagency Registry for Mechanically Assisted Circulatory Support
IPAH	idiopathic pulmonary arterial hypertension
IR	insulin resistance
IRIS	immediate risk stratification improves survival
ISHLT	International Society for Heart and Lung Transplantation
ITAMS	immune-receptor tyrosine based activation motifs
IVC	inferior vena cava
IVUS	intravascular ultrasound
JNK	jun N-terminal kinases
JVP	jugular venous pressure
KIR	killer immunoglobulin-like receptors
LA	left atrium
LAD	left anterior descending
LAO	left anterior oblique
LAP	left atrial pressure
LAS	lung allocation score
LBBB	left bundle branch block
LDH	lactate dehydrogenase
LFT	liver function test
LGE	late gadolinium enhancement
LIMA	left internal mammary artery
LM	lateral marginal
LV	left ventricle
LVAD	left ventricular assist device
LVEDP	left ventricular end-diastolic pressure
LVEDV	left ventricular end-diastolic volume
LVEF	left ventricular ejection fraction
LVFP	left ventricular filling pressure
LVH	left ventricular hypertrophy
LVOT	left ventricular outflow tract
LVP	left ventricular pacing
MAC	membrane attack complex
MAP	mean arterial pressure
MAPK	mitogen-activated protein kinase
MBL	mannose-binding lectin
MCS	mechanical circulatory support
MCV	middle cardiac vein
MHC	major histocompatibility complex
MI	myocardial infarction
MMF	mycophenolate mofetil
MPI	myocardial performance index
MPT	mitochondrial permeability transitions
MR	mitral regurgitation
MRS	magnetic resonance spectroscopy
MS	mitral stenosis
MSCT	multislice CT
MUGA	Multi Gated Acquisition Scan
MV	minute ventilation
MVR	mitral valve repair/replacement
MVV	maximum voluntary ventilation
NAION	nonarteritic anterior ischemic optic neuropathy
NAT	nucleic acid testing
NEM	necrotizing eosinophilic myocarditis
NFAT	nuclear factor of activated transcription
NHLBI	National Heart, Lung, and Blood Institute
NHR	nighttime heart rate
NIH	National Institutes of Health
NODM	new-onset diabetes mellitus
NPV	negative predictive value
NSAID	nonsteroidal anti-inflammatory drug
NYHA	New York Heart Association
OPCAB	off-pump coronary artery bypass
PA	pulmonary artery
PAC	pulmonary artery catheter
PAD	peripheral arterial disease
PAH	pulmonary arterial hypertension

PAM	patient advisory module
PAP	pulmonary artery pressure
PAWP	pulmonary arterial wedge pressure
PBMC	peripheral blood mononuclear cell
PCI	percutaneous coronary intervention
PCR	polymerase chain reaction
PCWP	pulmonary capillary wedge pressure
PDA	patent ductus arteriosus
PDA	posterior descending artery
PDGF	platelet-derived growth factor
PE	pulmonary embolism
PEA	peak endocardial acceleration
PEEP	positive end-expiratory pressure
PEP	pre-ejection period
PET	positron emission tomography
PFT	pulmonary function test
PH	pulmonary hypertension
PI	pulmonic insufficiency
PI	pulsatility index
PKA	*protein kinase A*
PKC	*protein kinase C*
PMA	phorbol myristate acetate
PND	paroxysmal nocturnal dyspnea
PPH	primary pulmonary hypertension
PR	pulmonary regurgitation
PRA	panel reactive antibody
PRES	posterior reversible encephalopathy syndrome
PS	pulmonic stenosis
PTLD	post-transplantation lymphoproliferative disorder
PVC	premature ventricular contraction
PVI	pulmonary vascular impedance
PVOD	pulmonary venous occlusive disease
PVR	pulmonary vascular resistance
QOL	quality of life
RA	right atrium
RAAS	renin–angiotensin–aldosterone system
RAP	right atrial pressure
RAVI	right atrial volume index
RBBB	right bundle branch block
RBC	red blood cells
RCA	right coronary artery
RCT	randomized controlled trial
RER	respiratory exchange ratio
RHC	right heart catheterization
RIMA	right internal mammary artery
RIP	receptor-interacting protein
RLC	regulatory light chain
ROC	receiver operating characteristic
RV	right ventricle
RVA	right ventricular apex
RVAD	right ventricular assist device
RVDP	right ventricular diastolic pressure
RVEF	right ventricular ejection fraction
RVFW	right ventricular free wall
RVMI	right ventricular myocardial infarction
RVOT	right ventricular outflow tract
RVSP	right ventricular systolic pressure
RVSWI	right ventricular stroke work index
RVWS	right ventricular wall stress
SAI	systolic area index
SCD	sudden cardiac death
SDI	systolic dyssynchrony index
SERCA	sarcoplasmic reticulum calcium ATPase
SFI	standard fluorescent intensity
SHF	second heart field; systolic heart failure
SM	sensor module
SMVT	sustained monomorphic ventricular tachycardia
SPECT	single photcon emission CT
SPI	solid-phase immunoassays
SR	sarcoplasmic reticulum; sinus rhythm
SSRI	selective serotonin reuptake inhibitor
STAR	speckle tracking and resynchronization
STE	speckle tracking echocardiography
STS	Society of Thoracic Surgeons
SV	stroke volume
SVC	superior vena cava
SVR	systemic vascular resistance
SVT	supraventricular tachycardia
SWI	stroke work index
TAC	transverse aortic constriction
TAH	total artificial heart
TAP	transporter associated with antigen processing
TAPSE	tricuspid annular plane systolic excursion
TARP	total atrial refractory period
TAVR	transcatheter aortic valve replacement
TCE	threshold-crossing event
TCR	T cell receptor
TDI	tissue Doppler imaging
TEE	transesophageal echocardiography
TNF	tumor necrosis factor
TOF	tetralogy of Fallot
TOR	target of rapamycin
TP	tachycardia pacing
TPG	transpulmonary gradient
TPR	total pulmonary resistance
TR	tricuspid regurgitation
TRP	transient receptor potential
TTE	transthoracic echocardiography
TV	tricuspid valve
TVM	tissue velocity mapping
UNOS	United Network for Organ Sharing
VA	ventricular arrhythmias
VAD	ventricular assist device
VCF	velocity of circumferential fiber
VEGF	vascular endothelial growth factor
VER	ventricular evoked response
VF	ventricular fibrillation
VIP	vasoactive intestinal peptide
VS	ventricular sensing
VSD	ventricular septal defect
VT	ventricular tachycardia
WHO	World Health Organization
WMA	wall motion abnormality

CHAPTER 1

Advanced heart failure in perspective

Marc A. Pfeffer MD PhD, Michael J. Domanski MD, and Mandeep R. Mehra MD

Introduction

Heart failure encompasses an extremely broad clinical syndrome which, despite its diverse etiologies, can uniformly lead to marked limitations in functional capacity with reduced quality and quantity of life. The syndrome is characterized by a constellation of signs and symptoms which are expressions of excessive intravascular volume and/or inadequate tissue perfusion.[1] Although multiple disorders of respiratory and renal function can also contribute to some of these signs and symptoms, an overarching inability of the heart to maintain adequate pump function without utilizing reserve mechanisms is fundamental for the diagnosis of heart failure.[2]

The reduction in the pump function of the heart may occur as the consequence of any of a multitude of abnormalities which distort the tightly coordinated aspects of the normally highly efficient cardiac performance. Impaired ventricular emptying (systolic dysfunction) is commonly characterized in clinical practice by reduced left ventricular ejection fraction. At the molecular level, this may result from any combination of either an intrinsic myofibrillar contractile defect (genetic or acquired) or loss of effective contractile mass from myocardial infarction, or myocarditis. However, disturbances in many other aspects of cardiac performance required for effective integrated cardiac function such as abnormal relaxation (lusitropy), inadequate coronary perfusion, electrical–mechanical dyssynchrony, arrhythmias, valvular stenosis or insufficiency, or commonly, combinations of these disorders that sufficiently impair the exquisitely integrated cardiac performance can result in the signs and symptoms of heart failure (Figure 1.1).

An evaluation during exercise may elicit more subtle abnormalities of cardiac function not apparent at rest to better delineate the connection of the heart to the clinical diagnosis of heart failure.[3] Even in the absence of an overt abnormality of cardiac structure of function, under extreme circumstances such as those produced by malignant hypertension or pheochromocytoma,[4,5,6,7] highly excessive loading conditions can exceed normal reserve capacity of the ventricle resulting in the transient appearance of heart failure in the context of intrinsically normal myocardial function. Many of the etiological pathways that precede the clinical appearance of symptomatic heart failure can be attributed to a less intense but more sustained hyperfunctional state imposed on the myocardium.[8]

An expanding number of genetic mutations encoding for a variety of cytoskeletal and mitochondrial abnormalities are being identified as causal factors for several dilated cardiomyopathies.[9] However, less well understood complex polygenetic environmental temporal interactions must currently be invoked for the vast majority of clinical heart failure, which is commonly preceded by hypertension and or coronary artery disease. The established concept of an initial adaptive (physiologic) hypertrophy where structural alterations are initially associated with an increased capacity to sustain these excessive workloads but can eventually lead to pathologic hypertrophy with an exhaustion of compensatory reserve and more overt cardiac dysfunction continues to be supported by longitudinal data.[8,10,11] In both experimental animal models and human studies a consistent temporal pattern has emerged that prolonged hyperfunction of a cardiac chamber can result in altered genotypic expression (shift towards a fetal or neonatal pattern) with a subsequent alteration in several cascades of signaling pathways that have been frequently identified in hypertrophied myocytes.[12,13,14] If sustained, these unfavorable molecular shifts lead to perturbations in calcium cycling, altered properties of β-adrenergic receptors, mitochondria, and key sarcomeric proteins (actin, myosin, titin), which have each been associated with the reduced contractile function observed in pathologic hypertrophy.[15,16,17,18] Imbalances in the signaling pathways for cell growth, cell death (apoptosis, necrosis, proteotoxicity), maladaptive autophagy, as well as the newly appreciated capacity to regenerate and repair, also appear to play important roles in the molecular mechanisms associated with this deterioration of cardiac performance[12,19,20,21] as well as perturbations of the histological balances in the relative tissue composition between myoctes, interstitial connective, and vascular elements.[22]

On a more macroscopic structural basis, sustained impairments in cardiac performance are also generally associated with enlargements of cardiac chambers often termed adverse ventricular remodeling. As opposed to acute distention, where the volume of the ventricle is increased due to raised filling pressure (operating on a higher portion of the pressure–volume curve), chronic dilatation or remodeling represents an actual structural change wherein the pressure–volume curve is shifted to the right with higher cavity volumes at the same filling pressure.[23] Distention is an effective short-term means of raising stroke volume by the Frank–Starling mechanism. Ventricular remodeling can also be considered as a mechanism of facilitating the restoration of stroke volume in the setting of loss of contractile function, since a structurally larger

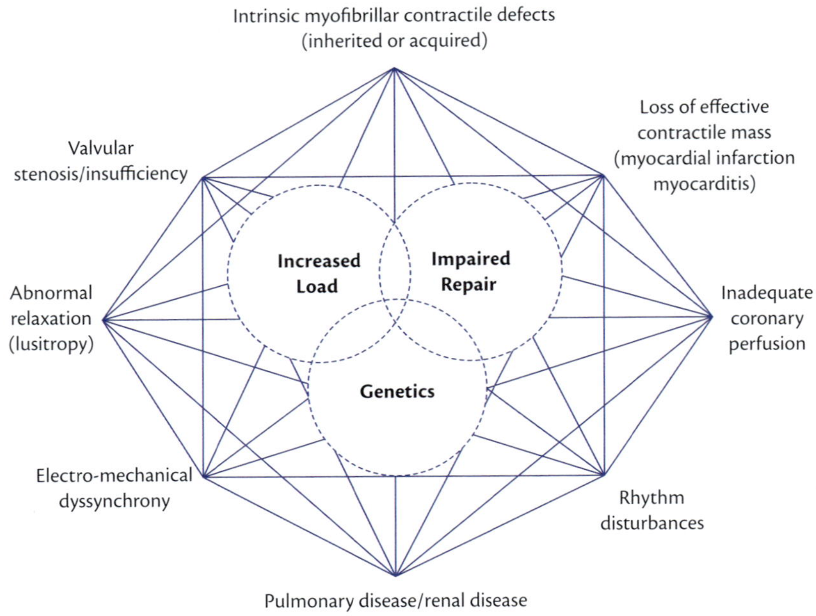

Fig. 1.1 Mosaic representation of the multifaceted aspects of cardiac performance that can contribute to cardiac dysfunction.

ventricular cavity requires less fractional shortening to eject a normal stroke volume.[24] However, based on the Laplace relationship, as a consequence of the larger radius, there is an important pathophysiologic offsetting increase in wall stress.[25] Some degree of structural ventricular enlargement may be considered as an adaptive mechanism to compensate for the loss of effective contractile tissue. The progressive nature of ventricular remodeling (a vicious cycle of enlargement begetting higher wall stress and more remodeling) makes this structural change maladaptive in the long run.[26,27,28]

Although the presence of abnormalities in any of the highly integrated aspects of cardiac performance or structure can be anticipated to result in heart failure, the converse is also true that similar findings can be present in asymptomatic individuals. Moreover, the degree of the cardiac performance abnormality is a limited predictor of symptoms or functional state.[29] Despite statistical associations between quantitative measures of cardiac function such as left ventricular ejection fraction (LVEF) and functional limitations (symptoms or exercise capacity) within large cohorts, these correlations are at best only modest.[30,31,32,33] Indeed, almost all of the abnormalities of cardiac performance can be identified to some extent in individuals with minimal or no symptoms. Just as experienced physicians are no longer surprised by patients with clinically important coronary or valvular heart disease who appear to have normal functional capacity, on an individual level, the finding of reduced LVEF or marked chamber enlargement does not in itself provide sufficient insight to permit a reliable estimate of functional status. Consider that some patients with heart failure and preserved ejection fraction (HFpEF) can be markedly symptomatic and limited, whereas a person with asymptomatic left ventricular dysfunction may have an excellent functional capacity despite an abnormal cardiac function and geometry. Acknowledging these limitations of structural and functional determinations on the assessment of functional capacity on an individual basis, in population studies the extent of these abnormalities have been consistently associated with a heightened risk for developing symptomatic heart failure and/or cardiovascular death.[34,35]

Crossing the clinical threshold from asymptomatic to symptomatic

NYHA classification system

Notwithstanding mechanistically diverse etiologies and the array of abnormalities of cardiac function as well as structure, it is the presence and magnitude of signs and symptoms that bestow some uniformity on both the diagnosis and prognosis across this broad syndrome encompassed by the clinical term heart failure. Since the diagnosis of heart failure covers such a broad range of severity from the compensated ambulatory fully functional to the bedridden mechanically supported patient, more refinement in categorization is needed. The time-honored New York Heart Association (NYHA) classification system was introduced in 1928 as a way of providing a description of an individual's physical limitations during the performance of daily activities.[36] The NYHA classification has consistently proven its value as a major instrument to not only assess disease severity but also provide important information regarding prognosis. The deceptively simple classification (class I, no symptoms or limitations; class II, mild shortness of breath during ordinary activities slightly limiting ordinary activities; class III, marked limitations with even less than ordinary activities but comfortable at rest; and class IV, severe limitations experiencing symptoms even at rest), continues to be an extremely useful and powerful tool to communicate disease severity for both the individual patient as well as cohorts in clinical trials, epidemiologic surveys, and administrative databases. Indeed, in everyday clinical parlance across the globe during exchange of clinical coverage and sign-out rounds, the description of a patient with heart failure is generally preceded by the designation of their NYHA class.

The very nature of the NYHA classification indicates that within the diagnosis of heart failure, there is a wide range of functional limitations. It is also well recognized that the NYHA class provides an important indicator of the likelihood for subsequent fatal and nonfatal heart failure events. All other factors being similar, a patient with NYHA class I or II would be anticipated to have a better life expectancy and fewer nonfatal heart-failure-related serious events than a comparable patient with more substantial limitations (NYHA III and IV).[37,38,39,40]

Experienced physicians, however, appreciate and understand the limitations of the subjective NYHA functional class and other symptom-based classification systems. An individual patient's status may fluctuate considerably. Fortunately, symptoms can frequently be mitigated with increases in physical capacity. Conversely, clinical condition can progressively or abruptly deteriorate. The NYHA classification figures prominently in all of the major stratification scores systems of heart failure prognosis,[37,38,39,40] and continues as the main severity categorization for the most recent European Society of Cardiology (ESC) guidelines for the diagnosis and treatment of acute and chronic heart failure.[41]

AHA/ACC guidelines

The American Heart Association/American College of Cardiology (AHA/ACC) guideline for the diagnosis and management of heart failure in adults, introduced in 2001, provided a new contextual framework to characterize this spectrum of heart failure and its treatments.[42] This four-stage (A, B, C, D) classification underscores the progressive nature of heart failure and additionally provides an important stage specific framework to consider opportunities for therapeutic interventions to lower the odds of both developing heart failure or progressing to the higher morbidity and mortality heart failure (Figure 1.2). This system was introduced in the setting of heart failure practice guidelines to improve the utilization of evidence-based approaches to prevent as well as manage heart failure. As such, it offers recommendations for therapies and goals in relation to disease severity and prognosis. The recommendations of the guidelines represent an attempt to better optimize the intensity of treatment considering risk/benefit assessments.[43,44]

Stages A and B designate those without signs and symptoms of heart failure and define "at-risk" populations. Although patients in these two stages would not be diagnosed as having heart failure, by highlighting two asymptomatic stages (A, at high risk for heart failure without structural heart disease; B, structural heart disease without signs or symptoms of heart failure), the task force committee appropriately emphasized that to a large extent heart failure should be considered a preventable disease. However, an effective population-based preventive strategy would require both improvements in detection of at-risk individuals along with greater implementation of proven deterrent approaches.[43]

For those at the lowest risk—stage A—the recommendations focus on nonpharmacologic lifestyle measures such as smoking cessation and, where appropriate, addressing obesity and encouraging more physical activity. These general wellness-promoting actions are of minimal risk as well as cost and are generally prudent approaches to lower the chances of developing heart failure (as well as atherosclerotic diseases). Identifying and effectively treating hypertension, diabetes, and lipid disorders are the earliest recommendations for long-term pharmacologic therapy, which for individuals in stage A, represent preventive measures for heart failure.[45,46,47,48,49,50,51,52]

The designation of stage B (structural heart disease but without signs or symptoms of heart failure) requires additional imaging

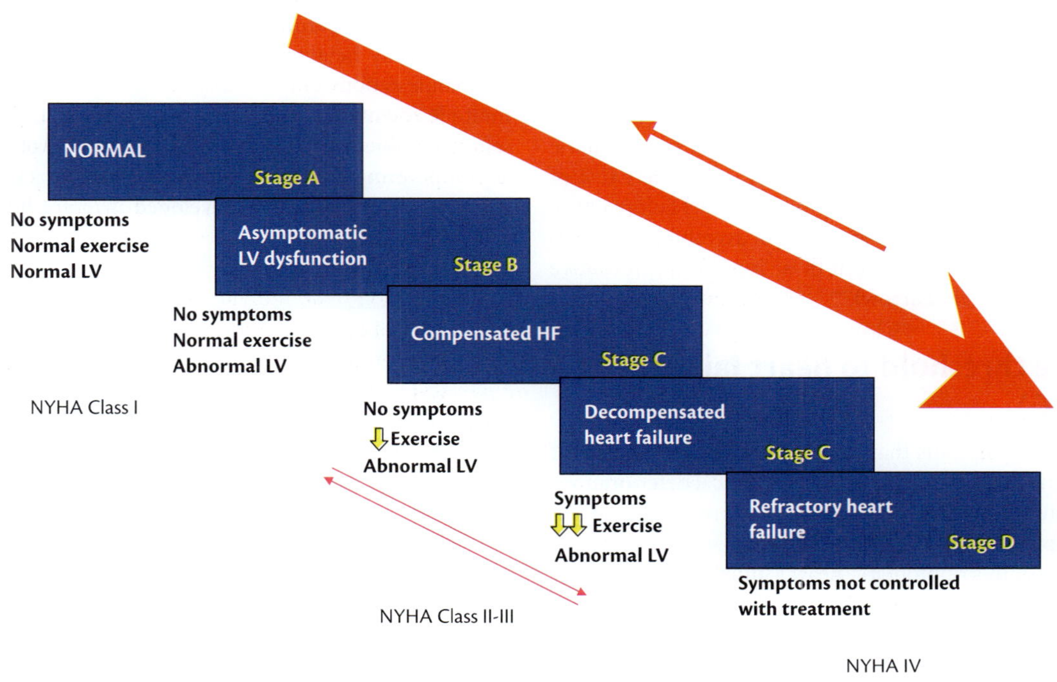

Fig. 1.2 Schematic depiction of the progression of heart failure using the ACC/AHA Guidelines for the Evaluation and Management of Heart Failure in the Adult. This adaptation superimposes NYHA functional class on the stages to emphasize that stages A and B represent asymptomatic conditions.

Adapted from Hunt SA, Baker DW, Chin MH, Cinquegrani MP, Feldmanmd AM, Francis GS, et al. ACC/AHA Guidelines for the Evaluation and Management of Chronic Heart Failure in the Adult: Executive Summary A Report of the American College of Cardiology/American Heart Association Task Force on Practice Guidelines (Committee to Revise the 1995 Guidelines for the Evaluation and Management of Heart Failure).

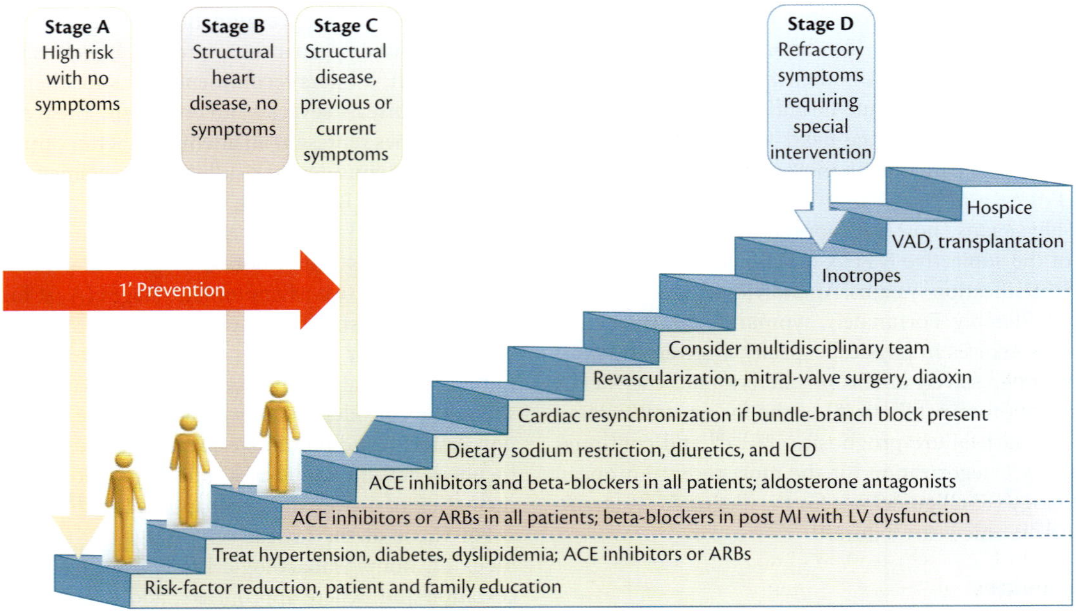

Fig. 1.3 Opportunities to prevent heart failure in AHA/ACC stages A and B.
Adapted from Jessup M, Brozena S. Heart failure. N Engl J Med 2003;348(20):2007–18.

or electrocardiographic evidence of a cardiac abnormality that augments the risk of developing heart failure. To a large extent, the justification for this additional screening for cardiac structural involvement stems from the results of both Studies Of Left Ventricular Dysfunction (SOLVD) Prevention and the Survival And Ventricular Enlargement (SAVE) trials, which both demonstrated that the strategy to identify and treat even asymptomatic persons with reduced LVEF with an angiotensin-converting enzyme inhibitor (ACEI), was effective in preventing the clinical appearance of heart failure and reducing mortality.[53,54] In the updated guidelines,[55] the higher risk of both heart failure and sudden unexpected death in stage B compared to A, coupled with clinical trial data demonstrating that interventions (ACEI, β-blockers and for some an implantable cardioverter defibrillator) can lower their risk of dying or progressing to developing symptomatic heart failure (stage C), further justified the additional screening of asymptomatic individuals to identify for the initiation of these long-term preventive interventions (Figure 1.3, red arrow).[56,57,58,59,60,61,62,63,64,65,66]

Crossing the threshold to heart failure (stage B to C)

Once the signs and symptoms that lead to the clinical diagnosis of heart failure are manifest, the risks for further clinical deteriorations and death escalate greatly. The marked negative prognostic impact of this crossing of the clinical threshold from asymptomatic ventricular dysfunction to symptomatic heart failure was also clearly demonstrated by the SOLVD investigators. The SOLVD program simultaneously conducted two of the pioneering randomized clinical trials comparing the differences in survival with use of an ACEI to placebo in subjects with reduced LVEF (<35%).[53,67] Enrollment into the SOLVD Treatment arm was predicated on physician-designated presence of symptomatic heart failure whereas in the concurrently conducted SOLVD Prevention, the entry criterion was the absence of a clinical diagnosis of heart failure. Since by design all patients had low LVEF, symptomatic status was the major difference between those enrolled in the Prevention and Treatment arms of SOLVD. The 1-year mortality rate in the asymptomatic left ventricular dysfunction Prevention group of approximately 4%, though much higher than anticipated from the general age- and sex-matched population, was still decisively better than for those classified as symptomatic. Indeed, the 12% annualized mortality rate of the Treatment cohort was nearly threefold higher than that of the low LVEF asymptomatic subjects in the Prevention arm of SOLVD (Figure 1.4).

This greatly heightened risk of death associated with the clinical manifestations of heart failure continues to be apparent within multiple recent clinical trials of diverse populations, even those not selecting subjects with reduced LVEF. In the Antihypertensive and Lipid-Lowering Treatment to Prevent Heart Attack Trial (ALLHAT), the 1761 participants that developed incident heart failure had a

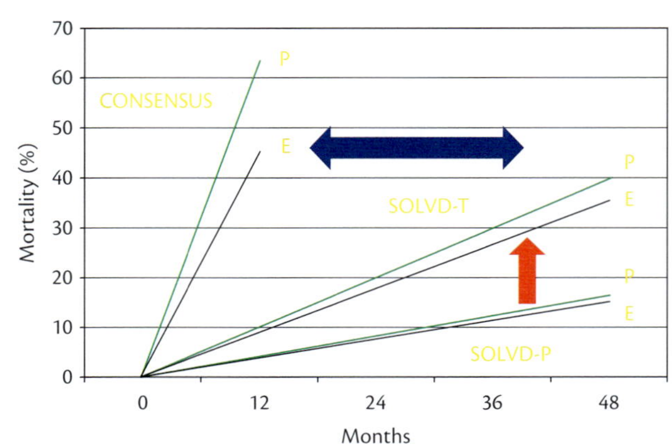

Fig. 1.4 Survival rate differences in asymptomatic people with left ventricular dysfunction[53] compared to symptomatic patients with same range of ejection fraction[67] indicated by the red arrow. Survival rate differences in trials of symptomatic heart failure patients are indicated by the blue arrow.[67,96]

nearly threefold risk of death compared to the other 31 043 with hypertension who did not, even with adjustments for several important demographic factors.[47] Similarly, within the population of patients with a prior myocardial infarction without a history of heart failure, enrolled in the Cholesterol And Recurrent Events (CARE) trial, the risk of death amongst 243 patients (6.3%) who developed heart failure during the 5 years of observation was eightfold higher than in the CARE patients who did not manifest heart failure.[68]

Survivors of a myocardial infarction (MI) represent an expanding reservoir of stage B candidates to develop incident heart failure (stage C). In the Framingham cohort, a history of a prior MI was associated with a 10-fold higher risk of manifesting heart failure.[69] Although hospital mortality of elderly patients (>65 years) experiencing a first myocardial infarction has declined in the last decade, over three-fourths of them develop heart failure or die within the subsequent 5 years.[70,71]

Even transient heart failure during an acute MI worsens prognosis. The clinical recognition of pulmonary congestion (rales) promptly emerged, in the early coronary care unit experiences, as one of the most important clinical discriminators for greater risk of death.[72,73] In the setting of an acute MI, even the transient appearance of clinical signs or symptoms consistent with pulmonary congestion (Killip 2 and higher) greatly augmented the risk of death or development of heart failure (Figure 1.5).[74] This worrisome intersection between MI and heart failure continues in the modern era and across the entire range of acute coronary syndromes.[75]

Measurements of circulating biomarkers, particularly the cardiac-derived markers of wall stress such as natriuretic peptides and troponin, as an indicator of myocyte necrosis have already added to the discriminative models for predicting the development of heart failure and death.[76,77,78,79,80] However, unlike LVEF, data demonstrating that the ascertainment of these biomarkers would lead to the detection of previously unidentified individuals who would derive benefits from a specific therapy are currently needed to justify this additional screening of asymptomatic individuals.[81]

Stage C: Structural heart disease with prior or current symptoms of heart failure

Though much of the burden of heart failure can be prevented or deferred, the reality is that symptomatic heart continues to be the dominant cardiovascular problem in elderly people.[82] Each year in the United States alone, over half a million new patients cross the threshold from stage B to C to become part of the 5 million living with the clinical diagnosis of symptomatic heart failure, double the prevalence of only 25 years ago.[83,84]

Although heart failure is seen in all age groups, it becomes increasingly, almost exponentially, more prevalent with advancing age (Figure 1.6).[82] In the Rotterdam study of a general population, heart failure was diagnosed in 1% individuals aged between 55 and 64 years, 3% from age 65 to 74 years, 7% from age 75 to 84 years, and over 10% for patients 85 years or age and over.[85] A US study of heart failure prevalence showed a similar increase with age, affecting more than 20% of those over 80 years of age. At 40 years of age, 1 in 9 men and 1 in 6 women can be anticipated to develop symptomatic heart failure (stage B to C) over their subsequent lifespan.[86]

Heart failure is therefore often considered a disease of aging attributed to the convergence of a number of contributing age-related disease processes such as coronary artery disease (more survivors of MI), hypertension, diabetes, and obesity. As a result of both its prevalence in the aging population and impact on the risk

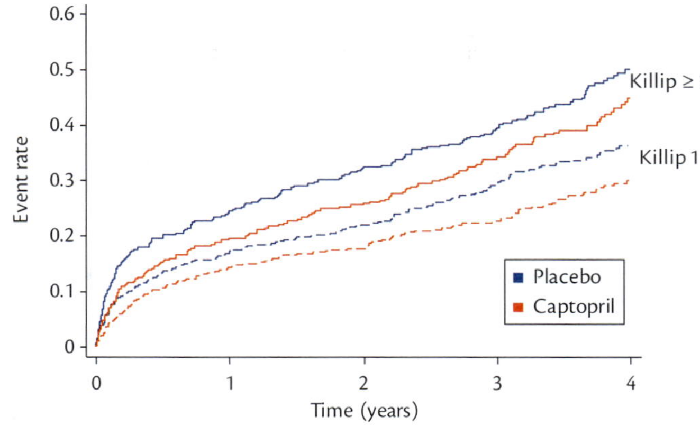

Fig. 1.5 Survival following myocardial infarction in those with (Killip ≥2) and without (Killip 1) pulmonary congestion, from the SAVE study.[54,74] The reduction in risk of death with randomization to captopril was observed in both groups.
Adapted from Moye LA, Pfeffer MA, Wun C, Davis BR, Geltman E, Hayes D, et al. Uniformity of captopril benefit in the SAVE study: Subgroup Analysis. European Heart Journal (1994);15(Suppl B):2-8 by permission of Oxford University Press.

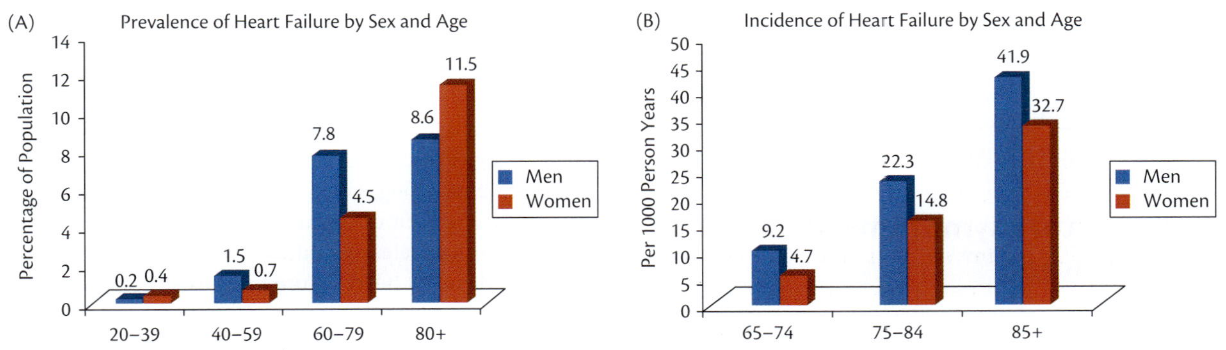

Fig. 1.6 Influence of age on prevalence (A) and incidence (B) of heart failure.
Adapted from Go AS, Mozaffarian D, Roger VL, Benjamin EJ, Berry JD, Borden WB, et al. Heart Disease and Stroke Statistics—2013 Update: A Report From the American Heart Association. Circulation 2013;127(1):e6-e245.

of developing heart failure, hypertension remains the most common underlying factor for heart failure on a population attributable basis.[87] Beyond the age of 70 years, heart failure is the most common reason for hospitalization.[84,88,89,90]

The devastating impact on prognosis, attending the development of heart failure symptoms, was well demonstrated by the classic population-based longitudinal cardiovascular epidemiologic studies. In the Framingham Heart Study, crossing the clinical threshold to the diagnosis of heart failure was associated with a 5-year mortality of ~50%.[91] Using a countrywide administrative database, Scottish investigators have shown that the 1-year mortality following a first hospitalization for heart failure, though improving, is still approximately 25%.[71] These, and many other comparisons of those with heart failure to their age- and sex-matched peers, provide powerful and consistent data regarding the medical and economic disease-related burdens across different countries.[41,92,93,94] However, within the diagnosis of heart failure, there is a well-recognized extremely broad spectrum of severity that must also be considered to gain fuller insights into the devastating personal as well as economic impacts of this clinical syndrome.[95] For example, in early clinical trials such as CONSENSUS,[96] the annualized mortality rate was approximately 50%, whereas in SOLVD-T[67] it was 10% (see Figure 1.4, blue arrow). Both groups are encompassed by stage C.

Despite this admittedly extensive range of severities under the unifying diagnosis of heart failure, the AHA/ACC Guidelines for the Diagnosis and Management of Heart Failure in Adults Committee choose to use only two stages to encompass all patients with symptomatic heart failure: C (structural heart disease with current or prior symptoms of heart failure) and D (refractory heart failure requiring specialized interventions) (see Figures 1.2 and 1.3). Fortunately, the vast majority of patients with symptomatic heart failure are classified in stage C rather than stage D. As with all prior stages, the goals of stage C are to build on prior strategies to prevent progression by adding appropriate use of evidenced-based therapies and devices to reduce symptoms and prolong survival. Over the past 30 years, compelling evidence from multiple high-quality randomized clinical outcome trials targeting these patients with reduced LVEF and symptomatic heart failure has resulted in proof that use of several classes of pharmacologic therapies and defibrillator/pacing devices can reduce episodes of clinical deterioration and/or prolong survival.[97] Several international societies have produced "practice guidelines" with evidence-graded recommendations.[41,43,94,98] The consistency of these authoritative documents and the relatively high number of grade 1A recommendations is a testament to the reliable evidence for improvements in clinical outcomes with multiple non-mutually-exclusive interventions (Chapter 8). Translating these discoveries into clinical practice has made a measurable positive impact.[43,99]

Stage D: Refractory symptoms requiring special intervention

Clinical status is of course not stagnant and apparently stable patients with heart failure may improve or experience a worsening of their symptoms. Often the adverse episodes or either chronic or acute decompensation can be addressed by adjustments in medical regimens. However, not infrequently, the consequences of either pulmonary congestion and/or hypoperfusion are so severe

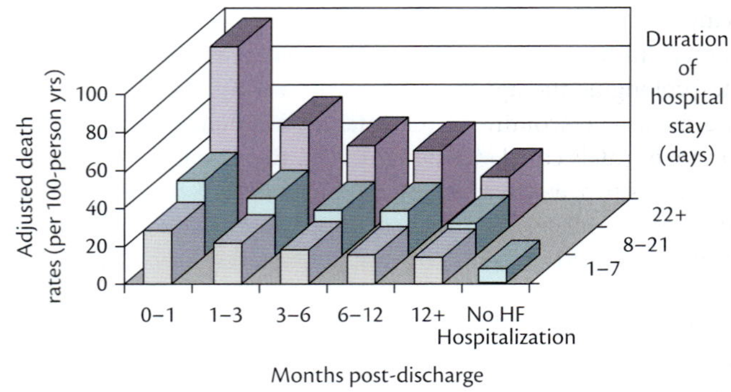

Fig. 1.7 The hazard of death is highest after a recent hospitalization for heart failure, and is exacerbated in those with a more prolonged stay compared to patients who are not hospitalized.

Data from the CHARM program: Braunwald E. The management of heart failure: the past, the present, and the future. Circulation: Heart Failure 2008;1(1):58–62.

and overall clinical status becomes so fragile that hospitalization is warranted. This inpatient care is considered necessary to provide the level of observation needed during this precarious period for the frequent medication adjustments made to manage symptoms and attempt to restore the patient to their prior baseline ambulatory activities. As the leading discharge diagnosis in the Medicare population, such heart failure-related hospitalizations are common.[84,88,89] These episodes of clinical deterioration requiring hospitalization are, unfortunately, much more than a bump in the road since they represent important clinical demarcations with lasting consequences (Figure 1.7).[100] Readmission and 30-day, all-cause, risk-standardized mortality rates are estimated at 24.56% and 11.17%, respectively.[101] Even within the hospitalized category, there are those who succumb to pump failure death, those patients who are managed with adjustments in their medications (stage C), and others who require ventilator and/or mechanical circulatory support to maintain adequate perfusion (stage D).

Refractory symptoms requiring special intervention (stage D) designates the most advanced severity of the AHA/ACC heart failure spectrum (see Figure 1.3). Terms like advanced, decompensated, recalcitrant, NYHA IV, end-stage, and refractory can all be used as descriptive adjectives before the words heart failure to effectively connote the extent, gravity, and precariousness of this most serious clinical condition. Others had previously highlighted that a significant minority of patients continue to do poorly despite conventional therapy; Adams and Zannad used a combination of poor functional status (NYHA III–IV), low LVEF (<30%) and limited exercise capacity (peak oxygen consumption <14 ml kg^{-1} min^{-1}) to identify and define an advanced heart failure cohort.[102] The study group of the Heart Failure Association of the ESC incorporated physical signs of congestion/poor perfusion, additional objective measurements, along with a history of a recent hospitalization for heart failure in their definition of advanced chronic heart failure.[41] Both definitions clearly indicate that these adverse conditions defining advanced heart failure must exist despite attempts to use and optimize proven therapies.

The AHA/ACC chose to incorporate the terms "refractory" and "requiring specialized interventions" to characterize this most worrisome of its categories of heart failure.[42,55] This important but fortunately small minority of patients who do not respond to the usual measures to alleviate their symptoms remain markedly symptomatic despite escalations in their medical therapy. Indeed, in many instances the disease progression is so severe that previous life-prolonging therapies are no longer hemodynamically tolerated and must be discontinued (Chapter 8). Many of these individuals cannot be safely cared for in the home setting and require extraordinary measures and support. That there is no absolute or uniformly accepted definition for this most severe category of heart failure is reminiscent of the citation from US Supreme Court Justice Potter Stewart "I know it when I see it" regarding hard-core pornography (Jacobellis v. Ohio, 378 U.S. 184, 1964).[103] For these patients with stage D heart failure, it may be more appropriate to add "and did not respond favorably to conventional therapies" to the justice's famous quote. Regardless of the precise definition of stage D heart failure, it is estimated that this group represents 2–5% of the symptomatic heart failure population in the US, which translates into approximately 200 000 individuals with advanced heart failure, and this number is anticipated to continue to grow.[82,84,104,105] The most recent ACCF/AHA guidelines offer some useful clinical features to identify these stage D patients (Table 1.1).[55]

This most challenging and fragile group of advanced heart failure patients disproportionately experiences the greatest healthcare burdens on individual, familial, and societal levels. An expanding number of healthcare providers have devoted their professional efforts to address the multiple challenges posed by these patients with stage D heart failure. The care for these most severely ill patients far exceeds that which can be expected to be offered by even the most capable and conscientious individual practitioner. Addressing these expanding needs has spawned new multidisciplinary teams. Consider how the advent of cardiac transplantation led major referral centers to garner the collective skills, expertise, and experience required to offer that resource-intensive service to "a significant minority" of highly selected patients. Subspecialists within cardiac surgery, cardiology, immunology, infectious diseases, nursing, and social services aligned within the selected institutions made the commitment to provide this extraordinary level of collective expertise and resources to offer cardiac transplantation.[106] It rapidly became apparent that the numbers of cardiac transplants performed at these specialized centers grossly underestimated the extent of the full clinical services rendered. Referrals to these multidisciplinary heart failure groups went beyond screening of potential transplant candidates. These self-selected teams rendered their specialized collective care to an expanding pool of advanced heart failure patients, many of whom were unlikely to become cardiac transplant recipients. As the patient populations being treated and the clinical services offered expanded, "advanced heart failure" rather than "transplant cardiology" became a better descriptor of the escalating medical activities of these affinity groups. Innovations in electrophysiological devices with randomized trials generating convincing evidence for morbidity and mortality benefits with the appropriate use of cardiac resynchronization therapy (CRT) and implantable cardioverter defibrillators (ICDs) fostered even greater collaborations with additional subspecialists (Chapters 9, 10, 11).[107,108,109,110,111] As the services of these groups specializing in the care of patients with advanced heart failure expanded, their referral base broadened well beyond potential candidates for cardiac transplantation.

Table 1.1 INTERMACS criteria which further discriminate patients with advanced heart failure beyond NYHA class

INTERMACS level	NYHA class	Shorthand
1	IV	"Crash and burn"
2	IV	"Sliding fast" on inotropes
3	IV	"Stable" on continuous inotropes
4	Ambulatory IV	Symptoms at rest
5	Ambulatory IV	"Housebound" Comfortable at rest, symptoms with minimal activity
6	IIIB	"Walking wounded" Meaningful activity limited
7	III	Advanced class III

Adapted from reference 115 (Stevenson LW, Pagani FD, Young JB, et al. INTERMACS profiles of advanced heart failure: the current picture. J Heart Lung Transplant 2009;28(6):535–41.)

An even clearer distinguishing feature of institutions committed to the care of patients with advanced heart failure was made by those centers that added the capability of offering relatively long-term mechanical circulatory support for the most hemodynamically compromised patients to their therapeutic armamentarium. The demonstration of improvements in both the quantity and quality of life with use of a pulsatile left ventricular assist device (LVAD) compared to optimized intensive medical therapy offered a strong impetus for the consolidation of the intense human and physical resources needed to effectively provide these highly specialized services.[112] The use of the LVAD as "destination therapy" for refractory patients, even those not considered candidates for cardiac transplantation, greatly expanded the population served by these advanced heart failure units. The more recent demonstration of further improvements in patient outcomes with the newer generation of nonpulsatile LVADs afforded even greater evidence for offering mechanical support for expanded number of stage D heart failure patients and the clinical workloads of these specialized centers.[113] The accompanying growth in services and referrals underscored that offering this level of care to patients with advanced heart failure requires an institutional team commitment exceeding what even the most talented and dedicated individual physicians could offer.

Advanced heart failure/heart transplantation as a distinct subspecialty

Patients with stage C heart failure are commonly encountered in medical practice and are most often treated by cardiologists, internists, or other healthcare providers. For this vast majority of heart failure patients, a physician well versed in the applicable guidelines with a background of knowledge and experience common to cardiovascular medicine training programs is appropriate and suitable.[114] However, the stage D patients, the 1–2% "refractory" individuals who remain incapacitated despite reasonable attempts with conventional therapies, are generally best served by the team approach offered at specialized advanced heart failure centers. Investigators cooperating on the Interagency Registry of Mechanically Assisted Circulatory Support (INTERMACS) report have offered a classification profile as a modern expansion for the NYHA class III–IV heart failure patients into seven categories.[115] As with the AHA/ACC stages, this "profiling" attempts to improve selection for the

Box 1.1 Clinical features useful for the identification of patients with stage D heart failure[55]

- Repeated (≥2) hospitalizations or Emergency Department visits for heart failure in the past year
- Progressive deterioration in renal function—e.g., rise in blood urea nitrogen (BUN) and creatinine
- Weight loss without other cause (e.g., cardiac cachexia)
- Intolerance to angiotensin converting enzyme (ACE) inhibitors due to hypotension and/or worsening renal function
- Intolerance to β-blockers due to worsening heart failure or hypotension
- Frequent systolic blood pressure <90 mmHg
- Persistent dyspnea with dressing or bathing requiring rest
- Inability to walk one block on the level ground due to dyspnea or fatigue
- Recent need to escalate diuretics to maintain volume status, often reaching daily furosemide equivalent dose >160 mg/day and/or use of supplemental metolazone therapy
- Progressive decline in serum sodium, usually to <133 mEq/L
- Frequent ICD shocks

expanding therapeutic approaches including mechanical circulatory support (Box 1.1). Titrating conventional therapies, deciding which patients are likely to benefit from revascularization, valve surgery, mechanical circulatory assistance, heart transplantation, and/or other "advanced" therapies including end-of-life care: all these are sensitive to individual patient preferences, requiring a definable body of knowledge, skills, and experience that are not generally sufficiently encountered even during a fellowship in cardiovascular medicine.[116]

As particular knowledge and experience is needed for the practice of interventional cardiology or electrophysiology, there is an analogous, though different, specialized body of knowledge and training needed to properly care for these fragile patients with advanced heart failure. The leadership of the Heart Failure Society of America provided the rationale, outlined the proficiencies, and advocated for this new subspecialty.[117] In the US, the American Board of Internal Medicine (ABIM) recognized this need for core competencies and training by formally establishing Advanced Heart Failure/Cardiac Transplantation as a subspecialty of Cardiovascular Diseases in 2010.[118,119]

With or without the imprint of the ABIM and whether or not other national organizations offer similar accreditation, the new challenges of providing and improving health care to the expanding population of patients with truly advanced heart failure has already led to important realignments of resources as well as training. Regardless of a certification process, there is general recognition and agreement that advanced heart failure is a clinical field of specialization which requires additional training and expertise beyond the experiences afforded in standard cardiology programs. This textbook is directed to this cadre of healthcare workers who have or are making this extraordinary commitment to dedicate their professional careers to improve the care and prognosis of patients with advanced heart failure.

References

1. Jessup M, Abraham WT, Casey DE, et al. 2009 focused update: ACCF/AHA Guidelines for the Diagnosis and Management of Heart Failure in Adults: a report of the American College of Cardiology Foundation/American Heart Association Task Force on Practice Guidelines: developed in collaboration with the International Society for Heart and Lung Transplantation. Circulation 2009;119(14):1977–2016.
2. Braunwald E, Ross Jr J, Sonnenblick E. Heart failure. In: Braunwald E, Ross Jr. J, Sonnenblick E, ed., Mechanisms of Contraction of the Failing Heart. Boston: Little, Brown; 1976, pp. 309–56.
3. Lele SS, Macfarlane D, Morrison S, et al. Determinants of exercise capacity in patients with coronary artery disease and mild to moderate systolic dysfunction: Role of heart rate and diastolic filling abnormalities. Eur Heart J 1996;17(2):204–12.
4. Dunn FG, De Carvalho JGR, Kem DC, et al. Pheochromocytoma crisis induced by saralasin. N Engl J Med 1976;295(11):605–7.
5. Szakacs JE CA. L-Norepinephrine myocarditis. Am J Clin Pathol 1958;30(5):425–34.
6. Van Vliet PD, Burchell HB, Titus JL. Focal myocarditis associated with pheochromocytoma. N Engl J Med 1966;274(20):1102–8.
7. Desai AS, Chutkow WA, Edelman E, et al. A crisis in late pregnancy. N Engl J Med 2009;361(23):2271–7.
8. Meerson FZ. Compensatory hyperfunction of the heart and cardiac insufficiency. Circ Res 1962;10(3):250–8.
9. McNally EM, Golbus JR, Puckelwartz MJ. Genetic mutations and mechanisms in dilated cardiomyopathy. J Clin Invest 2013;123(1):19–26.
10. Houser SR, Margulies KB, Murphy AM, et al. Animal models of heart failure: a scientific statement from the American Heart Association. Circ Res 2012;111(1):131–50.
11. Pfeffer MA, Pfeffer JM. Ventricular enlargement and reduced survival after myocardial infarction. Circulation 1987;75(5 Pt 2):IV93–7.
12. Hill JA, Olson EN. Cardiac plasticity. N Engl J Med 2008;358(13):1370–80.
13. Force T, Hajjar R, Del Monte F, et al. Signaling pathways mediating the response to hypertrophic stress in the heart. Gene Expr 1999;7(4–6):337–48.
14. van Berlo JH, Maillet M, Molkentin JD. Signaling effectors underlying pathologic growth and remodeling of the heart. J Clin Invest 2013;123(1):37–45.
15. van Der Velden J, Klein LJ, Zaremba R, et al. Effects of calcium, inorganic phosphate, and pH on isometric force in single skinned cardiomyocytes from donor and failing human hearts. Circulation 2001;104(10):1140–6.
16. Herman DS, Lam L, Taylor MR, et al. Truncations of titin causing dilated cardiomyopathy. N Engl J Med 2012;366(7):619–28.
17. Owen AA, Spinale FG. Myocardial basis for heart failure: role of the cardiac interstitium. In: Mann DL, ed., Heart Failure: A Companion to Braunwald's Heart Disease, 2nd ed. Philadelphia: Elsevier; 2010, pp. 73–84.
18. Marks AR. Calcium cycling proteins and heart failure: mechanisms and therapeutics. J Clin Invest 2013;123(1):46–52.
19. Willis MS, Patterson C. Proteotoxicity and cardiac dysfunction—Alzheimer's disease of the heart? N Engl J Med 2013;368(5):455–64.
20. Olivetti G, Abbi R, Quaini F, et al. Apoptosis in the failing human heart. N Engl J Med 1997;336(16):1131–41.
21. De Meyer GR, De Keulenaer GW, Martinet W. Role of autophagy in heart failure associated with aging. Heart Fail Rev 2010;15(5):423–30.
22. Sano M, Minamino T, Toko H, et al. p53-induced inhibition of Hif-1 causes cardiac dysfunction during pressure overload. Nature 2007;446(7134):444–8.

23. Borlaug BA, Kass DA. Invasive hemodynamic assessment in heart failure. Heart Fail Clin 2009;5(2):217–28.
24. Pfeffer MA, Braunwald E. Ventricular remodeilng after myocardial infarction. Experimental observations and clinical implications. Circulation 1990;81:1162–72.
25. Sandler H, Dodge HT. Left ventricular tension and stress in man. Circ Res 1963;13:91–104.
26. Grossman W, Jones D, McLaurin LP. Wall stress and patterns of hypertrophy in the human left ventricle. J Clin Invest 1975;56(1):56–64.
27. Hood WP, Rackley CE, Rolett EL. Wall stress in the normal and hypertrophied human left ventricle. Am J Cardiol 1968;22(4):550–8.
28. Fletcher PJ, Pfeffer JM, Pfeffer MA, Braunwald E. Left ventricular diastolic pressure-volume relations in rats with healed myocardial infarction. Effects on systolic function. Circ Res 1981;49(3):618–26.
29. Engler R, Ray R, Higgins CB, et al. Clinical assessment and follow-up of functional capacity in patients with chronic congestive cardiomyopathy. Am J Cardiol 1982;49(8):1832–7.
30. Aleksova A, Sabbadini G, Merlo M, et al. Natural history of dilated cardiomyopathy: from asymptomatic left ventricular dysfunction to heart failure—a subgroup analysis from the Trieste Cardiomyopathy Registry. J Cardiovasc Med 2009;10(9):699–705.
31. Rihal CS, Nishimura RA, Hatle LK, et al. Systolic and diastolic dysfunction in patients with clinical diagnosis of dilated cardiomyopathy. Relation to symptoms and prognosis. Circulation 1994;90(6):2772–9.
32. Pandhi J, Gottdiener JS, Bartz TM, et al. Comparison of characteristics and outcomes of asymptomatic versus symptomatic left ventricular dysfunction in subjects 65 years old or older (from the Cardiovascular Health Study). Am J Cardiol 2011;107(11):1667–74.
33. Yeboah J, Rodriguez CJ, Stacey B, et al. Prognosis of individuals with asymptomatic left ventricular systolic dysfunction in the multi-ethnic study of atherosclerosis (MESA). Circulation 2012;126(23):2713–19.
34. McDonagh TA, Morrison CE, Lawrence A, et al. Symptomatic and asymptomatic left-ventricular systolic dysfunction in an urban population. Lancet 1997;350(9081):829–33.
35. Wang TJ, Evans JC, Benjamin EJ, et al. Natural history of asymptomatic left ventricular systolic dysfunction in the community. Circulation 2003;108(8):977–82.
36. Criteria Committee of the New York Heart Association. Diseases of the Heart and Blood Vessels: Nomenclature and Criteria for Diagnosis, 6th edition, Boston: Little, Brown, 1928.
37. Levy WC, Mozaffarian D, Linker DT, et al. The Seattle Heart Failure Model: prediction of survival in heart failure. Circulation 2006;113(11):1424–33.
38. Senni M, Parrella P, De Maria R, et al. Predicting heart failure outcome from cardiac and comorbid conditions: The 3C-HF score. Int J Cardiol 2013;163(2):206–11.
39. Pocock SJ, Ariti CA, McMurray JJ, et al. Predicting survival in heart failure: a risk score based on 39 372 patients from 30 studies. Eur Heart J 2013;34(19):1404–13.
40. Aaronson KD, Schwartz JS, Chen T-M, et al. Development and prospective validation of a clinical index to predict survival in ambulatory patients referred for cardiac transplant evaluation. Circulation 1997;95(12):2660–7.
41. McMurray JJ, Adamopoulos S, Anker SD, et al. ESC Guidelines for the diagnosis and treatment of acute and chronic heart failure 2012: The Task Force for the Diagnosis and Treatment of Acute and Chronic Heart Failure 2012 of the European Society of Cardiology. Developed in collaboration with the Heart Failure Association (HFA) of the ESC. Eur Heart J 2012;33(14):1787–847.
42. Hunt SA, Baker DW, Chin MH, et al. ACC/AHA Guidelines for the evaluation and management of chronic heart failure in the adult: executive summary. A report of the American College of Cardiology/American Heart Association Task Force on Practice Guidelines (Committee to Revise the 1995 Guidelines for the Evaluation and Management of Heart Failure). Circulation 2001;104(24):2996–3007.
43. Hunt SA, Abraham WT, Chin MH, et al. 2009 focused update incorporated into the ACC/AHA 2005 guidelines for the diagnosis and management of heart failure in adults. A report of the American College of Cardiology Foundation/American Heart Association Task Force on Practice Guidelines developed in collaboration with the International Society for Heart and Lung Transplantation. J Am Coll Cardiol 2009;53(15):e1–90.
44. Bonow RO, Ganiats TG, Beam CT, et al. ACCF/AHA/AMA-PCPI 2011 performance measures for adults with heart failure: a report of the American College of Cardiology Foundation/American Heart Association Task Force on Performance Measures and the American Medical Association-Physician Consortium for Performance Improvement. Circulation 2012;125(19):2382–401.
45. Psaty BM, Lumley T, Furberg CD, et al. Health outcomes associated with various antihypertensive therapies used as first-line agents: a network meta-analysis. JAMA 2003;289(19):2534–44.
46. Beckett NS, Peters R, Fletcher AE, et al. Treatment of hypertension in patients 80 years of age or older. N Engl J Med 2008;358(18):1887–98.
47. Davis BR, Kostis JB, Simpson LM, et al. Heart failure with preserved and reduced left ventricular ejection fraction in the antihypertensive and lipid-lowering treatment to prevent heart attack trial. Circulation 2008;118(22):2259–67.
48. Kjekshus J, Pedersen TR, Olsson AG, Faergeman O, Pyorala K. The effects of simvastatin on the incidence of heart failure in patients with coronary heart disease. J Card Fail 1997;3(4):249–54.
49. Scirica BM, Morrow DA, Cannon CP, et al. Intensive statin therapy and the risk of hospitalization for heart failure after an acute coronary syndrome in the PROVE IT-TIMI 22 study. J Am Coll Cardiol 2006;47(11):2326–31.
50. de Lemos JA, Blazing MA, Wiviott SD, et al. Early intensive vs a delayed conservative simvastatin strategy in patients with acute coronary syndromes: phase Z of the A to Z trial. JAMA 2004;292(11):1307–16.
51. Khush KK, Waters DD, Bittner V, et al. Effect of high-dose atorvastatin on hospitalizations for heart failure: subgroup analysis of the Treating to New Targets (TNT) study. Circulation 2007;115(5):576–83.
52. Strandberg TE, Holme I, Faergeman O, et al. Comparative effect of atorvastatin (80 mg) versus simvastatin (20 to 40 mg) in preventing hospitalizations for heart failure in patients with previous myocardial infarction. Am J Cardiol 2009;103(10):1381–5.
53. SOLVD Investigators. Effect of enalapril on mortality and the development of heart failure in asymptomatic patients with reduced left ventricular ejection fractions. N Engl J Med 1992;327:685–91.
54. Pfeffer MA, Braunwald E, Moyé LA, et al. Effect of captopril on mortality and morbidity in patients with left ventricular dysfunction after myocardial infarction. Results of the survival and ventricular enlargement trial. The SAVE Investigators. N Engl J Med 1992;327:669–77.
55. Yancy CW, Jessup M, Bozkurt B. 2013 ACCF/AHA guideline for the management of heart failure: a report of the American College of Cardiology Foundation/American Heart Association Task Force on Practice Guidelines. Circulation 2013;128(16):e240–327.
56. Jong P, Yusuf S, Rousseau MF, et al. Effect of enalapril on 12-year survival and life expectancy in patients with left ventricular systolic dysfunction: a follow-up study. Lancet 2003;361(9372):1843–8.
57. Arnold JM, Yusuf S, Young J, et al. Prevention of heart failure in patients in the Heart Outcomes Prevention Evaluation (HOPE) study. Circulation 2003;107(9):1284–90.
58. Fox KM; EUROPA Investigators. Efficacy of perindopril in reduction of cardiovascular events among patients with stable coronary artery disease: randomised, double-blind, placebo-controlled, multicentre trial (the EUROPA study). Lancet 2003;362(9386):782–8.
59. Lewis EF, Solomon SD, Jablonski KA, et al. Predictors of heart failure in patients with stable coronary artery disease: a PEACE study. Circ Heart Fail 2009;2(3):209–16.
60. Dargie HJ. Effect of carvedilol on outcome after myocardial infarction in patients with left-ventricular dysfunction: the CAPRICORN randomised trial. Lancet 2001;357(9266):1385–90.
61. Colucci WS, Kolias TJ, Adams KF, et al. Metoprolol reverses left ventricular remodeling in patients with asymptomatic systolic

dysfunction: the reversal of ventricular remodeling with Toprol-XL (REVERT) trial. Circulation 2007;116(1):49–56.
62. Moss AJ, Zareba W, Hall WJ, et al. Prophylactic implantation of a defibrillator in patients with myocardial infarction and reduced ejection fraction. N Engl J Med 2002;346(12):877–83.
63. He J, Ogden LG, Bazzano LA, et al. Risk factors for congestive heart failure in US men and women: NHANES I epidemiologic follow-up study. Arch Intern Med 2001;161(7):996–1002.
64. Schocken DD, Benjamin EJ, Fonarow GC, et al. Prevention of heart failure: a scientific statement from the American Heart Association Councils on Epidemiology and Prevention, Clinical Cardiology, Cardiovascular Nursing, and High Blood Pressure Research; Quality of Care and Outcomes Research Interdisciplinary Working Group; and Functional Genomics and Translational Biology Interdisciplinary Working Group. Circulation 2008;117(19):2544–65.
65. Butler J, Kalogeropoulos A, Georgiopoulou V, et al. Incident heart failure prediction in the elderly: the health ABC heart failure score. Circ Heart Fail 2008;1(2):125–33.
66. Jessup M, Brozena S. Heart failure. N Engl J Med 2003;348(20):2007–18.
67. SOLVD Investigators. Effect of enalapril on survival in patients with reduced left ventricular ejection fractions and congestive heart failure. N Engl J Med 1991;325(5):293–302.
68. Lewis EF, Moye LA, Rouleau JL, et al. Predictors of late development of heart failure in stable survivors of myocardial infarction. J Am Coll Cardiol 2003;42(8):1446–53.
69. Velagaleti RS, Pencina MJ, Murabito JM, et al. Long-term trends in the incidence of heart failure after myocardial infarction. Circulation 2008;118(20):2057–62.
70. Ezekowitz JA, Kaul P, Bakal JA, et al. Declining in-hospital mortality and increasing heart failure incidence in elderly patients with first myocardial infarction. J Am Coll Cardiol 2009;53(1):13–20.
71. Jhund PS, Macintyre K, Simpson CR, et al. Long-term trends in first hospitalization for heart failure and subsequent survival between 1986 and 2003: a population study of 5.1 million people. Circulation 2009;119(4):515–23.
72. Wolk MJ, Scheidt S, Killip T. Heart failure complicating acute myocardial infarction. Circulation 1972;45(5):1125–38.
73. Norris RM, Bensley KE, Caughey DE, Scott PJ. Hospital mortality in acute myocardial infarction. Br Med J 1968;3(5611):143–6.
74. Moye LA, Pfeffer MA, Wun C, et al. Uniformity of captopril benefit in the SAVE study: Subgroup Analysis. Eur Heart J 1994;15(Suppl B):2–8.
75. Steg PG, Dabbous OH, Feldman LJ, et al. Determinants and prognostic impact of heart failure complicating acute coronary syndromes: observations from the Global Registry of Acute Coronary Events (GRACE). Circulation 2004;109(4):494–9.
76. Sabatine MS, Morrow DA, de Lemos JA, et al. Evaluation of multiple biomarkers of cardiovascular stress for risk prediction and guiding medical therapy in patients with stable coronary disease. Circulation 2012;125(2):233–40.
77. Omland T, Sabatine MS, Jablonski KA, et al. Prognostic value of B-Type natriuretic peptides in patients with stable coronary artery disease: the PEACE Trial. J Am Coll Cardiol 2007;50(3):205–14.
78. Dunn FG, Ichikawa I, Pfeffer JM, et al. Renal and systemic hemodyanic effects of synthetic atrial natriuretic peptide in the anesthetized rat. Circ Res 1986;59:237–46.
79. deFilippi CR, de Lemos JA, Christenson RH, et al. Association of serial measures of cardiac troponin T using a sensitive assay with incident heart failure and cardiovascular mortality in older adults. JAMA 2010;304(22):2494–502.
80. Velagaleti RS, Gona P, Larson MG, et al. Multimarker approach for the prediction of heart failure incidence in the community. Circulation 2010;122(17):1700–6.
81. Ky B, French B, Levy WC, et al. Multiple biomarkers for risk prediction in chronic heart failure. Circ Heart Fail 2012;5(2):183–90.
82. Go AS, Mozaffarian D, Roger VL, et al. Heart disease and stroke statistics—2013 update: a report from the American Heart Association. Circulation 2013;127(1):e6–245.
83. Heidenreich PA, Trogdon JG, Khavjou OA, et al. Forecasting the future of cardiovascular disease in the United States: a policy statement from the American Heart Association. Circulation 2011;123(8):933–44.
84. Heidenreich PA, Albert NM, Allen LA, et al. Forecasting the impact of heart failure in the United States: a policy statement from the American Heart Association. Circ Heart Fail 2013;6(3):606–19.
85. Bleumink GS, Knetsch AM, Sturkenboom MCJM, et al. Quantifying the heart failure epidemic: prevalence, incidence rate, lifetime risk and prognosis of heart failure: The Rotterdam Study. Eur Heart J 2004;25(18):1614–19.
86. Lloyd-Jones DM, Larson MG, Leip EP, et al. Lifetime risk for developing congestive heart failure: the Framingham Heart Study. Circulation 2002;106(24):3068–72.
87. Levy D, Larson MG, Vasan RS, et al. THe progression from hypertension to congestive heart failure. JAMA 1996;275(20):1557–62.
88. Chen J, Normand ST, Wang Y, Krumholz HM. National and regional trends in heart failure hospitalization and mortality rates for medicare beneficiaries, 1998–2008. JAMA 2011;306(15):1669–78.
89. Zannad F, Agrinier N, Alla F. Heart failure burden and therapy. Europace 2009;11 Suppl 5:v1–9.
90. Dunlay SM, Shah ND, Shi Q, et al. Lifetime costs of medical care after heart failure diagnosis. Circ Cardiovasc Qual Outcomes 2011;4(1):68–75.
91. Levy D, Kenchaiah S, Larson MG, et al. Long-term trends in the incidence of and survival with heart failure. N Engl J Med 2002;347(18):1397–402.
92. Laribi S, Aouba A, Nikolaou M, et al. Trends in death attributed to heart failure over the past two decades in Europe. Eur J Heart Fail 2012;14(3):234–9.
93. Cowie MR, Fox KF, Wood DA, et al. Hospitalization of patients with heart failure. A population-based study. Eur Heart J 2002;23(11):877–85.
94. McKelvie RS, Moe GW, Cheung A, et al. The 2011 Canadian Cardiovascular Society heart failure management guidelines update: focus on sleep apnea, renal dysfunction, mechanical circulatory support, and palliative care. Can J Cardiol 2011;27(3):319–38.
95. Moser DK, Yamokoski L, Sun JL, et al. Improvement in health-related quality of life after hospitalization predicts event-free survival in patients with advanced heart failure. J Card Fail 2009;15(9):763–9.
96. CONSENSUS Trial Study Group. Effects of enalapril on mortality in severe congestive heart failure. Results of the COoperative North Scandinavian ENalapril SUrvival Study (CONSENSUS). N Engl J Med 1987;316(23):1429–35.
97. Braunwald E. Heart failure. JACC Heart Fail 2013;1(1):1–20.
98. Heart Failure Society of America, Lindenfeld J, Albert NM, et al. HFSA 2010 Comprehensive Heart Failure Practice Guideline. J Card Fail 2010;16(6):e1–194.
99. Braunwald E. The management of heart failure: the past, the present, and the future. Circ Heart Fail 2008;1(1):58–62.
100. Solomon SD, Dobson J, Pocock S, et al. Influence of nonfatal hospitalization for heart failure on subsequent mortality in patients with chronic heart failure. Circulation 2007;116(13):1482–7.
101. Krumholz HM, Lin Z, Keenan PS, et al. Relationship between hospital readmission and mortality rates for patients hospitalized with acute myocardial infarction, heart failure, or pneumonia. JAMA 2013;309(6):587–93.
102. Adams KF, Jr., Zannad F. Clinical definition and epidemiology of advanced heart failure. Am Heart J 1998;135(6 Pt 2 Su):S204–15.
103. Jacobellis v. Ohio, 378 U.S. 184.
104. Ammar KA, Jacobsen SJ, Mahoney DW, et al. Prevalence and prognostic significance of heart failure stages: application of the American College of Cardiology/American Heart Association heart failure staging criteria in the community. Circulation 2007;115(12):1563–70.
105. Costanzo MR, Mills RM, Wynne J. Characteristics of "Stage D" heart failure: insights from the Acute Decompensated Heart Failure

National Registry Longitudinal Module (ADHERE LM). Am Heart J 2008;155(2):341–9.
106. DiBardino DJ. The history and development of cardiac transplantation. Tex Heart Inst J 1999;26(3):198–205.
107. Bardy GH, Lee KL, Mark DB, et al. Amiodarone or an implantable cardioverter-defibrillator for congestive heart failure. N Engl J Med 2005;352(3):225–37.
108. Bristow MR, Saxon LA, Boehmer J, et al. Cardiac-resynchronization therapy with or without an implantable defibrillator in advanced chronic heart failure. N Engl J Med 2004;350(21):2140–50.
109. Cleland JG, Daubert JC, Erdmann E, et al. The effect of cardiac resynchronization on morbidity and mortality in heart failure. N Engl J Med 2005;352(15):1539–49.
110. Moss AJ, Hall WJ, Cannom DS, et al. Cardiac-resynchronization therapy for the prevention of heart-failure events. N Engl J Med 2009;361(14):1329–38.
111. Tang AS, Wells GA, Talajic M, et al. Cardiac-resynchronization therapy for mild-to-moderate heart failure. N Engl J Med 2010;363(25):2385–95.
112. Rose EA, Gelijns AC, Moskowitz AJ, et al. Long-term use of a left ventricular assist device for end-stage heart failure. N Engl J Med 2001;345(20):1435–43.
113. Slaughter MS, Rogers JG, Milano CA, et al. Advanced heart failure treated with continuous-flow left ventricular assist device. N Engl J Med 2009;361(23):2241–51.
114. Schou M, Gustafsson F, Videbaek L, et al. Extended heart failure clinic follow-up in low-risk patients: a randomized clinical trial (NorthStar). Eur Heart J 2013;34(6):432–42.
115. Stevenson LW, Pagani FD, Young JB, et al. INTERMACS profiles of advanced heart failure: the current picture. J Heart Lung Transplant 2009;28(6):535–41.
116. Allen LA, Stevenson LW, Grady KL, et al. Decision making in advanced heart failure: a scientific statement from the American Heart Association. Circulation 2012;125(15):1928–52.
117. Konstam MA, Executive Council of the Heart Failure Society of America. Heart failure training: a call for an integrative, patient-focused approach to an emerging cardiology subspecialty. J Am Coll Cardiol 2004;44(7):1361–2.
118. Konstam MA, Jessup M, Francis GS, et al. Advanced heart failure and transplant cardiology: a subspecialty is born. J Am Coll Cardiol 2009;53(10):834–6.
119. <http://www.abim.org/specialty/advanced-heart-failure-transplant-cardiology.aspx>.

CHAPTER 2

Cell biology of heart failure

Kenneth B. Margulies MD and
J. Eduardo Rame MD MPhil

Introduction

Though the syndrome of congestive heart failure (CHF) can arise from a variety of different pathologic circumstances, this syndrome is always characterized by (indeed defined by) deterioration of cardiac pump function. Cardiac myocytes are the only cells in the heart capable of the cyclic active force generation and relaxation required for the pump function of the heart. Based on current estimates, the normal adult human left ventricle (LV) is comprised of more than 4 billion cardiac myocytes.[1] In many etiologies of heart failure, there is a reduction in this normal number of cardiac myocytes within the heart. This reduction may occur via a sudden ischemic event triggering myocardial necrosis or via alternative cell death pathways, such as apoptosis and autophagy, resulting from chronic pathologic stress. In addition to quantitative changes of cardiac myocytes (generally reductions), the syndrome of heart failure is consistently associated with qualitative changes in the cardiac myocytes.

Pathologic myocardial remodeling describes the multifaceted process in which gross changes in the morphology of the heart are accompanied by a variety of ultimately maladaptive changes at the tissue, cellular, and subcellular levels in response to disease-associated changes in biomechanical and biochemical stimuli. At the organ level, characteristics of remodeling typically include increases in myocardial mass, changes in the ratio of wall thickness to chamber volume, and other shape changes that can affect pump function, energy utilization, and the risk of unfavorable clinical sequelae including valvular dysfunction, heart failure, arrhythmias, and thromboembolism. In patients with LV systolic dysfunction, pathologic remodeling typically includes an increase in LV chamber volume, a transition from the normal elliptical shape of the LV to a more globular, spherical shape, and a decreased ejection fraction (LVEF). At the cellular level, the myocytes become longer and changes in calcium handling and β-adrenergic signaling cause changes in contractility and reductions in contractile reserve. These pathologic abnormalities in cellular morphology and function are also associated with, and often driven by, changes in intracellular signaling and energy metabolism. In many instances, adaptations to chronic biomechanical and neurohumoral stress or changes in availability of key substrates elicit activation of one or more cell death pathways that may further propagate the myocardial dysfunction and heart failure syndrome.

Though there is ongoing debate about which changes might be adaptive versus maladaptive, the qualitative changes in cardiac myocytes in failing hearts ultimately involve virtually every aspect of cell biology and profoundly impact both organ-level remodeling and the pump function of failing hearts. To better elucidate these important processes and the therapeutic opportunities they provide, this chapter describes the triggers, phenomena, and mechanisms associated with the transitions away from normal cardiac myocyte structure and function during pathologic remodeling of the heart. In many cases these transitions involve an increase in cell and organ size, referred to as pathologic hypertrophy. This chapter considers morphologic adaptations of cardiac myocytes, the regulation of cardiac contractility, cardiac metabolism, and alternative cell death pathways activated in failing hearts. In each section, we consider both normal biology and the molecular determinants and signaling pathways contributing to pathologic adaptations, and highlight opportunities for salutary therapeutic interventions. Finally, we highlight the reversibility of cardiac myocyte hypertrophy and dysfunction that has been demonstrated in in recent years. These reverse remodeling phenomena demonstrate the substantial plasticity of the severely failing heart, provide insights into factors driving and sustaining pathologic adaptations and attest to the potential benefit of therapeutic interventions targeting the failing heart.

Cardiac myocyte hypertrophy

Normal cardiac myocyte morphology

The billions of cardiac myocytes and other cell types within the heart, the cardiac conduction system, the full coronary vascular tree, and the extracellular matrix are arranged in a complex, three-dimensional structure that is well-suited to the primary function of the heart, namely contraction and relaxation to promote efficient pumping of blood to the lungs (RV) and other organs (LV). Within this complex structure, individual cardiac myocytes are arranged as an integrated syncytium such that each myocyte is in contact with several other myocytes, other cell types, multiple capillaries and an extracellular matrix that helps maintain structural integrity and coordinated contraction. As illustrated in Figure 2.1,[2] cardiac myocytes are generally rod-shaped striated cells with surface irregularities that form step-offs at the locations of contact with other cardiac myocytes. Within an individual adult heart there is great variation among the size of the constituent cardiac myocytes, which range from 50 to over 200 μm in length, from 10 to 50 μm in width and from 7500 to over 40 000 μm^3 in volume.[3] Across a variety of mammalian species, the *average* length/width ratio of normal cardiac myocytes is fairly consistent, between 7/1

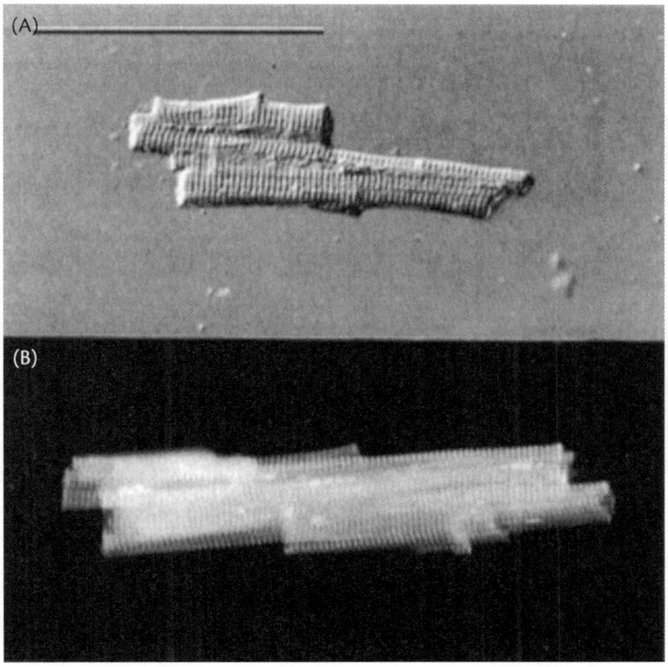

Fig. 2.1 (A) Typical isolated cardiac myocyte from a nonfailing human left ventricle. Nomarski optics; bar = 100 μm. (B) Isolated myocyte from the left ventricle of a patient with ischemic cardiomyopathy. Cell is labeled with rhodamine–phalloidin to show actin (same magnification as panel a).
Gerdes AM, Kellerman SE, Moore JA, Muffly KE, Clark LC, Reaves PY, Malec KB, McKeown PP, Schocken DD. Structural remodeling of cardiac myocytes in patients with ischemic cardiomyopathy. Circulation. 1992; 86(2):426–30.

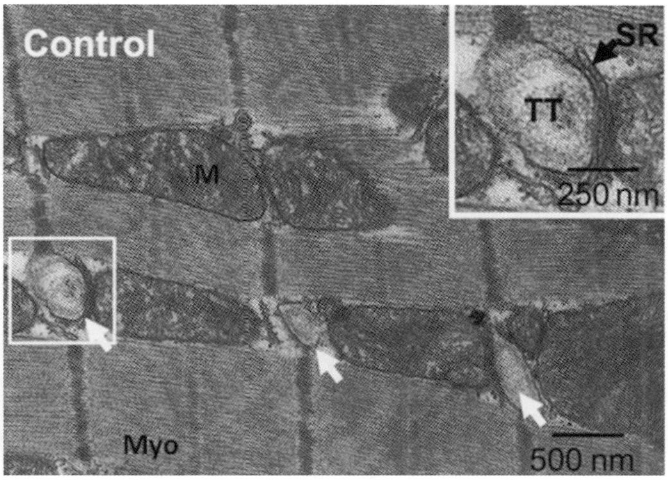

Fig. 2.2 Ultrastructural characterization of cardiac myocytes.
Zhang HB1, Li RC, Xu M, Xu SM, La YS, Wu HD, Xie XJ, Gao W, Ye H, Zhang YY, Meng X, Wang SQ. Ultrastructural uncoupling between T-tubules and sarcoplasmic reticulum in human heart failure. Cardiovasc Res. 2013 May 1;98(2):269–76.

and 9/1, despite wide differences in the number of cardiac myocytes within the heart. In addition, the cross-sections of most cardiac myocytes are elliptical rather than round. As shown in Figure 2.2,[4] ultrastructural characterization of cardiac myocytes[5] reveals that the striated appearance of cardiac myocytes is derived from a repeating pattern of sarcomeres that are defined by the partially overlapping thick and thin myofilaments responsible for muscle shortening and force generation. Myofibrils comprise nearly half of the volume of mature cardiac myocytes, and an additional 35% of the volume is occupied by mitochondria that provide the chemical energy required for cardiac pump function. Ultrastructural examination also reveals extensive invaginations, called T-tubules, in the myocyte cell surface that allow the plasma membrane, and voltage-gated ion channels, to have access to the interior of the cardiac myocytes. T-tubules, in turn, are closely approximated to the intracellular sarcoplasmic reticulum where large intracellular stores of Ca^{2+} are released and resequestered to activate and deactivate myofilament interactions, as discussed below.

Abnormal cardiac myocyte morphology

Though normal adult cardiac myocytes exhibit considerable variation in size and shape, there are characteristic changes observed in diseased hearts that contribute to cardiac remodeling at the whole-organ level. For example, cardiac myocytes from dilated failing human hearts due to either ischemic or nonischemic cardiomyopathy exhibit nearly a 50% increase in average myocyte length but only a 20% increase in average cell width and no significant change in average cell thickness.[3] As cardiac myocyte lengthening occurs, there is no change in average sarcomere length, indicating that sarcomeres are added in series to produce the increase in average myocyte length. Because disproportionate cardiac myocyte lengthening is a fundamental contributor to decreases in relative wall thickness, and associated increases in wall stress, the addition of sarcomeres in series represents a potential driving mechanism for progression of cardiac overload and dysfunction over time.

In contrast, in hearts with concentric hypertrophy with normal chamber size due to aortic stenosis or hypertension, there is no significant increase in average myocyte length, but myocyte cross-sectional area is nearly double what is observed in normal hearts.[6,7,8] However, when hypertensive rats progress to heart failure and decompensation with chamber dilation, length steadily increases in parallel with the increases in chamber volume.[6] Observing that the initial increase in relative wall thickness in response to sustained increases in systolic pressure loading effectively normalizes systolic wall stress, Grossman and colleagues speculated that this type of hypertrophy is adaptive.[9] However, this concept of adaptive hypertrophy is challenged by subsequent studies in which transgenic mice incapable of developing concentric hypertrophy exhibited improved cardiac function and better survival despite significantly greater wall stress following sustained pressure overload induced by aortic banding.[10]

Physiologic hypertrophic signaling in myocardium

Several different signaling pathways have been implicated in driving cardiac myocyte hypertrophy, but their relative contributions remain uncertain. Nevertheless, there is strong evidence that the hypertrophy of cardiac myocytes that occurs during maturation, pregnancy or following chronic exercise training, labeled "physiologic hypertrophy," involves signaling pathways that are distinct from those involved in the responses to pressure overload or myocardial infarction, labeled "pathologic hypertrophy," as illustrated in Figure 2.3.[11] Most importantly, at the organ level, cardiac function associated with physiologic hypertrophy is essentially normal, or even enhanced,[12] and associated with enhanced capacity for both oxidative and glycolytic metabolism that is distinct from

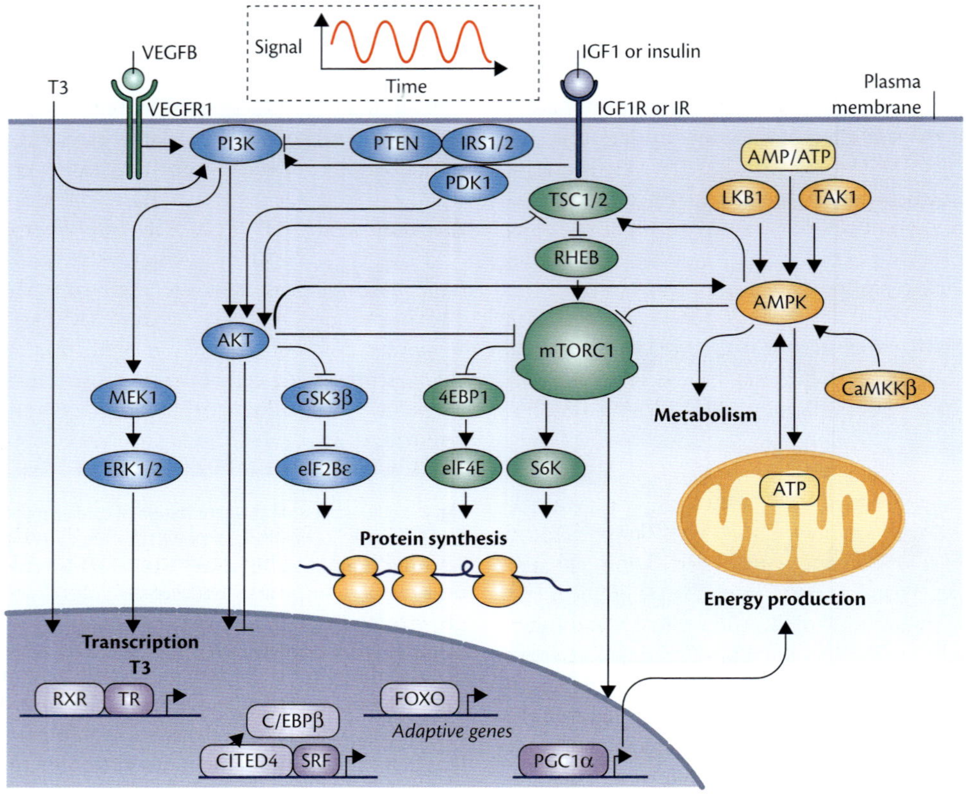

Fig. 2.3 Physiologic hypertrophy is an adaptive form of cardiac hypertrophy. The figure depicts central signaling pathways of physiologic hypertrophy discussed in the text. Physiologic hypertrophy is initiated by intermittent signals of triiodothyronine (T3), vascular endothelial growth factor B (VEGFB), insulin, and insulin-like growth factor 1 (IGF1), as illustrated by the oscillating curve. The growth hormones activate membrane-localized tyrosine kinase receptors (VEGF receptor 1 (VEGFR1), IGF1 receptor (IGF1R), or insulin receptor (IR)) and nuclear receptors (thyroid hormone receptor (TR)), which trigger intracellular signaling pathways specific to physiologic hypertrophy. These signaling pathways regulate the transcription of adaptive genes, protein synthesis, metabolism, and energy production. The growth signals centre on common signaling branches controlled by ERK1/2, PI3K, AKT, and mTOR complex 1 (mTORC1), whereas AMPK governs metabolic adaptive reprogramming. 4EBP1, eukaryotic translation initiation factor 4E-binding protein 1; C/EBPβ, CCAAT/enhancer binding protein-β; CaMKKβ, calcium/calmodulin-dependent protein kinase kinase-β; CITED4, CBP/p300 interacting transactivator 4; eIF2Bε, eukaryotic translation initiation factor 2Bε; FOXO, forkhead box O; GSK3β, glycogen synthase kinase 3β; IRS1/2, insulin receptor substrate 1 or 2; LKB1, liver kinase B1; PDK1, phosphoinositide-dependent protein kinase 1; PGC1α, peroxisome proliferator-activated receptor-γ coactivator 1α; RHEB, RAS homologue enriched in brain; RXR, retinoic acid receptor; S6K, S6 kinase; SRF, serum response factor; TAK1, transforming growth factor β-activated kinase 1; TSC1/2, tuberous sclerosis complex 1 or 2.

the impaired contractile reserve and increased dependence on glycolytic metabolism characteristic of pathologic myocardial hypertrophy.[13] The fact that maturation, exercise, and pregnancy trigger functional manifestations that are qualitatively different from those observed following pathologic stress indicates that there is a distinct set of physiologic sensing and signaling pathways involved with physiologic hypertrophy. As reviewed by Maillet et al., physiologic hypertrophy appears to be initiated by thyroid hormone, insulin, growth hormone, and insulin-like growth factor (IGF1),[11] with thyroid hormone and IGF1 most clearly involved with early postnatal maturational heart growth,[14,15] and insulin signaling involved with maintaining nonpathologic patterns of gene expression and metabolism.[11]

Growth hormone and IGF1 appear to be particularly important for exercise-induced, physiologic cardiac hypertrophy. In compelling studies using mouse models, Wilkins and colleagues demonstrated that IGF1 signaling through phosphoinositide 3-kinase and Akt mediate the physiologic cardiac hypertrophy associated with exercise.[11,16] Indeed, in transgenic mice, overexpression of the IGF1 receptor without exercise-induced cardiac hypertrophy was characterized by an increase in cardiac myocyte volume, absence of histopathology, and increased systolic function at 3 and 10 months of age.[17] Conversely, mice with IGF receptor deletion were resistant to exercise-induced hypertrophy.[18] In fact, IGF1 signaling is actively suppressed in response to pathologic stimuli such as chronic pressure overload and myocardial infarction.[11,16] These results strongly support the centrality of IGF1-dependent signaling to the physiologic growth of the heart.

Pathologic cardiac myocyte hypertrophy

A variety of factors can trigger pathologic cardiac myocyte hypertrophy with features that are distinct from the physiologic hypertrophy associated with exercise or pregnancy. The factors capable of triggering pathologic hypertrophy include biomechanical overload (either increased preload or afterload), neurohumoral mediators, and inflammation. Among neurohumoral mediators, those particularly implicated in triggering pathologic cardiac myocyte growth include catecholamines, angiotensin II, and endothelin. Among inflammatory cytokines most implicated in cardiac myocyte hypertrophy are interleukins IL-1β and IL-6 and tumor necrosis factor alpha (TNFα).[19,20] In many clinical situations, these factors can coexist and overlap, with more than one alternative pathway being activated at the same time, such as when neurohumoral activation triggers vasoconstriction and increased afterload or inflammatory responses in addition to their direct effects on cardiac myocyte growth. Nevertheless, in the next few sections we will separately consider the mechanosensing and signaling involved with sustained biomechanical overload and the agonist-triggered signaling involved with sustained stimulation by neurohumoral or inflammatory mediators. Of note, several of these signaling pathways affect not only cell growth and cell shape, but also affect characteristic pathologic features of hypertrophied and failing cardiac myocytes including contractile dysfunction, abnormal gene expression, metabolic abnormalities, and the activation of cellular death pathways.

Transduction of biomechanical overload

The factor most consistently linked with pathologic cardiac myocyte hypertrophy in clinical settings is sustained biomechanical overload, such as occurs in patients with hypertension, valvular heart disease (inducing excessive preload and/or afterload), and antecedent myocardial infarction (MI). In the case of MI, the surviving myocytes are subjected to increased biomechanical stress as a consequence of expansion and extension of the infarction producing increased wall stress and the requirement of maintaining adequate pump function despite a substantial reduction in myocyte number. In general, the severity of biomechanical overload is correlated with the severity of pathologic hypertrophy manifested as increased myocardial mass at the organ level and increased cardiac myocyte size at the or cellular level.

There are multiple mechanosensing systems that may regulate physiologic and pathologic hypertrophy through direct load-sensing mechanisms within cardiomyocytes. For example, stretch-activated, transient receptor potential (TRP) ion channels that permit passage of calcium and other cations could trigger activation of calcium-dependent myocyte growth processes. In particular, the TRPC1 and TRPC6 isoforms have been directly implicated in regulating cardiac hypertrophy in response to mechanical stretch.[21,22] Accordingly, ligands for these receptors represent a potential target for regulating upstream responses to biomechanical overload. Because they are attached to both myocytes and the extracellular matrix components like fibronectin, collagen and laminin, integrins are another family of mechnosensing proteins that could mediate stretch-induced signaling in myocytes directly or via interactions with neighboring fibroblasts. Finally, several sarcomeric proteins are potential candidates for primary mechanosensing involved with growth signaling in cardiac myocytes, including muscle LIM protein (MLP), telethonin, myopalladin, palladin, actinin-associated LIM protein (ALP), cardiac ankyrin repeat protein (CARP), ankyrin, nebulette, obscurin, and titin. Of these, the giant molecule titin is a particularly interesting candidate because it directly regulates the distention of sarcomeres and binds many other sarcomeric proteins and regulators. In fact, recent reports indicate that titin mutations may account for as many as 25% of familial dilated cardiomyopathies.[23]

β-Adrenergic signaling in cardiac myocyte hypertrophy

Despite its essential role in augmenting cardiac output exercise and other acute physiologic stress settings, sympathetic activation and β-adrenergic signaling has distinctly pathologic effects on cardiac myocyte structure, function, and gene expression. β-Adrenergic receptors are a subclass of G-protein-coupled receptors that trigger activation of adenylyl cyclase, generation of cAMP, and phosphorylation of intracellular target proteins via protein kinase A (PKA) [24] Both in-vitro studies in isolated cardiac myocytes[25] and in-vivo studies employing transgenic mice with overexpression of the cardiac β1-adrenergic receptor,[26] Gs,[27] and PKA[28] demonstrate that this classical signaling cascade triggers growth of cardiac myocytes. Though the details of downstream events remains uncertain, there is strong evidence supporting the involvement of the cAMP response binding protein (CREB) and the cAMP response element modulator (CREM) as mediators of the gene expression changes producing cellular hypertrophy in response to sustained β-adrenergic signaling within cardiac myocytes.[24,29] The clinical importance of cardiac myocyte hypertrophy mediated through β_1-AR signaling is supported by the well-established cardioprotective effects of β-blockers. The salutary effects of the new class of biased β-arrestin agonists that block the classical adenyl cyclase/cAMP/PKA signaling downstream of the β1-AR, but agonize the cardioprotective β-arrestin-dependent transactivation of epidermal growth factor receptor (EGFR) signaling also support the pathogenic role of sustained catecholamine stimulation.[30]

Calcium-dependent signaling in cardiac myocyte hypertrophy

Another effect of chronic β_1-AR stimulation is an increase in intracellular Ca^{2+} that itself activates downstream signaling factors including calcineurin and calmodulin-dependent protein kinase II (CaMKII) (see Figure 2.1). Calcineurin is a protein phosphatase that dephosphorylates the nuclear factor of activated transcription (NFAT) to trigger its translocation to the nucleus where it is a potent activator of numerous prohypertrophic genes.[31] Interestingly, the same studies demonstrating that exercise induces IGF1-mediated physiologic hypertrophy also found that exercise is associated with *suppression* of calcineurin–NFAT signaling. Conversely, chronic pressure overload or MI induce calcineurin–NFAT activation with suppression of IGF1 signaling. Constitutive activation of calcineurin in transgenic mice produces massive cardiac hypertrophy,[16] whereas a mouse lacking a gene encoding the catalytic subunit of calcineurin (CnAβ) has substantially reduced hypertrophy in response to pressure overload or infusion of cathecholamines or angiotensin II.[32] From a therapeutic standpoint, adenovirus-mediated gene transfer of endogenous calcineurin inhibitors like Cabin/Cain that inhibit cardiac calcineurin activity likewise reduce hypertrophy in response to pressure overload without reducing aortic pressure.[33]

There is also increasing evidence implicating the multifunctional CaMKII as a central mediator in cardiac myocyte hypertrophy. As recently reviewed,[34] CaMKII is a serine–threonine kinase that has a wide variety of actions within the heart including effects on action potential waveshape and arrhythmogenesis, excitation–contraction coupling, transcriptional regulation of myocyte growth, and cardiac myocyte apoptosis pathways. Though there are several isoforms of CaMKII, the predominant form of CaMKII in myocardium appears to be CaMKIIδ. Because CaMKII is activated in response to signals generated through several different G-protein-coupled receptors (GPCRs), it has a key role in mediating the hypertrophic effects of humoral agents such as norepinephrine (NE), phenylephrine (PE), and endothelin (ET-1). This activation occurs through Ca^{2+} release from nuclear stores sensitive to inositol trisphosphate (InsP3).[35]

Both in-vitro data using neonatal rat myocytes and transgenic mouse models strongly support a pivotal role for CaMKII in mediating the effects of GPCR agonists on cardiac myocyte hypertrophy.[34] Moreover, rapid and sustained CaMKII activation via GPCR activation is also triggered by transverse aortic constriction (TAC) in mice suggesting that this pathway is involved in load-induced cardiac myocyte hypertrophy.[36] Further mechanistic studies have demonstrated that the hypertrophic effects of either CaMKIIδB or δC isoforms are mediated by transactivation of myocyte enhancer factor 2 (*MEF2*) gene expression and histone deacetylase 4 (HDAC4) translocation from nucleus to cytoplasm, indicating that either isoform can stimulate HDAC4 phosphorylation but only the CaMKIIδC isoform is involved with changes in cardiac myocyte Ca^{2+} handling.[37] In fact, preclinical studies employing pharmacologic inhibition of calmodulin/CaMKIIδB activity reported improved cardiac function in mice subjected to TAC in association with correction of the imbalance between NCX1 and SERCA2 that is otherwise observed in this model and in humans with severe heart failure.[38]

MAPK signaling in cardiac myocyte hypertrophy

Mitogen-activated protein kinase (MAPK) cascades are highly conserved intracellular signal transduction pathways with diverse developmental and regulatory functions in the heart. MAPKs are typically divided into four major subfamilies, namely extracellular signal-regulated kinases (ERK1/2), c-Jun N-terminal kinases (JNK), p38 MAP kinases, and ERK5 kinase. As shown in Figure 2.4,[39] for each subfamily there is a three-tiered kinase cascade in which a MAPK kinase kinase activates a MAPK kinase which, in turn, activates the MAPK through serial phosphorylation. As well reviewed,[39] ERK1/2 is activated by various stimuli including growth factors, serum, phorbol esters, GPCRs, inflammatory cytokines, and microtubule disorganization.[40,41] ERK5 is activated by these same factors and also by oxidative stress and UV irradiation.[42] JNK and p38 are stress-activated kinases that respond most robustly to inflammatory cytokines and cellular stresses such as heat shock, hyperosmolarity, ischemia–reperfusion, UV radiation, oxidizing agents, DNA damage, and endoplasmic reticulum (ER) stress,[43,44] and less intensely by growth factors and GPCRs.

Each MAPK family has been implicated in cardiac myocyte hypertrophy, but definitive evidence supporting a central role has varied. For ERK1/2, overexpression and correlative approaches have implicated a role in cardiac hypertrophy,[39] but Purcell et al. found that reduced in ERK activity is not sufficient to prevent hypertrophy in response to various forms of hypertrophic stimuli in vivo.[45] For JNK, studies have been even more conflicting and the composite data from in-vitro and in-vivo studies suggests that JNK signaling tends to be antihypertrophic by excluding NFAT from the nucleus and upregulating JunD.[39] For p38, targeted activation of p38 in vivo did not induce cardiac hypertrophy.[46] On the other hand, there is fairly compelling data supporting a role for ERK5 in promoting eccentric cardiac hypertrophy. In-vitro studies indicated that activation of ERK5 signaling induces elongation of cultured myocytes and increase in serial sarcomere assembly, while blockade of ERK5 signaling prevented cellular elongation.[47] The unique role for ERK5 in this particular type of cell hypertrophy is supported by in-vivo studies in which transgenic overexpression of the MEK5β splice variant,[47] but not MEK5α,[48] induces ventricular thinning and dilation without a loss of cells consistent with

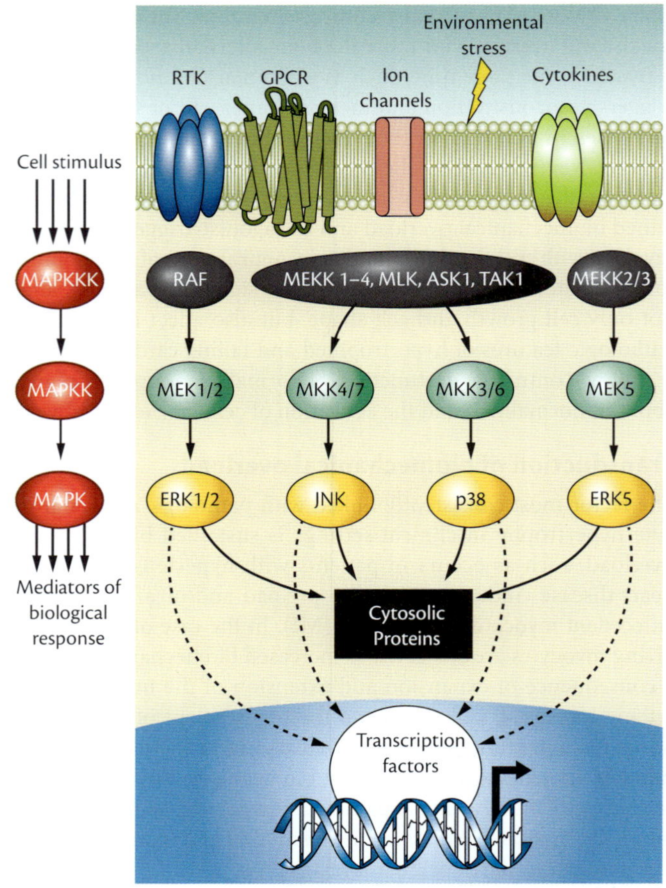

Fig. 2.4 Canonical mitogen-activated protein kinase (MAPK) signaling. MAPKs are prototypically activated by canonical three-tiered sequential phosphorylation events. The most well-known MAPKKK and MAPKK are listed for each MAPK; however, this is only a small representation of all identified upstream kinases. Furthermore, multiple steps may exist between the cell stimulus and activation of the MAPKKK and between activation of the MAPK and the biological response.
Based on Rose BA, Force T, Wang Y. Mitogen-activated protein kinase signaling in the heart: angels versus demons in a heart-breaking tale. Physiol Rev. 2010; 90(4):1507–46.

eccentric hypertrophy. Further extending these studies, recent studies in a canine model of mitral regurgitation have also reported increased activated ERK5 in caveolae as eccentric hypertrophy develops.[49] Thus, despite significant variation among the MAPK pathways, there is increasing support for a functionally significant role for ERK5 signaling in eccentric hypertrophy that may be targetable via specific inhibitors.[39]

Protein kinase C signaling in cardiac hypertrophy

Protein kinase C (PKC) is a family of serine–threonine protein kinases. In cardiac myocytes, PKC signaling is typically initiated by binding of specific plasma membrane GPCRs by endogenous ligands such as angiotensin II (AngII), phenylephrine (PE), and endothelin-1 (ET1) or exogenous agonists like phorbol myristate acetate (PMA). There are over a dozen different PKC isozymes that are grouped into different subtypes based on whether their signaling depends on diacylglycerol (DAG), calcium, or neither. Several PKC isoforms are expressed in heart, but there are significant interspecies differences that may affect the applicability of findings from one species to another.[50] In humans, the calcium-dependent isozymes α, βI, and βIIPKC, reside predominantly in the ventricle, δ

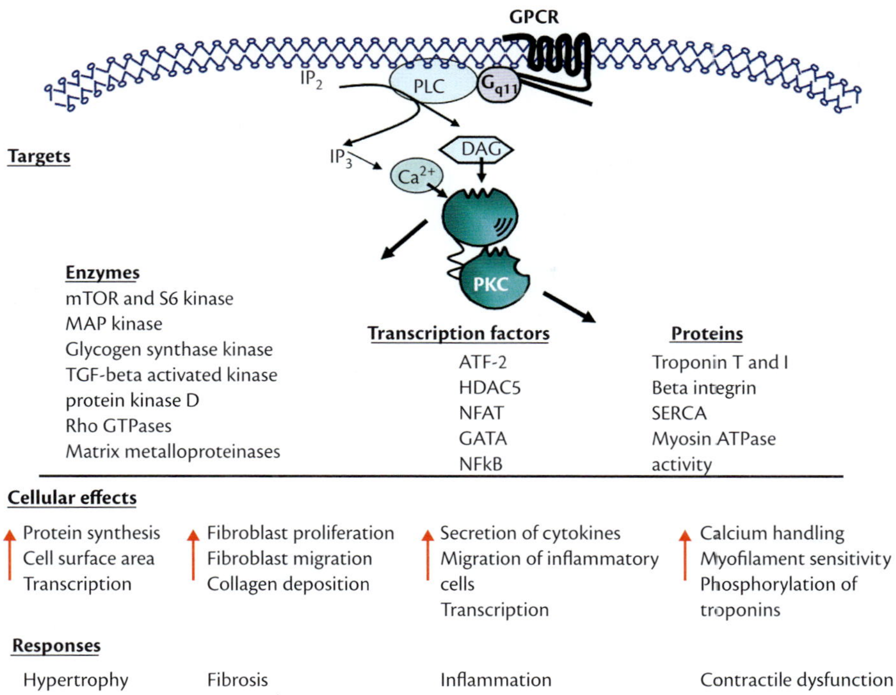

Fig. 2.5 Schematic protein kinase C (PKC) isozyme signaling pathways and downstream targets in the heart. The activation of different PKC isozymes contributes to the establishment of heart failure through phosphorylation of isozyme-selective substrates in the failing heart.

Palaniyandi SS, Sun L, Ferreira JC, Mochly-Rosen D. Protein kinase C in heart failure: a therapeutic target? Cardiovascular Research 2009; 82(2):229–39, by permission of Oxford University Press.

and ζPKC are expressed in the atria, and ε and λPKC are expressed in all chambers.[51]

As illustrated in Figure 2.5,[50] the actions of PKC-mediated signaling in the myocardium are quite diverse and include promotion of pathologic cardiac myocyte hypertrophy and impaired contractility along with inflammation and fibrosis mediated through other cell types. Coactivation of multiple GPCR agonists, interspecies differences, and the coexistence of many different PKC isozymes have challenged efforts to precisely define the PKC signaling most important in transducing cardiac hypertrophy in humans. Stimulation by AngII, PE, or ET1 induces PKC-dependent cardiac myocyte hypertrophy in neonatal rat cardiac myocytes.[50] Studies using more specific PKC agonists demonstrate that the α, βI, βII, and εPKC isozymes induce hypertrophy in this in-vitro model.[50] In in-vivo studies, myocardial dysfunction due to αPKC activation has been demonstrated in mouse models of heart failure, and αPKC knockout strategies have induced both reduced hypertrophy and improved contractility in mice.[52,53] In humans, αPKC is upregulated in the severe hypertrophy associated with chronic aortic stenosis.[51] However, in advanced dilated cardiomyopathy, there is marked activation of βPKC without αPKC activation.[51,54] In hypertensive rats, sustained treatment with a selective βIIPKC-specific inhibitor, βIIV5-3, prolonged survival and delayed the transition from compensated hypertrophy to cardiac dysfunction.[55] Complementary studies in diabetic rats, reported that selective PKCβ inhibition with the orally active agent ruboxistaurin substantially reduced cardiac myocyte cross-sectional area and overall heart hypertrophy in association with reductions in oxidative stress produced by inhibiting NADPH oxidase activation.[56] Thus, in humans, βPKC inhibition represents a promising approach for ameliorating pathologic hypertrophy and dysfunction in diseased hearts.

Basis of normal cardiac myocyte contractility

Normal excitation–contraction coupling and calcium cycling

Cardiac myocytes are excitable cells in which plasma membrane depolarization triggers a cascade of intracellular events collectively referred to as excitation–contraction coupling. In normal myocytes, cyclic increases and decreases in the level of free intracellular [Ca^{2+}], referred to as the Ca^{2+} transient, have a major impact on the rate and magnitude of both cellular contraction and relaxation. With every contraction, the Ca^{2+} transient is derived from two sources: movements of Ca^{2+} in and out of the myocyte and quantitatively larger movements of Ca^{2+} in and out of the sarcoplasmic reticulum (SR) within each myocyte. These movements of Ca^{2+} proceed in an orderly sequence referred to as calcium-induced calcium release. This process is triggered by depolarization of the myocyte plasma membrane during the action potential and begins with Ca^{2+} influx through voltage-sensitive L-type Ca^{2+} channels (LTCC) on the cell membrane. Extracellular Ca^{2+} enters myocytes through these channels and accumulates in a restricted intracellular space between the plasma membrane T-tubules and a portion of the SR that is rich in a Ca^{2+}-sensitive channel called the ryanodine receptor (RyR). Increased Ca^{2+} in this space triggers RyR opening and releases a large quantity of sequested Ca^{2+} from the SR into the cytoplasm where it, in turn, activates myofilament

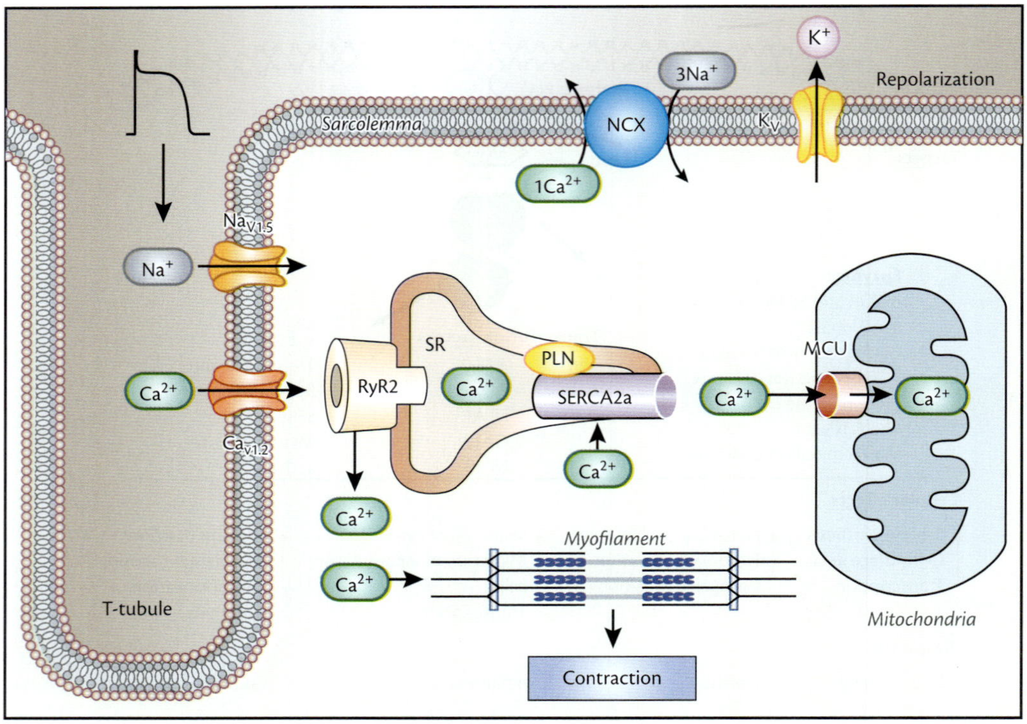

Fig. 2.6 Ca^{2+} homeostasis and excitation–contraction coupling (ECC). The ECC process is initiated when an action potential (AP) excites the myocyte cell membrane (sarcolemma) along its transverse tubules. This depolarization rapidly opens voltage-gated Na^+ channels (mostly $Na_V1.5$) that further depolarize the cell membrane, allowing opening of voltage-gated Ca^{2+} channels (mostly $Ca_V1.2$). Inward Ca^{2+} current triggers opening of ryanodine receptor 2 (RyR2) channels by a Ca^{2+}-induced Ca^{2+} release process, resulting in coordinated release of sarcoplasmic reticulum (SR) Ca^{2+} that contributes the major portion of the myofilament-activating increase in $[Ca^{2+}]_i$. The Ca^{2+} released from the SR binds to troponin C of the troponin–tropomyosin complex on the actin filaments in sarcomeres, facilitating formation of cross-bridges between actin and myosin and myocardial contraction. Voltage-gated K^+ channels open to allow an outward current that favors AP repolarization, establishing conditions required for relaxation. Relaxation occurs when Ca^{2+} is taken back up into the SR through the action of the SR Ca^{2+} ATPase SERCA2a and is extruded from the cell by the sarcolemmal Na^+ and Ca^{2+} exchanger (NCX). SERCA2a is constrained by phospholamban (PLN) under resting conditions.

Luo M, Anderson ME. Mechanisms of altered Ca^{2+} handling in heart failure. Circulation Research 2013; 113(6):690–708.

cross-bridge cycling and myocyte contraction (cellular systole). As the plasma membrane repolarizes during the latter portion of the action potential, Ca^{2+} entry via the LTCC and Ca^{2+} release via the RyR cease, and processes of Ca^{2+} efflux and SR Ca^{2+} reuptake serve to reestablish baseline conditions. In this cellular diastole, the great majority of Ca^{2+} that entered the cell via the LTCC channel leaves the cell via the sodium–calcium exchanger (NCX) while the Ca^{2+} released from the SR via the RyR is pumped back into the SR via the sarcoplasmic reticulum Ca-ATPase (SERCA). These movements of Ca^{2+} are illustrated in Figure 2.6.[57] The amplitude and duration of the Ca^{2+} transient is regulated to modulate the rate, magnitude and duration of contraction. SR Ca^{2+} release is induced and graded by Ca^{2+} influx, through L-type Ca^{2+} channels.[58] The magnitude of SR Ca^{2+} release is also determined by the amount of Ca^{2+} stored in the SR.[59,60]

Normal contractile protein structure and function

Within each sarcomere, there are two major contractile elements: the thick filament, made up mainly of myosin and associated proteins, and the thin filament containing actin, tropomyosin, and the troponin complex, as illustrated in Figure 2.7.[61] Ultimately, the movement of these filaments with respect to one another is responsible for cardiac myocyte shortening, cardiac muscle force generation, and ejection of blood from the heart to the body. The thick filament protruding from the M-line consists of myosin, titin, and myosin-binding protein C (C-protein). Cardiac muscle myosin is comprised of the constituent proteins myosin heavy chain (MHC), essential light chain (ELC or MLC-1), and regulatory light chain (RLC or MLC-2). The hexagonal cross-section of the thick filament is ideally suited for its interaction with six neighboring thin filaments. Filamentous actin (F-actin) is formed by polymerization of actin monomers. Two tropomyosin (Tm) strands and the troponin complex together regulate the affinity of F-actin for the myosin heads that drives the power stroke for sarcomere shortening. Actomyosin ATPase, the key enzyme driving cross-bridge cycling, is regulated by the troponin complex. The troponin complex, in turn, is a heterotrimer composed of the following distinct gene products: troponin C (TnC), the Ca^{2+} receptor; troponin I (TnI), an inhibitor of the actin–myosin interaction that shuttles between tight binding to actin and tight binding to the Ca^{2+}-bound TnC; and troponin T (TnT), a tropomyosin binding component. The position of tropomyosin, as regulated by TnT, is ultimately the major determinant of the actin–myosin cross-bridge interaction. In systole, increased Ca^{2+} binding to TnC leads to conformational changes, including a movement of tropomyosin away from the F-actin groove toward a more peripheral location that exposes the myosin binding site and permits cross-bridge formation. During diastole, decreases in cytosolic Ca^{2+} reverse the conformational changes of systole resulting in marked reductions in, and a weakening of, actin–myosin cross-bridges.[62] More detailed descriptions

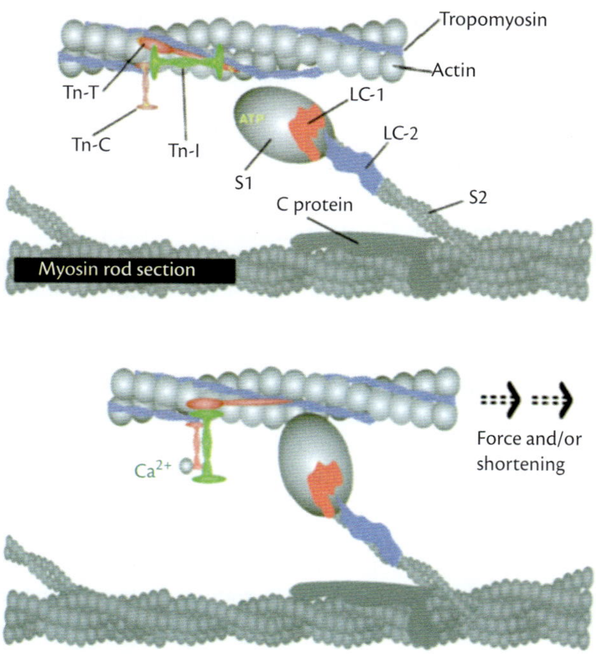

Fig. 2.7 Sarcomere structure and cross-bridge cycling. The major proteins that are involved in contractile activation and regulation are shown in diastole (top panel) and systole (bottom panel). The thin filament is composed of actin, tropomyosin, and the heterotrimer troponin (composed of the troponins Tn-T, Tn-C, and Tn-I). The thick filament is composed of myosin, an asymmetric dimer composed of a globular head portion (S1), a hinged stalk region (S2), and a rod section. The S1portion of myosin contains both theATP hydrolysis domain and the actin binding domain. The S1portion is also associated with two heterodimers, light chains 1 and 2 (LC-1 and LC-2). The myosin rod section also contains the myosin-binding protein C (C-protein); it has a 1–7 myosin stoichiometry. Calcium binding to Tn-C induces a conformational rearrangement in Tn-C, causing the Tn-C:Tn-I association to strengthen while at the same time weakening the Tn-I:Tn-T association; movement of tropomyosin exposes a myosin binding site on actin allowing cross-bridge formation to take place. This results in force development and/or shortening of the sarcomere. Tn-I and C-protein are substrates for protein kinase A (PKA); Tn-I, Tn-T, LC-2, and C-protein are substrates for protein kinase C (PKC).

Reprinted from Journal of Biomechanics Vol. 36 Issue 5, de Tombe PP, Cardiac myofilaments: mechanics and regulation, 721–30, copyright (2003) with permission from Elsevier.

of the complex molecular dynamics regulating cross-bridge cycling and force generation by cardiac myocytes are reviewed elsewhere.[62]

The normal relationship between the extracellular Ca^{2+} concentration and myocardial force generated is sigmoidal, as shown in Figure 2.8.[63] The maximal slope of the Ca^{2+}–force relationship is often referred to as the Hill coefficient. Prior studies demonstrate that motifs within the C-terminal region of cTnI play a central role in negatively regulating cooperativity such that either natural mutations or purposeful deletions in this region induce increases in cooperative binding between the myosin head and the thin filament.[64] Decreases in myofilament calcium-sensitivity are reflected by a shift to the right, such that equivalent force is generated with more extracellular calcium, while increases in calcium sensitivity are reflected by a shift to the left (equivalent force generated with less calcium). As discussed below, the main modulators of myofilament calcium sensitivity under physiologic conditions are the resting sarcomere length and the phosphorylation states of key sarcomeric proteins. Interactions between actin and myosin

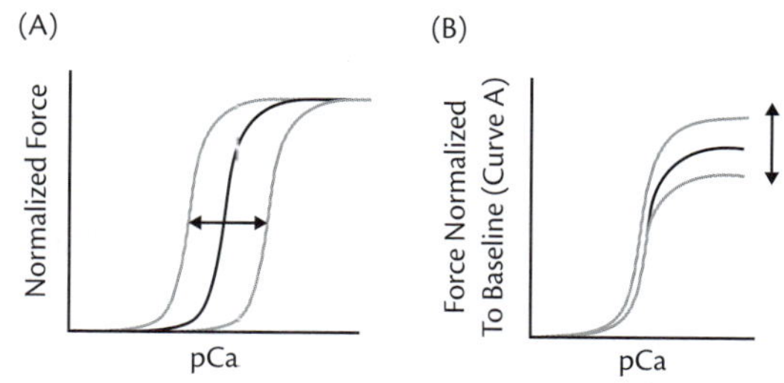

Fig. 2.8 (A) Baseline (dark l ne) force–calcium relationship with left or right shift (light lines) indicating increased (left) and decreased (right) calcium sensitivity of the myofilament. The calcium sensitivity of the myofilament is determined by the ratio of the on-rate and off-rate of calcium binding to troponin C. As the on-rate is determined largely by diffusion, modulation of the off-rate is the mechanism whereby calcium sensitivity can be altered. With a slowed off-rate, the calcium sensitivity of the myofilament is increased so that there is increased force generated at a given level of intracellular calcium. As this does not affect cross-bridges, maximal force is not changed. Interventions that affect troponin C calcium binding and also the interactions between troponin and tropomyosin can alter calcium sensitivity. (B) Force is normalized to baseline to quantify increased or decreased maximal force production with the light shaded lines. This can be achieved by altering the number of cross-bridges, the force produced per cross-bridge, or the number of active force-producing cross-bridges.

MacGowan GA. Cardiovasc Drugs and Therapy 2005, 203–10, Springer.

are further regulated by other contractile proteins, such as MLC, C-protein and the large elastic protein titin. For both the troponin complex and these other sarcomere-associated proteins, increasing evidence indicates that the balance of kinase-mediated phosphorylation and phosphatase-mediated dephosphorylation has a substantial impact on calcium sensitivity in health and disease.

Cardiac myocyte contractile reserve

A fundamental feature of normal cardiac contractility at the organ level is the ability to augment contractility under conditions of increased demand. In contrast to the capacity for partial muscle activation of skeletal muscles, the entire heart contracts with every beat, so that graded contractility must be derived from changes in the contractility of individual cardiac myocytes. In human cardiac myocytes and muscle preparations, acute increases in force generation can occur via increases in stimulation frequency, β-adrenergic stimulation, and increases in resting sarcomere length (the basis for the Frank–Starling relation). Accordingly, myocyte contractility must be evaluated over a broad range of conditions (varying muscle length, loading conditions, beating frequency, concentration of Ca^{2+} and sympathetic amines) because contractile properties can be similar in normal and failing muscles under basal conditions, whereas their responses to inotropic stimuli (frequency of contraction, $[Ca^{2+}]$, increased preload, and catecholamines) are very different.[65,66,67,68]

The force–frequency response

The ability to increase myocardial contractility in response to increased stimulation frequency represents a key mechanism for cardiac adaptation to acute increases in workload,[69] as typically occurs during exercise or other physiologic stress. Indeed, increased contractile force upon faster pacing rates (i.e., a positive force–frequency response/relationship (FFR)) is observed in normal hearts from all large mammals, including humans, but not in rodents. In general, the basis for a positive FFR begins with an increase in overall Ca^{2+} entry into the cell via the LTCC as a result of more channel openings in any given time period and a frequency-dependent increase in the calcium current (I_{Ca}) via phosphorylation by Ca^{2+}/calmodulin-dependent protein kinase (Ca/CaMK).[70,71] As long as increased Ca^{2+} entry per unit time is effectively sequestered into the SR, there will be a greater SR Ca^{2+} load, increased Ca^{2+} release, increased Ca^{2+} transient amplitude, and increased myofilament force generation during subsequent depolarizations. Consistent with this mechanism, SR calcium load does not increase with increased stimulation frequency in mouse and rat hearts, and a flat FFR is observed in these animals.[72] Other factors that have been implicated as regulators or contributors to the FFR are rate-dependent changes in NCX-mediated transport, Ca/CaM-dependent PLB phosphylation, and myofilament Ca sensitivity.[69] Moreover, though the FFR is a characteristic that is derived from cardiac myocytes or muscle preparations during constant preload,[73] some studies demonstrate that the slope of the FFR is modulated by preload, with steeper slopes observed at higher preloads in normal myocardium.[74]

Adrenergic regulation of cardiac myocyte contractility

Changes in cardiac myocyte contractility in response to β-adrenergic receptor stimulation is a central component of the integrated sympathetic nervous system response to acute physiologic stress, including exercise. Both norepinephrine released from cardiac sympathetic nerve endings and epinephrine release by the adrenal gland can bind β-adrenergic receptors on cardiac myocytes and rapidly (within seconds) trigger changes in cardiac myocyte contractility and relaxation dynamics. There are three subtypes of β-adrenergic receptors in the heart: β_1, β_2, and β_3. Of these, β_1 and β_2 regulate contractility directly. Binding to the relatively abundant β_1-adrenergic receptors activates the G_s-adenylyl cyclase (AC)-cAMP-protein kinase A (PKA) signaling cascade. In ventricular myocytes, PKA-mediated phosphorylation targets the LTCC, RyR, phospholamban, troponin I, and cardiac C-protein. Phosphoryation of the three Ca^{2+} handling proteins (LTCC, RyR, and PLB) favors increases in the Ca^{2+} transient amplitude while reduced inhibition of SERCA after PLB phosphorylation accelerates the rate of Ca^{2+} transient decay. Together, these changes favor the stronger and faster contractions needed in the setting of physiologic stress and associated faster heart rates resulting from β_1-mediated effects on the SA node. The less abundant β_2-adrenergic receptors on cardiac myocytes couple to both G_s and the pertussis toxin (PTX)-sensitive G_i proteins.[75,76] The β_2-adrenergic-G_i signaling has negative effects on AC activity, cAMP synthesis, PKA activation, and the inotropic response mediated by G_s.

Length-dependent increases in myocardial force production

Normal cardiac muscle exhibits increased contractile performance as preload or resting sarcomere length is increased. This phenomenon includes a rapid increase in developed force that is mainly attributable to increases in myofilament calcium sensitivity[77] and is the basis for the Frank–Starling relationship. Following sustained increases in preload, there is also a delayed (10–15 minutes) further increase in myocardial force generation (the slow force response) associated with an increase in the $[Ca^{2+}]_i$ transient amplitude[78] that is the basis of the Anrep effect in the intact heart. Together, these length-dependent mechanisms represent essential physiologic regulators of cardiac pump function in vivo. Despite its undisputed importance, the mechanisms underlying the length-dependence of calcium sensitivity have been controversial. One proposed mechanism is that the number of interacting cross-bridges is related to the degree of overlap of thick and thin filaments. However, the large increases in force observed with relatively small length changes suggest that other mechanisms are quantitatively more important.[79] For example, studies by Cazola et al. have supported a potential role for both the giant elastic protein titin[80] and C-protein in converting altered passive tension to changes in Ca^{2+} sensitivity. Additional studies have implicated the PKC phosphorylation site in cTnI as a modulator of length-dependent augmentation of contractility in cardiac sarcomeres.[81] Together, these findings suggest that signaling pathways involving troponin, C-protein and titin, rather than simply spatial relationships between actin and myosin, have a predominating influence on the magnitude of increased force generation in response to increases in sarcomere length. The intracellular basis for the slow force response has also been uncertain, with the most recent reviews affirming a central role for autocrine/paracrine mechanisms that activate redox-sensitive kinases, sodium-hydrogen exchanger (NHE1) activation, and reverse-mode sodium–calcium exchange promoting increased $[Ca^{2+}]_i$ transient amplitude.[82,83] Both animal models and studies examining severely failing human hearts (available through cardiac transplantation) suggest that the Frank–Starling mechanism intact in the failing heart but there is a reduction in the slow force response.[84,85]

Molecular basis of abnormal calcium cycling

In most circumstances, intrinsic defects in cardiac myocyte Ca^{2+} handling and/or alterations in myofilament Ca^{2+} sensitivity and shortening dynamics are centrally involved in the dysfunctional characteristics of the failing heart. This section highlights studies implicating abnormalities in cardiac myocyte Ca^{2+} handling while the next section considers disease-associated abnormalities in cardiac myocyte contractile proteins and molecules and processes involved in their functional regulation.

With respect to Ca^{2+} cycling, early studies by Gwathmey et al. using human myocardial preparations[86] demonstrated alterations in the cardiac myocyte Ca^{2+} transient, and stimulated subsequent research on the role of deranged Ca^{2+} homeostasis in the mechanical abnormalities of the failing heart. Fairly consistent changes in Ca^{2+} handling have been observed in studies using large and small animal models of CHF and in failing human heart muscles and myocytes, as previously reviewed.[87,88] Another general observation supported by numerous studies examining Ca^{2+} handling in failing myocardium is that the functional differences between nonfailing and failing preparations are magnified by acute stress conditions that normally lead to increased contractility, such as increased heart rate and increased β-adrenergic stimulation. As highlighted in the next few paragraphs, and illustrated in Figure 2.9,[89] changes in the abundance or activity of any of the key Ca^{2+} regulatory proteins can contribute to abnormal Ca^{2+} transients in the failing heart and many of these have also been linked to impairments in rate-dependent and adrenergic-dependent contractile reserve.

L-type Ca^{2+} channel

The L-type Ca^{2+} channel (LTCC) opening during plasma membrane depolarization and the resultant Ca^{2+} influx ($I_{Ca,L}$)

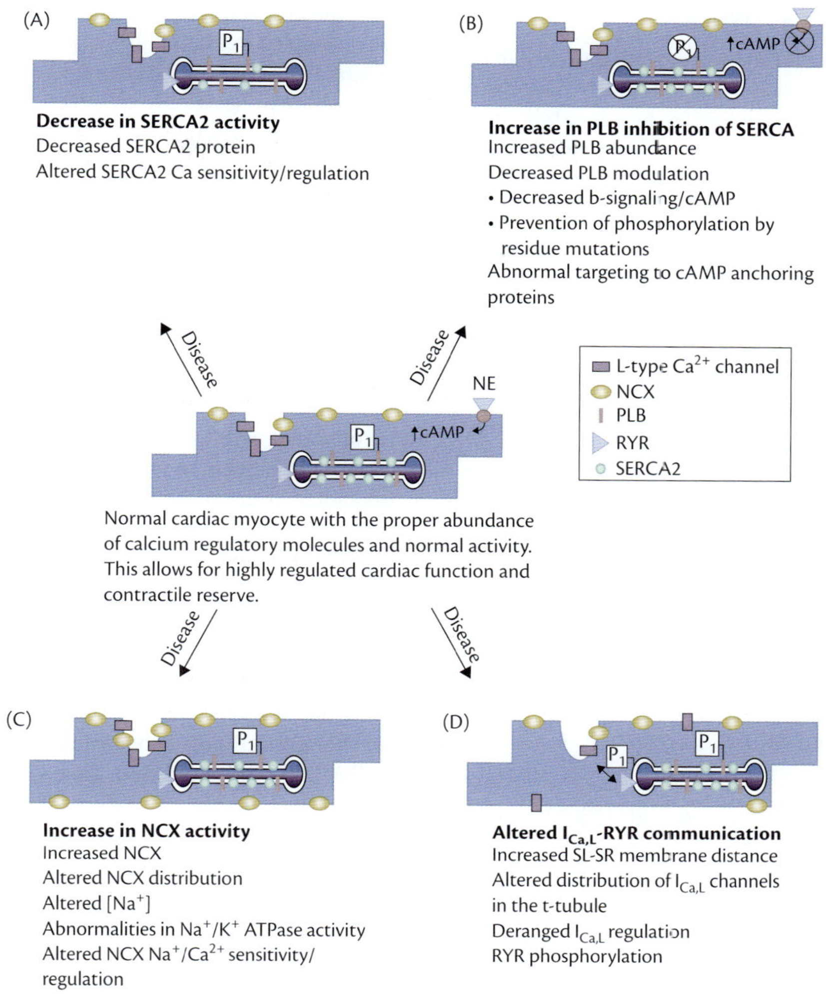

Fig. 2.9 Potential contributors to deranged Ca^{2+} homeostasis in CHF. (A) Decreased abundance of SERCA2 protein could explain reduced sarcoplasmic reticulum (SR) Ca^{2+} loading and slow decay of the Ca^{2+} transient in congestive heart failure. Alterations in SERCA2 protein due to phosphorylation or other modifications needs to be explored. (B) SR function could be depressed in CHF because of increased expression of PLN (which could inhibit SERCA2) or from abnormal phosphorylation of PLN (which relieves the inhibition). (C) Increased abundance of NCX (activity) could increase Ca^{2+} efflux during early phases of the Ca^{2+} transient and deplete SR calcium stores. Slow decay of the calcium transient could involve Ca^{2+} influx via reverse-mode NCX. NCX function in CHF could also be abnormal because of increased $[Na^+]_i$ or changes in the transporter distribution in surface and t-tubular membranes. (D) Reduced SR Ca^{2+} release in CHF could result from altered junctional microarchitecture, changes in L-type Ca^{2+} channel distribution, or dysfunctional phosphorylation of the RyR release channels.

contributes to the plateau phase of the action potential, directly elevates cytoplasmic $[Ca^{2+}]$, and induces SR Ca^{2+} release.[90] Ca^{2+} influx via the L-type Ca^{2+} current is also an important source of Ca^{2+} to maintain and modify the amount of Ca^{2+} stored in the SR [91] Reductions in the number of these Ca^{2+} channels, abnormal localization, or abnormal activity could explain many aspects of disrupted Ca^{2+} homeostasis in CHF. Extending studies in failing canine myocytes,[92] Chen et al demonstrated that the density of the LTCC is reduced in failing human myocytes but the Ca^{2+} current is maintained by increased PKA-mediated phosphorylation of the channels, which increase their activity.[93] Because the LTCC was largely phosphorylated in the basal state, sympathetic agonists had little ability to increase the current further. Therefore, blunted adrenergic effects on myocyte contractility are likely to involve a failure to increase Ca^{2+} influx and increase SR Ca^{2+} loading. These ideas are supported by experiments in which the open probability of single Ca^{2+} channels from failing human ventricular myocytes was shown to be increased, consistent with increased phosphorylation.[94] One study has shown that $I_{Ca,L}$ decreases more in failing than in normal myocytes when the beating frequency is increased.[95] These results also suggest that rate-related reduction of $I_{Ca,L}$ may be an important component of disrupted rate-dependent regulation of contractility in CHF.

Ryanodine receptor

Ca^{2+}-induced opening of the RyR allows Ca^{2+} to be released from the SR with each contraction. The Marks laboratory has pioneered the idea that RyR dysfunction, due to PKA-mediated hyperphosphorylation of RyR, is involved in dysregulated Ca^{2+} in human heart failure.[96] Though studies disagree about the relative importance of PKA-mediated hyperphosphorylation versus CaMKII-mediated phosphorylation,[97,98,99] most have shown RyR dysfunction in CHF.[100] Several studies have also implicated RyR dysfunction in arrhythmias.[101,102,103,104,105]

Sarcoplasmic reticulum Ca ATPase

Most studies have found that SR Ca^{2+} uptake rate is slowed in heart failure and this can lead to increased diastolic Ca^{2+} (diastolic dysfunction) and reduced SR Ca^{2+} storage (reduced systolic performance). Because reuptake of Ca^{2+} into the SR by SERCA affects both the amount available for subsequent release and the rate of myofilament relaxation, SERCA is a particularly important contributor to cellular calcium homeostasis. While several studies have reported reduced SERCA mRNA or protein abundance in failing human hearts, other studies that did not observe reduced SERCa protein abundance or Ca^{2+} uptake rates in failing human hearts[106,107] suggest that derangements in cellular Ca^{2+} handling in human myocytes are not always caused by a reduction in the abundance of SERCA. Another possibility is that changes in the functional inhibition of SERCA by an associated protein, phospholamban (PLN), might account for changes in SERCA-mediated Ca^{2+} reuptake into the SR. Studies in which SERCA overexpression prevented heart failure in susceptible transgenic mouse models[108,109,110] suggest that an inability of the SR to take up and store Ca^{2+} is a critical factor in heart failure induction and progression. The concept that therapeutic SERCA overexpression may have clinical efficacy was supported by a phase 1 clinical trial[111] and is being further examined in the CUPID 2b Trial (ClinicalTrials.gov, NCT01643330).

Phospholamban

PLN is a SR protein that directly interacts with SERCA and functionally inhibits SERCA-mediated Ca^{2+} transport. Phosphorylation of PLN by either protein kinase A or Ca^{2+}-calmodulin-dependent protein kinase[112] reduces the inhibitory effect of PLN on SERCA, increases the decay rate of the Ca^{2+} transient, and increased the amount of Ca^{2+} stored in the SR. Under normal circumstances, increased sympathetic nervous system activity associated with exercise or other physiologic stress triggers PLB phosphorylation and contributes to the increased contractility and relaxation rate required to increase cardiac output and faster heart rates. Either a higher PLN/SERCa ratio or reduced PLN phosphorylation could reduce SR Ca^{2+} transport without involving a change in SERCA protein.[113] Moreover, mouse studies indicate that genetic manipulations to induce decreases in PLN abundance produced similar benefit to that observed with SERCA overexpression.[114,115] However, humans with analogous PLN mutations that reduce the inhibitory effects of PLN on SERCA have cardiac dysfunction and premature death,[116] so there seem to be species differences between mice and humans that reduce the attractiveness of PLN inhibition as a therapeutic target in patients with heart failure.

Sodium–calcium exchanger (NCX)

The sodium–calcium exchanger (NCX) is a plasma membrane ion transporter that moves both sodium and calcium ions in and out of cardiac myocytes depending on their concentration gradients and the membrane potential. At the normal resting potential of −80 mV, and with normal concentrations of intracellular Na^{+}, there is sufficient energy in the Na^{+} electrochemical gradient to remove Ca^{2+} from the cell via NCX (termed *forward-mode NCX*). This is the principal mechanism for Ca^{2+} efflux in cardiac myocytes[88] and serves to balance the Ca^{2+} influx via the LTCC that triggers calcium-induced Ca^{2+} release. When the membrane potential is depolarized and/or intracellular Na increases, the energy in the Ca^{2+} electrochemical gradient can be sufficient to produce Ca^{2+} entry coupled to Na^{+} efflux via *reverse-mode NCX*.[117] Most studies of human myocardium have found increases in NCX abundance in failing human hearts.[118,119,120] This increase and prolonged action potential duration appear to contribute to the slowed decay of the Ca^{2+} transient in failing human myocytes due to Ca^{2+} influx during the action potential plateau (reverse-mode NCX). Then, upon repolarization, increased NCX function in forward mode (Ca^{2+} out) results in functional competition with SERCA such that more Ca^{2+} removed from the cytoplasm via NCX results in reduced SERCA-mediated SR Ca^{2+} loading. This construct suggests that the ratio of NCX to SERCA abundance and transport, regardless of the cause, is an important determinant of both the peak of the Ca^{2+} transient and the rate of Ca^{2+} transient decay.[121] This model is consistent with the observation that defects in isolated myocyte contractility are more pronounced during increases in stimulation frequency, as discussed below.

Pathologic frequency-dependent responses

Because augmenting force during increased stimulation frequency normally depends on augmenting Ca^{2+} transient amplitude, it is not surprising that changes in calcium-handling proteins are associated with defects in the FFR in failing hearts. When CHF is severe, such as in end-stage human heart failure, peak systolic Ca^{2+} and force (or shortening) is close to normal only at very slow pacing rates. As the beating rate is increased, there is either no change or a decrease in peak systolic Ca^{2+} and force of contraction (negative FFR) in the failing heart.[86,122] There is an associated increase in diastolic Ca^{2+} with increased heart rate.[122] These results strongly support the hypothesis that changes in cellular Ca^{2+} handling are a final common pathway for progressive deterioration of cardiac pump function in CHF. Pieske et al. first demonstrated that the flattened (or negative) FFR of failing human ventricular myocytes results from the fact that SR Ca^{2+} loading does not increase normally with stimulation rate.[123] In turn, the inability to increase SR Ca^{2+} load during higher stimulation frequencies seems to reflect the changes in the ratio of SERCA and NCX abundance and Ca^{2+} transport, as noted above. Specifically, decreases in the ratio of SERCa/NCX abundance are associated with a negative force–frequency relationship in the failing human heart.[124] When this activity ratio is decreased, the peak systolic Ca^{2+} will be blunted because forward-mode NCX will eliminate Ca^{2+} from the cytoplasm.[125] This "balance of activity" hypothesis is further supported by blunted FFR following adenovirus-mediated increases in NCX abundance[126] and enhanced FFR after either increasing in SERCA expression[127] or antagonizing PLN[128] in isolated cardiac myocytes. The changes in Ca^{2+} handling are also likely to be critically involved in the arrhythmias,[129,130] metabolic disturbances, activation of cell death pathways,[131,132,133,134] and hypertrophy[135] in advanced heart failure. This hypothesis is also supported by preclinical studies in animal models in which the transition from compensated hypertrophy to CHF coincides with the time that myocytes first lose their ability to maintain physiologic levels of systolic and diastolic Ca^{2+}.[136]

Pathologic adrenergic responses

In contrast to acute, short-term physiologic stress, heart failure results in persistent stimulation of β_1- and β_2-adrenergic receptors with a variety of distinct consequences for cardiac myocyte biology. For example, sustained stimulation of β_1-adrenergic receptors triggers cardiomyocyte hypertrophy[137] and maladaptive cardiac remodeling in vivo[26,138] by a CaMKII-dependent mechanism.[139] In addition, β_1-adrenergic-activated CaMKII signaling is involved in catecholamine-induced apoptosis (programmed cell death). In contrast to the cardiotoxic effects of persistent β_1-adrenergic activation, persistent β_2-adrenergic stimulation appears to be cardioprotective. Beneficial effects of persistent β_2-adrenergic signaling are mediated by β_2-adrenergic–G_i coupling which activates a distinct PI3K-Akt cell survival pathway.[140] Although beneficial in terms of cardiomyocyte viability, the protective effect of β_2-adrenergic activity comes at the cost of compromised contractile support. Another factor reducing contractile responses to endogenous and exogenous catecholamines in heart failure is a reduction in the abundance of β_1-adrenergic receptors,[141,142] with no change in β_2-adrenergic receptors.[143] This selective downregulation of β_1-adrenergic response is often associated with an upregulation of G_i and an enhanced β_2-adrenergic–G_i signaling.[144,145]

In heart failure, the signaling efficiency of β_1-adrenergic receptors is also reduced by an increase in the expression of a specific G-protein receptor kinase (βARK),[146] which results in the internalization of the β_1 receptor via endocytosis.[147] βARK-mediated desensitization of β_2-adrenergic receptors leads to reduced contractile responses to adrenergic agonists, but appears to be protective against excessive sympathetic stimulation during heart failure.[148,149] Together with the blunted force–frequency responses highlighted above, the multilevel abnormalities in β-adrenergic signaling indicate that in advanced heart failure, overall myocardial "contractile reserve" is severely depressed, even if basal contractility is maintained. These fundamental changes in muscle performance and regulation can explain the poor pump function, reduced exercise capacity, and tachycardia intolerance of the failing human heart. Studies demonstrating reduced contractile reserve in patients with heart failure and preserved LVEF suggest that some or all of these cellular defects may apply to failing hearts without obvious systolic dysfunction at rest.[150,151]

In rodent models of heart failure, upregulation of βARK[146,152] and G_i proteins[144,145,153] have been implicated as causal factors in the development of heart failure and both myocardial ischemia and hypertension have been associated with elevated GRK2 expression and activity.[154,155] However, the net balance of beneficial versus detrimental effects of reduced β-receptor abundance, altered β_1/β_2-subtype distribution and βARK-mediated desensitization in humans remains uncertain. As recently reviewed,[156] the resolution of this uncertainty, particularly in the setting of β-blocker therapy, which itself affects β_2-adrenergic signaling, has important implications for new drug development.

The studies summarized above support the idea that abnormal Ca^{2+} handling and the associated defects in frequency-dependent and β_1-adrenergic-mediated contractile reserve are closely associated with the progression of pump dysfunction and symptoms among patients with heart failure. However, available evidence does not implicate a single molecular defect as the cause for abnormal cardiac myocyte Ca^{2+} homeostasis. Rather, it appears that changes in the interaction of multiple Ca^{2+} regulatory proteins combine with multilevel abnormalities in β-adrenergic signaling to produce a significant impairment of contractile reserve that likely contributes to impaired exercise tolerance among patients with heart failure. Moreover, it appears that the severity of the derangements in Ca^{2+} handling and adrenergic signaling increases with the severity of heart failure. In this context, the critical question remains: Is the generalized blunting of Ca^{2+} handling in heart failure a reactive response that helps reduce Ca^{2+} overload and the associated activation of cell death signaling and arrhythmias, or are these changes maladaptive responses that drive the progression of the syndrome? The answer to this question is currently uncertain, but may ultimately be defined by clinical outcomes following interventions that restore normal Ca^{2+} handling and adrenergic stimulation in the CHF environment.

Targeting Ca cycling defects with S100A1

S100A1 is an EF-hand Ca^{2+} sensor protein that affects cardiomyocyte Ca^{2+} homeostasis and the subsequent regulation of excitability, contractile performance, energy metabolism, hypertrophic growth, and cell survival.[157] Its expression is progressively downregulated in failing myocardium.[158] Supporting the functional importance of S100A1, cardiac-specific S100A1 deletion accelerated the progression to heart failure after MI in mice,[159] whereas restoration of S100A1 expression via intracoronary adenoviral gene delivery to failing rat hearts normalized contractile performance.[160] Moreover, an adenovirus construct inducing overexpression of S100A1 in isolated human cardiac myocytes from severely failing hearts improves failing cardiomyocyte fractional shortening, relaxation rates, and Ca^{2+} transients compared with control cells.[161] Moreover, increased S100A1 expression improves both rate-dependent and β-adrenergic-mediated contractile reserve, while ameliorating markers of abnormal energy metabolism in isolated cardiomyocytes and mitochondria from failing hearts. Although details of the molecular mechanism of S100A1's actions remains uncertain, there is data to support direct interaction of S100A1 with SR and mitochondrial proteins (i.e., RyR, SERCA, and F1-ATPase)[162] and the interaction between the sarcomeric proteins titin and cardiac actin.[163] These findings suggest that S100A1 is a promising therapeutic target in human heart failure.[157]

Abnormalities in sarcomeric proteins

Alterations in cardiac myofilament dynamics can contribute to reduced cardiac pump function in a variety of ways that are relevant to both acute and chronic heart failure. Accordingly, we will consider how naturally occurring mutations, transgenic manipulations, and disease-associated modifications to sarcomeric proteins demonstrate their physiologic and pathophysiologic importance. This section also highlights how post-translational regulation of myofilament activity via phosphorylation affects cardiac performance in the setting of acute and chronic cardiac insults.

Heart failure due to sarcomeric protein mutations

As summarized in Box 2.1,[164] naturally occurring mutations in a wide variety of genes have been shown to produce hereditable cardiomyopathies. Identification of a genetic cause is most frequent for hypertrophic cardiomyopathies, with more than 1000 distinct heritable mutations identified as capable of inducing increases in wall thickness in the absence of increased hemodynamic load.[165,166] Most of these are mutations that affect a single nucleotide within the coding region of a cardiac myocyte sarcomeric protein and exhibit autosomal dominant inheritance with variable penetrance. In dilated cardiomyopathies with less distinctive morphologies,

Box 2.1 Sarcomeric protein mutations causing cardiomyopathy in humans

Mutations associated with a familial dilated cardiomyopathy

Affecting force generation/regulation

- Actin, α, cardiac muscle 1
- Myosin, heavy chain 7, cardiac muscle, β
- Troponin T type 2 (cardiac)
- Troponin I type 3 (cardiac)
- Troponin C type 1 (slow)

Affecting force transduction/mechanosensing

- Titin
- Dystrophin
- Sarcoglycan, Δ (35-kDa dystrophin-associated protein)
- Desmin

Mutations associated with a familial hypertrophic cardiomyopathy

- Myosin, heavy chain 7, cardiac muscle, β
- Myosin-binding protein C, cardiac
- Troponin T type 2 (cardiac)
- Troponin I type 3 (cardiac)
- Tropomyosin 1 (α)
- Myosin, light chain 2, regulatory, cardiac, slow
- Myosin, light chain 3, alkali; ventricular, skeletal, slow
- Actin, α, cardiac muscle 1

Modified from Cahill, T.J., H. Ashrafian, and H. Watkins, Genetic cardiomyopathies causing heart failure. Circulation Research, 2013. 113(6): p. 660–75.

recent analyses suggest that more than 30% of cases are directly caused by single-gene mutations. However, a smaller fraction of hereditary dilated cardiomyopathies are due to sarcomeric protein mutations, with mutations in various other gene families also capable of producing this phenotype.[167] Box 2.1 also demonstrates that alternative point mutations within a given gene can be associated with very different phenotypic features depending of the exact location of the mutation. For example, mutations involving cardiac isoforms of α-actin, myosin-binding protein C, MHC 7, titin, and troponin T can each cause hypertrophic cardiomyopathy, dilated cardiomyopathy, or LV noncompaction cardiomyopathy, depending on the specific mutation. It is likely that the morphologic and functional impact of a particular allelic mutation is the result of secondary adaptations to the initial mutation.[167] For example, one specific mutation affecting myofilament Ca^{2+} sensitivity may trigger a compensatory concentric hypertrophy and be associated with a primary diastolic abnormality, while another mutation affecting cross-bridge cycling may alter force transmission and be manifested as a dilated cardiomyopathy phenotype with systolic dysfunction. Fortunately, the ability to create an animal model analogue of mutations producing inherited cardiomyopathies is permitting the investigation of how particular sarcomeric protein domains regulate myocyte contractility.

Isoform switches of sarcomeric proteins in failing hearts

While studies of patients with familial cardiomyopathies demonstrate how single allelic mutations affecting sarcomeric proteins can be sufficient to induce profound phenotypic manifestations, such disease-causing mutations represent only a small fraction of the functionally important changes in sarcomeric proteins observed in failing hearts. In contrast, recent studies have increasingly identified pathologic changes in myofilament isoforms that are relatively common and may be functionally significant. Among the reported changes in contractile protein isoforms in failing human hearts, the MHC isoform switch is the most widely appreciated and best studied. Normal adult rat hearts express almost exclusively the alpha isoform of myosin heavy chain (α-MHC) while rats with experimental heart failure develop an almost complete conversion to β-MHC that is analogous to the situation in the fetal heart.[168] Thus, the switch from α-MHC to β-MHC in the hypertrophied or failing heart is referred to as a "fetal isoform switch." In failing human hearts, multiple studies have reported qualitatively similar, but quantitatively lesser, shifts with α-MHC expression decreasing from 5–15% in the normal myocardium to 0–2% in the failing human myocardium.[169] Other studies, using animals with experimental hypothyroidism and in-vitro constructs, have demonstrated that such relatively small shifts in α-MHC abundance can be functionally significant, with greater α-MHC expression allowing faster contraction.[170] Using a similar approach, Metzger and coworkers also showed that increased β-MHC was associated with a decrease in myofilament calcium sensitivity.[171] Additional studies have demonstrated that a highly conserved microRNA (miR-208) encoded by an intron of α-myosin heavy chain (*MHC*) gene plays a pivotal role in regulating the balance of α- and β-MHC in experimental hypothyroidism and pressure overload.[172] Interestingly, miRNA-208 knockout mice unable to upregulate β-MHC were resistant to hypertrophy and fibrosis during chronic pressure overload, but developed age-dependent defects in sarcomere structure and cardiac performance. Accordingly, these studies suggest that the pathologic α- to β-MHC isoform switch might have an adaptive role in the setting of sustained hemodynamic overload.

Analogous shifts to fetal isoforms during heart failure have also been observed for other contractile proteins. For example, smooth muscle α-actin is expressed during cardiac myogenesis, absent in normal adult heart and re-expressed following experimental pressure overload in rats or dilated cardiomyopathy in humans.[173] Pathologic expression of an atrial isoform of the cardiac myosin essential light chain (cMLC-1) in the RV of patients with tetralogy of Fallot was positively correlated with shortening velocity at a variety of different afterloads.[174] Similar correlations between atrial MLC content and contractility have been reported in patients with hypertrophic cardiomyopathy.[175] Because the ventricular expression of the atrial MLC-1 expression is linked with faster rates of contraction, the findings conform to the concept that "pathologic" isoform switches in failing hearts may be adaptive. More recently, developmental isoform switches have also been observed for titin, the large elastic filament that plays a prominent role in regulating

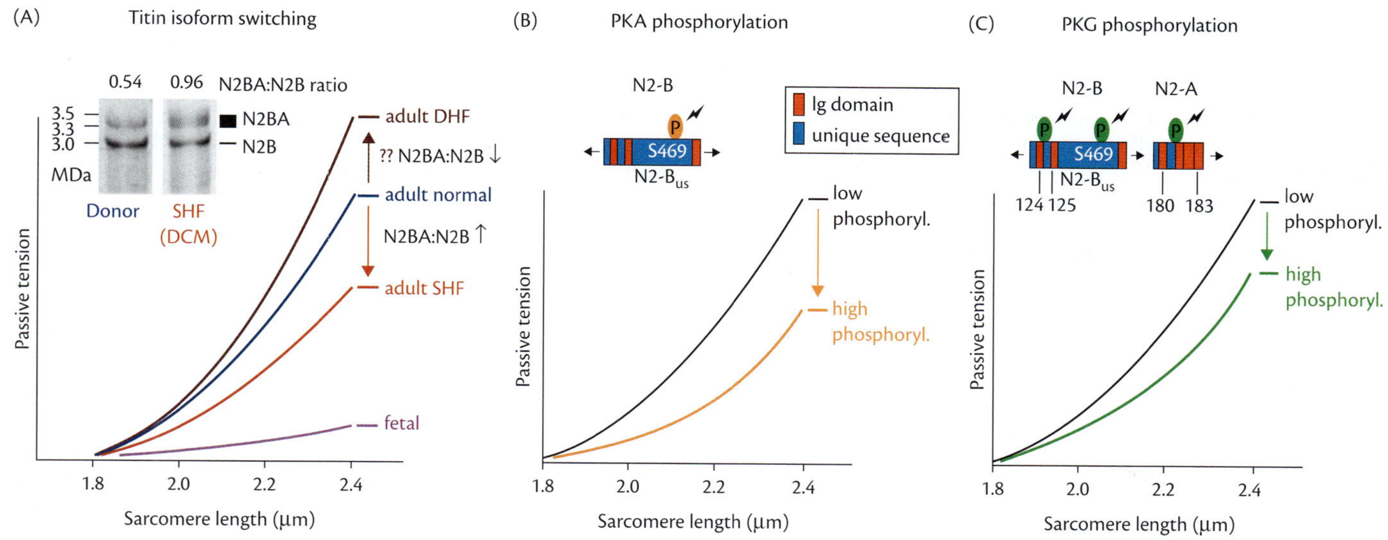

Fig. 2.10 Ways to modulate the passive tension of cardiac myocytes through alterations in titin stiffness. Shown are exemplary passive sarcomere length–tension relationships of cardiac myofibrils. DCM, dilated cardiomyopathy; DHF, diastolic heart failure; I24, I25, I80, I83, I-band titin Ig-domains; N2-Bus, unique sequence insertion of the cardiac N2-B titin domain; S469, serine residue 469 of the human N2-Bus; SHF, systolic heart failure.

myocyte passive tension. As illustrated in panel A of Figure 2.10,[176] the longer, more compliant titin isoform (N2BA) predominates in cardiac myocytes of the developing heart.[177] After birth, there is a transition to greater representation of the stiffer N2B isoform which ultimately becomes the dominant isoform in the LV. In the setting of advanced systolic heart failure with a severely reduced ejection fraction, there is a relative increase in the N2BA isoform associated with reduced myofibrillar stiffness.[178] On the other hand, in patients with heart failure and preserved ejection fraction, a lower N2BA:N2B ratio is associated with a severe increase in stiffness.[179] Despite these interesting results, the fact that multiple isoform shifts typically occur concurrently in the same muscle preparation presents a challenge to the interpretation of the overall functional significance of isoform switches in human myocardium.

PKA phosphorylation of sarcomeric proteins

Phosphorylation and other post-translational modifications of sarcomeric proteins mediate significant and important functional effects on myocardial contractility and relaxation dynamics. The best studied of these dynamics is the regulation of contractility by PKA-mediated phosphorylation of several myocyte proteins following β-adrenergic stimulation. Specifically, combined with phosphorylation of the LTCC, RyR, and PLN, PKA-mediated phosphorylation of key myofibrillar proteins permits the inotropy and faster relaxation required for achievement of enhanced stroke volume and faster heart rates required during physiologic stress. Under normal circumstances, increased adrenergic stimulation leads to *decreased* myofibrillar calcium sensitivity via PKA-dependent phosphorylation of TnI and C-protein.[180,181] PKA-dependent phosphorylation of the N-terminal region of cardiac TnI[182] lowers the affinity of TnC for Ca^{2+}. PKA-dependent phosphorylation of C-protein results in enhanced force generation[183] and accelerates actin–myosin cross-bridge kinetics to augment contractile performance both in vitro and in vivo.[184] Under loaded conditions, the net effect of TnI and C-protein phosphorylation via PKA is increased force-generating capacity and increased absolute power output, likely reflecting a predominating effect of C-protein on cross-bridge cycling.[185,186]

Recognizing that the syndrome of heart failure is characterized by chronic increases in cardiac adrenergic stimulation, several groups have examined the state of PKA-mediated regulation of myofibrillar function in failing human hearts and animal models of heart failure. Despite the potential effect of increased TnI phosphorylation to decrease Ca^{2+} sensitivity, greater myofibrillar Ca^{2+} sensitivity has been reported in failing mouse, rat, dog, pig, and human hearts compared with nonfailing controls.[187] In each of these models, there was an intact or enhanced response to direct (receptor-independent) PKA stimulation in vitro and a decreased level of in-vivo TnI phosphorylation despite increased ambient adrenergic tone, suggesting uncoupling of the adrenergic stimulation cascade. In interspecies comparisons, it is noteworthy that the greatest degree of enhanced Ca^{2+} sensitivity and uncoupling was observed in failing human myocardium, with rodent models of heart failure tending to substantially underestimate the defects. Consistent with these findings, several investigators have demonstrated reduced baseline phosphorylation of TnI and C-protein in failing human hearts compared with nonfailing controls.[187,188]

PKC phosphorylation of sarcomeric proteins

Many cellular actions of vasoactive peptides like angiotensin II and endothelin are mediated via PKC-dependent signaling processes. Gwathmey and Hajjar demonstrated that PKC-dependent phosphorylation reduces the peak force development and the slope of the Ca^{2+}/force relationship in both failing and nonfailing human myocardium, consistent with PKC-mediated reductions in Ca^{2+} sensitivity.[189] These studies were complemented by studies demonstrating that phosphorylation of both TnI and/or TnT by direct PKC stimulation causes inhibition of Mg ATPase activity.[190] Using transgenic mice lacking sites for PKC-mediated phosphorylation of troponin, Noland and coworkers demonstrated that phosphorylation of cardiac TnI at Ser-43/Ser-45 is responsible for PKC-mediated decreases in Ca^{2+} sensitivity while cTnI phosphorylation at Ser-23/Ser-24 is responsible for regulation of actomyosin MgATPase.[191] Extending these findings to humans, Noguchi et al. linked PKC phosphorylation of thin filaments from failing human hearts to decreased maximal force development despite increased shortening velocity, while van der Velden et al. reported a PKC-mediated decrease in Ca^{2+} sensitivity with minimal effects on peak force development.[192] Together, these studies demonstrated that intact PKC-dependent phosphorylation of both cTnI and cTnT improve diastolic function in failing human myocardium in which PKA-mediated TnI phosphorylation is decreased. These studies also implicate specific upregulation of PKC-α and PKC-β isoforms as contributors to increased PKC-dependent activity in heart failure, with reduced expression of these isoforms observed after left ventricular assist device (LVAD) support.

Titin phosphorylation and passive properties of myocytes

Though heart failure is consistently associated with a positive relationship between preload and contractility, the passive stiffness of the myocardium regulates preload-dependent contractility in vivo. In failing human myocardium, a greater increase in resting tension is typically required to achieve any given increment in muscle length (increased diastolic stiffness) so that the ratio of increased developed force to increased passive force is decreased. Though changes in the extracellular matrix (e.g., fibrosis) may also modulate myocardial stiffness, increased passive stiffness of cardiac myocytes themselves is observed in hearts with severely reduced systolic dysfunction.[187] In fact, phosphorylation via either a cAMP/PKA-dependent mechanism[193] or cGMP/PKG-dependent signaling[194] may alter titin's contribution to cardiac myocyte passive stiffness in failing hearts, as illustrated in panels B and C of Figure 2.10. In contrast to the titin isoform switches discussed above, these adaptations can occur on a beat-to-beat basis. Under normal circumstances, the decrease in passive tension induced by titin phosphorylation is greater following PKA phosphorylation than following PKG phosphorylation.[195] In this context, the observation that increased myocyte passive stiffness with systolic dysfunction can be prevented by direct PKA activation supports a role for impaired adrenergic signaling as an underlying mechanism for this pathophysiologic defect.[187] Other studies suggest that defects in adrenergic signaling contribute even more to increased myocyte passive stiffness in failing hearts with preserved ejection fraction.[196,197] Defects in PKG-mediated titin phosphorylation, as is activated by nitric oxide or natriuretic peptides (ANP and BNP), have likewise been implicated as contributing to increased myocyte passive stiffness in failing human and canine hearts.[194] In these studies, reductions in both PKA- and PKG-dependent titin phosphorylation were observed in failing hearts compared with non-failing controls. These studies raise the therapeutic possibility that pathologic increases in myocardial stiffness could be prevented by interventions that enhance PKA- or PKG-dependent signaling in failing hearts. Supporting this possibility, two separate groups have demonstrated that sustained inhibition of cGMP proteolysis via phosphodiesterase (PDE)-5 inhibition improves indices LV diastolic function in murine hearts.[198,199] Recent evidence indicating that PDE-9 degrades intracellular cGMP stimulated by natriuretic peptides,[200] suggests that PDE-9 inhibitors might likewise augment diastolic function via enhanced titin phosphorylation.

Limited proteolysis of contractile proteins

Another potentially important post-translational modification of contractile proteins contributing to contractile dysfunction is proteolysis of myofilaments themselves or key regulatory proteins. The myocardium is particularly ischemia-sensitive, and myocardial contractile proteins manifest structural changes after only 10 minutes of ex-vivo warm ischemia.[201] Indeed, the phenomenon of myocardial stunning, when sustained contractile dysfunction is induced by a transient ischemic insult, has been strongly linked to limited proteolysis of contractile proteins by studies demonstrating intact cytosolic Ca^{2+} transients in association with a severe contractile defects and decreased thin-filament Ca^{2+} sensitivity and time-dependent degradation of cTnI.[202] With more severe ischemia, there is release of TnI fragments (e.g., TnI_{1-193}) from myocytes enabling detection of myonecrosis by plasma assays. Building on these observations, some investigators have suggested that limited proteolysis of myofibrils with associated changes in Ca^{2+} sensitivity and force generation could be an important initiating or propagating pathophysiologic process within the failing heart.[203] For example, significantly elevated preload can induce limited TnI proteolysis, via activation of μ-calpains, even in the absence of frank ischemia.[204] These findings suggest the hypothesis that sustained increases in LV end-diastolic pressure, as often observed in patients with advanced heart failure, could contribute to contractile dysfunction via thin-filament proteolysis. Observations that overexpression of heat shock protein 27 protects cTnI, cTnT, and other sarcomeric proteins against proteolysis during transient ischemia or acute calcium overload suggest potential therapeutic opportunities.[205]

Abnormalities of cardiac metabolism

The heart consumes more energy per gram than any other organ, and myocardial metabolic demands are further increased in the setting of heart failure by pathologic hypertrophy, increased wall stress, neurohormonal stimulation, and vasoconstriction. Even in the absence of acute coronary insufficiency, an increasing body of literature supports the concept of the failing heart as an energy-starved organ.[206,207,208] With limited abilities to store ATP in the form of glycogen and phosphocreatine (PCr), the normal and failing heart is continuously dependent on ATP synthesis to maintain the force generation, myofibrillar relaxation, and ionic homeostasis involved in excitation–contraction coupling. Cardiac and skeletal muscles have endogenous systems of adaptation to physiologic challenges such as exercise and immobility. Central in this adaptation is the flexible metabolic circuitry that is capable of switching preferred energy substrates and regulating pathways of oxidative and non-oxidative energy transduction to optimally adapt to physiologic demands.

The metabolic derangements in failing hearts include myocardial insulin resistance, mitochondrial dysfunction, weight loss leading to cardiac cachexia in the more advanced stages, and myocardial energetic failure associated with a downregulation of lipid metabolism. There is a general shift from fatty acids to glucose as the primary energy substrate in association with decreased oxidative phosphorylation, and dysregulated systems of ATP transfer.[209] In this section we review the programs of metabolic adaptation that have been linked to pathologic myocardial hypertrophy and chronic systolic heart.

Metabolic adaptation in cardiac hypertrophy

Several animal models and studies in humans have identified that pathologic cardiac hypertrophy is associated with a reduction in fatty acid oxidation and increased glucose utilization, consistent with a reinduction or recapitulation of the "fetal metabolic program." In pathologic cardiac hypertrophy, changes in transcription factors such as PPARα and cofactors such as PGC-1α induce a reduction in fatty acid oxidation due to downregulation of proteins involved with fatty acid transport[208] and utilization,[210,211,212,213] and cardiac metabolism becomes more dependent upon glucose metabolism. In a swine model of moderate left ventricular hypertrophy (LVH), although no difference in glucose or free fatty acid (FFA) uptake was present in the basal state, increased myocardial workload with dobutamine stimulation significantly increased glucose uptake in LVH, as evidenced by increases in both glucose oxidation and anaerobic glycolysis.[214] In humans, myocardial fatty acid oxidation as measured in vivo with positron emission tomography (PET) was independently associated with LV mass and hypertensive LVH.[215,216] Another study, evaluating high-energy phosphate metabolism in patients with LVH using a ^{31}P magnetic resonance spectroscopy (MRS) technique measuring ATP flux through the creatine kinase (CK) systems in the human heart, identified a 30% reduction in the net ATP flux through CK in LVH and a 65% reduction in patients with LVH and a diagnosis of CHF, suggesting that a deficit in myocardial energy transfer may contribute in the transition from LVH to failure.[217]

Metabolic adaptation in systolic heart failure

Under resting conditions, the failing heart shifts fuel use toward greater glucose use and lower FFA oxidation. In the failing myocardium, glucose uptake and utilization increase and fatty acid uptake and oxidation decrease. The changes in myocardial gene expression associated with this shift in metabolism constitute part of the recapitulation of the "fetal gene program" which has been identified as a signature of pathologic cardiac hypertrophy.[218,219] This preferential dependence on carbohydrate metabolism has been attributed to the efficiency of glucose oxidation in the generation of high-energy phosphates; however, other mechanisms such as nonselective downregulation of genes governing myocardial FFA metabolism induced by epigenetic factors such as the ER stress response could also be present. For instance, one study identified that a downregulation of adult gene transcripts (such as GLUT4) rather than an increase in the transcripts constituting the fetal program could explain the switch to a "fetal pattern".[219] Several studies have identified downregulation of enzymes involved in fatty acid oxidation in explanted myocardium from patients with advanced heart failure at the time of cardiac transplantation. Studies in hypertensive rats transitioning to heart failure found that mRNA levels for fatty acid oxidation genes were downregulated (>70%) during both the LVH and heart failure stages in the SHHF rats compared with controls. However, the activity of medium-chain acyl-CoA dehydrogenase, which catalyzes a rate-limiting step in fatty acid oxidation, was not significantly reduced until the failure stage.[220] In a canine rapid pacing model of heart failure, a decreased myocardial uptake and oxidation of FFAs was associated with a decrease in the transcriptional control of the FFA oxidation program via the nuclear receptor retinoid X receptor α (RXRα).[211] Studies measuring FFA oxidation with PET in dilated cardiomyopathy identified a decrease in FFA uptake but no difference in the FFA oxidation constant in chronic heart failure patients as compared to nonfailing control subjects.[221] However, among the cardiomyopathy patients, individuals with the lowest LVEF actually had the highest FFA uptake and oxidation. This observation of increased FFA utilization through mass action could explain discrepant results of in-vivo cardiac metabolism in heart failure.[222]

Myocardial insulin resistance limits both glucose uptake and oxidation and impairs the heart's ability to generate much-needed ATP, especially in the presence of impaired FFA uptake and oxidation, as described above. In a canine model of pacing-induced heart failure, one study provided the first evidence of myocardial and whole-body insulin resistance associated with progressive LV dysfunction and identified impaired myocardial insulin signaling with decreased activation of *Akt-1* and translocation of GLUT-4.[223] This animal model demonstrated the metabolic phenotype of disease progression in heart failure, identifying increased serum FFA and whole-body insulin resistance (Figure 2.11) in the more advanced stage of this syndrome. These studies also support clinical observations of decreased glucose tolerance in advanced cardiomyopathy patients and preserved insulin sensitivity as a prognostic factor in human heart failure.[224,225] Indeed, independent of diabetes, chronic heart failure patients with decreased insulin sensitivity have a worse prognosis. In human dilated cardiomyopathy, Neglia et al. identified preferential utilization of carbohydrates, but a markedly impaired ability to increase glucose uptake during the physiologic stress of atrial pacing (no change in glucose uptake over a 15-minute period) as compared to control subjects who exhibited the expected increase in glucose uptake (twofold increased from baseline) during stress.[226] This study clearly demonstrates that, in heart failure, the loss of the flexible metabolic phenotype characteristic of the normal myocardium is physiologically limiting and detrimental.

Cardiac metabolism in diabetes and obesity

In the case of diabetes and diet-induced obesity, excess lipid accumulation in the heart has been implicated in the pathogenesis of myocardial dysfunction. Under normal circumstances, there is minimal lipid drop accumulation within cardiac myocytes, indicating that uptake and oxidation are well balanced. However, pathologic lipid accumulation has been reported in the hearts of patients with diabetes and the metabolic syndrome.[227,228] These findings have suggested that cardiac steatosis is part of a syndrome of end-organ dysfunction which results from the dysregulated lipid metabolism in obesity which also includes nonalcoholic fatty liver disease, increased intramyocellular lipid accumulation in skeletal muscle with impaired insulin signaling, and pancreatic β-cell dysfunction and apoptosis progressing to diabetes mellitus. Certainly, manipulation of a specific metabolic targets can result in cardiac lipid droplet accumulation and so-called lipotoxicity.[229,230] In translational studies in humans, advanced heart failure patients with diet-induced obesity or diabetes mellitus were found to have increased intramyocardial triglyceride levels at the time of cardiac transplantation—a phenotype that has been recapitulated in several animal models of obesity and diabetes, including the Zucker diabetic rodent model.[227] It was postulated that the combination of impaired myocardial FFA oxidation combined with the increased

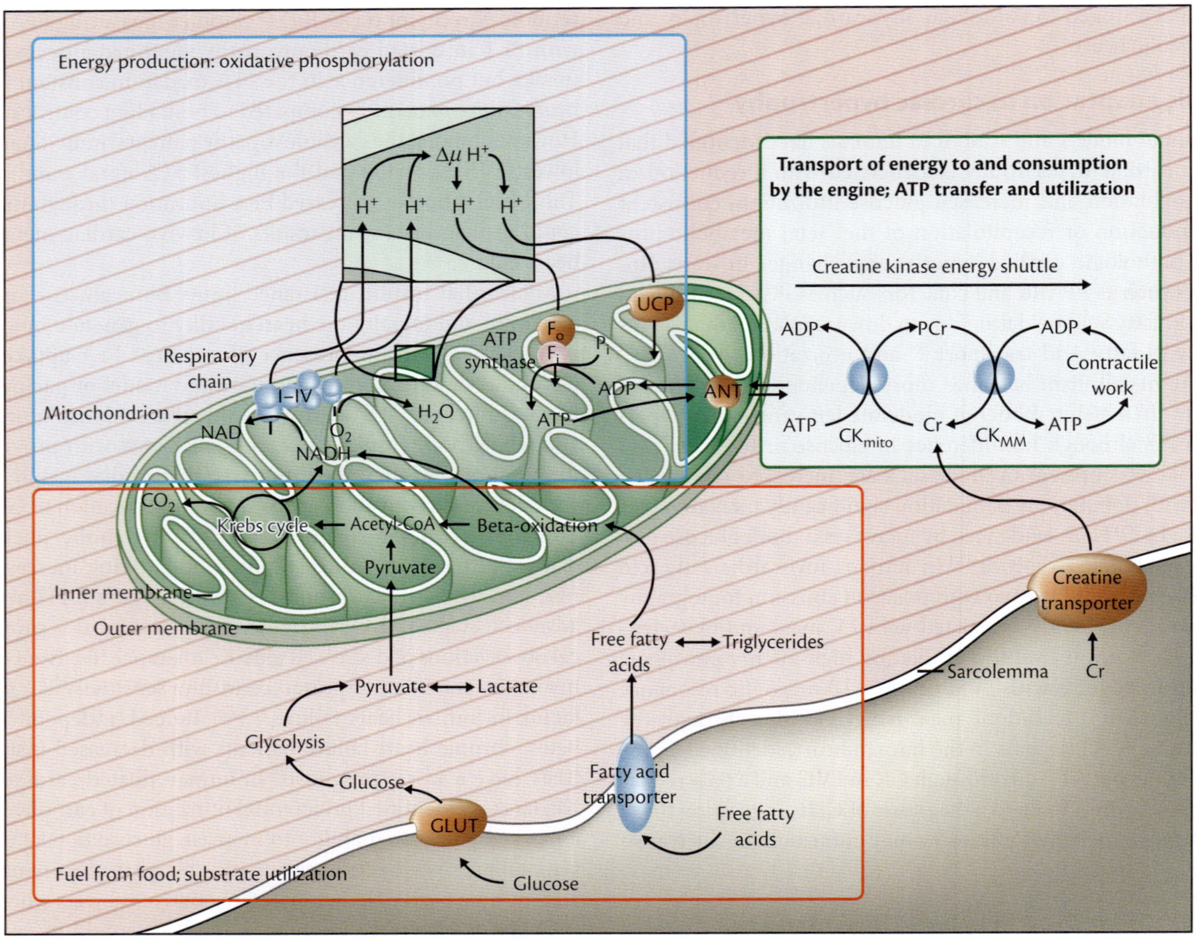

Fig. 2.11 Cardiac energy metabolism has three components. The first is substrate utilization (outlined in red), the cellular uptake of substrates, and their breakdown by β-oxidation and glycolysis; these processes result in the formation of acetyl coenzyme A (CoA), which is fed into the Krebs cycle and produces NADH and carbon dioxide (CO_2). The second component is oxidative phosphorylation (outlined in blue), the production of energy. Respiratory-chain complexes I–IV transfer electrons from NADH to oxygen, thereby creating a proton electrochemical gradient ($\Delta\mu$ H^+) across the inner mitochondrial membrane as well as NAD and water. This gradient drives the F_1,F_o ATP synthase, which produces ATP by phosphorylating ADP. Uncoupling proteins (UCPs) cause mitochondria to produce heat rather than ATP. The third component is energy transfer and utilization (outlined in green), the transport of energy to and consumption by myofibrillar ATPase and other ATP-consuming reactions, such as sarcolemmal and sarcoplasmic reticulum ion pumps. ATP transfer is achieved by the CK energy shuttle. Creatine, which is not produced in the heart, is taken up by the creatine transporter. ANT, adenine nucleotide translocase; CK_{mito}, mitochondrial creatine kinase isoenzyme; CK_{MM}, myofibrillar creatine kinase isoenzyme; Cr, free creatine; GLUT, glucose transporter; PCr, phosphocreatine; P_i, inorganic phosphate.

delivery of FFA in diabetic and obese patients accounted for the intramyocardial lipid overload associated with myocardial dysfunction. By distinguishing neutral lipid species such as triacylglycerides (TAGs) from toxic lipid intermediates such as diacylglycerols (DAGs) and ceramides in the myocardium of patients with end-stage heart failure, a more recent study was able to demonstrate a decrease in TAGs and an increase in the lipotoxic DAGs and ceramide species in comparison to nonfailing controls.[231] Furthermore, this study postulated that the accumulation of these toxic lipid intermediates could play a role in decreased activation of insulin signaling in the myocardium of end-stage human heart failure via increased activation of PKC, thus linking the lipotoxicity hypothesis to myocardial insulin resistance.

A major challenge to the lipotoxicity hypothesis is the body of evidence pointing to chronic heart failure as an energy-starved state and the failing heart as an "engine out of fuel."[232] Recent data generated from an untargeted lipidomic survey in myocardium from lean, nonischemic, and nondiabetic end-stage heart failure patients undergoing orthotopic heart transplantation has demonstrated that the vast majority of differentially present lipid species—including DAGs and ceramides—are significantly decreased in comparison to lean, nondiabetic, nonfailing control subjects.[233]

Studies investigating another component of cardiac energetic failure, deranged ATP transfer from the mitochondria to the myofibrillar elements where biomechanic transduction takes place, have also supported the "engine out of fuel" hypothesis. Human and animal studies of high-energy phosphate metabolism by ^{31}P MRS have consistently demonstrated impaired ATP transfer and utilization implicating significant deficits in the CK system in heart failure.[208,234,235,236,237] These studies have identified a decreased of PCr:ATP ratio, an index of available energetic flux in the heart. This index has been correlated with LVEF and NYHA class, and has been shown to be a strong predictor of mortality in patients with dilated cardiomyopathy.[236] Moreover, alterations in myocardial mitochondria,[238,239,240] including increased mitochondrial free radical production, oxidative stress, and alterations in the electron transfers chain, further impair ATP synthesis and cytosolic CK, thereby inhibiting energy transfer to myofibrils. The metabolic shifts that occur during progressive heart failure are summarized in Figure 2.11.[232]

Although no established heart failure therapy directly addresses abnormal myocardial metabolism and energetics, phenomena such as ischemic preconditioning and myocardial hibernation are now recognized to be native cardioprotective mechanisms that have metabolic adaptation and compensations at their core. In hibernation, ATP synthesis is reduced and contractility declines so that mitochondrial integrity is maintained and cell death avoided.[241,242] Conversely, it is probable that the adverse long-term effects of direct positive inotropes derive from their exacerbation of unfavorable myocardial energetics and oxidative stress. Based on these observations, therapies designed to increase glucose uptake by overcoming insulin resistance or by reducing oxidative stress and preserving mitochondrial integrity hold promise for improving myocardial energetics and preventing the progression of contractile abnormalities.

Targeting metabolic defects with GLP-1

Glucagon-like peptide-1 (GLP-1) is a naturally occurring incretin peptide that enhances cellular glucose uptake by stimulating insulin secretion and enhancing insulin sensitivity in target tissues.[243] In normal physiology, endogenous GLP-1 is implicated in the control of appetite and satiety.[244,245,246,247] Administration of exogenous GLP-1 as a continuous infusion in patients with type 2 diabetes causes an impressive increase in insulin sensitivity in both skeletal muscle and adipose tissue, with substantial improvements in insulin-mediated glucose uptake.[248,249] Importantly, the insulin-stimulating actions of GLP-1 cease at glucose levels below 4 mM (72 mg/dl) which mitigates the risk of hypoglycemia.[246,248,250] GLP-1 also promotes increased glucose uptake in target tissues via mechanisms independent of insulin.[250,251] Receptors for GLP-1 have been identified in rodent[252] and human[253] myocardium, thereby identifying myocardium as a direct target for GLP-1 action. Based on these observations, the FIGHT Study is an ongoing phase 2 evaluation of the efficacy of the GLP-1 agonist liraglutide as a potential therapy for patients with advanced heart failure with or without diabetes (ClinicalTrials.gov, NCT01800968).

Cell death pathways

Though the dogma that there is no capacity for new cardiac myocyte formation in the adult heart has been challenged in recent years, there remains a broad consensus that the native capacity for new myocyte formation is limited. In this context, mechanisms of cardiac myocyte death represent important drivers of both reduced cardiac pump function and pathological hypertrophy. In fact, cell death appears to be a feature of most etiologies of heart failure. In ischemic heart disease, where a critical loss of blood flow and tissue oxygenization often triggers extensive, sometimes acute, cardiac myocyte necrosis, other cell death mechanisms, namely apoptosis and autophagy, have recently been identified. In chronic heart failure, it appears that apoptosis and autophagy are even more prominent and increasingly well understood.[254] This understanding, in turn, is creating opportunities for therapeutic interventions aimed at maintaining cell number, as will be highlighted below.

At the outset, it should be noted that there is some controversy about what constitutes cell death and even more dispute about the specificity, sensitivity, and reversibility of particular phenomena associated with cardiac myocyte cell death. Highlighting the imperfect correlations between biochemical cell death characteristics and ultrastructural findings and the lack of definitive ultrastructural demonstration of apoptosis in failing human hearts, one recent review concluded that the very existence of cardiac myocyte apoptosis in heart failure remains controversial.[255] While this is an extreme position, the potential for situational and mechanistic overlap among alternative death mechanisms merits caution in interpreting the emerging biology of these processes. Features that unequivocally indicate irreversible cell death include loss of plasma membrane integrity, cellular fragmentation, and phagocytosis by neighboring cells. Other parameters, such as permeability of the inner or outer mitochondrial cell membranes, indicate serious injury but may not always induce cell death. Beyond the related question of reversibility versus irreversibility, another important distinction relevant to all mechanisms of cardiac myocyte death is whether the process is programmed and genetically regulated or merely a passive response to an environmental stress. In this regard, while both apoptosis and autophagy have long been recognized as having definable molecular mechanisms regulating their responses to stress, more recent studies suggest that at least some facets of cardiac myocyte necrosis are programmed. Such programs may play a role even in situations of cell death traditionally considered passive, such as trauma or major ischemic injury.[254]

Apoptosis

Apoptosis is a highly conserved cellular process involving active regulation of cell death under particular circumstances. During postnatal life, apoptosis in extracardiac cells is an essential feature of tissue homeostasis or for clearance of damaged or transformed cells, but apoptosis in adult cardiac myocytes is a pathologic process. As illustrated in Figure 2.12,[254] there are two main apoptotic pathways: the "extrinsic" pathway uses cell surface receptors and the "intrinsic" pathway does not. The majority of apoptotic stimuli such as nutrient deprivation, hypoxia, oxidative stress, DNA damage, or response to chemical or physical toxins proceed via a so-called intrinsic pathway of apoptosis. These proapoptotic stimuli ultimately converge at the mitochondria and the ER to initiate diverse intracellular responses as part of the "programmed cell death" associated with apoptosis. Death signals are transduced to the mitochondria and ER by two classes of proapoptotic B cell leukemia/lymphoma-2 (Bcl-2) proteins: Bax and BH3-only proteins.[256] Apoptotic stimuli induce activation of Bax and its translocation from the cytosol to the mitochondria and ER.[257,258] via transcriptional mechanisms, post-translational modifications and association with other proteins. The translocation of Bax and BH3-only proteins to the mitochondria triggers recruitment of additional mediators and ultimately leads to permeabilization of the outer mitochondrial membrane and release of several apoptogens into the cytosol to mediate and amplify the downstream facets of cellular apoptosis. For example, when cytochrome *c* (part of the electron transport chain in oxidative phosphorylation) is released into the cytosol it amplifies and propagates the apoptotic process

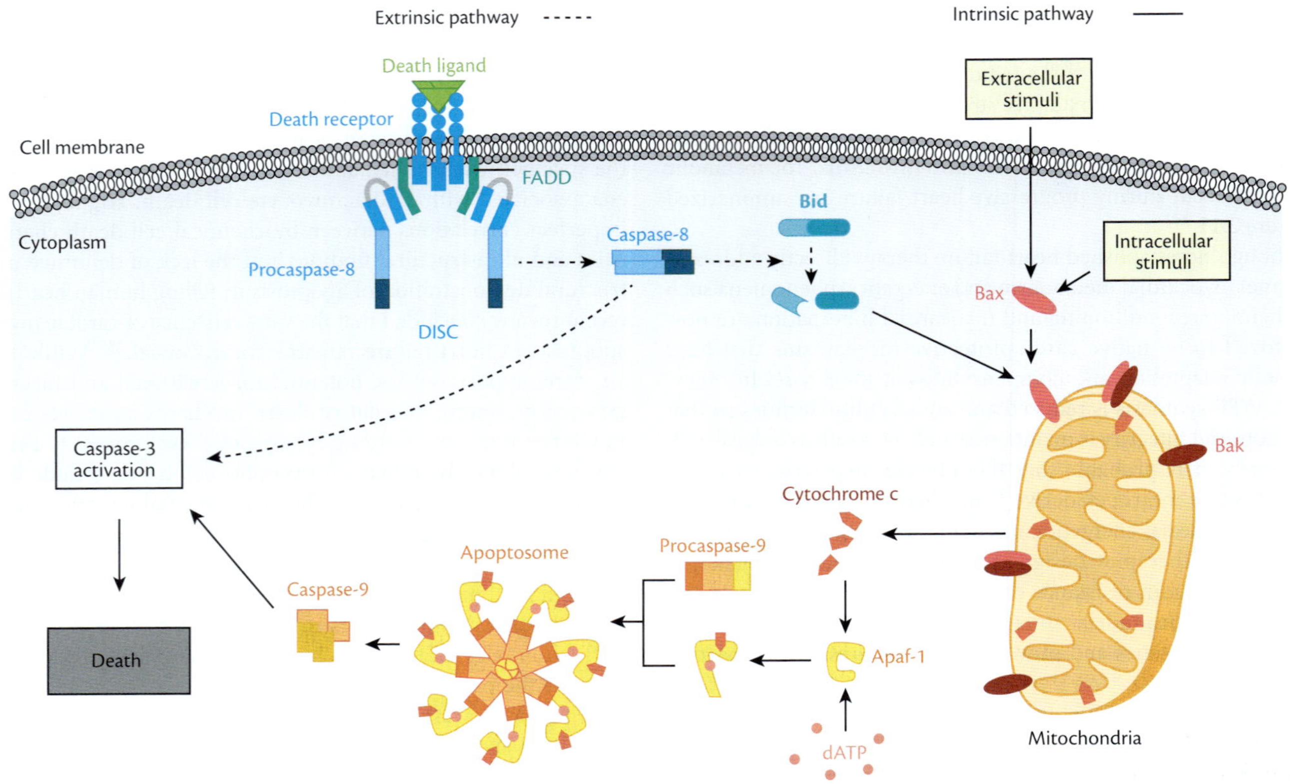

Fig. 2.12 Apoptosis pathways. Apoptosis is mediated by an extrinsic pathway involving cell surface death receptors and by an intrinsic pathway that utilizes the mitochondria and endoplasmic reticulum (ER). The extrinsic pathway is activated by binding of death ligand to its receptor, which triggers formation of the DISC. Caspase-8 is activated by forced proximity within the DISC and then cleaves and activates downstream procaspases. Caspase-8 can also cleave the BH3-only protein Bid, the carboxyl portion of which translocates to the mitochondria to trigger apoptotic mitochondrial events. The intrinsic pathway is activated by diverse biological, chemical, and physical stimuli. These signals are transduced to the mitochondria and ER (not shown) by proapoptotic Bcl-2 proteins: Bax (a multidomain protein) and BH3-only proteins. These death signals trigger the release of apoptogens from the mitochondria into the cytosol, one of which, cytochrome *c*, is depicted here. Cytosolic cytochrome *c* triggers the formation of a second multiprotein complex, the apoptosome, in which procaspase-9 undergoes activation. Caspase-9 then cleaves and activates downstream procaspases. Downstream caspases cleave several hundred cellular proteins to bring about the apoptotic death of the cell.
Whelan RS, Kaplinskiy V, Kitsis RN. Cell death in the pathogenesis of heart disease: mechanisms and significance. Annu Rev Physiol. 2010;72:19–44.

through a series of specific molecular interactions, including some that activate downstream caspases that are also involved with the extrinsic pathway.

The extrinsic apoptosis pathway involves cell surface death receptors, such as Fas or other TNFα superfamily receptors, which are activated by soluble or cell-bound ligands to trigger an intracellular signaling cascade involving proteases called caspases, which hydrolyze peptide bonds following aspartic acid residues. Sequential activation of upstream and downstream caspases ultimately induces death by cleaving hundreds of structural and regulatory proteins. In addition, caspases may amplify apoptotic signaling by activating other proapoptotic mediators.[259,260] The extrinsic pathway usually requires amplification at the mitochondria with processes and mediators that overlap with the intrinsic pathway. Indeed, there are multiple connections between the pathways that serve to amplify signals, increase the efficiency of killing, and promote stereotyped downstream characteristics of associated with apoptosis. In general, these characteristics together represent a more confined process of cell death that invokes less inflammation than would be observed with necrosis.

In the absence of widespread myocardial ischemia or infarction, during which great numbers of cardiac myocytes undergo apoptosis over a short period of time, rates of apoptosis in the hearts of patients with end-stage dilated cardiomyopathy are 0.08–0.25% compared with 0.001–0.002% in controls.[261,262] Nevertheless, transgenic mice with caspase-8 mutations causing similarly low levels of apoptosis (0.023%) developed a severe dilated cardiomyopathy over 8 weeks, died within 2–6 months, and could be rescued by administration of a caspase inhibitor.[263] Such studies support the potential functional significance of low-level apoptosis reported in failing human hearts.

A variety of endogenous inhibitors of apoptosis and small-molecule targets provide a potential basis for antiapoptotic therapeutics and have been examined in the setting of acute ischemia–reperfusion (I-R) injury. Endogenous antiapoptotic molecules include the Bcl-2 proteins, such as Bcl-2 and Bcl-xL (blocks mitochondrial apoptogen release), XIAP (inhibits activated caspases), and ARC (inhibits both the extrinsic and intrinsic pathways). In mice, either cardiac-specific overexpression of anti-apoptotic Bcl-2[264,265] or ablation of the proapoptotic Bax substantially reduces infarct size, cardiac myocyte apoptosis, and cardiac dysfunction following I-R injury.[266,267] Likewise, cardiac-specific transgenic overexpression of cIAP2 reduces infarct size following I-R of isolated perfused hearts.[268] In one study, transgenic overexpression of ARC decreased infarct size following I-R.[269] Adenoviral transduction of constitutively active Akt, which can inactivate multiple apoptotic mediators, into the myocardium also reduces cardiac myocyte apoptosis, infarct size, and cardiac dysfunction following I-R.[270,271] UCF-101, a small-molecule inhibitor of serine protease activity, also reduces infarct size following I-R.[272,273] Indeed, a variety of multicaspase inhibitors have substantially reduced infarct size in rodents following I-R.[274,275,276,277]

Autophagy

As recently reviewed,[278] autophagy, is a highly conserved catabolic process in which cellular constituents undergo intracellular degradation as a prosurvival mechanism to provides a source of energy under stress conditions. In autophagy, organelles and macromolecules to be recycled are partitioned within a double-membrane structures (autophagosomes) that fuse with lysosomes to initiate degradation. As illustrated in Figure 2.13,[278] autophagy proceeds through a well-choreographed sequence involving discrete signaling modules encoded by specific autophagy genes (ATGs). Under nutrient-rich conditions, the level of cardiac myocytes autophagy is low. However, during starvation or ischemia, the AMP-sensitive kinase (AMPK) phosphorylates ULK1/2 to initiate autophagosome formation. A critical late step in the process is the autophagosome–lysosome fusion that depends on the lysosomal membrane protein LAMP2 and the small GTPase RAB7.[279]

In addition to starvation,[280] both ischemia and I-R stress trigger autophagy both in vivo and in vitro.[281,282] AMPK is the pathway most strongly implicated in ischemia-triggered autophagy. The beneficial role of AMPK-mediated autophagy is supported by studies demonstrating that mice expressing dominant-negative AMPK in cardiac myocytes exhibit an attenuated autophagic response to ischemia with larger infarct size.[283] Conversely, pharmacological AMPK activators, including metformin and AICAR, mediate protection against subsequent ischemia via the so-called late preconditioning.[284,285] Beyond AMPK, studies using ATG-deficient mice[286,287] and naturally occurring human mutations[288] support the assertion that the low basal level of autophagy present in the heart exerts a favorable housekeeping role that helps preserve cardiac myocyte function by assuring protein and organelle "quality control."[278]

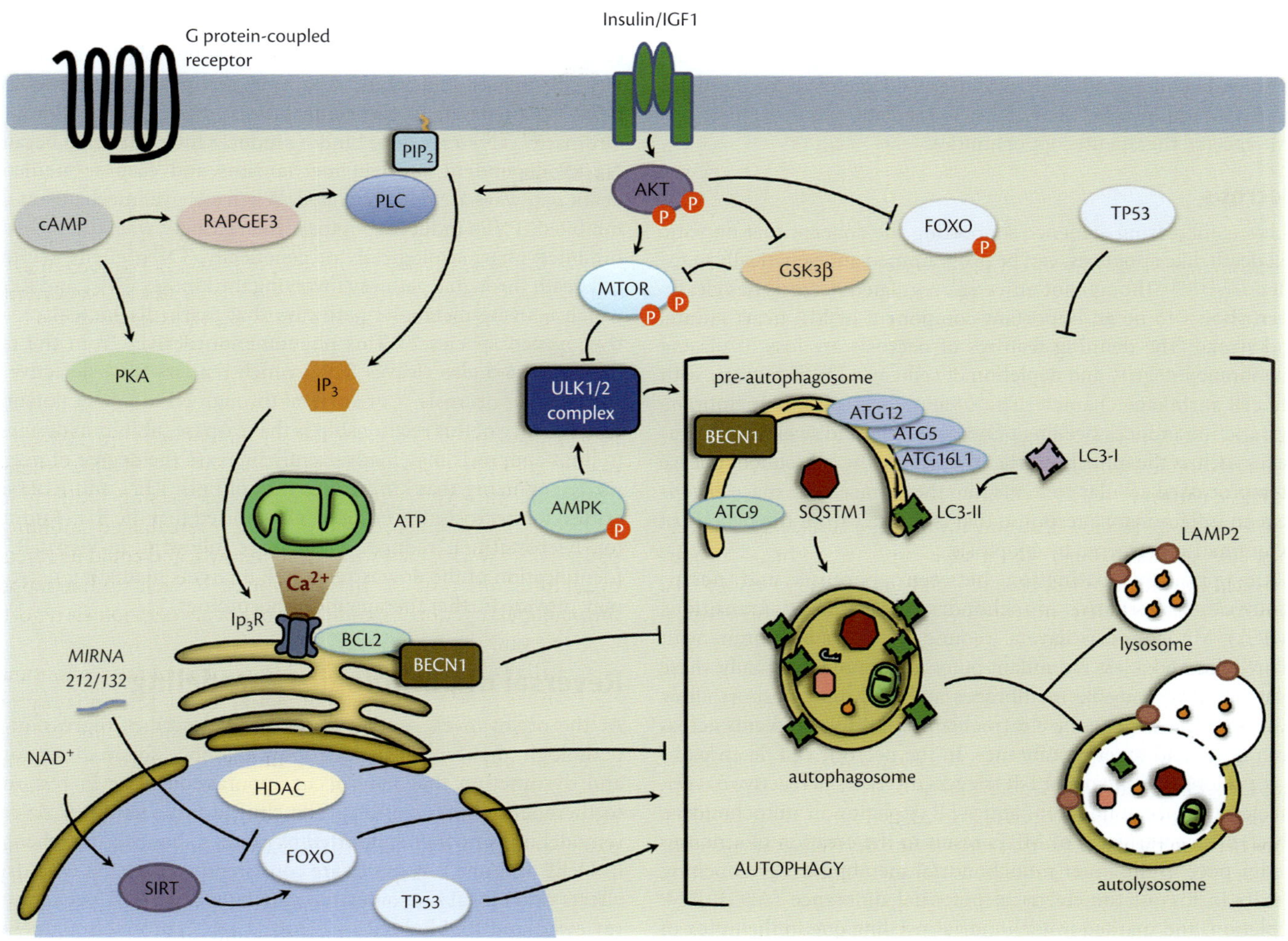

Fig. 2.13 Simplified scheme of the major cellular pathways governing autophagic responses in cardiomyocytes. Arrows denote stimulation, and T-shaped indicators denote inhibition.

Cardiovascular autophagy: Concepts, controversies and perspectives, Lavandero S, Troncoso R, Rothermel BA, Martinet W, Sadoshima J, Hill JA, Autophagy. 2013, Taylor and Francis Ltd, reprinted by permission of the publisher.

Reperfusion following ischemia triggers an even greater degree of autophagy, but autophagy following I-R is mechanistically distinct compared with ischemia alone. For example, autophagy following I-R is induced by a variety of intracellular triggers associated with reperfusion, including oxidative stress, mitochondrial damage, calcium overload, and ER stress,[289] and I-R associated autophagy is associated with beclin-1 upregulation and AMPK inactivation [281] Beclin-1, a BH3 member of the Bcl-2 gene family involved with regulation of apoptosis, can drive the autophagic process.[290] Though Bcl-2 is an antiapoptotic protein, it binds to beclin-1, suppressing beclin-1's ability to trigger autophagy.[291] Most importantly, autophagy following I-R is less clearly beneficial in that inhibition of beclin-1 in mice lessens the cell injury and cardiac dysfunction induced by I-R stress[283] and reduces both autophagy and pathological hypertrophy associated with chronic pressure overload. Moreover, beclin-1 overexpression enhances the severity of load-induced pathological hypertrophy.[292] From a therapeutic perspective, the mixed impact of cardiac autophagy is challenging: while a basal level of autophagy is essential and moderate activation of autophagy during caloric restriction or brief ischemia is beneficial, activation of autophagy with I-R stress or sustained pressure overload is generally detrimental. Development of clinically feasible strategies that selectively block detrimental autophagy without impairing beneficial autophagy would represent promising cell protective modality for failing hearts. In this regard, the overlap between beclin-1-mediated autophagy and members of the Bcl-2 family, best known for their ability to regulate apoptosis, may provide specific therapeutic opportunities.

Necrosis

There is increasing evidence supporting the concept that necrotic cell death, like apoptosis, can be programmed and genetically regulated.[293,294,295] Though not universal, regulated necrosis has clearly been shown to be an important component of MI, heart failure, and stroke. The defining features of necrosis are loss of plasma membrane integrity and depletion of cellular ATP. In contrast with the cell shrinkage characteristic of apoptosis, plasma membrane dysfunction induces swelling of necrotic cells and swelling of organelles such as the mitochondria. In necrosis, the subsequent release of unprocessed cellular contents into the extracellular space engenders an inflammatory response that is distinct from the paucity of inflammation triggered by apoptosis.

An important distinction between apoptosis and necrosis involves alternative mitochondrial permeability transitions (MPTs). Mitochondria have a "redundant" inner membrane with many folds and a less redundant outer membrane. Normally, these relatively impermeable membranes and electron transport allow mitochondria to generate electrochemical proton gradients across both inner and outer membranes. In the necrotic cell death pathway, prolonged ischemia or I-R triggers increases in reactive oxygen species, Ca^{2+} accumulation, and ATP depletion in mitochondria. These primary triggers of MPTs result in the creation of a nonselective pore in the inner mitochondrial membrane. Pore opening results in loss of the electrical potential difference ($\Delta\psi_m$), ATP depletion, and marked mitochondrial swelling due to the influx of water into the mitochondrial matrix. Thus, mitochondrial swelling is a hallmark of necrotic cell death. When the inner mitochondrial membrane swells sufficiently to rupture the nonredundant outer membrane, there is an uncontrolled release of mitochondrial apoptogens into the cytosol, which is distinct from the more selective outer membrane permeabilization that occurs during classic apoptosis. In fact, mitochondrial shrinkage, rather than swelling, is observed in apoptosis. Some have suggested that quantitative and qualitative features of MPTs will determine cell fate, such that minimal MPTs may allow cell recovery, moderate MPTs may trigger cell death, and severe MPTs will trigger necrosis.[296] Though the molecular features of the MPT pore remain uncertain, both gain- and loss-of-function studies demonstrate that cyclophilin D regulates pore opening.[297] Though cells lacking cyclophilin D are resistant to Ca^{2+}-induced swelling (necrosis), they remain sensitive to apoptosis via Bax. Thus, cyclophilin D represents a key switch affecting the mode of cell death in response to calcium overload and oxidative stress.[297,298,299] The potential relevance of cyclophilin to heart failure, rather than just ischemic injury, is supported by studies in which deletion of cyclophilin D rescued intracellular Ca^{2+} overload, myocyte necrosis, and heart failure induced by overexpression of the L-type Ca^{2+} channel β2a subunit in cardiac myocytes, while overexpression of antiapoptotic Bcl-2 did not prevent heart failure.[134] These studies support the potential of programmed necrosis to induce heart failure and highlight the potential therapeutic role of targeting cyclophilin D.

As the molecular dynamics regulating necrosis become apparent, interesting interrelationships between alternative cell fates are emerging. Outside the cardiovascular system, Holler et al. characterized a caspase-independent pathway that produces necrotic cell death via a separate receptor-interacting protein (RIP) pathway.[300] Ordinarily, TNFα receptor binding induces little cell death because NF-κB-dependent survival mechanisms and caspase-mediated death pathways are both activated. When survival mechanisms are inhibited, TNFα induces apoptosis. Interestingly, when caspases are inhibited pharmacologically or genetically, TNFα elicits necrotic cell death through a pathway involving the kinases RIP-1 and RIP3, which activate metabolic pathways that markedly increase reactive oxygen species.[301] This phenomenon derives from the fact that caspase-8 also cleaves RIP1, which renders RIP1 defective to signal either necrosis[293] or survival through NF-κB.[302] A potential consequence of this relationship is that caspase inhibition designed to limit apoptosis may inadvertently increase the degree of necrosis. Recognizing that kinase activities of both RIP1 and RIP3 are critical for necrosis,[300,303] Lim et al. reported that the RIP-1 inhibitor, necrostatin-1, reduced infarct size following in-vivo I-R.[304] Identification of the downstream RIP-3 targets mediating necrosis may provide further therapeutic opportunities.

Reversal of pathologic remodeling

At the organ level, reverse remodeling describes regression of pathologic myocardial hypertrophy, chamber shape distortions, and dysfunction that may occur spontaneously or in response to therapeutic interventions. The clinical importance of reverse remodeling is further supported by studies showing that changes in LVEF and/or LV volumes are consistently correlated with drug effects on clinical outcomes in heart failure trials.[305] As recently reviewed and highlighted in Figure 2.14,[306] reverse remodeling can be seen in diverse clinical settings. In response to amelioration of a sustaining etiology of heart failure, such as ischemia, chronic pressure or volume overload, electromechanical dyssynchrony, endocrinopathies, or toxic exposures, reverse remodeling proves

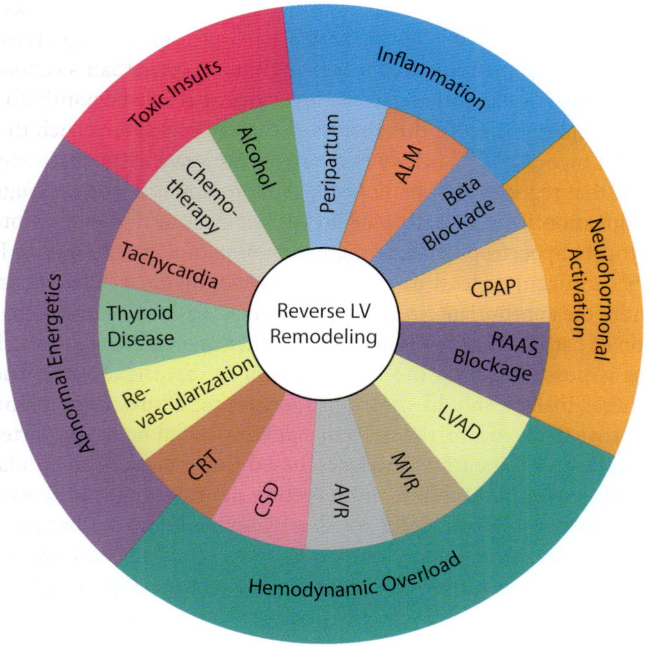

Fig. 2.14 Reverse remodeling is observed in a variety of clinical settings, as shown in the middle ring of the diagram. The segments illustrated in the outermost ring highlight the pathophysiological processes implicated by reverse remodeling in each particular clinical setting. ALM, acute lymphocytic myocarditis; AVR, aortic valve replacement; CPAP, continuous positive airway pressure; CRT, cardiac resynchronization therapy; CSD, cardiac support device; LVAD, left ventricular assist device; MVR, mitral valve repair/replacement; RAAS, renin–angiotensin–aldosterone system.

Hellawell JL, Margulies KB. Myocardial reverse remodeling. Cardiovasc Therapeutics. 2012; 30(3):172–81, Wiley.

the pathogenic nature of these stresses. Likewise, repeated demonstration of reverse remodeling (and favorable clinical outcomes) following treatment with β-adrenergic blockers[307,308,309,310,311,312] and renin–angiotensin system antagonists[313,314,315] demonstrates the maladaptive potential associated with sustained activation of these neurohormonal systems.[306] These observations also support a more general concept of myocardial plasticity and adaptability. Indeed, the concept of intrinsic plasticity is further reinforced by cases of spontaneous reverse remodeling, as is sometimes seen in cases of severe peripartum cardiomyopathy[316] and acute lymphocytic myocarditis.[317,318,319] Together, these observations underscore the remarkable potential for cardiac myocyte plasticity and link this adaptability to the overall trajectory of heart failure outcomes.

It appears that nearly all of the features of reverse remodeling at the organ level are paralleled by adaptations in cardiac myocytes.[306] In humans, most of the data indicating that myocyte remodeling is the predominant basis for organ-level remodeling is derived from the clinical situation in which patients with severe heart failure require circulatory support with a LVAD prior to heart transplantation.[3,320,321,322] Because LVAD support induces sustained reductions in both preload and afterload[323] and progressive decreases in pathological neurohormonal activation,[324] this intervention simultaneously ameliorates two fundamental drivers of pathological myocardial hypertrophy. Moreover, LVAD support as a bridge to heart transplantation permits multilevel explorations of the impact of these factors on the myocardium and its constituent cardiac myocytes. In many cases, analysis of the myocardial specimen removed from the LV apex at LVAD implantation provides a unique opportunity for a paired tissue-level comparison before and after a therapeutic intervention. This portal into the adaptability of diseased human myocardium has been exploited in numerous inquiries over the past two decades, and the remainder of this section highlights the insights into reverse remodeling gleaned from these diverse studies.

Regression of pathological hypertrophy

Studies from multiple laboratories demonstrate that LVAD support induces regression, but not full recovery, of many abnormalities characteristic of failing human cardiac myocytes.[325,326,327] As reviewed elsewhere, LVAD support reverses pathological myocyte hypertrophy with decreases in average cardiac myocyte size and reductions in cell length and cross-sectional dimensions,[3,328,329,330,331,332] but no evidence of myocyte atrophy. Associated with consistent, though incomplete, regression of pathological cardiac myocyte hypertrophy, several studies have observed decreases in ERK signaling in LVAD-supported hearts.[333,334,335] One of these studies linked LVAD-induced reductions in ERK activity to decreases in Akt and increases in glycogen synthase kinase (GSK-3-β) and demonstrated that either unloading of Langendorf-perfused mouse hearts or discontinuation of cyclic stretch-induced equivalent changes in ERK, Akt, and GSK-3-β.[334] These findings are consistent with a role for ERK signaling in transducing changes in biomechanical load during LVAD support. Though there have also been isolated reports of shifts in p38 and JNK MAPK pathways following LVAD support,[333] and membrane-associated PKCα,[336] studies to date have not linked regression of hypertrophy during LVAD support to changes in calcium-dependent signaling.

Improvements in contractile defects

LVAD support improves basal contractility as measured in isolated cardiac myocytes[339] or cardiac muscle strips.[120,332,337,338] LVAD support also induces improvements in both frequency-dependent contractile reserve[120,332,337,339] and β-adrenergic contractile responsiveness.[338,330,340] These studies support the concept that cardiac myocyte calcium cycling and the functional balance of key calcium-handling proteins are the major determinant of the FFR.[120,330] Specifically, tissue analyses after LVAD support demonstrate regression of pathologic increases in sodium–calcium exchanger protein abundance and function[120] and increases in the abundance of SERCA,[120,332,341,342,343] LTCC,[93] and RyR.[344] Improved β-adrenergic responsiveness after LVAD support is associated with increased β-adrenergic receptor density.[338,340,344,345] In addition, sustained LVAD support is associated with shortening of pathologically prolonged myocyte action potential duration.[320] As a composite, these studies support the general hypothesis that many myocardial abnormalities observed in failing hearts are a direct or indirect consequence of increased myocardial wall stress and sustained neurohumoral activation. The primacy of hemodynamic unloading as the driving factor is supported by studies showing greater regression of cellular hypertrophy and improvements in contractile reserve in the unloaded LV myocardium compared with the less unloaded RV myocardium.[332]

Metabolic recovery

Though incompletely characterized, the metabolic adaptations to sustained LVAD support indicate significant plasticity at this level. An early study focusing on metabolically relevant transcripts reported normalized expression of uncoupling protein following LVAD support, but little change in the reductions of the glucose transporters GLUT-1 and GLUT-4 associated with advanced heart failure.[346] Nevertheless, other studies showed improved mitochondrial respiratory function[347] and improved nitric oxide-mediated regulation of mitochondrial respiration.[348] Extending these studies, Chokshi et al. reported decreases in myocardial insulin resistance with improved insulin-dependent signaling based on phosphorylation of Akt and FOXO. These studies also documented increased expression of genes implicated in lipid metabolism (*CD36, CPT1, ACO*) and reduced levels of potentially toxic lipid intermediates, ceramide, and diacylglycerol following sustained LVAD support.[336] LVAD-associated improvements in reduced glucose metabolism have also been demonstrated using NMR spectroscopy.[349] Taken together, these studies suggest that defects in glucose utilization and mitochondrial function associated with advanced heart failure tend to be improved with sustained LVAD support though the completeness of recovery is undefined.

Deactivation of death pathways

Most studies exploring LVAD-induced changes in cardiac myocyte death pathways have found decreased rates of cardiac myocyte apoptosis.[333,334,350,351,352,353] Several of these studies have linked reductions in cardiac myocyte apoptosis to reduced expression of inflammatory cytokines within the LVAD-supported heart.[333,351,353] In addition, there has been one report of reduced expression of beclin-1 and several autophagy-related genes following LVAD support.[354]

Observations during reverse remodeling of the myocardium permit several important generalizations. The fact that myocardial unloading is one of the most potent triggers for reverse remodeling demonstrates that overload is a major factor sustaining pathological hypertrophy. At the same time, there are multiple levels of evidence supporting the importance of excess β-adrenergic stimulation as another important factor sustaining pathological cardiac remodeling. Tissue-based studies of LVAD-supported hearts also support the hypothesis that the potential for myocardial reverse structural and functional remodeling is retained even in severely diseased hearts. Nevertheless, despite a great deal of plasticity, it is safe to say that few pathological features of the failing heart truly normalize with LVAD support or other interventions. The incompleteness of cellular recovery is particularly well supported by studies demonstrating that less than 1% of the consistently abnormal transcripts in failing hearts normalize after LVAD support based on whole-genome mRNA profiling.[355,356] In fact, the degree of structural and functional recovery observed in many cases is remarkable given how few genes are actually normalized. One likely explanation for this is that the generalized complexity and adaptability of cardiac myocytes allow many possible combinations of the same elements—so-called "good enough solutions"—for achieving a phenotype that can meet physiological demands.[357]

Conclusions

Despite the tremendous and increasingly appreciated complexity of the normal and diseased cardiac myocytes as reviewed above, one theme emerging from this review of cardiac myocyte cell biology is that myocardial plasticity is clearly bidirectional at many levels, such that regression of pathological abnormalities is as possible as progression. This is clearly true for pathological cardiac and cardiac myocyte hypertrophy where regression of pathological abnormalities can occur at least as rapidly as development of hypertrophy under the appropriate circumstances. It is also apparent that regression of pathological hypertrophy and other myocardial abnormalities is possible across the full spectrum of disease severity. This general insight should motivate therapeutic efforts designed to improve the myocardial defects that develop in failing hearts. Given that most of the current evidence-based therapeutic strategies for patients with heart failure are targeting neurohumoral activation and vasoconstriction, there are clearly many opportunities to further improve heart failure outcomes by targeting the increasingly well-characterized molecular pathways that shape the phenotypes of failing hearts.

Moreover, because myocardial structure and function are integrated at many levels, either dysfunction or improvements in one aspect of myocardial phenotype can indirectly trigger dramatic changes in other facets of myocardial biology. With respect to defects, this principal is especially well illustrated by disease-causing mutations in which a single nucleotide switch can affect the dynamics of myocardial force generation and, over time, have profound effects on both cardiac function and morphology. On the other hand, because increases in myocardial wall stress are both a consequence of disproportionate cell lengthening and also a fundamental driver of further pathological signaling and activation of cell death pathways, an intervention that ameliorates disproportionate cell lengthening and/or LV dilation may fundamentally alter the trajectory of both the cellular and organ-level features of cardiac remodeling. Integration is also apparent in the diverse effects on cellular phenotype that key signaling pathways regulate and transduce during the cellular adaptations in heart failure. As a result, an intervention that favorably affects β-adrenergic signal transduction might have direct and potent effects on contractility, metabolism and cell death pathways and indirect effects on cell growth, inflammation and other signaling cascades. An additional corollary of this integration is that therapeutic strategies ultimately need to be proven effective in intact animal models, including large-animal models, because insights from reductionist systems and rodent models have not proven sufficiently robust to predict clinical responses.

References

1. Mollova M, Bersell K, Walsh S, et al. Cardiomyocyte proliferation contributes to heart growth in young humans. Proc Natl Acad Sci U S A 2013;110(4):1446–51.
2. Gerdes AM, et al. Structural remodeling of cardiac myocytes in patients with ischemic cardiomyopathy. Circulation 1992;86(2):426–30.
3. Zafeiridis A, et al. Regression of cellular hypertrophy after left ventricular assist device support. Circulation 1998;98(7):656–62.
4. Hayashi T, et al. Three-dimensional electron microscopy reveals new details of membrane systems for Ca^{2+} signaling in the heart. J Cell Sci 2009;122(Pt 7):1005–13.

5. Legato MJ, The correlation of ultrastructure and function in the mammalian myocardial cell. Prog Cardiovasc Dis 1969;11(5):391–409.
6. Onodera T, et al. Maladaptive remodeling of cardiac myocyte shape begins long before failure in hypertension. Hypertension 1998;32(4):753–7.
7. Maron BJ, Ferrans VJ, Roberts WC. Myocardial ultrastructure in patients with chronic aortic valve disease. Am J Cardiol 1975;35(5):725–39.
8. Hess OM, et al. Diastolic function and myocardial structure in patients with myocardial hypertrophy. Special reference to normalized viscoelastic data. Circulation 1981;63(2):360–71.
9. Grossman W, Jones D, McLaurin LP. Wall stress and patterns of hypertrophy in the human left ventricle. J Clin Invest 1975;56(1):56–64.
10. Esposito G, et al. Genetic alterations that inhibit in vivo pressure-overload hypertrophy prevent cardiac dysfunction despite increased wall stress. Circulation 2002;105(1):85–92.
11. Maillet M, van Berlo JH, Molkentin JD. Molecular basis of physiological heart growth: fundamental concepts and new players. Nat Rev Mol Cell Biol 2013;14(1):38–48.
12. Pluim BM, et al. The athlete's heart. A meta-analysis of cardiac structure and function. Circulation 2000;101(3):336–44.
13. Abel ED, Doenst T. Mitochondrial adaptations to physiological vs. pathological cardiac hypertrophy. Cardiovasc Res 2011;90(2):234–42.
14. Kenessey A, Ojamaa K. Thyroid hormone stimulates protein synthesis in the cardiomyocyte by activating the Akt-mTOR and p70S6K pathways. J Biol Chem 2006;281(30): 20666–72.
15. Baker J, et al. Role of insulin-like growth factors in embryonic and postnatal growth. Cell 1993;75(1):73–82.
16. Wilkins BJ, et al. Calcineurin/NFAT coupling participates in pathological, but not physiological, cardiac hypertrophy. Circ Res 2004;94(1):110–18.
17. McMullen JR, et al. The insulin-like growth factor 1 receptor induces physiological heart growth via the phosphoinositide 3-kinase(p110alpha) pathway. J Biol Chem 2004;279(6):4782–93.
18. Kim J, et al. Insulin-like growth factor I receptor signaling is required for exercise-induced cardiac hypertrophy. Mol Endocrinol 2008;22(11):2531–43.
19. Szabo-Fresnais N, et al. A new regulation of IL-6 production in adult cardiomyocytes by beta-adrenergic and IL-1 beta receptors and induction of cellular hypertrophy by IL-6 trans-signalling. Cell Signal 2010;22(7):1143–52.
20. Gullestad L, et al. Inflammatory cytokines in heart failure: mediators and markers. Cardiology 2012;122(1):23–35.
21. Spassova MA, et al. A common mechanism underlies stretch activation and receptor activation of TRPC6 channels. Proc Natl Acad Sci U S A 2006;103(44):16586–91.
22. Seth M, et al. TRPC1 channels are critical for hypertrophic signaling in the heart. Circ Res 2009;105(10):1023–30.
23. Herman DS, Lam L, Taylor MR, et al. Truncations of titin causing dilated cardiomyopathy. N Engl J Med 366(7):619–28.
24. Fu Y, Xiao H, Zhang Y. Beta-adrenoceptor signaling pathways mediate cardiac pathological remodeling. Front Biosci (Elite Ed) 2012;4:1625–37.
25. Morisco C, et al. Beta-adrenergic cardiac hypertrophy is mediated primarily by the beta(1)-subtype in the rat heart. J Mol Cell Cardiol 2001;33(3):561–73.
26. Bisognano JD, et al. Myocardial-directed overexpression of the human beta(1)-adrenergic receptor in transgenic mice. J Mol Cell Cardiol 2000;32(5):817–30.
27. Gaudin C, et al. Overexpression of Gs alpha protein in the hearts of transgenic mice. J Clin Invest 1995;95(4):1676–83.
28. Antos CL, et al. Dilated cardiomyopathy and sudden death resulting from constitutive activation of protein kinase A. Circ Res 2001;89(11):997–1004.
29. Lewin G, et al. Critical role of transcription factor cyclic AMP response element modulator in beta1-adrenoceptor-mediated cardiac dysfunction. Circulation 2009;119(1):79–88.
30. Noma T, et al. Beta-arrestin-mediated beta1-adrenergic receptor transactivation of the EGFR confers cardioprotection. J Clin Invest 2007;117(9):2445–58.
31. Molkentin JD, et al. A calcineurin-dependent transcriptional pathway for cardiac hypertrophy. Cell 1998;93(2):215–28.
32. Bueno OF, et al. Impaired cardiac hypertrophic response in calcineurin Abeta-deficient mice. Proc Natl Acad Sci U S A 2002;99(7):4586–91.
33. De Windt LJ, et al. Targeted inhibition of calcineurin attenuates cardiac hypertrophy in vivo. Proc Natl Acad Sci U S A 2001;98(6):3322–7.
34. Anderson ME, Brown JH, Bers DM. CaMKII in myocardial hypertrophy and heart failure. J Mol Cell Cardiol. 51(4):468–73.
35. Wu X, et al. Local InsP3-dependent perinuclear Ca^{2+} signaling in cardiac myocyte excitation-transcription coupling. J Clin Invest 2006;116(3):675–82.
36. Colomer JM, et al. Pressure overload selectively up-regulates Ca^{2+}/calmodulin-dependent protein kinase II in vivo. Mol Endocrinol 2003;17(2):183–92.
37. Zhang T, et al. CaMKIIdelta isoforms differentially affect calcium handling but similarly regulate HDAC/MEF2 transcriptional responses. J Biol Chem 2007;282(48):35078–87.
38. Lu YM, et al. CaMKIIδB mediates aberrant NCX1 expression and the imbalance of NCX1/SERCA in transverse aortic constriction-induced failing heart. PLoS One 2011;6(9):e24724.
39. Rose BA, Force T, Wang Y. Mitogen-activated protein kinase signaling in the heart: angels versus demons in a heart-breaking tale. Physiol Rev 2010;90(4):1507–46.
40. Goldsmith ZG, Dhanasekaran DN. G protein regulation of MAPK networks. Oncogene 2007;26(22):3122–42.
41. McKay MM, Morrison DK, Integrating signals from RTKs to ERK/MAPK. Oncogene 2007;26(22):3113–21.
42. Hayashi M, Lee JD. Role of the BMK1/ERK5 signaling pathway: lessons from knockout mice. J Mol Med (Berl) 2004;82(12):800–8.
43. Bogoyevitch MA. The isoform-specific functions of the c-Jun N-terminal Kinases (JNKs): differences revealed by gene targeting. Bioessays 2006;28(9):923–34.
44. Raman M, Chen W, Cobb MH. Differential regulation and properties of MAPKs. Oncogene 2007;26(22):3100–12.
45. Purcell NH, et al. Genetic inhibition of cardiac ERK1/2 promotes stress-induced apoptosis and heart failure but has no effect on hypertrophy in vivo. Proc Natl Acad Sci U S A 2007;104(35):14074–9.
46. Liao P, et al. The in vivo role of p38 MAP kinases in cardiac remodeling and restrictive cardiomyopathy. Proc Natl Acad Sci U S A 2001;98(21):12283–8.
47. Nicol RL, et al. Activated MEK5 induces serial assembly of sarcomeres and eccentric cardiac hypertrophy. EMBO J 2001;20(11):2757–67.
48. Cameron SJ, et al. Activation of big MAP kinase 1 (BMK1/ERK5) inhibits cardiac injury after myocardial ischemia and reperfusion. FEBS Lett 2004;566(1–3):255–60.
49. Liu Y, et al. Volume overload induces differential spatiotemporal regulation of myocardial soluble guanylyl cyclase in eccentric hypertrophy and heart failure. J Mol Cell Cardiol 2013;60:72–83.
50. Palaniyandi SS, et al. Protein kinase C in heart failure: a therapeutic target? Cardiovasc Res 2009;82(2):229–39.
51. Simonis G, et al. Protein kinase C in the human heart: differential regulation of the isoforms in aortic stenosis or dilated cardiomyopathy. Mol Cell Biochem 2007;305(1–2):103–11.
52. Braz JC, et al. PKC-alpha regulates cardiac contractility and propensity toward heart failure. Nat Med 2004;10(3):248–54.
53. Belin RJ, et al. Augmented protein kinase C-alpha-induced myofilament protein phosphorylation contributes to myofilament dysfunction in experimental congestive heart failure. Circ Res 2007;101(2): 195–204.
54. Bowling N, et al. Increased protein kinase C activity and expression of Ca^{2+}-sensitive isoforms in the failing human heart. Circulation 1999;99(3):384–91.
55. Ferreira JC, Koyanagi T, Palaniyandi SS, et al. Pharmacological inhibition of βIIPKC is cardioprotective in late-stage hypertrophy. J Mol Cell Cardiol 2011;51(6):980–7.

56. Liu Y, Lei S, Gao X, et al. PKCβ inhibition with ruboxistaurin reduces oxidative stress and attenuates left ventricular hypertrophy and dysfunction in rats with streptozotocin-induced diabetes. Clin Sci (Lond) 2012;122(4):161–73.
57. Luo M, Anderson ME, Mechanisms of altered Ca^{2+} handling in heart failure. Circ Res 2013;113(6):690–708.
58. Mattiello JA, et al. Contribution of reverse-mode sodium-calcium exchange to contractions in failing human left ventricular myocytes. Cardiovasc Res 1998;37(2):424–31.
59. Bassani JW, Yuan W, Bers DM. Fractional SR Ca release is regulated by trigger Ca and SR Ca content in cardiac myocytes. Am J Physiol 1995;268(5 Pt 1):C1313–19.
60. Quaile MP, et al. Reduced sarcoplasmic reticulum Ca^{2+} load mediates impaired contractile reserve in right ventricular pressure overload. J Mol Cell Cardiol 2007;43(5):552–63.
61. de Tombe PP. Cardiac myofilaments: mechanics and regulation. J Biomech 2003;36(5):721–30.
62. Solaro RJ, Rarick HM. Troponin and tropomyosin: proteins that switch on and tune in the activity of cardiac myofilaments. Circ Res 1998;83(5):471–80.
63. MacGowan GA. The myofilament force-calcium relationship as a target for positive inotropic therapy in congestive heart failure. Cardiovasc Drugs Ther 2005 19(3):203–10.
64. Engel PL, et al. Identification of a region of troponin I important in signaling cross-bridge-dependent activation of cardiac myofilaments. J Biol Chem 2007;282(1):183–93.
65. Hasenfuss G, Pieske B. Calcium cycling in congestive heart failure. J Mol Cell Cardiol 2002;34(8):951–69.
66. Houser SR, et al. Functional properties of failing human ventricular myocytes. Trends Cardiovasc Med 2000;10(3):101–7.
67. Houser SR, Piacentino V 3rd, Weisser J. Abnormalities of calcium cycling in the hypertrophied and failing heart. J Mol Cell Cardiol 2000;32(9):1595–607.
68. Hasenfuss G. Alterations of calcium-regulatory proteins in heart failure. Cardiovasc Res 1998;37(2):279–89.
69. Palomeque J, Vila Petroff MG, Mattiazzi A. Pacing staircase phenomenon in the heart: from Bodwitch to the XXI century. Heart Lung Circ 2004;13(4):410–20.
70. Anderson ME, et al. Multifunctional Ca^{2+}/calmodulin-dependent protein kinase mediates Ca^{2+}-induced enhancement of the L-type Ca^{2+} current in rabbit ventricular myocytes. Circ Res 1994;75(5):854–61.
71. Dzhura I, et al. Calmodulin kinase determines calcium-dependent facilitation of L-type calcium channels. Nat Cell Biol 2000;2(3):173–7.
72. Maier LS, Pieske B, Allen DG. Influence of stimulation frequency on Na^+i and contractile function in Langendorff-perfused rat heart. Am J Physiol 1997;273(3 Pt 2):H1246–54.
73. Kort AA, Capogrossi MC, Lakatta EG. Frequency, amplitude, and propagation velocity of spontaneous Ca1964;-dependent contractile waves in intact adult rat cardiac muscle and isolated myocytes. Circ Res 1985;57(6):844–55.
74. Petre RE, et al. Sex-based differences in myocardial contractile reserve. Am J Physiol Regul Integr Comp Physiol 2007;292(2):R810–18.
75. Xiao RP, Ji X, Lakatta EG. Functional coupling of the beta 2-adrenoceptor to a pertussis toxin-sensitive G protein in cardiac myocytes. Mol Pharmacol 1995;47(2):322–9.
76. Xiao RP, et al. Beta 2-adrenergic receptor-stimulated increase in cAMP in rat heart cells is not coupled to changes in Ca^{2+} dynamics, contractility, or phospholamban phosphorylation. J Biol Chem 1994;269(29): 19151–6.
77. Hibberd MG, Jewell BR. Calcium- and length-dependent force production in rat ventricular muscle. J Physiol 1982;329:527–40.
78. Allen DG, Kurihara S. The effects of muscle length on intracellular calcium transients in mammalian cardiac muscle. J Physiol 1982;327:79–94.
79. Allen DG, Kentish JC. The cellular basis of the length-tension relation in cardiac muscle. J Mol Cell Cardiol 1985;17(9):821–40.
80. Cazorla O, et al. Titin-based modulation of calcium sensitivity of active tension in mouse skinned cardiac myocytes. Circ Res 2001;88(10):1028–35.
81. Tachampa K, et al. Cardiac troponin I threonine 144: role in myofilament length dependent activation. Circ Res 2007;101(11):1081–3.
82. Cingolani HE, Pérez NG, Cingolani OH, Ennis IL. The Anrep effect: 100 years later. Am J Physiol Heart Circ Physiol 2013;304(2):H175–82.
83. Prosser BL, Khairallah RJ, Ziman AP, et al. X-ROS signaling in the heart and skeletal muscle: stretch-dependent local ROS regulates $[Ca^{2+}]$i. J Mol Cell Cardiol 2013;58:172–81.
84. Holubarsch C, et al. Existence of the Frank-Starling mechanism in the failing human heart. Investigations on the organ, tissue, and sarcomere levels. Circulation 1996;94(4):683–9.
85. von Lewinski D, et al. Reduced stretch-induced force response in failing human myocardium caused by impaired Na^+-contraction coupling. Circ Heart Fail 2009;2(1):47–55.
86. Gwathmey JK, et al. Abnormal intracellular calcium handling in myocardium from patients with end-stage heart failure. Circ Res 1987;61(1):70–6.
87. Houser SR, Margulies KB. Is depressed myocyte contractility centrally involved in heart failure? Circ Res 2003;92(4):350–8.
88. Bers DM. Altered cardiac myocyte Ca regulation in heart failure. Physiology (Bethesda) 2006;21:380–7.
89. Margulies KB, Houser SR, Cellular basis for heart failure. In: Mann DL, ed., Heart Failure: A Companion to Braunwald's Heart Disease. St. Louis, MO: Elsevier; 2011, pp. 32–47.
90. Weber CR, et al. Na^+-Ca^{2+} exchange current and submembrane Ca^{2+} during the cardiac action potential. Circ Res 2002;90(2):182–9.
91. Weber CR, et al. Calcium influx via I(NCX) is favored in failing human ventricular myocytes. Ann N Y Acad Sci 2002;976:478–9.
92. He J, et al. Reduction in density of transverse tubules and L-type Ca^{2+} channels in canine tachycardia-induced heart failure. Cardiovasc Res 2001;49(2):298–307.
93. Chen X, et al. L-type Ca^{2+} channel density and regulation are altered in failing human ventricular myocytes and recover after support with mechanical assist devices. Circ Res 2002;91(6):517–24.
94. Schroder F, et al. Increased availability and open probability of single L-type calcium channels from failing compared with nonfailing human ventricle. Circulation 1998;98(10):969–76.
95. Sipido KR, et al. Frequency dependence of Ca^{2+} release from the sarcoplasmic reticulum in human ventricular myocytes from end-stage heart failure. Cardiovasc Res 1998;37(2):478–88.
96. Marx SO, et al. PKA Phosphorylation dissociates FKBP12.6 from the calcium release channel (ryanodine receptor): defective regulation in failing hearts. Cell 2000;101(4):365–376.
97. Wehrens XH, et al. Ryanodine receptor/calcium release channel PKA phosphorylation: a critical mediator of heart failure progression. Proc Natl Acad Sci U S A 2006;103(3):511–18.
98. Eisner DA, et al. What role does modulation of the ryanodine receptor play in cardiac inotropy and arrhythmogenesis? J Mol Cell Cardiol 2009;46(4):474–81.
99. Tateishi H, et al. Defective domain-domain interactions within the ryanodine receptor as a critical cause of diastolic Ca^{2+} leak in failing hearts. Cardiovasc Res 2009;81(3):536–45.
100. Chelu MG, et al. Calmodulin kinase II-mediated sarcoplasmic reticulum Ca^{2+} leak promotes atrial fibrillation in mice. J Clin Invest 2009;119(7):1940–51.
101. Uchinoumi H, Yano M, Suetomi T, et al. Catecholaminergic polymorphic ventricular tachycardia is caused by mutation-linked defective conformational regulation of the ryanodine receptor. Circ Res 2010;106(8):1413–24.
102. Eisner DA, et al. From the ryanodine receptor to cardiac arrhythmias. Circ J 2009;73(9):1561–7.
103. Belevych AE, et al. Redox modification of ryanodine receptors underlies calcium alternans in a canine model of sudden cardiac death. Cardiovasc Res 2009;84(3):387–95.

104. MacLennan DH, Chen SR. Store overload-induced Ca^{2+} release as a triggering mechanism for CPVT and MH episodes caused by mutations in RYR and CASQ genes. J Physiol 2009;587(Pt 13):3113–15.
105. Chen W, Wasserstrom JA, Shiferaw Y. Role of coupled gating between cardiac ryanodine receptors in the genesis of triggered arrhythmias. Am J Physiol Heart Circ Physiol 2009;297(1):H171–80.
106. Schwinger RH, et al. Unchanged protein levels of SERCA II and phospholamban but reduced Ca^{2+} uptake and Ca^{2+}-ATPase activity of cardiac sarcoplasmic reticulum from dilated cardiomyopathy patients compared with patients with nonfailing hearts. Circulation 1995;92(11):3220–8.
107. Movsesian MA, Bristow MR, Krall J. Ca^{2+} uptake by cardiac sarcoplasmic reticulum from patients with idiopathic dilated cardiomyopathy. Circ Res 1989;65(4):1141–4.
108. Muller OJ, et al. Transgenic rat hearts overexpressing SERCA2a show improved contractility under baseline conditions and pressure overload. Cardiovasc Res 2003;59(2):380–9.
109. Ito K, et al. Transgenic expression of sarcoplasmic reticulum Ca^{2+} ATPase modifies the transition from hypertrophy to early heart failure. Circ Res 2001;89(5):422–9.
110. Miyamoto MI, et al. Adenoviral gene transfer of SERCA2a improves left-ventricular function in aortic-banded rats in transition to heart failure. Proc Natl Acad Sci U S A 2000;97(2):793–8.
111. Jessup M, Greenberg B, Mancini D, et al. Calcium Upregulation by Percutaneous Administration of Gene Therapy in Cardiac Disease (CUPID): a phase 2 trial of intracoronary gene therapy of sarcoplasmic reticulum Ca^{2+}-ATPase in patients with advanced heart failure. Circulation 2011;124(3):304–13.
112. Kirchberger MA, Tada M, Katz AM. Adenosine 3′:5′-monophos phate-dependent protein kinase-catalyzed phosphorylation reaction and its relationship to calcium transport in cardiac sarcoplasmic reticulum. J Biol Chem 1974;249(19):6166–73.
113. Kubo H, et al. Patients with end-stage congestive heart failure treated with beta-adrenergic receptor antagonists have improved ventricular myocyte calcium regulatory protein abundance. Circulation 2001;104(9):1012–18.
114. MacLennan DH, Kranias EG. Phospholamban: a crucial regulator of cardiac contractility. Nat Rev Mol Cell Biol 2003;4(7):566–77.
115. Minamisawa S, et al. Chronic phospholamban-sarcoplasmic reticulum calcium ATPase interaction is the critical calcium cycling defect in dilated cardiomyopathy. Cell 1999;99(3):313–22.
116. DeWitt MM, et al. Phospholamban R14 deletion results in late-onset, mild, hereditary dilated cardiomyopathy. J Am Coll Cardiol 2006;48(7):1396–8.
117. Eisner DA, Lederer WJ, Vaughan-Jones RD. The quantitative relationship between twitch tension and intracellular sodium activity in sheep cardiac Purkinje fibres. J Physiol 1984;355:251–66.
118. Flesch M, et al. Evidence for functional relevance of an enhanced expression of the Na^+-Ca^{2+} exchanger in failing human myocardium. Circulation 1996;94(5):992–1002.
119. Studer R, et al. Gene expression of the cardiac Na^+-Ca^{2+} exchanger in end-stage human heart failure. Circ Res 1994;75(3):443–53.
120. Chaudhary KW, et al. Altered myocardial Ca^{2+} cycling after left ventricular assist device support in the failing human heart. J Am Coll Cardiol 2004;44(4):837–45.
121. Hasenfuss G, et al. Relation between myocardial function and expression of sarcoplasmic reticulum Ca^{2+}-ATPase in failing and nonfailing human myocardium. Circ Res 1994;75(3):434–42.
122. Davies CH, et al. Reduced contraction and altered frequency response of isolated ventricular myocytes from patients with heart failure. Circulation 1995;92(9):2540–9.
123. Pieske B, et al. Ca^{2+} handling and sarcoplasmic reticulum Ca^{2+} content in isolated failing and nonfailing human myocardium. Circ Res 1999;85(1):38–46.
124. Hasenfuss G, et al. Relation between myocardial function and expression of sarcoplasmic reticulum Ca^{2+}-ATPase in failing and nonfailing human myocardium. Circ Res 1994;75(3):434–42.
125. Schmidt U, et al. Human heart failure: cAMP stimulation of SR Ca^{2+}-ATPase activity and phosphorylation level of phospholamban. Am J Physiol 1999;277(2 Pt 2):H474–80.
126. Schillinger W, et al. Impaired contractile performance of cultured rabbit ventricular myocytes after adenoviral gene transfer of Na^+-Ca^{2+} exchanger. Circ Res 2000;87(7):581–7.
127. del Monte F, et al. Restoration of contractile function in isolated cardiomyocytes from failing human hearts by gene transfer of SERCA2a. Circulation 1999;100(23):2308–11.
128. Ziolo MT, et al. Adenoviral gene transfer of mutant phospholamban rescues contractile dysfunction in failing rabbit myocytes with relatively preserved SERCA function. Circ Res 2005;96(8):815–17.
129. Antoons G, et al. Cellular basis for triggered ventricular arrhythmias that occur in the setting of compensated hypertrophy and heart failure: considerations for diagnosis and treatment. J Electrocardiol 2007;40(6 Suppl):S8–14.
130. Desantiago J, et al. Arrhythmogenic effects of beta2-adrenergic stimulation in the failing heart are attributable to enhanced sarcoplasmic reticulum Ca load. Circ Res 2008;102(11):1389–97.
131. Chakir K, et al. Reversal of global apoptosis and regional stress kinase activation by cardiac resynchronization. Circulation 2008;117(11):1369–77.
132. Chen X, et al. Ca^{2+} influx-induced sarcoplasmic reticulum Ca^{2+} overload causes mitochondrial-dependent apoptosis in ventricular myocytes. Circ Res 2005;97(10):1009–17.
133. Diwan A, et al. Endoplasmic reticulum-mitochondria crosstalk in NIX-mediated murine cell death. J Clin Invest 2009;119(1): p 203–12.
134. Nakayama H, et al. Ca^{2+}- and mitochondrial-dependent cardiomyocyte necrosis as a primary mediator of heart failure. J Clin Invest 2007;117(9):2431–44.
135. Molkentin JD. Dichotomy of Ca^{2+} in the heart: contraction versus intracellular signaling. J Clin Invest 2006;116(3):623–6.
136. Kiss E, et al. Differential changes in cardiac phospholamban and sarcoplasmic reticular Ca^{2+}-ATPase protein levels. Effects on Ca^{2+} transport and mechanics in compensated pressure-overload hypertrophy and congestive heart failure. Circ Res 1995;77(4):759–64.
137. Sucharov CC, et al. A beta1-adrenergic receptor CaM kinase II-dependent pathway mediates cardiac myocyte fetal gene induction. Am J Physiol Heart Circ Physiol 2006;291(3):H1299–308.
138. Engelhardt S, et al. Progressive hypertrophy and heart failure in beta1-adrenergic receptor transgenic mice. Proc Natl Acad Sci U S A 1999;96(12):7059–64.
139. Zhu WZ, et al. Linkage of beta1-adrenergic stimulation to apoptotic heart cell death through protein kinase A-independent activation of Ca^{2+}/calmodulin kinase II. J Clin Invest 2003;111(5):617–25.
140. Zhu WZ, et al. Dual modulation of cell survival and cell death by beta(2)-adrenergic signaling in adult mouse cardiac myocytes. Proc Natl Acad Sci U S A 2001;98(4):1607–12.
141. Bristow MR, et al. Beta 1- and beta 2-adrenergic-receptor subpopulations in nonfailing and failing human ventricular myocardium: coupling of both receptor subtypes to muscle contraction and selective beta 1-receptor down-regulation in heart failure. Circ Res 1986;59(3):297–309.
142. Bristow MR, et al. Reduced beta 1 receptor messenger RNA abundance in the failing human heart. J Clin Invest 1993;92(6):2737–45.
143. Bristow MR, et al. Beta 1- and beta 2-adrenergic receptor-mediated adenylate cyclase stimulation in nonfailing and failing human ventricular myocardium. Mol Pharmacol 1989;35(3):295–303.
144. Bohm M, et al. Radioimmunochemical quantification of Gi alpha in right and left ventricles from patients with ischaemic and dilated cardiomyopathy and predominant left ventricular failure. J Mol Cell Cardiol 1994;26(2):133–49.
145. Feldman AM, et al. Increase of the 40,000-mol wt pertussis toxin substrate (G protein) in the failing human heart. J Clin Invest 1988;82(1):189–97.
146. Ungerer M, et al. Altered expression of beta-adrenergic receptor kinase and beta 1-adrenergic receptors in the failing human heart. Circulation 1993;87(2):454–63.

147. Lefkowitz RJ, G protein-coupled receptors. III. New roles for receptor kinases and beta-arrestins in receptor signaling and desensitization. J Biol Chem 1998;273(30):18677–80.
148. Faulx MD, et al. Strain-dependent beta-adrenergic receptor function influences myocardial responses to isoproterenol stimulation in mice. Am J Physiol Heart Circ Physiol 2005;289(1):H30–6.
149. Liggett SB, et al. A GRK5 polymorphism that inhibits beta-adrenergic receptor signaling is protective in heart failure. Nat Med 2008;14(5):510–17.
150. Norman HS, et al. Decreased cardiac functional reserve in heart failure with preserved systolic function. J Card Fail 2011;17(4):301–8.
151. Phan TT, et al. Heart failure with preserved ejection fraction is characterized by dynamic impairment of active relaxation and contraction of the left ventricle on exercise and associated with myocardial energy deficiency. J Am Coll Cardiol 2009;54(5):402–9.
152. Ungerer M, et al. Expression of beta-arrestins and beta-adrenergic receptor kinases in the failing human heart. Circ Res 1994;74(2): 206–13.
153. Xiao RP, et al. Coupling of beta2-adrenoceptor to Gi proteins and its physiological relevance in murine cardiac myocytes. Circ Res 1999;84(1):43–52.
154. Ungerer M, et al. Activation of beta-adrenergic receptor kinase during myocardial ischemia. Circ Res 1996;79(3):455–60.
155. Gros R, et al. G-protein-coupled receptor kinase activity is increased in hypertension. J Clin Invest 1997;99(9): 2087–93.
156. Woo AY, Xiao RP. β-Adrenergic receptor subtype signaling in heart: from bench to bedside. Acta Pharmacol Sin 2012;33(3):335–41.
157. Rohde D, et al. S100A1 gene therapy for heart failure: a novel strategy on the verge of clinical trials. J Mol Cell Cardiol 2011;50(5):777–84.
158. Remppis A, et al. Altered expression of the Ca^{2+}-binding protein S100A1 in human cardiomyopathy. Biochim Biophys Acta 1996;1313(3):253–7.
159. Most P, et al. Cardiac S100A1 protein levels determine contractile performance and propensity toward heart failure after myocardial infarction. Circulation 2006;114(12):1258–68.
160. Most P, et al. Cardiac adenoviral S100A1 gene delivery rescues failing myocardium. J Clin Invest 2004;114(11):1550–63.
161. Brinks H, et al. S100A1 genetically targeted therapy reverses dysfunction of human failing cardiomyocytes. J Am Coll Cardiol 2011;58(9):966–73.
162. Volkers M, et al. S100A1: a regulator of striated muscle sarcoplasmic reticulum Ca^{2+} handling, sarcomeric, and mitochondrial function. J Biomed Biotechnol 2010;2010:178614.
163. Fukushima H, Chung CS, Granzier H. Titin-isoform dependence of titin-actin interaction and its regulation by S100A1/Ca^{2+} in skinned myocardium. J Biomed Biotechnol 2010;2010:727239.
164. Cahill TJ, Ashrafian H, Watkins H. Genetic cardiomyopathies causing heart failure. Circ Res 2013;113(6):660–75.
165. Alcalai R, Seidman JG, Seidman CE. Genetic basis of hypertrophic cardiomyopathy: from bench to the clinics. J Cardiovasc Electrophysiol 2008 19(1):104–10.
166. Seidman CE, Seidman JG. Identifying sarcomere gene mutations in hypertrophic cardiomyopathy: a personal history. Circ Res 2011;108(6):743–50.
167. Kamisago M, et al. Mutations in sarcomere protein genes as a cause of dilated cardiomyopathy. N Engl J Med 2000;343(23):1688–96.
168. Ojamaa K, et al. Thyroid hormone effects on cardiac gene expression independent of cardiac growth and protein synthesis. Am J Physiol 1992;263(3 Pt 1):E534–40.
169. Miyata S, et al. Myosin heavy chain isoform expression in the failing and nonfailing human heart. Circ Res 2000;86(4):386–90.
170. Korte FS, et al. Power output is linearly related to MyHC content in rat skinned myocytes and isolated working hearts. Am J Physiol Heart Circ Physiol 2005;289(2):H801–12.
171. Metzger JM, et al. Effects of myosin heavy chain isoform switching on Ca^{2+}-activated tension development in single adult cardiac myocytes. Circ Res 1999;84(11):1310–17.
172. van Rooij E, et al. Control of stress-dependent cardiac growth and gene expression by a microRNA. Science 2007;316(5824):575–9.
173. Adachi S, et al. Skeletal and smooth muscle alpha-actin mRNA in endomyocardial biopsy samples of dilated cardiomyopathy patients. Life Sci 1998;63(20):1779–91.
174. Morano M, et al. Regulation of human heart contractility by essential myosin light chain isoforms. J Clin Invest 1996;98(2):467–73.
175. Ritter O, et al. Expression of atrial myosin light chains but not alpha-myosin heavy chains is correlated in vivo with increased ventricular function in patients with hypertrophic obstructive cardiomyopathy. J Mol Med 1999;77(9):677–85.
176. Kruger M, Linke WA. Titin-based mechanical signalling in normal and failing myocardium. J Mol Cell Cardiol 2009;46(4):490–8.
177. Lahmers S, et al. Developmental control of titin isoform expression and passive stiffness in fetal and neonatal myocardium. Circ Res 2004;94(4):505–13.
178. Makarenko I, et al. Passive stiffness changes caused by upregulation of compliant titin isoforms in human dilated cardiomyopathy hearts. Circ Res 2004;95(7):708–16.
179. van Heerebeek L, et al. Myocardial structure and function differ in systolic and diastolic heart failure. Circulation 2006;113(16):1966–73.
180. Wolff MR, et al. Myofibrillar calcium sensitivity of isometric tension is increased in human dilated cardiomyopathies: role of altered beta-adrenergically mediated protein phosphorylation. J Clin Invest 1996;98(1):167–76.
181. Cazorla O, et al. Length and protein kinase A modulations of myocytes in cardiac myosin binding protein C-deficient mice. Cardiovasc Res 2006;69(2):370–80.
182. Kentish JC, et al. Phosphorylation of troponin I by protein kinase A accelerates relaxation and crossbridge cycle kinetics in mouse ventricular muscle. Circ Res 2001;88(10):1059–65.
183. Kulikovskaya I, et al. Effect of MyBP-C binding to actin on contractility in heart muscle. J Gen Physiol 2003;122(6):761–74.
184. Watson JD. The human genome revealed. Genome Res 2001;11(11):1803–4.
185. Care A, et al. MicroRNA-133 controls cardiac hypertrophy. Nat Med 2007;13(5):613–18.
186. Herron TJ, Korte FS, McDonald KS. Power output is increased after phosphorylation of myofibrillar proteins in rat skinned cardiac myocytes. Circ Res 2001;89(12):1184–90.
187. Hamdani N, et al. Myofilament dysfunction in cardiac disease from mice to men. J Muscle Res Cell Motil 2008;29(6–8):189–201.
188. Zakhary DR, et al. Protein kinase A (PKA)-dependent troponin-I phosphorylation and PKA regulatory subunits are decreased in human dilated cardiomyopathy. Circulation 1999;99(4):505–10.
189. Hajjar RJ, et al. Myofilament calcium regulation in human myocardium. Circulation 2000;101(14):1679–85.
190. Noland TA, Jr., Raynor RL, Kuo JF. Identification of sites phosphorylated in bovine cardiac troponin I and troponin T by protein kinase C and comparative substrate activity of synthetic peptides containing the phosphorylation sites. J Biol Chem 1989;264(34):20778–85.
191. Noland TA, Jr., et al. Cardiac troponin I mutants. Phosphorylation by protein kinases C and A and regulation of Ca^{2+}-stimulated MgATPase of reconstituted actomyosin S-1. J Biol Chem 1995;270(43):25445–54.
192. van der Velden J, et al. Functional effects of protein kinase C-mediated myofilament phosphorylation in human myocardium. Cardiovasc Res 2006;69(4):876–87.
193. Yamasaki R, et al. Protein kinase A phosphorylates titin's cardiac-specific N2B domain and reduces passive tension in rat cardiac myocytes. Circ Res 2002;90(11):1181–8.
194. Ji R, et al. MicroRNA expression signature and antisense-mediated depletion reveal an essential role of MicroRNA in vascular neointimal lesion formation. Circ Res 2007;100(11):1579–88.
195. Palanisamy N, Ateeq B, Kalyana-Sundaram S, et al. Rearrangements of the RAF kinase pathway in prostate cancer, gastric cancer and melanoma. Nat Med 2010;16(7):793–8.

196. Morrow DA, Braunwald E. Future of biomarkers in acute coronary syndromes: moving toward a multimarker strategy. Circulation 2003;108(3):250–2.
197. Park PJ. ChIP-seq: advantages and challenges of a maturing technology. Nat Rev Genet 2009;10(10):669–80.
198. Gerszten RE, Wang TJ. The search for new cardiovascular biomarkers. Nature 2008;451(7181):949–52.
199. Lewis GD, Farrell L, Wood MJ, et al. Metabolic signatures of exercise in human plasma. Sci Transl Med 2010;2(33):33ra37.
200. de Vente J, Markerink-van Ittersum M, Vles JS. ANP-mediated cGMP signaling and phosphodiesterase inhibition in the rat cervical spinal cord. J Chem Neuroanat 2006;31(4):263–74.
201. Hein S, Scheffold T, Schaper J. Ischemia induces early changes to cytoskeletal and contractile proteins in diseased human myocardium. J Thorac Cardiovasc Surg 1995;110(1):89–98.
202. Gao WD, et al. Relationship between intracellular calcium and contractile force in stunned myocardium. Direct evidence for decreased myofilament Ca^{2+} responsiveness and altered diastolic function in intact ventricular muscle. Circ Res 1995;76(6):1036–48.
203. Weber C, Schober A, Zernecke A. MicroRNAs in arterial remodelling, inflammation and atherosclerosis. Curr Drug Targets 2010;11(8):950–6.
204. Feng J, et al. Preload induces troponin I degradation independently of myocardial ischemia. Circulation 2001;103(16): 2035–7.
205. Lu XY, et al. Overexpression of heat shock protein 27 protects against ischaemia/reperfusion-induced cardiac dysfunction via stabilization of troponin I and T. Cardiovasc Res 2008;79(3):500–8.
206. Wu F, Zhang J, Beard DA. Experimentally observed phenomena on cardiac energetics in heart failure emerge from simulations of cardiac metabolism. Proc Natl Acad Sci U S A 2009;106(17):7143–8.
207. Ingwall JS, Weiss RG. Is the failing heart energy starved? On using chemical energy to support cardiac function. Circ Res 2004;95(2):135–45.
208. Weiss RG, Gerstenblith G, Bottomley PA. ATP flux through creatine kinase in the normal, stressed, and failing human heart. Proc Natl Acad Sci U S A 2005;102(3):808–13.
209. Rame JE. Chronic heart failure: a reversible metabolic syndrome? Circulation 2012;125(23):2809–11.
210. O'Donnell JM, et al. The absence of endogenous lipid oxidation in early stage heart failure exposes limits in lipid storage and turnover. J Mol Cell Cardiol 2008;44(2):315–22.
211. Osorio JC, et al. Impaired myocardial fatty acid oxidation and reduced protein expression of retinoid X receptor-alpha in pacing-induced heart failure. Circulation 2002;106(5):606–12.
212. Stanley WC, Recchia FA, Lopaschuk GD. Myocardial substrate metabolism in the normal and failing heart. Physiol Rev 2005;85(3):1093–129.
213. Sorokina N, et al. Recruitment of compensatory pathways to sustain oxidative flux with reduced carnitine palmitoyltransferase I activity characterizes inefficiency in energy metabolism in hypertrophied hearts. Circulation 2007;115(15):2033–41.
214. Massie BM, et al. Myocardial high-energy phosphate and substrate metabolism in swine with moderate left ventricular hypertrophy. Circulation 1995;91(6):1814–23.
215. de las Fuentes L, et al. Myocardial fatty acid metabolism: independent predictor of left ventricular mass in hypertensive heart disease. Hypertension 2003;41(1):83–7.
216. de las Fuentes L, et al. Hypertensive left ventricular hypertrophy is associated with abnormal myocardial fatty acid metabolism and myocardial efficiency. J Nucl Cardiol 2006;13(3):369–77.
217. Smith CS, et al. Altered creatine kinase adenosine triphosphate kinetics in failing hypertrophied human myocardium. Circulation 2006;114(11):1151–8.
218. Bishop SP, Altschuld RA. Increased glycolytic metabolism in cardiac hypertrophy and congestive failure. Am J Physiol 1970;218(1):153–9.
219. Razeghi P, et al. Metabolic gene expression in fetal and failing human heart. Circulation 2001;104(24):2923–31.
220. Sack MN, et al. Fatty acid oxidation enzyme gene expression is downregulated in the failing heart. Circulation 1996;94(11):2837–42.
221. Tuunanen H, et al. Decreased myocardial free fatty acid uptake in patients with idiopathic dilated cardiomyopathy: evidence of relationship with insulin resistance and left ventricular dysfunction. J Card Fail 2006;12(8):644–52.
222. Asano K, et al. Altered expression of endothelin receptors in failing human left ventricles. J Mol Cell Cardiol 2002;34(7):833–46.
223. Nikolaidis LA, et al. The development of myocardial insulin resistance in conscious dogs with advanced dilated cardiomyopathy. Cardiovasc Res 2004;61(2):297–306.
224. Doehner W, et al. Impaired insulin sensitivity as an independent risk factor for mortality in patients with stable chronic heart failure. J Am Coll Cardiol 2005;46(6):1019–26.
225. Witteles RM, et al. Insulin resistance in idiopathic dilated cardiomyopathy: a possible etiologic link. J Am Coll Cardiol 2004;44(1):78–81.
226. Neglia D, et al. Impaired myocardial metabolic reserve and substrate selection flexibility during stress in patients with idiopathic dilated cardiomyopathy. Am J Physiol Heart Circ Physiol 2007;293(6):H3270–8.
227. Sharma S, et al. Intramyocardial lipid accumulation in the failing human heart resembles the lipotoxic rat heart. FASEB J 2004;18(14):1692–700.
228. McGavock JM, et al. Cardiac steatosis in diabetes mellitus: a 1H-magnetic resonance spectroscopy study. Circulation 2007;116(10):1170–5.
229. Kim JK, et al. Tissue-specific overexpression of lipoprotein lipase causes tissue-specific insulin resistance. Proc Natl Acad Sci U S A 2001;98(13):7522–7.
230. Yokoyama M, et al. Apolipoprotein B production reduces lipotoxic cardiomyopathy: studies in heart-specific lipoprotein lipase transgenic mouse. J Biol Chem 2004;279(6):4204–11.
231. Chokshi A, et al. Ventricular assist device implantation corrects myocardial lipotoxicity, reverses insulin resistance, and normalizes cardiac metabolism in patients with advanced heart failure. Circulation 2012;125(23):2844–53.
232. Neubauer S. The failing heart—an engine out of fuel. N Engl J Med 2007;356(11):1140–51.
233. Bedi CKM, Margulies K, Blair I, Rame JE. Intramyocardial lipid dysregulation in end stage human heart failure. American Heart Association Basic Cardiovascular Science Meeting 2013.
234. Hardy CJ, et al. Altered myocardial high-energy phosphate metabolites in patients with dilated cardiomyopathy. Am Heart J 1991;122(3 Pt 1):795–801.
235. Lamb HJ, et al. Diastolic dysfunction in hypertensive heart disease is associated with altered myocardial metabolism. Circulation 1999;99(17):2261–7.
236. Neubauer S, et al. Myocardial phosphocreatine-to-ATP ratio is a predictor of mortality in patients with dilated cardiomyopathy. Circulation 1997;96(7):2190–6.
237. Neubauer S, et al. Contributions of 31P-magnetic resonance spectroscopy to the understanding of dilated heart muscle disease. Eur Heart J 1995;16 Suppl O:115–18.
238. Rosca MG, Hoppel CL. Mitochondria in heart failure. Cardiovasc Res 2010;88(1):40–50.
239. Bugger H, Abel ED. Mitochondria in the diabetic heart. Cardiovasc Res 2010;88(2):229–40.
240. Chen L, Knowlton AA. Mitochondria and heart failure: new insights into an energetic problem. Minerva Cardioangiol 2010; 58(2):213–29.
241. Thomas S, McFalls EO. Hibernating myocardium: a mitochondrial adaptation that may be destined to heart failure. J Cardiovasc Transl Res 2008;1(4):328–31.
242. Bito V, et al. Reduced force generating capacity in myocytes from chronically ischemic, hibernating myocardium. Circ Res 2007;100(2):229–37.
243. Fields AV, et al. Glucagon-like peptide-1 and myocardial protection: more than glycemic control. Clin Cardiol 2009;32(5):236–43.

244. Drucker DJ, Minireview: the glucagon-like peptides. Endocrinology 2001;142(2):521–7.
245. Drucker DJ, Biological actions and therapeutic potential of the glucagon-like peptides. Gastroenterology 2002;122(2):531–44.
246. Perfetti R, Merkel P. Glucagon-like peptide-1: a major regulator of pancreatic beta-cell function. Eur J Endocrinol 2000;143(6):717–25.
247. Doyle ME, Egan JM. Glucagon-like peptide-1. Recent Prog Horm Res 2001;56:377–99.
248. Egan JM, et al. Glucagon-like peptide-1 augments insulin-mediated glucose uptake in the obese state. J Clin Endocrinol Metab 2002;87(8):3768–73.
249. Meneilly GS, et al. Glucagon-like peptide-1 (7-37) augments insulin-mediated glucose uptake in elderly patients with diabetes. J Gerontol A Biol Sci Med Sci 2001;56(11):M681–5.
250. Meneilly GS, et al. Effect of glucagon-like peptide 1 on non-insulin-mediated glucose uptake in the elderly patient with diabetes. Diabetes Care 2001;24(11):1951–6.
251. Bhashyam S, Fields AV, Patterson B, et al. Glucagon-like peptide-1 increases myocardial glucose uptake via p38alpha MAP kinase-mediated, nitric oxide-dependent mechanisms in conscious dogs with dilated cardiomyopathy. Circ Heart Fail 2010;3(4):512–21.
252. Bullock BP, Heller RS, Habener JF. Tissue distribution of messenger ribonucleic acid encoding the rat glucagon-like peptide-1 receptor. Endocrinology 1996;137(7):2968–78.
253. Wei Y, Mojsov S. Distribution of GLP-1 and PACAP receptors in human tissues. Acta Physiol Scand 1996;157(3):355–7.
254. Whelan RS, Kaplinskiy V, Kitsis RN. Cell death in the pathogenesis of heart disease: mechanisms and significance. Annu Rev Physiol 2010;72: 19–44.
255. Takemura G, et al. Cardiomyocyte apoptosis in the failing heart—a critical review from definition and classification of cell death. Int J Cardiol 2013;167(6):2373–86.
256. Youle RJ, Strasser A. The BCL-2 protein family: opposing activities that mediate cell death. Nat Rev Mol Cell Biol 2008;9(1):47–59.
257. Nechushtan A, et al. Conformation of the Bax C-terminus regulates subcellular location and cell death. EMBO J 1999;18(9):2330–41.
258. Zong WX, et al. Bax and Bak can localize to the endoplasmic reticulum to initiate apoptosis. J Cell Biol 2003;162(1):59–69.
259. Cardone MH, et al. The regulation of anoikis: MEKK-1 activation requires cleavage by caspases. Cell 1997;90(2):315–23.
260. Li H, et al. Cleavage of BID by caspase 8 mediates the mitochondrial damage in the Fas pathway of apoptosis. Cell 1998;94(4):491–501.
261. Olivetti G, et al. Apoptosis in the failing human heart. N Engl J Med 1997;336(16):1131–41.
262. Saraste A, et al. Cardiomyocyte apoptosis and progression of heart failure to transplantation. Eur J Clin Invest 1999;29(5):380–6.
263. Wencker D, et al. A mechanistic role for cardiac myocyte apoptosis in heart failure. J Clin Invest 2003;111(10):1497–504.
264. Brocheriou V, et al. Cardiac functional improvement by a human Bcl-2 transgene in a mouse model of ischemia/reperfusion injury. J Gene Med 2000;2(5):326–33.
265. Chen Z, et al. Overexpression of Bcl-2 attenuates apoptosis and protects against myocardial I/R injury in transgenic mice. Am J Physiol Heart Circ Physiol 2001;280(5):H2313–20.
266. Hochhauser E, et al. Bax ablation protects against myocardial ischemia-reperfusion injury in transgenic mice. Am J Physiol Heart Circ Physiol 2003;284(6):H2351–9.
267. Hochhauser E, et al. Bax deficiency reduces infarct size and improves long-term function after myocardial infarction. Cell Biochem Biophys 2007;47(1):11–20.
268. Chua CC, et al. Overexpression of IAP-2 attenuates apoptosis and protects against myocardial ischemia/reperfusion injury in transgenic mice. Biochim Biophys Acta 2007;1773(4):577–83.
269. Pyo JO, et al. Protection of cardiomyocytes from ischemic/hypoxic cell death via Drbp1 and pMe2GlyDH in cardio-specific ARC transgenic mice. J Biol Chem 2008;283(45):30707–14.
270. Matsui T, et al. Akt activation preserves cardiac function and prevents injury after transient cardiac ischemia in vivo. Circulation 2001;104(3):330–5.
271. Fujio Y, et al. Akt promotes survival of cardiomyocytes in vitro and protects against ischemia-reperfusion injury in mouse heart. Circulation 2000;101(6):660–7.
272. Liu HR, et al. Role of Omi/HtrA2 in apoptotic cell death after myocardial ischemia and reperfusion. Circulation 2005;111(1):90–6.
273. Bhuiyan MS, Fukunaga K. Inhibition of HtrA2/Omi ameliorates heart dysfunction following ischemia/reperfusion injury in rat heart in vivo. Eur J Pharmacol 2007;557(2–3):168–77.
274. Yaoita H, et al. Attenuation of ischemia/reperfusion injury in rats by a caspase inhibitor. Circulation 1998;97(3):276–81.
275. Huang JQ, et al. In vivo myocardial infarct size reduction by a caspase inhibitor administered after the onset of ischemia. Eur J Pharmacol 2000;402(1–2):139–42.
276. Holly TA, et al. Caspase inhibition reduces myocyte cell death induced by myocardial ischemia and reperfusion in vivo. J Mol Cell Cardiol 1999;31(9):1709–15.
277. Yang W, et al. MX1013, a dipeptide caspase inhibitor with potent in vivo antiapoptotic activity. Br J Pharmacol 2003;140(2):402–12.
278. Lavandero S, et al. Cardiovascular autophagy: Concepts, controversies and perspectives. Autophagy 2013;9(10):1455–66.
279. Chen Y, Klionsky DJ. The regulation of autophagy—unanswered questions. J Cell Sci. 124(Pt 2):161–70.
280. Wohlgemuth SE, et al. Autophagy in the heart and liver during normal aging and calorie restriction. Rejuvenation Res 2007;10(3):281–92.
281. Matsui Y, et al. Distinct roles of autophagy in the heart during ischemia and reperfusion: roles of AMP-activated protein kinase and Beclin 1 in mediating autophagy. Circ Res 2007;100(6):914–22.
282. Yan L, et al. Autophagy in chronically ischemic myocardium. Proc Natl Acad Sci U S A 2005;102(39):13807–12.
283. Russell RR, 3rd, et al. AMP-activated protein kinase mediates ischemic glucose uptake and prevents postischemic cardiac dysfunction, apoptosis, and injury. J Clin Invest 2004;114(4):495–503.
284. Solskov L, et al. Metformin induces cardioprotection against ischaemia/reperfusion injury in the rat heart 24 hours after administration. Basic Clin Pharmacol Toxicol 2008;103(1):82–7.
285. Kristiansen SB, et al. 5-Aminoimidazole-4-carboxamide-1-beta-D-ribofuranoside increases myocardial glucose uptake during reperfusion and induces late pre-conditioning: potential role of AMP-activated protein kinase. Basic Clin Pharmacol Toxicol 2009;105(1):10–16.
286. Nakai A, et al. The role of autophagy in cardiomyocytes in the basal state and in response to hemodynamic stress. Nat Med 2007;13(5):619–24.
287. Taneike M, et al. Inhibition of autophagy in the heart induces age-related cardiomyopathy. Autophagy 2010;6(5):600–6.
288. Maron BJ, et al. Clinical outcome and phenotypic expression in LAMP2 cardiomyopathy. JAMA 2009;301(12):1253–9.
289. Gustafsson AB, Gottlieb RA. Autophagy in ischemic heart disease. Circ Res 2009;104(2):150–8.
290. Valentim L, et al. Urocortin inhibits Beclin1-mediated autophagic cell death in cardiac myocytes exposed to ischaemia/reperfusion injury. J Mol Cell Cardiol 2006;40(6):846–52.
291. Pattingre S, et al. Bcl-2 antiapoptotic proteins inhibit Beclin 1-dependent autophagy. Cell 2005;122(6):927–39.
292. Zhu H, et al. Cardiac autophagy is a maladaptive response to hemodynamic stress. J Clin Invest 2007;117(7):1782–93.
293. Chan FK, et al. A role for tumor necrosis factor receptor-2 and receptor-interacting protein in programmed necrosis and antiviral responses. J Biol Chem 2003;278(51):51613–21.
294. Van de Velde C, et al. BNIP3 and genetic control of necrosis-like cell death through the mitochondrial permeability transition pore. Mol Cell Biol 2000;20(15):5454–68.

295. Mughal W, Dhingra R, Kirshenbaum LA. Striking a balance: autophagy, apoptosis, and necrosis in a normal and failing heart. Curr Hypertens Rep 2012;14(6):540–7.
296. Honda HM, Ping P. Mitochondrial permeability transition in cardiac cell injury and death. Cardiovasc Drugs Ther 2006 20(6):425–32.
297. Baines CP, et al. Loss of cyclophilin D reveals a critical role for mitochondrial permeability transition in cell death. Nature 2005;434(7033):658–62.
298. Nakagawa T, et al. Cyclophilin D-dependent mitochondrial permeability transition regulates some necrotic but not apoptotic cell death. Nature 2005;434(7033):652–8.
299. Schinzel AC, et al. Cyclophilin D is a component of mitochondrial permeability transition and mediates neuronal cell death after focal cerebral ischemia. Proc Natl Acad Sci U S A 2005;102(34):12005–10.
300. Holler N, et al. Fas triggers an alternative, caspase-8-independent cell death pathway using the kinase RIP as effector molecule. Nat Immunol 2000;1(6):489–95.
301. Zhang DW, et al. RIP3, an energy metabolism regulator that switches TNF-induced cell death from apoptosis to necrosis. Science 2009;325(5938):332–6.
302. Lin Y, et al. Cleavage of the death domain kinase RIP by caspase-8 prompts TNF-induced apoptosis. Genes Dev 1999;13(19):2514–26.
303. He S, et al. Receptor interacting protein kinase-3 determines cellular necrotic response to TNF-alpha. Cell 2009;137(6):1100–11.
304. Lim SY, et al. The cardioprotective effect of necrostatin requires the cyclophilin-D component of the mitochondrial permeability transition pore. Cardiovasc Drugs Ther 2007;21(6):467–9.
305. Konstam MA, Reliability of ventricular remodeling as a surrogate for use in conjunction with clinical outcomes in heart failure. Am J Cardiol 2005;96(6):867–71.
306. Hellawell JL, Margulies KB. Myocardial reverse remodeling. Cardiovasc Ther 2012;30(3):172–81.
307. Domanski MJ, et al. A comparative analysis of the results from 4 trials of beta-blocker therapy for heart failure: BEST, CIBIS-II, MERIT-HF, and COPERNICUS. J Card Fail 2003;9(5):354–63.
308. McKelvie RS, et al. Comparison of candesartan, enalapril, and their combination in congestive heart failure: randomized evaluation of strategies for left ventricular dysfunction (RESOLVD) pilot study. The RESOLVD Pilot Study Investigators. Circulation 1999;100(10):1056–64.
309. Doughty RN, et al. Left ventricular remodeling with carvedilol in patients with congestive heart failure due to ischemic heart disease. Australia-New Zealand Heart Failure Research Collaborative Group. J Am Coll Cardiol 1997;29(5):1060–6.
310. Palazzuoli A, et al. Effects of carvedilol on left ventricular remodeling and systolic function in elderly patients with heart failure. Eur J Heart Fail 2002;4(6):765–70.
311. Bristow MR, et al. Carvedilol produces dose-related improvements in left ventricular function and survival in subjects with chronic heart failure. MOCHA Investigators. Circulation 1996;94(11):2807–16.
312. Torp-Pedersen C, et al. Effects of metoprolol and carvedilol on cause-specific mortality and morbidity in patients with chronic heart failure—COMET. Am Heart J 2005;149(2):370–6.
313. Wong M, et al. Valsartan benefits left ventricular structure and function in heart failure: Val-HeFT echocardiographic study. J Am Coll Cardiol 2002;40(5):970–5.
314. Granger CB, et al. Effects of candesartan in patients with chronic heart failure and reduced left-ventricular systolic function intolerant to angiotensin-converting-enzyme inhibitors: the CHARM-Alternative trial. Lancet 2003;362(9386):772–6.
315. Chan AK, et al. Aldosterone receptor antagonism induces reverse remodeling when added to angiotensin receptor blockade in chronic heart failure. J Am Coll Cardiol 2007;50(7):591–6.
316. Abboud J, et al. Peripartum cardiomyopathy: a comprehensive review. Int J Cardiol 2007;118(3):295–303.
317. McCarthy RE, 3rd, et al. Long-term outcome of fulminant myocarditis as compared with acute (nonfulminant) myocarditis. N Engl J Med 2000;342(10):690–5.
318. Kodama M, et al. Early and long-term mortality of the clinical subtypes of myocarditis. Jpn Circ J 2001;65(11):961–4.
319. Chau EM, et al. Treatment and outcome of biopsy-proven fulminant myocarditis in adults. Int J Cardiol 2006;110(3):405–6.
320. Harding JD, et al. Electrophysiological alterations after mechanical circulatory support in patients with advanced cardiac failure. Circulation 2001;104(11):1241–7.
321. Klotz S, et al. Mechanical unloading during left ventricular assist device support increases left ventricular collagen cross-linking and myocardial stiffness. Circulation 2005;112(3):364–74.
322. Maybaum S, et al. Cardiac improvement during mechanical circulatory support: a prospective multicenter study of the LVAD Working Group. Circulation 2007;115(19):2497–505.
323. Nakatani S, et al. Prediction of right ventricular dysfunction after left ventricular assist device implantation. Circulation 1996;94(9 Suppl):II216–21.
324. James KB, et al. Effect of the implantable left ventricular assist device on neuroendocrine activation in heart failure. Circulation 1995;92(9 Suppl):II191–5.
325. Burkhoff D, Klotz S, Mancini DM. LVAD-induced reverse remodeling: basic and clinical implications for myocardial recovery. J Card Fail 2006;12(3):227–39.
326. Drakos SG, Kfoury AG, Selzman CH, et al. Left ventricular assist device unloading effects on myocardial structure and function: current status of the field and call for action. Curr Opin Cardiol 2011;26(3):245–55.
327. Birks EJ. Molecular changes after left ventricular assist device support for heart failure. Circ Res 2013;113(6):777–91.
328. Altemose GT, et al. Altered myocardial phenotype after mechanical support in human beings with advanced cardiomyopathy. J Heart Lung Transplant 1997;15(7):765–73.
329. de Jonge N, et al. Left ventricular assist device in end-stage heart failure: persistence of structural myocyte damage after unloading. An immunohistochemical analysis of the contractile myofilaments. J Am Coll Cardiol 2002;39(6):963–9.
330. Terracciano CM, et al. Changes in sarcolemmal Ca entry and sarcoplasmic reticulum Ca content in ventricular myocytes from patients with end-stage heart failure following myocardial recovery after combined pharmacological and ventricular assist device therapy. Eur Heart J 2003;24(14):1329–39.
331. Khan T, et al. Dobutamine stress echocardiography predicts myocardial improvement in patients supported by left ventricular assist devices (LVADs): hemodynamic and histologic evidence of improvement before LVAD explantation. J Heart Lung Transplant 2003;22(2):137–46.
332. Barbone A, et al. Comparison of right and left ventricular responses to left ventricular assist device support in patients with severe heart failure: a primary role of mechanical unloading underlying reverse remodeling. Circulation 2001;104(6):670–5.
333. Flesch M, et al. Differential regulation of mitogen-activated protein kinases in the failing human heart in response to mechanical unloading. Circulation 2001;104(19):2273–6.
334. Baba HA, et al. Dynamic regulation of MEK/Erks and Akt/GSK-3beta in human end-stage heart failure after left ventricular mechanical support: myocardial mechanotransduction-sensitivity as a possible molecular mechanism. Cardiovasc Res 2003;59(2):390–9.
335. Huebert RC, et al. Identification and regulation of Sprouty1, a negative inhibitor of the ERK cascade, in the human heart. Physiol Genomics 2004;18(3):284–9.
336. Chokshi A, Drosatos K, Cheema FH, et al. Ventricular assist device implantation corrects myocardial lipotoxicity, reverses insulin resistance, and normalizes cardiac metabolism in patients with advanced heart failure. Circulation 2012;125(23):2844–53.

337. Heerdt PM, et al. Chronic unloading by left ventricular assist device reverses contractile dysfunction and alters gene expression in end-stage heart failure. Circulation 2000;102(22):2713–19.
338. Ogletree-Hughes ML, et al. Mechanical unloading restores beta-adrenergic responsiveness and reverses receptor downregulation in the failing human heart. Circulation 2001;104(8):881–6.
339. Dipla K, et al. Myocyte recovery after mechanical circulatory support in humans with end-stage heart failure. Circulation 1998;97(23):2316–22.
340. Klotz S, et al. Left ventricular assist device support normalizes left and right ventricular beta-adrenergic pathway properties. J Am Coll Cardiol 2005;45(5):668–76.
341. Ogletree ML, Sweet WE, Talerico C, et al. Duration of left ventricular assist device support: Effects on abnormal calcium cycling and functional recovery in the failing human heart. J Heart Lung Transplant 2010;29(5):554–61.
342. Madigan JD, et al. Time course of reverse remodeling of the left ventricle during support with a left ventricular assist device. J Thorac Cardiovasc Surg 2001;121(5):902–8.
343. Terracciano CM, et al. Clinical recovery from end-stage heart failure using left-ventricular assist device and pharmacological therapy correlates with increased sarcoplasmic reticulum calcium content but not with regression of cellular hypertrophy. Circulation 2004;109(19):2263–5.
344. Marx SO, et al. PKA phosphorylation dissociates FKBP12.6 from the calcium release channel (ryanodine receptor): defective regulation in failing hearts. Cell 2000;101(4):365–76.
345. Bick RJ, et al. Left ventricular unloading with an assist device results in receptor relocalization as well as increased beta-adrenergic receptor numbers: are these changes indications for outcome? J Card Surg 2005 20(4):332–6.
346. Razeghi P, et al. Downregulation of metabolic gene expression in failing human heart before and after mechanical unloading. Cardiology 2002;97(4):203–9.
347. Lee SH, et al. Improvement of myocardial mitochondrial function after hemodynamic support with left ventricular assist devices in patients with heart failure. J Thorac Cardiovasc Surg 1998;116(2):344–9.
348. Mital S, et al. Left ventricular assist device implantation augments nitric oxide dependent control of mitochondrial respiration in failing human hearts. J Am Coll Cardiol 2000;36(6):1897–902.
349. Weitzel LB, et al. Left ventricular assist device effects on metabolic substrates in the failing heart. PLoS One. 8(4):e60292.
350. Effect of metoprolol CR/XL in chronic heart failure: Metoprolol CR/XL Randomised Intervention Trial in Congestive Heart Failure (MERIT-HF). Lancet 1999;353(9169):2001–7.
351. de Jonge N, et al. Cardiomyocyte death in patients with end-stage heart failure before and after support with a left ventricular assist device: low incidence of apoptosis despite ubiquitous mediators. J Heart Lung Transplant 2003;22(9):1028–36.
352. Patten RD, et al. Ventricular assist device therapy normalizes inducible nitric oxide synthase expression and reduces cardiomyocyte apoptosis in the failing human heart. J Am Coll Cardiol 2005;45(9):1419–24.
353. Hattori T, Effect of mechanical assist devices for ischemic myocardial damage-cardiomyocyte apoptosis and TNFalpha. Ann Thorac Cardiovasc Surg 2003;9(4):233–40.
354. Kassiotis C, et al. Markers of autophagy are downregulated in failing human heart after mechanical unloading. Circulation 2009;120(11 Suppl):S191–7.
355. Margulies KB, et al. Mixed messages: transcription patterns in failing and recovering human myocardium. Circ Res 2005;96(5):592–9.
356. Matkovich SJ, et al. Reciprocal regulation of myocardial microRNAs and messenger RNA in human cardiomyopathy and reversal of the microRNA signature by biomechanical support. Circulation 2009;119(9):1263–71.
357. Weiss JN, Karma A, MacLellan WR, et al. "Good enough solutions" and the genetics of complex diseases. Circ Res 2012;111(4):493–504.

CHAPTER 3

Physiology and hemodynamic assessment of the failing heart: Current knowledge and unmet needs for advanced heart failure

J. Julia Shin MD, Mandeep R. Mehra MD, and Ileana L. Piña MD MPH

Introduction

Heart failure (HF) is one of the most significant health care problems in the United States (US). There are more than 5 million people in the US who carry a diagnosis of HF. In addition, acute decompensated heart failure (ADHF) is the leading cause of hospitalizations among patients older than 65 years.[1] Readmission rates for HF remain consistently high, approaching 50% at 6 months.[2] The majority of ADHF admissions are due to symptoms of volume overload[3] and readmissions to the hospital after the index diagnosis are frequently related to inadequate removal of excess intravascular volume during the previous hospitalization or failure to apply evidence-based therapies. The identification of volume overload and fluid congestion in a HF patient depends on the clinical skills and judgment of the clinician and on the individual characteristics of the patient. Accurate assessment of both intravascular volume and the hemodynamic profile of the patient is crucial to decreasing the morbidity and mortality associated with ADHF. Recent clinical trials studying routine hemodynamic assessment of the HF patient have not shown benefit, and care is often delivered according to the personal experience of the treating physician.[4]

Definition of advanced heart failure

By definition, HF is a hemodynamic problem, or more precisely, a syndrome caused by a multisystem disorder that involves the heart, kidneys, skeletal muscle, and sympathetic nervous system. HF leads to overstimulation of the sympathetic nervous system resulting in an intricate constellation of neurohormonal changes. Despite a common clinical presentation, the etiologies of HF are diverse. A concise definition of advanced HF is challenging because there is no single, objective parameter that defines advanced HF. Rather, the entity encompasses multiple factors including the length of time that the syndrome has been manifest, multiple objective criteria of worsening ventricular function, and symptoms, among others. For example, it would be inappropriate to assign a label of advanced HF to a patient who has not received evidence-based therapies or one in whom adherence problems with diet or medications precipitate frequent hospitalization. Therefore, the diagnosis of advanced HF requires consideration of the overall clinical context. Experts may agree on defining advanced HF in a patient who has had multiple readmissions, deterioration in symptoms, and worsening ventricular size/function, in spite of optimal medical and device therapy. The diagnosis may also be applicable to a patient who is truly unable to tolerate optimal medications at optimal doses due to marked side effects, such as symptomatic hypotension, and who is thus refractory to pharmacologic therapy. There are many models that predict outcome over time using a series of clinical parameters, e.g., the Seattle Heart Failure Score.[5]

The stages of HF, as defined by the AHA/ACC guidelines (see Chapter 1) describe the progression of HF and include a stage C time where the patient may become compensated and even improve considerably.[6] Some patients, however, continue to have marked symptoms in spite of good care and deteriorate to stage D where the use of healthcare services, and corresponding costs, can become considerable.[7] Cardiac transplantation provides the only known "cure" of advanced HF but resources and donor hearts are limited and thus this precious resource cannot be available to all. Recent advances in mechanical circulatory support offer other options for patients with advanced HF whose disease has progressed despite optimal medical and device therapies.

HF may be due to either systolic or diastolic dysfunction of the left (or right) ventricle. While both systolic and diastolic failure of the left ventricle (LV) are characterized by elevated LV filling pressures, the underlying hemodynamic mechanisms differ considerably. For example, in systolic dysfunction (HFrEF) the slope of the pressure–volume relationship between myocardial fiber length and force generated is reduced. Filling pressures are increased and stroke volume and cardiac output may be compromised. In diastolic dysfunction heart failure (HFpEF) the end-systolic volume of the LV is preserved, but there is an increase in diastolic pressure at any given volume due to a decrease in ventricular compliance. Both systolic and diastolic HF cause congestive symptoms. The assessment and monitoring of the hemodynamic status in this complicated group of patients with HF remains challenging.[8] Nonetheless, a thorough history and physical examination are needed tools to relate findings to the hemodynamic status of the patient. In this chapter we review some noninvasive and invasive approaches to assessing the hemodynamic profile of the advanced HF patient and describe practical approaches to patient evaluation.

Physiology of the failing heart

Etiology

Although patients with advanced HF have many similarities in presentation, symptoms, and physical examination findings, individual etiologies differ. The most common etiologies include ischemia with or without a previous myocardial infarction (MI), hypertension, and valvular disorders.

Myocardial infarction

MI is an excellent model of ventricular remodeling since the timing of the insult is acute and known. Postinfarct remodeling was initially studied in animal models that followed the sequence of events from coronary ligation to the development of HF.[9] Studies of patients with MI have included those where an intervention such as pharmacologic therapy or cell therapy has been used to delay or reverse the remodeling process. Studies performed prior to the era of early revascularization describe the sequence of hemodynamic events that can culminate in acute decompensated HF. Not all patients, however, remodel adversely, nor is the sequence of decompensation universal in timing across patient groups. Clinicians are poorly equipped to determine a priori which patients who will remodel quickly and decompensate acutely or during their hospitalization. To better understand the advanced HF patient who has an ischemic postinfarction physiology, it is useful to review the remodeling process with its compensations and ultimate loss or exaggeration of compensatory mechanisms that can insidiously lead the patient to the advanced stage of HF.[10] The progression from early to late remodeling may take months or years and its true trajectory may be difficult to measure because patients can remain asymptomatic secondary to the many compensatory mechanisms. Thus, using hemodynamics, we can compare early changes and the late appearance of these in the more advanced patient. Hemodynamics are the window to understanding the dynamic process of development of advanced HF.

Thomas and colleagues mapped the hemodynamic course of nine patients who suffered MIs.[11,12] Notably, these observations were made prior to the use of renin–angiotensin–aldosterone system (RAAS) system blocking agents, such as angiotensin converting enzyme inhibitors (ACEIs) and therefore demonstrate the untreated cardiovascular response. Although there was significant variability in the early (i.e., 1–3 day) response, the trends by day 6 were similar (see Figure 3.1). Heart rate changes paralleled drops in cardiac output in four patients and others failed to mount a tachycardic response to drops in cardiac output. After day 3, the heart rate remained constant. Cardiac output also varied, with the lowest occurring in a patient with a previous MI and another who had an extension of the then current infarct. In patients in whom the cardiac output dropped, the blood pressure also dropped with an increase in peripheral vascular resistance. As noted in Figure 3.1, by day 6 the cardiac output had either plateaued or increased in most of the patients. As cardiac output rose, there was a parallel clinical improvement. By day 6 brachial blood pressure had increased in the majority of patients.

Since the cardiac output normalizes by day 6 without a major increase in heart rate, the stroke volume must have increased. Indeed, that is the case and although variability of stroke volume occurs early, there is a gradual increase after day 6. This observation parallels that of Konstam et al. using data from the Studies of Left Ventricular Dysfunction (SOLVD) trial. The patients on placebo exhibited an increasing LV end-diastolic volume whereas those receiving enalapril therapy had a blunted increase in stroke volume.[13] The patients in SOLVD had established HF and therefore, this was a chronic, more advanced phase of class II–III (Figure 3.2). Similar results were found in the Studies of Ventricular Enlargement (SAVE) trial up to 1 year post MI (Figure 3.3).[14]

Thus, one of the hallmarks of the transition to advanced HF is a progressively increasing LV end-diastolic volume (LVEDV) with an apparent normalization of cardiac output and an increase in stroke volume. This seemingly "benign" remodeling process may leave patients asymptomatic and it is therefore not surprising that many patients present with symptoms and have developed an advanced state without significant alterations in blood pressure. The extent of the LV volume increase is a determinant of poor outcomes, as shown in Figure 3.4. Similarly, the difference between symptomatic and asymptomatic HF may be attributed to the increase in LVEDV eventually culminating in symptoms of congestion.

Hypertension

Long-standing chronic systemic arterial hypertension can lead to diastolic and systolic HF due to increased workload on the heart. Systolic pressure appears to be a more important factor than diastolic pressure in causing changes in LV geometry and function.[15] Left ventricular hypertrophy (LVH) is the characteristic change that occurs due to chronically increased systemic blood pressure. LVH maintains normal systolic wall stress and stroke volume in the setting of increased afterload. While the hypertrophy is initially a physiologic response to increased afterload, over time the response leads to pathologic dysfunction of the heart.[16] In fact, the presence of LVH predicts the development of future HF.[17] Increased systemic arterial pressures results in increased cardiac wall stress and this causes the myocardium to hypertrophy. This is an adaptive response in an attempt to maintain normal wall tension in the setting of increased LV pressure. Over time, however, this leads to structural changes and myocardial fibrosis that contributes to dysfunction of the heart.

A chronic increase in systolic wall tension of the LV causes hypertrophy of individual myocardial cells. This cause increased work for the LV that, over time, results in progressive diastolic and systolic dysfunction and ultimately to clinical HF.[16,18] As the heart remodels pathologically in the face of chronically increased wall stress, increased interstitial fibrosis leads to loss of compliance and diastolic dysfunction or decreased lusitropy: that is, the

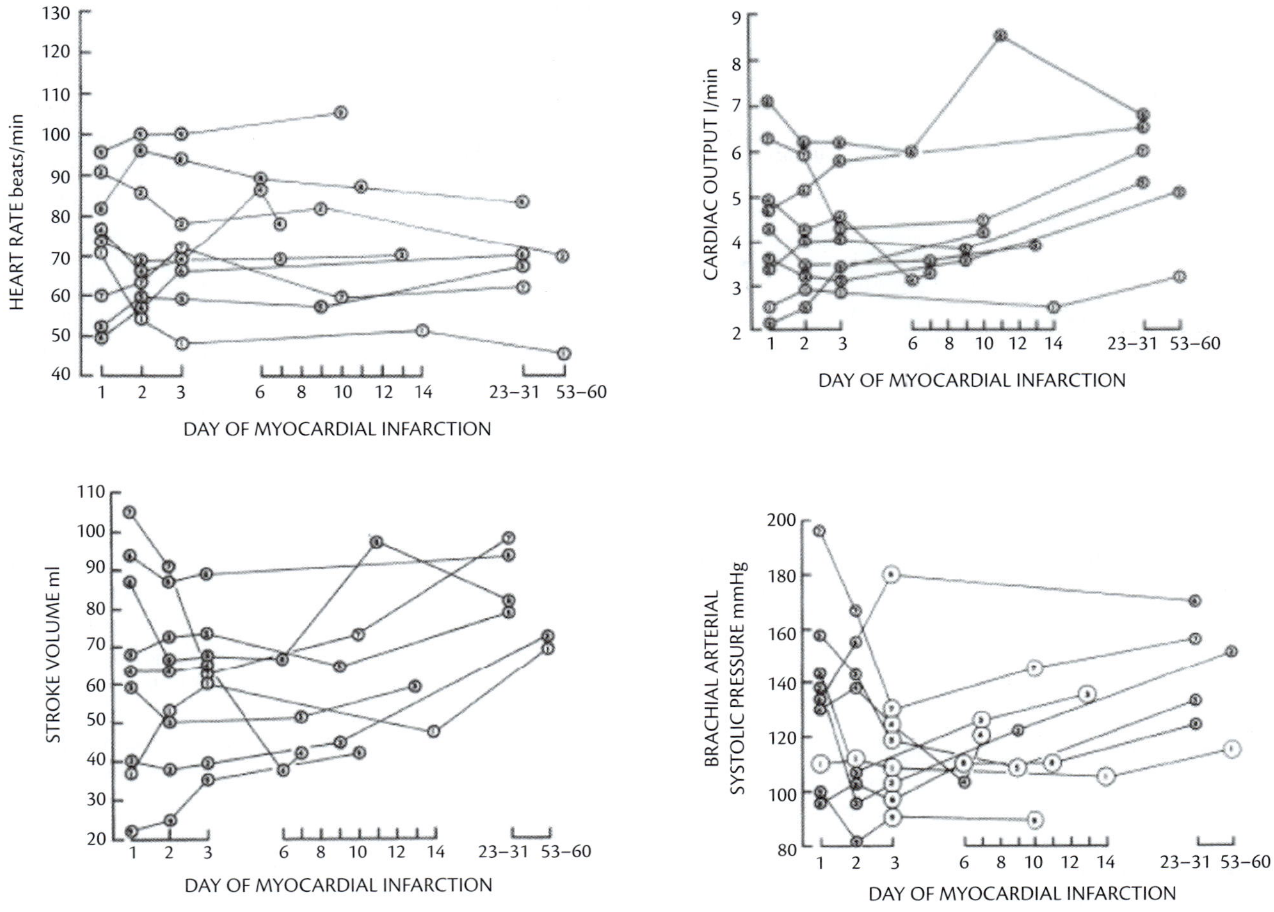

Fig. 3.1 The hemodynamics of the first 2 weeks after a myocardial infarction.

Thomas et al, Hemodynamic Changes in Patients with Acute: Myocardial Infarction, Circulation. 1965;31:811–823.

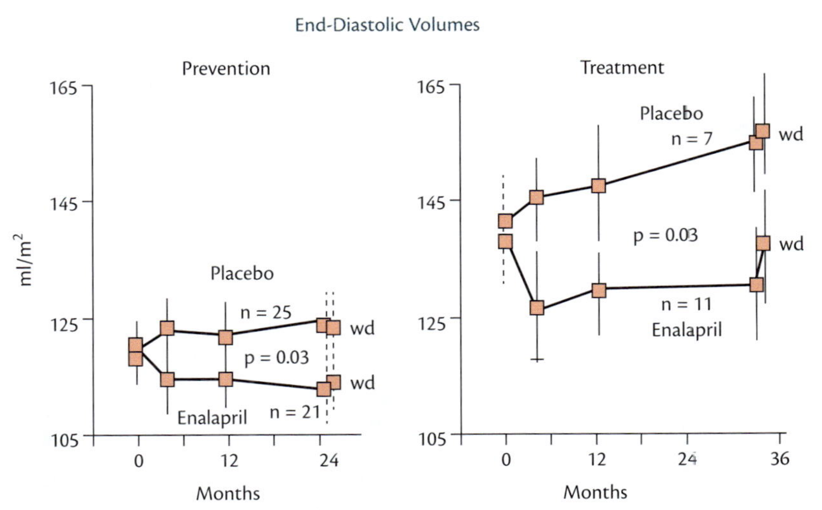

Fig. 3.2 Effects of angiotensin converting enzyme(ACE) inhibitor on ventricular volumes. Changes in left ventricular enc-diastolic volume over time in asymptomatic (Prevention) and symptomatic (Treatment) patients with decreased left ventricular ejection fraction (LVEF) while randomized to placebo or enalapril, from the SOLVD (Studies of Left Ventricular Dysfunction) trials. During long-term follow-up, patients randomized to placebo demonstrate evidence of progressive increase in left ventricular end-diastolic volume, whereas those randomized to enalapril showed reductions in left ventricular volume. wd = restudy after withdrawal of placebo or enalapril.

Reprinted from Journal of the American College of Cardiology: Cardiovascular Imaging, Vol 4, Issue 1, Konstam, M et al., Left Ventricular Remodeling in Heart Failure: Current Concepts in Clinical Significance and Assessment, 98–108, copyright (2011) with permission from Elsevier.

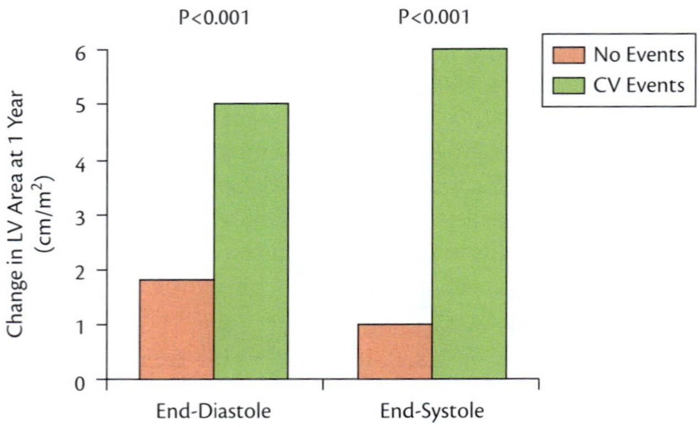

Fig. 3.3 Longitudinal ventricular dilation and prognosis. Changes in left ventricular (LV) area at end-systole and end-diastole over 1 year in patients after myocardial infarction with baseline left ventricular dysfunction, from the SAVE (Studies of Ventricular Enlargement) trial, compared in patients who sustained versus those who did not sustain adverse cardiovascular (CV) events. Patients experiencing events had a significantly greater increase in areas (i.e., more adverse remodeling) compared with those who had no events.

inability of the ventricle to "relax" normally. The increase in fibrosis is compounded by myocyte injury and necrosis as a result of being chronically overworked. Chronically elevated systolic blood pressure ultimately leads to LVH, which, if combined with abnormal cardiac remodeling, can lead to both diastolic and systolic dysfunction. Hypertension frequently interacts with other risk factors for heart disease, such as neurohormonal or sympathetic nervous system activation, synergistically increasing the risk of developing HF.

Valvular disease

Like systemic hypertension, valvular heart disease results in a hemodynamic load on the heart. In severe aortic stenosis, obstruction to LV outflow causes a pressure overload that results in concentric myocardial hypertrophy and the maladaptations described above for hypertensive heart disease.[19,20,21] In contrast to the ventricular dysfunction that can result from increased workload in chronic hypertension and aortic stenosis, however, regurgitant valvular disease can lead to HF due to volume overload. Over time, the chronic volume overload causes myocardial cell death and fibrosis, leading to systolic HF. In chronic aortic insufficiency, eccentric myocardial hypertrophy (versus concentric myocardial hypertrophy as seen in hypertensive heart disease) initially enables the ventricle to accommodate a compensatory increase in stroke volume consequent to regurgitant flow. An increase in myocyte length allows for an increase in LV volume, which thereby increases stroke volume. This enables the addition of regurgitant volume to be accommodated by the LV at a lower filling pressure. In this manner, chronic aortic regurgitation can actually be well tolerated because of the compensation that affords normal filling pressures and cardiac output. Myocyte hypertrophy results from the loading conditions.[22,23] As previously described, hypertrophy serves to normalize wall stress, but progresses to myocyte death and fibrosis, leading to both diastolic and systolic failure of the LV.

In contrast to aortic regurgitation, mitral regurgitation leads to volume overload of both the left atrium (LA) and LV. Acute mitral regurgitation causes pulmonary congestion due to an increase in LA pressure and a decrease in cardiac output due to a loss of "forward" flow. The volume overload of the LV causes the same pathophysiologic changes as for chronic aortic regurgitation, with eccentric hypertrophy of myocardial cells to accommodate the increase in end-diastolic volume at a normal pressure.[24] While the

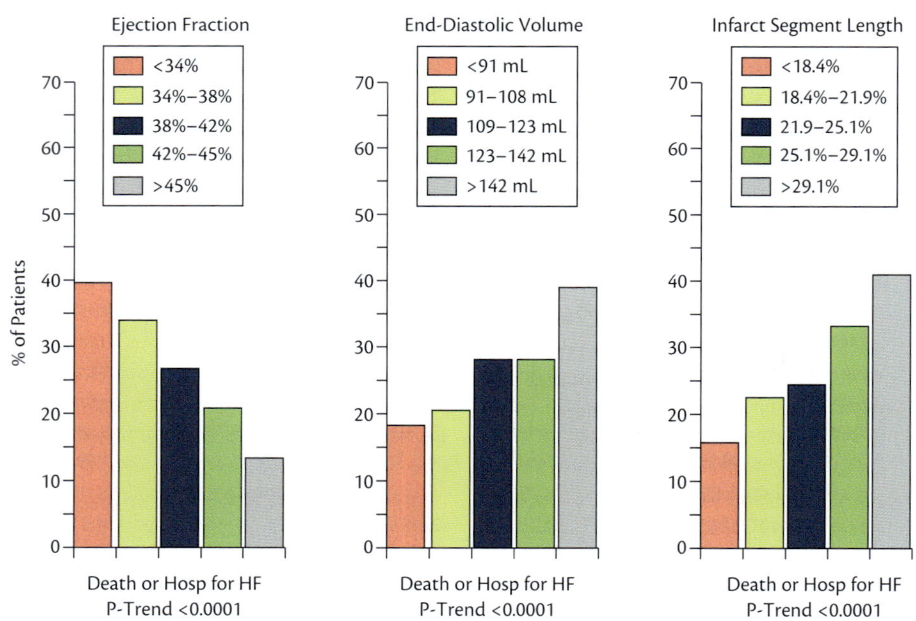

Fig. 3.4 Ventricular measurements and prognosis. Relationship between echocardiographic parameters, ejection fraction, end-diastolic volume, and infarct segment length, and the combined outcome of death or hospitalization for heart failure (HF) after myocardial infarction.

total stroke volume is increased in mitral regurgitation because the LV is ejecting through the aortic valve and also into the relatively low-pressure LA, forward stroke volume is usually not normal. When the regurgitant fraction becomes high, chronic volume overload of the LV results, eccentric cardiac hypertrophy (increase in cell length to accommodate an increase in ventricular volume) occurs, and ultimately LV dysfunction results. This is compounded by activation of the sympathetic nervous system that amplifies fibrosis. The final pathologic endpoint in both chronic aortic and mitral regurgitation is an increase in afterload from LV dysfunction that propagates adverse changes ventricular geometry.[24]

Neurohormonal activation

Regardless of etiology, the result is adverse LV remodeling that leads to systolic failure (impaired myocardial contraction, HFrEF) or diastolic failure (abnormal myocardial relaxation, HFpEF). Both systolic and diastolic HF lead to intravascular volume overload and congestion, which is a characteristic feature for patients who present with ADHF. Increased intracardiac filling pressures, reduced cardiac output, exaggerated peripheral vasoconstriction, and impaired diuresis from cardiorenal syndrome are significant factors in advanced HF that result in volume overload. Renal sodium and water retention by the kidneys in patients with ADHF results in an increase in total blood volume. Elevations in LV and/or right ventricular (RV) filling pressures cause the symptoms and signs of HF such as dyspnea, orthopnea, elevated jugular venous pressure (JVP), pulmonary rales, hepatomegaly, and peripheral edema. A decrease in cardiac output and excessive peripheral vasoconstriction lead to other signs and symptoms of HF such as cool extremities, worsening renal function, hypotension, and mental status changes. The pathophysiologic changes that occur in HF lead to a cyclical detrimental process by which activation of the neurohormonal system further exacerbates volume overload and myocardial dysfunction. In normal patients, an increase in total blood volume should result in an increase in sodium and water excretion by the kidneys. The opposite occurs in patients with advanced HF due to several maladaptive mechanisms.[25] In general, a decrease in cardiac output causes deficiencies in the arterial circulation despite an increase in the total blood volume of the patient. The attenuated arterial circulation to the kidneys results in a maladaptive renal response in ADHF, namely, excessive neurohormonal activation of the RAAS and the sympathetic nervous system.[26] Arterial baroreceptors sense a decrease in arterial circulation and increases adrenergic output from the central nervous system, with resultant activation of the RAAS. Both adrenergic stimulation and an increase in circulating angiotensin II cause the renal proximal tubular epithelium to reabsorb sodium and decrease sodium delivery to the collecting duct. An increase in circulating angiotensin II and aldosterone also increases cardiac remodeling and fibrosis. Neurohormonal activation also directly increases systemic vascular resistance, thus increasing cardiac afterload,[27] which further decreases cardiac output. Neurohumoral stimulation in ADHF also causes the release of arginine vasopressin (AVP) through a baroreceptor-mediated mechanism.[28,29,30] AVP activation of the V2 vasopressin receptor in the collecting ducts of the kidneys causes water retention and is the major factor leading to a characteristic hyponatremia associated with advanced HF.[31] Furthermore, stimulation of the V1a vasopressin receptors of the peripheral vasculature activates vascular smooth muscle, thus leading to an increase in cardiac preload and afterload. Neurohormonal activation also results in tachycardia, which is detrimental in advanced HF by increasing oxygen demand of the myocardium and decreasing diastolic filling time.

Hemodynamic derangements

The hemodynamic abnormalities that can occur in advanced HF include increased central venous pressure, increased right atrial (RA) and RV pressures, pulmonary hypertension, increased LA and LV pressures, low cardiac output, and elevated systemic vascular resistance. More recently, the measurement of biomarkers has also helped to distinguish the more advanced HF patient who has higher levels of the natriuretic hormones B-type natriuretic peptide (BNP) and N-terminal pro-BNP (NT-pro-BNP) and signs of myocardial damage with higher levels of troponin.[32]

Patient assessment

Approach to the advanced heart failure patient

It is critically important to differentiate a truly advanced HF patient from one who has a brief excursion into decompensation due to an easily resolvable event, such as discontinuation of chronic therapy or dietary indiscretion. The truly advanced patient is one who in spite of optimal medical therapy or expert attempts to optimize fails and whose ventricular function continues to deteriorate in spite of therapy and who now has frequent hospitalizations.[3] The physiology and hemodynamics of these patients show sign of severe adverse remodeling with ventricular dilation, wall thinning, and decreasing ejection fraction. Many may exhibit functional mitral regurgitation with or without pulmonary hypertension. Pulmonary hypertension may be present and severe; RV dysfunction may occur with peripheral edema, ascites, and pleural effusions. Although symptom progression is helpful in diagnosis, the early dyspnea resolves fairly quickly with diuretic administration. A complete medical history and physical examination remain the key to the initial assessment of a patient with advanced HF and can help elucidate the clinical hemodynamic profile of the patient.

History

The components of a HF history and physical examination exhibit a wide range of specificities and sensitivities in regard to accurately determining the presence or absence of intravascular congestion.

Dyspnea is the most common presenting symptom for a patient with ADHF.[33] Dyspnea in HF is usually due to congestion of the pulmonary vasculature from an increase in pulmonary capillary wedge pressure (PCWP) as a result of LV dysfunction. Dyspnea can also often be of noncardiac origin, however, and this symptom is not particularly sensitive or specific for ADHF. A prior history of HF, MI, or coronary disease increases the likelihood that the presenting symptom of dyspnea is actually due to ADHF.[34] Patients with advanced HF often present with gradual worsening of symptoms, usually on exertion, leading to dyspnea at rest. Others report fatigue with activity requiring periods of rest during an ordinary day. In these patients, activities of daily living seem difficult to sustain. Fatigue of this type is associated with low cardiac output. Symptoms elicited with activity soon become troublesome at night with orthopnea. The symptom of orthopnea appears to be a more sensitive and specific symptom of ADHF than dyspnea. In the Evaluation Study of Congestive Heart Failure and Pulmonary Artery Catheterization Effectiveness (ESCAPE) trial, orthopnea

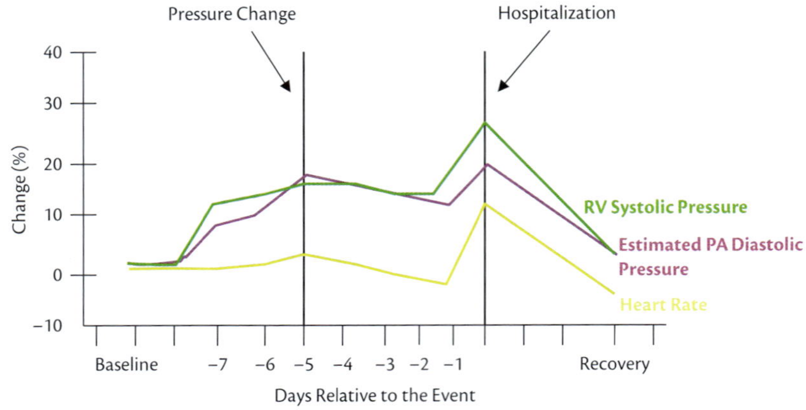

Fig. 3.5 Congestion precedes hospitalization.
Adapted from Journal of the American College of Cardiology, Vol 41, Issue 4, Adamson PB et al., p565–571 copyright (2003) with permission from Elsevier.

was independently associated with a PCWP of 28 mmHg or more.[35] Furthermore, persistent orthopnea is associated with higher rates of rehospitalization for ADHF.[36]

Alternatively, the patient may present with a rapid change from clinical stability to instability often heralded by an acute event, such as initiation of atrial fibrillation, discontinuation of stable chronic medical therapy, or acute ischemia. It has been noted in device trials that intracardiac pressure changes often precede an episode of decompensation (Figure 3.5). Paroxysmal nocturnal dyspnea, often described in the advanced patient, may not be readily recognizable to the patient but a close relative or partner may find these symptoms, including apnea, very disturbing. Although this presentation with reverse remodeling has been attributed to low ejection fraction (EF) patients (HFrEF), these signs and symptoms are as likely to occur in patients with preserved EF (HFpEF). A thorough history will help clarify the timing of decompensation in terms of being slowly worsening or abrupt in onset.

Two aspects of the history are critical in the care of the advanced patient: etiology of the syndrome and reasons for decompensation. A history of MI or previous revascularization will certainly bring an ischemic etiology into focus. Ischemia may be present even in the absence of classical chest pain. If the patient has risk factors for coronary artery disease but has not had angiography, it should be considered during the workup. The background leading to decompensation is especially important in patients who have had a significant period of stability only to destabilize. Patients often know what the reason for their decompensation is, and a careful, thoughtful, interview is often revealing.

Patients should be queried about recent discontinuation of evidence-based therapy, such as ACEI, which may also precipitate worsening symptoms. Concomitant use of contraindicated drugs, such as nonsteroidal anti-inflammatory therapy of calcium channel blocking agents, should be part of the history. Common reasons for decompensation are shown in Box 3.1. In elderly people, anemia can occur insidiously and lead to worsening HF. Intercurrent infections, whether respiratory or urinary, can also be in the background of a decompensation episode.

Physical examination

Assessment of two important parameters should be included in every patient assessment: volume and output. An evaluation of HF symptoms is the first step in the assessment of volume and hemodynamic status of the patient.

In the absence of insertion of a Swan–Ganz catheter, the physical examination provides an estimate of hemodynamics in the advanced patient. Volume assessment should include determination of the JVP, findings of ascites, peripheral edema, presence of effusions. JVP reflects RA pressure and has a strong correlation with invasive measurements of central venous pressure (CVP)[37] and PCWP in patients with advanced HF.[38] In the ESCAPE trial, for example, an elevated JVP correlated well with a PCWP above 22 mmHg.[35] Multiple studies have shown that elevated JVP is an accurate predictor of high PCWP[39,40] and is thus an important component of the physical examination in assessing a patient with ADHF. Accurately assessing JVP takes training and practice (Figure 3.6). Careful examination of jugular venous pulsation can also provide clues to specific abnormalities of the heart, such as tricuspid regurgitation (accentuated “v” wave); Kussmaul sign (failure of inspiratory fall of venous pressure), which is seen in RV failure or decreased myocardial compliance; pulmonary hypertension (large a-wave); or atrial fibrillation (absent a-wave).

Box 3.1 Common causes of decompensation

- Poor compliance:
  - Dietary (sodium, fluid)
  - Medications
- Alcohol abuse
- Hypertension
- Ischemia
- Arrhythmias
- Infections
- Anemia
- Thyroid disease
- Iatrogenic
- Over-the-counter drugs

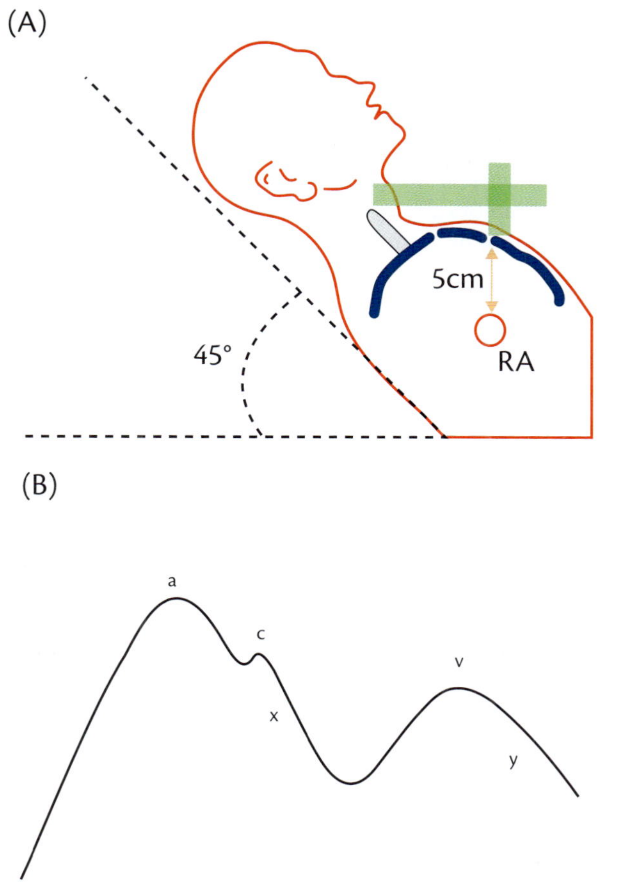

Fig. 3.6 (A) Height of venous column and jugular venous waves. (B) Venous waves as detected in the jugular venous examination. a, atrial contraction; c, ventricular contraction and resulting bulging of tricuspid into the right atrium during isovolumetric contraction;v, atrial venous filling; x descent, atrial relaxation with the tricuspid valve moving downward; y descent, filling of the ventricle after tricuspid opening.

It is important to note, however, that patients may have clear lung fields in the presence of volume overload. Weight gain without an increase in appetite may also be a sign of volume increase. The presence of a third heart sound (S3) is also a sensitive marker for elevated intracardiac filling pressures,[39] but may not be very specific.[41] Other physical examination findings such as peripheral edema and pulmonary rales show a wide range of sensitivity and specificity for determining the presence of elevated cardiac filling pressures,[39,42] and both signs can be due to noncardiac causes. Lower-extremity edema, for example, can be caused by disorders of the hepatic, renal, or vascular systems and is not specific to ADHF. Rales, when present, have good specificity for the presence of pulmonary congestion, but the majority of patients with ADHF do not have rales on lung examination due to an increase in lymphatic drainage and chronic compensation of the pulmonary vasculature.[41] The absence of rales, therefore, should not be taken as an absence of pulmonary edema in a patient presenting with ADHF.

Since a drop in cardiac output is compensated by an increase in peripheral vascular constriction, extremities may be cool and clammy, a narrow pulse pressure measured, perioral cyanosis or nail bed cyanosis. and symptoms of difficulty concentrating are notable. Other symptoms can include claudication, muscle weakness, lightheadedness or syncope, and cognitive impairment. It is important to identify poor perfusion because this is associated with worse survival in patients with ADHF.[43]

If ventricular dilation is significant with remodeling, mitral regurgitation follows and subsequent pulmonary hypertension with an augmented pulmonary component of S2 (P2). Eventually, tricuspid regurgitation will lead to RV failure and increasing symptoms of right sided volume with peripheral edema, ascites and pleural effusions. Pulmonary hypertension may be insidious and echocardiography can identify high RV systolic pressures,

Initial assessment

Laboratory testing can also aid in the initial assessment of the decompensated HF patient. For example, the natriuretic peptides BNP and NT-pro-BNP are released in response to increased myocardial volume/pressure loading and wall stress and have been shown to improve diagnostic accuracy of the congested patient in ADHF.[44] In the future biomarkers may help determine extent of fibrosis or inflammation. Creatinine correlates to clinical outcomes in ADHF, but is of limited utility as a diagnostic aid or as a marker of congestion in ADHF.[45] Nonetheless, it is important to obtain blood urea nitrogen (BUN) and creatinine levels at baseline as well as a serum potassium. These values will be critical when the decision is made to initiate aldosterone antagonist therapy. Hyponatremia is a powerful predictor of poor outcomes and also a sign of increased neurohormonal activity. It is important to measure hemoglobin and compare, if possible to a previous value. As noted above, a drop in hemoglobin may initiate an episode of decompensation. Underlying hypothyroidism may present as a low-output cardiomyopathy and this diagnosis is easily eliminated by a baseline thyroid profile including TSH.

Chest radiography remains a routine test in evaluating a patient with ADHF. But, while signs of pulmonary congestion by chest radiography are reasonably specific, they are relatively insensitive, as many patients with hemodynamic confirmation of elevated intracardiac filling pressures will have clear chest radiographs.[42] Often patients with known chronic HF can present with upper respiratory infections including pneumonia and the sequence of symptom worsening by etiology is often difficult: did the pulmonary infection precede a decompensation, or develop later?

Echocardiography

Echocardiography is a useful tool for the noninvasive assessment of a hemodynamic profile in a patient with ADHF and is discussed in detail elsewhere in this textbook. Echocardiography is useful in assessing cardiac structure and function, including valvular structure and function and the presence or absence of valvular disease. Ventricular filling pressures and pulmonary artery pressures can be estimated.

Invasive hemodynamic assessment

The gold standard of hemodynamic assessment in a patient with ADHF remains right heart catheterization (RHC) with a pulmonary artery catheter (PAC). RHC can be used to assess hemodynamic status, to measure intracardiac filling pressures and cardiac output, and to monitor the response to therapy in patients who have advanced HF. However, the use of invasive hemodynamic measurements routinely for all patients with ADHF remains controversial. Earlier reports suggested that therapy guided by continuous RHC monitoring was safe and led to greater reductions in filling pressures.[50] Other studies, however, had shown that patients managed with PACs had a significantly increased 30-day mortality, higher hospital costs, and longer lengths of stay.[51] This report resulted in overall concerns and fears about using PACs even in the most experienced critical care units. Because of these discrepancies, the ESCAPE trial was designed to be the first prospectively randomized and controlled multicenter trial to evaluate the use of the PAC in hospitalized patients with advanced HF.[52] The intent of this study was to determine if the addition of PAC-guided or "tailored" therapy to clinical assessment would improve patient outcomes by reducing mortality and rehospitalizations, as compared to therapy guided by clinical assessment alone in patients with ADHF. A total of 433 patients were enrolled and randomly assigned to the clinical assessment group, for which therapeutic decisions were guided by clinical assessment alone, or to the PAC group, where therapy was guided by clinical assessment in addition to the hemodynamic data provided by continuous invasive hemodynamic monitoring. Both groups reported an improvement in the symptoms and signs of congestion, but there was no statistical difference in the primary endpoint of total number of days alive out of the hospital in the first 6 months after enrollment. Furthermore, the PAC group had a higher rate of procedure-related adverse events such as infection. This trial showed that tailored therapy by continuous invasive hemodynamic monitoring in hospitalized ADHF patients did not provide additional benefit in survival or future hospitalizations when compared to clinical assessment alone. It is important to note, however, that patients whose management required a PAC for clinical management, such as those with worsening renal failure or who required intravenous inotropic agents for clinical stabilization, were excluded from the ESCAPE study. Generalization of the ESCAPE trial results to all HF patients should be avoided. RHC still possesses an important role in the assessment and treatment of ADHF, such as for the patient whose volume status cannot be accurately assessed from clinical assessment alone, or for the patient who does not respond to or deteriorates despite management based on initial clinical assessment. The PAC also definitely provides the necessary assessment of pulmonary vascular resistance and reactivity of the pulmonary vascular bed in patients with pulmonary hypertension and those who are being considered for cardiac transplantation and/or placement of mechanical circulatory support devices. The American Heart Association/American College of Cardiology (AHA/ACC) guidelines on the diagnosis and management of chronic HF in the adult support the use of the PAC to guide therapy in selected patients with refractory end-stage HF, and in those patients with pulmonary hypertension or as part of cardiac transplant evaluation.[53]

Other potential, but not proven, methods of invasive hemodynamic assessment in the decompensated HF patient includes the use of a central venous catheter to continuously assess CVP or to obtain oxygen saturations of blood from the superior vena cava as an approximation of mixed venous oxygen saturation for the calculation of cardiac output by the Fick method.

The development of novel implantable devices, such as those that measure LA pressure or pulmonary pressures, offer a tantalizing methodology to assess hemodynamics chronically with the intent to reduce overt decompensation[54] or to target specific treatments. The role of these devices in truly allowing prevention of events remains somewhat controversial[55] and is addressed specifically later in the chapter.

Hemodynamics of cardiorenal syndrome

The presence of renal impairment is common in patients with ADHF and renal dysfunction is an independent risk factor for morbidity and mortality in these patients.[56,57] The term "cardiorenal syndrome" (CRS) is now used to describe the pathophysiologic interdependence of the cardiac and renal systems in HF.[58] While CRS can simplistically be described as a hemodynamic phenomenon, it cannot be entirely explained by the traditional argument that poor arterial flow due to low cardiac output leads to worsening renal function in HF patients. Indeed, worsening renal function in ADHF may not correlate with reduced LV ejection fraction (LVEF) or low cardiac output at all.[45,59] While a decrease in myocardial function results in predictable hemodynamic derangements such as low cardiac output and decreased arterial perfusion, these abnormalities are compensated by mechanisms of sodium retention and vasoconstriction via activation of the sympathetic nervous system and the RAAS in a maladaptive cycle (described earlier in the chapter), whereby increasing preload and afterload leads to worsening cardiac and renal function.

The only hemodynamic parameter that has been strongly associated with worsening renal function is high CVP. High CVP leads to high renal vein pressure, and renal dysfunction is more likely to result from high renal vein pressure than due to hypoperfusion from low cardiac output.[60] Indeed, the reduction of renal vein congestion by diuresis is a mechanism proposed to explain an improvement in renal function during clinical management for patients in ADHF. Patients admitted with ADHF commonly experience worsening renal function early in their hospital course, even when they are still volume overloaded.[61] Although overdiuresis can eventually play a role in renal dysfunction by depleting intravascular volume, prerenal physiology does not likely play a large role in the early development of CRS. While aggressive diuresis can result in an increase in serum creatinine, this appears to be a transient worsening in renal function without an overall impact on patient outcomes.[62]

Implantable monitors

There are several devices that can be implanted subcutaneously, like a permanent pacemaker, and continuously monitor the hemodynamic status of the patient. These devices, called implantable hemodynamic monitors (IHM), have been developed to provide ambulatory hemodynamic data that can be accessed remotely. Several of these devices are described in this chapter. The data obtained from IHMs can potentially assist in the diagnosis of vascular congestion in patients with HF and guide in treatment. One such device, the Chronicle IHM (Medtronic, Minneapolis, MN) was implanted subcutaneously, similar to a permanent pacemaker, into the pectoral region. A transvenous lead in the RV outflow tract monitored heart rate and RV systolic and diastolic pressures and demonstrated good correlation with data obtained by RHC.[63] This device was evaluated in the Chronicle Offers Management to Patients with Advanced Signs and Symptoms of Heart Failure (COMPASS-HF) study, which showed a 21% reduction of all HF-related events when the hemodynamic information from the monitor was used to guide patient management, but this difference was not statistically significant.[54] Furthermore, New York Heart Association (NYHA) class IV patients did not show a reduction in hospitalization events. A post-hoc analysis showed a statistically significant 36% reduction of the time to first hospitalization for

ADHF in the Chronicle group for NYHA class III. This device did not receive approval from the US Food and Drug Administration (FDA). Although the COMPASS trial did not achieve its original endpoint, it did allow a view into decompensation, in that the pressures were rising days before a symptomatic decompensation occurred and that weight was not reliable for these episodes. The treatment of choice in COMPASS was a diuretic. However, diuresis alone may not be the appropriate response to rising pulmonary pressures. An ongoing trial, Reducing Events in Patients with Chronic Heart Failure (REDUCEhf), is evaluating the effect of the Chronicle ICD (a dual ICD and IHM) in reducing HF-related events and mortality.

The HeartPOD device (St Jude Medical, St Paul, MN) is another IHM that is subcutaneously implanted and can provide measures of LA pressure by a transseptal approach. In the initial pilot study, use of this device to tailor HF therapy seemed to improve LV function and prolong survival free of ADHF, without compromising renal function or posing other important safety issues.[64] The HeartPOD device is currently being evaluated in a randomized trial to elucidate its value in monitor-guided therapy.

Implantable devices can also measure intrathoracic bioimpedance, which indirectly provides an assessment of cardiac output and intravascular volume status, with the theory that lower impedance indicates greater intrathoracic fluid volume. These devices can also theoretically estimate cardiac output by synchronizing fluid volume changes with heart rate. The cardiac output measurements seem to correlate well with an assessment of cardiac output obtained by RHC[65] and may be useful in monitoring response to therapeutic interventions.[66] The OptiVol Fluid Status Monitoring System (Medtronic, Minneapolis, MN) was initially shown to identify patients at a higher risk of HF hospitalization by alerting the clinician to rising impedance,[67] but subsequent trials show that the device may not improve HF outcomes.[68] The use of IHM devices remains controversial, as does the appropriate medical therapy response to worsening hemodynamics in the absence of overt decompensation. This field remains widely open to further explicit clinical trials. The implantation and device costs should be justifiable based on reductions in costly hospitalizations. The cost effectiveness of these devices remains to be proven.

Noninvasive cardiac output monitors

Several devices have been developed that may be useful in the noninvasive assessment of cardiac output (CO), although validation studies have provided mixed results.[69,70] For example, CO can be calculated by the carbon dioxide (CO_2) partial rebreathing technique using the modified Fick equation. NICO (Respironics, Murraysville, PA) is one such device that uses this principle to measure CO. This device measures end-tidal CO_2 partial pressure obtained during a nonrebreathing period and compares that with CO_2 partial pressure obtained during a subsequent rebreathing period. The ratio of the change in end-tidal CO_2 and CO_2 elimination after a brief period of partial rebreathing estimates CO.[71]

Pulse contour analysis to calculate CO is based on the relationship between blood pressure, stroke volume (SV), arterial compliance, and systemic vascular resistance (SVR). The SV or CO can be calculated from the arterial pressure waveform if the arterial compliance and SVR are known. Standard bioimpedance systems administer an electric current of known amplitude and frequency across the thorax. These systems then measure changes in voltage, or the amplitude of the returning signal compared with the injected signal. The ratio between voltage and current amplitudes measures resistance across the thorax and this varies in proportion to the amount of fluid in the lungs. Despite a sound theory, however, bioimpedance has limitations in clinical practice. For example, in the Bioimpedence CardioGraphy (BIG) substudy of the ESCAPE trial, there was a poor agreement between thoracic electrical bioimpedance and invasively measure hemodynamic profiles.[72] The NICOM device (Cheetah Medical, Portland, OR) is another device that measures transthoracic bioreactance. The CO as measured by this device has been shown to correlate with that measured by thermodilution.[73] A variety of noninvasive methods have been developed to estimate CO, but insufficient data are available at this time to demonstrate that these monitoring devices improve clinical outcomes.

Cardiopulmonary exercise testing in advanced heart failure

The cardiopulmonary system functions as a single gas exchange unit between the environment and the organism's cells. In a steady state, "external respiration" equals "internal respiration" meaning that respiratory oxygen uptake ($\dot{V}O_2$) and carbon dioxide outflow ($\dot{V}CO_2$) is equivalent to oxygen utilization ($\dot{Q}O_2$) and carbon dioxide production ($\dot{Q}CO_2$), respectively, at the cellular level.[74] Cardiopulmonary exercise testing (CPET) can directly measure $\dot{V}O_2$, $\dot{V}CO_2$, air flow (minute ventilation $\dot{V}_e$, tidal volume, and respiratory rate) using a metabolic cart (Figure 3.7). Numerous physiological parameters can be deduced from CPET (Box 3.2).

CPET is designed to (1) assess functional capacity, (2) evaluate the underlying cause of symptom expression (dyspnea and fatigue), and (3) ascertain prognosis. Assessment of physiological parameters during exercise provocation can differentiate symptoms caused by circulatory defects from those due to pulmonary disease or deconditioning.

A simple diagnostic algorithm

An abnormally low peak oxygen uptake (Pk$\dot{V}O_2$) is defined as less than 85% of that predicted for age and gender. A normal anaerobic threshold (AT) is ≥60% of the predicted Pk$\dot{V}O_2$, while an AT less than 40% of the predicted peak $\dot{V}O_2$ is considered pathognomic of underlying circulatory failure, provided the effort applied is optimal. A respiratory exchange ratio (RER) of less than 1.1 (particularly <1.0) in the absence of other metabolic abnormalities suggests poor effort, anxiety, or mild disease.[75] A reduced breathing reserve (BR) (<30%) is indicative of ventilatory impairment. Ventilatory impairment is often accompanied by exercise related arterial desaturation, suggesting lung impairment. When peak ventilation during exercise approaches or exceeds maximal voluntary ventilation (MVV), defined as the maximum volume of air that can be voluntarily expired at rest in 1 minute, a pulmonary cause is likely contributing to symptoms of dyspnea.[76] Normal individuals and even those with mild chronic obstructive lung disease, are able to maintain minute ventilation ($\dot{V}_E$) that is around 70% of the maximum voluntary ventilation. Thus, an increase of $\dot{V}_E$:MVV to over 0.7 indicates a pulmonary mechanical limit to exercise. The most commonly encountered cause for this in clinical practice is severe chronic obstructive lung disease, parenchymal lung disease, or abnormality in the chest wall.

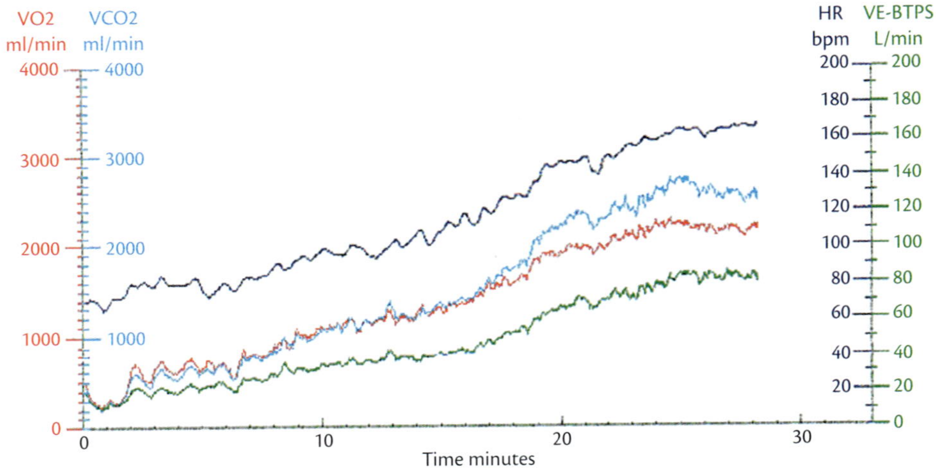

Fig. 3.7 Image from CPET exercise testing system showing exercise time vs. $\dot{V}O_2$, $\dot{V}CO_2$, minute ventilation ($\dot{V}_E$), and heart rate directly measured.

Technical considerations

CPET data accuracy requires a skilled technician who pays attention to meticulous data accrual, appropriate encouragement and teaching of the patient, and avoidance of system leaks (breathing around mouthpiece, nasal breathing, or sampling line leaks). $\dot{V}O_2$ is now commonly used as an endpoint in HF clinical investigations.[77] An increase in Pk$\dot{V}O_2$ of 1 mL kg^{-1} min^{-1} correlates with a 69-second gain in treadmill exercise time, improvement in functional capacity, and improved cardiovascular outcomes.[78] Accuracy of the technique is critical and a Pk$\dot{V}O_2$ value may be effort dependent. Therefore, some investigators have advocated against using this parameter but instead focusing on the AT, considered to be a more reproducible and effort-independent parameter in HF patients undergoing serial testing.[79] If AT is not achieved, the $\dot{V}_e/\dot{V}CO_2$ slope may be used to reliably predict outcomes.[80,81] Heart failure patients with very limited exercise tolerance (e.g., resulting from low-threshold angina) may require an exercise surrogate of Pk$\dot{V}O_2$ for risk stratification. In these patients, the change in $\dot{V}_E/\dot{V}CO_2$ ratio during early exercise predicts Pk$\dot{V}O_2$ and prognosis. A decrease in $\dot{V}_e/\dot{V}CO_2$ of less than 10% early in exercise predicts a Pk$\dot{V}O_2$ of less than 14 mL kg^{-1} min^{-1} and poor outcome in patients with HF.[81]

Box 3.2 Physiological parameters analyzed by CPET

- **Peak oxygen uptake (Pk$\dot{V}O_2$):** The highest $\dot{V}O_2$ achieved during CPET at or near peak exercise. Reported as a weight-adjusted parameter in ml kg^{-1} min^{-1}. $\dot{V}O_2$ = (heart rate × stroke volume) × (arteriovenous O_2 content difference).
- **Breathing reserve (BR):** The reserve capacity of the ventilatory system, calculated as 1 minus the ratio of peak exercise minute ventilation ($\dot{V}_E$) to maximal voluntary ventilation (MVV). A normal value would be ≥30% (similarly, a $\dot{V}_E$/MVV >0.7 would reflect pathology).
- **Oxygen saturation (SpO_2):** The percentage of hemoglobin that is saturated with oxygen. Typically measured by pulse oximetry.
- **O_2 pulse:** The amount of O_2 consumed from the volume of blood delivered to tissues by each heartbeat. Calculated as $\dot{V}O_2$/heart rate.
- **Ventilation/carbon dioxide production ratio ($\dot{V}_E/\dot{V}CO_2$):** Also known as the ventilatory equivalent for CO_2, this represents a respiratory control function that reflects ventilatory efficiency.
- **Peak $\dot{V}O_2$ lean:** Peak oxygen uptake adjusted for lean body mass. Reported as a lean body weight-adjusted parameter in mL kg^{-1} min^{-1}.
- **Anaerobic threshold (AT):** The highest oxygen uptake attained without a sustained increase in blood lactate concentration and lactate/pyruvate ratio. Reported as a weight-adjusted parameter in mL kg^{-1} min^{-1}.
- **Respiratory exchange ratio (RER):** the respiratory quotient, defined as the ratio of $\dot{V}CO_2$ to $\dot{V}O_2$. When ≥1.1, indicates adequacy of effort.

CPET and prognosis in advanced heart failure

In the Veterans Administration Heart Failure Trial (V-HeFT), the mortality rate of patients with a $\dot{V}O_{2\,max}$ 14.5 mL kg^{-1} min^{-1} or less was twice as high as for those whose $\dot{V}O_{2\,max}$ exceeded this threshold.[82] In HF patients referred for cardiac transplantation, Mancini and colleagues determined that a Pk$\dot{V}O_2$ of less than 14 kg^{-1} min^{-1} was a reliable predictor of poor survival and the need for transplantation.[83] Importantly, transplantation could be deferred in patients whose Pk$\dot{V}O_2$ was greater than 14 kg^{-1} min^{-1}, a group whose survival exceeded that of patients undergoing heart transplantation in that early era. Using an absolute dichotomous threshold may have some general applicability but may require modification in situations such as obesity, use of β-blockers or cardiac resynchronization therapy, or in very young patients.[84] In those with HF who tolerate a β-blocker, a cutoff for peak $\dot{V}O_2$ of 12 ml kg^{-1} min^{-1} or less suggests that prognosis can be improved by heart transplantation.[84] Typically, the disparity in prognostic usefulness is seen in the grey zone of intermediate levels of Pk$\dot{V}O_2$ (10–18 ml kg^{-1} min^{-1}) in certain clinical conditions such as women or obese patients with HF. This has led to more sophisticated analyses to better discriminate among these groups and many laboratories have evaluated alternative indices such as percentage of predicted Pk $\dot{V}O_2$, ventilation/CO_2 production ratio and slope, O_2

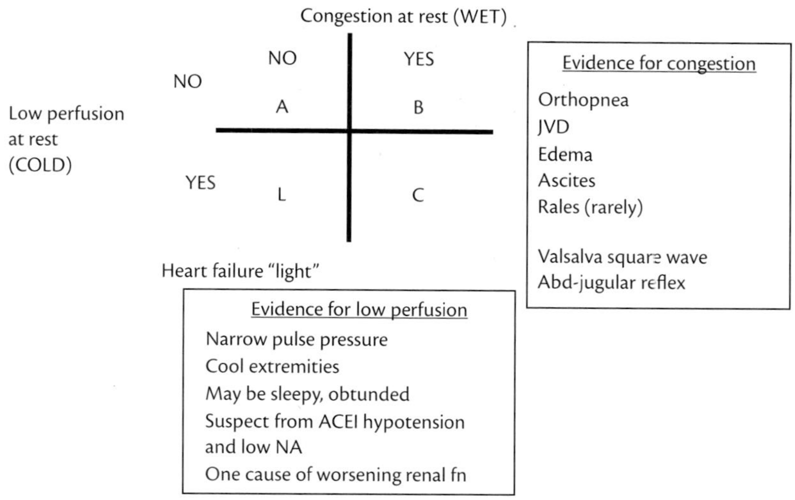

Fig. 3.8 Four hemodynamic profiles based on evidence of resting congestion and/or hypoperfusion.
Stevenson LN, Tailored Therapy to Hemodynamic Goals for Advanced Heart Failure, 1999, Wiley.

consumption recovery, and O_2 pulse.[85] However, it has been noted that even among these parameters, there is sufficient variability.

A fundamental understanding of O_2 consumption explains heterogeneity in predictive accuracy of CPET in unique clinical conditions such as the obese HF patients. Body fat is "metabolically inert," consumes essentially no oxygen, and can represent a significant portion of total weight. Yet, Pk$\dot{V}O_2$ is reported by a total weight correction, not accounting for the considerable variability in body composition among patients with HF. It has been demonstrated that correcting Pk$\dot{V}O_2$ for lean body mass (Pk$\dot{V}O_2$lean) provides a better discriminator of outcome than total weight-adjusted values. In HF patients, a Pk$\dot{V}O_2$lean cutoff of 19 ml kg^{-1} min^{-1} may provide a more robust parameter of prognosis than the total weight-adjusted figure of 14 ml kg^{-1} min^{-1}.[86] Thus, body fat using the three-site skin-fold method can be measured before each CPET study to calculate lean body mass. Using lean body mass adjustments, previously observed disparities between genders and in obese patients can be eliminated. A peak O_2 pulse (cutoff value 10 mL/beat), especially when corrected for lean body mass (cutoff value 14 mL/beat), can predict prognosis in patients with chronic systolic HF.[87]

Invasive CPET

Unlike the noninvasive CPET described above, an invasive CPET uses pulmonary artery and radial artery catheters to measure hemodynamics and allows for comprehensive tissue O_2 extraction analyses. It thus allows for a more detailed evaluation of the cardiopulmonary bases of symptoms by additionally allowing categorization of entities such as exercise-induced pulmonary hypertension, exercise-induced HF with preserved ejection fraction, and a less well-known entity recently described, called preload failure.[88] In preload failure, the maximal exercise-induced CO is decreased without a concomitant increase in right heart or pulmonary vascular pressures.[88] The complexity and elaborate setup required for this form of testing makes it less feasible for routine assessment.

Treatment by hemodynamic profiles

Standard therapies for ADHF include vasodilators, diuretics, and neurohormonal modifying drugs. The information obtained by a careful history and physical examination allows the clinician to assign a hemodynamic profile to the patient, as first described by Stevenson,[89] which designates the patient to a "wet" or "dry" category based on evidence of congestion (e.g., orthopnea, JVD, edema, and ascites) and a "warm" or "cold" category based on signs of poor perfusion (e.g., narrow pulse pressure, cold extremities, and poor mentation) (Figure 3.8). The initial therapeutic strategies should be based on the hemodynamic profile assigned to the patient. For example, "wet and warm" patients usually respond well to diuresis and afterload and volume reduction. "Cold and wet" patients, however, may need inotropic therapy to enhance perfusion or vasodilatation if the SVR is high, and may benefit from a tailored therapeutic approach with invasive hemodynamic monitoring (see ESCAPE trial[52]). These hemodynamic profiles not only guide treatment strategies, but also are predictive of patient outcomes in ADHF.[43] Inotropes are known to increase mortality. However, in severe ADHF, inotropic therapy may be sometimes warranted. It is important to realize that patients requiring inotropic therapy may have worse survival either from the inherent disease or from the inotrope itself.[90,91]

Conclusions

The ability to accurately assess the hemodynamic profile in patients with ADHF is important to provide appropriate treatment and decrease rates of rehospitalization and death. Volume overload and congestion (pulmonary or systemic) are among the most complex of pathologic processes in the management of ADHF. Various mechanisms contribute to hemodynamic derangements in HF, of which neurohormonal activation likely plays a key role. The pathophysiology is complex, involving neurohormonal and other cellular modulators as well as an interaction between the heart and kidneys. Alleviating congestion to ensure symptomatic relief remains the fundamental goal of therapy to improve forward flow and diminish congestion. Although the pathophysiology and hemodynamic profile of the ADHF patient is better understood, there remains a paucity of convincing clinical trial evidence to determine the best course of therapy. ADHF remains one of the unmet clinical needs in the arena of HF care.

References

1. Roger VL, Go AS, Lloyd-Jones DM, et al. Executive summary: heart disease and stroke statistics—2012 update: a report from the American Heart Association. Circulation 2012;125:188–97.
2. Fonarow GC, Heywood JT, Heidenreich PA, et al. Temporal trends in clinical characteristics, treatments, and outcomes for heart failure hospitalizations 2002 to 2004: findings from Acute Decompensated Heart Failure National Registry (ADHERE). Am Heart J 2007;153:1021–28.
3. Adams KF, Jr., Fonarow GC, Emerman CL, et al. Characteristics and outcomes of patients hospitalized for heart failure in the United States: rationale, design, and preliminary observations from the first 100,000 cases in the Acute Decompensated Heart Failure National Registry (ADHERE). Am Heart J 2005;149:209–16.
4. O'Connor CM, Starling RC, Hernandez AF, et al. Effect of nesiritide in patients with acute decompensated heart failure. N Engl J Med 2011;365:32–43.
5. Levy WC, Mozaffarian D, Linker DT, et al. The Seattle Heart Failure Model: prediction of survival in heart failure. Circulation 2006;113:1424–33.
6. Yancy CW, Jessup M, Bozkurt B, et al. 2013 ACCF/AHA Guideline for the Management of Heart Failure: A Report of the American College of Cardiology Foundation/American Heart Association Task Force on Practice Guidelines. Circulation 2013;62(16):e147–239.
7. Jessup M, Abraham WT, Casey DE, et al. Focused Update: ACCF/AHA Guidelines for the Diagnosis and Management of Heart Failure in Adults. A Report of the American College of Cardiology Foundation/ American Heart Association Task Force on Practice Guidelines. Circulation 2009;119(14):1977–2016.
8. Leier CV. Invasive hemodynamic monitoring the aftermath of the ESCAPE trial. Cardiol Clin 2007;25:565–71.
9. Pfeffer JM, Pfeffer MA, Fletcher PJ, Braunwald E. Progressive ventricular remodeling in rat with myocardial infarction. Am J Physiol 1991;260:H1406–14.
10. Shen Y, Hendricks A, Zhang S, Kazis LE. VHA enrollees' health care coverage and use of care. Med Care Res Rev 2003;60:253–67.
11. Thomas M, Malmcrona R, Shillingford J. Hemodynamic changes in patients with acute myocardial infarction. Circulation 1965;31:811–23.
12. Thomas M. Haemodynamics after acute myocardial infarction. Schweiz Med Wochenschr 1972;102:1818–24.
13. Konstam MA, Kronenberg MW, Rousseau MF, et al. Effects of the angiotensin converting enzyme inhibitor enalapril on the long-term progression of left ventricular dilatation in patients with asymptomatic systolic dysfunction. SOLVD (Studies of Left Ventricular Dysfunction) Investigators. Circulation 1993;88:2277–83.
14. Pfeffer MA. The Survival and Ventricular Enlargement (SAVE) study: rationale and perspective. Herz 1993;18(Suppl 1):430–5.
15. Papademetriou V, Devereux RB, Narayan P, et al. Similar effects of isolated systolic and combined hypertension on left ventricular geometry and function: the LIFE Study. Am J Hypertens 2001;14:768–74.
16. Grossman W, Jones D, McLaurin LP. Wall stress and patterns of hypertrophy in the human left ventricle. J Clin Invest 1975;56:56–64.
17. Palmieri V, Wachtell K, Gerdts E, et al. Left ventricular function and hemodynamic features of inappropriate left ventricular hypertrophy in patients with systemic hypertension: the LIFE study. Am Heart J 2001;141:784–91.
18. Vasan RS, Levy D. The role of hypertension in the pathogenesis of heart failure. A clinical mechanistic overview. Arch Intern Med 1996;156:1789–96.
19. Sasayama S, Ross J, Jr., Franklin D, et al. Adaptations of the left ventricle to chronic pressure overload. Circ Res 1976;38:172–78.
20. Murakami T, Hess OM, Gage JE, et al. Diastolic filling dynamics in patients with aortic stenosis. Circulation 1986;73:1162–74.
21. Villari B, Campbell SE, Hess OM, et al. Influence of collagen network on left ventricular systolic and diastolic function in aortic valve disease. J Am Coll Cardiol 1993;22:1477–84.
22. Wisenbaugh T, Spann JF, Carabello BA. Differences in myocardial performance and load between patients with similar amounts of chronic aortic versus chronic mitral regurgitation. J Am Coll Cardiol 1984;3:916–23.
23. Taniguchi K, Nakano S, Kawashima Y, et al. Left ventricular ejection performance, wall stress, and contractile state in aortic regurgitation before and after aortic valve replacement. Circulation 1990;82:798–807.
24. Carabello BA. Mitral regurgitation: basic physiologic principles. Mod Concepts Cardiovasc Disease 1988;57:53–58.
25. Schrier RW, Abraham WT. Hormones and hemodynamics in heart failure. N Engl J Med 1999;341:577–85.
26. Packer M. The neurohormonal hypothesis: a theory to explain the mechanism of disease progression in heart failure. J Am Coll Cardiol 1992;20:248–54.
27. Unger T, Li J. The role of the renin-angiotensin-aldosterone system in heart failure. J Renin Angiotensin Aldosterone Syst 2004;5(Suppl 1):S7–10.
28. Schrier RW, Reid IA, Berl T, Earley LE. Parasympathetic pathways, renin secretion and vasopressin release. Clin Sci Mol Med 1975;48:83–89.
29. Schrier RW, Berl T. Nonosmolar factors affecting renal water excretion (first of two parts). N Engl J Med 1975;292:81–88.
30. Schrier RW, Berl T, Harbottle JA, McDonald KM. Catecholamines and renal water excretion. Nephron 1975;15:186–96.
31. Szatalowicz VL, Arnold PE, Chaimovitz C, et al. Radioimmunoassay of plasma arginine vasopressin in hyponatremic patients with congestive heart failure. N Engl J Med 1981;305:263–66.
32. Troughton RW, Richards AM. BNP for clinical monitoring of heart failure. Heart Fail Clin 2006;2:333–43.
33. Fonarow GC, Abraham WT, Albert NM, et al. Organized Program to Initiate Lifesaving Treatment in Hospitalized Patients with Heart Failure (OPTIMIZE-HF): rationale and design. Am Heart J 2004;148:43–51.
34. Wang CS, FitzGerald JM, Schulzer M, et al. Does this dyspneic patient in the emergency department have congestive heart failure? JAMA 2005;294:1944–56.
35. Drazner MH, Hellkamp AS, Leier CV, et al. Value of clinician assessment of hemodynamics in advanced heart failure: the ESCAPE trial. Circ Heart Fail 2008;1:170–177.
36. Beck DS, Mielniczuk L, Laberge M, et al. Persistent orthopnea and the prognosis of patients in the heart failure clinic. Congest Heart Fail 2004;10:177–80.
37. Vinayak AG, Levitt J, Gehlbach B, et al. Usefulness of the external jugular vein examination in detecting abnormal central venous pressure in critically ill patients. Arch Intern Med 2006;166:2132–37.
38. Drazner MH, Hamilton MA, Fonarow G, et al. Relationship between right and left-sided filling pressures in 1000 patients with advanced heart failure. J Heart Lung Transplant 1999;18:1126–32.
39. Butman SM, Ewy GA, Standen JR, et al. Bedside cardiovascular examination in patients with severe chronic heart failure: importance of rest or inducible jugular venous distension. J Am Coll Cardiol 1993;22:968–74.
40. Badgett RG, Lucey CR, Mulrow CD. Can the clinical examination diagnose left-sided heart failure in adults? JAMA 1997;277:1712–19.
41. Stevenson LW, Perloff JK. The limited reliability of physical signs for estimating hemodynamics in chronic heart failure. JAMA 1989;261:884–88.
42. Chakko S, Woska D, Martinez H, et al. Clinical, radiographic, and hemodynamic correlations in chronic congestive heart failure: conflicting results may lead to inappropriate care. Am J Med 1991;90:353–59.
43. Nohria A, Tsang SW, Fang JC, et al. Clinical assessment identifies hemodynamic profiles that predict outcomes in patients admitted with heart failure. J Am Coll Cardiol 2003;41:1797–804.
44. Worster A, Balion CM, Hill SA, et al. Diagnostic accuracy of BNP and NT-proBNP in patients presenting to acute care settings with dyspnea: a systematic review. Clin Biochem 2008;41:250–259.

45. Nohria A, Hasselblad V, Stebbins A, et al. Cardiorenal interactions: insights from the ESCAPE trial. J Am Coll Cardiol 2008;51:1268–74.
46. Kircher BJ, Himelman RB, Schiller NB. Noninvasive estimation of right atrial pressure from the inspiratory collapse of the inferior vena cava. Am J Cardiol 1990;66:493–96.
47. Berger M, Haimowitz A, Van Tosh A, et al. Quantitative assessment of pulmonary hypertension in patients with tricuspid regurgitation using continuous wave Doppler ultrasound. J Am Coll Cardiol 1985;6:359–65.
48. Nagueh SF, Middleton KJ, Kopelen HA, et al. Doppler tissue imaging: a noninvasive technique for evaluation of left ventricular relaxation and estimation of filling pressures. J Am Coll Cardiol 1997;30:1527–33.
49. Abbas AE, Fortuin FD, Schiller NB, et al. A simple method for noninvasive estimation of pulmonary vascular resistance. J Am Coll Cardiol 2003;41:1021–27.
50. Stevenson LW. Tailored therapy to hemodynamic goals for advanced heart failure. Eur J Heart Fail 1999;1:251–57.
51. Connors AF, Jr., Speroff T, Dawson NV, et al. The effectiveness of right heart catheterization in the initial care of critically ill patients. SUPPORT Investigators. JAMA 1996;276:889–97.
52. Binanay C, Califf RM, Hasselblad V, et al. Evaluation study of congestive heart failure and pulmonary artery catheterization effectiveness: the ESCAPE trial. JAMA 2005;294:1625–33.
53. Hunt SA, Abraham WT, Chin MH, Feldman AM, Francis GS, Ganiats TG et al. 2009 focused update incorporated into the ACC/AHA 2005 Guidelines for the Diagnosis and Management of Heart Failure in Adults. A Report of the American College of Cardiology Foundation/American Heart Association Task Force on Practice Guidelines. Circulation 2009;53(15):e1–e90.
54. Bourge RC, Abraham WT, Adamson PB, et al. Randomized controlled trial of an implantable continuous hemodynamic monitor in patients with advanced heart failure: the COMPASS-HF study. J Am Coll Cardiol 2008;51:1073–79.
55. Abraham WT, Adamson PB, Bourge RC, et al. Wireless pulmonary artery haemodynamic monitoring in chronic heart failure: a randomised controlled trial. Lancet 2011;377:658–66.
56. Hillege HL, Nitsch D, Pfeffer MA, et al. Renal function as a predictor of outcome in a broad spectrum of patients with heart failure. Circulation 2006;113:671–78.
57. Dries DL, Exner DV, Domanski MJ, et al. The prognostic implications of renal insufficiency in asymptomatic and symptomatic patients with left ventricular systolic dysfunction. J Am Coll Cardiol 2000;35:681–89.
58. Ronco C, Haapio M, House AA, et al. Cardiorenal syndrome. J Am Coll Cardiol 2008;52:1527–39.
59. Heywood JT, Fonarow GC, Costanzo MR, et al. High prevalence of renal dysfunction and its impact on outcome in 118,465 patients hospitalized with acute decompensated heart failure: a report from the ADHERE database. J Card Fail 2007;13:422–30.
60. Mullens W, Abrahams Z, Francis GS, et al. Importance of venous congestion for worsening of renal function in advanced decompensated heart failure. J Am Coll Cardiol 2009;53:589–96.
61. Gottlieb SS, Brater DC, Thomas I, et al. BG9719 (CVT-124), an A1 adenosine receptor antagonist, protects against the decline in renal function observed with diuretic therapy. Circulation 2002;105:1348–53.
62. Felker GM, Lee KL, Bull DA, et al. Diuretic strategies in patients with acute decompensated heart failure. N Engl J Med 2011;364:797–805.
63. Magalski A, Adamson P, Gadler F, et al. Continuous ambulatory right heart pressure measurements with an implantable hemodynamic monitor: a multicenter, 12-month follow-up study of patients with chronic heart failure. J Card Fail 2002;8:63–70.
64. Ritzema J, Troughton R, Melton I, et al. Physician-directed patient self-management of left atrial pressure in advanced chronic heart failure. Circulation 2010;121:1086–95.
65. Drazner MH, Thompson B, Rosenberg PB, et al. Comparison of impedance cardiography with invasive hemodynamic measurements in patients with heart failure secondary to ischemic or nonischemic cardiomyopathy. Am J Cardiol 2002;89:993–95.
66. Peacock WF, Summers RL, Vogel J, Emerman CE. Impact of impedance cardiography on diagnosis and therapy of emergent dyspnea: the ED-IMPACT trial. Acad Emerg Med 2006;13:365–71.
67. Whellan DJ, Ousdigian KT, Al Khatib SM, et al. Combined heart failure device diagnostics identify patients at higher risk of subsequent heart failure hospitalizations: results from PARTNERS HF (Program to Access and Review Trending Information and Evaluate Correlation to Symptoms in Patients With Heart Failure) study. J Am Coll Cardiol 2010;55:1803–10.
68. van Veldhuisen DJ, Braunschweig F, Conraads V, et al. Intrathoracic impedance monitoring, audible patient alerts, and outcome in patients with heart failure. Circulation 2011;124:1719–26.
69. Rocco M, Spadetta G, Morelli A, et al. A comparative evaluation of thermodilution and partial CO_2 rebreathing techniques for cardiac output assessment in critically ill patients during assisted ventilation. Intensive Care Med 2004;30:82–7.
70. Nilsson LB, Eldrup N, Berthelsen PG. Lack of agreement between thermodilution and carbon dioxide-rebreathing cardiac output. Acta Anaesthesiol Scand 2001;45:680–5.
71. Jaffe MB. Partial CO_2 rebreathing cardiac output—operating principles of the NICO system. J Clin Monit Comput 1999;15:387–401.
72. Kamath SA, Drazner MH, Tasissa G, et al. Correlation of impedance cardiography with invasive hemodynamic measurements in patients with advanced heart failure: the BioImpedance CardioGraphy (BIG) substudy of the Evaluation Study of Congestive Heart Failure and Pulmonary Artery Catheterization Effectiveness (ESCAPE) Trial. Am Heart J 2009;158:217–23.
73. Dickstein K, Cohen-Solal A, Filippatos G, et al. ESC Guidelines for the diagnosis and treatment of acute and chronic heart failure 2008: the Task Force for the Diagnosis and Treatment of Acute and Chronic Heart Failure 2008 of the European Society of Cardiology. Developed in collaboration with the Heart Failure Association of the ESC (HFA) and endorsed by the European Society of Intensive Care Medicine (ESICM). Eur Heart J 2008;29:2388–442.
74. Milani RV, Lavie CJ, Mehra MR, Ventura HO. Understanding the basics of cardiopulmonary exercise testing. Mayo Clin Proc 2006;81(12):1603–11.
75. Milani RV, Lavie CJ, Mehra MR. Cardiopulmonary exercise testing: how do we differentiate the cause of dyspnea? Circulation 2004;110(4):e27–3.
76. Medoff BD, Oelberg DA, Kanarek DJ, Systrom DM. Breathing reserve at the lactate threshold to differentiate a pulmonary mechanical from cardiovascular limit to exercise. Chest 1998;113:913–18.
77. Bensimhon DR1, Leifer ES, Ellis SJ, et al.; HF-ACTION Trial Investigators. Reproducibility of peak oxygen uptake and other cardiopulmonary exercise testing parameters in patients with heart failure (from the Heart Failure and A Controlled Trial Investigating Outcomes of exercise traiNing). Am J Cardiol 2008;102(6):712–17.
78. Wilson JR1, Hanamanthu S, Chomsky DB, Davis SF. Relationship between exertional symptoms and functional capacity in patients with heart failure. J Am Coll Cardiol 1999;33(7):1943–7.
79. Piña IL1, Karalis DG. Comparison of four exercise protocols using anaerobic threshold measurement of functional capacity in congestive heart failure. Am J Cardiol 1990;65(18):1269–71.
80. Guazzi M. Abnormalities in cardiopulmonary exercise testing ventilatory parameters in heart failure: pathophysiology and clinical usefulness. Curr Heart Fail Rep 2014;11(1):80–7.
81. Milani RV, Mehra MR, Reddy TK, et al. Ventilation/carbon dioxide production ratio in early exercise predicts poor functional capacity in congestive heart failure. Heart 1996;76(5):393–6.
82. Cohn JN, Johnson GR, Shabetai R, et al. Ejection fraction, peak exercise oxygen consumption, cardiothoracic ratio, ventricular arrhythmias, and plasma norepinephrine as determinants of prognosis in heart failure. The V-HeFT VA Cooperative Studies Group. Circulation 1993;87(6 Suppl):VI5–16.

83. Mancini DM, Eisen H, Kussmaul W, et al. Value of peak exercise oxygen consumption for optimal timing of cardiac transplantation in ambulatory patients with heart failure. Circulation 1991;83:778–86.
84. Mehra MR, Kobashigawa J, Starling R, et al. Listing criteria for heart transplantation: International Society for Heart and Lung Transplantation guidelines for the care of cardiac transplant candidates—2006. J Heart Lung Transplant 2006;25(9):1024–42.
85. Robbins M, Francis G, Pashkow FJ, et al. Ventilatory and heart rate responses to exercise better predictors of heart failure mortality than peak oxygen consumption. Circulation 1999;100(24):2411–17.
86. Osman AF, Mehra MR, Lavie CJ, et al. The incremental prognostic importance of body fat adjusted peak oxygen consumption in chronic heart failure. J Am Coll Cardiol 2000;36(7):2126–31.
87. Lavie CJ, Milani RV, Mehra MR. Peak exercise oxygen pulse and prognosis in chronic heart failure. Am J Cardiol 2004;93(5):588–93.
88. Maron BA, Cockrill BA, Waxman AB, Systrom DM. The invasive cardiopulmonary exercise test. Circulation 2013;127(10):1157–64.
89. Stevenson LW. Tailored therapy before transplantation for treatment of advanced heart failure: effective use of vasodilators and diuretics. J Heart Lung Transplant 1991;10:468–76.
90. Gheorghiade M, Gattis WA, Klein L. OPTIME in CHF trial: rethinking the use of inotropes in the management of worsening chronic heart failure resulting in hospitalization. Eur J Heart Fail 2003;5:9–12.
91. Adams KF, Jr., Fonarow GC, Emerman CL, et al. Characteristics and outcomes of patients hospitalized for heart failure in the United States: rationale, design, and preliminary observations from the first 100,000 cases in the Acute Decompensated Heart Failure National Registry (ADHERE). Am Heart J 2005;149:209–16.

CHAPTER 4

Transplantation immunology

James F. George PhD

Introduction

It is now well known that the tendency of most reasonably complex organisms, especially mammals, to reject transplants of vascularized and nonvascularized organs is due to an immune response. How this was determined is discussed later in the chapter, but for now it is worthwhile to carefully examine what the ultimate function of the immune response is in biological terms. On this planet, humans, which are an integrated collection of living cells acting in concert for mutual support and survival, live within in a biological milieu in which they must maintain self-integrity. That is, the human organism must be able to maintain itself as a distinct entity and it must prevent other organisms from consuming it for food. This entity we can call "self," which can be definitively distinguished by the genome that resides within it. Other living things, possessing a different genome, can be called "nonself." This definition of nonself, notably, also includes other members of the same species which, although genomes within a species are highly similar, remain unique. Thus, at the most basic level, we can define the function of the immune system as the maintenance of self-integrity. This function is a complex task because a single complete failure results in a loss of homeostasis and consumption of the body as food by other organisms. The immune system must be able to discriminate self from nonself in order to eliminate or isolate organisms that gain entry into the body without causing collateral damage (or at least irreparable damage). In terms of organ transplantation, then, a heart originating from another genetically distinct individual is therefore nonself and, according to these definitions, merits attention by the immune system as a potential threat. Thus, these core functions constitute the functional basis of the immune response, and this is why, except under highly specific circumstances, the immune system will destroy a transplanted heart unless steps are taken to inhibit its response to the heart. How the immune system works in the context of transplantation is the subject of this chapter. It is assumed that the reader understands the basic principles of biology and knows the locations, but not necessarily the function, of the primary and secondary lymphoid organs. We begin with a more in-depth discussion of what the immune system does in the context of solid organ transplantation and then proceed with a detailed explanation of the anatomy of the immune system and how it works.

General terminology

In any discussion of a complex system, the discussants must agree on the terminology that is used to describe the parts of the system and its functional characteristics. Important words include the following:

- *Antigen*—Usually, but not always a protein; can exist inside or outside a cell. All molecules capable of eliciting an immune response are termed antigens and are considered to be the driving force of immune responses.
- *Activation*—A change in the functional state of a cell, such as a lymphocyte or a dendritic cell, from a relatively inactive or quiescent state to one in which the cell actively participates in some functional pathway. The activation state can be detected by changes in morphology, gene transcription, or changes in the expression of surface molecules.
- *Signal*—When a cell surface receptor contacts its respective ligand, the information that such contact has taken place propagates into the interior of the cell through a series of biochemical events, ultimately resulting in some functional change.
- *Proliferation*—Many cells, especially lymphocytes, will multiply when activated. Usually, this results in a relatively rare cell, which might have the capability of reacting to a particular antigen, becoming much less rare, a process also called *amplification*.
- *Differentiation*—A process in which a cell changes its morphology and gene expression to the point where it can no longer be considered the same cell type. For example, B cells differentiate into antibody-secreting plasma cells.

What is an immune response?

The characteristics of an immune response, as we understand it, were defined in the late 19th and early 20th centuries through observations of the appearance of factors in the blood serum that would protect against disease. It had been known for well over a millennium that those who survived infections during plagues did not reacquire the disease and could minister to those who were sick with the same illness. The first observations of the basis for such protection were made when it was found that protection from a disease could be transferred by blood serum from one individual to another. Through such observations and many others during the early 20th century, the most basic characteristics of immunity were defined. A typical immune response that might be followed would be production of antibodies against a specific organism or antigen.

The basic phenomenology and immunologic basis of transplantation was determined by the man widely regarded as the father of transplant immunology, Sir Peter Medawar. He observed patterns of skin graft rejection in a burn patient during World War II that suggested that graft rejection was due to an immune response:[1] *inducibility*, meaning a response took place only after a graft was applied; *memory*—a second exposure to a graft from the same individual resulted in a quicker, stronger, and longer-lasting response; and *specificity*—meaning that the host could distinguish between

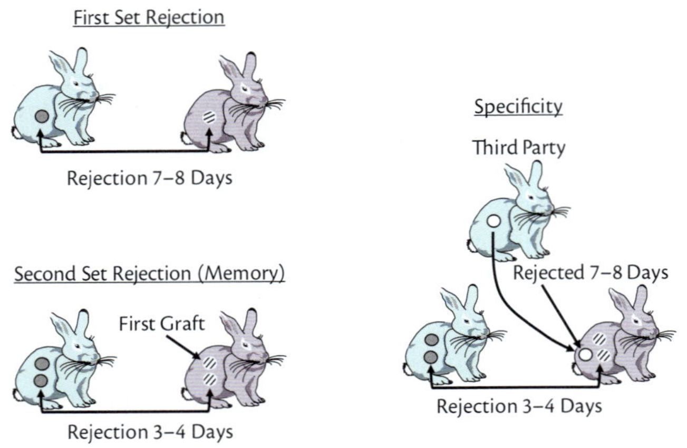

Fig. 4.1 Medawar's experiments that defined the immunologic basis of solid organ allograft rejection. Animals receiving a second graft from the same donor rejected it more quickly than the first (memory). If a graft from another rabbit, genetically unrelated to the original donor and recipient, was applied at the same time, it was not rejected faster than the first graft (specificity). These experiments showed evidence of memory and specificity, hallmarks of an acquired immune response.

grafts from one individual or another. He later performed more detailed studies in rabbits.[2] The results of these studies are worth describing in detail because they define the basic phenomenology of solid organ allograft rejection. A schematic of the results of these studies is shown in Figure 4.1. In these experiments, skin grafts transferred from one individual to another of the same species are rejected in 7–10 days. The grafts heal-in, become vascularized within the first few days, then become necrotic and drop off. Notably, if a second graft is applied from the same donor, it is rejected much more quickly, in 3–5 days, which is indicative of immunologic memory. Lastly, Medawar and colleagues showed that if a graft from a genetically unrelated, third-party animal was applied at the same time as the second graft, it was rejected in 7–10 days even if it was located proximally to the secondary graft. This showed that the host could distinguish between tissues originating from two different individuals (specificity). From these results, Medawar and colleagues concluded that graft rejection was due to an immune response, therefore making the conceptual breakthrough that gave rise to the science of transplantation immunology. The concepts of memory and specificity, in particular, form the basis of our thinking regarding transplant rejection. The rejection of solid organ grafts is a function of genetic differences between donor and recipient and, as we will show, these differences are largely defined by human leukocyte antigens (HLA). A memory response, also called an anemnestic response, is central to the issue of sensitization, which is discussed in the context of heart transplantation in Chapter 16.

In clinical heart transplantation, the phenomenology of acute graft rejection is somewhat different because no one transplants a heart without protecting it with immunosuppressive drugs. A rejecting graft is infiltrated with mononuclear cells, followed by cytoarchitectural disruption with myocyte and endothelial cell death, ultimately resulting in hemodynamic compromise. Subsequent sections of this chapter detail the molecular and cellular events that take place as the immune system detects the presence of a transplanted organ and then mobilizes a response.

Components and anatomy of the immune system

The immune system, like every other integrated system in the body, is not just a collection of cells, but consists of a series of interconnected microenvironments through which cellular components reside or traverse. A transplanted organ is one such microenvironment connected via the peripheral blood and indirectly through surrounding lymphatic vessels to the peripheral lymphoid organs—i.e., the lymph nodes, spleen, Peyer's patches, and gut-associated lymphoid tissue (GALT). The cells in these microenvironments and how they cooperate are key to understanding how the immune response works. Table 4.1 lists these cell types, major subpopulations, their distributions and major functions.

In the context of immune responses, two lineages bear special mention: T cells and B cells. As noted in Table 4.1, each of these lymphoid populations are key cells in specific antigen recognition by virtue of highly unique antigen receptors on their surfaces. On T cells, this structure is called the T cell receptor and, among newly arisen T cells, it is essentially unique for each T cell, with the ability to bind to a unique combination of an antigenic peptide complexed with a host HLA molecule. If a T cell for a given antigen is unique, it is therefore rare, so the secondary lymphoid organs are structured in such a way that relatively rare cells can come into contact with the respective antigen for which they are specific.

Given the functions of immunity, the systems involved in the implementation of these functions are distributed throughout the body. Antigen-presenting cells (APCs), primarily dendritic cells and macrophages, are present in most tissues, and provide a scanning function by constantly sampling and integrating signals from their surrounding environment. T cells can also be found in tissues and the blood, especially in the presence of inflammation, but

Table 4.1 Cells of the immune system

Cell type	Function	Markers[a]
T cell	Regulation, anti-virus and anti-fungal responses	CD3, CD4, CD8
NK cell	Innate immunity	CD56
B cell	Soluble antigen detection, plasma cell precursor	CD19, CD20, CD72, immunoglobulin, HLA II
Plasma cell	Antibody secretion	CD38, CD138
Macrophage	Phagocytosis, antigen presentation	CD68, F4/80, HLA II, CD16, CD14
Dendritic cell	Antigen presentation	HLA II, CD303. CD1c, CD141
Neutrophil	Phagocytosis, bactericidal mechanisms	CD66a, CD66c, CD68, CD15
Eosinophil	Killing of antibody-coated parasites	CD15
Basophil	Unknown	CD68, CD123, FcεR1
Mast cell	Release of histamine and other agents	CD88

[a] Some markers delineate subsets.

tend to congregate in the secondary lymphoid organs, primarily the lymph nodes and spleen, where they can meet APCs bearing processed antigens for which they are specific. The primary function of the secondary (or peripheral) lymphoid organs is to trap antigen or antigen-bearing cells in order to provide a location where cellular elements of the adaptive immune response can encounter antigens, and to provide an environment in which cells of the immune system can communicate or cooperate. Figure 4.2 shows the anatomical relationships of the primary and secondary lymphoid organs, as well major organs and the lymphatic system. The primary lymphoid organs are the bone marrow and the thymus. The bone marrow gives rise to precursors of all the cell types listed in Table 4.1. A subset of these precursors also travels to the thymus where they develop into T cells, which are selected to recognize antigenic peptides complexed to HLA molecules. The secondary lymphoid organs are located throughout the body. The lymph nodes (Figure 4.3) collect extracellular fluid via the lymphatic vessels, which eventually return the extracellular fluid, or lymph, to the blood. The cells in the lymph nodes, B and T lymphocytes, APCs, and other support cells and structures are organized. Histological sections show germinal centers, which contain B cells undergoing proliferation and differentiation. Germinal centers are sites where T cells, B cells, and APCs cooperate. The spleen contains similar structures, but also is the site of senescent red cell disposal (red pulp). It contains a large number of macrophages. Lymphocytes surround the arterioles in a periarteriolar sheath (which also contains dendritic cells), which is proximal to a B cell corona. A marginal zone rich in dendritic cells surrounds the whole structure. These cells, and the structures around them, constitute the milieu in which immune responses are generated.

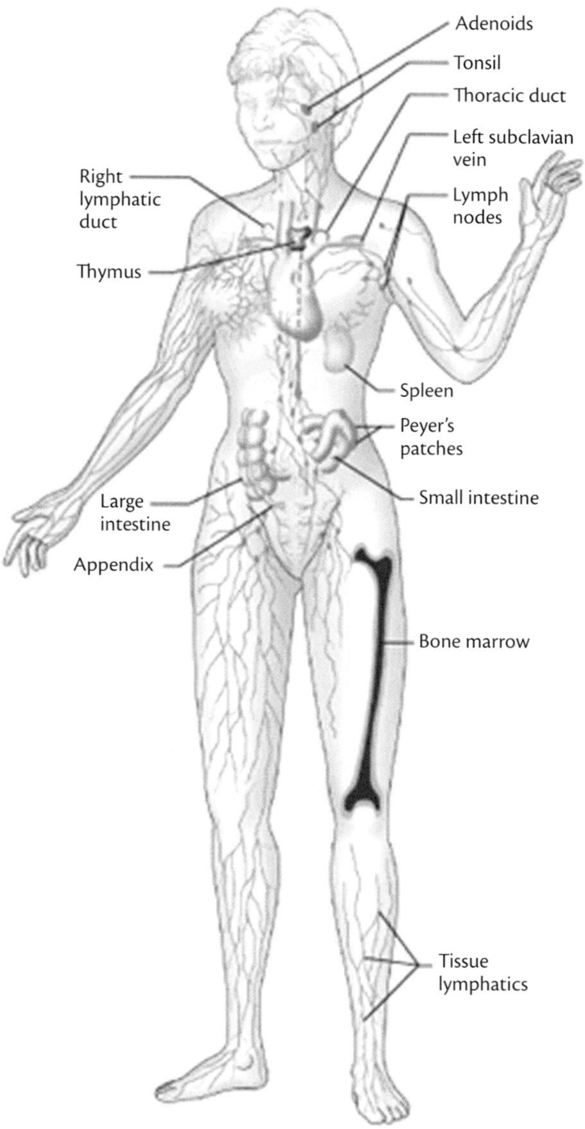

Fig. 4.2 The distribution of primary and secondary lymphoid organs and lymphatics. Immune cells arise from the bone marrow and circulate throughout the body. The secondary lymphoid organs, such as the lymph nodes, spleen, and Peyer's patches are structurally organized to facilitate immune cell interactions.
Reprinted with permission of WH Freeman, Kuby Immunology, Kindt, Thomas J and Goldsby, Richard A, copyright 2006.

Recognition of donor antigens

What does the immune system "see" when the transplanted organ is revascularized in the host? As we noted in the description of Medawar's original work, the immune response is a function of the genetic relatedness of donor and recipient and, furthermore, one individual can be distinguished from another. It follows then that there are structures recognized by the immune system that are unique for each individual, or at least highly diverse. These structures are HLA molecules, which are unique in their ability to complex with short antigenic peptides and in their extreme polymorphism (variations in amino acid sequence) within the human population. HLA molecules play such an integral role in immune regulation, as well as serving as targets of anti-graft responses, that concepts concerning immune regulation and immune recognition can be difficult to distinguish. To facilitate understanding, we first discuss the structure of the HLA molecules, the genetic basis

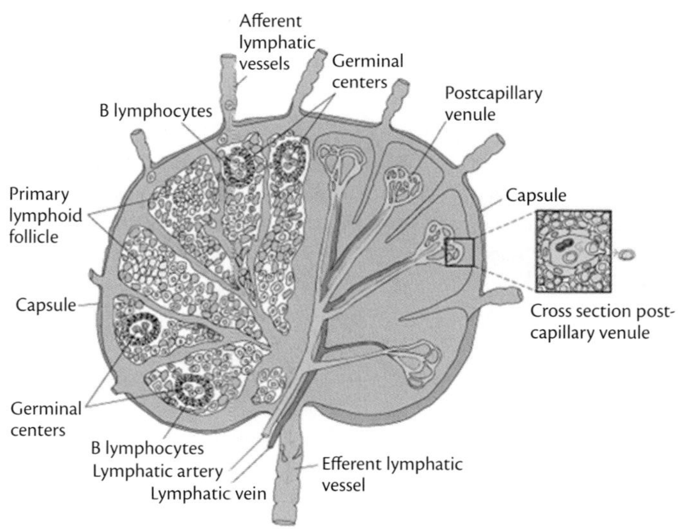

Fig. 4.3 Schematic of the structure of a lymph node, a secondary lymphoid organ in which cooperation between cells takes place. The cells in the lymph nodes, B and T lymphocytes, antigen-presenting cells, and other support cells and structures are organized into three-dimensional structures that enhance cellular cooperation and increase the probability that relatively rare clonal lymphocyte populations will encounter antigen-presenting cells and each other.

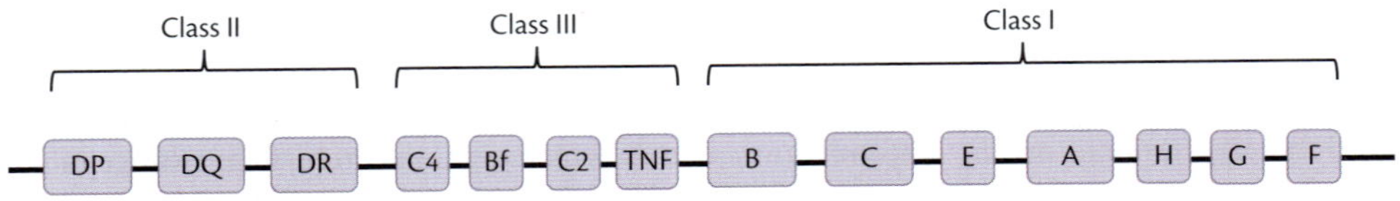

Fig. 4.4 Schematic of the human HLA gene complex (not to scale).

of their polymorphism, and why they are polymorphic in terms of their biological role.

HLA molecules

HLA molecules are coded by a complex of genes called the major histocompatibility complex (MHC) on the short arm of chromosome 6, hence many investigators also use the term MHC antigens. As shown in Figure 4.4, there are a number of genes within the human HLA locus, which can also be divided into classes, depending on their structure and tissue distribution. Many of these genes are highly polymorphic, with a large number of alleles distributed within the human population. The alleles exhibit small variations in nucleotide sequence resulting in changes in amino acid sequence, while retaining the same overall structure. Since there are many genes within the HLA locus, each with many alleles in the population, the number of possible combinations of different HLA alleles in the population is very large. The A locus, for example, has more than 50 commonly inherited alleles, with new uncommon ones still being discovered. It is this polymorphism that is the ultimate driving force of allograft rejection. Given the large number of possible allele combinations, it is highly unusual that two randomly selected individuals will have identical HLA alleles.

The three-dimensional structure of HLA molecules along with the effects of polymorphism is important for their function. Figure 4.5 shows a three-dimensional view of an HLA molecule from the "top" perspective as the molecule sits on the cell surface.

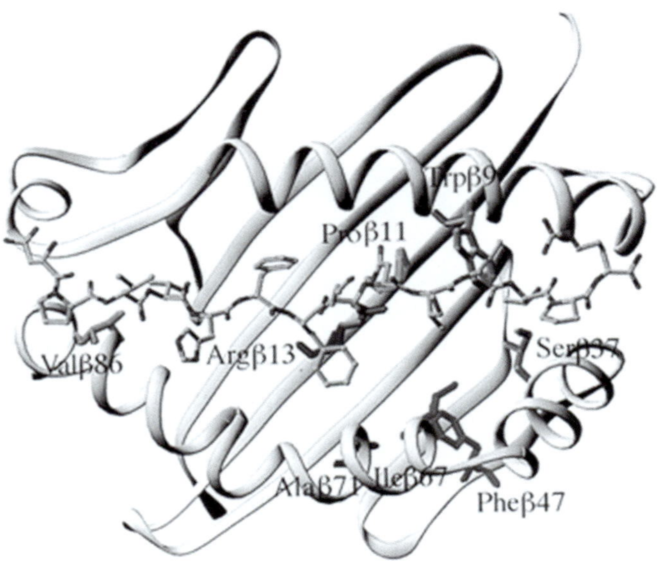

Fig. 4.5 Three-dimensional ribbon model of an HLA class II (DR2) molecule. A myelin basic protein peptide is depicted in the peptide-binding groove as a ball and stick model. Note that the peptide-binding groove consists of two α helices underlain by a β-pleated sheet.

Smith K J et al. J Exp Med 1998;188:1511-1520, used with permission from Rockefeller University Press.

The molecule contains a distinct groove formed by two α helices underlaid by a β-pleated sheet. Within this groove lies a peptide, noncovalently bound, that can originate from proteins in the interior or exterior of the cell. The peptide is variable: individual HLA molecules coded by the same gene on a single cell can contain a variety of different peptides. The peptides that reside within these grooves constitute a molecular sample of molecules that exist within the interior or exterior of the cell.

HLA proteins are divided into groups called class I, class Ib, class II, and class III. Class I and class II molecules are the most relevant to transplantation. They have similar overall structures with a peptide-binding groove, but are different in the origins of the peptides that tend to inhabit the groove (the biochemical pathways involved in loading a peptide into the groove are different), and differ in their distribution among cell types throughout the body.

Class I

The classical human HLA molecules that are routinely typed at most centers are called A, B, and C. HLA class I is expressed by nearly all nucleated cells, although the level of expression (i.e., the number of molecules expressed on the cell surface) can vary widely according to cell type. Also, exposure to soluble factors, such as interferon-γ, can modulate expression. There are more than 50 alleles for the HLA-A gene, more than 75 for HLA-B, and more than 30 for HLA-C. HLA class I proteins are composed of two chains: a 44 kDa highly polymorphic α-chain and a 12 kDa non-polymorphic β-chain, called β_2-microglobulin, coded by a gene on chromosome 15. The α-chain contains three domains called α_1, α_2, and α_3 as well as a transmembrane and cytoplasmic domain (Figure 4.6). The α_3 domain is relatively constant, and interacts with the β_2-microglobulin chain. The polymorphic regions of the HLA class I molecules are largely within the α_1 and α_2 domains, which constitute the peptide-binding portions of the molecule.

Class Ib

Class Ib molecules are smaller, but similar in structure to class I and also associate with β_2-microglobulin. These include HLA-E, HLA-F, and HLA-G. They are not thought to play a significant role in allograft rejection and are not distributed in the same manner as class I. HLA-H and HLA-J appear to be pseudo-genes so they are not expressed at all.

Class II

HLA class II molecules are not as widely distributed, being found primarily on cells involved in antigen presentation: dendritic cells, monocytes/macrophages, B cells and, under specific conditions, endothelial cells. They consist of a 33–35 kDa α chain and a 26–28 kDa β chain which are noncovalently associated. The α chain contains an α_1 and α_2 domain and the β chain contains a β_1 and β_2 domain (Figure 4.6). The most relevant HLA class II molecules to organ transplantation are HLA-DR, HLA-DP, and HLA-DQ. These molecules also contain a peptide groove except that, in contrast to HLA class I molecules, the peptide groove has open ends allowing the accommodation of somewhat longer peptides.

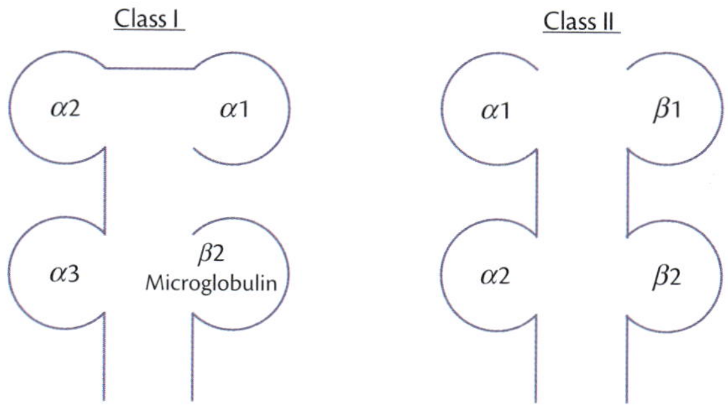

Fig. 4.6 Schematic structures of HLA class I and class II molecules. HLA class I molecules, expressed on all nucleated cells, consist of an α chain with three immunoglobulin-like domains. The α_3 domain is noncovalently associated with β_2-microglobulin. HLA class II molecules, expressed on antigen-presenting cells, are heterodimers consisting of an α and β chain, each with two immunoglobulin-like domains. Most of the polymorphisms found in HLA class I and class II molecules are found in the α and β chains respectively.

Class III

These molecules have a variety of functions and include complement components (e.g. factor B and C2), tumor necrosis factor-α, and heat shock proteins. They do not have direct involvement in antigen presentation.

Antigen processing

Endogenous pathway

The peptides that are loaded into the peptide-bonding grooves of MHC class I molecules primarily come from the interior of the cell upon which the molecules reside. The loading of peptides into HLA molecules is called antigen processing, a process in which a whole or partial protein molecule is broken into peptides of a specific size range before loading into the peptide-binding groove of the HLA class I molecule. Since the peptides in class I molecules mostly come from the cellular interior, the process has been called the endogenous pathway because the site of peptide generation is in the cytosol and peptide loading occurs in the endoplasmic reticulum (ER). In general, neither of these cellular compartments encounters material from endocytic compartments, which contain materials from outside the cell. This segregation means that MHC class I molecules usually will not contain materials obtained by phagocytosis. So in the case of viral infection, HLA class I molecules of a virus-infected cell will contain viral peptides and can therefore be targeted by cytotoxic T lymphocytes. But cells which have simply phagocytosed virus-infected cells but are not infected will not be targeted, which minimizes bystander effects. It is important to note that antigen presentation pathways operate continuously, so in the absence of foreign antigens, essentially all HLA molecules will contain peptides from self proteins. So antigen processing does not distinguish self from nonself. In the endogenous pathway, therefore, the HLA molecules contain a representative sample of the interior of the cell.

Proteins continuously undergo turnover within the cytoplasm. They are degraded into peptides by a large structure composed of 14 subsets organized into a roughly cylindrical structure of rings (Figure 4.7). This structure, called a proteasome, produces the small peptides that are ultimately loaded into HLA class I molecules. The peptides are moved into the ER in an ATP-dependent fashion by the TAP (transporter associated with antigen processing) protein. In the ER, HLA class I molecules are assembled, assisted by the

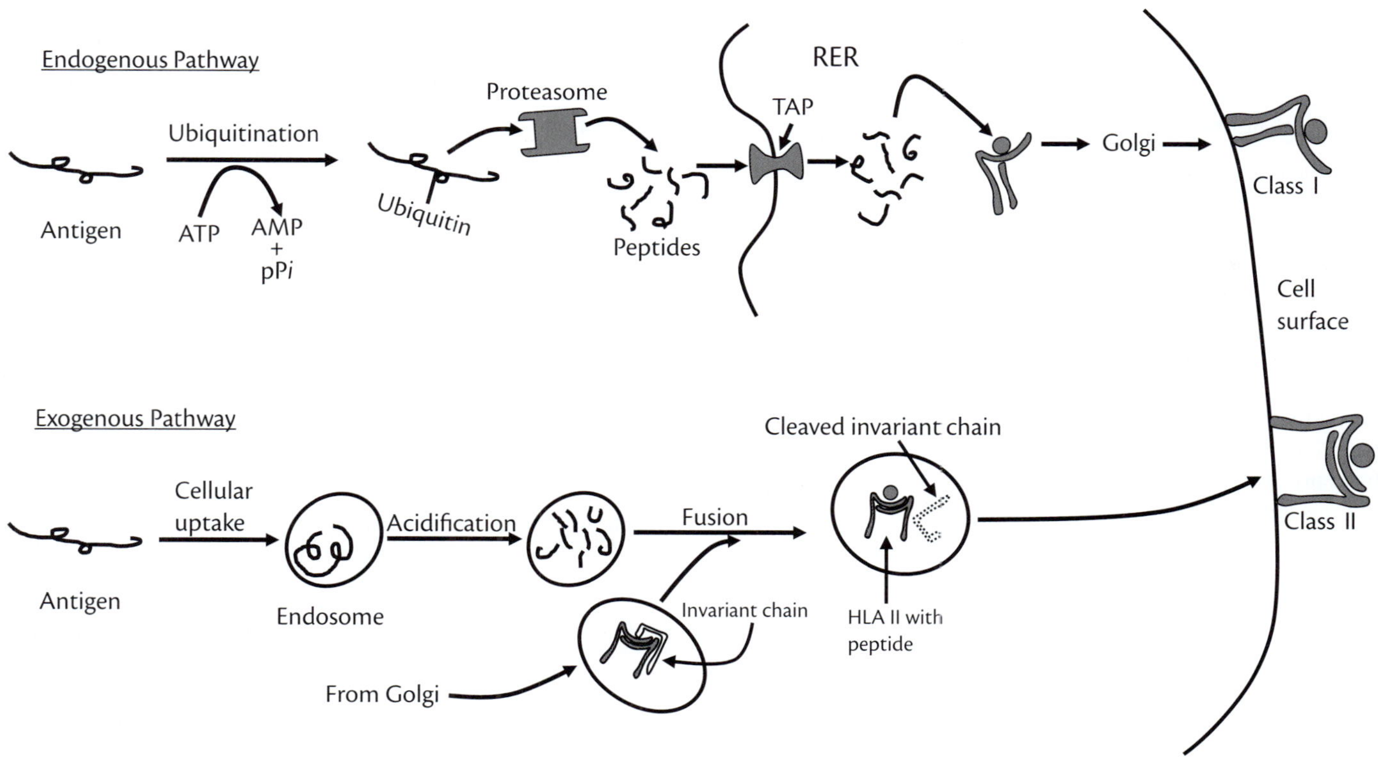

Fig. 4.7 Antigen processing. There are two distinct pathways for antigen processing. The exogenous pathway, which processes antigens from outside the cell, loads peptides into the peptide-binding groove of HLA class II molecules. The endogenous pathway primarily processes antigens from inside the cell and loads peptides into HLA class I molecules. This pathway results in HLA class I molecules bearing a "molecular signature" of the interior of the cell.

action of a variety of chaperone proteins. When the peptide is loaded into the HLA class I molecule, the molecule is then exported from the ER and proceeds to the cell surface via the Golgi complex.

Exogenous pathway

Antigens originating from the exterior of the cell are processed via the exogenous pathway. Dendritic cells and macrophages internalize antigens by phagocytosis, endocytosis, or pinocytosis, and B cells internalize antigens via receptor (immunoglobulin)-mediated endocytosis. The vesicles containing the internalized materials are shuttled to increasingly acidic compartments containing acid-dependent hydrolases in which antigens are degraded into peptides, mostly 13–18 amino acids in length.

HLA class II molecules are synthesized within the rough ER (see Figure 4.7) where they noncovalently associate with invariant chains, which occupy the peptide-bending groove. The invariant chain blocks the peptide-binding groove, which prevents peptides from occupying the site before a processed peptide is loaded into it. The N-terminal portion of the invariant chain guides the assembled HLA molecule to the Golgi apparatus and to the endocytic vesicles that contain peptides from the external environment. The invariant chain is degraded when the molecular complex is joined to the endocytic cellular compartment, leaving a fragment in the peptide-binding groove called class II associated invariant chain peptide (CLIP). A second class-II-like molecule, called HLA-DM, causes the release of the CLIP, allowing loading of an exogenous peptide into the HLA class II peptide-binding groove. HLA-DM, like other HLA class II molecules, is composed of α and β chains, but is not expressed on the cell surface. It is primarily found within cytoplasmic vesicles. Once the HLA class II molecule is fully assembled and loaded, it is exported to the plasma membrane where it is available for binding by T cell antigen receptors.

The division of the exogenous and endogenous pathways is not absolute. Peptides from exogenous antigens can be found in class II molecules. The clearest examples of this phenomenon have been found in dendritic cells.

How the presence of both donor and recipient HLA molecules affects the transplant recipient

It is important to remember that the transplant recipient contains both donor cells and recipient cells, each likely expressing distinct HLA class I molecules, and among APCs, distinct HLA class II molecules. Since HLA molecules are highly polymorphic (i.e., distinct among individuals) they constitute the most important donor antigens to which the recipient immune system will react. Therefore, one of the most important populations of peptides observed in the peptide-binding grooves of recipient HLA molecules are derived from processed *donor* HLA molecules. Transplant immunologists call this *indirect* antigen presentation: when peptides derived from HLA molecules of donor cells are presented within (in the context of) recipient HLA molecules. Immunologists often call this "nominal antigen presentation" because it constitutes the normal pathway by which all antigens are presented. However, transplant biologists have also found that recipient T cells will also recognize and react to intact, unprocessed *donor* HLA molecules on the surfaces of donor cells, a phenomenon called *direct* antigen presentation. This is important for two reasons. The first is that intact HLA antigens exist on the vascular endothelium of the donor organ as well as any APCs that are carried over to the recipient within the donor organ. Therefore, there is a substantial and persistent source of intact donor HLA molecules, especially early post-transplant when the relatively short-lived, terminally differentiated APCs still exist within the recipient. The second is that a large proportion of recipient T cells are capable of reacting to intact donor HLA antigens. This means that the proportion of T cells responding to intact donor antigen can be one to two orders of magnitude higher than the proportion of T cells that respond to normally processed donor peptides.[3,4] Therefore responses to donor antigens via the direct pathway are very strong and appear to be predominant early post-transplant before donor-derived APCs, which are largely terminally differentiated, expire.

Central functions of HLA

Since heart transplantation is an artificial situation, it is clear that the biologic function of HLA is not to drive allograft rejection. However, we can discern these central functions of HLA molecules, as well as their associated antigen presentation machinery, when we consider their properties as discussed earlier. These properties are:

- high polymorphism such that a complete set of identical HLA molecules between individuals is very rare
- the structure of the molecules are such that they always carry a solvent-accessible peptide derived from the interior (class I) or exterior (class II) of the cell, therefore providing a sample of the environment inside or outside the cell
- during development, T cells are selected so that they only recognize antigens as peptides complexed with HLA molecules except for intact *donor* HLA molecules, which are a special case.

Since T cells only recognize antigens in the peptide-binding groove of HLA molecules, they therefore will only recognize antigens on the surfaces of other cells, which means T cells do not bind free antigens. Virus-specific killer T cells, then, will only "see" virus presented by HLA class I molecules on virus-infected cells. In an individual infected with a virus, especially during viremia, this characteristic can mean the difference between resolving or not resolving an infection. The key to resolving virus infections is the elimination of virus-infected virus-producing cells. T cells that reacted with free virus would be unable to perform this function, and would likely be saturated during viremia.

For providing regulatory functions, this restriction to recognizing antigenic peptides also assures T cells cooperate with relevant B cells. B cells bind free antigen via surface immunoglobulin receptors, process them, and then present them on the surface where they can be "seen" by T cells of the appropriate specificity. Notably, since HLA molecules are polymorphic (not exactly the same in different individuals), the three-dimensional structure of the antigen peptide–HLA complex is not the same in all individuals. For infectious organisms, this means evolving the means to evade the immune response in one individual or a group of individuals does not guarantee evasion of the immune response in all individuals in the population: that is, it reduces the likelihood that a single infectious agent can wipe out an entire population. Diversity therefore enhances species survival.

T cells and the T cell receptor

In the previous section, we alluded to recognition of the HLA–peptide complex by T cells. During their development in the thymus, T cells are selected such that only those that recognize HLA–peptide complexes are allowed to survive. Those that recognize self HLA antigens alone (dangerous) or do not recognize them at all (useless) are not allowed to leave the thymus. The recognition of HLA–antigen is conferred by the T cell receptor (TCR). This receptor merits special attention because it, along with the HLA locus, is central to the phenomena of cardiac allograft rejection.

The ligand for the TCR is HLA–antigen. Given that the number of different peptides that could be potentially incorporated into HLA molecules is extremely large, it follows that the number of distinct ligands is very large (diverse). To accommodate such diversity, a receptor must be able to bind a large array of different ligands or, alternatively, the structure of the receptor itself must also be diverse. The former characteristic would preclude specificity, which is not consistent with observations of the phenomena of transplant rejection (remember Sir Peter Medawar's experiments). So therefore the TCR structure must be diverse. Those who originally deduced that antigen receptors must be highly diverse also realized that there must be a mechanism to generate the diversity of recognition structures the TCR must have. It was also found that the TCR expressed by any newly developed, resting T cell is essentially uniquely specific for a particular antigen. Each unique, specific T cell is called a *clone*. Each clone can give rise to daughter clones, each bearing the same specificity, a characteristic that is important after a primary immune response is initiated. Estimates of the number of possible TCRs (and therefore uniquely specific T cells) are as high as 10^{15}. Therefore, each individual bears a pool of T cells, which contains a large array of specificities. The consequence of this large array is that a T cell of a particular specificity is rare. So one of the first things to occur after T cells encounter antigen is that they proliferate, a process called clonal expansion.

The TCR belongs to a group of proteins designated the immunoglobulin superfamily because of both structural and amino acid similarities. The proteins in this superfamily contain immunoglobulin domains, regions 70–110 amino acids long that have a degree of homology with immunoglobulin variable or constant region domains. These domains characteristically contain cysteine residues that connect a disulfide-bonded loop of 55–75 amino acids.

The part of the TCR that contacts the HLA–peptide complex is a heterodimer consisting of an α chain of 40–60 kDa and a β chain of 40–50 kDa. There is also a smaller subpopulation of T cells in which HLA–peptides are bound by γ and δ chains coded by distinct genes rather than α and β chains. The α and β chains each contain a variable region, designated such because the amino acid sequence of the region is generated by combinatorial rearrangement of gene segments. The rearrangement of these gene segments is imprecise, which further increases the variability of the sequence of amino acids. This is the same process in which diversity is generated in antibody molecules (see Box 4.1).

The antigen-binding portion of the TCR is associated with the CD3 complex (Figure 4.9), a group of connected membrane-bound proteins that is required for expression of the TCR on the cell surface and transduces a signal to the interior of the cell when the TCR heterodimer is bound by HLA–peptide or the complex is cross-linked by something else. Cross-linking of the TCR–CD3 complex can occur after administration of anti-thymocyte globulin or other polyclonal or monoclonal antibodies that contain specificities for the TCR. This can result in system-wide release of soluble proinflammatory proteins (cytokines).

T cell function

T cells serve two broad roles under which they perform a variety of overlapping subfunctions. In one role, they serve as *effector cells*, which can be defined as cells that participate directly in elimination or sequestration of antigen. One example is cytotoxic T lymphocytes (CTL), which can directly lyse cells bearing the HLA–peptide for which they are specific. T cells can also secrete cytokines that can directly affect the function or viability of target cells. They also serve to regulate the function and differentiation of other cells through cell-to-cell contact and through secretion of regulatory factors, such as interleukin 2 (IL-2). The classification of T cells within these roles is not absolute. It is possible for some cells to perform multiple functions or to switch roles. Also, depending on how an author defines effector cells, the reader may find functionally similar cells classified differently in the literature. T cells regulate antigen-specific immune responses and they are also capable of effector functions such as killing virus-infected cells. The functional characteristics of an individual T cell results from the integration of multiple signals in addition to the initiating event, which is the ligation of the TCR by HLA–peptide on an APC. These signals can come in the form of ligation of surface receptors or soluble factors, and these are dependent on the local microenvironment in which the T cell exists, such as a lymph node or a site of inflammation. T cells are highly mobile and circulate throughout the body. Therefore, events affecting T cell activation are not necessarily colocalized.

T cell activation

T cell activation is a process in which a T cell leaves a quiescent, resting state and engages in a process involving a complex series of biochemical cascades leading to the synthesis of new gene products, ultimately resulting in entry into the cell cycle. Proliferation, or clonal expansion, is necessary for a single T cell clone to exert regulation or effector functions in the immune response. Resting T cells that have not previously encountered their specific antigen (also called naive T cells) require at least two distinct signals before activation takes place.

The first signal is the engagement of the TCR by its complementary antigenic peptide–MHC complex. This results in a series of biochemical events which, in concert with a second signal, result in alterations in gene transcription in the nucleus. These biochemical events collectively constitute a *signal*. As described earlier in this chapter, the TCR consists of an antigen–MHC binding heterodimer associated with the group of proteins called CD3. When the TCR is engaged, a signaling complex is formed in which the TCR associates with either CD4 (MHC class II specific TCRs) or CD8 (class I specific TCRs) coreceptors. These coreceptors bring a tyrosine kinase, p56 *lck*, into the proximity of immune-receptor tyrosine based activation motifs which are then phosphorylated. This initiates a cascade of phosphorylation events proceeding down a number of distinct biochemical (signaling) pathways. For this signal to result in T cell activation, the cell must also receive a second signal. The second signal is a simultaneous or subsequent, non-antigen-specific costimulating signal provided by the APC primarily through engagement of CD28 on the T cell by members of the B7 family of molecules on the APC. There are two types of B7 molecules: B7-1 and B7-2, each of which has distinct cytoplasmic domains. These are constitutively expressed on dendritic cells, but are inducible on macrophages. In addition to CD28, the

Box 4.1 Antigen receptor gene rearrangement

In elementary genetics we are taught that one gene codes for one protein. However, it is well known that antigen receptors are extremely diverse for both B cells and T cells, such that a corresponding T cell or B cell can be found for nearly any foreign antigen. If each possible T cell or B cell receptor was coded by a unique, complete gene, then coverage of the number of potential antigenic specificities could easily take up the entire genome.

Characterization of both the T cell receptor and immunoglobulin gene loci shows the mechanism by which a sufficiently diverse array of different antigen receptors can be generated. Antigen receptor genes are assembled from gene segments. During B cell development, one of 30 short gene segments, called diversity (D) segments, is joined to one of 6 possible joining (J) gene segments. The gene rearrangement occurs by removal of the intervening genomic DNA between the D and J gene segments (Figure 4.8). How particular gene segments are chosen is not well understood, but evidence shows that it is not completely random.[46,47,48,49,50,51,52] To complete the gene the concatenated DJ segments are then joined to one of many variable region gene segments.[53,54,55] The light chain is assembled in a similar manner except there are no diversity gene segments.

This combinatorial diversity is enhanced because the joining of the gene segments is imprecise. Individual nucleotides are removed and added to the gene segments during the rearrangement process.[56,57]

T cell receptor genes are rearranged in a similar manner. Unique to the immunoglobulin genes, however, is that rearranged immunoglobulin V-regions can mutate (somatic mutation). This drives the process of *affinity maturation* where the affinity of the antibodies generated in response to a particular antigen increases over time.[58,59] A base change in an immunoglobulin gene can result in an increase or a decrease in affinity as well as changing the specificity of an antibody entirely. In the latter case, the B cells undergo apoptosis. Therefore B cells binding antigen with high affinity tend to accumulate.

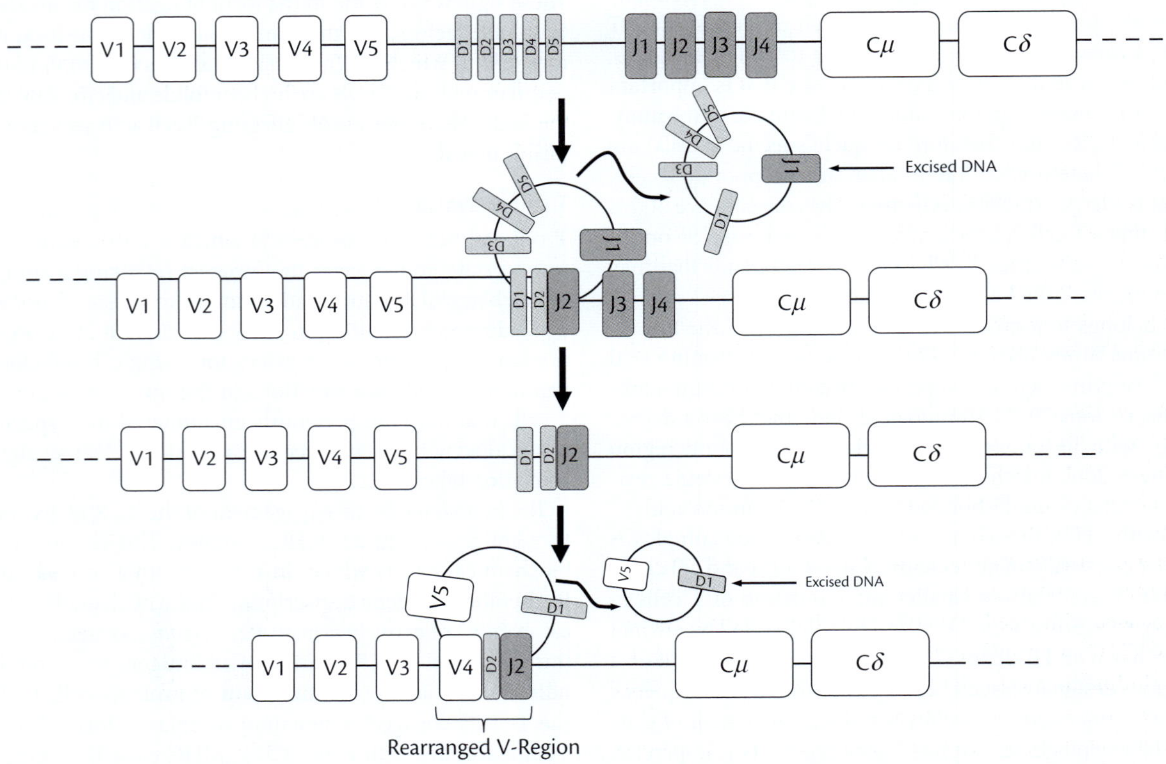

Fig. 4.8 Immunoglobulin (Ig) heavy chain variable region gene rearrangement. Diversity in the antigen-binding portion of Ig molecules is generated by combinatorial rearrangement of gene segments termed V (variable), D (diversity), and J (joining). The gene segments rearrange by looping out the DNA that lies between the two rearranging gene segments. Light chains rearrange in a similar manner except that they do not have D segments. Additional diversity is generated by random addition of bases into the gene segment junctions during rearrangement. The same process of rearrangement takes place for TCR genes. V, D, and J segments for the β chain and V-J segments form the α chain. There is no somatic hypermutation or equivalent to class switching in the T cell receptor locus.

B7 molecules will also bind a molecule on T cells called CTLA-4. CD28 and CTLA-4 are antagonistic such that engagement of CD28 promotes T cell activation, but engagement of CTLA-4 inhibits it. It is believed that CTLA-4, which is virtually absent on resting T cells, limits T cell activation. Its absence in mice results in uncontrolled proliferation, lymphadenopathy, and death. If a T cell encounters antigen–HLA without a costimulatory signal, the encounter can result in *clonal anergy*, a state in which the T cell will not respond to subsequent antigen stimulation.

After signal 1 and signal 2, a T cell will enter the cell cycle and at the same time will begin transcribing the IL-2 gene and also increase the number of IL-2 receptors on the cell surface. The costimulatory signal results in an increase in the half-life of IL-2 mRNA as well, so the increased transcription and half-life results

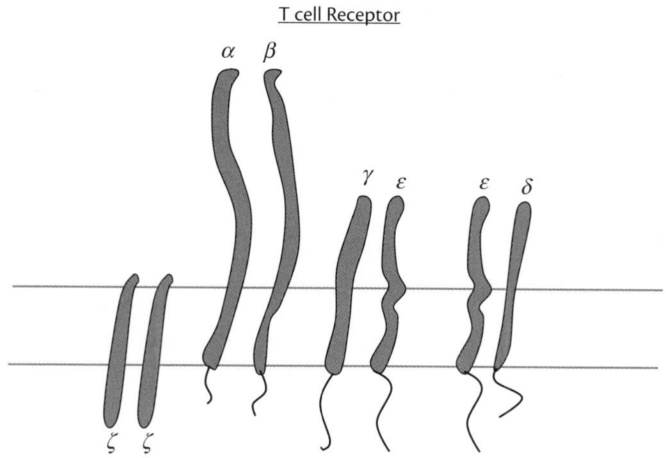

Fig. 4.9 The T cell receptor (TCR) complex. The part of the TCR that contacts the HLA–peptide complex is a heterodimer consisting of an α chain and a β chain. The α and β chains each contain a variable region, designated such because the amino acid sequence of the region is generated by combinatorial rearrangement of gene segments. The antigen-binding portion of the TCR is associated with the CD3 complex, which consists of εδ chains and the εγ chains. The α and β chains along with CD3 are associated with a ζζ homodimer which resides mostly within the interior of the cell. Many monoclonal antibodies used for visualizing T cells are specific for the ε chain.

in an increase in IL-2 local amounts by two orders of magnitude. The IL-2 binds to the IL-2 receptor (also called CD-25), inducing the cell to proliferate and subsequent generations to differentiate into effector cells or memory cells. Fully activated T cells will divide 2–3 times a day for about 4–5 days, their numbers increasing by 2^n where n is the number of generations. If we assume 15 generations of a single cell, the final result would be 32 768, an increase of 4 orders of magnitude.

Depending on the local environment, T cells can differentiate into different subpopulations with distinct functional characteristics. One such subpopulation, called the TH1 subset, secretes IL-2, IFN-γ, and TNFβ and is considered proinflammatory, favoring the generation of CTLs and recruitment of other proinflammatory cell lineages. Another subpopulation, called the TH2 subset, does not favor inflammation and secretes IL-4, IL-5, IL-6, and IL-10. This subset is associated with B cell activation and differentiation. A third subset, called TH17, is proinflammatory. TH17 cells produce IL-17, IL-17F, and IL-22. These cells also facilitate differentiation of other T cells into another subset called regulatory T cells (Treg), which are CD4+ cells that express high levels of the IL-2 receptor. One of the signature markers of Treg cells is expression of the transcription factor forkhead box P3 (FOXP3). Treg cells, as the name implies, are associated with immune regulation and can strongly suppress T cell-mediated responses in an antigen-specific manner.

B cells

Both the TCR and antibody molecules confer specificity to the adaptive immune response. TCRs, after selection in the thymus, only bind antigen on the surface of other cells in conjunction with HLA class I or class II. Antibodies, also called immunoglobulins, will bind to free antigen and also exist in soluble form. They are secreted in quantity by *plasma cells*, which ultimately arise from B lymphocytes (B cells). B cells are so named because they were originally found to arise from a specialized tissue called the bursa of Fabricius in the chicken. No such organ exists in mammals, whose B cells are generated in the bone marrow.

Immunoglobulins bound to the B cell surface serve as the antigen-sensing portion of B cell antigen receptors. B cell antigen receptors are composed of immunoglobulin bound to CD79a/CD79b through which signals are propagated into the interior of the cell via multiple molecular pathways.

Immunoglobulin molecules are composed of a heavy chain and a light chain linked together to form a complete molecule. Each heavy and light chain pair contains an antigen-binding region, so each antibody molecule has two binding sites (Figure 4.10). The end of the molecule where the heavy and light chains are joined together forms the antigen-binding region and is called the variable region because the amino acid sequence in this region is different for each B cell clone. How this variable amino acid sequence is generated is discussed in Box 4.1. The other end of the immunoglobulin molecule is formed from the heavy chains and is called the constant region. The heavy chain constant regions constitute the effector portion of secreted immunoglobulins and form the basis of classification of them into groups called *isotypes* named (in order of abundance in the circulation) IgG, IgA, IgM, IgD, and IgE. There are four subtypes of IgG (IgG1 through IgG4) and two subtypes of IgA (IgA1 and IgA2). The isotype of an antibody molecule determines the range of effector functions in which it can participate. Some cells express receptors that bind specific immunoglobulin isotypes, which can assist in the clearance of bacterial infections. Some isotypes also fix complement (discussed later in the chapter). Portions of the immunoglobulin molecule are also named according to fractions produced by digestion with specific proteolytic enzymes. The antigen-binding portion of the molecule with the constant region

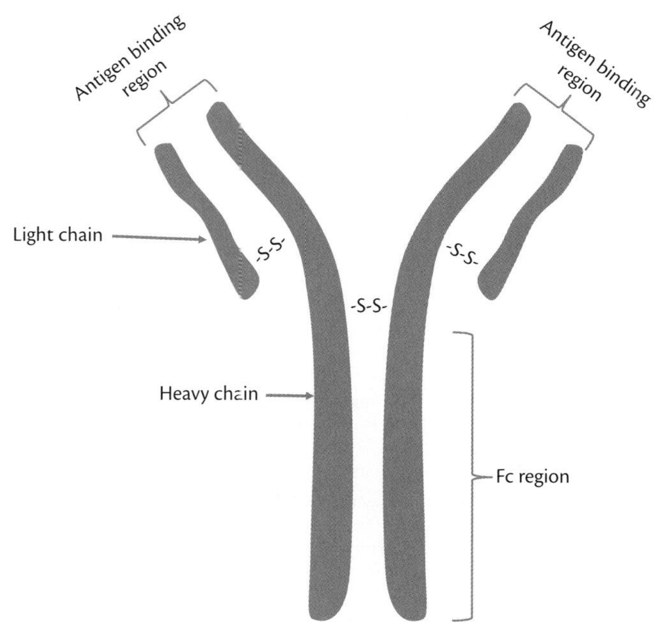

Fig. 4.10 Schematic of an immunoglobulin molecule. The molecule consists of two pairs of a heavy and light chain covalently bound together by disulfide bonds. It is divalent, with each antigen-binding region formed by a light chain and a heavy chain. The two heavy chains also form the Fc region, which effectively constitutes the effector end of the molecule. Many immune cells have receptors for immunoglobulin Fc regions.

removed is called the F(ab)′ or F(ab)″ fragment, depending on whether it is monovalent or divalent, respectively. The portion of the antibody molecule formed by the constant regions is also called the Fc region.

Characteristics of antibody responses

The structure of the antibody molecules and their classification into isotypes based on that structure is discussed in the previous section. Since antibodies are secreted into the serum and bind to antigens in an unmodified form, they can be readily detected. In heart transplantation, the most relevant antibody specificities are those directed towards donor HLA. Whether an individual has been previously exposed to a specific HLA molecule will strongly influence the kinetics and characteristics of an antibody response after exposure to an antigen. The response upon first exposure to antigen results from activation of naive B cells and T cells, but a secondary response is the product of memory lymphocytes.

Upon first exposure to a foreign antigen, an individual generates a primary humoral response. At the cellular level, this begins with activation of B cells followed by their clonal expansion and differentiation into antibody-secreting plasma cells and memory B cells. The production of antibody the first time a particular antigen is encountered is called a primary response. This begins with a lag period, where no antibody is produced for a period of several days, after which the quantity of antibody detected in the serum will increase logarithmically, then plateau, and finally decline (Figure 4.11). The plateau duration depends on a number of variables, including persistence of the antigen. In transplantation, the antigen is obviously never cleared. The first antibodies detected in a primary response are IgM. This is followed by IgG antibodies of increasing quantity and specificity. Upon second exposure to the same antigen, the response arises after a much shorter lag period. The total amount of antibody produced is much greater with a higher proportion consisting of IgG, and the plateau period lasts longer. This quicker, stronger, and longer-lasting response is a function of memory B cells. Memory B cells arise during a primary humoral response. They have a lower threshold of activation than naive B cells. A significant reason for the strength of the secondary response is that the number (frequency) of memory B cells specific for a given antigen is much higher than naive B cells, which are relatively rare.

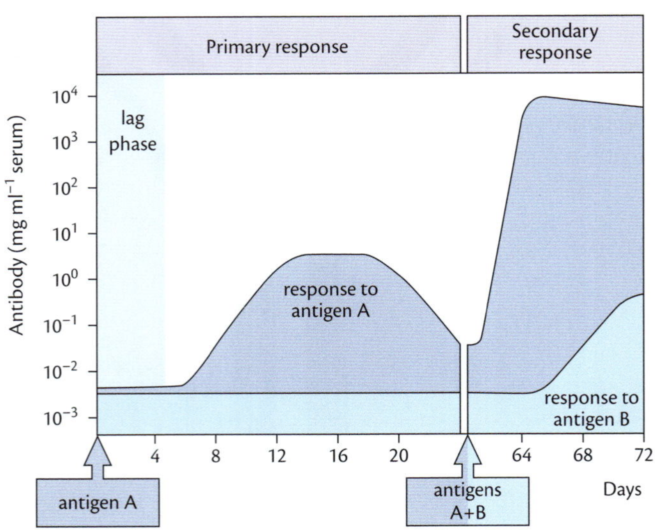

Fig. 4.11 The kinetics of antibody production in response to antigen. A second exposure to the same antigen results in a shorter lag period and a stronger, longer-lasting antibody response. In the secondary response, the predominant isotype changes from IgM to IgG.

Isotype switching

As noted in the previous section, the first antibodies produced are IgM. The initial IgM antibodies are of lower affinity than those produced later, but they efficiently activate complement. IgG antibodies of the same or similar specificity are produced when *isotype switching* occurs, a process in which the same variable region is switched to a different constant region within the immunoglobulin gene, a process called *switch recombination*. This results in a change in the effector functions of the antibody. CD4+ T cells regulate isotype switching, a process requiring cell-to-cell contact in which the T cell engages CD40 on B cells. The process of isotype switching begins about 6 days following B cell activation in vivo.[5] IgG becomes the dominant isotype in the extracellular spaces and in the peripheral blood circulation. IgA is the predominant isotype in the mucosa. The specific isotype switch that takes place in a B cell is dependent on a number of cellular signals, such as those mediated by cytokines.

NK cells

In 1975, two groups reported a population of large granular lymphocytes that lysed, apparently spontaneously, tumor cell lines in vitro.[6,7] The cells were named natural killer (NK) cells because no prior immunization was necessary and the killing of target cells did not appear to be HLA-restricted. It has since been learned that NK cells are important in innate immunity, consisting of an important line of defense against viral infections before effective, antigen-specific viral immune responses can be generated. NK cells can also mediate *antibody-dependent cellular cytotoxicity* in which they can attach to antibody-coated cells via Fc receptors and kill them. While not thought to be a dominant force in solid organ transplant rejection, NK cells can be very important for hematopoietic cell grafts as exemplified by the phenomenon of "hybrid resistance" in mice. NK cells mediate rejection of parental hematopoietic grafts transplanted into F1 offspring even though the F1 mice express the parental antigens.

NK cells possess two general types of receptors. The first, lectin-like receptors, are structurally similar to receptors that bind carbohydrates, even though they bind proteins. The second type is immunoglobulin-like receptors, termed killer immunoglobulin-like receptors, which bind HLA-B or HLA-C molecules. NK cells tend to kill target cells expressing abnormal levels of HLA molecules, especially those in which expression is abnormally low. NK cells express both activating and inhibitory receptors. Activating receptors, most with unknown ligands, signal the NK cell to kill the target cell. Inhibitory receptors, which typically bind class I HLA, inhibit killing. The activating signal will predominate if HLA class levels are abnormally low.

Cytokines

We can define cytokines as secreted proteins that alter the behavior or properties of cells and/or recruit cells from other locations.

Table 4.2 Major cytokines relevant to transplantation

Cytokine	Sources	Biological activity
IL-1α	Macrophages, epithelial cells	T cell and macrophage activation
IL-2	T cells	T cell activation and proliferation
IL-4	T cells, mast cells	B cell activation, downregulation of Th1 cells
IL-6	T cells, macrophages, epithelial cells	Acute-phase protein production, T and B cell growth
IL-8 (chemokine)	Macrophages, endothelial cells, others	Neutrophil chemotaxis
IL-10	T cells, macrophages	Downregulation of macrophage function
IL-12	T cells, macrophages	Differentiation of Th1 cells, activation of NK cells
IL-17	T cells, Th17 cells	Recruitment of monocytes and neutrophils
IL-23	Dendritic cells, macrophages	Induction of Th17 cells
IFN-γ	T cells, NK cells	Macrophage activation, increased HLA expression, Ig class switch
TNFα	T cells, macrophages, NK cells	Endothelial activation, proinflammatory
TGF-β	Monocytes, T cells, others	Fibrosis, inhibition of T cell proliferation, anti-inflammatory

In general, cytokines are not like hormones and act over relatively short distances. High concentrations are not typically found in the circulation in normal circumstances because they tend to have short half-lives. The term "cytokines" encompasses a complex array of proteins with an extremely wide range of functional activities. To complicate matters further, the functional effects of a given cytokine often depend on the target cell type or the functional state of the target cell type. This means that the nomenclature for cytokines can be confusing, with many of them named after the biological activity noted upon their discovery (e.g. tumor necrosis factor). In 1979, a nomenclature system was established in which cytokines are designated by the term "interleukin" followed by a number. T cell growth factor, for example, was renamed as interleukin 2 (IL-2). In transplantation, the cytokines that have received the most attention are those found to be involved in inflammation and fibrosis. These cytokines are often discussed in the transplant literature (see Table 4.2), so some of the major cytokines merit discussion here.

Interleukin 2

IL-2 is a T cell growth factor important for T cell activation and proliferation. The receptor for IL-2 (IL-2R, also called CD-25) is the target for humanized monoclonal antibodies used routinely in cardiac transplantation. The IL-2 receptor consists of three subunits termed α, β, and γ. When a T cell is activated, it synthesizes the α chain of the IL-2R, which subsequently complexes with the β and γ chains to form the complete high-affinity IL-2R structure for expression on the cell surface.[8,9,10] Upon activation, a T cell makes IL-2. Costimulatory signals, such as ligation of CD28, also result in stabilization of IL-2 mRNA, which further increases the available bioactive IL-2. The IL-2 is secreted; affecting cells in the surrounding environment, but also binds to the IL-2R of the cell that secreted it, a process called *autocrine stimulation*. IL-2 is regulated at the level of transcription. The promoter region of the IL-2 gene contains elements that bind transcription factors that are part of proinflammatory signaling pathways as well as those associated with specific immunity.

Interleukin 6

IL-6 is an example of a pleiotropic cytokine. Several research groups discovered it, each assigning it a unique name and activity.[11] They discovered they were studying the same molecule after they cloned it and determined its sequence. It is secreted by a wide variety of cell types including T cells and macrophages, and induces a number of acute-phase proteins. Since it is associated with the acute-phase response, it is induced by a variety of stressful events and is usually elevated after cardiac surgery. It is a 26 kDa protein with a number of biological activities including induction of B cell differentiation into plasma cells, activation of macrophages and NK cells, regulation of T cell activation, and differentiation into different functional subpopulations.

Tumor necrosis factor

In its active form, tumor necrosis factor (TNF) is a 52 kDa trimer with three identical 17 kDa chains.[12,13,14,15] It belongs to the TNF-ligand superfamily, which are type II membrane proteins (an intracellular N-terminus, extracellular C-terminus with a single transmembrane region). As implied by the name, TNF was discovered as a soluble factor induced by endotoxin in mice that could cause necrosis of sarcomas. It has since been determined to be both proinflammatory and cytotoxic in vitro. It is secreted by a wide variety of cell types, including macrophages, T cells, and smooth muscle cells[15] in response to other proinflammatory mediators (e.g., IL-1) including itself.[12,16] TNF is also a primary factor involved in cachexia.[17]

Interferon-γ

Interferon-γ (IFN-γ) was first discovered as a factor secreted by T cells that inhibited viral replication.[18] It is secreted by T cells and NK cells. It can facilitate antigen presentation by increasing expression of HLA class I and class II molecules, an activity that can also be exerted on vascular endothelial cells,[19,20,21] which is of potential importance for an anti-graft immune response. IFN-γ is a potent proinflammatory cytokine as an activator of macrophages and monocytes. This tends to induce increased production of reactive oxygen species and nitrogen intermediates.

Interleukin 17

IL-17 has recently been described as an important cytokine in chronic inflammation and autoimmunity.[22,23] It increases chemokine production in a number of tissues, resulting in recruitment of cells involved in control of extracellular pathogens. It is secreted by a specialized subset of T cells (TH17 cells) and NK cells. Molecules involved in the induction of TH17 cells in humans include TGF-β, IL-6, and IL-23.[24,25]

Adhesion molecules

An important part of immune function is the traffic of cells into particular tissues. For example, T cells can be recruited into particular tissues through the action of adhesion molecules. Observations of cells moving through blood vessels show that cells alternately stick and release from the vessel walls, resulting in a rolling action. During inflammation, the density of adhesion molecules will increase and undergo changes in distribution causing the cells to stick or adhere to the vessel wall. The cells can then migrate through the vessel into the surrounding tissue. So adhesion molecules regulate how leukocytes home and are retained in tissues in response to activation of local or systemic immune responses. *Integrins* generally hold cells in position by anchoring to the extracellular matrix. *Selectins* and members of the *immunoglobulin superfamily* are involved in cell-to-cell adhesion.

Integrins

Integrins are heterodimers. Each chain in the heterodimer can be identified by a different monoclonal antibody. There are two families of integrins: the β1 family is primarily involved in cell–matrix adhesion and the β2 family is more directly involved in specific immune and inflammatory responses. For example, high-affinity binding of a leukocyte can depend on an integrin called LFA-1 (leukocyte function associated antigen, also called CD11a/CD18) and another called Mac-1 (CD11b/CD 18). These integrins bind to ICAM-1 (CD54), a member of the immunoglobulin superfamily that is expressed on endothelial cells and can be upregulated by proinflammatory stimuli.[26,27,28] The integrins allow the cell to adhere to vascular endothelium long enough to migrate through the vessel wall into the surrounding tissue, a process called *diapedesis* (Figure 4.12).

Selectins

Selectins are important in attaching leukocytes to the vascular endothelium to the extent that they tend to roll along the length of the vessel wall.[26,29,30] They bind to carbohydrate moieties on the surfaces of other cells. L-selectins (CD62L) are primarily found on lymphocytes and facilitate lymphocyte homing to the lymph nodes. E-selectins are expressed by activated endothelial cells after exposure to a proinflammatory stimulus such as TNFα or lipopolysaccharide.[31,32,33] P-selectin is similarly upregulated after a proinflammatory stimulus, but very quickly because it is stored within granules called Weibel–Palade bodies,[34,35] which are translated to the plasma membrane immediately after a stimulus such as IL-1, TNF, or IFN-γ.[31] Both P-selectin and E-selectin, by mediating rolling of leukocytes along the vessel wall, effectively allow them to "scan" the vessel wall until they stick to a region where a proinflammatory stimulus causes greater adhesion, at which time rolling stops.

Immunoglobulin superfamily adhesion molecules

Adhesion molecules in this family facilitate diapedesis, the process in which leukocytes traverse through the vessel wall (see Figure 4.12).

- LFA-2 is found on T cells, thymocytes, and NK cells. It binds to CD58 (LFA-3) and is involved in T cell activation.
- ICAM can be found on several cell types and binds to LFA-2. It is found on dendritic cells and endothelial cells. LFA-1 on cytotoxic T cells binds to ICAM-1 on target cells, increasing their adhesion to the target cells.
- VCAM binds to the integrin VLA-4. It is expressed on activated endothelial cells, dendritic cells, macrophages, myoblasts, and bone marrow fibroblasts. VCAM is important for recruitment of leukocytes to regions of inflammation.
- PECAM also facilitates diapedesis. It is expressed at the functions of endothelial cells as well as on platelets and leukocytes.

These adhesion molecules can be important in rejection episodes because the cytokines elaborated during rejection increase the density of adhesion molecules.[36,37]

Complement

The complement system is a major effector component of the humoral immune system and it is also a major component of the innate immune system.

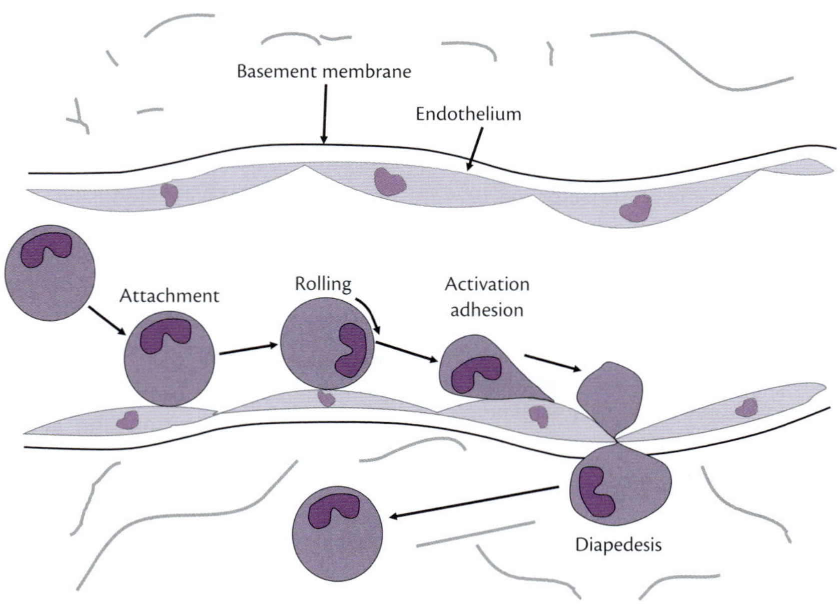

Fig. 4.12 The progression of white blood cells through the peripheral circulation is a function of the affinity of their attachment to the vascular endothelium. When injury or inflammation occurs in an area, the endothelial cells increase expression of adhesion molecules. Instead of continuing to roll along the vascular endothelium, the cells adhere more tightly and then migrate into the parenchymal tissue, a process called diapedesis.

So far in this chapter we have considered the mechanisms of specific, adaptive immune responses: T cell-mediated responses and antibody responses, both of which are important in prevention and clearance of infections as well as transplant rejection. Since these responses are adaptive, they take time to develop to their full potential, on the order of days to weeks. Other immune subsystems have evolved which are more effective for immediate threats, with reaction times of seconds to minutes.

Complement is one such subsystem. It consists of an array of proteins found in the circulation in sufficient quantities that a reaction can take place without prior protein synthesis and secretion. In transplantation, the most spectacular manifestation of complement activation is hyperacute rejection. Hyperacute rejection can occur after transplantation if there is a blood-type mismatch (eg. AB→O) or if cross-species transplants are performed. In each case, preformed anti-donor antibodies are present which, upon revascularization of the graft, bind to the vascular endothelium and activate the complement pathway. This reaction can occur with extreme speed, destroying the organ almost immediately.

Complement pathways

There are three pathways of complement activation. The first, called the classical pathway, usually begins with antibody binding to a cellular target, followed by "fixing" of complement, resulting in initiation of the complement cascade. The second pathway is called the alternative pathway. It does not require antibodies, and is activated by a variety of foreign surfaces including lipopolysaccharide on bacteria and fungi (Figure 4.13). These pathways converge at a common point.

The third pathway is the lectin pathway, which is activated by binding of mannose-binding lectin (MBL) of mannose residues on carbohydrates or glycoproteins. These pathways converge at a common point, which is the formation of the membrane attack complex (MAC) that results in the loss of membrane integrity on the cell on which the MAC is formed.

Classical pathway

Activation of the classical pathway is antibody dependent. It begins with binding of antibody to soluble antigen, forming immune complexes, or with binding of antibody to a cellular target (a donor cell or bacterial cell). Only specific classes or subclasses of antibodies can activate complement. In humans, they are IgM, IgG1, IgG2, and IgG3, but not IgG4.

When IgM binds antigen, conformational changes take place in the Fc region (the constant portion of the heavy chain). The IgM molecule is different than other isotypes because it forms a pentamer, which when bound, forms a so-called stable configuration that exposes three sites capable of binding the initial component of the classical complement pathway, C1q. Each C1 component must bind at least two Fc regions to form a stable complex. Therefore, a single pentameric IgM molecule can activate complement, but at least two monomeric IgG molecules must bind in close proximity. Once this cross-linking occurs, Cl becomes enzymatically active as a protease of which two other complement components, C4 and C2, are its substrate (see Figure 4.13). Each of these is cleaved into two fragments. One fragment from each component, C4b and C2a, combine to form *C3 convertase*. The other fragment of C4, C4a, is an *anaphylatoxin*, which does not participate in direct lysis, but potentiates inflammation through action on both immune and nonimmune cells. The next complement component in the pathway, C3, is where both the classical and alternative pathways converge. The C3 convertase cleaves C3 into two fragments, C3a and C3b. Note that this is the result of enzymatic activity. Therefore, each C3 convertase molecule can generate more than 200 C3b molecules, the next active component, providing exponential amplification. C3b can combine with the C3 convertase to form C5 convertase, which leads to formation of the membrane attack complex (MAC). C3b can also coat other cells, making them more susceptible to phagocytosis, a process called *opsonization*.

One other component merits further attention because of its importance in clinical diagnosis of antibody-mediated rejection. After C4 is converted to C4b and C4a, C4b is also converted to C4d. C4d can covalently bind to endothelial and basement membranes where it can remain attached for long periods of time, therefore serving as a marker for complement activation in tissue such as a donor heart. It is also presumptive evidence of current or prior deposition of anti-donor antibodies.

Alternative pathway

The alternative pathway is considered part of the innate immune system because it has no requirement for antibody. This pathway

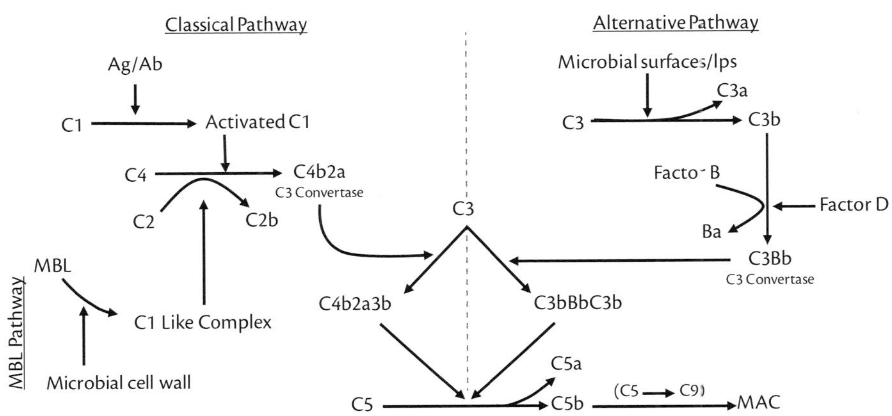

Fig. 4.13 The complement system can provide an immediate defense against organisms that gain access to the interior of the body. The two most active pathways are the classical pathway, which is antibody dependent, and the alternative pathway, which can activate immediately upon encounter with surfaces bearing a range of molecular patterns. Each of these pathways converges at C3, shown in the center of the diagram. Once C5 convertase is formed, the pathway proceeds to formation of the membrane attack complex (MAC), resulting in pores in the plasma membrane.

is activated on the basis of structural differences on the cell surface. C3, by itself, is relatively stable, but it is subject to hydrolysis, exposing new binding sites, which allows it to bind to cell surfaces, including host cells. On host cells, it is usually rapidly inactivated, so the reaction does not proceed. But on foreign surfaces such as bacteria, the C3b fragment remains on the cell surface much longer. This C3b then binds a serum protein called factor B. Factor B then exposes a site that allows another protein, factor D, to cleave factor B resulting in a C3 convertase (C3bBb). Properdin, a serum protein, stabilizes the C3 convertase. The C3 convertase catalyzes the formation of C3bBb3b, a C5 convertase with same activity as the C5 convertase generated by the classical pathway.

Membrane attack complex (MAC)

Both the alternative and classical pathways, as well as the MBL pathway, lead to the formation of the MAC. The MAC forms large channels in the cell membrane, essentially destroying the cell. Like the pathways leading to the formation of C5 convertases, the formation of the MAC results from a cascade of complement component activity. The C5 convertase cleaves C5, forming C5a and C5b. C5b binds to the cell membrane, which forms the initiation point of the MAC. This is stabilized by components C7, C8, and C9, which react sequentially in this complex ultimately forming a tubular structure that creates a pore in the cell membrane. Osmotic and electrolyte integrity is lost and the cell dies.

In transplantation, complement activation is a serious event, typically initiated by anti-donor antibodies. However, once the classical pathway is activated, it is also supplemented by the alternative pathway, which can actually generate the bulk of complement activity. The consequences of complement activation, at one extreme, can be wholesale destruction of the donor organ through direct lysis and loss of vascular integrity, an exceedingly rare event in clinical transplantation. Even relatively low levels of complement activation result in the generation of complement components that, although they may not contribute to the formation of MACs, have proinflammatory activity resulting in deleterious effects. C3a, for example has a number of activities, including enhancement of mast cell, basophil, and eosinophil degranulation as well as chemotaxis of leukocytes. Hence in the second decade of the 21st century there is increasing attention on the detection of these components. C4d, as noted earlier, is used as a marker of antibody-mediated rejection because of its persistence in tissue.

Activation of the immune response after heart transplantation

Before transplantation, there are events and factors that can affect subsequent events. Some of these factors include the extent of ischemia-reperfusion injury in the donor heart, the number of HLA mismatches between donor and recipient, age of the recipient, and presence or absence of particular viruses (e.g., Epstein–Barr virus or cytomegalovirus). From the perspective of the host immune response, the initial event is the implantation of the donor heart: specifically, it is the removal of the cross-clamp allowing entry of recipient blood into the heart and release of donor materials into the recipient circulation. Early post-transplant, the materials released from the heart will be donor cells, some of which will be APCs, cellular fragments, soluble proteins, exosomes, and other particles. Once this occurs, a number of cellular and molecular events are set in motion that, if allowed to proceed unchecked, will result in complete destruction of the donor organ within days, a process called *allograft rejection*. The pathological features resulting from allograft rejection, their identification, and prevention or treatment with immunosuppressive drugs are the basis of clinical practice in heart transplantation.

Recognition of the donor heart

The moment of removal of the cross-clamp after transplantation of the donor heart is when the host immune system detects the presence of nonself tissue within the body. Materials leaving the heart are flushed into the peripheral circulation (defined here as circulating blood and lymph). Some of the material leaving the heart will bear donor HLA antigens that are different than those of the host. Some of this material will be APCs from the donor, as well as cellular fragments with HLA antigens on them and in nanoparticulate or soluble form. In minutes, donor antigens in these forms begin to be taken up by host phagocytic cells, especially macrophages and dendritic cells, which are present at highest density in the spleen and lymph nodes. Kupffer cells in the liver also take up a considerable amount of material, but the role of these cells in heart transplantation is not known. Lymph nodes are very efficient at retaining antigen that passes into them via the afferent lymphatic vessels (see Figure 4.3). They can retain up to 90% of antigen that arrives in soluble form, in antigen–antibody complexes, and as antigen in dendritic cells and macrophages. The lymph nodes, spleen and gut associated lymphoid tissue (GALT) provide a microenvironment optimal for APCs to come into contact with T cells that traffic through the lymph node. In lymph nodes, dendritic cells enter from the periphery into the paracortex that is populated by T cells, macrophages, and interdigitating dendritic cells (IDCs). The IDCs, as well as other dendritic cells, constantly internalize molecules and particles form the surrounding environment and present them on their surfaces. Dendritic cells and IDCs have extremely large surface areas. IDCs have especially long cytoplasmic "arms" extending through the lymph node, contacting as many as 200 T cells at the same time. If any T cell within the lymphoid organ is specific for one of the donor HLA antigens, it is very likely to come into contact with an APC, which will present the donor antigen along with other requisite signals and activate the T cell. If a T cell does not encounter an antigen for which it is specific, it will not be retained in the lymph node. Instead, it will leave the lymph node via the efferent lymphatic vessels in the medulla and re-enter the circulation via the thoracic duct or enter another lymph node. T cells are highly mobile,[38] as are NK cells,[39,40] neutrophils,[41,42] monocytes,[43] and B cells.[44,45] Therefore, T cells scan the environment and may be retained in a particular location depending on the signals in the local environment. Naive T cells enter the lymph nodes from the blood via specialized high endothelial venules. Memory T cells enter lymph nodes via the afferent lymph, which drains into the paracortex.

In transplantation, donor antigen also makes its way into the secondary lymphoid organs on donor APCs. This can be in the form of dendritic cells or macrophages formerly residing within the graft interstitium or circulation. It can also be in the form of other cell types, such as vascular endothelial cells which have upregulated HLA molecules on their surfaces and been shed into the circulation.

Presentation of donor antigens

While antigen presentation and T cell activation have been previously discussed in general terms, they merit special attention in the

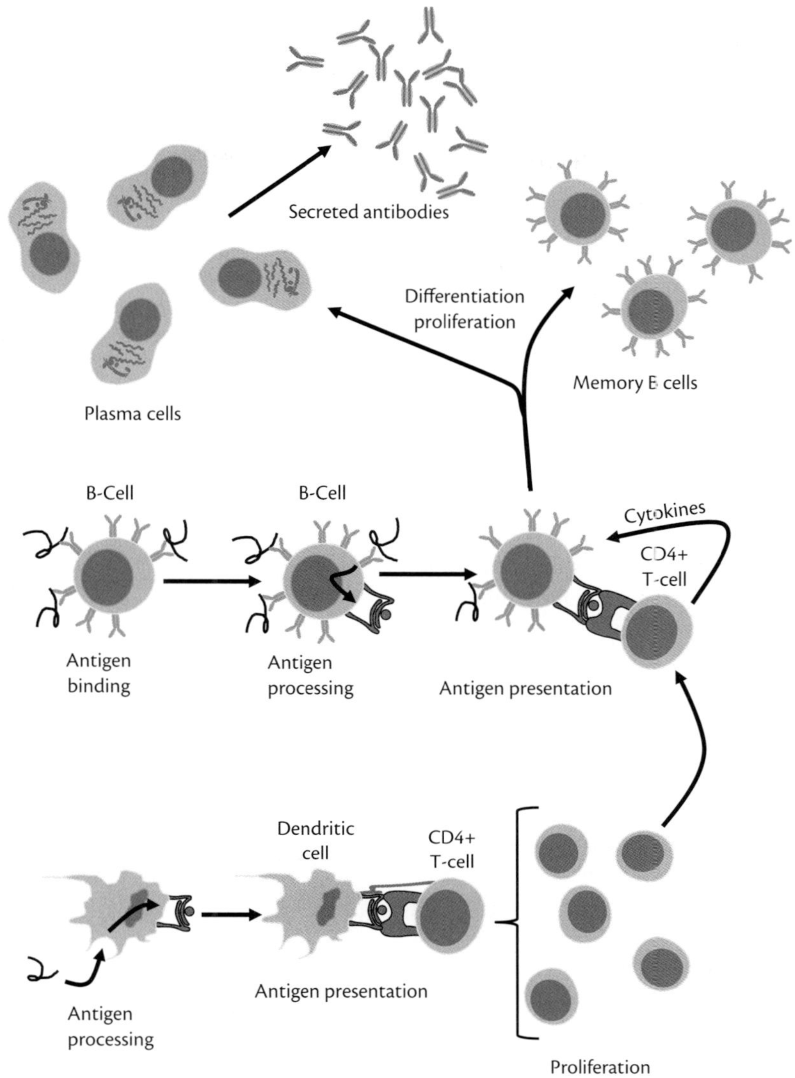

Fig. 4.14 Cellular mechanisms of antibody generation. Antibody generation is the result of cellular cooperation between antigen-presenting cells (APCs), T cells, and B cells. APCs ingest antigen, process it, and present it to a T cell of the appropriate specificity. The T cell becomes activated and clonally expands. The resulting T cells differentiate into functional subsets, which include T cells capable of facilitating B cell activation. B cells bind antigen via immunoglobulin receptors, internalize it, process it, and present it to activated T cells. In this way, B cells will only interact with T cells specific for the same antigen. Through signal exchange via surface receptors and soluble factors, B cells proliferate and differentiate into memory B cells and plasma cells. Plasma cells secrete large amounts of antibody into the circulation.

context of heart transplantation. In the transplantation literature one often sees the terms "direct" and "indirect" antigen presentation or allorecognition. As noted earlier, APCs originating from the donor can enter the recipient circulation. These cells express intact, unprocessed donor HLA molecules. Host T cells are "educated" or selected to recognize host HLA molecules incorporating a nonself peptide, yet a large number of host T cells will recognize unprocessed donor HLA molecules, and the peptide that resides within the peptide-binding groove of the HLA molecule is often unimportant. This phenomenon is called *direct recognition*. Notably, the frequency of host T cells that recognize antigen in this manner is 10–100-fold higher than those that recognize antigen in the "normal" manner, i.e., as a peptide complexed with self HLA.[3,4] Because of this, responses driven through the direct pathway can be remarkably strong, even without prior immunization. Since APCs are terminally differentiated cells arising from the bone marrow, the number of donor APCs in the host declines over time. Many have speculated that this could be the reason for the rapid decline in the frequency of rejection in the first year post-transplantation. *Indirect recognition* is the "normal" mode of recognition in which donor HLA molecules are processed by recipient APCs and presented as peptides complexed with recipient HLA molecules.

Once recognition of donor HLA antigens has taken place, the molecular and cellular events described earlier as T cell activation take place, culminating in clonal expansion and differentiation of T cells into various effector subsets, many of which will find their way into the graft parenchyma. There they can exert direct cytotoxicity and mediate inflammation. T cells that remain in the lymph node can cooperate with B cells so that they can differentiate into antibody-producing plasma cells, undergo class switching, and produce antibodies of higher affinity for donor antigen. Figure 4.14 shows a global model of the events so far discussed, showing how both free antigen and their cell-bound processed peptides drive the specific immune response. Immunosuppressive drugs largely target these pathways and therefore tend to inhibit humoral immunity as well, albeit less effectively. At the time of writing, only one drug targets plasma cells directly.

The role of innate immunity

During the process of transplantation, from organ procurement to implantation, the donor organ is subject to stress resulting from a number of variables including events taking place in the donor, ischemic time, and technical issues during implantation. These events can strongly influence the host immune system, especially early post-transplant. A large component of these early responses is the innate immune system, so called because it is largely based on pattern recognition and is much less specific than adaptive immunity. Innate immunity can provide immediate or nearly immediate defense. Complement is one part of innate immunity, providing nearly immediate defense when activated via the alternative or lectin pathways. Many cell types, such as neutrophils, macrophages, and dendritic cells express invariant pattern recognition receptors that enable detection of repetitive structural units on pathogens. Such receptors can also detect damage-associated molecular patterns on heat shock proteins and other damage-related molecules such as heparan sulfate. There are several families of pattern recognition receptors, including Toll-like receptors (TLR), C-type lectin receptors, and a variety of cytoplasmic receptors. Thus, innate immunity can be triggered by an array of molecules associated with tissue damage. The signals from these receptors result in upregulation of genes and secretion of proinflammatory proteins, many of which can augment specific immunity. The secreted molecules include IL-1, IL-6, TNF, and chemokines, which attract other cells to the site. Interferons can upregulate HLA molecules, augmenting the specific immune response. This process will begin immediately after implantation and it will occur even if there is no genetic disparity between donor and recipient.

Concluding remarks

Since the immunologic basis of solid organ transplant rejection was discovered in the mid-20th century, the science of transplantation immunology has been an active and dynamic field of study. However, clinical heart transplantation, pioneered by Shumway and colleagues, only began to be widely accepted after the introduction of cyclosporin, a calcineurin inhibitor that targets T cell activation. The clinical inhibition of calcineurin in combination with other drugs is discussed in Chapter 17. Based on our knowledge of the mechanisms of cell-mediated immune responses, new classes of drugs such as those that block costimulation or block the IL-2 receptor have become available, giving physicians more options for treating rejection and for maintenance immunosuppression. Future advances in transplantation immunology are characteristically difficult to predict. Based on discoveries in immunology, especially in the area of chronic inflammation, one can speculate that significant advances may be made with respect to the role of innate immunity in transplant rejection and to alternative strategies for induction of operational tolerance to the donor organ.

References

1. Gibson T, Medawar PB. The fate of skin homografts in man. J Anat 1943;77(Pt 4):299–310.
2. Medawar PB. The behaviour and fate of skin autografts and skin homografts in rabbits: A report to the War Wounds Committee of the Medical Research Council. J Anat 1944;78(Pt 5):176–99.
3. Liu Z, et al. Contribution of direct and indirect recognition pathways to T cell alloreactivity. J Exp Med 1993;177(6):1643–50.
4. Ansari AA, et al. Indirect presentation of donor histocompatibility antigens contributes to the allogeneic response against human cardiac myocytes. J Heart Lung Transplant 1992;11(3 Pt 1):467–77; discussion 477–8.
5. Stavnezer J, Immunoglobulin class switching. Curr Opin Immunol 1996;8(2):199–205.
6. Kiessling R, et al. Genetic variation of in vitro cytolytic activity and in vivo rejection potential of non-immunized semi-syngeneic mice against a mouse lymphoma line. Int J Cancer 1975;15(6):933–40.
7. Kiessling R, et al. Killer cells: a functional comparison between natural, immune T-cell and antibody-dependent in vitro systems. J Exp Med 1976;143(4):772–80.
8. Theze J, Alzari PM, Bertoglio J. Interleukin 2 and its receptors: recent advances and new immunological functions. Immunol Today 1996;17(10):481–6.
9. Sugamura K, et al. The interleukin-2 receptor gamma chain: its role in the multiple cytokine receptor complexes and T cell development in XSCID. Annu Rev Immunol 1996;14:179–205.
10. Gaulton GN, Williamson P. Interleukin-2 and the interleukin-2 receptor complex. Chem Immunol 1994;59:91–114.
11. Van Damme J, et al. Purification and characterization of human fibroblast-derived hybridoma growth factor identical to T-cell-derived B-cell stimulatory factor-2 (interleukin-6). Eur J Biochem 1987;168(3):543–50.
12. Spies T, et al. Genes for the tumor necrosis factors alpha and beta are linked to the human major histocompatibility complex. Proc Natl Acad Sci U S A 1986;83(22):8699–702.
13. Jones EY, Stuart DI, Walker NP. Structure of tumour necrosis factor. Nature 1989;338(6212):225–8.
14. Eck MJ, Sprang SR. The structure of tumor necrosis factor-alpha at 2.6 A resolution. Implications for receptor binding. J Biol Chem 1989;264(29):17595–605.
15. Barbara JA, Van Ostade X, Lopez A. Tumour necrosis factor-alpha (TNF-alpha): the good, the bad and potentially very effective. Immunol Cell Biol 1996;74(5):434–43.
16. Tracey KJ, Cerami A. Tumor necrosis factor: a pleiotropic cytokine and therapeutic target. Annu Rev Med 1994;45:491–503.
17. Beutler B, et al. Purification of cachectin, a lipoprotein lipase-suppressing hormone secreted by endotoxin-induced RAW 264.7 cells. J Exp Med 1985;161(5):984–95.
18. Weissenbach J, et al. Two interferon mRNAs in human fibroblasts: in vitro translation and Escherichia coli cloning studies. Proc Natl Acad Sci U S A 1980;77(12):7152–6.
19. McDouall RM, et al. MHC class II expression on human heart microvascular endothelial cells: exquisite sensitivity to interferon-gamma and natural killer cells. Transplantation 1997;64(8):1175–80.
20. Leszczynski D. Interleukin-1 alpha inhibits the effects of gamma-interferon and tumor necrosis factor alpha on the expression of the major histocompatibility antigens by the rat endothelium. Am J Pathol 1990;136(1):229–37.
21. Groenewegen G, et al. Effect of cyclosporine on MHC class II antigen expression on arterial and venous endothelium in vitro. Transplantation 1985;40(1):21–5.
22. Yao Z, et al. Herpesvirus Saimiri encodes a new cytokine, IL-17, which binds to a novel cytokine receptor. Immunity 1995;3(6):811–21.
23. Yao Z, et al. Human IL-17: a novel cytokine derived from T cells. J Immunol 1995;155(12):5483–6.
24. Gaffen SL. Structure and signalling in the IL-17 receptor family. Nat Rev Immunol 2009;9(8):556–67.
25. Gaffen SL. Recent advances in the IL-17 cytokine family. Curr Opin Immunol 2011;23(5):613–19.

26. Hogg N, Landis RC. Adhesion molecules in cell interactions. Curr Opin Immunol 1993;5(3):383–90.
27. Berlin C, et al. Alpha 4 integrins mediate lymphocyte attachment and rolling under physiologic flow. Cell 1995;80(3):413–22.
28. Bates PA, et al. Leukocyte integrin activation. Pathol Biol (Paris) 1992;40(8):785–8.
29. Stewart M, Thiel M, Hogg N. Leukocyte integrins. Curr Opin Cell Biol 1995;7(5):690–6.
30. Springer TA. Traffic signals on endothelium for lymphocyte recirculation and leukocyte emigration. Annu Rev Physiol 1995;57:827–72.
31. Luscinskas FW, Ding H, Lichtman AH. P-selectin and vascular cell adhesion molecule 1 mediate rolling and arrest, respectively, of CD4+ T lymphocytes on tumor necrosis factor alpha-activated vascular endothelium under flow. J Exp Med 1995;181(3):1179–86.
32. Klein CL, et al. Comparative studies on vascular endothelium in vitro. 3. Effects of cytokines on the expression of E-selectin, ICAM-1 and VCAM-1 by cultured human endothelial cells obtained from different passages. Pathobiology 1995;63(2):83–92.
33. Klein CL, et al. Comparative studies on vascular endothelium in vitro. I. Cytokine effects on the expression of adhesion molecules by human umbilical vein, saphenous vein and femoral artery endothelial cells. Pathobiology 1994;62(4):199–208.
34. Wagner DD. The Weibel-Palade body: the storage granule for von Willebrand factor and P-selectin. Thromb Haemost 1993;70(1):105–10.
35. Dole VS, et al. Activated platelets induce Weibel-Palade-body secretion and leukocyte rolling in vivo: role of P-selectin. Blood 2005;106(7):2334–9.
36. Taylor PM, et al. Induction of vascular adhesion molecules during rejection of human cardiac allografts. Transplantation 1992;54(3):451–7.
37. Ruan XM, et al. Cytokine expression and endothelial cell and lymphocyte activation in human cardiac allograft rejection: an immunohistochemical study of endomyocardial biopsy samples. J Heart Lung Transplant 1992;11(6):1110–15.
38. Germain RN, Robey EA, Cahalan MD. A decade of imaging cellular motility and interaction dynamics in the immune system. Science 2012;336(6089):1676–81.
39. Celli S, Albert ML, Bousso P. Visualizing the innate and adaptive immune responses underlying allograft rejection by two-photon microscopy. Nat Med 2011;17(6):744–9.
40. Garrod KR, et al. Natural killer cells actively patrol peripheral lymph nodes forming stable conjugates to eliminate MHC-mismatched targets. Proc Natl Acad Sci U S A 2007;104(29):12081–6.
41. Chtanova T, et al. Dynamics of neutrophil migration in lymph nodes during infection. Immunity 2008;29(3):487–96.
42. Peters NC, et al. In vivo imaging reveals an essential role for neutrophils in leishmaniasis transmitted by sand flies. Science 2008;321(5891):970–4.
43. Auffray C, et al. Monitoring of blood vessels and tissues by a population of monocytes with patrolling behavior. Science 2007;317(5838):666–70.
44. Cahalan MD, et al. Two-photon tissue imaging: seeing the immune system in a fresh light. Nat Rev Immunol 2002;2(11):872–80.
45. Wei SH, et al. Two-photon imaging in intact lymphoid tissue. Adv Exp Med Biol 2002;512: 203–8.
46. Schroeder HW, Jr., et al. Developmental regulation of the human antibody repertoire. Ann N Y Acad Sci 1995;764:242–60.
47. Zemlin M, et al. Regulation and chance in the ontogeny of B and T cell antigen receptor repertoires. Immunol Res 2002;26(1–3):265–78.
48. George JF, Jr., Schroeder HW, Jr. Developmental regulation of D beta reading frame and junctional diversity in T cell receptor-beta transcripts from human thymus. J Immunol 1992;148(4):1230–9.
49. Borst J, et al. Non-random expression of T cell receptor gamma and delta variable gene segments in functional T lymphocyte clones from human peripheral blood. Eur J Immunol 1989 19(9):1559–68.
50. Milstein C, et al. Non-random features of the repertoire expressed by the members of one V kappa gene family and of the V-J recombination. Eur J Immunol 1992;22(6):1627–34.
51. Feeney AJ, Tang A, Ogwaro KM. B-cell repertoire formation: role of the recombination signal sequence in non-random V segment utilization. Immunol Rev 2000;175:59–69.
52. Alt FW, et al. Ordered rearrangement of immunoglobulin heavy chain variable region segments. EMBO J 1984;3(6):1209–19.
53. Cook GP, et al. A map of the human immunoglobulin VH locus completed by analysis of the telomeric region of chromosome 14q. Nat Genet 1994;7(2):162–8.
54. Tomlinson IM, et al. Human immunoglobulin VH and D segments on chromosomes 15q11.2 and 16p11.2. Hum Mol Genet 1994;3(6):853–60.
55. Seidman JG, et al. Multiple related immunoglobulin variable-region genes identified by cloning and sequence analysis. Proc Natl Acad Sci U S A 1978;75(8):3881–5.
56. Desiderio SV, et al. Insertion of N regions into heavy-chain genes is correlated with expression of terminal deoxytransferase in B cells. Nature 1984;311(5988):752–5.
57. Alt FW, Baltimore D. Joining of immunoglobulin heavy chain gene segments: implications from a chromosome with evidence of three D-JH fusions. Proc Natl Acad Sci U S A 1982;79(13):4118–22.
58. Kim S, et al. Antibody diversity: somatic hypermutation of rearranged VH genes. Cell 1981;27(3 Pt 2):573–81.
59. Berek C, Milstein C. Mutation drift and repertoire shift in the maturation of the immune response. Immunol Rev 1987;96:23–41.

CHAPTER 5

Implantable devices for cardiovascular monitoring

Max J. Liebo MD and W. H. Wilson Tang MD

Introduction

Despite major advancements in treatment and management, heart failure (HF) remains the most common indication for hospitalization in Americans over 65 years of age and is associated with the highest readmission rates of any medical condition (27% at 30 days, 44% at 6 months).[1,2,3] Not only do these hospitalizations strongly influence the progression of left ventricular (LV) dysfunction, they account for up to 70% of the total cost of HF[4] and thus represent an important target to reduce both individual morbidity and mortality as well as societal costs. Conventional HF management approaches focusing on the development of symptoms and changes in weight have proven inadequate in limiting these hospital admissions, and clinicians have started to look for novel means to ameliorate the growing epidemic. Despite their proven efficacy, structured telephone support programs have failed to achieve widespread use, in part due to resource intensiveness but—perhaps more importantly—due to overreliance on motivated patients and antiquated markers of disease. Over the last few decades many new implantable sensor technologies have emerged, and capabilities for remote monitoring of HF patients have increased dramatically. Many of these advances have stemmed from the increased prophylactic and therapeutic utilization of cardiovascular implantable electronic devices (CIEDs), including implantable cardioverter defibrillator (ICD) and cardiac resynchronization therapy (CRT), while others have developed as stand-alone devices, including implantable hemodynamic monitors (IHM). All have offered new insights into the pathophysiology of HF decompensations and illuminated novel targets that might facilitate more timely therapeutic intervention and better stave off overt decompensations, hospitalizations, and disease progression. While these implantable sensor technologies have the potential to significantly enhance the clinician's armamentarium, many of the modalities are only in their infancy and will require further investigation and experience to standardize their use and identify their place in HF management. Similarly, these new technologies promise to generate vast amounts of data, and equally sophisticated triage systems will need to evolve in order to prevent overloading already overburdened clinicians. In this chapter we begin by discussing the pathophysiology around the transition from chronic stable to acute decompensated heart failure (ADHF) from the point of view of the implantable sensors, then proceed to describe the different types of implantable cardiac monitoring devices and remote monitoring systems, and end with a discussion regarding the strategies for utilizing these implantable monitors in clinical practice along with their present limitations and a view to the future.

Pathophysiologic insights derived from sensor technology

Given that over 90% of HF hospitalizations are characterized by excess intravascular volume and uncontrolled pulmonary and systemic congestion,[5] current HF guidelines emphasize the importance of daily volume assessment and vigilant attention to the signs and symptoms of HF. However, while highly specific, signs of volume overload (including an increase in body weight) have been shown to have poor sensitivity (<20%) for detecting incipient exacerbations,[6] and it is clear that most clinical decompensations do not start at the moment a patient's weight changes or symptoms develop.[7] Recent clinical studies with implantable devices have provided new insights into the pathophysiology of the transition from chronic compensated HF to ADHF, and these insights are highlighted in Figure 5.1.

In patients with systolic or diastolic HF the earliest measureable change in a physiologic parameter seems to be a small but consistent increase in cardiac filling pressures that begins up to 24–30 days before the event.[8,9,10] This rise in filling pressures is similar in patients with systolic and diastolic HF and likely results from very small increases in intravascular volume due to gradual accumulation, vascular redistribution, and/or alterations in vascular tone.[9,10,11,12] As the body attempts to maintain homeostasis autonomic dysregulation ensues, manifested primarily by vagal withdrawal and sympathetic dominance that lead to a decrease in heart rate variability (HRV) that is detectable up to 21 days before hospitalization.[12,13] The increased filling pressures and autonomic maladaptation can then lead to a more substantial increase in fluid accumulation and/or vascular redistribution that is detectable by intrathoracic impedance measurements as early as 18 days before admission.[14] Finally, overt clinical symptoms and an increase in total body weight may become detectable by the patient around 1 week prior to admission.[15]

While the described timeline of physiologic alterations associated with HF decompensation (see Figure 5.1) suggests early detection is practical and straightforward, it is important to note that the clinical studies and trials evaluating IHMs and electrophysiologic variables revealed wide changes during regular daily activities, physical exercise, and changes in body position that are likely "normal biological variations," and as such not

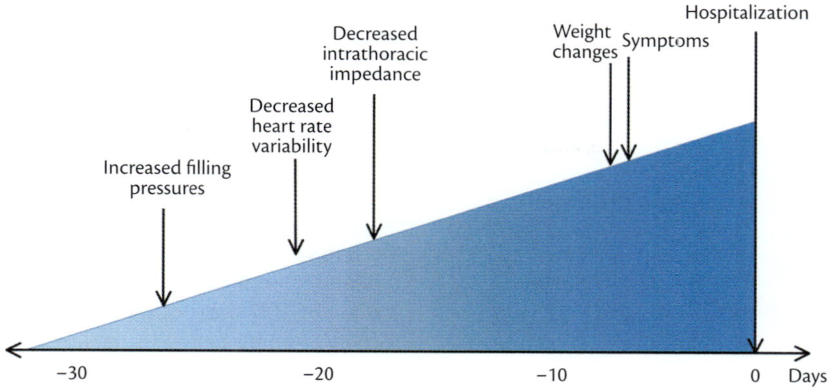

Fig. 5.1 Pathophysiology (and potential therapeutic targets) from the perspective of implantable sensors during the transition from chronic stable to acute decompensated HF.

Modified from Adamson, PB. Current Heart Failure Reports 2009;6:287–292, Springer.

every rise in cardiac filling pressures or reduction in intrathoracic impedance or HRV is an indicator of incipient ADHF.[16,17] Moreover, the described timeline delineates the average point at which a significant change in each parameter has been reported, and not every individual patient will necessarily follow the timeline in the same manner when transitioning from stable to decompensated HF.

General assumptions

Before delving into each individual sensor technology and physiologic parameter in detail, it is important to consider the general assumptions being made when applying any of these diagnostic devices to patient management:

- Device-based diagnostics measure physiologic signals that are indicative of physiologic derangements.
- The fidelity and biological variability of such measurements are within the ranges of an acceptable "confidence interval" for therapeutic decision-making.
- There are changes in therapeutic approaches that can be based on differences in measurements.
- There are systems of care that can ultimately implement this "care loop."

In many ways these assumptions are not unique to implantable monitoring devices and are already a part of everyday clinical medicine. For example, most clinicians recognize and accept the variability of home blood-pressure monitoring and are comfortable using it to make decisions as we have studies telling us how to react and respond to these numbers, albeit inaccurate and in an asynchronous communications manner. The difference with implantable devices and remote monitoring technology, and what poses the greatest challenge to their translation at this time, is that we lack a commensurate level of experience. Only through further investigation and additional "field testing" will we learn how to best utilize these technologies and feel comfortable integrating them into clinical practice. The following sections thus focus not only on the science and rationale behind implantable sensors and the biological parameters they monitor but also describe the present state of evidence for their incorporation into the management of patients with HF.

Electrophysiologic parameters

The recent increase in utilization of CIEDs in patients with HF has provided an opportunity to monitor a growing number of electrophysiologic parameters that may aid in the management of HF patients. In addition to their therapeutic and life-saving functions, these devices provide continuous monitoring of heart rhythm, device therapy (percent biventricular pacing, anti-tachycardia pacing, and ICD shocks), heart rate, and HRV that can be analyzed by the clinician during routine follow-up office visits or transmitted from the patient's home to a central server for remote follow-up (discussed later in the chapter). Attention to each of these parameters (summarized in Table 5.1) may play an important role in predicting and preventing episodes of ADHF, and consequently they have become subjects of growing interest and investigation.

Heart rhythm and device therapy

Among patients with HF, atrial and ventricular dysrrhythmias—i.e., atrial tachycardia (AT), atrial fibrillation (AF), premature ventricular complexes (PVC), and ventricular tachycardia (VT)—are quite common. As many as 20–35% of patients hospitalized for ADHF have AT or AF as their presenting rhythm, and registry data suggest these dysrrhythmias are a precipitating factor in over 13% of HF admissions.[18,19] Contemporary CIEDs continuously monitor AT/AF burden as well as their corresponding ventricular rates with high accuracy,[20] and recent studies have demonstrated that device-detected AT/AF is associated with a poor prognosis, increased HF hospitalizations, and increased death.[21] It is also clear that newly recognized AT/AF (particularly when associated with poor rate control) is a strong independent predictor of increased cardiovascular hospitalization,[22,23] and that rapid AF can have a particularly deleterious effect on patients undergoing CRT by reducing the overall time spent biventricular pacing.[24] Ventricular tachyarrhythmias and both appropriate and inappropriate ICD shocks are also associated with worse long-term prognosis, increased HF events, and death;[25,26] even high PVC burden is an established independent risk predictor of death in patients with chronic HF.[27] Consequently the presence of these arrhythmias and their effect on device therapy have been incorporated into a number of CIED diagnostic algorithms developed for the purpose of risk stratification in the advanced HF population (see Table 5.2). While there have been no studies to date that specifically evaluate how a change in cardiac rhythm or HF management based

Table 5.1 Parameters continuously monitored by contemporary cardiac implantable electronic devices

Parameter	Description	Sign of worsening HF
Atrial fibrillation		
Duration	Trends the total time spent in AF on a daily basis	New-onset AF Increased AF burden
Ventricular rate	Trends the average daily ventricular rate occurring during AF	Poorly controlled ventricular rates
Ventricular arrhythmias		
Device therapy	Records frequency and duration of VT/VF episodes	VT/VF may precipitate or be a sign of worsening HF
ATP/ICD shocks	Records episodes of ATP, appropriate, and inappropriate shocks	Increased ATP and ICD shocks
Percent BiV pacing	Records the percentage of time each day spent ventricularly pacing	Reduction in time spent BiV pacing
HR		
Mean HR	Trends baseline HR	Increase in HR
NHR	Trends average resting HR while patient sleeps	Increase in NHR
Heart rate variability	Trends daily average of the standard deviations of 5-minute median atrial-to-atrial depolarization intervals (SDAAM). HRV is not computed if > 80% of time is AP/AT/AF	HRV decreases as vagal input is withdrawn and autonomic outflow becomes more sympathetic dominant
Patient activity	Accelerometer-detected anteroposterior motion of the chest wall quantifies patient activity levels (ACT)	Decrease in ACT
Intrathoracic impedance	Trends the average daily impedance, reference baseline impedance, and their cumulative negative difference (FI)	Reduction in impedance As intrathoracic fluid increases, average daily impedance decreases below the reference impedance and the FI increases

ACT, activity counts; AF, atrial fibrillation; AP, atrial paced; AT, atrial tachycardia; ATP, anti-tachycardia pacing; BiV, biventricular; FI, fluid index; HR, heart rate; HRV, heart rate variability; ICD, implantable cardioverter defibrillator; NHR, night heart rate; VF, ventricular fibrillation; VT, ventricular tachycardia.

on CIED-identified dysrrhythmias affects HF outcomes, the current evidence strongly supports its prognostic value in risk-stratifying HF patients, and better attention toward and treatment of these dysrrhythmias does indeed appear warranted.

Heart rate

Perhaps the simplest biological parameter continuously monitored by CIEDs is heart rate; even the earliest-generation devices have the capability of trending the intrinsic and/or paced heart rate over time. Intrinsic heart rate is under the control of the autonomic nervous system (ANS), and an increase in both resting and mean heart rate is one of the earliest signs of stress on the cardiovascular system or the body in general. It is no surprise then that an elevated resting heart rate has been associated with increased mortality in patients with HF,[28] and when trended over time with an implanted device can identify patients with suboptimal HF control who are at increased short-term and long-term risk for destabilization, decompensation, and adverse HF events/outcomes.

Contemporary studies evaluating the sensitivity and predictive value of CIED diagnostics for adverse HF events have included a variety of simple heart rate parameters (resting heart rate, nighttime heart rate [NHR], and mean heart rate), the reported sensitivity of which ranges widely (14–70%) depending on which parameter is evaluated, what threshold and duration for "elevated heart rate" are used (typically >80–90 bpm for NHR or an "increase" in resting/mean heart rate from a few days to >1 week preceding the HF event), and what primary outcomes are evaluated (worsening HF, hospital admission for ADHF, or hospital admission for any cardiovascular event).[29,30,31] While an increase in mean resting heart rate and 24-hour heart rate within 7 days was the most reliable predictor of HF-rehospitalization in one study,[29] and NHR has been demonstrated to be a significant univariate predictor of 30-day HF readmissions (HR 2.5, CI 1.2–5.1, $p = 0.011$) in another recent study,[32] neither has consistently been identified as an independent predictor of HF events; rather, they appear to be most incremental when combined with other CIED diagnostic parameters. A few studies have evaluated the effect of improved HF management, namely via implementation of CRT, on resting and mean heart rates demonstrating significant reductions in both parameters in patients that respond well to resynchronization therapy.[33]

Heart rate variability

Another heart rate parameter derived from CIED data that can provide insight into the body's physiologic state is HRV. As previously mentioned, heart rate is controlled by the ANS which continuously receives afferent nerve information from baroreceptors in the aorta and cardiopulmonary areas and, via its efferent sympathetic and parasympathetic arms, constantly adjusts heart rate, contractility, and vasomotor tone in order to maintain homeostasis. Most of the beat-to-beat variation in heart rate (commonly encountered as respiratory sinus arrhythmia) is due to parasympathetic vagal tone;[34] however, when the cardiovascular system is in a diseased or decompensated state, autonomic dysregulation ensues manifested primarily by vagal withdrawal, sympathetic dominance, and a resultant decrease in HRV. While much of the literature on HRV comes from point-in-time investigations comparing R-R intervals obtained from electrocardiograms and Holter monitors before and during disease states,[27,35] the incorporation of HRV algorithms into contemporary CIEDs has recently made it possible to continuously monitor these values and trend them over time.

The most common algorithm for computing HRV using implanted monitoring devices calculates the standard deviation of the 5-minute median atrial sensed A-A intervals (SDAAM) and then records an averaged daily SDAAM every 24 hours for trending purposes. Because this measurement of HRV is dependent on small autonomic alterations in the intrinsic sinus nodal activity, episodes of AT, AF, and atrial pacing are typically excluded from analysis if they exceed 80% of the 24-hour period. Less commonly the R-R

Table 5.2 Trials evaluating combined device diagnostics for risk stratification of patients with heart failure

Study, author (year)	Study design	Study population	*n*	Device diagnostic parameters	Primary endpoint	Results
Perego et al. (2008)	Multicenter, prospective, observational	NYHA II (40%) NYHA III (57%) CRT-D	558	1. Intrathoracic impedance TCE (FI 60 Ω d) 2. Patient activity (ACT <30 min) 3. Tachyarrhythmia events (AT and VT) 4. NHR (>90 bpm) 5. HRV (<80 ms)	Adjudicated HF hospitalization	TCE, patient activity, and HRV were all independently associated with increased risk for HF hospitalization
OFFISER, Small et al. (2009)	Multicenter, retrospective	NYHA II (17%) NYHA III (79%) CRT-D	326	1. Intrathoracic impedance TCE (FI 60 Ω d) 2. Patient activity (<30 min) 3. HRV (<80 ms) 4. NHR (>90 bpm)	Adjudicated HF hospitalization	TCE frequency (OR 1.352, $p < 0.001$) and NHR (OR 1.007, $p < 0.001$) only independent risk factors
PARTNERS-HF, Whellan et al. (2010)	Multicenter, prospective, observational	NYHA III CRT-D	694	1. Intrathoracic impedance TCE with very high FI (100 Ω·d) 2. Any two: • High FI (60 Ω d) • Patient activity (<1 h over 1 wk) • NHR (>85 bpm × 7 d) • HRV (<60 ms × 5 d) • AF duration (≥ 6 h in one day) • AF + RVR (ave HR ≥ 90 bpm ≥1 d) • % CRT (BiV pacing < 90% for 5 of 7 d) • ICD shocks (≥shock)	Adjudicated HF hospitalizations within 30 days	Combined HF device algorithm (HR 5.5, 95% CI 3.4 to 8.8, $p < 0.0001$) significantly identified increased risk beyond intrathoracic impedance alone (HR 2.7, $p < 0.0001$)
Home-CARE, Sack et al. (2011)	Multicenter, prospective, observational	NYHA II (15%) NYHA III (75%) NHYA IV (8.5%) CRT-D	377	1. 24 hour mean heart rate 2. Resting heart rate 3. Patient activity 4. RV apical impedance 5. Number of PVCs 6. Enhanced predictors • HRV • Painless shock impedance	Adjudicated CV hospitalization (worse HF 52%, arrhythmias 20%, chest pain 9%, syncope 5%) within 30 days	Combined device diagnostic sensitivity 65%, specificity 99.5%, with 1.8 FP per patient year, PPV 7.8, and NPV 99.9%
Whellan et al. (2013)	Multicenter, retrospective	NYHA II-III ICD/CRT-D	166	1. Intrathoracic impedance TCE (FI 60 Ω·d) 2. Any AF diagnostic • duration ≥ 6 h ≥ 1 d • Ave HR ≥ 90 bpm ≥ 1 d • BiV pacing £90% 3. NHR (> 80 ≥ 1 d) 4. HRV	Rehospitalization for HF within 30 d	Impedance, AF, AF + RVR, reduced CRT, and high NHR were significant univariate predictors. HRV was not

ACT, activity counts; AF, atrial fibrillation; AT, arial tachyarrhythmia; BiV, biventricular; CRT, cardiac resynchronization therapy; CRT-D, cardiac resynchronization therapy implantable cardioverter defibrillator device; FI, fluid index; FP, false positive; HR, heart rate; HRV, heart rate variability; ICD, implantable cardioverter defibrillator; NHR, night heart rate; NPV, negative predictive value; NYHA,New York Heart Association functional class; PPV, positive predictive value; RVR, rapid ventricular response; TCE, threshold-crossing event; VT, ventricular tachyarrhythmia.

interval obtained from the right ventricular (RV) electrode is utilized for calculating HRV. Additional algorithms have been devised to assist in the trending of SDAAM data over time (akin to those devised for monitoring changes in intrathoracic impedance, discussed later). After excluding the first 4 weeks following implantation of the device to allow patients to return to their normal lifestyle following surgery, an adaptive reference baseline is computed for the individual patient based on their preceding SDAAM values. The measured daily SDAAM is then compared to the adaptive reference SDAAM, and any negative difference is accumulated based on its magnitude and duration until it crosses an arbitrary threshold programmed into the CIED.[13]

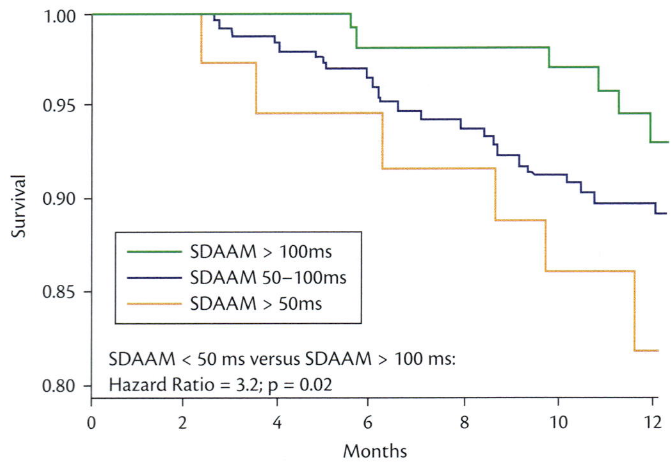

Fig. 5.2 Heart rate variability and all-cause mortality. Kaplan–Meier survival curves based on average heart rate variability (SDAAM) tertiles as measured from weeks 5 to 8 after device implantation.

Adamson et al. Continuous autonomic assessment in patients with symptomatic heart failure: prognostic value of heart rate variability measured by an implantable cardiac resynchronization device. Circulation 2004;110:2389–94.

The evidence supporting use of HRV data for managing HF patients has been steadily growing, and over the past decade a number of studies have demonstrated both short-term[27] and long-term[13] prognostic value of absolute SDAAM values (low <50 ms, intermediate 50–100 ms, high >100 ms) with respect to HF hospitalizations and survival (see Figure 5.2). A decrease in HRV has 50–70% sensitivity for HF hospitalizations,[13,31] and trending of SDAAM values has shown that these changes in HRV occur weeks before patients note changes in body weight, signs, and/or symptoms heralding HF decompensation and hospital admissions.[13] Other studies have demonstrated that improvements in HRV with a shift away from sympathetic dominance seem to occur earlier and be even more robust than the improvements in resting and mean heart rate following implementation of CRT.[33,36] Like other electrophysiologic parameters obtained from CIEDs, HRV data can be reviewed by the clinician during regular office visits to assist with risk stratification and prognostication, and/or can be remotely downloaded over the internet intermittently for the purpose of early identification of potential HF decompensations.

Patient activity and minute ventilation

Another objective physiologic parameter that can be continuously monitored by CIEDs is patient activity (see Table 5.1). Originally incorporated into CIEDs to modulate rate-adaptive pacing, capacitive accelerometers have subsequently been recognized as a means of tracking patient activity levels as a marker of their functional status. The accelerometer works by sensing anteroposterior motion of the chest wall and accumulating the total number of activity counts each minute, and various algorithms have been developed to quantify and trend these activity counts in terms of steps per minute or a mean daily workload. Clinicians can then program the device with an arbitrary threshold whereby a minute that contains a sufficient number of counts above or below that threshold (typically equal to walking 70 steps/min) is considered "active" or "inactive," respectively. As HF patients transition from chronic stable to ADHF it is reasonable to think their activity levels would decrease. Moreover, it is reasonable to think that small decreases in patient activity levels might be detectable by the accelerometer before the patients themselves note any decline in their function. The value of this novel metric has been evaluated in a number of combined CIED diagnostic studies, though given substantial variability in the definitions and thresholds used, its true predictive ability remains unclear. While low patient activity was one of the most common findings (second only to intrathoracic impedance) in two of the larger studies to evaluate combined CIED diagnostics in patients hospitalized for HF,[30,37] it was the least predictive of six parameters tested (with a disappointing 23% sensitivity) in another study.[31] While patient activity has not been demonstrated to be a robust independent predictor, it does appear to be an integral part of combined CIED diagnostic algorithms for risk stratification and prediction of HF events (Table 5.2).

Another objective parameter that has variably been used to provide information regarding functional status is minute ventilation (MV). As with accelerometers, impedance MV sensors were initially designed and incorporated into CIEDs for the purpose of modulating rate-adaptive pacing. By sensing small changes in thoracic impedance throughout the respiratory cycle, these sensors are capable of measuring respiratory rate and tidal volume from which MV can be calculated, and several clinical studies have shown high correlation between impedance MV and the actual MV measured by a cardiopulmonary system.[38,39] Observational studies have demonstrated that MV is significantly higher both at rest and with activity in patients with HF as compared to controls, and in at least one small study an increase in MV was predictive of HF hospitalizations with a sensitivity of 88%, specificity 94%, positive predictive value 71% (0.55 false positives per patient year), and negative predictive value 98%.[40] Unfortunately impedance MV sensors are not as commonly employed as accelerometers in contemporary CIEDs and thus have so far been the subject of limited research. Consequently they are not currently incorporated into any of the contemporary HF device diagnostic algorithms.

Intrathoracic impedance

Impedance, denoted by the symbol Z and quantified in ohms (Ω) is a measure of the degree to which a medium or substance resists the flow of electrical current. The more resistance a substance has to current, the higher its impedance; conversely, the less resistance a substance has to current, the lower its impedance. Empirically, blood and fluid (65–150 Ω cm) provide much less resistance to current than thoracic tissue (200–5000 Ω cm),[41] and it has subsequently been demonstrated that increases in thoracic fluid volume and left heart filling pressures are associated with a measurable decrease in intrathoracic impedance.[14]

The principle of impedance has provided the basis for a number of diagnostic medical applications over the past half-century. As early as the 1940s it was recognized that beat-to-beat changes in impedance are related to pulsatile blood volume,[42] and by the 1970s impedance cardiography (ICG), measured by four external band electrodes placed on the bilateral neck and lower thorax ("band electrode method"), was established as a means of noninvasively estimating stroke volume, cardiac output, systemic vascular resistance, and intrathoracic fluid volume.[43,44] These classic ICG measurements have been fairly well validated[45] and effectively used to assist in the one-off selection and titration of medications for patients with hemodynamic derangements;[46] however, their utility for long-term or serial monitoring has ultimately been limited by the need for the patient to be on location for the test; confounding of sequential measurements related to variable electrode placement, temporal differences in skin moisture, blood composition, and body habitus; and the questionable accuracy and consistency of cardiac output measurements in late-stage HF patients.[47,48]

Coincident with the recent proliferation of CIEDs in the HF population, a more contemporary "implanted device-based method" for measuring intrathoracic impedance was developed. While initially incorporated into CIEDs to monitor lead integrity, impedance software has since been augmented to include algorithms capable of assessing thoracic fluid volume, and its implanted platform provides a number of advantages over classic ICG including the elimination of the confounding factors associated with external electrodes and the ability to detect changes in impedance trends over time.[47] CIEDs that are capable of measuring intrathoracic impedance do so by intermittently generating a characteristic low-level electrical current from the tip of one of the intracardiac pacing or defibrillator leads that travels across the thoracic organs toward the metallic casing ("can") of the device generator (Figure 5.3A). Various configurations have been tested, and the vector between the LV pacing lead and the can was associated with the fastest and greatest change in impedance upon inducing pulmonary congestion in a comparative animal model;[49] however, contemporary studies in humans have utilized the RV pacing lead ring or defibrillator coil,[14,30,37,50,51,52] and by convention this seems to be the vector most often used in clinical practice.

Regardless of which vector is utilized, the device obtains multiple intermittent impedance measurements over the course of the day to determine a single "average daily impedance" level. Initially after implantation the average daily impedance levels follow a predictable pattern with low levels immediately post-implant (presumably due to surgically related device pocket inflammation) that gradually increase and then plateau around 30 days. In order to facilitate management of impedance data and determine if a subsequent drop in impedance is relevant, several device-specific algorithms have been employed. Approximately 34 days post-implantation one such algorithm is initiated generating an individualized "reference impedance" based on the trends of the patient's recent average daily impedance levels. The reference impedance is essentially a patient-specific slow-moving average that provides a baseline against which future average daily impedance levels can be compared. Another algorithm, using the cumulative sum method, then calculates the "fluid index" (FI) by accumulating the negative difference between the average daily impedances and the reference impedance. This FI depends on both the magnitude (Ω) and duration (days) of the differences, and when the FI surpasses an arbitrary threshold (typically 60 Ω days), a "threshold-crossing event" (TCE) is detected (Figure 5.3B).

The predictive ability of TCEs has subsequently been evaluated by a number of studies, with mixed results. Early experience suggested the sensitivity of a TCE for HF hospitalizations or HF events was in the order of 60–76% with 0.2–1.9 unexplained detections per patient year and a positive predictive value of 60%;[14,50,51] however, two large follow-up studies have since demonstrated far lower sensitivities (20–42%) for HF hospitalization within 30 days and positive predictive values (4% and 38%) for HF hospitalizations and worsening HF, respectively.[31,52] A summary of these studies is provided in Table 5.3.[53] Given the slight differences in the

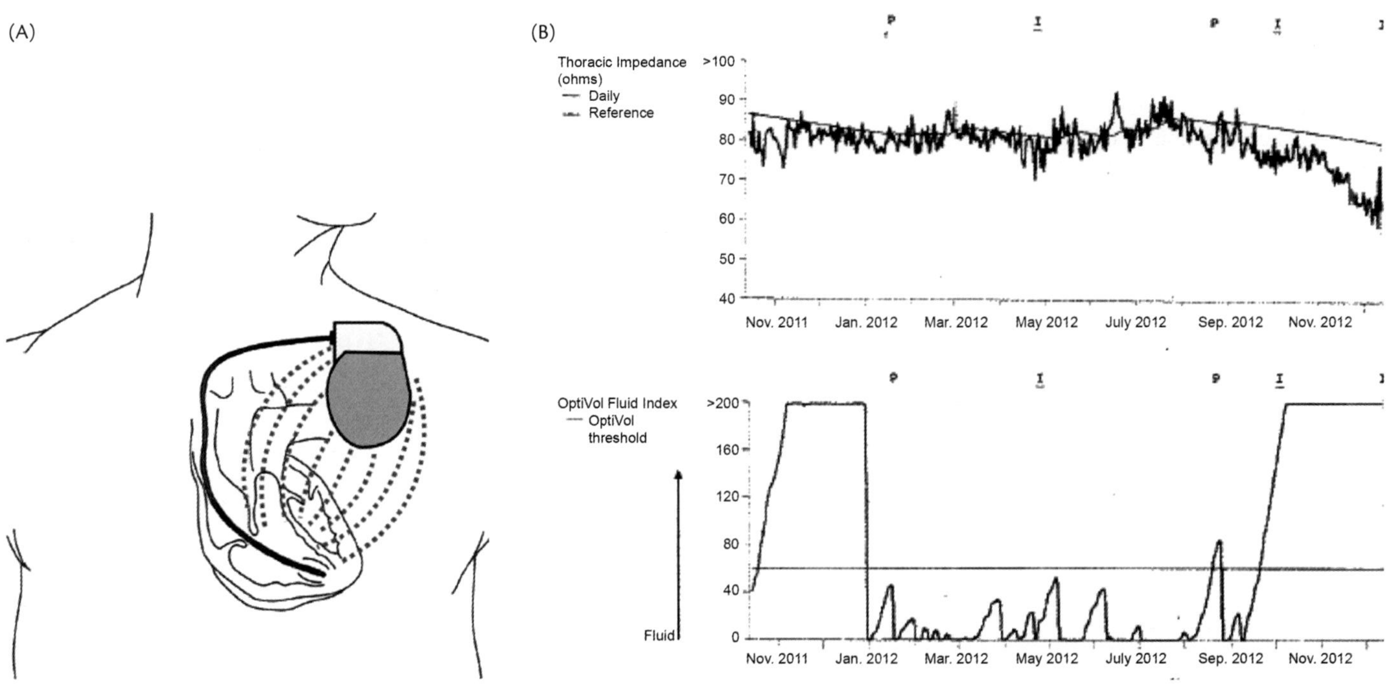

Fig. 5.3 Intrathoracic impedance measurement: (A) schematic of intrathoracic impedance measurement utilizing the implanted device method with the classic RV lead tip to device generator can configuration; (B) example of intrathoracic impedance changes and fluid index (FI) threshold crossing events in a patient that developed significant increase in atrial and ventricular dysrrhythmias associated with decompensated heart failure requiring hospitalization in November 2012.

Table 5.3 Studies evaluating the utility of intrathoracic impedance in predicting heart failure events

Study/author (year)	Design	Population	n	Study variable	Endpoint	Results
MIDHEFT, Yu et al. (2005)	Single center, prospective, observational, double blind	NYHA III (91%), HFpEF (24%) with ICD	33	1. FI (60 Ω·d) 2. Impedance	1. HF hospitalization within 30 days 2. PCWP	1. TCE sensitivity 76.9%, unexplained detection rate 1.5 per patient year 2. Z inversely correlated to PCWP
European InSync Sentry Observational study, Vollmann et al. (2007)	Multicenter, prospective, observational, unblinded	NYHA II-IV with ICD/CRT-D	373	FI (60 Ω·d)	HF deterioration within 14 days	1. TCE sensitivity 60%, PPV 60% 2. Unexplained detection rate 0.2 per patient year 3. ↑ NYHA FC associated with ↑ true positives
FAST, Abraham et al. (2011)	Multicenter, prospective, observational, double blind	NYHA II-III (85%) with ICD/CRT-D	156	1. FI (60 Ω·d) 2. Body weight	Adjudicated HF events	1. TCE sensitivity 76% (vs. 22% for weight change) 2. Unexplained detection rate 1.9 per patient year (vs 4.3 for weight change)
SENSE-HF, Cowie et al. (2011)	Multicenter, prospective, observational, double blind	NYHA II-IV with ICD/CRT-D	501	FI (60 Ω·d)	1. Phase I (blinded): sensitivity for HF hospitalization within 30 days 2. Phase II (unblinded): PPV of TCE alert for worsening HF within 30 days	1. TCE sensitivity 20%, PPV 4% in Phase I 2. TCE PPV 38% in Phase II
OFISSER Study, Small et al. (2009)	Multicenter, retrospective	NYHA II (17%) NYHA III (79%) CRT-D	326	FI (60 Ω·d) 1. # of TCE 2. TCE burden (days)	Adjudicated HF hospitalization	1. Each TCE associated with 35% increased risk 2. Both # of TCE and days > threshold independently predictive
PARTNERS-HF, Whellen et al. (2010)	Multicenter, prospective, observational	NYHA III CRT-D	694	Combined HF device diagnostic algorithm including high FI (60 Ω·d) or very high FI (100 Ω·d)	HF hospitalization within 30 days	1. 2.7-fold increased risk for TCE at FI threshold = 60 Ω·d 2. 3.9-fold increased risk for TCE at FI threshold 100 Ω·d 3. 5.5-fold increased risk for combined device diagnostic algorithm
Catanzariti et al. (2009)	Multicenter, prospective, unblinded	NYHA 2.6 ± 0.5 with CRT-D	532	FI (60 Ω·d) 1. Alert ON 2. Alert OFF	1. HF hospitalization 2. Composite death, urgent HTX, or HF hospitalization	1. 7% in ON group vs 20% in OFF group (p <0.001) 2. Nonsignificant reduction in composite endpoint with ON group
DOT-HF, Braunschweig et al. (2011)	Multicenter, prospective, randomized, unblinded	NYHA II (60%) NYHA III (36%) ICD (18%) CRT-D (82%	335	1. Access arm: FI (60 Ω·d), alert ON, full access device diagnostics (save remote monitoring) 2. Control arm: Usual care	Composite all-cause mortality or HF hospitalization	1. Trial stopped early due to futility 2. Nonsignificant increase composite outcome in access arm (29% vs 20%, p = 0.06) driven by HF hospitalizations (HR 1.8, p = 0.02)

CRT-D, cardiac resynchronization therapy implantable cardioverter defibrillator device; FI, fluid index; HFpEF, heart failure with preserved ejection fraction; HTX, heart transplantation; ICD, implantable cardioverter defibrillator; NYHA New York Heart Association functional class; PCWP, pulmonary capillary wedge pressure; PPV, positive predictive value; TCE, threshold-crossing event; Z, impedance.

Modified from Samara et al. Device monitoring strategies in acute heart failure syndromes. Heart Failure Review 2011;16:491–502.

methodologies of these studies, the true predictive value of a TCE remains somewhat unclear.

Generally speaking there are two main ways clinicians can follow and utilize impedance trends in the management of HF patients. The simplest approach appears to be performing periodic device interrogations at the time of routine scheduled follow-up clinic visits for the purpose of risk stratification. The occurrence of TCEs has been associated with both increased short-term adverse HF events[30,54] and long-term morbidity and mortality[55] and thus identifies a group of patients at higher risk who may benefit from increased vigilance and HF therapies. In the largest impedance cohort analyzed to date (21 217 patients with an ICD or CRT-D [51%] device), TCEs that occurred within the first 6 months of implantation were associated with a dose-dependent increased risk of morbidity and mortality independent of AF or ICD shocks (2.15-fold increased risk of all-cause mortality, p <0.0001) (Figure 5.4). In the same study a stabilization of impedance trends (with a reduction in the frequency of TCEs after the first 6 months) was associated with a significant mortality risk reduction (HR 0.48, p <0.001).[55] In addition to supporting its value in risk stratification, these findings also suggest impedance trends and the presence or absence of TCEs may be used to evaluate the effectiveness of HF therapy, a concept that was recently highlighted by a small study that demonstrated TCEs within the first 6 months following initiation of CRT identified patients that did not respond to CRT, whereas the group that lacked TCEs during the same time period had significant improvements in BNP levels, LV dimensions, and LVEF.[56]

In addition to their value in risk stratification, TCEs have been shown to be a more sensitive (76% vs. 22%)[50] and earlier predictor (up to 15 days on average)[14] of incipient HF decompensations than changes in body weight or the development of symptoms, respectively. While perhaps more time consuming than performing the occasional device interrogation in clinic, activating the device's remote monitoring capabilities and enabling the audible patient alert function to warn when a TCE has occurred makes it possible for the clinician to follow impedance trends more closely

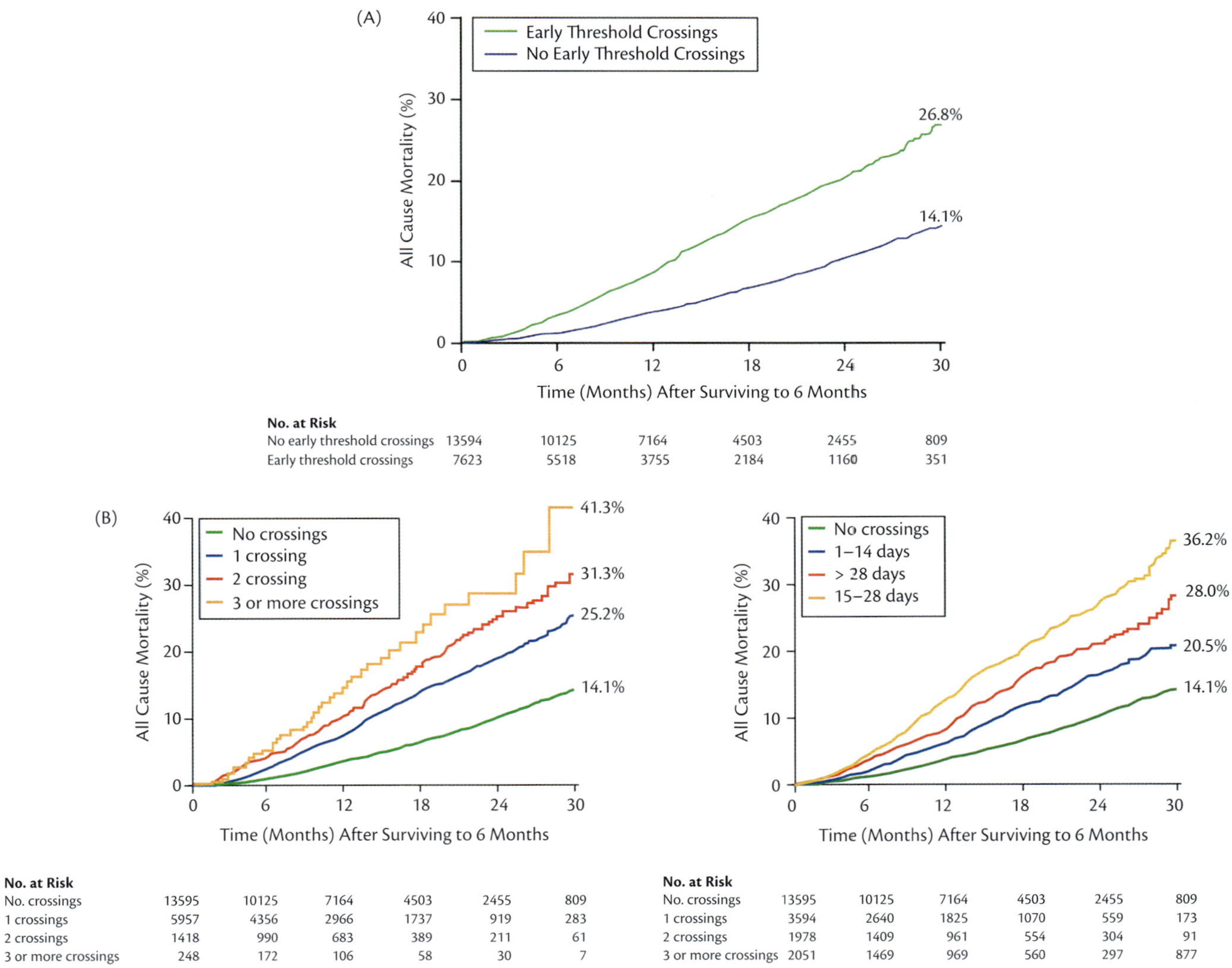

Fig. 5.4 Intrathoracic impedance threshold crossings and long-term survival: (A) association of fluid index (FI) threshold-crossing within the first 6 months of device implantation with all-cause mortality; (B) association of number and duration of FI threshold crossings with all-cause mortality.

Tang et al. Threshold crossing of device-based intrathoracic impedance trends identifies relatively increased mortality risk. European Heart Journal 2012;33:2189–96 by permission of Oxford University Press.

and potentially identify subclinical congestion before HF hospitalization becomes imminent. This hypothesis has been recently evaluated, and like the studies evaluating the predictive value of TCEs, results have been mixed (also summarized in Table 5.2). While an initial observational study demonstrated remote monitoring and audible patient alerts (enabled vs. disabled) were associated with a significant reduction in hospital admissions (7% vs. 20%, $p < 0.001$),[57] the two prospective randomized controlled trials (RCTs) to evaluate the effect of audible alert guided management have recently been stopped prematurely due to futility, with the intervention arms actually demonstrating a significant increase in healthcare utilization compared to the usual care control arms.[37,58] It is notable that these randomized trials did not allow for remote monitoring follow-up and by design required patients to present to clinic for further evaluation whenever an alert was triggered.[37] As the excess healthcare utilization (both unplanned office visits and hospitalizations) in the intervention arm was largely triggered by TCE alerts in the absence of clinical signs or symptoms of HF and the investigators were not given any instruction on how to proceed with these evaluations, it is unclear to what extent physician unfamiliarity with the new technology played a role in the overall results. Still, this phenomenon is notable in and of itself as it highlights an issue inherent to all forms of intracardiac monitoring (and all forms of diagnostic testing for that matter): obtaining the information is only half the battle; how we synthesize that information and what we do with it is just as important for any new technology to be effective.

Intrathoracic impedance technology has a number of additional limitations. For one, though it has been clearly correlated to intracardiac filling pressures and intrathoracic fluid volume, the exact source of the impedance signal in humans remains incompletely understood.[47] Its specificity for worsening HF is diminished by other conditions that increase intrathoracic fluid (e.g., pulmonary infections) or interfere with lead integrity (e.g., lead dislodgement), but universally raising nominal FI thresholds (in order to increase specificity) would likely reduce its sensitivity, which has already been shown to miss a substantial number of clinical HF events (55% of false negatives in one observational study were associated with an increase in FI below the programmed threshold).[51] Modified impedance algorithms[59] and individualized nominal TCE thresholds have been proposed as ways to improve overall accuracy and will be the focus of future investigations, but for now it appears the greatest value of impedance trends remains in the risk stratification of patients with advanced HF.

Implantable hemodynamic monitors

While alterations in the physiologic parameters measured by CIEDs (including intrathoracic impedance) can provide useful markers for worsening HF and pulmonary congestion, they do so essentially as surrogates for the elevated ventricular filling pressures that are in and of themselves pathognomonic for decompensated HF. Regardless of the precipitant, all causes of acute HF share the common pathway of elevated intracardiac filling pressures, and in this way elevated filling pressures are essential for decompensated HF. Moreover, as changes in filling pressures seem to occur earlier than any other measurable parameter during the transition from chronic stable to ADHF (see Figure 5.1),[9,10] they represent an ideal therapeutic target to reverse the process before hospitalization becomes imminent. For these reasons a permanent implanted sensor that reliably and accurately monitors ventricular filling pressures has long been considered the Holy Grail in the management of patients with advanced HF.

Over the past two decades a number of IHMs utilizing various monitoring sites, pressure-transducer technologies, implantation platforms, and means of power and data management have been developed and investigated to this end. Their attributes are summarized in Table 5.4.

The first developed IHM system (Chronicle, Medtronic Inc, Minneapolis, MN, USA; Figure 5.5A) consists of three components: (1) an implanted programmable memory system, (2) a modified unipolar passive fixation pacemaker lead with a pressure sensor incorporated near its tip, and (3) an external pressure reference device (EPR) carried separately by the patient that corrects for the surrounding barometric pressure. The programmable memory system (consisting of of a lithium–manganese dioxide power source, integrated circuitry, piezoelectric activity sensor, and a radiofrequency transmission coil hermetically sealed in a titanium can similar in size to the pulse generator of a pacemaker) is implanted subcutaneously in the prepectoral area, and the transvenous pressure-sensor lead is positioned in the RV outflow tract (RVOT) using standard pacemaker implantation techniques. The pressure sensor uses the principle of variable conductance to measure absolute pressures throughout the cardiac cycle specifically obtaining values corresponding to the onset of the R-wave (RV diastolic pressure [RVDP]), maximum pressure (RV systolic pressure [RVSP]), and the pressure at the maximum rate of pressure increase ($+dP/dt$) that has been validated to be an accurate estimate of pulmonary artery diastolic pressure (ePAD). The relationship between these pressures is demonstrated in Figure 5.5B. For patients without significant pulmonary vascular disease, ePAD provides a useful clinical estimate of pulmonary capillary wedge pressure (PCWP) and LV diastolic pressure (LVEDP).[60] While the device measures all of these pressures continuously, it ultimately stores a smaller dataset of median values (as well as the 6th and 94th percentiles) based on a programmable interval (typically set to 8 minutes). The data is then transmitted by the patient using a home monitor/interrogation device via telephone line to a secure online server that can be accessed by clinicians using conventional internet access.

Clinical studies evaluating this IHM in both patients with systolic and diastolic HF have shown it to be safe, well-tolerated, and accurate[61,62,63] with the nighttime minimum pressures correlating best with the supine resting pressures obtained during clinic visits.[17] Subsequent analyses demonstrated that the product of ePAD pressure and time ($P \times T$) is best associated with the transition to ADHF,[8] and an automated change detection algorithm based on the cumulative sum method (similar to those used to calculate the FI from impedance data, see Figure 5.5C) demonstrated 83% sensitivity for detecting this transition with a false-positive rate of 4.1 per patient year.[64] Unfortunately the first prospective RCT to evaluate the value of this RV pressure sensor in the management of chronic HF patients did not achieve its primary endpoint due to a nonsignificant 21% reduction ($p = 0.33$) of HF-related events in the intervention arm, though a post-hoc analysis did demonstrate a significant 36% reduction in time to first hospitalization.[65] With nearly 90% of patients completing the 6 months follow-up there were no reported pressure-sensor failures; however, 8% suffered a

Table 5.4 Implantable hemodynamic monitors currently under investigation

Device (manufacturer)	Pressure measured	Implantation platform	Pressure transduction	Power	Data management	Studies—design and results
Chronicle (Medtronic Inc, Minneapolis, MN)	Absolute RVSP, RVDP, ePAD	Prepectoral device; lead transvenously positioned in RVOT	Variable capacitance	Lithium manganese dioxide	Continuous storage; RF wand interrogation, transmit to server via telephone line, data available via Internet	COMPASS-HF ◆ 274 NYHA III-IV pts (HFrEF & HFpEF) ◆ Multicenter, prospective, RCT ◆ primary endpoint not met ◆ Nonsignificant 21% reduction in HFE ◆ Time to first HFE was reduced (p = 0.03)
RemonCHF (Boston Scientific Corp, Natick, MA)	Absolute PASP, PADP	Sensor with self-expanding nitinol stent placed in right PA via RHC	Variable capacitance	Recharged by acoustic coupling	No data storage in device; US sensor activates device and records 10-s waveform transmission	PAPIRUS II ◆ 31 NYHA III-IV pts ◆ Multicenter, prospective, Phase I study ◆ Safe and feasible
HeartPOD (St. Jude Medical, St. Paul, MN)	Absolute LAP	Prepectoral device; LA transeptal lead	Variable capacitance	No battery; electromechanical coupling	No data storage in device; RF interrogation with PAM, data uploaded in clinic at follow-up visits and used by patient for dynamic therapy	HOMEOSTASIS ◆ 40 NYHA III-IV pts ◆ Multicenter, prospective, observational, open-label registry ◆ Unblinded after first 3 months ◆ Increase ACEI dose (37%) and BB dose (40%) (p <0.001) ◆ Decrease in loop diuretic dose (27%) ◆ Mean LAP decreased 17.6 to 14.8 mmHg (p = 0.03) ◆ HF events less frequent after first 3 months (HR 0.16, p = 0.012) ◆ Survival free of ADHF 61% at 3 yrs
CardioMEMS (CardioMEMS Inc., Atlanta, GA)	Absolute PASP, PADP	Sensor with two nitinol wire loops to prevent distal embolization placed in PA via RHC	Inductive capacitance resonant circuit	No battery; electromechanical coupling	No data storage in device; antenna activates device and records pressures in real time	CHAMPION ◆ 550 NYHA III pts ◆ Multicenter, prospective, RCT ◆ Freedom from device complications 98.6% ◆ 39% reduction in HF hospitalizations (p <0.0001) ◆ Vasodilators were main treatment strategy

ACEI, angiotensin converting enzyme inhibitor; ADHF, acute decompensated heart failure; BB, beta-blocker; ePAD, estimated pulmonary artery diastolic pressure; HFE, heart failure event; HFpEF, heart failure with preserved ejection fraction; HFrEF, heart failure with reduced ejection fraction; LA, left atrium; LAP, left atrial pressure; NYHA, New York Heart Association functional class; PA, pulmonary artery; PADP, pulmonary artery diastolic pressure; PAM, personal advisory module; PASP, pulmonary artery systolic pressure; RCT, randomized controlled trial; RF, radiofrequency; RHC, right heart catheterization; RVDP, right ventricular diastolic pressure; RVOT, right ventricular outflow tract; RVSP, right ventricular systolic pressure; US, ultrasound.

Modified from Samara et al. Device monitoring strategies in acute heart failure syndromes. Heart Failure Review 2011;16:491–502.

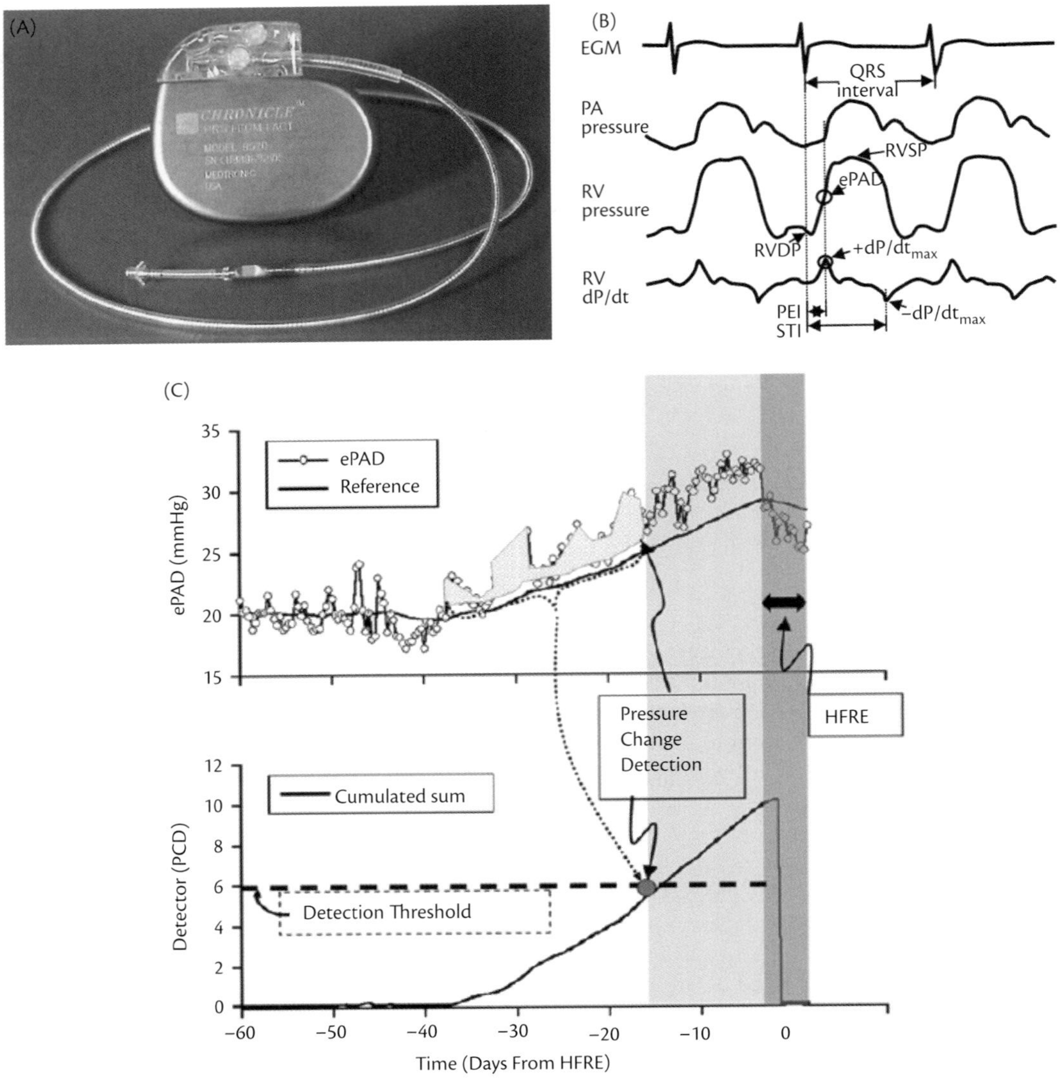

Fig. 5.5 Chronicle implantable hemodynamic monitoring system: (A) programmable memory system with tip-mounted pressure sensor lead; (B) schematic of RV pressure, *dP/dt*, and ePAD measurements; (C) schematic for ePAD pressure change detection algorithm.

Figures 1 and 2 from Magalski et al. Continuous ambulatory right heart pressure measurements with an implantable hemodynamic monitor: a multicenter, 12-month follow-up of patients with chronic heart failure. Journal of Cardiac Failure 2002;8:63-70 (ISSN: 1071-9164, DOI: 10.1054/jcaf.2002.32373). Figure 1 from Adamson et al. Hemodynamic factors associated with acute decompensated heart failure: part 2--use in automated detection. Journal of Cardiac Failure 2011;17:366-373 (ISSN: 1071-9164, DOI: 10.1016/j.cardfail.2011.01.011)

system-related complication, most of which were due to lead dislodgement that required repositioning or replacement.[65] The only other major RCT evaluating this technology was recently halted prematurely by the manufacturer due to issues related to lead integrity. While initial studies demonstrated good durability of the sensor lead out to 12 months,[62] 4-year follow-up data indicated a 4% single-source lead failure rate, and it was determined that it would not be possible to remanufacture the lead in a timely enough manner to continue the trial.[66] It is likely that the positioning of the lead in the RVOT subjects it to considerable mechanical and flow-related stress, and it is clear that further investigation and modification will be necessary before the device is ready for widespread use.

Two relatively newer IHM devices developed in recent years have some important advantages when compared to the Chronicle system. For one, their sensors are positioned in a branch of the pulmonary artery (CardioMEMS®, CardioMEMS Inc., Atlanta, GA, USA) or the left atrium (HeartPOD, St. Jude Medical, St. Paul, MN, USA) which not only allows for a more direct measurement of cardiac filling pressures but also avoids subjecting the sensor to the high mechanical and flow-related stresses inherent to the RVOT. Another important difference is that these newer IHMs are powered via electromechanical coupling with their external (interrogation) components and do not require batteries, which at least theoretically eliminates the need for future change-outs.

The HeartPOD IHM system (Figure 5.6) has four components: (1) an implantable left atrial pressure (LAP) sensor, (2) a subcutaneous antenna coil, (3) an external patient advisory module (PAM), and (4) the clinician's personal computer software. The LAP sensor is a modified pacemaker lead with a 3 × 7-mm hermetically sealed sensor module containing a titanium-encapsulated pressure-transducer membrane and circuitry for measuring and communicating LAP, temperature, and intracardiac electrograms (IEGM). Its distal (sensing) end is implanted into the atrial septum oriented toward the left atrium and affixed with folding nitinol

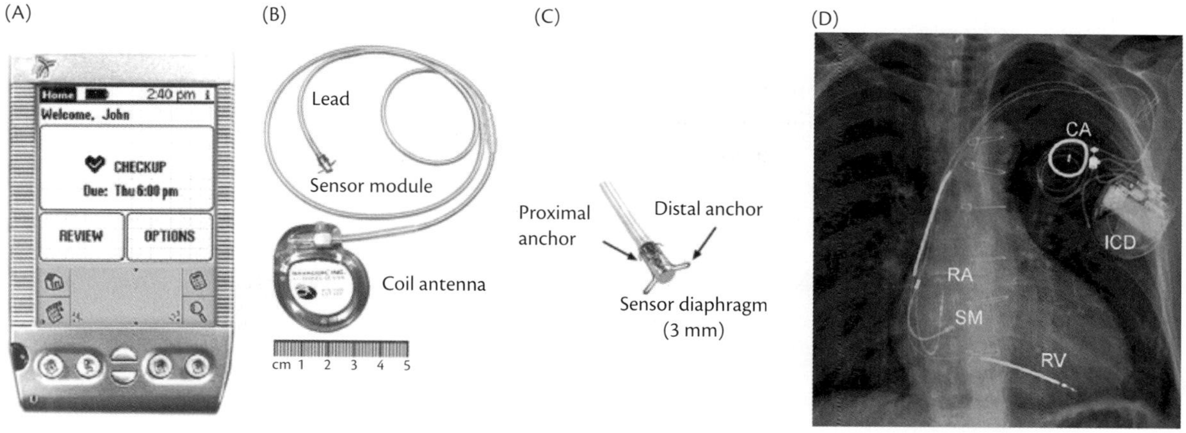

Fig. 5.6 HeartPOD implantable hemodynamic monitoring system: (A) handheld patient advisory module (PAM); (B) subcutaneous antennae (CA) with transvenous, transeptal, tip-mounted pressure sensor lead; (C) magnified view of sensor module (SM) with septal anchor-fixation system; (D) anteroposterior chest radiograph demonstrating position of SM in relation to right atrial (RA) and right ventricular (RV) leads associated with an implantable cardioverter defibrillator (ICD).
Ritzema et al. Physician-directed patient self-management of left atrial pressure in advanced chronic heart failure. Circulation 2010;121:1086–95.

anchors using standard transeptal puncture equipment and technique; its proximal end is connected to the subcutaneous antenna coil which is buried in its own pocket, typically in the prepectoral area or lower rectus abdominus sheath. The implanted device is then powered up and interrogated via electromechanical coupling (128-kHz radiofrequency wireless signal) with the external PAM that contains an external pressure sensor to correct absolute LAPs for atmospheric pressure. Interrogated LAP values as well as high-fidelity physiologic waveforms (LAP and IEGMs) are stored in the PAM for immediate viewing by the patient and/or later download by the clinician. The PAM is programmed to alert the patient with reminders to take medications and can be enabled to recommend real-time diuretic dose adjustments based on an individualized, dynamic LAP sliding-scale regimen designed by the clinician.

The initial experience with the HeartPOD was positive in that it demonstrated that implantation was safe, direct LAPs correlated closely with invasive RHC, and there were no device-related complications or device failures at 3 months.[67] Longer-term follow-up results have recently been reported with a respectable 95% freedom from device failure at 2 years falling off to 88% freedom from failure at 4 years, and the causes of failure were apparently identified and mitigated, with a 100% freedom from device failure in the last 41 consecutive patients implanted ($p = 0.005$).[68] The subsequent multicenter, prospective, open-label registry evaluating a physician-directed patient self-management program has also produced encouraging results. After a 3-month blinded run-in phase, LAP measurements were used to tailor pharmacotherapy in two ways: "static therapies" were adjusted based on the individual's long-term LAP trends, and "dynamic therapies" were adjusted immediately in response to individual LAP measurements. By the end of the trial patients had significantly uptitrated their neurohormonal blockers, showed a trend toward lower diuretic doses, and had small but significant improvements in their NYHA class, LVEF, symptoms, and quality of life. Three-year survival without decompensation was an impressive 61%, and HF events were less frequent once LAP measurements were unblinded (HR 0.16, 95% CI 0.04–0.68, $p = 0.012$). Ultimately mean daily LAP decreased from 17.6 mmHg during the first 3 months to 14.8 mmHg during pressure-guided therapy ($p = 0.003$) with a 67% reduction in the frequency of LAP in excess of 25 mmHg ($p < 0.001$).[69] The first prospective RCT to evaluate the efficacy of HeartPOD is currently enrolling patients.[70]

Unlike the Chronicle and HeartPOD IHM systems, the CardioMEMS heart sensor (Figure 5.7) is not associated with any leads or subcutaneously implanted devices. Consisting of a three-dimensional coil and a pressure-sensitive capacitor encased in a hermetically sealed silica capsule, the CardioMEMS device is a wireless, battery-less sensor with two nitinol loop anchors that secure it in a branch pulmonary artery following deployment during RHC. The coil and capacitor form an electrical circuit that resonates at a specific characteristic frequency and is altered only by changes in the surrounding pressures. The device is both powered and interrogated via electromechanical coupling with an external antenna that contains an atmospheric barometer to automatically subtract the ambient pressure from the absolute pressure measured by the implanted sensor. Early studies showed the device was safe, well-tolerated, and accurate when compared to invasive RHC pressures,[71,72] and in a large multicenter prospective, RCT it met its primary endpoint with a 37% reduction in HF-related hospitalizations ($p < 0.0001$).[73] Additionally, the treatment arm was associated with a greater reduction in mean pulmonary artery pressure, greater number of changes in HF medications, more days alive outside the hospital, and better quality of life.[73] A subsequent subgroup analysis of patients with preserved EF (LVEF >40%) demonstrated pulmonary artery pressure guided management was associated with a 50% reduction in HF hospitalizations compared to standard heart failure care over an average blinded follow-up of 17.6 months,[84] and in the summer of 2015 the CardioMEMS heart failure system became the first and only IHM to date to be approved by the US Food and Drug Administration (FDA) for commercial use.

Additional sensor technologies

Additional implantable sensor technologies have been developed to measure a number of other physiologic variables including cardiac output and peak endocardial acceleration. By incorporating a ratiometric reflectance oximeter (capable of emitting and detecting red and infrared photodiodes) into the tip of a modified RV pacing lead, mixed venous oxygen saturation can be semi-noninvasively

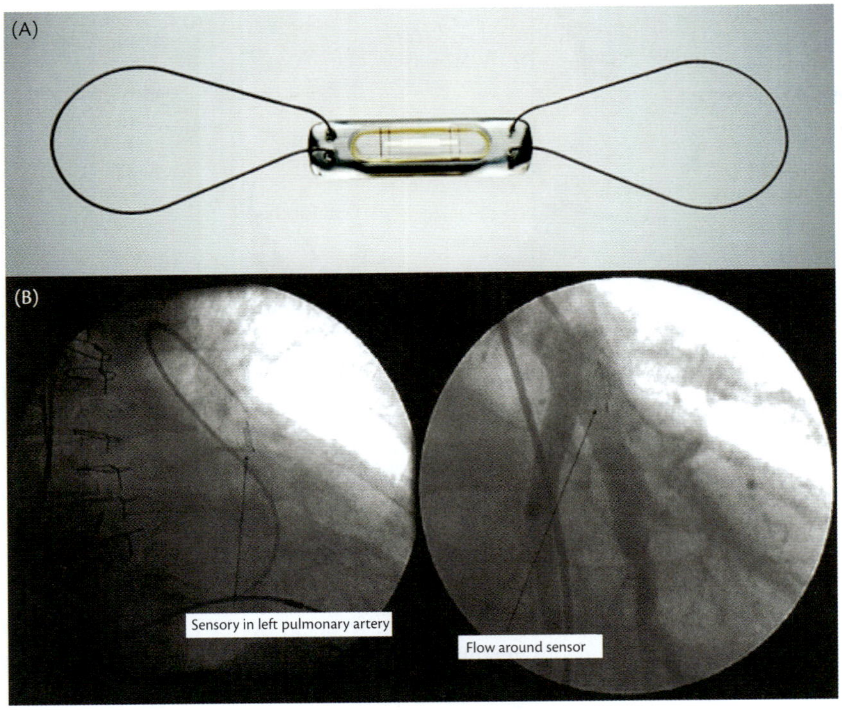

Fig. 5.7 CardioMEMS pulmonary artery pressure sensor: (A) leadless, wireless pressure sensor with two nitinol anchors; (B) fluoroscopic image demonstrating placement of pressure sensor in branch of left pulmonary artery.

measured and used to calculate cardiac output according to the Fick principle. Studies as early as the mid 1990s have compared these semi-noninvasive oxygen saturations and cardiac outputs with invasive pulmonary artery catheter measurements and demonstrated their accuracy and stability over both the short and long term.[74,75,76] However, while mixed venous oxygen saturation and cardiac output can be instrumental in the titration of vasoactive and diuretic medications in the inpatient setting, ventricular filling pressures and pulmonary congestion have become the favored therapeutic targets for outpatients, and consequently the implantable oxygen saturation sensor is not commonly used at present.

Another notable sensor that has been around since the mid 1990s utilizes an implantable lead tip-mounted microaccelerometer to measure the maximum amplitude of vibrations produced by the first heart sound and determine peak endocardial acceleration (PEA).[77] These measurements of PEA correlate well with myocardial contractility (*dP/dt*) and have recently become the subject of much interest as a means of optimizing atrioventricular timing in CRT.[78]

Remote monitoring systems

The recent advancements in sensor technology and CIED monitoring capabilities described up to this point have in many ways been promoted by and coincident with equally important advancements in the infrastructure for accommodating large data transfers and facilitating effective data management systems. Over the past decade each major device company has developed its own platform for remote transmission and management of data essential to connecting what has been coined the "circle of home HF management" paradigm (Figure 5.8).[79] While each of these remote monitoring systems is in varying phases of development, clinical investigation, and medical application, they all operate along the same general principals: (1) the implanted device is equipped with a micro-antennae that communicates with a portable or stationary external device known as the patient transmitter, (2) data obtained by the patient transmitter is transferred via standard analog telephone line or wireless cellular phone transmission to a central database on a secure online server, and (3) data processing facilities integrated with the central database can trigger a quick alert for the physician via phone call, email, fax, or SMS text message depending on the clinical urgency of the event. Key differences in the remote monitoring systems are related to the parameters monitored, the level of patient involvement in transmissions, the frequency of transmissions, and the impact of daily monitoring on battery longevity. The key attributes of each of the FDA-approved remote monitoring platforms is summarized in Table 5.5.[80]

Strategies for using implantable monitors

As outlined thus far, the proliferation of CIED HF diagnostics and the development of stand-alone IHMs has offered clinicians an unprecedented wealth of new information in patients with advanced HF; the next step is to determine strategies for how to best implement this data into patient disease management. As alluded to in the previous discussion on intrathoracic impedance, there are essentially two main ways one can utilize the information obtained from implantable monitors. The first way, via periodic face-to-face device interrogations during routine follow-up, is to assess long-term device diagnostic trends in order to better risk-stratify patients and identify those who may benefit from more aggressive therapy and a higher degree of vigilance, perhaps even

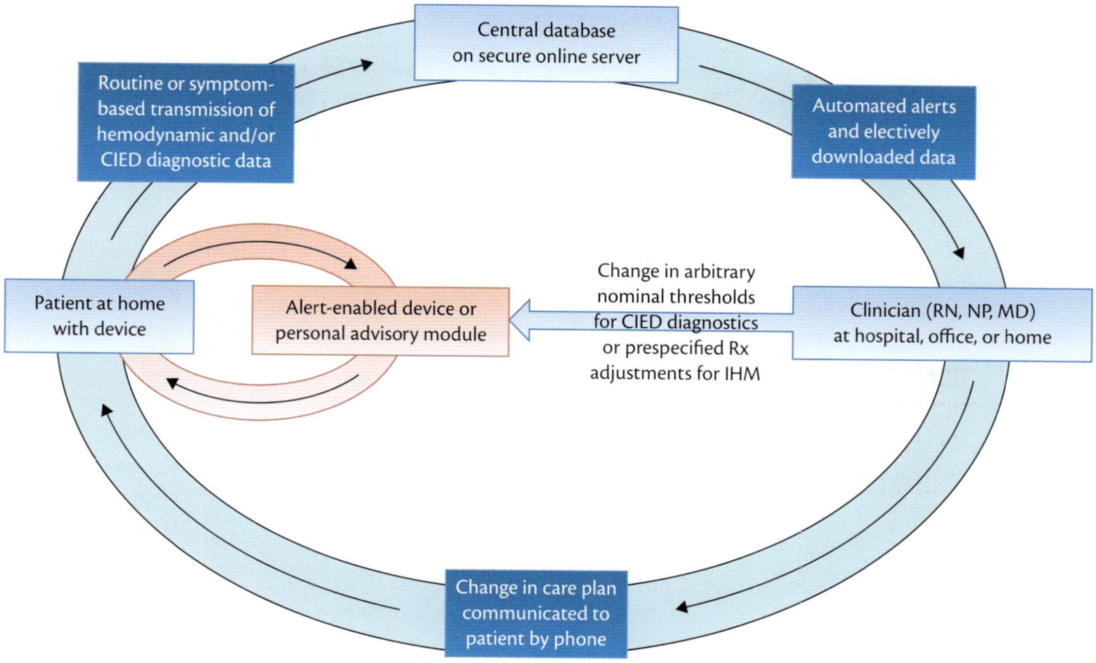

Fig. 5.8 Circle of home management in heart failure: simplified schematic demonstrating the flow of information and potential treatment pathways related to implantable monitoring devices. CIED, cardiac implantable electronic device; IHM, implantable hemodynamic monitor; MD, medical doctor; PA, physician assistance; RN, registered nurse; Rx, medication.

additional monitoring devices (i.e., IHMs). A number of studies have investigated the value of intrathoracic impedance, HRV, and combined HF device diagnostic algorithms for this purpose, and ample evidence now exists to support their role in risk stratification for both future HF events[13,30,31,32,54] and mortality[27,47] (see Tables 5.2 and 5.3).

The other strategy for utilizing CIED diagnostics in HF patients is to activate the audible alerts, enable remote monitoring, and perform more frequent device interrogations, either on a fixed schedule (e.g., monthly) or in response to alerts, with the goal of detecting incipient decompensations earlier in their course in order to facilitate more timely therapy and ultimately reduce HF hospitalizations, morbidity, and mortality. This strategy requires a complex sequence of events: (1) measurement of a parameter that is accurate for worsening HF, (2) timely transmission and interpretation of the data, and (3) rapid implementation of a successful intervention. Errors or time delays at any point along this "sensor–effector" care loop (the circle of home HF management) will lead to a decrement in the success of this strategy. So, despite evidence from observational studies that characteristic changes in CIED diagnostics (namely reductions in intrathoracic impedance and HRV) may be detectable weeks prior to overt decompensation,[11,13,14] the trials that have evaluated the effect of CIED diagnostics-guided management on subsequent HF events have not been as positive.[37,57] Potential reasons for this include the variable accuracy of the measurements (and subsequent physician uncertainty of what to do with the data) in addition to the incomplete incorporation of the available technology and a lack of standardized algorithms for guiding subsequent patient management. Notably, the first large-scale RCT to evaluate the effect of device diagnostics-guided management on HF outcomes did not allow for use of remote monitoring or remote transmissions of device data, and the activation of audible patient alerts inevitably led to an increase in the primary endpoint of healthcare utilization in the intervention arm.[37] Had remote monitoring been made available to the investigators, the excess clinic visits and hospital admissions might have been averted. Indeed, another recent RCT demonstrated that the remote monitoring use was associated with a significant 35% reduction in healthcare utilization (emergency department and unscheduled, urgent office visits), decreased time till data review (1.4 days vs. 24.8 days, $p < 0.001$), and an improvement in quality of life scores for HF patients with ICD or CRT-D devices.[81]

In contrast to the variable sensitivity and accuracy of CIED HF diagnostic surrogates, IHMs (namely the CardioMEMS pulmonary artery pressure sensor and HeartPOD direct LAP monitor) accurately measure ventricular filling pressures that are both highly sensitive and specific for worsening HF.[67,71,72] These attributes make them well suited to implement a strategy of early detection, and based on the growing evidence that IHM-guided management leads to reduced HF hospitalizations [69,73] one such device has already been FDA approved for clinical use.

Limitations of the current evidence

As indicated throughout the preceding sections of this chapter, the current evidence in support of implantable sensors and remote monitoring systems has several limitations. Even when stratified into groups, the bulk of existing studies are largely observational in nature, and the information analyzed is often not directing patient care. These group summaries then have little bearing on the monitoring and therapeutic tailoring of individual patients, and while useful for demonstrating the value of implantable monitors for risk stratification and prediction of HF events, these studies have not been helpful in determining their value for guiding patient

Table 5.5 Summary of current FDA-approved remote monitoring platforms

	Home monitoring (Biotronik; Berlin, Germany)	**Merlin.net Patient Care Network (St. Jude Medical; St. Paul, MN)**	**CareLink Network (Medtronic, Inc; Minneapolis, MN)**	**Latitude patient management system (Boston Scientific Corporation; Natic, MA)**
FDA approval (year)	2001	2003	2005	2006
Available in	PM, CRT, ICD	PM, CRT, ICD	PM, CRT, ICD	CRT, ICD
Electrophysiology parameters	Device info (battery life, lead integrity, etc.), HR/HRV, AT/AF + V rate, VT/VF, device therapy, IEGM, % pacing, % CRT	Device info (battery life, lead integrity, etc.), HR/HRV, AT/AF + V rate, VT/VF, device therapy, IEGM, % pacing, % CRT	Device info (battery life, lead integrity, etc.), HR/HRV, AT/AF + V rate, VT/VF, device therapy, IEGM, % pacing, % CRT	Device info (battery life, lead integrity, etc.), HR/HRV, AT/AF + V rate, VT/VF, device therapy, IEGM, % pacing, % CRT
Additional parameters	Patient activity	Patient activity, CorVue impedance monitoring	Patient activity, OptiVol impedance monitoring	Patient activity; integrated weight, BP, and HF Sx log
Transmitter	CardioMessenger (portable)	Merlin@home (stationary)	CareLink Home Monitor (stationary)	Latitude Communicator (stationary)
Patient participation	Active or passive (wireless)	Active (wand-operated) or passive (wireless)	Active (wand-operated) or passive (wireless)	Active (wand-operated) or passive (wireless)
Frequency of transmission	Daily (fixed time), event activated (immediate), and patient activated	Scheduled (£ ≤21 days) and patient activated	Scheduled and patient activated	Scheduled (typically every week) and patient activated
Long range transmission	Analog landline or GSM network	Analog landline or GSM network	Analog landline or GSM network	Analog landline
Patient alert	CardioMessenger call-back light	Vibration alert	Audible alert	Audible alert
Data storage	Home monitoring service center	Merlin.net	PaceART	Latitude
Alert notification	Text message, email, fax	Email, fax	Text message, email	Phone, email, fax
Integration with EMR	Software available	Software available	Software available	Software available
Impact of daily monitoring on battery longevity	Low	High	High	High
Practice-based interrogator	None available	Merlin On-Demand	CardioSite	None available

AF, atrial fibrillation; AT, atrial tachycardia; CRT, cardiac resynchronization therapy; EMR, electronic medical record; FDA, US Food and Drug Administration; GSM, Global System for Mobile Communication; HR, heart rate; HRV, heart rate variability; ICD, implantable cardioverter defibrillator; IEGM, intracardiac electrogram; PM, pacemaker; V rate, ventricular rate; VF, ventricular fibrillation; VT, ventricular tachycardia.

Modified from Jung et al., Journal of Interventional Cardiac Electrophysiology 2008;23:73–85, Springer.

Sources of information (last accessed December 27, 2012): Biotronik, <http://www.biotronik-healthservices.com; Boston Scientific: <http://www.aboutlatitude.com; Medtronic, <http://www.medtronic.com; St. Jude Medical, <http://www.sjm.com/devices.

management. Unfortunately the few trials that have attempted to directly assess the value of CIED diagnostics-guided management have suffered from a lack of systems to accommodate the new workflow, and to date the only implanted sensor technology to show a significant benefit on HF outcomes (namely hospitalizations) in a large randomized intervention study is the CardioMEMS pulmonary artery sensor.

Financial and medicolegal aspects

Filtering relevant information from the vast amount of data generated by implantable devices and remote monitoring systems is time consuming and not without significant financial cost or medicolegal concerns.

As the number of patients with HF, utilization of CIEDs, and thus the total number of potential candidates for remote monitoring continue to grow, it is clear that sophisticated triage systems will be necessary to make this management strategy timely and effective. Even if data collection is limited to "alarm" conditions, the implementation of remote monitoring programs for this population will likely require an increase in midlevel HF personnel and/or the development of dedicated around-the-clock telemonitoring centers,[82] neither of which would be without substantial cost. Unfortunately, despite the creation of Current Procedural Terminology (CPT®) billing codes for remote monitoring, the present reimbursement policies for telemedicine remain far from standardized and in many states and countries do not even exist; until there is more evidence supporting the concept that these resources improve the care of HF patients and reduce HF outcomes in a cost-effective manner, this inopportune fact is unlikely to change.

Moreover, as with all new technologies, there is a steep learning curve, and many healthcare providers including cardiology professionals and subspecialists are not comfortable utilizing these resources at the present time. This issue, which will only improve with further education and active participatory experience, is likely to require improved incentives (e.g., consistent reimbursement schemes) before widespread use is possible. As such, the importance of improving the predictive ability of the information generated by implantable devices, development of reliable algorithms to guide management based on this information, and ultimately the demonstration that these strategies are efficacious and cost-effective cannot be overestimated.

Finally, it is also important to consider the legal ramifications of remote monitoring. While the establishment of around-the-clock telemonitoring centers and direct incorporation of remote monitoring data into the appropriate electronic medical records may minimize time delays or the risk of missing important remotely transmitted events altogether, a number of additional risks exist inherent to the storage of patient information in central databases. While none of the secure internet server databases have been breached to date, with the right technical expertise it is at least theoretically possible that they could be hacked, and consequently ongoing security measures will be necessary to ensure the preservation of patient privacy and to prevent the possibility of unauthorized and even potentially malicious remote manipulation of implantable devices.[83]

Future considerations

Given the present paucity of evidence that implantable monitoring technologies significantly improve outcomes, it remains yet unclear if these strategies will live up to their full potential. The heterogeneous nature of HF and subsequent decompensation events presents a significant obstacle, and the possible reasons for the equivocal results identified thus far include variable patient selection, variable accuracy of implantable sensor diagnostics, an incomplete understanding of exactly what we are measuring, and a lack of standardized management guidelines.

Future research will need to focus on which patients are most appropriate for these devices. If IHMs do in fact demonstrate unequivocal reductions in HF morbidity (namely rehospitalizations) and mortality, one strategy may be to selectively implant them in patients who have the highest risk for HF events based on established and novel risk stratification models that might include biomarkers (e.g., NT pro-BNP), frequent intrathoracic impedance TCEs, and of course rehospitalizations.

Future studies will also need to focus on how to best shorten the sensor–effector care loop with the ultimate goal of patient self-management akin to the way a diabetic patient manages their blood sugar. Notably, the HeartPOD direct LAP monitor has already begun testing this strategy. It has even been proposed that the biosensors of the future might close the loop entirely by effecting therapeutic changes automatically without any immediate input from the patient or clinician. Clearly the field of HF is in a state of flux right now, and nowhere is it more apparent than with the new implantable biosensor technologies that look to revolutionize HF management strategies.

Conclusions

The emergence of novel biosensor technologies incorporated into implantable devices has made available unprecedented information regarding the dynamic physiologic changes of HF in the ambulatory setting with little to no reliance on patient compliance. Accessing this information during routine follow-up and via remote monitoring allows clinicians to better assess HF status over long periods of time and has demonstrated value in risk stratification and prediction for future HF events. A dearth of randomized, blinded, clinical trials evaluating the utility of remotely-monitored, HF parameter-guided management strategies leaves its overall effect on outcomes unclear, and consequently healthcare providers and the medical establishment have yet to fully accept this new HF management paradigm. While implantable devices and remote monitoring systems will undoubtedly play an important role in a comprehensive approach to outpatient HF management, much of their acceptance is still dependent on further technological refinement, development of infrastructure and systems to facilitate the timely transmission, triage, and integration of the data, and ultimately the demonstration of improved outcomes.

References

1. Roger VL, Go AS, Lloyd-Jones DM, et al. Heart Disease and Stroke Statistics—2012 update: a report from the American Heart Association. Circulation 2012;125:e20–220.
2. Jencks SF, Williams MV, Coleman EA, et al. Rehospitalizations among patients in the Medicare fee-for-service program. N Engl J Med 2009;360:1418–28.
3. Krumholz HM, Parent EM, Tu N, et al. Readmission after hospitalization for congestive heart failure among Medicare beneficiaries. Arch Intern Med 1997;157:99–104.
4. Lee WC, Chavez YE, Baker T, et al. Economic burden of heart failure: a summary of recent literature. Heart Lung 2004;33:362–71.
5. Fonarow GC, Abraham WT, Albert NM, et al. Factors identified as precipitating hospital admissions for heart failure and clinical outcomes: findings from OPTIMIZE-HF. Arch Int Med 2008;168:847–54.
6. Lewin J, Ledwidge M, O'Loughlin C, et al. Clinical deterioration in established heart failure: what is the value of BNP and weight gain in aiding diagnosis?. Eur J Heart Fail 2002;2:953–7.
7. Friedman MM Older adults' symptoms and their duration before hospitalization for heart failure. Heart Lung 1997;26:169–76.
8. Zile MR, Adamson PB, Yong KC, et al. Hemodynamic factors associated with acute decompensated heart failure: part 1—insights into pathophysiology. J Cardiac Fail 2011;17:282–91.
9. Zile MR, Bennett TD, St. John Sutton M, et al. Transition from chronic compensated to acute decompensated heart failure. Pathophysiologic insights obtained from continuous monitoring of intracardiac pressures. Circulation 2008;118:1433–41.
10. Vanderheyden M, Houben R, Verstreken S, et al. Continuous monitoring of intrathoracic impedance and right ventricular pressures in patients with heart failure. Circ Heart Fail 2010;3:370–7.
11. Fallick C, Sobotka PA, Dunlap ME Sympathetically mediated changes in capacitance: redistribution of the venous reservoir as a cause of decompensation. Circ Heart Fail 2011;4:669–75.
12. Adamson PB Pathophysiology of the transition from chronic compensated and acute decompensated heart failure: new insights from continuous monitoring devices. Curr Heart Fail Rep 2009;6:287–92.
13. Adamson PB, Smith AL, Abraham WT, et al. Continuous autonomic assessment in patients with symptomatic heart failure: prognostic value of heart rate variability measured by an implanted cardiac resynchronization device. Circulation 2004;110:2389–94.

14. Yu CM, Wang L, Chau E, et al. Intrathoracic impedance monitoring in patients with heart failure. Circulation 2005;112:841–8.
15. Chaudhry SI, Wang Y, Concato J, et al. Patterns of weight change preceding hospitalization for heart failure. Circulation 2007;116:1549–54.
16. Ohlsson A, Steinhaus D, Kjellstrom B, et al. Central hemodynamic responses during serial exercise tests in heart failure patients using hemodynamic monitors. Eur J Heart Fail 2003;5:253–9.
17. Adamson PB, Kjellstrom B, Braunschweig F, et al. Ambulatory hemodynamic monitoring from an implanted device: components of continuous 24-hour pressures that correlate to supine resting conditions and acute right heart catheterization. Congest Heart Fail 2006;12:14–19.
18. DiMarco JP Atrial fibrillation and acute decompensated heart failure. Circ Heart Fail 2009;2:72–73.
19. Fonarrow GC, Abraham WT, Albert NM, et al. Factors identified as precipitating hospital admissions for heart failure and clinical outcomes. Arch Intern Med 2008;168:847–54.
20. Swerdlow CD, Schsls W, Dijkman B, et al. Detection of atrial fibrillation and flutter by a dual-chamber implantable cardioverter-defibrillator. Circulation 2000;101:878–85.
21. Santini M, Gasparini M, Landolina M, et al. Device-detected atrial tachyarrhythmias predict adverse outcome in real-world patients with implantable biventricular defibrillators. J Am Coll Cardiol 2011;57:167–72.
22. Willems R, Morck ML, Exner DV, et al. Ventricular high-rate episodes in pacemaker diagnostics identify a high-risk subgroup of patients with tachy-brady syndrome. Heart Rhythm 2004;1:414–21.
23. Ousdigian KT, Johnson WB, Koehler JL, et al. Newly recognized atrial tachyarrhythmias are fairly common and increase the risk of supraventricular shocks and cardiovascular hospitalizations in ICD patients [abstract]. Heart Rhythm 2006;3:S162.
24. Knight BP, Desai A, Coman J, et al. Long-term retention of cardiac resynchronization pacing. J Am Coll Cardiol 2004;44:72–7.
25. Poole JE, Johnson GW, Hellkamp AS, et al. Prognostic importance of defibrillator shocks in patients with heart failure. N Eng J Med 2008;359:1009–17.
26. Goldenberg I, Moss AJ, Hall WJ, et al. Causes and consequences of heart failure after prophylactic implantation of a defibrillator in the multicenter automatic defibrillator implantation trial II. Circulation 2006;113:2810–17.
27. La Rovere MT, Pinna GD, Maestri R, et al. Short-term heart rate variability strongly predicts sudden cardiac death in chronic heart failure patients. Circulation 2003;107:565–70.
28. Fosbol EL, Seibaek M, Brendorp B, et al. Long-term prognostic importance of resting heart rate in patients with left ventricular dysfunction in connection with either heart failure or myocardial infarction: the DIAMOND study. Int J Cardiol 2006;140:279–86.
29. Ellery S, Pakrashi T, Paul V, et al. Predicting mortality and rehospitalization in heart failure patients with Home Monitoring—the Home CARE pilot study. Clin Res Cardiol 2006;95:S3:29–35.
30. Whellan DJ, Ousdigian KT, Al-Khatib SM, et al. Combined heart failure device diagnostics identify patients at higher risk of subsequent heart failure hospitalizations: results from PARTNERS HF study. J Am Coll Cardiol 2010;55:1803–10.
31. Sack S, Wende CM, Nagele H, et al. Potential value of automated daily screening of cardiac resynchronization therapy defibrillator diagnostics for prediction of major cardiovascular events: results from Home-CARE (Home Monitoring in Cardiac Resynchronization Therapy) study. Eur J Heart Fail 2011;13:1019–27.
32. Whellan DJ, Sarkar S, Koehler J, et al. Development of a method to risk stratify patients with heart failure for 30-day readmission using implantable device diagnostics. Am J Cardiol 2013;111:79–84.
33. Fantoni C, Raffa S, Regoli F, et al. Cardiac resynchronization therapy improves heart rate profile and heart rate variability of patients with moderate to severe heart failure. J Am Coll Cardiol 2005;46:1875–82.
34. Katona PG and Jih, F. Respiratory sinus arrhythmia: noninvasive measure of parasympathetic cardiac control. J Appl Physiol 2002;39:801–5.
35. Aronson D, Mittleman MA, Burger AJ. Measures of heart period variability as predictors of mortality in hospitalized patients with decompensated congestive heart failure. Am J Cardiol 2004;93:59–63.
36. Adamson PB, Kleckner KJ, VanHout WL, et al., Cardiac resynchronization therapy improves heart rate variability in patients with symptomatic heart failure. Circulation 2003;108:266–9.
37. Van Veldhuisen DJ, Braunschweig F, Conraads V, et al. for the DOT-HF Investigators. Intrathoracic impedance monitoring, audible patient alerts, and outcome in patients with heart failure. Circulation 2011;124:1719–26.
38. Kay GN, Bubien RS, Epstein AE, et al. Rate-modulated cardiac pacing based on transthoracic impedance measurements of minute ventilation: correlation with exercise gas exchange. J Am Coll Cardiol 1989;14:1283–9.
39. Cole CR, Jenson DN, Cho Y, et al. Correlation of impedance minute ventilation with measured minute ventilation in a rate-responsive pacemaker. PACE 2001;24:989–93.
40. Page E, Cazeau S, Ritter P, et al. Physiological approach to monitor patients in congestive heart failure: application of a new implantable device-based asystem to monitor daily life activity and ventilation. Europace 2007;9:687–93.
41. Summers RL, Shoemaker WC, Peacock WF, et al. Bench to bedside: electrophysiologic and clinical principles of noninvasive hemodynamic monitoring using impedance cardiography. Acad Emerg Med 2003;10:669–80.
42. Nyboer J, Bango S, Barnett A, et al. Radiocardiograms: electrical impedance changes of the heart in realation to electrocardiograms and heart sounds. J Clin Invest 1940;19:773.
43. Denniston JC, Maher JT, Reeves JT, et al. Measurement of cardiac output by electrical impedance at rest and during exercise. J Appl Physiol 1976;40:91–5.
44. Luepker RV, Michael JR, Warbasse JR Transthoracic electrical impedance; quantitative evaluation of a non-invasive measure of thoracic fluid volume. Am Heart J 2973;85:83–93.
45. De Maria AN, Raisinghani, A. Comparative overview of cardiac output measurement methods: has impedance cardiography come of age? Congest Heart Fail 2000;6:60–73.
46. Taler SJ, Textor SC, Augustine JE. Resistant hypertension: comparing hemodynamic management to specialist care. Hypertension 2002;39:982–8.
47. Tang WHW, Tong W. Measuring impedance in congestive heart failure: current options and clinical applications. Am Heart J 2009;157:402–11.
48. Kamath SA, Drazner MH, Tasissa G, et al. Correlation of impedance cardiography with invasive hemodynamic measurements in patients with advanced heart failure: the BioImpedance CardioGraphy (BIG) substudy of the Evaluation Study of Congestive Heart Failure and Pulmonary Artery Catheterization Effectiveness (ESCAPE) Trial. Am Heart J 2009;158:217–23.
49. Khoury DS, Naware M, Siou J, et al. Ambulatory monitoring of congestive heart failure by multiple bioelectric impedance vectors. J Am Coll Cardiol 2009;53:1075–81.
50. Abraham WT, Compton S, Haas G, et al. Intrathoracic impedance vs daily weight monitoring for predicting worsening heart failure events: resulst of the fluid accumulation status trial (FAST). Congest Heart Fail 2011;17:51–5.
51. Vollmann D, Nagele H, Schauerte P, et al. Clinical utility of intrathoracic impedance monitoring to alert patients with an implanted device of deteriorating chronic heart failure. Eur Heart J 2007;28:1835–40.
52. Conraads VM, Tavazzi L, Santini M, et al. Sensitivity and positive predictive value of implantable intrathoracic impedance monitoring as a predictor of heart failure hospitalizations: the SENSE-HF trial. Eur Heart J 2011;32:2266–73.
53. Samara MA, Tang WHW. Device monitoring strategies in acute heart failure syndromes. Heart Fail Rev 2011;16:491–502
54. Small RS, Wickemeyer W, Germany R, et al. Changes in intrathoracic impedance are associated with subsequent risk of hospitalizations for

acute decompensated heart failure: clinical utility of implanted device monitoring without a patient alert. J Cardiac Fail 2009;15:475–81.
55. Tang WHW., Warman EN, Johnson JW, et al. Threshold crossing of device-based intrathoracic impedance trends identifies relatively increased mortality risk. Eur Heart J 2012;33:2189–96.
56. Kaneshiro T, Suzuki H, Yamada S, et al. Intrathoracic impedance changes reflect reverse left ventricular remodeling in response to cardiac resynchronization therapy in chronic heart failure patients. Int Heart J 2012;53:249–52.
57. Catanzariti D, Lunati M, Landolina M, et al. Monitoring intrathoracic impedance with an implantable defibrillator reduces hospitalizations in patients with heart failure. PACE 2009;32:363–70.
58. Evaluation of Cardiac Compass With OptiVol in the Early Detection of Decompensation Events for Heart Failure (PRECEDE-HF). ClinicalTrials.gov, Accessed 1 Dec 2012.
59. Sarkar S, Hettrick DA, Koehler J, et al. Improved algorithm to detect fluid accumulation via intrathoracic impedance monitoring in heart failure patients with implantable devices. J Cardiac Fail 2011;17:569–76.
60. Reynolds DW, Bartelt N, Taepke R, et al. Measurement of pulmonary artery diastolic pressure from the right ventricle. J Am Coll Cardiol 1996;25:1176–82.
61. Steinhaus DM, Lemery R, Bresnahan DR Jr., et al. Initial experience with an implantable hemodynamic monitor. Circulation 1996;93:745–52.
62. Magalski A, Adamson P, Gadler F, et al. Continuous ambulatory right heart pressure measurements with an implantable hemodynamic monitor: a multicenter 12-month follow-up study of patients with chronic heart failure. J Card Fail 2002;8:63–70.
63. Ohlsson A, Kubo SH, Steinhaus D, et al. Continuous ambulatory monitoring of absolute right ventricular pressure and mixed venous oxygen saturation in patients with heart failure using an implantable haemodynamic monitor: results of a 1 year multicentre feasibility study. Eur Heart J 2001;22:942–54.
64. Adamson PB, Zile MR, Cho YK, et al. Hemodynamic factors associated with acute decompensated heart failure: part 2—use in automated detection. J Card Fail 2011;17:366–73.
65. Bourge RC, Abraham WT, Adamson PB, et al. Randomized controlled trial of an implantable continuous hemodynamic monitor in patients with advanced heart failure: the COMPASS-HF study. J Am Coll Cardiol 2008;51:1073–9.
66. Adamson PB, Gold MR, Bennett T, et al. Continuous hemodynamic monitoring in patients with mild to moderate heart failure: results from the reducing decompensation events utilizing intracardiac pressures in patients with heart failure (REDUCE HF) trial. Congest Heart Fail 2011;17:248–54.
67. Ritzema J, Melton IC, Richards AM, et al. Direct left atrial pressure monitoring in ambulatory heart failure patients: initial experience with a new permanent implantable device. Circulation 2007;116:2952–9.
68. Troughton RW, Ritzema J, Eigler NL, et al. Direct left atrial pressure monitoring in severe heart failure: long-term sensor performance. J Cardiovasc Trans Res 2011;4:3–13.
69. Ritzema J, Troughton R, Melton I, on behalf of the HOMEOSTASIS study group. Physician-directed patient management of left atrial pressure in advanced chronic heart failure. Circulation 2010;121:1086–95.
70. Left atrial pressure monitoring to optimize heart failure therapy (LAPTOP-HF). ClinicalTrials.gov Accessed 1 Dec 2012.
71. Verdejo HE, Castro PF, Concepcion R, et al. Comparison of a radiofrequency-based wireless pressure sensor to swan-ganz catheter and echocardiography for ambulatory assessment of pulmonary artery pressure in heart failure. J Am Coll Cardiol 2007;50:2375–82.
72. Castro PF, Concepcion R, Bourge RC, et al. A wireless pressure sensor for monitoring pulmonary artery pressure in advanced heart failure: initial experience. J Heart Lung Transplant 2007;26:85–8.
73. Abraham WT, Adamson PB, Bourge RC, et al. Wireless pulmonary artery haemodynamic monitoring in chronic heart failure: a randomized controlled trial. Lancet 2011;377:658–66.
74. Ohlsson A, Bennett T, Ottenhoff F, et al. Long-term recording of cardiac output via an implantable haemodynamic monitoring device. Eur Heart J 1996;17:1902–10.
75. Ohlsson A, Kubo SH, Steinhaus D, et al. Continuous ambulatory monitoring of absolute right ventricular pressure and mixed venous oxygen saturation in patients with heart failure using an implantable haemodynamic monitor. Eur Heart J 2001;22:942–54.
76. Kjellstrom B, Linde C, Bennett T, et al. Six years follow-up of an implantable SvO2 sensor in the right ventricle. Eur J Heart Fail 2004;6:627–34.
77. Rickards AF, Bombardini T, Corbucci G, et al. An implantable intracardiac accelerometer for monitoring myocardial contractility. The multicenter PEA study group. Pacing Clin Electrophysiol 1996;19:2066–71.
78. Ritter P, Delnoy PP, Padeletti L, et al. A randomized pilot study of optimization of cardiac resynchronization therapy in sinus rhythm patients using a peak endocardial acceleration sensor vs standard methods. Europace 2012;14:1324–33.
79. Desai AS, Stevenson LW Connecting the circle from home to heart-failure disease management. N Engl J Med 2010;363:2364–7.
80. Jung W, Rillig A, Birkemeyer R, et al. Advances in remote monitoring of implantable pacemakers, cardioverter defibrillators and cardiac resynchronization therapy systems. J Interv Card Electrophysiol 2008;23:73–85.
81. Landolina M, Perego GB, Lunati M, et al. Remote monitoring reduces healthcare use and improves quality of care in heart failure patients with implantable defibrillators: the evolution of management strategies of heart failure patients with implantable defibrillators (EVOLVO) study. Circulation 2012;125:2985–92.
82. Anker SD, Koehler F, Abraham WT, et al. Telemedicine in remote management of patients with heart failure. Lancet 2011;378:731–9.
83. Burri H, Senouf, D. Remote monitoring and follow-up of pacemakers and implantable cardioverter defibrillators. Europace 2009;11:701–9.
84. Adamson PB, Abraham WT, Bourge RC, et al. Wireless pulmonary artery pressure monitoring guides management to reduce decompensation in heart failure with preserved ejection fraction. Circ Heart Fail 2014;7:935–44.

CHAPTER 6

Endomyocardial biopsy in the failing heart

Michael J. Domanski MD, Mark Halushka MD, and Sean P. Pinney MD

Introduction

Endomyocardial biopsy (EMB) enables direct microscopic examination of the myocardium. The clinical application of EMB generally falls into one of two broad categories: (1) surveillance for rejection of a transplanted heart and (2) diagnosis of cardiomyopathy, including supporting chemotherapy decisions when direct examination of tissue provides risk assessment not otherwise available.

By far the most common indication for EMB is following patients for post-transplant immune rejection. Although newer serum-based evaluations based on gene activation have potential usefulness, there is still no acceptable noninvasive approach to diagnosing rejection that is superior to the EMB. Thus, EMB-based surveillance remains, for the present a medical necessity. As a result, the procedure is commonly (and safely) performed in cardiac transplant centers.

In contrast, EMB is infrequently used in general cardiology practice in spite of the high incidence and prevalence of cardiomyopathy. The reasons for this include (1) etiology can often be determined without the need to examine cardiac tissue; (2) histologic findings are similar and nonspecific in many patients with ventricular dysfunction and so a specific diagnosis is not frequently obtained by tissue examination; and (3) for many causes of cardiomyopathy, therapy specific to etiology is not available, thus limiting treatment to that of heart failure syndrome physiology (neurohumoral antagonists, diuretics, etc). Another factor contributing to infrequent use is unfamiliarity among clinicians regarding when EMB is useful in the management of cardiomyopathy patients.

Recent guidelines[1] seek to clarify the role of EMB in routine cardiology practice. They offer clinicians advice regarding when EMB should be performed based on the clinical presentation, which is what a physician is actually confronted with in the patient care setting. These guidelines are very useful and should be part of the knowledge repertoire of heart failure physicians. However, the absence of randomized clinical trials data results in mostly class II recommendations. Indeed, even in the 2 (of 14) clinical scenarios that carry class I recommendations for EMB, the recommendations are based on thoughtful analysis rather than randomized trials. Also, while the notion of using clinical presentation to assess the likelihood that EMB will aid in decision-making, the scenarios stop short of offering a comprehensive set of principles applicable to all patients.

So, while the guidelines are helpful in organizing an approach to deciding when to use EMB, considerable clinical judgment remains necessary. A central goal of this chapter is to develop, from first principles, a rationale for the use of EMB that guides decision-making regardless of whether or not the patient's presentation precisely fits one of the guideline scenarios.

We begin with a discussion of the diagnosis of cardiomyopathies that references the various guideline scenarios, followed by a discussion of EMB for rejection surveillance after cardiac transplantation. Finally, we review the technical aspects of EMB.

Diagnosis of cardiomyopathies

The current guidelines for the role of EMB in the management of cardiovascular disease were a joint scientific statement of the major cardiovascular societies[1] and are summarized in Table 6.1. EMB is generally considered in the workup of cardiomyopathy only when other means of diagnosis fail to yield an etiology *and* when knowing the etiology would materially affect patient management. To allow a pathologist the best chance of making a diagnosis, careful consideration must be made at the time of biopsy to collect tissue for the proper studies (e.g., light microscopy, electron microscopy, viral PCR) (Tables 6.2 and 6.3).

Heart failure associated with reduced ejection fraction (Scenarios 1, 2, 3, 4, 9, 10)

When a patient presents with sudden-onset heart failure (starting within about 2 weeks of presentation) with hemodynamic compromise and the etiology remains obscure after conventional study (Scenario 1), myocarditis is suspected. EMB is indicated because management is likely to vary depending on the tissue diagnosis. The most common specific diagnoses that would alter therapy in this time frame are any variant of myocarditis. Of particular concern, with a sudden onset of heart failure, is giant cell myocarditis (see next paragraph). Lymphocytic and eosinophilic myocarditis are also identified with increased frequency in this time frame owing to their ability to cause acute heart failure. Even when these diseases are present, due to the patchy nature of inflammatory processes, an EMB is able to make a specific diagnosis in this time frame only approximately one-third of the time.[2] Thus, the absence of a definitive histologic diagnosis does not exclude the possibility of myocarditis.

Table 6.1 Summary of guideline scenarios

Scenario number	Clinical scenario	Class of recommendation (I, IIa, IIb, III)	Level of evidence (A, B, C)
1	New-onset HF of <2 *weeks* duration associated with a normal-sized or dilated LV and hemodynamic compromise	I	B
2	New-onset HF of 2 *weeks to 3 months* duration associated with a dilated LV and new ventricular arrhythmias, second- or third-degree heart block, or failure to respond to usual care within 1–2 weeks	I	B
3	HF of >3 *months* duration associated with a dilated LV and new ventricular arrhythmias, second- or third-degree heart block, or failure to respond to usual care within 1–2 weeks	IIa	C
4	Heart failure associated with a DCM of any duration asscciated with suspected allergic reaction and/or eosinophilia	IIa	C
5	HF associated with suspected anthracycline cardiomyopathy	IIa	C
6	HF associated with unexplained restrictive cardiomyopathy	IIa	C
7	Suspected cardiac tumors	la	C
8	Unexplained cardiomyopathy in children	la	C
9	New-onset HF of 2 *weeks to 3 months* duration associated with a dilated LV, without new ventricular arrhythmias or second- or third-degree heart block, that responds to usual care within 1–2 weeks	ib	B
10	HF of >3 *months* duration associated with a dilated LV, without new ventricular arrhythmias or second- or third-degree heart block, that responds to usual care within 1–2 weeks	IIb	C
11	Heart failure associated with unexplained HCM	IIb	C
12	Suspected ARVD/C	IIb	C
13	Unexplained ventricular arrhythmias	IIb	C
14	Unexplained atrial fibrillation	III	C

ARVD/C, arrhythmogenic right ventricular dysplasia/cardiomyopathy; DCM, dilated cardiomyopathy; HCM, hypertrophic cardiomyopathy; HF, heat failure; LV, left ventricle.

Cooper L, Baughman K, Feldman A, et al. The role of endomyocardial biopsy in the management of cardiovascular disease. Circulation 2007. 116:2116–2233.

Table 6.2 A typical distribution of EMBx tissues for processing based on clinical scenarios. Collection of tissues for clinical harvesting

Clinical scenario	LM	EM	IF	NuAc
New-onset heart failure <3 months	+	+		+
Heart failure >3 months duration	+	+		
Heart failure with DCM	+			
Heart failure associated with anthracycline use	+	+		
Heart failure associated with RCM	+	+	+	
Suspected cardiac tumors	+	+		
Cardiomyopathy in children	+	+		+
Heart failure associated with HCM	+	+		
Suspected ARVD/C	+			
Plasma cell dyscrasia and cardiac symptoms	+	+	+	

ARVD/C, right ventricular arrythymogenic dysplasia/cardiomyopathy; DCM, dilated cardiomyopathy; EM, electron microscopy; HCM, hypertrophic cardiomyopathy; IF, immunofluorescence; LM, light microscopy; PCR, viral PCR studies; RCM, restrictive cardiomyopathy.

Reprinted from Cardiovascular Pathology, 21(1), Stone JR et al., Recommendations for processing cardiovascular surgical pathology specimens: a consensus statement from the Standards and Definitions Committee of the Society for Cardiovascular Pathology and the Association for European Cardiovascular Pathology, 2–16, copyright (2012) with permission from Elsevier.

Giant cell myocarditis (GCM)[3] is a rare disease characterized by the presence of an intense lymphocytic infiltrate, giant cells, and myocardial necrosis (Figure 6.1). An EMB has a sensitivity of about 80% for making this diagnosis. Patients present with heart failure and frequently with ventricular tachyarrhythmias and/or conduction abnormalities. The disease may occur in the setting of thymoma[4] or other autoimmune disease[1] and has also been associated with drug hypersensitivity.[5] Survival is improved with

Table 6.3 Diagnoses that can be rendered based upon different sources of material for histopathologic review

Study	Possible diagnosis
Light microscopy	Myocarditis, giant cell myocarditis, amyloidosis, sarcoidosis, ARVC, hemochromatosis, iron overload, cardiac tumor
Electron microscopy	Fabry disease, hydroxychloroquine cardiotoxicity, chemotherapeutic cardiotoxicity, mitochondrial myopathy, glycogen storage disease, amyloidosis, desmin cardiomyopathy
Immunofluorescence	Nonamyloidotic light-chain deposition disease
Nucleic acid study (viral PCR)	Myocarditis

ARVC, right ventricular arrythymogenic cardiomyopathy.

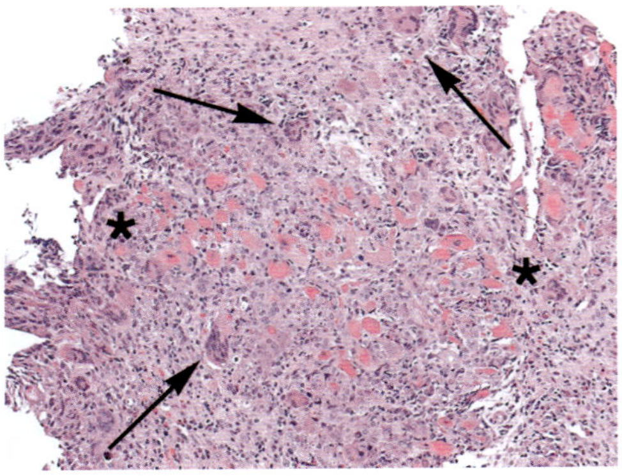

Fig. 6.1 Giant cell myocarditis. Arrows point to giant cells and residual myocytes are seen between the stars (H&E, ×64).

immunosuppression but the prognosis remains poor and transplantation is the treatment of choice. GCM can, however, recur following transplantation.

Lymphocytic myocarditis (Figure 6.2) represents almost 90% of the cases of acute myocarditis and presents with a typical lymphocytic infiltrate and myocardial injury.[1] Often at biopsy, frank myocardial necrosis is not observed but clusters of lymphocytes are seen. This histopathologic appearance has been termed "borderline myocarditis" in the Dallas Criteria nomenclature. Myocarditis is seen at biopsy in approximately 50% of cases. While these patients may present in cardiogenic shock, the prognosis is generally good as long as they receive hemodynamic support. No drug therapy has been shown to be effective.[6]

Necrotizing eosinophilic myocarditis (NEM) is an extremely rare entity that presents with a diffuse eosinophilic infiltrate associated with diffuse myocardial necrosis.[7] NEM is frequently preceded by a viral illness. Peripheral eosinophilia is present but may disappear later in the course. In addition to supportive therapy, these patients are treated with immunosuppression but there is little data on effectiveness, prognosis remains poor, and listing for transplant is indicated when the diagnosis is made.

NEM is distinguished from hypersensitivity myocarditis (HSM) which may be (rarely) associated with eosinophilia, rash and/or fever and is a diagnosis more likely seen in the setting of Scenario 4. Previously unsuspected HSM occurs in between 5% and 10% of explanted hearts of patients in whom the diagnosis was not suspected on clinical grounds.[8] Drugs, particularly those started recently, are potential culprits but HSM can also occur in the setting hypereosinophilic syndrome, parasite infestation, or malignancy.[1,9]

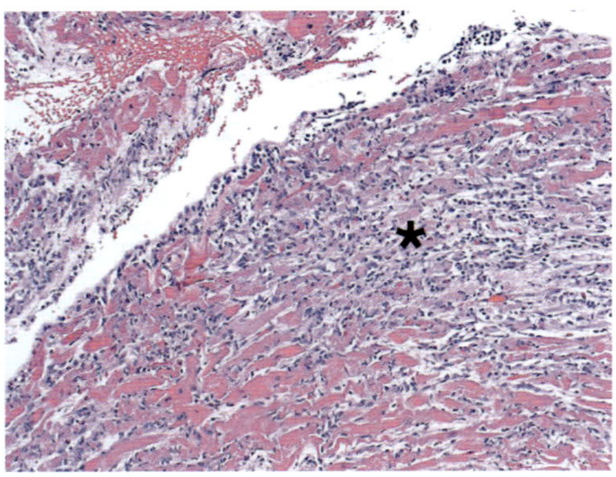

Fig. 6.2 Lymphocytic myocarditis. A heavy inflammatory cell infiltrate is seen around the * (H&E, ×64).

HSM is associated with an interstitial infiltrate of lymphocytes and eosinophils but not with myocardial necrosis. Treatment is corticosteroids for immunosuppression and removal of the precipitating agent. Identifying hypersensitivity as a cause for heart failure is particularly important because it prompts both immunosuppression and a search for, and removal of, the offending agent.

With a longer duration of heart failure of 2 weeks to 3 months, other specific diagnoses are expected (Scenarios 2, 3, 9, 10). Myocarditis is still prevalent at this point in time, often appearing as more chronic active, with increased fibrosis. Chronic diseases such as cardiac sarcoidosis, genetic diseases, iron overload, or even hydroxychloroquine toxicity may be seen.

Sarcoid heart disease (Figure 6.3) is characterized by the presence of noncaseating granulomas giant cells, and fibrosis of the myocardium.[1] Cardiac involvement is most often asymptomatic but may result in heart failure, high-grade conduction delays, and ventricular tachyarrhythmias.[1,10,11] EMB is successful in finding granulomas in only approximately 10–25% of biopsies because of the patchy nature and left-sided and septal dominance of the disease. When sarcoidosis is suspected, the pathologist should be encouraged to "exhaust the block" to search for a granuloma. Nonrandomized studies suggest that corticosteroid treatment improves outcome, particularly when instituted before the development of widespread fibrosis.[10]

Sarcoid heart disease may have an acute (Scenarios 1, 2) or subacute (with symptom onset in the preceding approximately 3 months) (Scenario 3) presentation unresponsive to usual medical therapy. Sarcoid heart disease should be also be suspected in patients with heart failure of unexplained etiology associated with the onset of ventricular tachyarrhythmias or high-grade conduction blocks.[1]

Patients with a subacute presentation (2 weeks to 3 months—Scenario 2) who have heart failure poorly responsive to therapy or who develop ventricular tachyarrhythmias are liable to have the same set of diagnoses as Scenario 1, and EMB is indicated in these patients.

So, a clinical presentation characterized by sudden onset of hemodynamic compromise or onset in recent months poorly responsive to medical therapy or associated with ventricular tachyarrhythmias or high-grade conduction disturbances merits EMB to delineate etiology.

In contrast, for patients who present with a dilated cardiomyopathy of any but the shortest duration (>2 weeks in the guidelines) without ventricular tachyarrhythmias or high-grade heart block and who respond to standard treatment of fluid overload (Scenarios 9, 10), EMB rarely results in a diagnosis that affects management and is thus not recommended. This is particularly the case for patients with a history of years of chronic heart failure, including those presenting with acute decompensation.

Heart failure associated with restrictive, infiltrative, and hypertrophic cardiomyopathies (Scenarios 6, 11, 12)

Restrictive physiology is characterized by impaired relaxation in diastole. While impaired relaxation is present in ventricles with systolic dysfunction, restriction can occur in the setting of normal

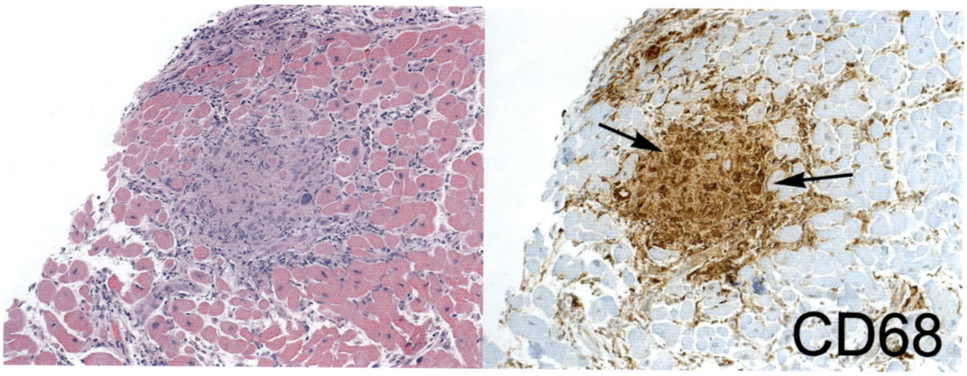

Fig. 6.3 Sarcoidosis. A well-circumscribed granuloma is seen (H&E, ×64). The histiocytes and giant cells (arrows) are highlighted by a CD68 immunohistochemical stain (×64).

systolic function or can be the dominant cause of congestion in patients with mixed systolic and diastolic dysfunction. For some entities, specific treatment is available or prognostic information can be adduced, placing a premium on definitive diagnosis. When etiology remains obscure following routine workup, EMB becomes critical to diagnosis. Tables 6.2 and 6.3 list entities that cause restrictive cardiomyopathy. When symptomatic heart failure is associated with restrictive physiology or unexplained hypertrophy is present and the diagnosis cannot otherwise be inferred, EMB may be useful (Scenarios 6, 11). See Box 6.1.

In patients with idiopathic restriction, or when restrictive physiology results from hypertrophy associated with hypertension, EMB findings are nonspecific. For the infiltrative cardiomyopathies, on the other hand, EMB can offer definitive diagnosis.[12]

Amyloid heart disease is an important example. Cardiac amyloidosis (Figure 6.4) may accompany plasma cell dyscrasias or be the result of the deposition of transthyretin. Nearly 100% of cases of cardiac amyloidosis causing symptoms are detected by EMB, due to the diffuse nature of the disease. Laser capture microdissection with mass spectrometry has become the gold standard to type amyloid. Although the prognosis for patients with amyloidosis is poor, with shorter survival for light-chain disease,[12] the type of amyloidosis affects available treatment. For patients with nonfamilial transthyretin deposition no specific treatment is available, while for the familial form liver transplantation can abort further deposition. Patients with plasma cell dyscrasias are treated with alkylating agents.

Fabry disease is an X-linked recessive disorder in which a deficiency of α-galactosidase A results in deposition of glycolsphyngolipids causing a restrictive cardiomyopathy. Serum α-galactosidase A level is low and EMB is diagnostic, though rarely necessary. Enzyme replacement offers definitive treatment.[12]

Hemochromatosis is another example of a treatable cause of cardiomyopathy that can cause restrictive physiology.[12] Iron is deposited in the myocardium and other tissues either because of an autosomal recessive disorder in iron uptake or in exposure to excessive iron through transfusion or diet, and results in elevated ferritin and transferrin saturation. This diagnosis is also uniformly made on EMB when present, due to the diffuse nature of the disease, and MRI can elucidate the severity of body iron overload. Other causes of iron overload, such as liver or renal failure, can cause a similar histologic picture, requiring clinical correlation (Figure 6.5). Treatment by phlebotomy or chelation is effective.

Hence, in the setting of restrictive cardiomyopathy or in the setting of unexplained hypertrophy, where etiology remains unclear after routine diagnostic workup, EMB can make the diagnosis and offers important prognostic information. Because most diseases that cause restrictive cardiomyopathy are diagnosed at a high rate

Box 6.1 Selected restrictive cardiomyopathies

- Idiopathic restrictive cardiomyopathy
- Hypertension
- Amyloid
- Hemochromatosis
- Sarcoidosis
- Hypertrophic cardiomyopathy
- Scleroderma
- Hypereosinophilic syndrome
- Fabry disease
- Radiation fibrosis
- Storage diseases

Box 6.2 Grading system for acute cellular rejection

Grade	Signs
0R	No rejection
1R	Interstitial or perivascular infiltrate with no more than one focus of myocyte damage
2R	Two or more foci of infiltrate with myocyte damage
3R	Diffuse infiltrate with multifocal myocyte damage; may have associated edema, hemorrhage, and vasculitis

Adapted from Journal of Heart and Lung Transplantation, Vol 24, Issue 11, Stewart S et al., Revision of the 1990 Working Formulation for the Standardization of Nomenclature in the Diagnosis of Heart Rejection, 1710–1720, copyright (2005) with permission from Elsevier.

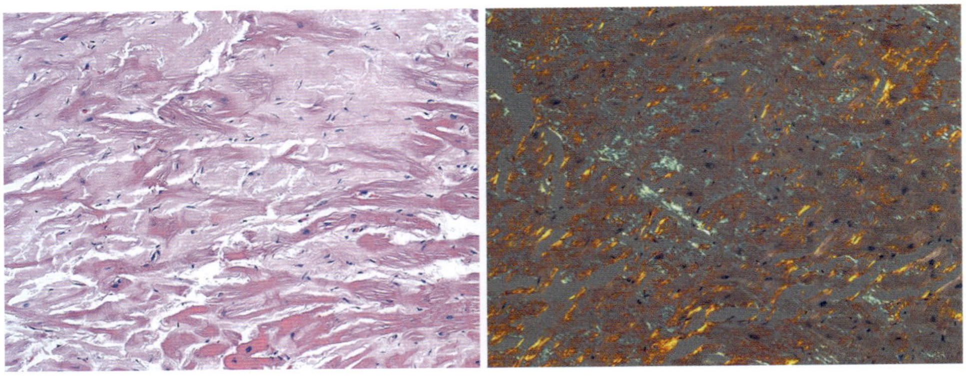

Fig. 6.4 Amyloidosis. Pale pink amorphous material separates the myocytes (H&E, ×64). A Congo red stain displays apple-green birefringence (×64).

(~100% accuracy), when a biopsy is nondiagnostic the clinician should reconsider constrictive disease and focus attention on the pericardium. Imaging modalities such as echocardiography and MRI elucidate structure and function but are limited in providing a definitive diagnosis.

Guiding chemotherapy to prevent heart failure

For the most part, chemotherapy dosing decisions are made on the basis of known risks associated with cumulative dose and by following for changes in myocardial function. However, in patients who may benefit from additional doses of medication despite exceeding a cumulative dose guideline, the technique can be useful in deciding whether to proceed.

EMB is considered to be the most sensitive technique for diagnosis of cardiac toxicity associated with chemotherapy agents (Scenario 5).[1] Chemotherapeutic toxicity to myocardial cells results in characteristic ultrastructural alterations on electron microscopy including patchy myofibrillar dropout, dilatation of sarcoplasmic tubules, and accumulation of lysosomes within the cytoplasm of the myofiber; a grading system has been developed that is based on the percent of cells in the biopsy specimen showing damage (1 if <5%, 2 if 5–35% and 3 if >35%).[13,14] The score appears valuable in predicting risk of heart failure with continuing medication. For instance, a score of 1.5 or more has been associated with a greater than 20% chance of heart failure with additional chemotherapy.[14]

Summary of endomyocardial biopsy for diagnosis of cardiomyopathies

The reader is referred to Table 6.1 and the scientific statement on the role of endomyocardial biopsy in the management of cardiovascular disease,[1] which provides information on the guidelines for EMB for cardiomyopathy diagnosis. In the foregoing we have tried provide a series of principles that encompass the scenarios in the guidelines and also provide a basis for judgment in cases where the scenarios do not precisely apply. To summarize:

- EMB is useful when the etiology of a cardiomyopathy would affect management or provide a clear prognosis *and* when the diagnosis cannot be obtained by routine diagnostic testing.
- We propose that clinical presentation suggests that therapeutically or prognostically useful information is likely in the following settings:
    - Patients with acute onset (first few weeks—2 weeks in the guidelines) of hemodynamically compromising left ventricular dysfunction
    - Patients with recent onset (a few months—3 months in the guidelines) of heart failure refractory to usual treatment or associated with the development of new-onset ventricular tachyarrhythmias or high-grade conduction delays in the setting of left ventricular dysfunction
    - Patients with unexplained restrictive or infiltrative cardiomyopathies.

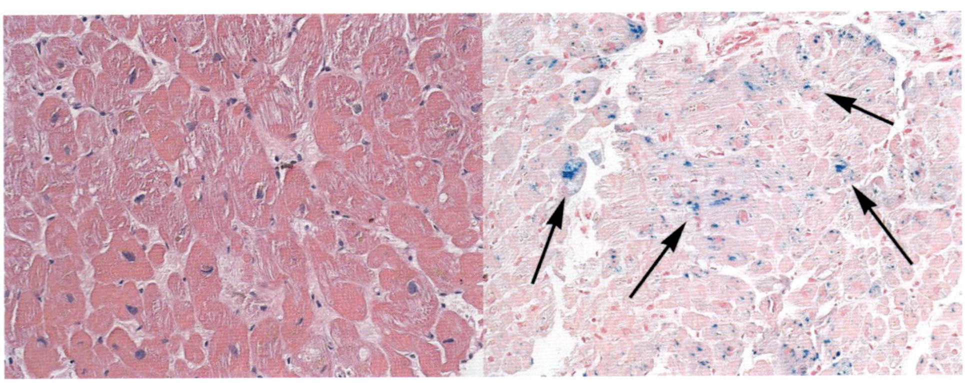

Fig. 6.5 Hemachromatosis or iron overload is difficult to appreciate on an H&E stain, but is clearly evident on a Prussian blue stain (×100).

- EMB may be useful in the setting of unexplained ventricular tachyarrhythmias.
- EMB offers the most specific guidance in making a decision about whether to proceed to a higher than usual dose of chemotherapy when the decision depends on the risk of heart failure or when there is a need for more chemotherapy and there is a question about a causative role of chemotherapy in causing a patient's cardiomyopathy.
- EMB is unlikely to yield useful information in patients with long-standing dilated cardiomyopathies or in those with atrial tachyarrhythmias.
- EMB considerations in children are similar to those in adults (Scenario 8).

Endomyocardial biopsy for post-transplant rejection assessment

Cardiac allograft rejection occurs in 21–30% of patients in the first year after transplant and less frequently thereafter, becoming unusual after the fifth year[15,16,17] Most episodes of rejection are cellular but humoral rejection can occur and grading scales have been developed to describe severity. Importantly, most rejection episodes are discovered on routine surveillance biopsies rather than as a result of presenting with symptoms. Treatment is based on a weighing of rejection type, the state of left ventricular function, and signs and symptoms. Table 6.1 shows an example of a schema for initial treatment based on biopsy result and clinical presentation. For the present, routine EMB is the gold standard for the diagnosis of rejection.

Cellular rejection

EMB is performed as surveillance for both cellular and humoral (antibody-mediated) rejection. Cellular rejection is a predominantly T-cell mediated infiltration and destruction of cardiac myocytes. When the amount of inflammation is high, other inflammatory cells such as B cells, eosinophils, and neutrophils may contribute to the infiltrate.

A variety of histopathologic changes can be seen on EMB in heart transplant patients. In the early years of transplant surveillance, a variety of grading schemes were developed incorporating a number of these features. Ultimately, in 1990, under the leadership of Margaret Billingham and the International Society for Heart and Lung Transplantation, a uniform and standardized grading system was developed.[18] These criteria were revised in 2005, although many centers continue to report on the basis of the 1990 criteria (Box 6.2).[19,20] These grading systems are based upon identifying an inflammatory infiltrate and myocyte injury.

The current grading scheme (ISHLT-2005) has four levels of classification (Table 6.4). The absence of any inflammation is reported as grade 0R—no rejection (R stands for revised). The presence of any pattern of lymphocytic infiltrate and up to a single focus of myocyte injury is considered mild rejection (grade 1R). Multiple foci (two or more) of myocyte injury is indicative of moderate rejection (grade 2R). In moderate rejection, in addition to lymphocytes, occasionally eosinophils and neutrophils can be seen. Severe rejection is seen histopathologically as a heavy inflammatory process with diffuse myocyte injury that can include edema and hemorrhage (grade 3R) (Figure 6.6).

Table 6.4 Initial treatment of rejection

Normal EF	Reduced EF	Heart failure/shock
Cellular		
1R: No treatment	Steroid + taper	1R, 2R, 3R, AMR 1
2R: Steroid + taper		Steroid
		Cytolytic
		Plasmapheresis
		IVIg
		Rituximab
		Hemod support
Humoral		
AMR 0, 1: No treatment	AMR 1: Steroid + taper	Steroid
		Cytolytic
		Plasmapheresis
		IVIg
		Rituximab
		Hemod support

The treatment of transplant patients based on these diagnostic categories is generally consistent among institutions. Almost all transplant centers will leave unchanged, or reduce, the pharmaceutical treatment of a patient with a grade 0R or 1R. Again, almost all centers will treat, by adding additional therapy, any patient with a diagnosis of 2R or 3R. The main variation between centers is the handling of biopsies that show a single focus of myocyte injury. Some centers treat this value as rejection akin to a grade 2R.[21] Other centers increase surveillance of the patient but do not alter treatment therapy. Still other centers do nothing in the setting of this diagnosis.[22]

Antibody-mediated rejection

Antibody-mediated rejection (AMR) has slowly gained acceptance as a cause of cardiac failure, primarily due to the work of M. Elizabeth Hammond.[23] Despite a few outliers, most institutions report very low levels of AMR in their transplant populations.[24] In AMR, antibodies to HLA and other antigens are increased and attack the heart as foreign. A number of risk factors for AMR have been described including female sex, multiparity, prior major surgery, blood transfusions, prior use of OKT3 monoclonal antibody, elevated pretransplant panel reactive antibodies, positive donor-specific crossmatch, cytomegalovirus infection, and the use of left ventricular assist devices.[25] The standard anti-rejection medications treat cellular rejection, not AMR. So the finding of AMR results in the need for alternative therapies.

The earliest descriptions of AMR were histological changes: macrophages filling the lumens of blood vessels, endothelial cell swelling, blebbing, and tissue edema (Figure 6.7). These findings, however, do not have very robust sensitivity or specificity.[26] A number of immunoglobulins and members of the complement cascade have been evaluated for their ability to discriminate AMR.[27] Despite a wide range of stains that have been tried, most institutions now

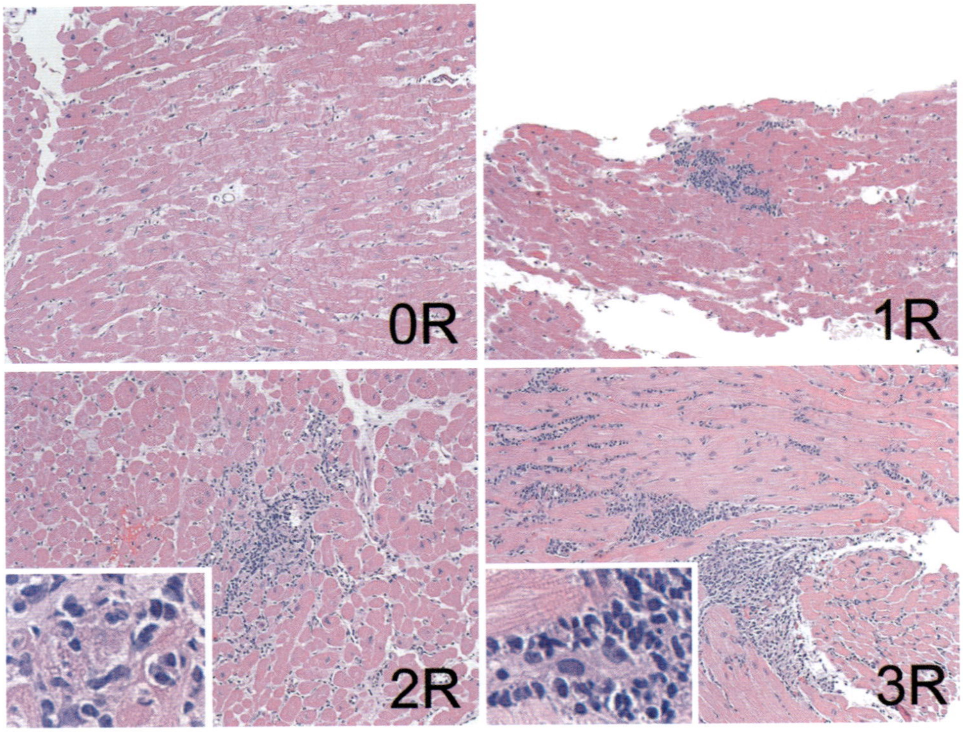

Fig. 6.6 Features of cardiac rejection: 0R, no inflammatory infiltrate; 1R, no myocyte injury; 2R, multifocal myocyte injury (inset) is present; 3R, diffuse multifocal myocyte injury.

evaluate the complement split product C4d as a marker of AMR by either immunofluorescence or immunohistochemistry.[24] These staining methods perform fairly equally.[28] Many institutions augment C4d with C3d, which appears to better predict AMR outcomes (Figure 6.7).[29]

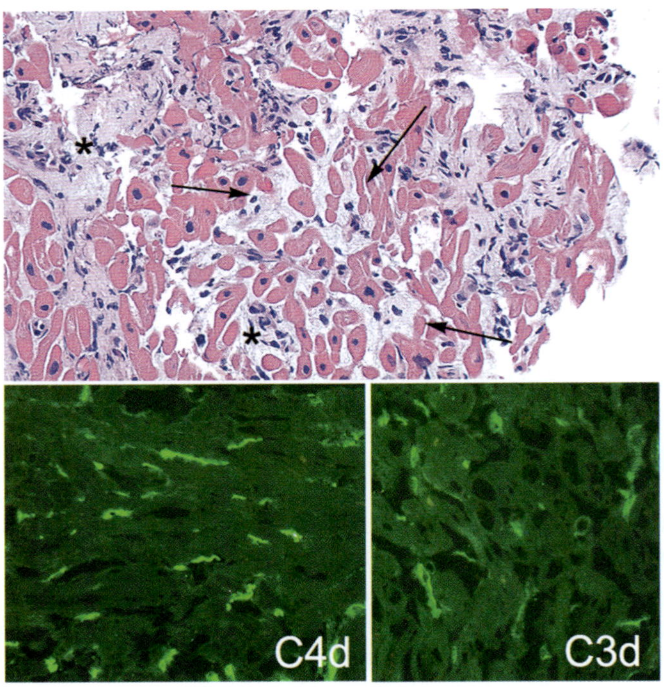

Fig. 6.7 Antibody-mediated rejection: edema (arrows) and increased inflammatory cells (*) in and around blood vessels are seen (×100). Endothelial cells are highlighted by C4d and C3d immunofluorescent staining.

Recently, consensus has been reached regarding the determination of AMR on EMB (Table 6.5).[30] When the diagnosis of AMR is made on histopathologic tissues, it is called pAMR. If histological features are present in the absence of C4d positivity, it is termed pAMR 1(H+). C4d positivity alone is termed pAMR 1 (I+). When both features are present it is called pAMR 2, and when it is severe enough to cause hemorrhage and edema, it is called pAMR 3. At this time it is unknown how this classification scheme correlates with the need to treat or with patient outcome. One recent study in a pediatric population showed no change in all-cause mortality regardless of the pAMR diagnosis.[31] Also unsettled is any consensus on how often to perform C4d staining and whether a pAMR is sufficient to initiate treatment in the absence of other positive data.

Quilty lesions

There are several histopathologic findings one can see on a transplant EMB in addition to describing cellular and antibody-mediated effects. One of the most common findings is a Quilty lesion, or Quilty effect, seen in around 14% of EMB (Figure 6.8). This collection, predominantly of lymphocytes, is mostly an endocardial surface lesion named after the first patient in which it was described. It is a mimicker of rejection and peri-Quilty myocyte injury can be seen at the borders of infiltrative Quilty lesions. Quilty lesions can generally be discriminated from rejection by their increased ratio of B lymphocytes to T lymphocytes, increased vascularity, increased fibrosis, and (when present), the presence of CD21by IHC.[32,33] The clinical significance of Quilty lesions remains an enigma with both positive and negative studies linking the presence of Quilty lesions to AMR, transplant vasculopathy, cellular rejection, and microvascular disease.[34,35,36,37]

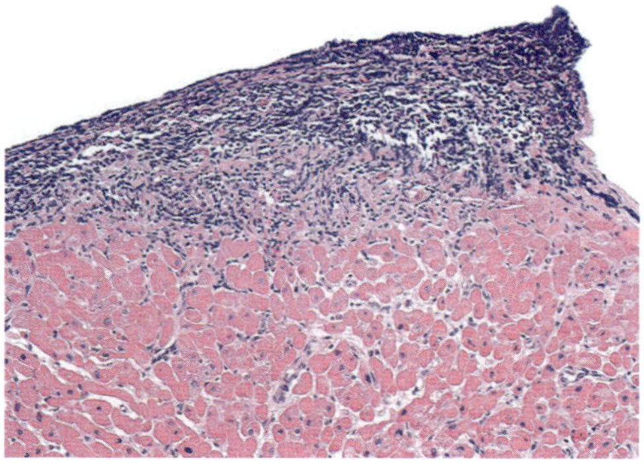

Fig. 6.8 Quilty lesion (H&E, ×64).

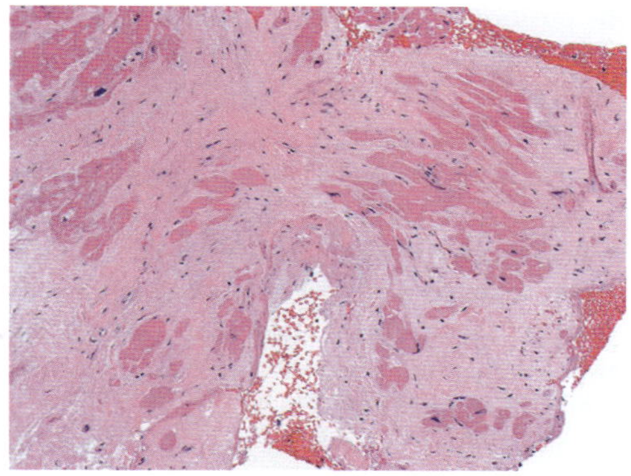

Fig. 6.10 Previous biopsy site showing dense fibrosis, rare inflammatory cells, and disarray of myocytes.

Peritransplant injury

In the early transplant period, a common finding is peritransplant ischemic (preservation procurement) injury (Figure 6.9). This injury changes its histologic appearance as the tissue goes through the healing process. Often at the first biopsy, ischemic injury is noted as collections of anucleate myocytes with wavy fibers and hematoxylin and eosin (H&E) staining that varies from the adjacent viable cells. By 2 weeks, a macrophage infiltrate appears and has begun clearing the dead myocytes. By 4 weeks, ischemic injury is generally noted by pigment-laden macrophages and loose connective tissue where myocytes should have been. Ischemic injury is easily observed by C4d staining, where dead myocytes are strongly stained due to the activation of the complement cascade. Ischemic injury can be a mimicker of cellular rejection, so in the first month post-transplant it is important not to over-interpret this as rejection. Ischemic injury is most noticeable around 2–4 weeks post-transplant and may vary based on the preservation solution.[38,39]

Previous biopsy site

Another common finding on transplant surveillance EMB is scar and organized thrombi associated with a previous biopsy site. In many transplant recipients, the bioptome tends to go to the same place on the interventricular septum. If it has been a short time from the previous biopsy (£2 months), then the biopsy site can be cellular, undergoing reparative processes. It may have overlying thrombus material that is moderately to well organized. An older biopsy site may consist of dense collagen, with poorly oriented myocytes and some inflammatory cells within the fibrosis.

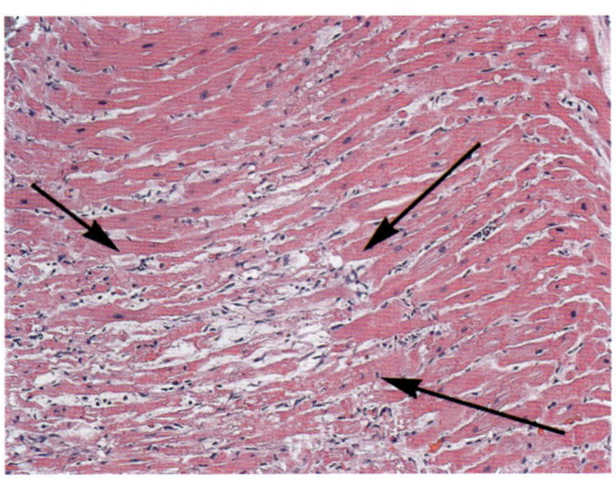

Fig. 6.9 Peritransplant injury. The arrow highlights an area of ischemic injury.

Inflammation in a fibrotic scar is another mimicker of rejection but should not be graded as such (Figure 6.10).

Tumors and infections

Transplant recipients are immunosuppressed and therefore at increased risk of tumors and infections. Skin and solid organ tumors are significantly increased among heart transplant recipients. Post-transplant lymphoproliferative disorder (PTLD) is reported in 2–10% of patients, but is exceedingly rare in the heart.[40] It is strongly associated with an Epstein–Barr virus (EBV) infection. PTLD would appear as a heterogeneous or monomorphic lymphocytic infiltrate with predominantly B cell lymphocytes and EBV positivity by in-situ hybridization. The adjacent cells could be necrotic, making this histologic picture very difficult to distinguish from cellular rejection.[41]

Cytomegalovirus (CMV) infection, although common among transplant recipients, is also rarely noted on EMB. When it appears in the heart, it is more likely to be a primary infection rather than a recurrence. If seen, it is either noted as viral inclusions in endothelial cells without an inflammatory reaction or as viral inclusions in myocytes with a necrotizing myocarditis.[42]

Endomyocardial biopsy technique

Access for EMB is usually gained through the venous system. The right internal jugular (IJ) vein offers a direct approach to the right ventricle (RV), as do the femoral veins. A left subclavian vein approach can be used if incorporating a long venous sheath which can be positioned directly in the RV. Biopsy of the left ventricle through the arterial system is possible, but is usually avoided because of the risk of damaging the mitral valve chordae and producing mitral regurgitation. Because there is no safety difference between an IJ or femoral venous approach, the choice is usually based on patient and provider preference. Some argue that procedural and recovery times are shorter with an IJ approach whereas others prefer the comfort of a femoral approach.

EMB may be performed using fluoroscopy or echocardiography for guidance. The advantage of echocardiography is its easy applicability and the avoidance of radiation exposure for patient and provider alike. In appropriate instances, the use of echocardiography allows biopsies to be performed in the intensive care unit (ICU), obviating the need to transfer vulnerable patients to a catheterization laboratory. Echocardiography also allows direct visualization of bioptome positioning against the interventricular septum and away from tricuspid valve (TV) chordae, minimizing procedural complications. On the other hand, most centers employ fluoroscopy either with a portable C arm in a dedicated biopsy suite or in a cardiac catheterization laboratory. Fluoroscopy allows the direct visualization of the bioptome as it passes through the superior or inferior vena cava across the TV into the RV. Positioning the image intensifier from an anteroposterior (AP) to an left anterior oblique (LAO) projection allows for confirmation that the bioptome is directed toward the septum and away from the anterior wall, avoiding the risk of perforation of the RV.

Standard equipment consists of a venous access sheath and a bioptome. The original multi-use Scholten bioptome, fashioned from a forceps handle and long biotome, has given way to disposable single-use bioptomes. Typical bioptomes range in size from 5 to 7 French, with smaller devices being more flexible and larger ones procuring more adequately sized samples. Use of a 45 cm venous sheath positioned directly adjacent the RV septum over an 0.025 inch (0.64 mm) wire is particularly helpful in those cases where passing a bioptome across a "ledge" at the junction between the donor and recipient superior vena cava (SVC) is difficult. This setup also avoids any errant passage of the rigid bioptome across the suture line in the first few biopsies after transplantation. When taking a femoral venous approach, directing a long (70 cm) sheath into the RV may be facilitated by using an internal balloon-tipped catheter rather than the stiffer introducer.

EMB is a safe procedure with a serious complication rate of only 0.1%. Pneumothorax, ventricular arrhythmias, supraventricular arrhythmias, carotid artery puncture, venous hematoma, and heart block are all infrequent complications in experienced centers. RV perforation leading to tampanade and hemodynamic collapse is infrequently encountered. Although the rate of ventricular perforation is probably higher than assumed, rarely does tamponade develop since the potential space between myocardium and pericardium is frequently obliterated after transplantation. When present, tamponade may be detected first by the loss of the "y" descent in the central venous pressure (CVP) trace and later confirmed with echocardiography. TV injury with the subsequent development of chronic tricuspid regurgitation is common, but rarely requires surgical intervention. The adoption of less frequent protocol biopsies and early cessation of routine surveillance has decreased the incidence of chronic tricuspid regurgitation. Biopsying structures other than RV endocardium may be best avoided by confirming the bioptome's position by echocardiography or fluoroscopy and seeing PVCs on the ECG before opening the bioptome.

Pathologic processes and evidence of transplant rejection, when present, are heterogeneously distributed in the myocardium. As a result, a sufficient number of biopsy specimens is needed to achieve adequate sensitivity and specificity. Guidelines published on behalf of the ISHLT recommend at least three biopsy specimens containing at least 50% myocardium.[43] Prior data suggest that with three biopsy specimens there is only a 5% chance of missing mild rejection and 0% of missing moderate or severe rejection.[44] With four specimens, the chance of missing mild rejection falls to 2%.[45]

To avoid introducing artifacts, specimens should not be handled with a forceps or cut with a scalpel and should not be left in contact with normal saline or nonisosmotic solutions more than briefly.[46]

Endomyocardial samples placed into 10% phosphate-buffered formalin may be stained with hematoxylin and eosin or immunoshistochemical stains looking for complement degradation proteins (C4d and C3d) present in humoral rejection or CD68, a macrophage marker. Samples undergoing immunofluorescence should first be placed into OCT compound (Miles Inc., Diagnostics Division, Elkhart, IN, USA) and deep frozen.

References

1. Cooper L, Baughman K, Feldman A, et al. The role of endomyocardial biopsy in the management of cardiovascular disease. Circulation 2007;116:2116–233.
2. Bennett MK, Gilotra NA, Harrington C, et al. Evaluation of the role of endomyocardial biopsy in 851 patients with unexplained heart failure from 2000–2009. Circ Heart Fail 2013;6:676–84.
3. Cooper L, Barry G, Shebetai R, et al. Idiopathic giant cell myocarditis—natural history and treatment. N Engl J Med 1997;336:1860–6.
4. Kilgallen C, Jackson E, Sakomon R, et al. A case of giant cell myocarditis and malignant thymoma: a postmortem diagnosis by needle biopsy. Clin Cardiol 1998;21:48–51.
5. Daniels P, Berry G, Tazelaar H, et al. Giant cell myocarditis as a manifestation of drug hypersensitivity. Cardiovasc Pathol 2000;9:287–91.
6. Gupta S, Markham DW, Drazner MH, Mammen PP. Fulminant myocarditis. Nat Clin Pract Cardiovasc Med 2008;5:693–706.
7. DeMello D, Liapis H, Juveidini J, et al. Cardiac localization of eosinophil granule major basic protein in acute necrotizing myocarditis. N Engl J Med 1990;325:1542–5.
8. Hawkins E, Levine T, Goa S, et al. Hypersensitivity myocarditis in the explanted heart of transplant recipients: reappraisal of pathologic criteria and their clinical implications. Pathol Annual 1995;30 (Part 1) 287–304.
9. Taliercin C, Olney B, Lie J. Myocarditis related to drug hypersensitivity. Mayo Clin Proc 1985;60:463–8.
10. Litovsky SH, Burke AP, Virmani R. Giant cell myocarditis: an entity distinct from sarcoidosis characterized by multiphasic destruction by cytotoxic T cells and histiocytic giant cells. Mod Pathol 1996;9:1126–34.
11. Takado K, Ina Y, Yamamoto M, et al. Prognosis after pacemaker implantation in sarcoidosis in Japan: Clinical evaluation of corticosteroid treatment. Sarcoidosis 1994;11:113–17.
12. Hare J. The dilated, restrictive, and infiltrative cardiomypathies. In: Bonow RO, Mann DL, Zipes DP, and Libby P, ed., Braunwald's Heart Disease: A Textbook of Cardiovascular Medicine, 9th edition. Philadelphia, PA: Elsevier; 2012; pp. 1739–63.
13. Meinardi M, van der Graaf W, van Veldhuisen D, et al. Detection of anthracyclin-induced cardiotoxicity. Cancer Treat Rev 1999;25:237–47.
14. Macay B, Ever M, Carrasco C, et al. Assessment of anthracycline cardiomyopathy by endomyocardial biopsy. Ultrastructural Pathol 1994;18:203–11.
15. Lindenfeld J, Miller G, Shaker S, et al. Drug therapy in the heart transplant recipient: part 1: cardiac rejection and immunosuppressive drugs. Circulation 2004;110:3734–40.
16. Taylor D, Edwards L, Mohacsi P, et al. The registry of the International Society for Heart and Lung Transplantation: twentieth official adult heart transplant report—2003. J Heart Lung Transplant 2003;22:616–24.
17. Tan CD, Baldwin WM 3rd, Rodriguez ER. Update on cardiac transplantation. Arch Path Lab Med 2007; I31:1169–91.
18. Billingham ME, Cary NR, Hammond ME, et al. A working formulation for the standardization of nomenclature in the diagnosis of heart and lung rejection: Heart Rejection Study Group. The International Society for Heart Transplantation. J Heart Transplant 1990;9:587–93.
19. Stewart S, Winters GL, Fishbein MC, et al. Revision of the 1990 working formulation for the standardization of nomenclature in the diagnosis of heart rejection. J Heart Lung Transplant 2005;24:1710–20.

20. Maleszewski JJ, Kucirka LM, Segev DL, Halushka MK. Survey of current practice related to grading of rejection in cardiac transplant recipients in North America. Cardiovasc Pathol 2011;20:261–5.
21. Felkel TO, Smith AL, Reichenspurner HC, et al. Survival and incidence of acute rejection in heart transplant recipients undergoing successful withdrawal from steroid therapy. J Heart Lung Transplant 2002;21:530–9.
22. Fishbein MC, Bell G, Lones MA et al. Grade 2 cellular heart rejection: does it exist? J Heart Lung Transplant 1994;13:1051–7.
23. Hammond ME, Stehlik J, Snow G et al. Utility of histologic parameters in screening for antibody-mediated rejection of the cardiac allograft: a study of 3,170 biopsies. J Heart Lung Transplant 2005;24:2015–21.
24. Kucirka LM, Maleszewski JJ, Segev DL, Halushka MK. Survey of North American pathologist practices regarding antibody-mediated rejection in cardiac transplant biopsies. Cardiovasc Pathol 2011;20:132–8.
25. Almuti K, Haythe J, Dwyer E, et al. The changing pattern of humoral rejection in cardiac transplant recipients. Transplantation 2007;84:498–503.
26. Hammond ME, Stehlik J, Snow G, et al. Utility of histologic parameters in screening for antibody-mediated rejection of the cardiac allograft: a study of 3,170 biopsies. J Heart Lung Transplant 2005;24:2015–21.
27. Rodriguez ER, Skojec DV, Tan CD, et al. Antibody-mediated rejection in human cardiac allografts: evaluation of immunoglobulins and complement activation products C4d and C3d as markers. Am J Transplant 2005;5:2778–85.
28. Miller DV, Roden AC, Gamez JD, Tazelaar HD. Detection of C4d deposition in cardiac allografts: a comparative study of immunofluorescence and immunoperoxidase methods. Arch Pathol Lab Med 2010;134:1679–84.
29. Tan CD, Sokos GG, Pidwell DJ, et al. Correlation of donor-specific antibodies, complement and its regulators with graft dysfunction in cardiac antibody-mediated rejection. Am J Transplant 2009;9:2075–84.
30. Berry GJ, Angelini A, Burke MM, et al. The ISHLT working formulation for pathologic diagnosis of antibody-mediated rejection in heart transplantation: evolution and current status (2005–2011). J Heart Lung Transplant 2011;30:601–11.
31. Everitt MD, Hammond ME, Snow GL et al. Biopsy-diagnosed antibody-mediated rejection based on the proposed International Society for Heart and Lung Transplantation working formulation is associated with adverse cardiovascular outcomes after pediatric heart transplant. J Heart Lung Transplant 2012;31:686–93.
32. Gopal S, Narasimhan U, Day JD et al. The Quilty lesion enigma: focal apoptosis/necrosis and lymphocyte subsets in human cardiac allografts. Pathol Int 1998;48:191–8.
33. Sattar HA, Husain AN, Kim AY, Krausz T, et al. The presence of a CD21+ follicular dendritic cell network distinguishes invasive Quilty lesions from cardiac acute cellular rejection. Am J Surg Pathol 2006;30:1008–13.
34. Costanzo-Nordin MR, Winters GL, Fisher SG, et al. Endocardial infiltrates in the transplanted heart: clinical significance emerging from the analysis of 5026 endomyocardial biopsy specimens. J Heart Lung Transplant 1993;12:741–7.
35. Joshi A, Masek MA, Brown BW Jr, Weiss LM, Billingham ME. "Quilty" revisited: a 10-year perspective. Hum Pathol 1995;26:547–57.
36. Chu KE, Ho EK, de la Torre L, et al. The relationship of nodular endocardial infiltrates (Quilty lesions) to survival, patient age, anti-HLA antibodies, and coronary artery disease following heart transplantation. Cardiovasc Pathol 2005;14:219–24.
37. Hiemann NE, Knosalla C, Wellnhofer E, et al. Quilty indicates increased risk for microvasculopathy and poor survival after heart transplantation. J Heart Lung Transplant 2008;27:289–96.
38. Wasowska BA, Lee CY, Halushka MK, Baldwin WM 3rd. New concepts of complement in allorecognition and graft rejection. Cell Immunol 2007;248:18–30.
39. George TJ, Arnaoutakis GJ, Beaty CA, et al. A novel method of measuring cardiac preservation injury demonstrates University of Wisconsin solution is associated with less ischemic necrosis than Celsior in early cardiac allograft biopsy specimens. J Heart Lung Transplant 2012;31:410–18.
40. Khedmat H, Taheri S. Heart allograft involvement by posttransplant lymphoproliferative disorders: report from the PTLD. Int survey. Exp Clin Transplant 2011;9:258–64.
41. Nalesnik MA, Jaffe R, Starzl TE, et al. The pathology of posttransplant lymphoproliferative disorders occurring in the setting of cyclosporine A-prednisone immunosuppression. Am J Pathol 1988;133:173–92.
42. Arbustini E, Grasso M, Diegoli M, et al. Histopathologic and molecular profile of human cytomegalovirus infections in patients with heart transplants. Am J Clin Pathol 1992;98:205–13.
43. Stewart S, Winters G, Fishbein M, et al. Revision of the 1990 working formulation for the standardization of nomenclature in the diagnosis of heart rejection. J Heart Lung Transplant 2005;24:1710–20.
44. Billingham M, Cary N, Hammond M, et al. A working formulation for the standardization of nomenclature in the. Diagnosis of heart and lung rejection: Heart Rejection Study Group. The International Society for Heart Transplantation. Heart Transplant 1990;9:587–93.
45. Spiegelhalter D, Stovin P. An analysis of repeated biopsies following cardiac transplantation. Stat Med 1983;2:33–40.
46. Tan C, Baldwin W, Rodriguez R. Update on cardiac transplantation pathology. Arch Path Lab Med 2007;131:1169–91.

CHAPTER 7

Imaging in advanced heart failure

Mayank Kansal MD, Manish Bansal MD, Jagat Narula MD, and Partho P. Sengupta MD

Introduction

Imaging techniques play an indispensable role in the management of patients presenting with advanced heart failure (HF). From underlying etiopathological mechanisms to the severity and nature of HF, imaging provides a plethora of information that not only is critical to decision-making but has prognostic significance as well. Almost all therapeutic decisions in these patients, whether relating to medical therapy, surgery, or device therapy, are guided partly or wholly by information derived through imaging.

Echocardiography, nuclear imaging, and magnetic resonance techniques form the mainstay of imaging in HF. Due to its wider availability, ease of use, low cost, easy repeatability, and ability to provide comprehensive information about different elements of cardiac structure and function, echocardiography is the imaging test of choice in most patients with HF. Nuclear imaging and MRI have their own advantages but play largely a complementary role in HF patients. However, as discussed below, there are several indications for which they have incremental value over echocardiography, and are therefore preferred.

Echocardiography in heart failure

As mentioned above, echocardiography is the most widely used imaging modality in patients with HF. The applicability, reproducibility, and easy availability of echocardiography are well suited to the need for comprehensive noninvasive evaluation in these patients. Morphologic assessment of left ventricular (LV) dimensions and ejection fraction (EF) provides information that has prognostic and therapeutic implications. Doppler assessment of intracardiac hemodynamics allows for real-time assessment of volume status and stroke volume that can aid in medication titration. Patients in need of advanced HF therapies such as cardiac resynchronization therapy (CRT), implantable cardioverter defibrillator (ICD), ventricular assist devices (VADs), surgical correction of mitral regurgitation (MR), ventricular reconstruction surgery, or heart transplantation can be appropriately selected and followed serially to assess for complications as well as for improvement in cardiac function. Newer echocardiographic techniques such as strain and three-dimensional (3D) imaging enable echocardiography to provide further insights into cardiac morphology and function that will continue to aid in the assessment and management of patients with HF.

Assessment of intracardiac hemodynamics

Knowledge of the intracardiac hemodynamics in patients with HF is vital to facilitate appropriate management, both during the chronic, compensated phase as well as during acute decompensation. While a thorough physical examination is often helpful in getting an initial impression of the overall hemodynamic condition of the patient, it is limited in its ability to accurately characterize right- and left-sided filling pressures.[1,2] Direct measurement of filling pressures by an intracardiac catheter can provide more comprehensive and accurate hemodynamic data and remains the gold standard for this purpose. However, invasive hemodynamic monitoring is expensive and is associated with an appreciable risk of complications that may often outweigh the benefits derived.[3,4,5] In contrast, echocardiography can provide hemodynamic information comparable to that obtained by cardiac catheterization,[6] but without the risks of performing an invasive procedure. More importantly, the greatest advantage of echocardiography is to permit serial assessment of hemodynamics, as and when needed, which is particularly relevant to this patient population.

Stroke volume and cardiac output

During echocardiography, a combination of two-dimensional (2D) and Doppler imaging can provide a rapid and reliable estimate of the LV stroke volume and cardiac output.[7] The basic principle involved is that the flow through any structure within the cardiovascular systems is equal to the cross-sectional area of the structure and the distance traveled by the blood column during a given period of time (Figure 7.1). If the blood flow is constant, the distance can be easily calculated by multiplying flow velocity by time. However, in the cardiovascular system, blood flow is pulsatile and therefore instantaneous velocities need to be measured and integrated over time to obtain the corresponding distance value. Echocardiographically, this can be accomplished by manually tracing the outer border of the spectral Doppler velocity signal; the built-in software automatically provides the velocity–time integral (VTI; Figure 7.2). Multiplying the VTI by the cross-sectional area of the structure provides stroke volume through that structure and further multiplication by heart rate provides cardiac output.

With echocardiography, stroke volume and cardiac output can be measured across any cardiac structure that lends itself to an accurate measurement of the size and the blood velocity at that level. However, in practice, the LV outflow tract (LVOT) is the commonest site used for this purpose, for several reasons. The LVOT is easily visualized during echocardiography, its cross-section is nearly circular, and its size remains almost constant during the cardiac cycle. In addition, the blood flow through the LVOT is mostly laminar, which minimizes the chances of inadvertently sampling velocities that are not truly representative of the actual blood flow at that point. All these factors contribute to an accurate estimation of cardiac output at this level.

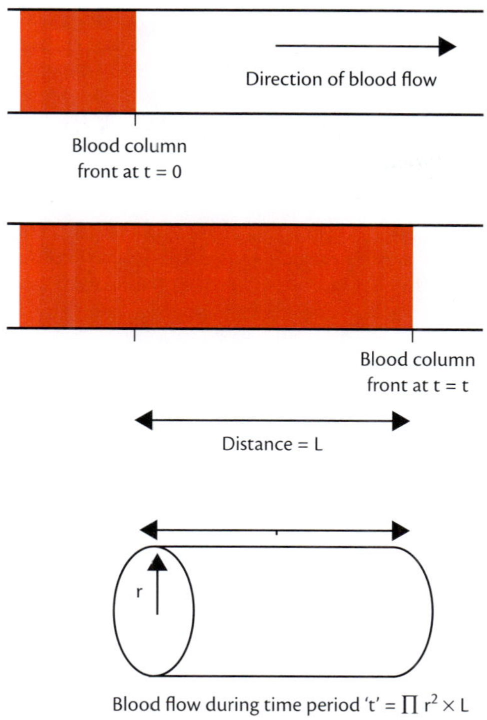

Fig. 7.1 The underlying principle of echocardiographic estimation of blood flow through the cardiovascular system. See text for details.

The LVOT area is calculated by measuring the LVOT diameter from the parasternal long-axis view (Figure 7.3). The LVOT diameter is measured as the distance between the insertion points or the hinge points of the two aortic valve leaflets during early systole when the valve leaflets are fully open. Care should be taken to obtain an accurate measurement because any error will be magnified when the cross-sectional area is calculated. To ensure this, the diameter should be measured 3–5 times, and the largest of these measurements should be used in the equation. Magnifying the image also helps to minimize any measurement error. The LVOT VTI is measured in the apical five-chamber view by placing the pulsed-wave sample volume in the LVOT, at a location roughly 5 mm proximal to the aortic valve (see Figure 7.3). The correct placement can be confirmed by the presence of the aortic valve closing click and the absence of the opening click on the spectral Doppler display. In addition, spectral broadening of the signal is minimal at this level, which also helps in confirming the correct positioning of the sample volume. After the spectral Doppler signal is obtained, the VTI is derived by tracing the outer border of the signal. The outer edge of the densest portion of the signal should be traced, and the dispersion outside of this dense signal (greatest at the peak velocity) should be ignored. All Doppler measurements should be obtained at a sweep speed of 50–100 mm/s, and the filter settings should be kept at low values. The measurements should be averaged over 3–5 cardiac cycles during sinus rhythm and over 5–10 cardiac cycles during atrial fibrillation.[7]

There are several circumstances in which the cardiac output measured at the LVOT may not be accurate or representative of true cardiac output. When the difficulties relate to accurate estimation of LVOT size and VTI, as in presence of significant LVOT obstruction, the measurements can be performed at the mitral valve or at the right ventricular outflow tract (RVOT), provided there is no significant MR or intracardiac shunt respectively. When performing these measurements on the right side of the heart, it is important to average the measurements over the entire respiratory cycle to account for the influence of respiration on the right side blood flow. Alternately, a non-Doppler method can also be used to measure stroke volume. The LV end-diastolic and end-systolic volumes are calculated using the modified Simpsons' method, as described below, and the difference between the two is the stroke volume. Of course, this latter method will not be applicable in presence of significant aortic regurgitation (AR) which is characterized by disproportionately increased LV cardiac output.

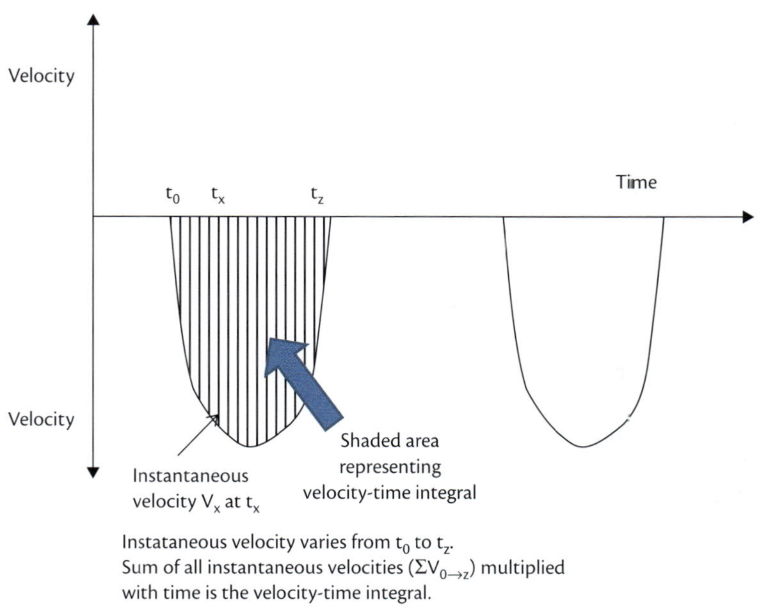

Fig. 7.2 Concept of velocity–time integral used for Doppler estimation of blood flow. See text for details.
Modified with permission from Feigenbaum H, Armstrong W, Ryan T, eds. Feigenbaum's Echocardiography. 6th ed. Philadelphia: Lippincott, Williams and Wilkins, 2005.

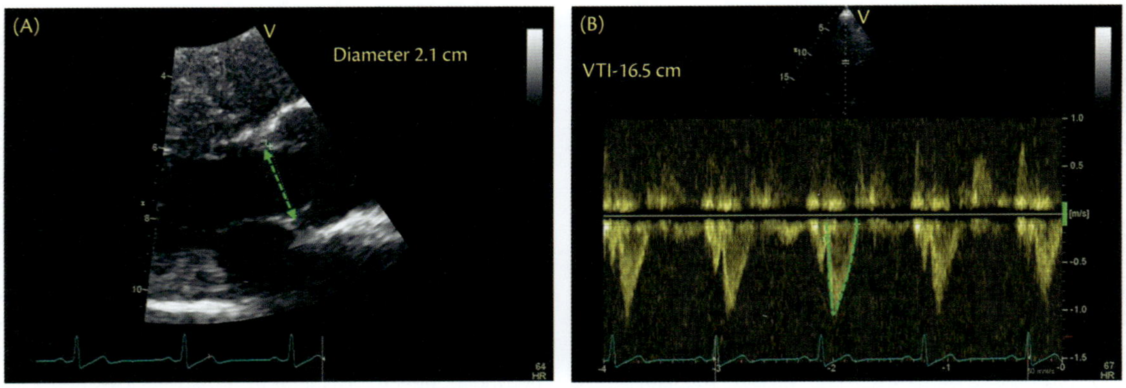

Stroke volume = cross-sectional area × VTI
= 0.785 × 2.1 × 2.1 × 16.5
= 57.1 ml
Cardiac output = stroke volume × heart rate
= 57.1 × 67
= 3.83 l/min

Fig. 7.3 Echocardiographic estimation of cardiac output at the left ventricular outflow tract (LVOT). (A) LVOT diameter is measured from parasternal long-axis view in mid-systole. (B) LVOT velocity–time integral (VTI) is measured using pulsed-wave Doppler in apical five-chamber view. See text for details.

Intracardiac pressures

Right heart filling pressures

Right-sided filling pressures can be estimated by measuring inferior vena cava (IVC) size and its collapsibility on inspiration (Figure 7.4).[8] An IVC 2.1 cm or less in size with more than 50% collapse with respiration corresponds to a mean right atrial (RA) pressure of 3 mmHg (range 0–5 mmHg), whereas a size greater than 2.1 cm with less than 50% collapse on inspiration indicates an RA pressure of 15 mmHg (range 10–20 mmHg). A small IVC without significant collapse or a large IVC with significant collapse corresponds to an RA pressure in the intermediate range (average 8 mmHg, range 5–10 mmHg). The IVC size should be measured just proximal to the junction of the hepatic veins that lie approximately 0.5 to 3.0 cm proximal to the ostium of the RA. Accurate assessment of IVC size and collapsibility is affected by several factors. Transducer positioning parallel to the axis of the IVC is necessary to avoid underestimation of IVC size. Additionally, young, healthy, and athletic individuals can have an enlarged IVC, in which case assessment of hepatic vein inflows can be used to further define the true RA pressure. In patients on mechanical ventilation, the positive intrathoracic pressure during inspiration will falsely reduce IVC collapsibility, precluding accurate assessment of RA pressure. Whenever there is uncertainty, additional indices of RA pressure should be obtained by examining right ventricle (RV) inflow pattern, tricuspid annular early diastolic velocity, hepatic vein flow pattern, etc.[8]

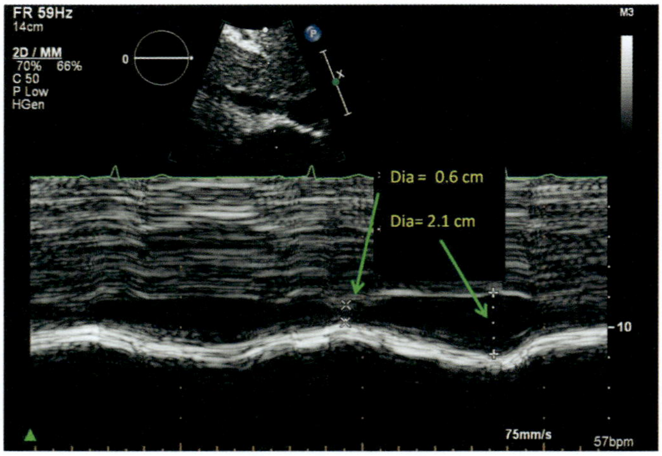

Fig. 7.4 Estimation of right atrial pressure (RAP) from inferior vena cava (IVC) size and collapsibility with inspiration. In this example, the IVC is dilated (2.1 cm) but collapses more than 50% on deep inspiration, suggesting mean RAP to be roughly 8 mmHg.

Pulmonary artery pressures

Echocardiography permits indirect estimation of almost all the different elements of pulmonary vascular hemodynamics including pulmonary artery (PA) systolic pressure (PASP), PA diastolic pressure, mean PA pressure, pulmonary capillary wedge pressure (PCWP), and pulmonary vascular resistance (PVR).[8]

PASP is usually estimated from the tricuspid regurgitation (TR) jet (Figure 7.5). The TR jet is a reflection of the peak pressure gradient between RV and RA during systole and therefore adding RA pressure to peak TR gradient provides an estimate of RV systolic pressure, which in absence of RVOT obstruction is same as PASP. The peak TR gradient is measured from TR jet velocity using the simplified Bernoulli equation ($\Delta P = 4v.^2$, where ΔP is the pressure gradient and v is the jet velocity) and the RA pressure is estimated from IVC, as described above. From this data, PASP can be calculated using the following equation:

$$\begin{aligned}\text{PASP} &= \text{RV systolic pressure}\\ &= 4\,(\text{Peak TR velocity})^2 + \text{mean RA pressure}\end{aligned}$$

However, interpretable TR waveforms are available only in approximately 80% of cases,[9] though they may be improved with the use of saline contrast.[8,10] Underestimation of TR velocities by nonparallel ultrasound interrogation or incomplete flow profiles are common errors, while overestimation of PASP may also happen due to overestimation of RA pressure or problems with the simplified

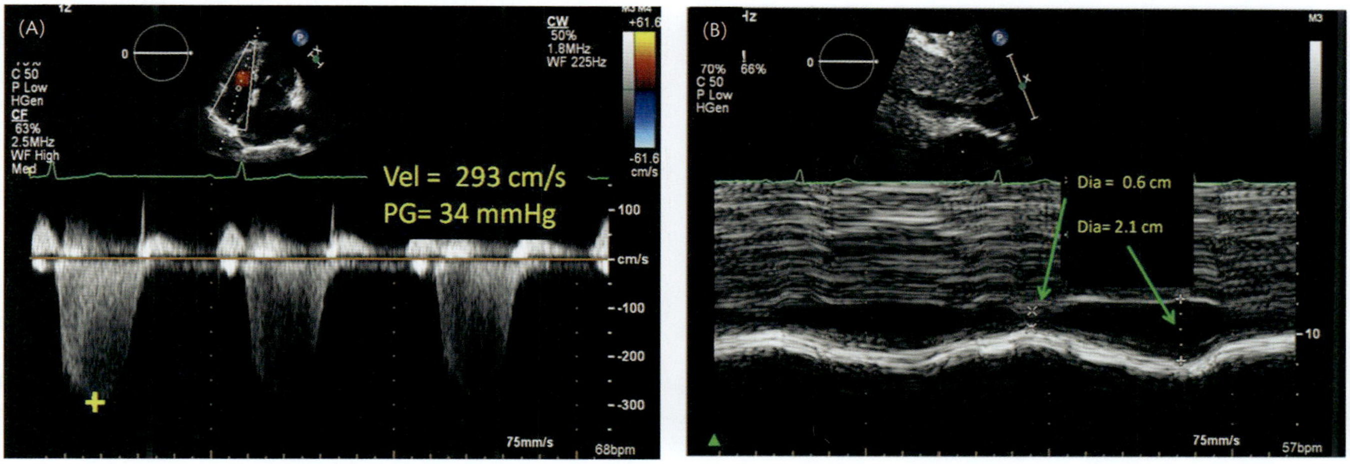

Pulmonary artery systolic pressure = Peak tricuspid regurgitation gradient + Mean right atrial pressure
= 34 + 8 = 42 mmHg

Fig. 7.5 Estimation of pulmonary artery or right ventricular systolic pressure from tricuspid regurgitation jet (A) and inferior vena cava (B). See text for details.

Bernoulli equation as a result of pressure recovery phenomena or changes in blood viscosity from anemia or hypoxemia.[11] A non-TR-dependent measurement utilizing the time from onset of PA flow to the peak of PA flow, also known as RVOT/PA acceleration time, has recently been shown to accurately quantitate peak PASP using the following equation:.[12]

$$\log\left[\text{PASP}\right] = -0.004(\text{PA acceleration time}) + 2.1 \text{ with an r value of } -0.95$$

where PASP is measured in mmHg and PA acceleration time in ms.

RVOT/PA acceleration time is measured from the basal short-axis view, by placing the pulsed-wave sample volume within the RVOT or just at the pulmonary valve annulus to obtain the RVOT jet velocity trace. The time from the onset of the trace to peak velocity is the acceleration time.

PA end-diastolic pressure can be calculated by measuring the pulmonary regurgitation (PR) end-diastolic velocity on Doppler interrogation of the PR jet. As PR is a reflection between the diastolic pressure gradient between the PA and the RV, adding the estimated RV end-diastolic pressure (which is similar to mean RA pressure in absence of RV inflow obstruction) to the PR end-diastolic gradient yields PA end-diastolic pressure as

$$\text{PA end-diastolic pressure} = \text{End-diastolic PR gradient} + \text{RV end-diastolic pressure, or}$$

$$\text{PA end-diastolic pressure} = 4 \times (\text{End-diastolic PR velocity})^2 + \text{mean RA pressure}$$

Unlike the PA systolic and diastolic pressures, it is not possible to estimate PA mean pressure directly on echocardiography and is therefore extrapolated from other indices. Numerous echocardiographic methods are available to estimate PA mean pressure that have been validated in different studies.

- *From PASP*: Chemla et al.,.[13] using cardiac catheterization, demonstrated that there was a linear relationship between PASP and the mean PA pressure, which could be expressed by the following regression equation:

$$\text{Mean PA pressure (mmHg)} = 0.61 \times \text{PASP (derived from TR velocity)} + 2 \text{ mmHg}$$

Subsequently, Friedberg et al.[14] proposed a similar formula by Doppler echocardiography, in a slightly different patient population:

$$\text{Mean PA pressure(mmHg)} = 0.69 \times \text{PASP} - 0.22$$

- *From the PR jet*: In this method, mean PA pressure is derived from the continuous-wave spectral trace of the PR jet using the simplified Bernoulli equation:

$$\text{Mean PA pressure} = 4 \times (\text{peak PR velocity})^2.$$

The addition of echocardiographically derived RA pressure has been shown to increase the accuracy of the peak PR estimate by this method from a mean of –8 mmHg to within +1 mmHg of catheterization-derived measurements.[15]

- *From RVOT acceleration time*: The mean PA pressure can be derived from the RVOT acceleration time, using the following regression equation (also known as Mahan's equation) which has been shown to correlate well with invasively derived values:.[16]

$$\text{Mean PA pressure} = 79 - (0.45 \times \text{RVOT acceleration time in msec})$$
(Figure 7.6)

When the acceleration time is less than 120 ms, the formula needs to be modified:.[17]

$$\text{Mean PA pressure} = 90 - (0.62 \times \text{RVOT acceleration time})$$

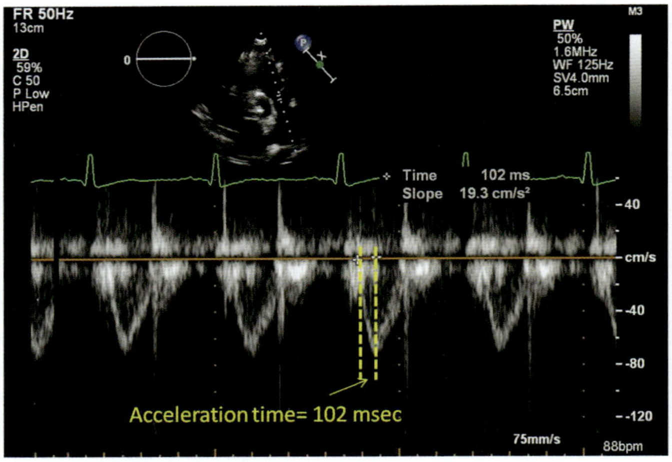

Mean PAP in mmHg = 79–(0.45 × RVOT acceleration time in msec)
Mean PAP = 79–0.45 × 102 = 79–45.9 = 33.1 mmHg

Fig. 7.6 Estimation of mean pulmonary artery pressure (PAP) from RVOT acceleration time.

Other investigators have proposed a different method for estimation of mean PA pressure from RVOT acceleration time:.[18]

$$\log_{10}(\text{mean PA pressure}) = -0.0068 \times \text{RVOT acceleration time} + 2.1$$

A simple rule of thumb from the above equations is that an acceleration time of less than 100 ms will imply presence of elevated mean PA pressure and can be used a rough indicator of pulmonary hypertension.

- *From the TR jet*: In a recent study, a novel method has been proposed for estimation of mean PA pressure from the TR jet.[19] It was found that mean PA pressure derived by adding RA pressure to the mean TR gradient approximated catheterization-derived mean PA pressure to an average difference of −1.6 mmHg.

PCWP is same as mean left atrium (LA) pressure and can be estimated as described in the next section.

Left heart filling pressures

The recently published guidelines by the American Society of Echocardiography have outlined the stepwise approach to estimation of left heart filling pressure in patients with and without LV systolic dysfunction.[20] In patients with LV systolic dysfunction, when mitral inflow *E/A*—the ratio of the mitral inflow early diastolic velocity (*E*) to late diastolic velocity (*A*)—is less than 1 and *E* is less than 50 cm/s, a normal LA pressure can be safely assumed (Figure 7.7). However, when the *E/A* ratio is ≥2 or mitral *E* deceleration time (*dtE*) is less than 150 ms, an increased LA pressure is assumed. In the intermediate situations, i.e., when *E/A* is greater than 1 but less than 2, or when it is less than 1 but with *E* greater than 50 cm/s, additional information needs to be obtained by assessing mitral annular early diastolic velocity (*e´*), mitral inflow propagation velocity (*Vp*), pulmonary vein flow pattern, especially the duration of *A* reversal (*Ar*), PASP, etc., and the presence of any of the following two abnormalities indicates elevated LV filling pressures:

- average *E*/*e´* ratio >15
- *E*/*Vp* ratio >2.5
- pulmonary veins systolic to diastolic ratio <1
- *Ar*–mitral *A* duration >30 ms
- PA systolic pressure >35 mmHg.

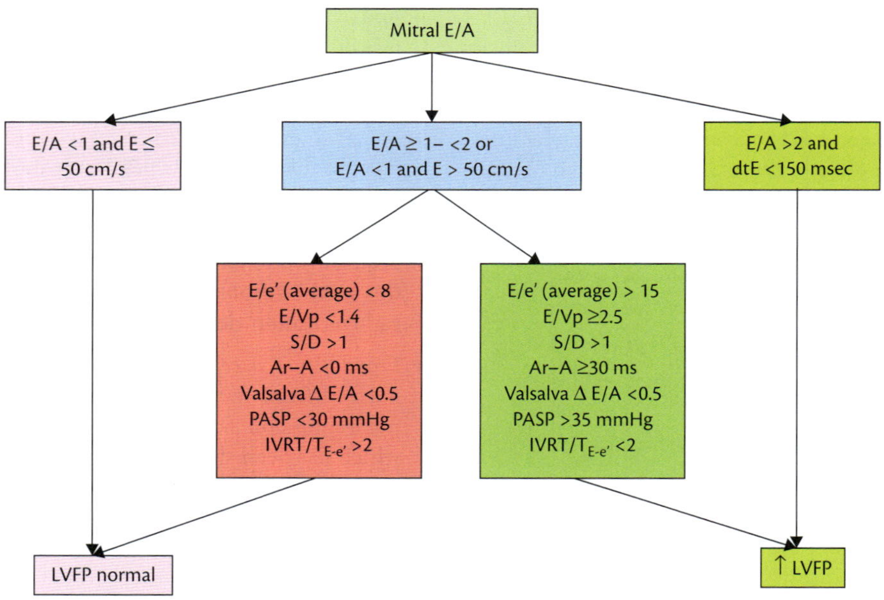

Fig. 7.7 Echocardiographic assessment of left ventricular filling pressure (LVFP) in presence of left ventricular systolic dysfunction. A, mitral inflow late diastolic velocity; Ar, atrial reversal in the pulmonary vein flow; D, pulmonary vein flow diastolic velocity; dtE, deceleration time of mitral inflow early diastolic velocity; E, mitral inflow early diastolic velocity; e', mitral annular early diastolic velocity; IVRT, isovolumic relaxation time; PASP, pulmonary artery systolic pressure; S, pulmonary vein flow systolic velocity; $T_{E\text{-}e'}$, time interval between the onset of mitral E and e' velocities, measured from the onset of QRS complex on ECG; Vp, mitral inflow propagation velocity.

The accuracy of this algorithm was tested in a recent study by Nagueh et al.[21] The algorithm was found to have 98% sensitivity and 91% specificity for identifying patients with increased PCWP on cardiac catheterization.

When a detailed assessment of all the different indices is not feasible for technical reasons or due to time constraints, the mitral *E/e'* alone appears to be the most informative. The *e'* needs to be measured both at the medial and lateral mitral annulus and the average value should be used. In the study by Nagueh et al.,[14] an average *E/e'* ratio greater than 15 alone had 89% sensitivity and 91% specificity for identifying patients with PCWP in excess of 15 mmHg.[21] In yet another recent study involving patients with severe HF, the echocardiographic measurements were compared with the direct measurement of LA pressure obtained using a permanently implanted monitoring device. In this study, an average *E/e'* demonstrated 96% specificity and 90% accuracy in detecting LA pressure in excess of 15 mmHg. It was also found that an *E/e'* of less than 12 essentially ruled out an elevated LA pressure with a sensitivity of 94%.[22]

To ensure accuracy of measurements, it is important to pay close attention to technical details while performing these measurements. At the same time, disease states that affect accuracy of these parameters should also be kept under consideration. For example, mitral inflow velocities can have lower accuracy in patients with mitral valve disease; pulmonary vein velocities have limitations in patients with atrioventricular block and arrhythmias; and tissue Doppler velocities are not reliable in normal subjects, in those with normal LVEF, and in patients with primary mitral valve disease, left bundle branch block, paced rhythms, or constrictive pericarditis.[20]

The LV filling pressure is perhaps the most important hemodynamic parameter in patients with HF. It not only facilitates titration of the pharmacological treatment according to the underlying hemodynamic status of the patient, but also provides important prognostic information. In a study involving 96 patients with chronic HF undergoing treatment on outpatient basis, medical management guided by Doppler echocardiography-based estimates of LV filling pressures and stroke volumes was compared with the standard practice. It was found that the echocardiography-guided treatment strategy resulted in significantly improved event-free survival compared to the conventional strategy (58.5% vs. 36.5%, $p = 0.04$) at a mean follow-up of 230 days, primarily driven by a significant decrease in first hospitalization.[23] The usefulness of LV filling pressures in guiding medical management in HF patients has been demonstrated in other studies as well, and numerous studies have demonstrated the excellent prognostic value of indices of LV filling pressure.[20,24,25,26] In patients with HF, pseudonormal or restrictive LV filling patterns are indicators of worse functional status as well as predictors of increased HF events.[25,26] Similarly, in patients with advanced HF, the mitral inflow (*dtE*) has been shown to be an independent multivariable predictor of HF hospitalization or death, with predictive accuracy superior to that of even LVEF.[24]

Vascular resistance

The measurement of systemic vascular resistance (SVR) is helpful in determining the mechanism of hemodynamic shock, whereas a similar measurement for the pulmonary circulation provides clues to the underlying mechanisms responsible for pulmonary hypertension and right HF. Echocardiographically, SVR and PVR can be estimated using Ohm's law, which states that the resistance across any vascular circuit is equal to the pressure gradient across the circuit divided by the flow. Therefore

$$\text{SVR} = (\text{Mean aortic pressure} - \text{mean RA pressure}) / \text{systemic blood flow, and}$$

$$\text{PVR} = (\text{Mean PA pressure} - \text{mean LA pressure}) / \text{pulmonary blood flow}$$

Mean systemic blood pressure is used as a surrogate for mean aortic pressure whereas all other values can be obtained by echocardiography as described above.

When the pressure gradient is measured in mmHg and cardiac output in L/min, the derived vascular resistance is in Wood units, which can be converted to dynes s cm.$^{-5}$ by multiplying by 80 or to MPa s m.$^{-3}$ by multiplying by 8.

Since accurate estimation of mean PA pressure on echocardiography is often challenging, an alternate method has been proposed which relies on TR jet and RVOT flow velocity:

$$\text{PVR (Wood units)} = [\text{Peak TR velocity (m/s)} / \text{RVOT VTI (cm)}] \times 10 + 0.16.$$

Left ventricular systolic function

LV systolic function is undoubtedly the most important determinant of outcomes in patients with HF and, along with LV volumes, is one of the most important factors guiding therapeutic decision-making in these patients. Multiple large clinical trials in chronic HF have demonstrated that LVEF and LV size are independently predictive of cardiac morbidity and mortality,[27,28,29,30] and accordingly, improvement in LV volumes and EF has been a key outcome measure when assessing efficacy of pharmacologic therapy in HF.[31] In the Cooperative New Scandinavian Enalapril Survival Study II (CONSENSUS II) evaluating the role of enalapril after acute myocardial infarction, end-systolic volume index and age were the only multivariable parameters that predicted functional class after 5 months of follow-up.[31,32] Similarly, β-blockers reduce morbidity and mortality in patients with chronic HF compared to placebo, with the magnitude of benefit correlating with reductions in end-diastolic and systolic dimensions and improvements in EF but not with the changes in symptom class.[32]

The pathological processes that affect the LV systolic function can involve the LV myocardium globally or regionally, and this distinction has both diagnostic and therapeutic implications. LV volumes and LVEF are the conventionally used measures of global LV systolic function whereas segmental wall motion analysis is the method for assessing regional LV systolic function.[33]

Global left ventricular systolic function

The simplest method for estimation of LV volumes is the cubed method which requires measurement of the minor-axis diameter of the LV.[33] The measurement can be obtained either by M-mode or 2D echocardiography in the parasternal long-axis view. While M-mode offers excellent temporal resolution, the alignment of the M-mode along the true minor axis of the LV is often challenging. Consequently, 2D echocardiography is being increasingly used for these measurements. The LV internal diameter needs to be measured both at end-diastole and at end-systole, identified as the frames showing the largest and the smallest LV cavity size, respectively. Once these dimensions are available, the LV volumes and EF can be calculated as

$$\text{LV cavity volume} = (\text{LVID})^3 \text{and}$$
$$\text{LVEF} = [(\text{LVID}_{\text{end-diastolic}})^3 - (\text{LVID}_{\text{end-systolic}})^3] / (\text{LVID}_{\text{end-diastolic}})^3$$

where LVID is the LV cavity internal dimension.

Though the above method is the easiest and the simplest for estimation of LV volumes and EF, it assumes LV to be contracting symmetrically and therefore cannot be applied in the presence of regional wall motion abnormalities. In addition, one must be careful to obtain accurate LV cavity size as any error in the measurement is magnified when the dimension is cubed to obtain the volume.

To overcome the problems related to distorted, nonsymmetrically contracting ventricles, the current guidelines recommend use of volumetric methods for estimation of LV cavity volumes and EF; the biplane Simpson method is the current gold standard for this purpose.[33] The Simpson method assumes the LV cavity to be a stack of disks of equal height, and the LV volume is calculated by summating the volumes of all the disks. In practice, this is accomplished by manually tracing the LV endocardial border in the apical four- and two-chamber views (Figure 7.8). The built-in software in the echocardiography equipment performs all the calculations to derive LV volumes and EF automatically. The greatest advantage of the Simpson method is that it remains applicable even when the LV is distorted. However, the accuracy of this method depends heavily on adequate visualization of the blood–endocardial interface. In difficult cases, the use of harmonic imaging and LV cavity contrast can help improve endocardial visualization and thus the accuracy of LVEF assessment. However, when LV cavity contrast is not available or cannot be used for any reason, the alternate area–length method can be used.[33] This method assumes LV to be bullet shaped and the LV volume is calculate using the following equation:

$$\text{LV volume} = 5\ \text{AL} / 6, \ (\text{Figure 7.9})$$

where A is the short-axis cross-sectional area of the LV at the mid-ventricular level and L is the LV cavity length in the apical four-chamber view. It should be remembered that when measuring the LV cavity short-axis area, papillary muscles are considered to be a part of the LV cavity and the endocardial border is traced from outside the papillary muscles.

Although the current guidelines recommend using one of the formal quantitative methods for estimation of LVEF, in practice LVEF is usually estimated by visual assessment only. Interestingly, for experienced users, this "eyeballing" method has been shown to have a high degree of accuracy and an excellent correlation with the formal quantitative estimates of LVEF.[34]

Regional left ventricular systolic function

The assessment of regional LV systolic function is performed by dividing the LV into 16 or 17 segments, as recommended by the American Society of Echocardiography, and visually assessing the extent of wall thickening in each of these segments (Figure 7.10).[33] Depending on the extent of wall thickening, the wall motion can be classified as normal, hypokinetic, akinetic, or dyskinetic. A formal scoring system is also available (normal, 1; hypokinetic, 2; akinetic, 3; and dyskinetic, 4) to provide a semiquantitative estimate of regional LV systolic function. Averaging the scores of all the evaluated segments provides a wall motion score index, which can be used as a surrogate for global LVEF. While performing wall motion analysis, it is important to be able to differentiate between actual wall thickening and endocardial motion as the latter can also result from tethering effects from the adjacent myocardial segments or by the translational movement of the heart, even in absence of actual myocardial contraction.

The wall motion analysis has major diagnostic and therapeutic implications. First, as coronary artery disease is by far the commonest condition affecting the LV in a regional manner, presence of regional wall motion abnormalities is considered to be virtually diagnostic of coronary artery disease. In addition, the distribution of wall motion abnormalities helps in identifying the affected coronary vascular territory. Second, the detection of myocardial ischemia and viability on echocardiography is based predominantly on wall motion analysis, performed initially at rest and

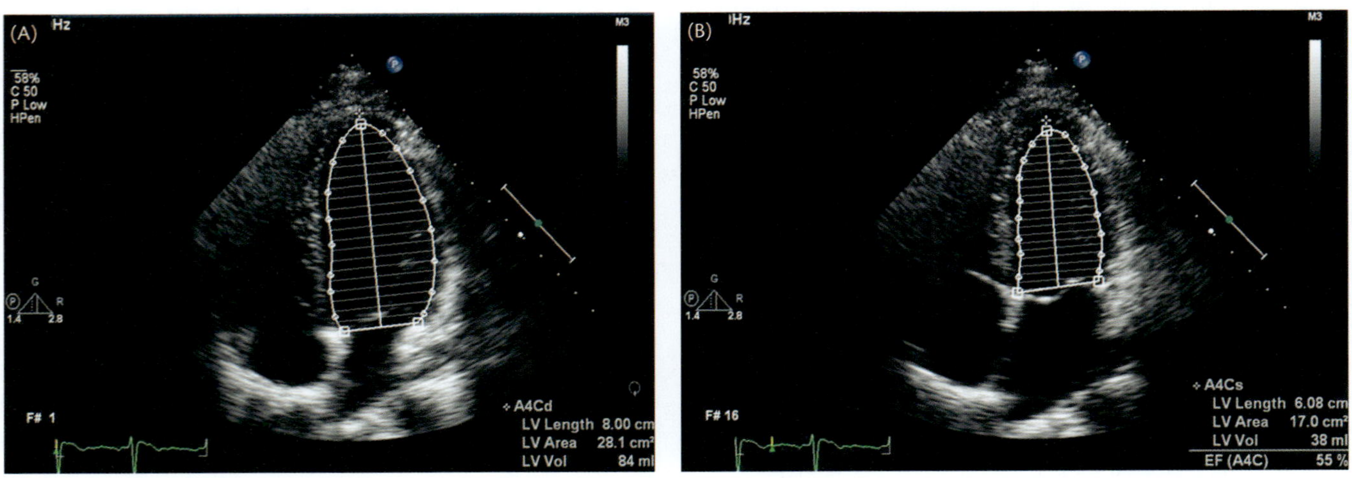

Fig. 7.8 Measurement of left ventricular volume and ejection fraction using the modified Simpson method. The endocardial border is traced at end-diastole and end-systole in both the apical four-chamber (A, B) and two-chamber views (not shown). The automated software divides the left ventricular cavity into a stack of disks of equal height and calculates volumes.

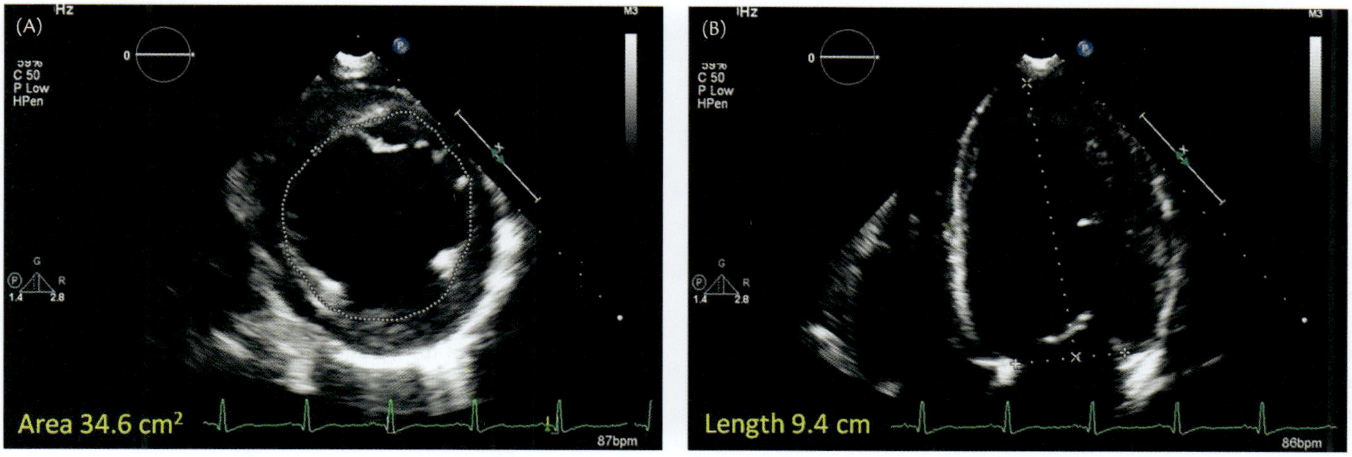

$$\text{Volume} = \frac{5 \times \text{area} \times \text{length}}{6}$$

$$= 5 \times 34.6 \times 9.4/6 \quad = 271 \text{ ml}$$

Fig. 7.9 Area–length method for estimation of left ventricular volumes and ejection fraction. The cross-sectional area of the left ventricular cavity is measured in mid-ventricular short-axis view (A) and the length is measured in the apical four-chamber view (B).

subsequently in response to exercise or pharmacological stress. Finally, in patients with significantly dilated LV, especially with aneurysms, an assessment of the aneurysm size, the extent of akinesia and/or dyskinesia, and extent of wall thinning are important findings required for planning appropriate ventricular reconstruction surgery.

Assessment of myocardial viability

Numerous studies have shown that in patients with ischemic, severe LV systolic dysfunction, an increment in the contractile performance of the LV following revascularization is associated with significantly improved morbidity and mortality compared to

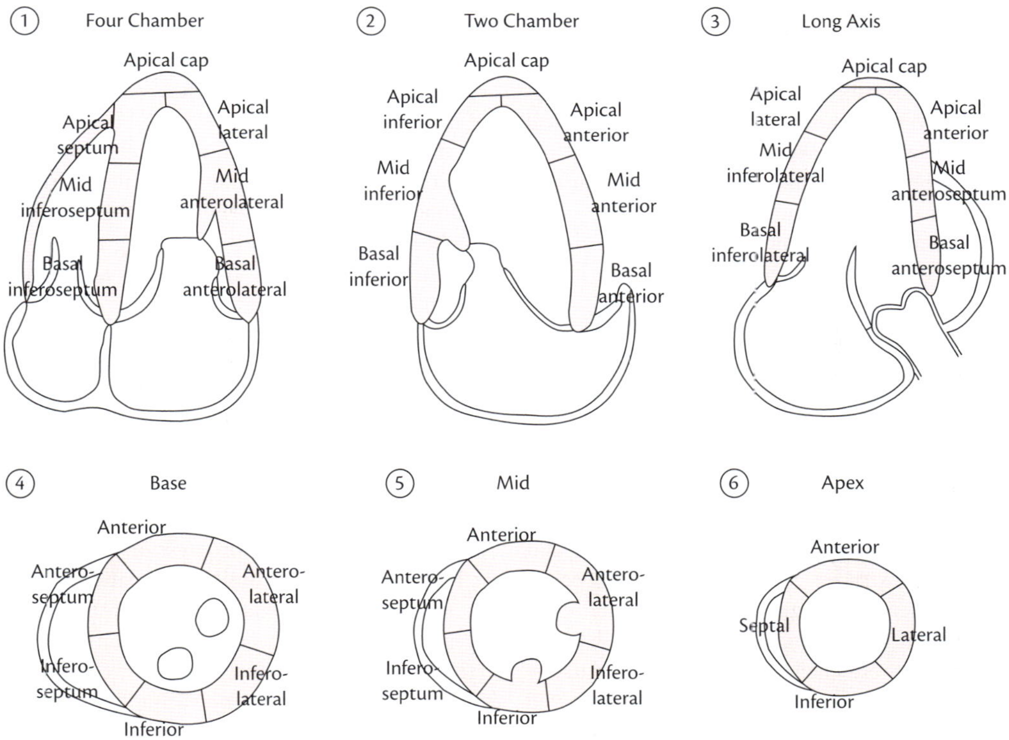

Fig. 7.10 The 17-segment model used for assessment of left ventricular regional systolic function.

Modified from Journal of the American Society of Echocardiography, 18, Lang RM, et al., Recommendations for chamber quantification: A report from the American Society of Echocardiography's Guidelines and Standards Committee and the Chamber Quantification Writing Group, developed in conjunction with the European Association of Echocardiography, a branch of the European Society of Cardiology.

medical therapy alone.[35,36,37] Consequently, recognition of such dysfunctional yet "viable" myocardium that has potential to recover following revascularization is an important goal of evaluation in patients with ischemic HF.

Echocardiography is a commonly employed modality for assessment of myocardial viability. The diastolic wall thickness at rest itself provides useful clues to the presence of viable myocardium. Myocardial thinning with a wall thickness of less than 6 mm has been shown to have a high degree of specificity for scar tissue and indicates lack of viability with a negative predictive value of 93%.[38] However, the positive predictive value of a relatively preserved wall thickness is poor (53%). It should be noted that these observations are applicable only after at least 4 months from myocardial infarction, to allow the healing process and scar formation to take place.

Dobutamine echocardiography is the most commonly used echocardiographic technique for assessment of myocardial viability and remains the echocardiographic gold standard for this purpose. Incremental doses of dobutamine are administered as an intravenous infusion, usually beginning at 2.5 or 5 μg kg.$^{-1}$ min.$^{-1}$ and increasing every 3 min to a maximum dose of 40 μg kg.$^{-1}$ min.$^{-1}$. The wall motion analysis is performed at baseline and is repeated at every stage during the dobutamine infusion. A viable ischemic myocardium is characterized by reduced contractility at rest that improves at low-dose dobutamine (typically 5–10 μg kg.$^{-1}$ min.$^{-1}$) and worsens again at peak dose (usually 30–40 μg kg.$^{-1}$ min.$^{-1}$). This biphasic response is the hallmark of myocardial viability and is the most accurate predictor of functional improvement after revascularization.[39] Occasionally, there is worsening even at low dose, implying severe ischemia. These segments also tend to improve after revascularization but the response rate is variable. In contrast, a uniphasic response characterized by sustained improvement in contractility at low- and peak-dose dobutamine indicates viable but nonischemic myocardium. In the acute setting, this is usually a manifestation of myocardial stunning and indicates high likelihood of spontaneous recovery, without the need for any surgical or percutaneous revascularization. However, in the chronic setting, this may just represent viable myocardium with overlying scar and no ischemia. These areas usually do not improve.

Several studies have compared wall motion analysis on dobutamine echocardiography with other nonechocardiographic methods for assessment of myocardial viability. A pooled analysis of 37 such studies found dobutamine echocardiography to be the most specific (81%) modality for prediction of functional recovery following revascularization. The sensitivity was also excellent (84%), albeit lower than the same for rest–redistribution thallium perfusion scintigraphy (90%).[40]

The major limitation with myocardial viability assessment on dobutamine echocardiography is that it is based on visual interpretation of wall motion, which is highly subjective and operator-dependent.[41] This subjective interpretation necessitates adequate expertise to ensure diagnostic accuracy and even for experienced operators it remains a source of interobserver variability.[41,42] To overcome these challenges, several quantitative approaches such as myocardial strain imaging have been evaluated as adjunct to wall motion analysis. The role of such techniques is discussed in greater detail in the subsequent sections.

Valvular heart disease

Valvular lesions are common but eminently treatable causes of HF. Aortic stenosis, AR, and MR, when significant and sustained for prolonged periods, produce LV systolic dysfunction resulting in systolic HF. In contrast, mitral stenosis does not cause significant LV systolic dysfunction but leads to the development of pulmonary venous and arterial hypertension with consequent right HF. Correction of these valvular anomalies, through surgical or nonsurgical intervention, is highly effective in relieving symptoms and, depending on the stage at which correction is performed, also leads to partial or complete resolution of the hemodynamic alterations. Therefore, the recognition and characterization of the valve disease in patients with HF has immense therapeutic value.[43]

Echocardiography is the most useful and the most informative diagnostic modality for evaluation of valve diseases.[44,45,46,47] It provides comprehensive information about the valve morphology, presence and severity of valvular dysfunction, its impact on intracardiac hemodynamics, status of the cardiac chambers and ventricular function, and any other structural or functional anomaly, if present. Such information is not only essential for determining the need and timing of the intervention but also helps in choosing the appropriate type of intervention—whether surgical or percutaneous and, if surgical, then whether valve repair or replacement.[43] In addition, intraprocedural transesophageal echocardiography (TEE) helps in guiding the repair procedure, checking the adequacy of repair once the procedure is complete, and excluding any residual defects or complications.[48,49] The recent advent of live 3D TEE has greatly enhanced the role of echocardiography for these indications.[48]

Unlike other valve lesions, MR has a unique place in the pathophysiology of HF. While organic MR is an important cause of HF, HF itself can lead to significant MR. This form of MR, which develops in the absence of any structural damage to the mitral valve apparatus, is known as functional MR. The apical and posterolateral displacement of the papillary muscles with consequent tethering of the mitral valve (MV) leaflets is the commonest mechanism responsible for functional MR, accounting for nearly three-fourth of all such cases (Figure 7.11).[50,51,52,53] In patients with HF, as the LV dilates, the papillary muscles get displaced away from the MV apparatus resulting in chordal traction which precludes adequate systolic closure of the mitral leaflets. Consequently, the mitral leaflets become tented and the resulting malcoaptation of the leaflets leads to MR. Global LV dilatation is not mandatory for the development of mitral leaflet tenting as the isolated, localized distortion of the basal infero-posterior segment of the LV itself can lead to tenting. However, in such cases, the posterior mitral leaflet is usually restricted to a greater extent producing asymmetrical tenting, unlike the more symmetrical tenting seen with uniform dilatation of the LV.[47] In addition to tenting, other factors such as dilatation of the mitral annulus, reduced contractile force of the LV, and intermittent myocardial and papillary muscle ischemia also contribute to the development and progression of functional MR.[51,52,53]

Functional MR is common in patients with HF with as many as 50% of these patients having at least some degree of MR.[54] The presence of MR in these patients contributes to the worsening of HF by adversely affecting the already compromised systolic performance of the LV and by increasing the severity of pulmonary congestion. Any degree of MR in patients with HF is associated with an adverse prognosis, with the risk increasing with the severity of MR.[55,56] Nevertheless, the appropriate management of functional MR remains highly controversial.[53,57] Myocardial revascularization alone fails to correct MR in the vast majority of patients and therefore surgical correction of MR is required at the time of coronary

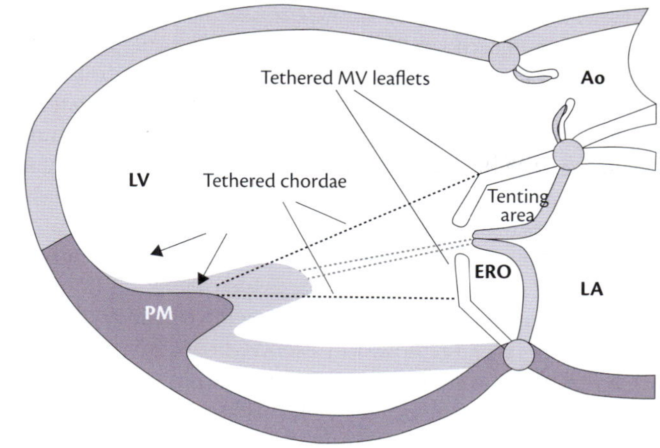

Fig. 7.11 Left ventricular remodeling resulting in papillary muscle displacement leading to mitral leaflet tenting and functional mitral regurgitation. Ao, aorta; ERO, effective regurgitant orifice; LA, left atrium; LV, left ventricle; MV, mitral valve; PM, papillary muscle.

Modified from American Journal of Medicine, 119, Bursi, F et al., Mitral regurgitation after myocardial infarction: A review, 103–112, copyright (2006) with permission from Elsevier.

artery bypass grafting if MR is moderate or severe.[58] Ring annuloplasty is the most commonly used surgical technique for correction of functional MR but the long-term results are usually inferior to those seen in patients with degenerative MR.[53,57] Several innovative techniques such as the Coapsys device, Alfieri stitch, and chordal resection have been evaluated as alternate approaches but have shown variable results.[53,57] More recently, percutaneous repair of functional MR has become possible using a technique similar to the Alfieri stitch. The long-term results of this procedure are still awaited.[59]

The management of MR in patients with LV dysfunction not requiring myocardial revascularization is even more controversial. Although mitral valve repair has been shown to improve quality of life in these patients, the overall survival seems to be unaffected due to the overriding influence of underlying LV systolic dysfunction on mortality.[60]

As for any other valve lesion, echocardiography is the most useful diagnostic modality for evaluation of functional MR also. However, the evaluation of functional MR presents several challenges. As the contractile force driving the MR in these cases is usually impaired, the regurgitant volume is usually smaller for the same degree of MR severity. Accordingly, the qualitative measures of MR severity such as MR jet area are usually misleading and a formal quantitative assessment is invariably needed. Effective regurgitant orifice area and regurgitant volume can be calculated using a proximal isovelocity surface area method. However, even on quantitative assessment, the threshold for diagnosing severe MR is lower for functional MR than for organic MR. In case of functional MR, an orifice area greater than 20 mm.^{2} or regurgitant volume greater than 30 ml indicates severe MR, whereas the cutoff values for the same are 30 mm.^{2} and 60 ml respectively for organic MR.[47,61] In addition to MR severity, echocardiography in these patients is also expected to provide detailed information about mitral valve geometry. Tenting height, tenting area, mitral annulus size, mitral leaflet length, chordal length, and interpapillary muscle distance need to be measured (Figure 7.12). Such information is not only helpful in planning repair but also predicts long-term outcome following mitral valve repair. For instance, a tenting height greater than 1 cm, tenting area 1.6 cm.^{2} or more, mitral annulus size 3.7 cm or more, or the presence of a complex MR jet predict increased risk of recurrence of MR following mitral valve repair.[62,63] Some echocardiography platforms allow detailed mitral valve quantification using live 3D TEE but the incremental value of such information in influencing long-term outcome is yet to be determined.

The role of stress echocardiography in the evaluation of functional MR is not clear. The effect of exercise on MR severity is variable and depends on a combination of factors such as presence of inducible ischemia, changes in LV cavity size with exercise, or alteration in mitral valve geometry. However, a significant increase in the severity of MR on exercise has been shown to be a poor prognostic marker and indicates the need to undertake mitral valve repair at the time of myocardial revascularization.[64] In contrast, dobutamine echocardiography may not be of much help in evaluation of functional MR as dobutamine administration often reduces

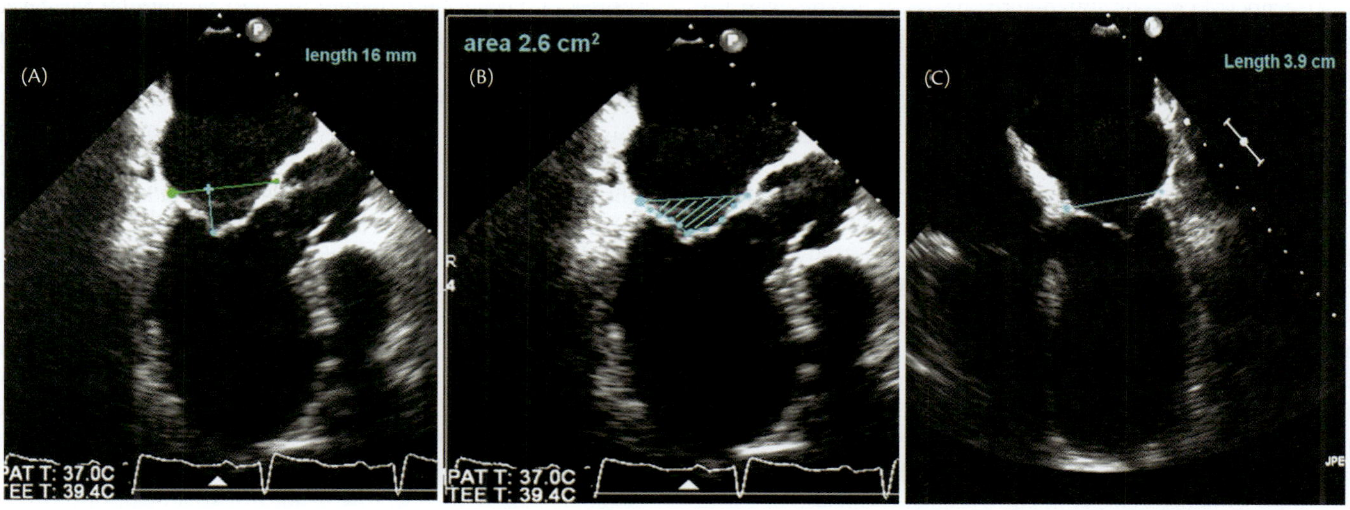

Fig. 7.12 Echocardiographic predictors of recurrence of mitral regurgitation following mitral valve repair for functional mitral regurgitation. Tenting height (A) and tenting area (B) are measured during systole from mid-esophageal long-axis view on transesophageal echocardiography or a corresponding view on transthoracic echocardiography. Similarly, mitral annular systolic diameter (C) can be measured either from mid-esophageal four-chamber view or apical four-chamber view.

the severity of MR by reducing afterload, without affecting the MV geometry.

Dyssynchrony assessment

Patients with advanced HF often have an intraventricular conduction defect (IVCD), which is an important determinant of morbidity and mortality in these patients.[65,66,67,68,69] The prevalence of IVCD increases with increasing severity of HF with almost 38% of patients with moderate to severe HF having evidence of IVCD.[69] The presence of IVCD results in asynchronous contraction of different segments of LV which compromises systolic function, adversely affects diastolic filling, and results in development and progression of MR. The ventricular filling is further compromised by the presence of atrioventricular dyssynchrony which often coexists in these patients. Accordingly, numerous trials have shown that the correction of intraventricular and atrioventricular dyssynchrony with the help of CRT reduces HF symptoms, increases exercise capacity, improves quality of life, and even reduces mortality.[70,71,72] Therefore, CRT is currently recommended in all patients with LVEF 35% or less and broad QRS (duration ≥120 ms) who continue to have HF symptoms despite optimum medical therapy.[73] However, a major limitation with CRT is that even when appropriately selected, nearly one-third of all patients undergoing CRT do not adequately respond to the therapy.[72] Though a number of mechanisms have been proposed to explain this lack of benefit with CRT, the absence of mechanical dyssynchrony despite the presence of IVCD appears to be one of the important mechanisms. It has been observed that electrical dyssynchrony as seen on surface ECG does not necessarily correlate with mechanical dyssynchrony, which is the real therapeutic target for CRT.[74,75,76] To overcome this limitation, several echocardiographic indices of mechanical dyssynchrony have been developed to improve patient selection for CRT.[77]

On echocardiography, three major components of cardiac dyssynchrony can be recognized: atrioventricular, interventricular, and intraventricular.[77] Of these, intraventricular dyssynchrony appears to be the most important determinant of the outcomes after CRT. Although a number of different methods are available for detection of intraventricular dyssynchrony, septal-posterior wall mechanical delay, difference in time to peak velocity, and systolic dyssynchrony index (SDI) have been evaluated most extensively (Figure 7.13). Septal-posterior wall mechanical delay is the time interval between the peak contraction of the anteroseptum and the posterior wall on M-mode echocardiography in the parasternal long- or short-axis view. A delay of more than 130 ms indicates presence of intraventricular dyssynchrony.[77,78,79] Addition of color tissue Doppler imaging to M-mode improves the ability to correctly identify the peak contraction and thus improves the accuracy of this technique. The time to peak systolic velocity is obtained using color tissue Doppler imaging, though older studies used pulsed-wave tissue Doppler imaging (TDI) also. Using color TDI, time interval from the onset of QRS to the peak systolic velocity is measured in each of the six basal or six basal plus six mid segments of the LV. A delay of 65 ms or more between any two opposing segments, or 100 ms or more between any two myocardial segments, indicates intraventricular dyssynchrony.[77,80,81,82,83] The standard deviation of the time to peak systolic velocity in all 12 segments can also be calculated and is known as SDI or Yu index. A value of 33 ms or more indicates intraventricular dyssynchrony and has been shown to be a more accurate predictor of response to CRT than many of the other parameters.[84,85] As described below, a similar measurement can be obtained from 3D echo also.[86,87]

Since most of the indices mentioned above were evaluated in small, single-center studies, a large, multicenter trial—the PROSPECT study—was performed to validate these indices and to identify the most accurate predictor of functional response to CRT. Unfortunately, this trial did not find any of the several echocardiographic indices to be accurate enough in predicting the response to CRT.[88] The findings of this trial greatly decreased interest in echocardiographic assessment of mechanical dyssynchrony.

Nevertheless, despite the disappointing results of the PROSPECT trial, there are several reasons why echocardiography continues to play an important role in the evaluation of HF patients undergoing CRT. First, the PROSPECT trial itself had several technical and design-related flaws which are likely to have contributed to the apparent failure of echocardiography in the prediction of CRT response.[89] Second, since the publication of the PROSPECT trial, many other measures of mechanical dyssynchrony have been developed which appear to be more robust than those previously studied. For example, radial dyssynchrony, defined as a delay of 130 ms or more in time to peak radial strain between mid posterior wall and mid anteroseptum on speckle tracking echocardiography (STE) has been shown to predict response to CRT with a high degree of accuracy (Figure 7.13).[90,91,92] Third, echocardiography helps in recognizing several additional features that are associated with poor response to CRT.[93] Excessive dilatation of the LV, presence of significant regional wall motion abnormalities, lack of myocardial viability, and presence of significant RV systolic dysfunction indicate high likelihood of nonresponse to CRT and may help in excluding patients who are unlikely to benefit from CRT. Fourth, echocardiography also helps in identifying the optimum site for LV lead placement.[92,94] In a recent study based on STE, the optimum site for LV lead placement was determined by a combination of delay in activation and the extent of scarring (assessed using radial strain). It was found that the best outcome was achieved when there was concordance between the actual site of LV lead placement and the optimum site predicted by echocardiography. In contrast, significant discordance between the two was associated with much worse echocardiographic and clinical outcomes.[94] Finally, echocardiography also helps in optimizing the biventricular pacemaker settings following device implantation.[95]

Role in patients receiving ventricular assist devices

Echocardiography performs a key role in the assessment and management of the patients undergoing implantation of left- and/or right-sided ventricular assist devices (LVAD and RVAD, respectively). VADs have been used as a bridge to transplant in patients with advanced HF, and more recently are being used as a bridge to recovery or as destination therapy. With the increasing use of VAD therapy, there is a need for accurate and comprehensive evaluation of the effects of VADs on cardiac function and physiology so as to enable the treating physicians to make appropriate management decisions as required. Echocardiography is helpful in evaluation of these patients at every step, extending from preoperative assessment to intraoperative evaluation to postoperative follow-up.

Comprehensive preoperative echocardiography prior to device implant is required to prevent potential complications after LVAD placement.[96,97,98,99,100] The site of inflow cannula placement at the LV apex and outflow cannula placement in the aorta should

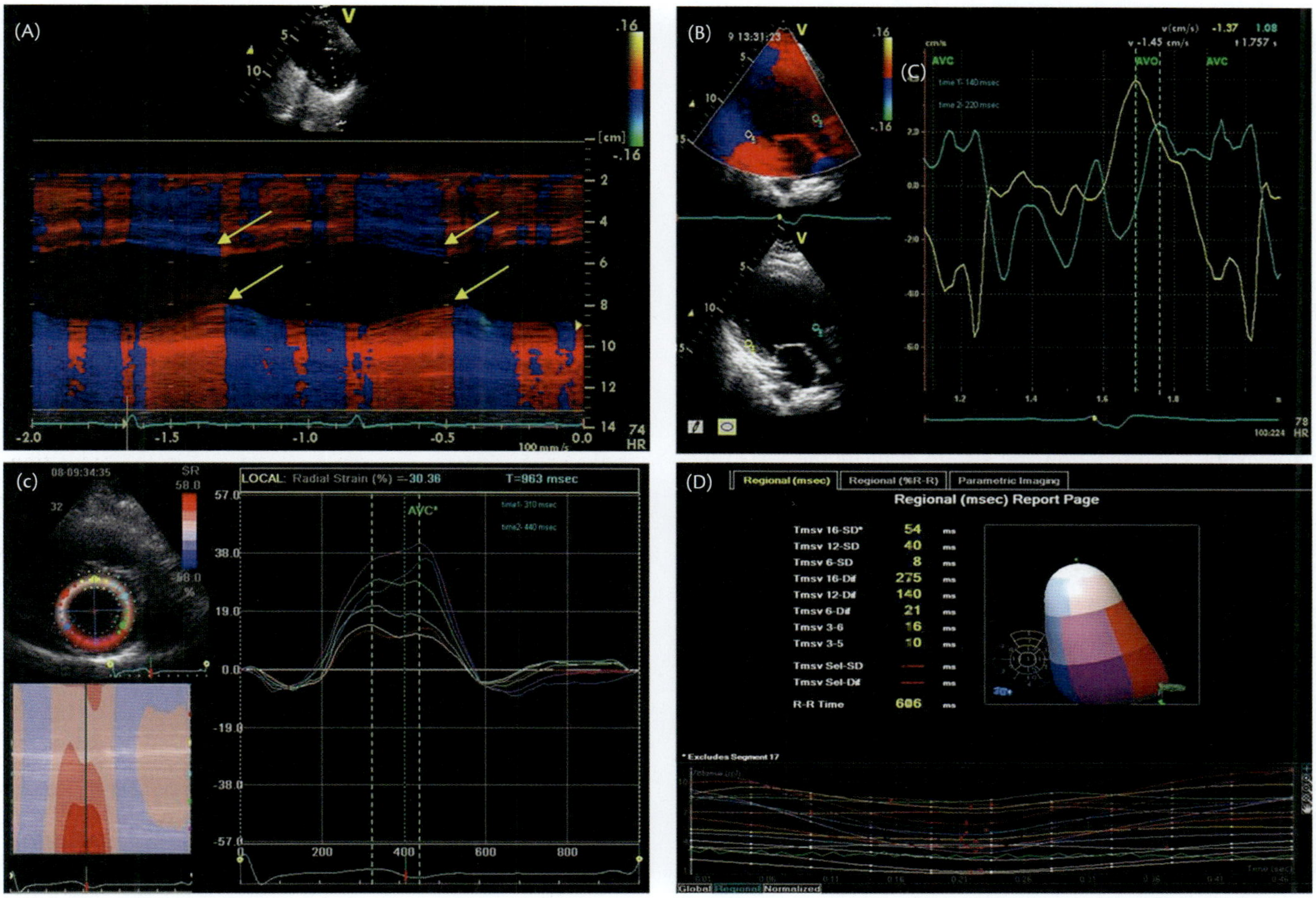

Fig. 7.13 Commonly used echocardiographic measures of intraventricular dyssynchrony. (A) Septal-posterior wall mechanical delay measured from parasternal short-axis view using color M-mode. (B) Delay in time to peak systolic velocity in opposing wall segments on color tissue Doppler imaging. (C) Radial dyssynchrony measured using speckle tracking echocardiography. (D) Systolic dyssynchrony index or Yu index measured with three-dimensional echocardiography.

be imaged for the presence of thrombus, atheroma, or aneurysm before insertion. The LV function and volumes should be assessed thoroughly to aid in appropriate device selection, as should RV function, as some patients may require placement of an RVAD as well. Severe RV enlargement, elevated PVR, RV systolic dysfunction, and significant TR are associated with RV failure in the setting of LVAD placement and should be recognized early.[101,102] The delayed placement of an RV assist device for RV failure after LVAD placement is associated with worse survival compared to early planned biventricular mechanical circulatory support, emphasizing the need for careful assessment of the right heart before LVAD insertion.[103] Traditionally, RV systolic function is typically assessed subjectively by visual estimation. However, quantitative methods are available and should be routinely used to provide more objective and accurate assessment of RV systolic function.[8] Tricuspid annular plane systolic excursion (TAPSE), fractional area change (FAC), and tricuspid annular systolic velocity by TDI are the commonly used measures of RV systolic function. TAPSE is an M-mode derived parameter and measures the distance the lateral tricuspid annulus moves during systole in the apical four-chamber view. A value of less than 16 mm suggests RV systolic dysfunction. FAC is the percentage change in the RV area from diastole to systole, measured in the apical four-chamber view. Normal RV FAC is 35% or more, with values less than 20% being associated with increased likelihood of RV failure after LVAD placement.[104] The tricuspid annular systolic velocity is obtained by placing the pulsed-wave TDI sample volume at the lateral tricuspid annulus. Values less than 10 cm/s are suggestive of RV dysfunction. More recently, STE-based longitudinal strain has also been used to assess RV systolic function and has been shown to be an independent predictor of RV failure in patients undergoing LVAD implantation. A peak strain cutoff of −9.6% predicted RV failure with 68% sensitivity and 76% specificity in these patients.[102]

Valvular pathology is equally important to assess preoperatively. AR may worsen after LVAD placement as a result of the active "pulling" of blood from the LV into the inflow cannula. This reduces cardiac output due to the run-off of blood delivered by the outflow cannula back into the LV instead of into the systemic circulation. Correction of the AR before LVAD placement will depend on the severity of regurgitation, with options including valve replacement and patch or primary suture closure.[104] It is important to note that in patients with advanced HF, the degree of AR is typically underestimated preoperatively due to high LV end-diastolic pressure and low aortic diastolic pressure. Re-evaluation during cardiopulmonary bypass at the time of LVAD implantation may unmask the true degree of regurgitation in such cases.

The presence of intracardiac shunting such as through a patent foramen ovale can be a cause of numerous complications after LVAD implantation and should also be looked for carefully. Decompression of the LV with lowering of LV and LA pressures can lead to a pressure gradient from RA to LA, facilitating right-to-left shunting. The shunting of blood from right to left can lead to systemic desaturation, or a paradoxical embolus that can cause LVAD obstruction or stroke. Careful inspection of the interatrial septum by color Doppler and agitated saline can detect shunts that need to be closed at the time of device insertion. In addition, perioperative TEE may increase the detection of small interatrial shunts not seen by conventional transthoracic echocardiogram (TTE), even with saline contrast.

After LVAD implantation, echocardiography can be used to assess the various expected and unexpected changes in the cardiac hemodynamics and function and also to evaluate the VAD functioning. A reduction in LV volumes by 40–50% and LV internal diameter by 20–30% suggests optimal unloading of the LV by the LVAD.[105,106,107] The aortic valve may demonstrate continuous mild aortic insufficiency from pre-existing valvular pathology and LVAD unloading of the LV. Alternatively, AR can also result from malcoaptation of the aortic leaflets occurring as a consequence of the elevated systemic pressure and distention of the proximal aortic root from LVAD outflow cannula flow. In contrast, functional MR may improve markedly as the previously globular LV now assumes a more normal prolate ellipsoid shape after pressure and volume unloading by an LVAD.[108] The geometric changes in the RV after LVAD placement are not as pronounced as they are for the LV. In a study on patients undergoing LVAD implantation, RV chamber size and function, as measured by FAC and TAPSE, remained unchanged for 6 months after LVAD implantation. However, there were improvements in TR severity and RV systolic pressure as a consequence of a fall in PVR following LVAD placement. Importantly, these hemodynamic improvements correlated with improved symptomatic status in these patients, while those who had deterioration in there right-sided hemodynamics fared much worse, underlying the importance of comprehensive right heart evaluation after LVAD.[109]

Inflow and outflow cannula should also be interrogated by echocardiography. Elevated inflow and/or outflow cannula velocities greater than 2 m/s suggest obstruction of flow from an incorrectly angled, kinked, or thrombosed cannula or graft.[110]

Role of newer techniques

Strain echocardiography

For decades, LVEF has been the most useful and the most commonly used measure of LV systolic function, and it remains so. An extensive database, originating from research studies as well as clinical experience, supports the utility and the robustness of LVEF for this purpose. However, LVEF as a measure of LV systolic function has several limitations whose clinical relevance is now being increasingly recognized. First, LVEF is not sensitive enough to detect early myocardial damage.[111,112,113] A substantial amount of myocardial damage has to occur before it can become apparent as a fall in LVEF. For the same reason, LVEF is also not a useful modality for detecting subtle changes in LV systolic function occurring either as a result of progression of the disease process or because of the effect of the treatment. Second, LVEF is highly load dependent and is not really a true measure of myocardial contractility. Third, LVEF is only a measure of global LV systolic function and thus represents an oversimplification of the complex multidimensional deformation of the myocardium that normally takes place during the cardiac cycle.[111] The newer technique of "strain imaging," more appropriately called "deformation imaging," measures the myocardial deformation directly and attempts to overcome many of the limitations of LVEF.[111,113]

When used in the context of myocardium, *strain* refers to the percent change in the length of a myocardial segment from its original length and is expressed as follows:

$$\text{Strain}\ (\%) = \Delta L / L_0,$$

where ΔL is the change in length and L_0 is the original length.

Strain rate is the speed at which deformation takes place and its units are 1/s or s^{-1}. By convention, a negative value of strain and strain rate denotes shortening whereas a positive value signifies lengthening. There are three normal or primary strains (longitudinal, radial, circumferential) and three shear strains (circumferential–longitudinal, circumferential–radial, longitudinal–radial). Circumferential–longitudinal shear strain is also known as rotational deformation, torsion, or twist.

On echocardiography, there are primarily two approaches to measure myocardial strain: TDI based and STE based.[113] The Doppler method uses velocity data that is converted to strain rate information and then subsequently to strain data. The Doppler-based technique has the advantage of providing superior temporal resolution, but is highly dependent on the angle of insonation. As a result, only longitudinal strain can be measured using the Doppler method. In contrast, STE is a gray-scale-based technique and uses a different approach to determine strain. Echocardiographic ultrasound imaging of the myocardium results in the appearance of natural acoustic markers, or "speckles" within the myocardium. The STE software recognizes these speckles and tracks them frame by frame, using the sum-of-absolute-differences algorithm. The information thus obtained is analyzed to resolve all the different components of myocardial deformation. Longitudinal strain is derived from the apical four-chamber, two-chamber, and three-chamber views whereas the short-axis views are used for deriving radial and circumferential strain, and rotation and torsion (Figure 7.14).[111,114]

There are certain physiological and technical differences among different forms of myocardial strain which are clinically relevant.[111,115] The longitudinal strain is determined predominantly by the subendocardial fibers whereas radial and circumferential strain and rotation are governed mainly by the midmyocardial and subepicardial fibers. As a result, owing to the greater vulnerability of the subendocardial fibers to pathological disturbances, longitudinal strain is the first to be compromised in disease processes; radial and circumferential strain are affected late in the course of disease when the myocardial damage has become more transmural. In addition, longitudinal strain is easier to measure, can be obtained by both TDI and STE, and is more reproducible than radial and circumferential strain. For these reasons, most of our knowledge about myocardial deformation has been derived using longitudinal strain only.

Strain imaging in heart failure

Myocardial strain imaging has numerous applications in patients with HF. As mentioned above, strain provides a quantitative measure of LV systolic function that is more objective and has the

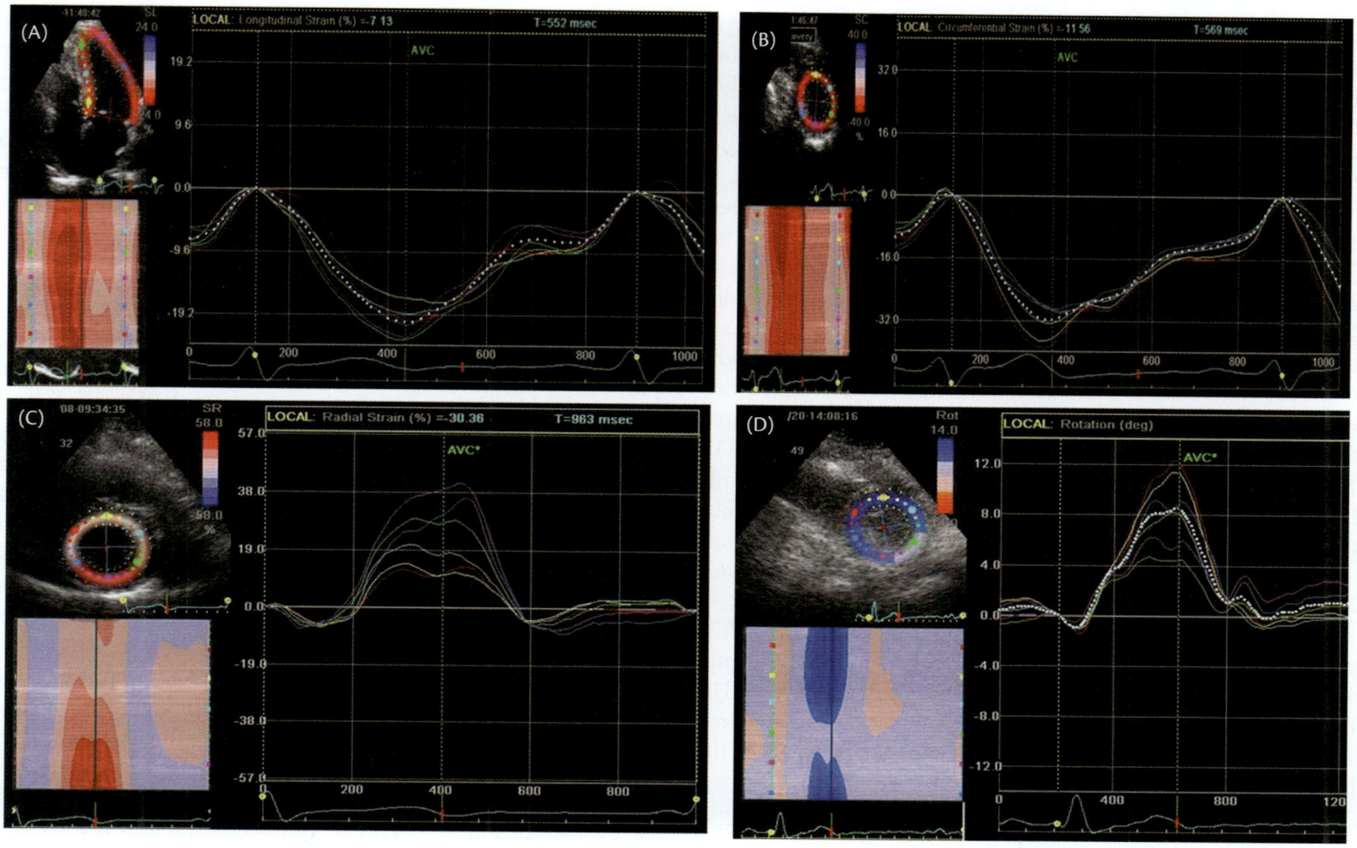

Fig. 7.14 Two-dimensional speckle tracking echocardiography for measurement of left ventricular strain and rotation. Longitudinal strain is measured from apical four-chamber (A), two-chamber, and three-chamber views whereas short-axis views are used for measurement of circumferential stain (B), radial strain (C), and rotation (D) and torsion.

capability to track subtle changes in myocardial contractile function. Global longitudinal strain has been successfully used as a surrogate for LVEF in a wide range of clinical conditions and has been shown to have better correlation with MRI-derived LVEF than conventional 2D echocardiography-based LVEF measurements.[33,116,117] Recently, innovative STE-based algorithms have been developed that allow semi-automatic and rapid assessment of LV systolic function with reasonable accuracy.[118,119] In addition, regional and global longitudinal strain has also been used for assessing the response to various therapeutic measures in patients with HF.[111,120]

In patients with ischemic HF, strain imaging helps in determining the transmural extent of the myocardial damage and in predicting myocardial viability.[121,122,123,124,125,126,127,128,129] The subendocardial infarcts are usually characterized by impairment of only longitudinal strain whereas transmural infarcts are associated with reduction of both longitudinal and circumferential strain.[121,122] This distinction is important, as a segment with transmurally more extensive myocardial damage is less likely to recover after revascularization. Even the longitudinal strain itself has been shown to be a predictor of myocardial viability and LV remodeling following an acute coronary event.[123,124,125,126,127] The lower global longitudinal strain values after myocardial infarction are associated with less likelihood of segmental or global functional recovery and a higher risk of adverse LV remodeling. Nonetheless, the most important role of strain imaging in assessment of myocardial viability is as an adjunct to wall motion analysis on dobutamine echocardiography. Both Doppler-based and STE-based longitudinal strain and strain rate have been shown to improve the accuracy of dobutamine echocardiography for prediction of functional recovery following myocardial revascularization.[128,129] However, Doppler-based strain appears to perform better than STE-based strain and strain rate for this purpose.[129]

Myocardial strain imaging has also been shown to have powerful prognostic value.[130,131] In a prospective study involving patients with acute HF, longitudinal and circumferential strains were compared with LVEF in predicting subsequent cardiac events. Interestingly, global circumferential strain was found to be the most powerful predictor of cardiac events, more so than even LVEF and longitudinal strain.[130] In yet another study involving 1060 patients with chronic ischemic LV dysfunction, baseline global longitudinal strain (GLS) was independently related to all-cause mortality and a combination of all-cause mortality and HF hospitalization.[131] Similarly, in a study of patients with dilated cardiomyopathy referred for heart transplantation, patients who deteriorated clinically had significantly lower longitudinal strain and strain rate at the time of referral compared to those who remained stable at 6 months of follow-up.[132] In the same study, late diastolic longitudinal strain rate provided the highest sensitivity and specificity for predicting rapid clinical deterioration (cutoff $<0.3\ s^{-1}$, sensitivity 94%, specificity 83%). Baseline GLS has also been shown to predict the likelihood of spontaneous or inducible ventricular tachycardia in patients with ischemic and nonischemic LV systolic dysfunction.[133,134,135]

Strain imaging has been employed to assess myocardial dyssynchrony also. As already discussed, STE-based radial dyssynchrony appears to be one of the most robust measures of myocardial dyssynchrony and a predictor of response to CRT.[90,91] A difference in peak radial strain of more than 130 ms between the anteroseptum and posterior wall by STE was first shown by Suffoletto et al. to correlate with improvement in LVEF after CRT.[90] The subsequent prospective multicenter Speckle Tracking and Resynchronization (STAR) study was the first large trial to assess the role of STE in predicting CRT response.[91] In this study, dyssynchrony on radial strain from the short-axis view was found to be strongly associated with long-term survival after CRT. Interestingly, patients who lacked baseline radial dyssynchrony prior to CRT had higher incidence of death, transplantation, or LVAD placement than those who had baseline dyssynchrony. In addition, as noted earlier, STE has been used to guide LV lead placement also.[92,94] It not only allows identification of the site of latest activation, but also permits simultaneous assessment of the extent of scarring. Together, such information can be of great help in choosing the optimum site for LV lead placement.

STE-based strain has been applied to the LA and RV also.[136] The assessment of the contractile function of these chambers is helpful in planning appropriate management strategy in patients with HF. For example, in patients undergoing LVAD placement, impaired longitudinal strain of the RV free wall can reliably predict the chances of RV failure during follow-up.[102]

Real-time 3D echocardiography

Real-time 3D echocardiography (RT3DE) was initially developed in the early 1990s, and over the past few years the technology has advanced to the point where it is readily available for regular clinical use. For patients with advanced HF, the clinical utility of RT3DE is an active area of investigation. Given the prognostic significance of LV volumes and EF, accurate assessment of these parameters in HF is vital. Transthoracic RT3DE has been shown to be reproducible, accurate, and superior to 2D echocardiography in the assessment of LV volumes,[137] and compares well to cardiac MRI and radionuclide imaging[137,138,139] for this purpose. Similarly, compared to traditional 2D echocardiography, the assessment of RV volumes and function is also improved with RT3DE.[140] However, whether RT3DE assessment of ventricular volumes and function has incremental value over 2D echocardiography in improving clinical outcomes in advance HF is yet to be determined.

The value of RT3D TEE for the assessment of valvular heart disease and for guiding surgical or percutaneous repair of the valve lesions has already been emphasized. In addition, RT3DE has also been applied to the assessment of LV dyssynchrony and to myocardial deformation imaging. As discussed earlier, 2D echocardiography and TDI have demonstrated variable results when used for the evaluation of mechanical dyssynchrony in order to improve patient selection for CRT. Given these limitations, many studies have evaluated the role of RT3DE in the assessment of ventricular dyssynchrony. Using 3D echocardiography, SDI can be calculated as the standard deviation of the time taken to reach minimum regional volume for each myocardial segment. The RT3DE-derived SDI has been shown to be comparable to or superior to TDI in the assessment of LV dyssynchrony and in predicting response to CRT.[86,87,141,142] In addition, RT3DE has also been shown to be superior to 2D imaging in determining the optimal LV pacing site.[143]

Finally, 3D echocardiography has also been applied to STE. 3DSTE permits comprehensive assessment of LV myocardial mechanics from a single 3D pyramidal volume dataset, as opposed to multiple thin slices required for the conventional 2D STE. Although 3DSTE appears to overcome many of the limitations of 2DSTE, particularly those related to through-plane motion, more work is still needed to establish its clinical utility over conventional 2D STE.[144,145,146]

Cardiovascular flow visualization

Recent insights gained from animal studies, in-vitro experiments, and clinical studies involving sophisticated echocardiographic and MRI techniques have revealed that, contrary to previously held beliefs, the blood flow within the cardiovascular system follows complex multidimensional flow patterns characterized by the formation of spiral or vortical flow streams.[147] These vortices form as a consequence of the opposing effects of the pressure-head driving the forward flow on one hand and the viscosity and the shear stress between the fluid layers and the containing boundaries trying to slow down the blood flow on the other hand. The formation of these vortices represents a unique mechanistic adaptation of the cardiovascular system that serves to minimize energy loss associated with the movement of the blood. For example, it is only because of this characteristic flow behavior that the blood entering the LV from the LA during diastole is swiftly redirected toward the LVOT, while at the same time preventing energy being completely lost during this process. It fact, it has been estimated that roughly 16 ± 8% of the kinetic energy of diastolic mitral flow is conserved to the end of diastole and carried over into the next beat.[148] From a functional standpoint, such a vortical flow pattern plays an important role in the maintenance of optimal systolic and diastolic performance of the LV, in normal functioning of the cardiac valves, and in maintenance of normal circulation through different segments of the cardiovascular system under a wide range of physiological and nonphysiological conditions.[147]

Recent technical advances have now enabled in-vivo visualization and characterization of these blood flow patterns. Velocity-encoded cardiac MRI and echocardiographic contrast particle imaging velocimetry appear to be the two most promising modalities for this purpose (Figure 7.15).[147] However, both these modalities are currently in their infancy and much evolution is still needed before they will be ready for regular clinical use. Nevertheless, the ability to analyze the intracardiac and intravascular flow patterns has opened up several potential clinical applications.[147,149,150,151,152] The analysis of blood flow patterns has been shown to be helpful in preclinical detection of LV systolic and diastolic dysfunction, in defining pathological mechanisms involved in hypertrophic cardiomyopathy (HCM), and in the evaluation of valvular diseases, guiding surgical repair of valve regurgitation, assessing myocardial dyssynchrony, and optimization of cardiac resynchronization devices.[149,150,151,152] Many of these applications are directly relevant to patients with advanced HF. In addition, the application of these blood flow visualization techniques to the atria may provide insights into atrial function/dysfunction in various congenital and acquired cardiac diseases and may help in stratifying risk of clot formation in these disease states.[153,154] Similarly, extension of this knowledge to the great arteries may be helpful in quantifying the risk of developing aortic dilatation, aortic dissection, pulmonary thromboembolism, pulmonary hypertension, etc.[155,156]

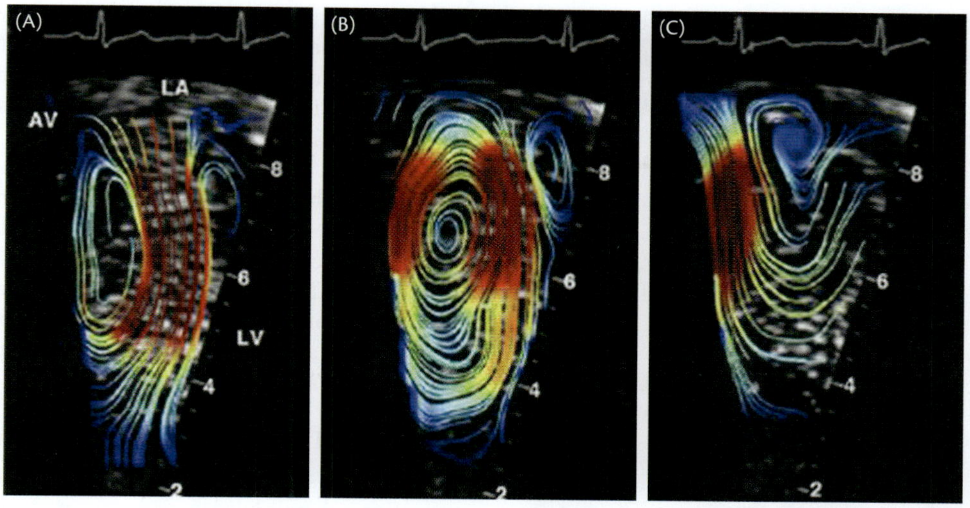

Fig. 7.15 Echocardiographic particle imaging velocimetry for intracardiac flow characterization. The flow is shown along the long-axis view of the left ventricle during (A) early diastole, (B) late diastole, and (C) the ejection phases of the cardiac cycle.

Modified from Journal of the American College of Cardiology: Cardiovascular Imaging, 5, Sengupta PP et al., Emerging trends in CV flow visualization, 305–316, copyright (2012) with permission from Elsevier.

Cardiac MRI in advanced heart failure

MRI was first described in 1971, but it was not until the advent of ECG-gated MRI in 1984 that it could be applied to the moving heart.[157] Since then, cardiac MRI has evolved to permit comprehensive assessment of myocardial structure, function, and perfusion. Its ability to permit assessment of cardiac dimensions, RV and LV function, valvular morphology and function, myocardial viability, and scar formation in a single scan without the use of ionizing radiation are some of its advantages over echocardiography, nuclear imaging, and CT. At the same time, cardiac MRI also allows tissue characterization, which has numerous diagnostic, prognostic, and therapeutic implications but is not possible with any of the other commonly used imaging modalities. These advantages, coupled with the accuracy and reproducibility of the measurements obtained by cardiac MRI, make it a model technique to evaluate therapeutic response as well as to guide management decisions in the complex HF patients.

Cardiac MRI techniques

Cardiac MRI images are obtained through the use of a magnetic gradient field switches that occur in the presence of a strong magnetic field, along with radiofrequency pulses and time-dependent data acquisition in precise orders known as "sequences." Radiofrequency pulses generated by a secondary external magnetic field excite the protons in the tissue to a higher energy state. The relaxation time of the protons from the excited state back to their equilibrium state is known as T1 and T2 relaxation, while the rate of T2 decay is known as T2*. With the use of various pulse sequences and parameters, image contrast patterns can be generated in different tissues dependent on T1, T2, and T2* relaxation times. Cine images of the moving heart in both the long-axis and short-axis planes are most commonly acquired during steady-state free precession sequences, which provide exceptional definition of the blood–tissue border. From these images, planimetry of the short-axis images along with summation of the slice volumes can accurately determine ventricular diastolic and systolic volumes, EF, and mass.[158] Due to the excellent definition of the blood–tissue border, volumetric assessment by cardiac MRI (CMR) is highly reproducible and correlates well with 3D echocardiography, though the former tends to underestimate volumes in most patients. Cine cardiac MRI is further used to detect regional wall motion changes during dobutamine stress testing for assessment of contractile reserve and inducible ischemia,[159] as well as for determination of atrial dimensions and volumes.[160] Compared to dobutamine echocardiography stress, dobutamine cardiac MRI has the added advantages of providing excellent visualization of wall motion without the limitations of acoustic windows or body habitus. Additional techniques such as tissue tagging and phase mapping, as well as strain encoding, allow for quantitation of myocardial velocity and strain, but are primarily research modalities at present.[161,162]

The use of intravenous contrast agents, most commonly gadolinium based, during cardiac MRI enables assessment of perfusion and scar imaging. The specific properties of gadolinium enhance the relaxation rates of water molecule protons, thereby shortening T1 and T2 times. At typical doses of gadolinium contrast agent, T1-weighted images produce positive contrast, while at very high doses or injection rate, T2*-weighting can produce negative contrast images. T1- and T2-weighted imaging sequences allow detection of the presence of gadolinium (positive or negative enhancement) in the myocardium and the blood pool in various normal and disease states. For first-pass perfusion imaging, vasodilator stress testing with adenosine, dipyrimadole, or regadenoson is performed while the passage of gadolinium contrast through the cardiac chambers and myocardium is followed. In areas of significantly diseased arteries less contrast enhancement is seen in the myocardium, producing an area of hypointense signal compared to areas with normal myocardial blood flow and contrast enhancement (Figure 7.16). With its high spatial resolution (usually <3 mm), perfusion cardiac MRI is able to identify even small regions of subendocardial perfusion defects.[163] For imaging myocardial injury and infarction, cardiac MRI takes advantage of the ability of gadolinium contrast to become distributed in areas of irreversible myocardial injury. T1-weighted images of the delayed washout

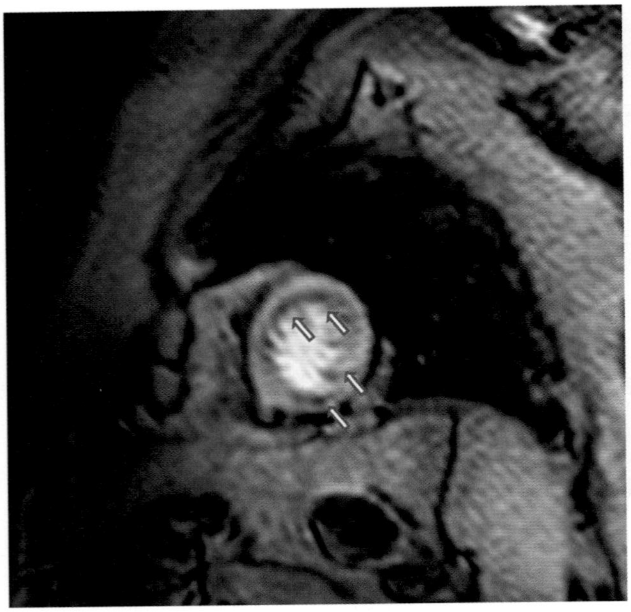

Fig. 7.16 Cardiac MRI stress image with gadolinium contrast enhancement demonstrating hyperintense signal in the myocardium but with a hypointense signal in the subendocardial septal, anterior and lateral walls (arrows) consistent with inducible ischemia in these areas.

of gadolinium from these areas show the presence of the contrast agent for a prolonged period of time after initial administration, known as late gadolinium enhancement (LGE) (Figure 7.17). After acute myocardial injury, cell death results in the release of gadolinium from the intracellular space into the extracellular space, while after chronic infarction, cell death and/or fibrosis leads to an increase in the extracellular space within the myocardium, allowing for a large distribution volume for gadolinium to accumulate in the interstitial space. Because of the high spatial resolution, LGE is able to detect even small areas of injury or infarction that can be missed by nuclear single-photon emission CT (SPECT) imaging.[164] This is particularly important since the presence of even small areas of myocardial infarct by LGE in patients without known ischemic disease correlates with increased morbidity.[165,166] Cardiac MRI can also detect the presence of edema that can be a feature of acute myocardial ischemia, even in the absence of irreversible injury seen by LGE.[167] T2-weighted images can demonstrate increased myocardial water content from increased influx that occurs in areas of ischemia. The presence of myocardial edema usually extends beyond the borders of irreversible injury seen by LGE after reperfusion of an acute myocardial infarction, representing an area of salvaged myocardium.[168]

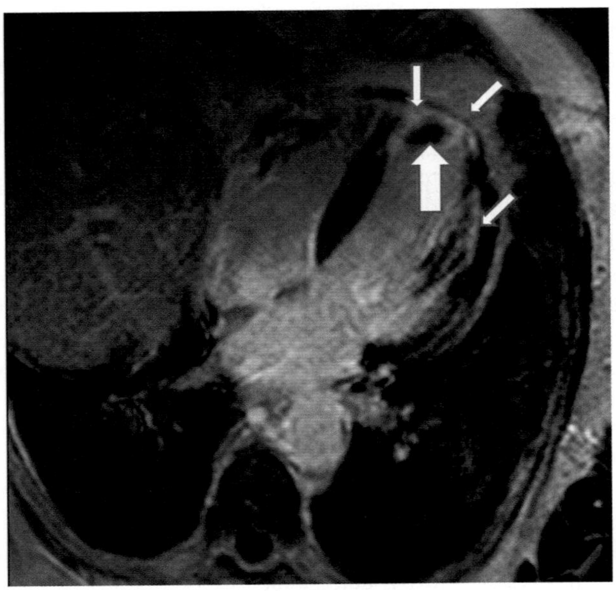

Fig. 7.17 Cardiac MRI image with late gadolinium enhancement imaging demonstrating a hyperintense signal in the apex and subendocardial anterolateral wall consistent with scar in these areas (thin arrows). The hypointense signal at the apex represents the presence of an apical thrombus (thick arrow).

Cardiac MRI in ischemic cardiomyopathy

Cardiac MRI is particularly useful in ischemic cardiomyopathy in evaluating ischemic burden, presence, or absence of viable myocardium, or presence of cardiac dyssynchrony, and for differentiating an ischemic from a nonischemic cardiomyopathy.

In ischemic LV dysfunction, cardiac MRI permits evaluation of the extent of ischemia and potential recovery of myocardial function after revascularization. Transmural extent of infarction by LGE is a reliable predictor of improvement in myocardial contractile function after coronary revascularization.[169,170] Severely hypokinetic or akinetic segments that have 0–25% transmural extent of scar have a high likelihood of recovery while more than 75% transmural scarring portends a poor chance of recovery (Figure 7.18).[170] However, the response rate in regions with intermediate LGE (~50%) is highly variable. In such cases, simultaneous assessment

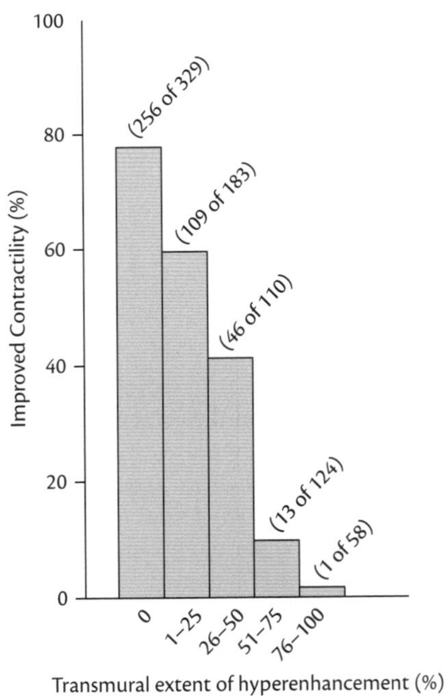

Fig. 7.18 Likelihood of improving segmental ventricular contraction after revascularization is decreased as transmural extent of late gadolinium enhancement by cardiac MRI, a measure of scarring, increases.

From New England Journal of Medicine, Kim RJ, Wu E, Rafael A, Chen EL, Parker MA, Simonetti O, et al. The use of contrast-enhanced magnetic resonance imaging to identify reversible myocardial dysfunction, 343:1445–1453, Copyright © (2000) Masachusetts Medical Society. Reprinted with permission from Massachusetts Medical Society.

of contractile reserve with the use of low-dose dobutamine MRI has been shown to improve the specificity for prediction of functional recovery by LGE.[171,172] While these studies have demonstrated that LGE by CMR can reliably predict segmental myocardial recovery, recovery of global LV function after revascularization is clinically a more relevant issue in patients with severe LV systolic dysfunction. Studies involving patients undergoing surgical revascularization have revealed that viability assessment on cardiac MRI can predict improvement in global LV systolic function also. It has been demonstrated that the patients with 10 or more segments of 50% or less transmural LGE on cardiac MRI show overall improvement in global LV function after revascularization.[173] A corollary to these findings is the prognostic value of LGE on cardiac MRI. In patients with advanced ischemic HF, the extent of myocardial scar as assessed by LGE on cardiac MRI has been shown to be associated with increased mortality or the need for cardiac transplantation.[174]

Cardiac MRI has also been evaluated for detection of cardiac dyssynchrony and to improve patient selection for CRT. Three techniques are currently used to assess dyssynchrony: cardiac MRI–myocardial tagging, phase-contrast tissue velocity mapping (TVM), and displacement encoding with stimulated echoes (DENSE). MRI–myocardial tagging is performed by creating a grid-like pattern on a myocardial image with the use of saturation pulses that are either parallel or perpendicular to the image slice. Deformation of the gridlines during systole and diastole can be measured to quantify myocardial motion (Figure 7.19). Similar to STE discussed earlier, myocardial tagging can assess deformation or strain in multiple directions including longitudinal, circumferential, radial, and rotational. Circumferential dyssynchrony by myocardial tagging has been shown to predict improvement in functional class and LVEF after CRT, but is limited by the specialized training and analysis time needed to obtain these measurements. In contrast, phase-contrast TVM is similar to echocardiographic TDI and encodes the velocity of the myocardium in a given direction. Although dyssynchrony assessment by TVM has shown to correlate with TDI measurements, the data assessing the ability of TVM to predict CRT response is currently lacking.[175,176] DENSE imaging is similar to TVM, but encodes displacement rather than velocity data. Traces of the endocardial and epicardial borders are used to compare the location of the myocardial segments at end-diastole and at end-systole, and systolic displacement is calculated from this data (Figure 7.20). Animal models have demonstrated that dyssynchrony measures by DENSE correlate with those obtained by tissue tagging, but the clinical utility of this modality for prediction of response to CRT in humans is yet to be reported.[177]

Besides dyssynchrony, scar location and quantification by LGE-CMR also helps in predicting response rates to CRT.[2,89,90,91,92] In ischemic cardiomyopathy, high total scar burden is associated

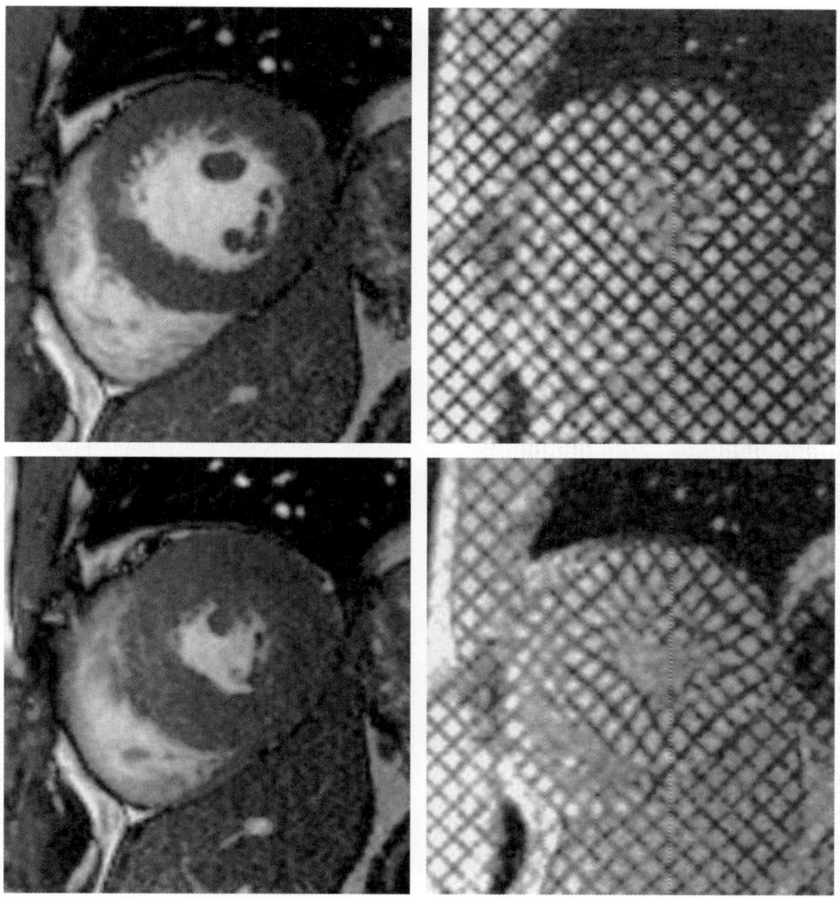

Fig. 7.19 Example of myocardial tagging by cardiac MRI. A grid is superimposed on the myocardium with the use of saturation pulses. Movement of the myocardium during systole and diastole is tracked and deformation of the grid lines can be used to quantify myocardium motion.
Modified from Cardiology Clinics, 25, White JA, Patel MR, The Role of Cardiovascular MRI in Heart Failure and the Cardiomyopathies 71–94, copyright (2007) with permission from Elsevier.

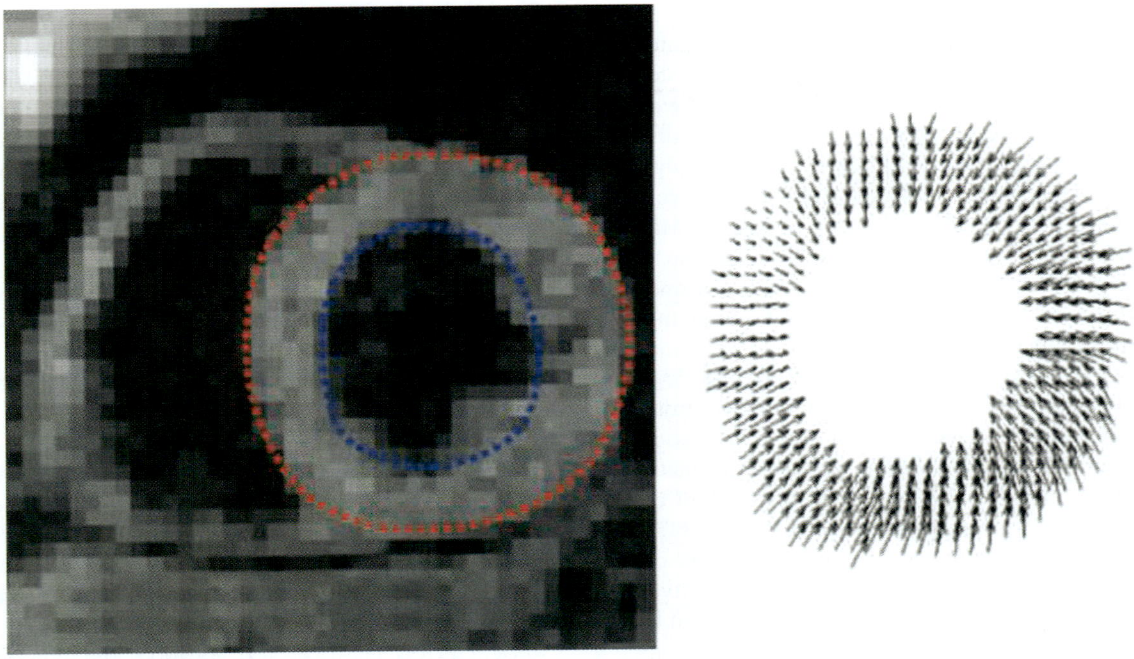

Fig. 7.20 Example of DENSE cardiac MRI. Endocardial and epicardial traces are placed (left image) and tracked from end-systole to end-diastole. A reconstructed images of the movement or displacement of the traces is shown (right image) from which wall motion abnormalities, dyssynchrony, and myocardial function can be evaluated.

with poor response to CRT.[178,179,180] A total scar burden cutoff value of 15% of the LV myocardium has been shown to predict response to CRT with high specificity and sensitivity (85% and 90%, respectively).[178] In addition to the overall extent, the location of scar is equally important. The presence of ischemic scar in the posterolateral wall, the preferred location for placement of the lateral LV lead, lowers response rates after biventricular pacing. In one study, the CRT responder rate was 83% in patients without posterolateral scar, and 47% in patients with posterolateral scar ($p < 0.0001$).[181] An added advantage of cardiac MRI is its ability to allow simultaneous assessment of cardiac venous anatomy, which in combination with the scar location data, may be able to improve lead positioning and outcomes. However, further studies are required to validate this approach.

Differentiation between ischemic and nonischemic cardiomyopathy

LGE on cardiac MRI permits detection of scar pattern that can differentiate between ischemic and nonischemic injury (Figure 7.21). The presence of subendocardial or transmural LGE supports a diagnosis of ischemic cardiomyopathy. In contrast, most nonischemic cardiomyopathies do not result in any LGE, while about 20% of dilated cardiomyopathy patients demonstrate patchy LGE, mostly in the mid-myocardium. Overall, when compared to coronary angiography, LGE on cardiac MRI has excellent sensitivity (98%), specificity (84%), and accuracy (93%) for differentiating ischemic from nonischemic cardiomyopathies. However, about 13–16% of patients with nonischemic cardiomyopathy, as determined by nonobstructive disease on cardiac catheterization, can have evidence of subendocardial or transmural scar on LGE cardiac MRI, suggestive of prior myocardial infarction.[182,183] This is more likely to be due to spontaneous recanalization of an occlusive coronary thrombus or severe coronary vasospasm than true nonischemic cardiomyopathy.[184]

Cardiac MRI in nonischemic cardiomyopathy

A significant portion of advanced HF patients have nonischemic cardiomyopathies, but identifying the underlying cause can be challenging in many cases. Understanding the specific pathology that results in LV dysfunction in these patients has strong prognostic as well as therapeutic implications. As compared to the patients with idiopathic cardiomyopathy, those with peripartum cardiomyopathy have better survival whereas those with cardiomyopathy due to infiltrative disorders, HIV infection, or doxorubicin toxicity have much worse outcomes.[185] Differentiation among these various etiologies can be difficult by conventional imaging techniques such as echocardiography and nuclear cardiology. However, cardiac MRI provides excellent tissue characterization not obtainable by other imaging modalities, and has a unique role to play in the evaluation of nonischemic cardiomyopathies.

Cardiac MRI in dilated cardiomyopathy

The LV enlargement and dysfunction seen in dilated cardiomyopathy can be due to multiple etiologies such as ischemic, inflammatory, or infiltrative diseases. Though echocardiography, angiography, and occasionally endomyocardial biopsy may allow for determination of the underlying etiology, tissue characterization by cardiac MRI may itself provide the diagnosis without the aid of complementary modalities. As noted earlier, LGE-CMR can reliable detect the presence of myocardial viability and scar formation, and can accurately determine if an ischemic injury has occurred by the presence of subendocardial or transmural scar pattern. In dilated cardiomyopathy, LGE typically demonstrates hyperenhancement in the midmyocardial layer of the LV, which can be seen in about

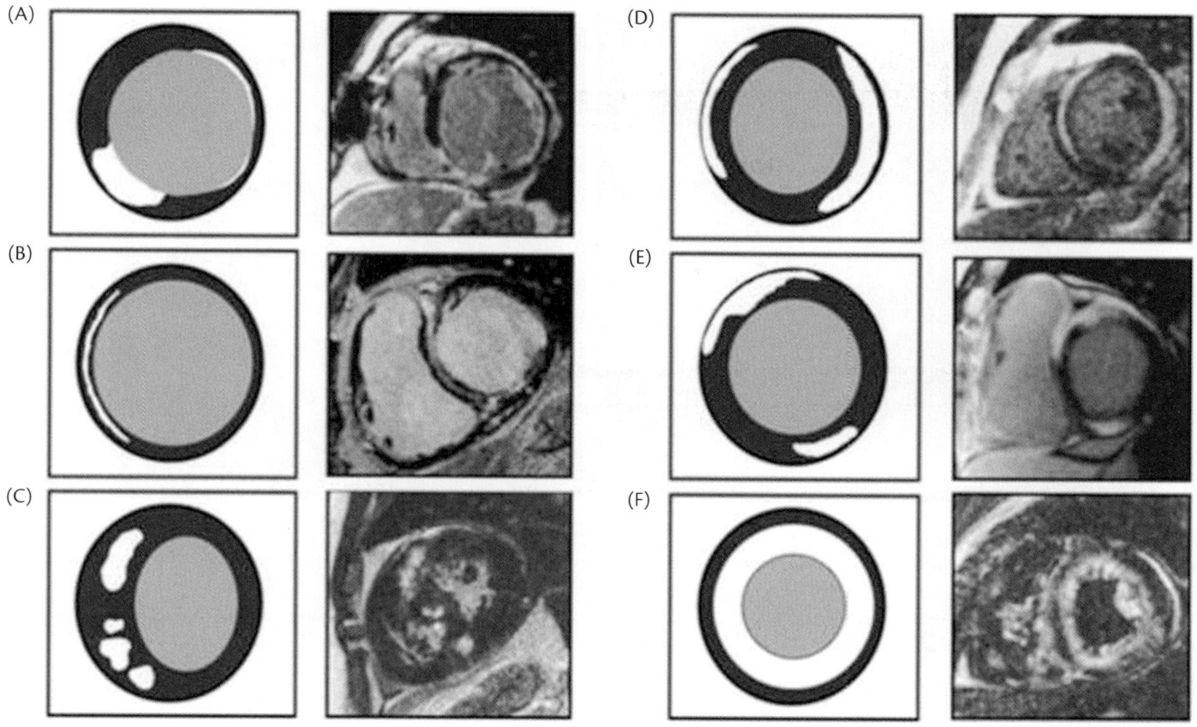

Fig. 7.21 Patterns of late gadolinium enhancement (LGE) that can be seen in different cardiomyopathies. (A) Ischemic cardiomyopathy: subendocardial scar in the lateral wall and transmural scar in inferoseptal wall. (B) Idiopathic dilated cardiomyopathy: midmyocardial wall scar in the basal septum. (C) Hypertrophic cardiomyopathy: septal wall with patchy LGE. (D) Myocarditis: epicardial and midmyocardial LGE in lateral and septal walls. (E) Sarcoidosis: dense epicardial and midmyocardial LGE in the anteroseptal and inferior walls. (F) Amyloidosis: diffuse LGE predominantly subendocardial and midmyocardial.

one-third of these patients.[186] However, assessing true fibrosis burden in these patients is often challenging. The qualitative assessment of LGE may not be reliable because of the typical diffuseness of collagen deposition in dilated cardiomyopathy. A newer technique employing T1-mapping can permit quantitative assessment of global myocardial fibrosis in these patients.[187] In this technique, T1 relaxation times are directly measured after administration of gadolinium contrast agent and the post-contrast T1 times correlate histologically to interstitial fibrosis.

Cardiac MRI also provides important prognostic information in dilated cardiomyopathy. The presence of LGE in dilated cardiomyopathy is associated with increased mortality and sudden cardiac death, independent of LVEF.[188] In a study of 101 patients with dilated cardiomyopathy, mid-wall fibrosis was seen in all 35 patients who experienced the primary outcome of all-cause mortality or hospitalization, while the risk of secondary endpoint of sudden cardiac death or ventricular tachycardia was also significantly increased in presence of mid-wall fibrosis compared to those with the evidence of myocardial fibrosis (hazard ratios 3.4 and 5.2, respectively). In another study involving nonischemic cardiomyopathy patients undergoing electrophysiological study, the transmural extent of mid-wall scaring correlated with the likelihood of ventricular tachycardia inducibility. Mid-wall fibrosis involving 26–75% of total wall thickness was highly predictive of inducible ventricular tachycardia.[189]

Cardiac MRI in hypertrophic cardiomyopathy

HCM is caused by mutations in sarcomeric proteins resulting in global or regional myocardial hypertrophy. With an estimated prevalence of 0.2% in the general population, HCM is the most common cause of sudden cardiac death in young patients, with an annual mortality rate of 1–6%.[190] Noninvasive imaging plays a key role in the diagnosis and management of HCM, with echocardiography being the primary modality for this purpose. However, cardiac MRI has recently emerged as an excellent complementary tool and may even be superior to echocardiography in certain aspects. Cardiac MRI is particularly useful when adequate visualization on echocardiography is difficult due to poor acoustic windows (Figure 7.22). In such cases, LV hypertrophy may be incorrectly characterized or may even be completely missed on echocardiography. In a study of 48 patients with suspected HCM who were imaged by both echocardiography and cardiac MRI, 3 of the patients (6%) were diagnosed to have phenotypic HCM by cardiac MRI but not by echocardiography.[191] LV mass can also be more accurately determined by cardiac MRI and may have prognostic implications. In a study of 264 patients with HCM assessed by cardiac MRI, 21% of patients had a normal overall LV mass despite having regional hypertrophy, demonstrating that increased LV mass was not a requirement for the diagnosis of HCM.[192] However, overall LV mass was a more sensitive predictor of outcome than maximal wall thickness, supporting the importance of accurate assessment of LV mass. Cardiac MRI also allows better delineation of papillary muscle anatomy. The presence of anteroapical papillary muscle displacement and hypermobile bifid papillary muscles can be easily identified on MRI. These papillary muscle abnormalities are usually associated with higher LVOT gradients that are independent of septal wall thickness,[193,194] and may at times necessitate

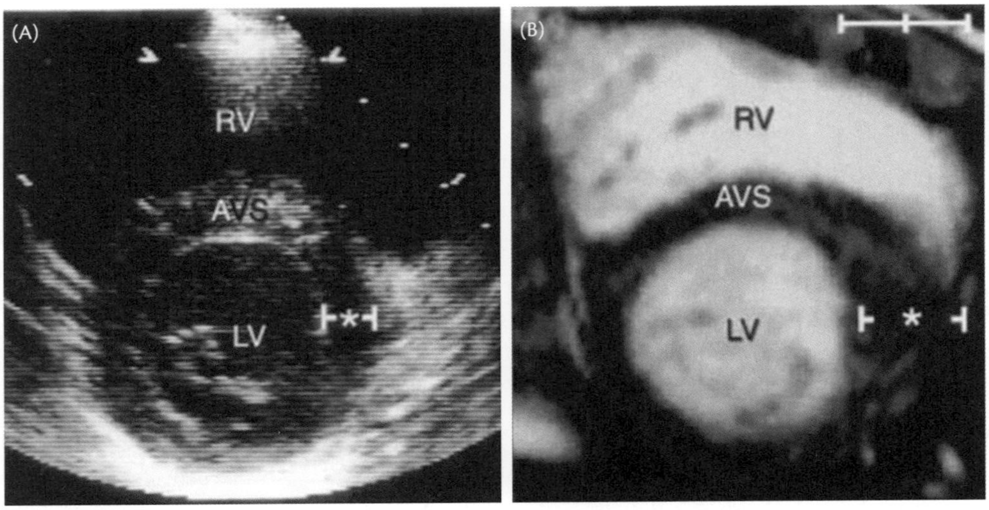

Fig. 7.22 Demonstration of a "missed" case of hypertrophy cardiomyopathy by echocardiogram that was recognized by cardiac MRI. In (A) the anterolateral wall at the level of the mitral valve was normal in measure. In the corresponding CMR image at the level of the mitral valve (B) in the same patient, the anterolateral wall measures 20 mm. AVS, anterior ventricular septum; LV, left ventricle; RV, right ventricle.

From Rickers C, Wilke NM, Jerosch-Herold M, Casey SA, Panse P, Panse N, Weil J, Zenovich AG, Maron BJ. Utility of cardiac magnetic resonance imaging in the diagnosis of hypertrophic cardiomyopathy. Circulation. 2005;112(6):855–61.

papillary muscle realignment without septal myectomy to relieve the obstruction.[195]

Identification of scar by LGE on cardiac MRI also provides valuable prognostic information in patients with HCM. Contrast-enhanced cardiac MRI studies in HCM patients have demonstrated that about 50% of these patients have evidence of LGE,[196,197] with a significant proportion of them demonstrating less than 10% LV wall scar by volume. Though commonly seen in HCM complicated by end-stage systolic dysfunction, presence of significant scar volume has also been demonstrated in patients with preserved LV function. The presence of scar by LGE in patients with HCM is associated with the presence of nonsustained ventricular tachycardia on ambulatory monitoring, a risk marker for sudden cardiac death in these patients.[198,199] In a prospective study of 220 HCM patients who were followed for clinical events after being evaluated by cardiac MRI, the presence of scar by LGE was associated with an odds ratio of 5.47 for all-cause mortality and 8.01 for cardiac mortality.[200] Similar findings have been noted in other several other studies.[197,198,201] However, most of these studies were limited by small sample size and larger and longer-term studies are needed to fully characterize the relevance of LGE in HCM in predicting risk for sudden cardiac death.[190]

Cardiac MRI in infiltrative cardiomyopathies

Cardiac MRI can provided diagnostic information in many types of infiltrative cardiomyopathies and may facilitate recognition of the underlying etiology, often challenging on echocardiography.

In cardiac amyloidosis, the expanded interstitial space from amyloid deposition can be readily identified by LGE and T1-mapping (Figure 7.23).[202,203] The LGE pattern can, however, be quite varied, including patchy or diffuse enhancement and even subendocardial or transmural enhancement. In addition to late enhancement, cardiac MRI will also detect increased wall thickness and mass of the LV or RV, presence of pericardial effusions, and enlarged atrial sizes, all of which support the diagnosis of cardiac amyloidosis.

In iron overload cardiomyopathy secondary to thalassemia, early stages can be treated with chelation therapy while chronic iron overload without chelation results in HF and has a poor prognosis.[204] Thus, determining when the iron content in the myocardium surpasses the normal storage capacity of myocardial transferrin and results in direct myocardial injury from non-transferrin-bound iron is vital in management of patients with thalassemia. The cardiac MRI technique T2*, the time constant of transverse magnetic relaxation, closely correlates inversely with myocardial iron levels and can help in quantifying total iron burden. Myocardial iron clearance can be measured by serial T2* imaging during chelation therapy to guide therapy and evaluate the effects on LV function.[205,206] This cardiac MRI method has provided for marked improvement in the management and survival of these patients,[204] as well as for monitoring the effects of pharmacologic treatment on iron content and LVEF.[205,206]

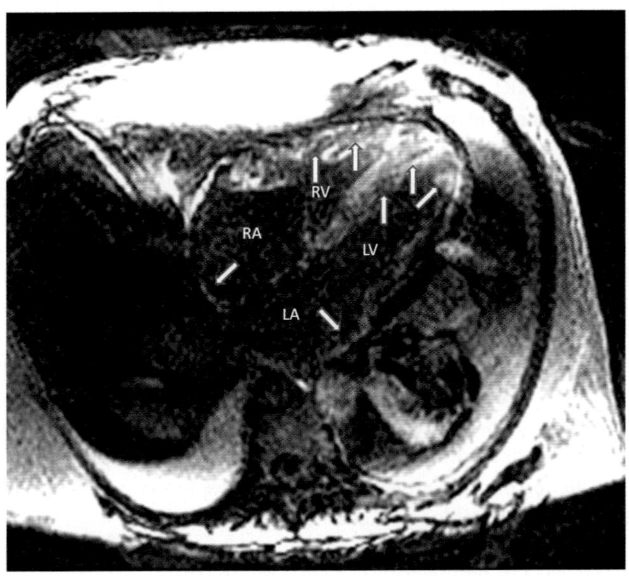

Fig. 7.23 Diffuse late gadolinium hyperenhancement seen in both ventricles and in the atria consistent with cardiac amyloid. LA, left atrium; LV, left ventricle; RA, right atrium; RV, right ventricle.

Fabry–Anderson disease is another cause of infiltrative cardiomyopathy that is often underdiagnosed. It is caused by an X-linked recessive deficiency in α-galactosidase that results in the intracellular accumulation of glycosphingolipids. The main cardiac finding, LVH, is often mistaken for HCM, leading to incorrect diagnosis. LGE on cardiac MRI can aid in differentiating Fabry–Anderson disease from the other causes of infiltrative cardiomyopathies. The typical pattern of scar distribution in Fabry–Anderson disease involves midmyocardial and epicardial layers in the basal inferolateral wall.[207] This pattern is distinguishable from that of HCM which typically involves the hypertrophied anteroseptal regions as well as RV insertion points.[208,209] Direct measurement of myocardial T2 relaxation time has also been proposed as a method for detecting the presence of excess glycosphingolipids in the myocardium. A study compared 12 patients with Fabry–Anderson disease with 12 HCM patients and 12 controls. It was found that the myocardial T2 relaxation time was significantly prolonged in patients with Fabry–Anderson disease compared to other groups, suggesting that MRI might be useful in diagnosing this disease.[210]

Cardiac MRI in inflammatory cardiomyopathies

Inflammation of the myocardial tissue, or myocarditis, is caused by a wide range of underlying etiologies including viral infection, immune mediated, drug or toxin related conditions, and even ischemic insults. The clinical presentation can also vary markedly, from subclinical to life-threatening illness. A large number of studies have shown contrast and noncontrast cardiac MRI to provide very high diagnostic accuracy in evaluating suspected myocarditis.[211,212,213,214,215,216,217,218,219,220] Inflammatory myocardial cell injury results in loss of intracellular water into the interstitial space. This myocardial edema can be sensitively detected by T2-weighed imaging as a hyperintense signal. Tissue inflammation also leads to regional vasodilatation and capillary leak. Early myocardial enhancement with gadolinium can be used to detect myocardial hyperemia and inflammation, supporting the presence of acute myocarditis in the appropriate clinical context. Further, as discussed earlier, LGE demonstrates irreversible myocardial injury that can also be seen in myocarditis. Several patterns of LGE can be seen including localized subepicardial, variably extending into the myocardium, as well as focal and multifocal patchy or diffuse distributions (Figure 7.24). Typically in myocarditis the subendocardium is not involved in a focal, isolated manner as seen in myocardial infarction. In practice, the combined use of all three diagnostic approaches (early gadolinium enhancement, LGE, and T2-weighted imaging) is recommended to achieve the best diagnostic accuracy for myocarditis. In patients with clinical suspected myocarditis, the presence of at least of two of the above three MRI abnormalities provides a diagnostic accuracy ranging from 73% to 85%.[213,216]

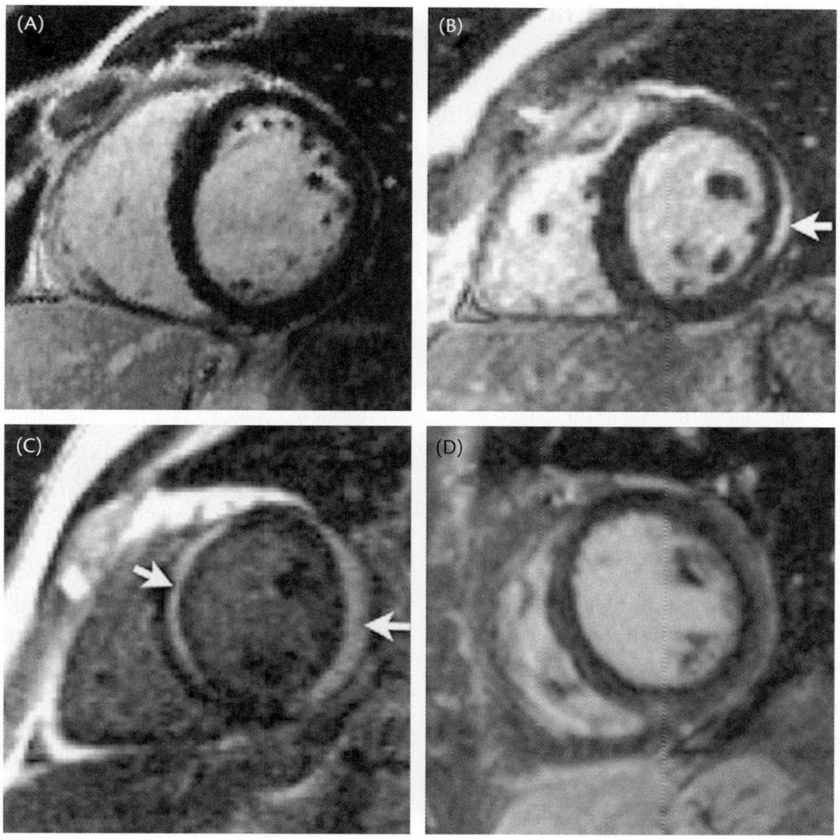

Fig. 7.24 Patterns of late gadolinium enhancement (LGE) seen in myocarditis. (A) No evidence of LGE; (B) lateral wall subepicardial LGE (arrow); (C) Septal midmyocardial LGE and lateral subepicardial and midmyocardial LGE (arrows); (D) Diffuse myocardial LGE enhancement of the midmyocardial and subepicardial regions.
Reprinted from Journal of the American College of Cardiology, 53(17), Friedrich MG et al., Cardiovascular magnetic resonance in myocarditis: A JACC White Paper, 1475-87, copyright (2009) with permission from Elsevier.

Sarcoidosis, a granulomatous inflammatory disease, can affect the heart in multisystemic cases and occasionally as isolated occurrences. Cardiac disease is associated with an adverse prognosis but is often not detected until autopsy, since early sarcoid involvement typically does not produce structural changes that can be appreciated on echocardiography. To this end, cardiac MRI allows for evaluation of subclinical cardiac dysfunction as well as evidence of myocardial granulomatous disease. T2-weighted images can detect presence of acute inflammation suggestive of active disease, while LGE can detect focal and diffuse areas of scar and fibrosis suggestive of chronic disease. Cardiac MRI may also be helpful in monitoring response to treatment. A small study of six patients receiving steroid treatment demonstrated that the changes in T2 and LGE images on serial exams correlated with clinical improvement or worsening.[221] The extent of LGE also correlates with LV size, severity of LV systolic dysfunction, and the presence of nonsustained ventricular tachycardia, which may explain the association of LGE with clinical outcomes. In a series of patients with cardiac sarcoid, presence of LGE was associated with a higher rate of adverse events (17.2% vs. 1.9% per year) compared to patients without LGE.[222] Sudden cardiac death has been reported to account for 30–65% of deaths in patients with cardiac sarcoid.[223] The presence of LGE on cardiac MRI is associated with ventricular arrhythmias and can help in risk stratification of these patients for sudden cardiac death. However, ongoing research will hopefully further refine the role of cardiac MRI for this purpose.

Nuclear imaging in advanced heart failure

While echocardiography and cardiac MRI provide vast amounts of structural and functional information helpful in diagnosis and management of HF patients, nuclear cardiac imaging still ranks as the most commonly employed modality for assessment of myocardial viability in these patients.[224] In addition, recent advances in nuclear imaging now also permit evaluation of several additional myocardial processes of potential therapeutic significance, such as sympathetic imaging for prediction of sudden cardiac death and ventricular arrhythmias. The greatest advantage of nuclear imaging is its ability to directly probe molecular myocardial processes that provides direct insights in to myocardial metabolism and function, not available with any other imaging modality.

Methodological aspects

There are two major types of nuclear imaging: SPECT and positron emission tomography (PET). Both these techniques employ a gamma camera to detect the emission of high-energy photons from an injectable radionuclide tracer. After injection and binding of the radionuclide to a region or tissue of interest such as the myocardium, acquisition of images from multiple planes or projections followed by tomographic reconstruction of the 2D imaging planes into a 3D dataset provides comprehensive information about regional myocardial perfusion and metabolism. Due to the wider availability of SPECT cameras and radiotracers along with the relatively straightforward acquisition protocols, SPECT imaging remains the most commonly employed nuclear imaging technique for cardiac purposes.

For SPECT myocardial perfusion imaging, the main radionuclides currently in use are 201-thallium (^{201}Tl) and 99 m-technetium ($^{99\,m}$Tc) (Table 7.1).[201] Thallium is a potassium analog and is transported across cell membranes by Na^+-K^+ ATPase. Since Na^+-K^+ ATPase-mediated transport is an energy-dependent process, ^{201}Tl can be taken up only by the cells that have preserved metabolic function. After an initial injection, cellular uptake of ^{201}Tl is directly proportional to the blood flow and therefore it is preferentially localized to myocardial regions with good blood supply. This initial distribution is then followed by a characteristic redistribution, mediated in part by differential washout and partly by cell-to-cell movement of ^{201}Tl through the Na^+-K^+ ATPase channel. Myocardial regions with good blood supply take up greater amount of ^{201}Tl initially but the subsequent washout is also faster from these regions. Conversely, in regions with compromised blood supply, the initial uptake of ^{201}Tl is lower but the washout is also gradual. As a result, the underperfused but viable areas show perfusion defects on initial imaging which are "refilled" on images obtained a few hours after the initial injection. This refilling of perfusion defects as a result of redistribution is the hallmark of viability on ^{201}Tl imaging. In contrast, in the nonviable segments, the initial perfusion defect does not show any refilling and remains irreversible or "fixed" over time (Figure 7.25).

Table 7.1 Comparison of technetium and thallium radiotracers for myocardial perfusion imaging using SPECT

	Technetium-99 m	Thallium-201
Dose	20–30 mCi	2–4 mCi
Photon energy	140 keV	69–83 keV
Half-life	6 hours	73 hours
Availability	Generator produced	Cyclotron produced
Image quality	Excellent	Relatively inferior
Cellular uptake	Passive diffusion driven by transmembrane electrochemical gradient, stored within mitochondria	Active uptake by Na^+-K^+ ATPase
Significant redistribution	No	Yes
Use in myocardial availability assessment	Not a preferred agent for this purpose Tracer uptake >50–60% of maximal uptake on rest imaging used as an evidence of viability	Preferred agent for this purpose Refilling of initial perfusion defects on delayed (4 or 24 hours) imaging indicates viability

The myocardial kinetics of $^{99\,m}$Tc-based tracers ($^{99\,m}$Tc-sestamibi and $^{99\,m}$Tc -tetrofosmin) are vastly different from those of ^{201}Tl. The uptake of $^{99\,m}$Tc by cells is through a passive diffusion process, which is driven by the transmembrane electrochemical gradient. As the maintenance of the this gradient requires energy, only viable cells take up $^{99\,m}$Tc. However, once inside the cells, $^{99\,m}$Tc is avidly retained by mitochondria and does not undergo any redistribution. This lack of redistribution limits its use as a SPECT tracer for myocardial viability assessment.

There are also other important differences in the physical properties of these two tracers that are relevant to myocardial perfusion imaging. ^{201}Tl emits lower-energy photons (80 keV) and has long half-life (73 hours) which limits the maximum dose that can be used. For both these reasons, the image quality with ^{201}Tl is usually

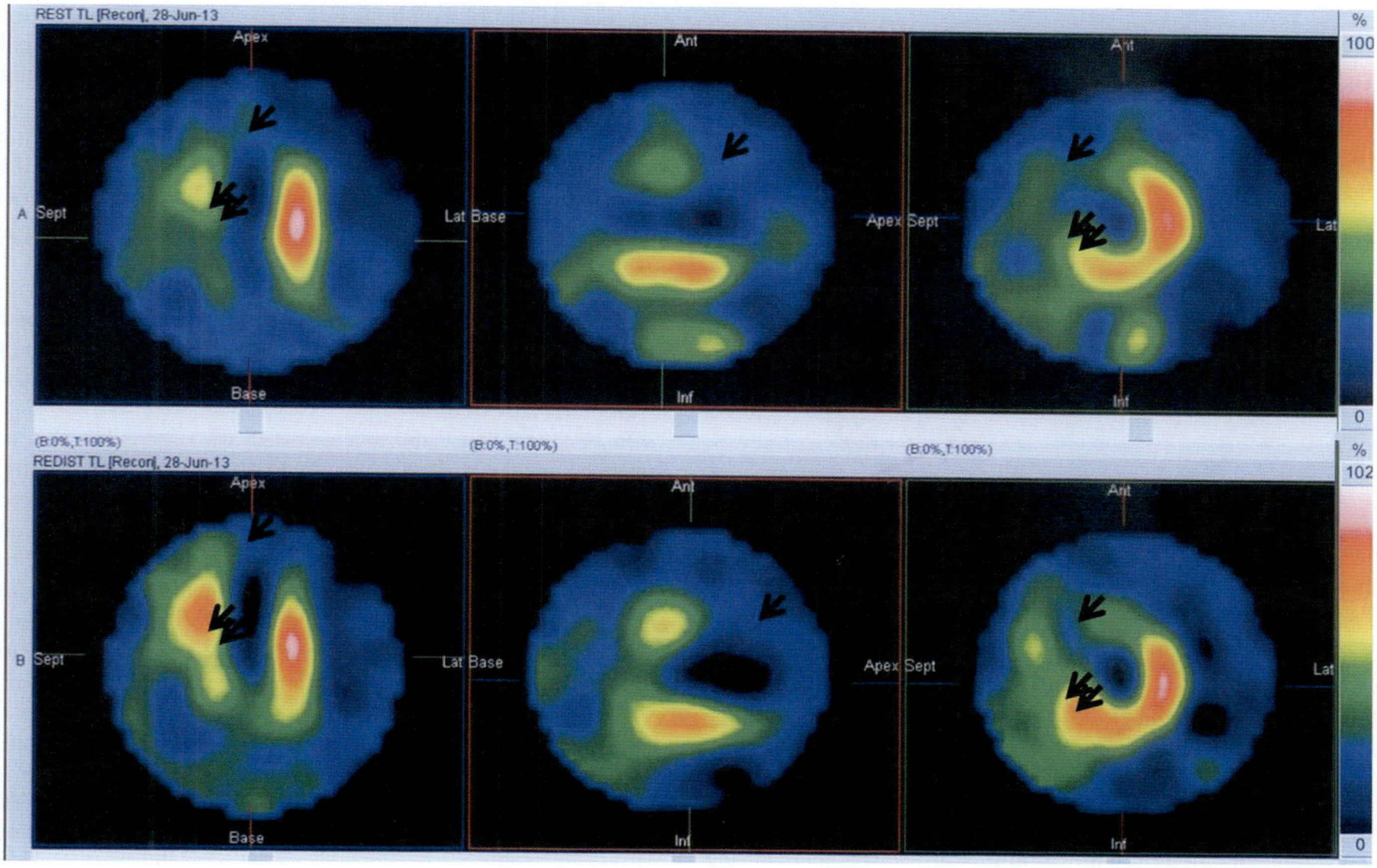

Fig. 7.25 Redistribution of thallium-201 as a marker of myocardial viability on SPECT imaging. The initial rest images are shown in the upper panel and the 3-hour redistribution images in the lower panel. There are large perfusion defects in the region of apex and apicoseptum which do not show any refilling on redistribution imaging (single arrows), indicating lack of viability ("fixed defect"). In contrast, there is significant refilling in the mid and basal portions of septum implying presence of viability (double arrows).

suboptimal. In contrast, the ^{99m}Tc-based tracers have shorter half-life (6 hours) and emit higher-energy photons (140 keV), both of which help toward excellent image quality.

Unlike SPECT imaging, PET scanning uses radioisotopes which are chemically identical to naturally occurring elements such as oxygen, nitrogen, or carbon, and therefore can be incorporated into molecules required for normal tissue functioning. Thus, ^{15}O-labeled water, ^{13}N-ammonia, and rubidium-82 (^{82}Rb) are used for myocardial perfusion assessment whereas ^{18}F-labeled 2-fluoro-2-deoxyglucose (FDG) is used for assessment of myocardial metabolism. ^{82}Rb and ^{13}N-ammonia are nondiffusible flow tracers that are retained in the myocardium as a function of blood flow and are not rapidly washed out from the myocardium as are diffusible tracers such as ^{15}O. Rubidium has properties similar to thallium and potassium and is actively taken up by the cells via Na^+-K^+ ATPase, whereas ^{13}N-ammonia is transported into the cells by passive diffusion and to a lesser extent by active Na^+-K^+ ATPase transport. The half-life of ^{82}Rb is 75 seconds and that of ^{13}N-ammonia is 10 minutes.

Unlike the SPECT tracers, PET tracers do not emit photons directly. Instead, they emit positrons that collide with electrons in the tissues to produce two high-energy (511 keV) photons. These two photons travel in exactly opposite directions and are simultaneously detected by two PET detectors situated directly opposite to each other (Figure 7.26). Such "coincidence detection" greatly improves the temporal and spatial resolution of PET imaging as compared to SPECT. Another major advantage of PET scanning is that it allows absolute quantification of myocardial perfusion and metabolism, unlike SPECT which provides only semiquantitative information. In patients with multivessel disease, uniformly reduced myocardial blood flow may be undetected by SPECT due to similar relative reduction in the perfusion, i.e., balanced ischemia, but can be detected by PET imaging. Similarly, quantitative assessment by PET may also allow detection of subtle abnormalities in blood flow, such as may be due to microvascular dysfunction, and can serve as a predictor of cardiovascular outcomes even in absence of obstructive CAD.[225,226]

In addition to the assessment of myocardial metabolism and perfusion, nuclear imaging can be used for assessment of ventricular systolic and diastolic functions also. ECG gating during SPECT perfusion studies is a standard practice that permits simultaneous assessment of myocardial contractile function. This not only allows measurement of LVEF but is also helpful in differentiating true perfusion defects from imaging artifacts. However, radionuclide ventriculography (RVG) has been the traditional nuclear imaging technique used for assessment of ventricular volumes and function. Unlike perfusion imaging, RVG employs blood pool labeling with radioisotopes followed by ECG-gated imaging to quantify

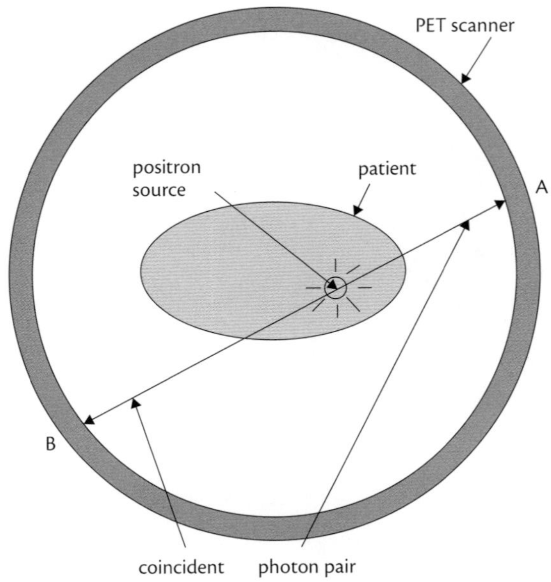

Fig. 7.26 An annihilation event produces a coincident photon pair that are directed 180° to each other during PET emission imaging. Detection of this coincident photon pair by the PET scanner allows for accurate localization and superior resolution.

Reprinted from Seminars in Nuclear Medicine, 33(3), Kinahan, Paul E et al., X-ray-based attenuation correction for positron emission tomography/computed tomography scanners, 166-79, copyright (2003) with permission from Elsevier.

the volume of blood present within the cardiac chambers during different phases of the cardiac cycle. There are two major types of RVG: equilibrium RVG, popularly known as multigated acquisition (MUGA) scan, and first-pass RVG. In case of equilibrium RVG, used mainly for studying the LV function, ^{99m}Tc-labeling is applied to albumin or red blood cells and ECG-gated scanning is performed from multiple projections. Counts obtained over several hundred cardiac cycles are summated to provide estimates of blood volumes within LV throughout the cardiac cycle. This information is then analyzed to derive information about LV systolic and diastolic functions.

The first-pass RVG is used mainly for assessment of RV systolic function. The most commonly used tracer for this purpose is ^{99m}Tc-labeled diethylenetriaminepentaacetic acid (DTPA), which is injected rapidly, followed by rapid scanning during the first few cardiac cycles as the tracer travels through different cardiac chambers. The temporal sequence of tracer flow provides separation between RV and LV and allows accurate assessment of RV systolic function.

Assessment of myocardial viability

There are several different nuclear imaging protocols for assessment of myocardial viability, with rest–redistribution ^{201}Tl imaging being the most standard one. The radioisotope is injected at rest, followed by scanning immediately thereafter and repeat scanning about 3–4 hours later. As discussed earlier, perfusion defects seen on initial scan that are refilled on the second scan indicate presence of myocardial viability (see Figure 7.26). In many patients, though, the redistribution may occur relatively slowly. In such patients, when no significant viability is apparent on early redistribution images, repeating the imaging at 24 hours (late redistribution) may be helpful by showing additional areas of viability. Another commonly encountered problem is the rapid washout of ^{201}Tl, resulting in substantial reduction in the amount of radioactivity within the myocardium by 4 hours. This precludes accurate detection of myocardial viability. In such cases, injecting an additional, small dose of radioisotope at rest may improve the ability to detect viable myocardium by raising blood levels of ^{201}Tl (rest–redistribution–reinjection) (Figure 7.27).

As mentioned previously, due to lack of redistribution, ^{99m}Tc is not the best suited radioisotope for assessment of myocardial viability. Nevertheless, in the dysfunctional segments, ^{99m}Tc uptake of 50–60% of maximal uptake, particularly after administration of sublingual nitroglycerine, has been used a criterion for viable myocardium in many studies.[227,228]

On PET imaging, viability is assessed using a combination of metabolic imaging, typically with ^{18}F-FDG and perfusion imaging, usually with ^{82}Rb or ^{13}N-ammonia. ^{18}F-FDG is transported into the myocardial cells through glucose transporters as a function of the rate of glucose metabolism. After metabolism in the cell to ^{18}F-FDG 6-phosphate, the tracer undergoes no further metabolism and is trapped within the cell due to its negative charge. Since only viable cells are able to take up glucose, the presence of ^{18}F-FDG in the myocardium serves as excellent marker of viability. Moreover, as ischemia is associated with progressive shifting of myocardial metabolism from fatty acid oxidation to glucose metabolism, ischemic cells often demonstrate enhanced glucose uptake compared to the nonischemic regions. Thus, a segment with preserved or enhanced glucose metabolism but reduced perfusion (defect "mismatch") indicates presence of ischemic, viable myocardium whereas a "matched" defect indicates lack of viability (Figure 7.28). Due to difficulties in procuring ^{82}Rb and ^{13}N-ammonia (the latter requiring an on-site cyclotron), many centers combine SPECT perfusion imaging, instead of PET perfusion imaging, with PET metabolic imaging for assessment of myocardial viability.

Nuclear imaging with SPECT or PET provides valuable diagnostic and prognostic information and has been shown to be helpful in guiding therapeutic decision-making in patients with HF. Most importantly, the evidence of myocardial ischemia and/or viability in patients with ischemic LV dysfunction predicts functional recovery and improved clinical outcomes following revascularization.[36,40,229] A meta-analysis of 24 nonrandomized studies (that also included dobutamine echocardiography) documented a profound mortality benefit with revascularization in patients with ischemic HF when there was evidence of viability on at least one of the various imaging studies.[36] In these patients, medical management alone was associated with significantly increased risk of death, which was even greater than the risk seen in those without evidence of viability. In contrast, both medical management and revascularization were associated with similar survival rates in patients without evidence of significant myocardial viability. These findings were also confirmed in a more recent meta-analysis by Inaba et al.[229] These investigators also estimated that roughly 22–44% viable myocardium was required to result in survival benefit with revascularization.

Multiple mechanisms have been proposed to explain the survival benefit seen with revascularization in patients with ischemic viable myocardium. Improvement in LVEF is considered to be the most important determinant of improved outcomes following revascularization.[230] An absolute increment of

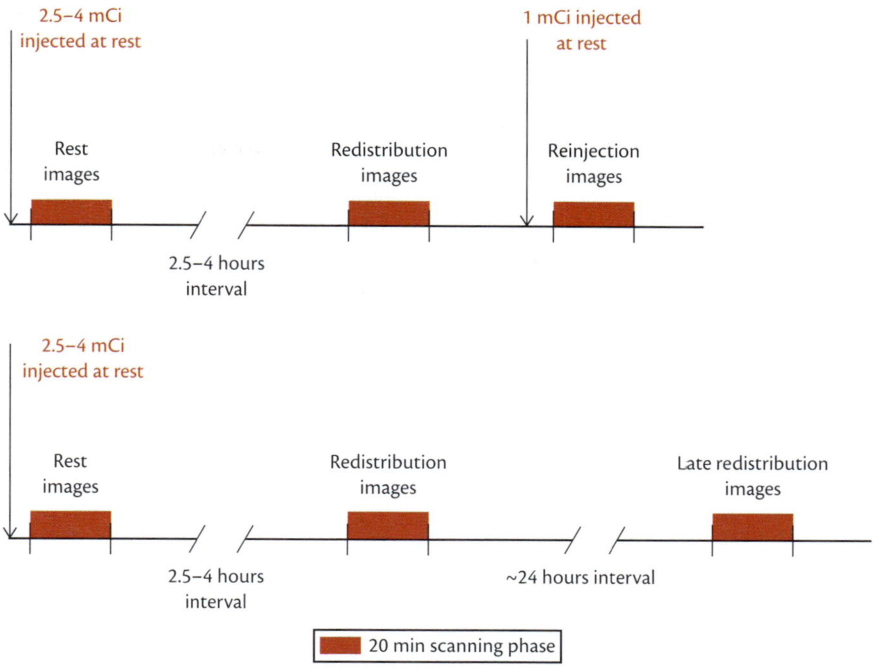

Fig. 7.27 Commonly used thallium-201 perfusion scintigraphy protocols for assessment of myocardial viability using SPECT imaging. The radioisotope is injected at rest, followed immediately by initial scanning and a repeat scan 3–4 hours later (rest–redistribution imaging). In some patients, when initial redistribution images do not show any refilling, reinjection of smaller dose of radioisotope followed by another scanning (rest–redistribution–reinjection; upper panel) or delayed scanning at 24 hours (rest–redistribution–late redistribution; lower panel) may help in detecting myocardial viability.

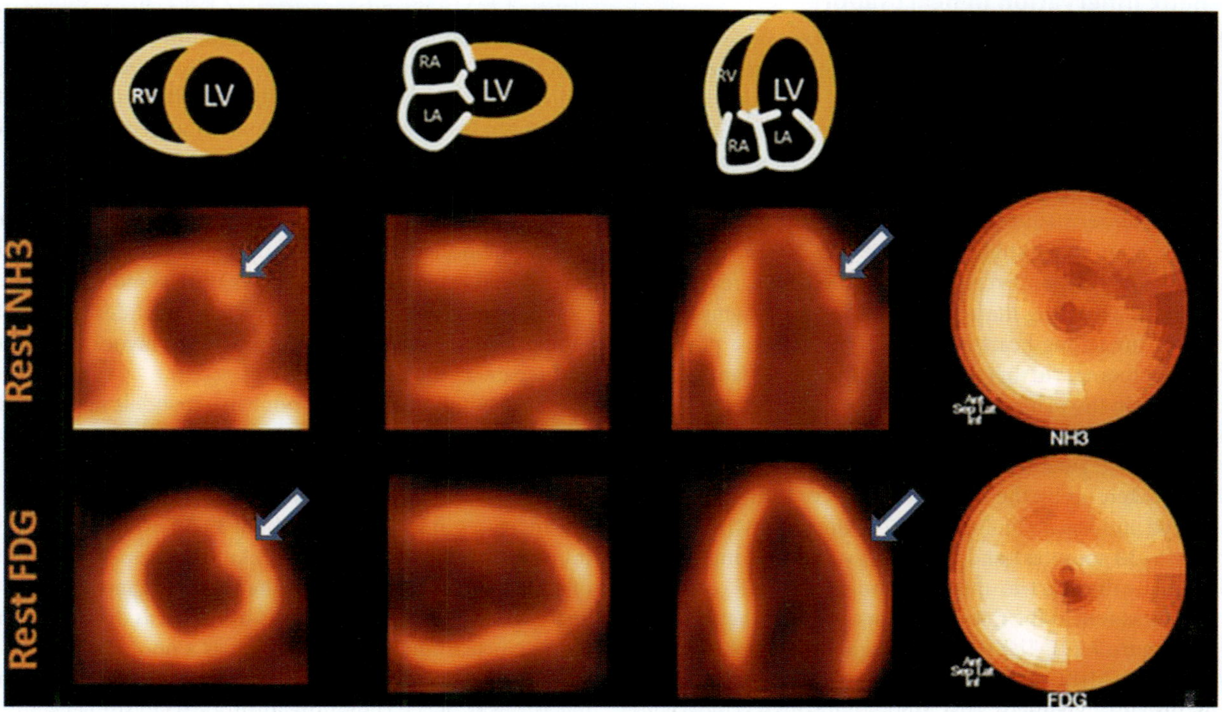

Fig. 7.28 Resting ^{13}N-ammonia perfusion and resting ^{18}F-FDG uptake in short- and long-axis views in a patient undergoing viability assessment. The anterolateral wall (arrows) demonstrates decreased perfusion with ^{13}N-ammonia at rest with uptake of ^{18}F-FDG consistent with hypoperfused but viable myocardium.

Adapted from Rischpler C, Nekolla S, Schwaiger M. PET and SPECT in heart failure. Curr Cardiol Rep. (2013) 15(3):337, Springer.

at least 5% in LVEF is considered to be significant and has been used as the criterion to define functional recovery. Using this definition, most studies have demonstrated that roughly 36–88% of patients with evidence of viability show improvement in LVEF following revascularization.[231,232] However, an increase in LVEF is not always apparent after revascularization although it may not necessarily be associated with lack of clinical benefits.[233] Some of the previous studies have shown similar cardiac outcomes after revascularization irrespective of improvement in LVEF,[233] suggesting beneficial effects of revascularization extend beyond just increase in LVEF alone.

Several studies have compared the accuracy of different imaging techniques for prediction of functional recovery following revascularization. A pooled analysis of 37 such studies demonstrated that among all different imaging modalities,[201] Tl rest–redistribution imaging had the highest sensitivity (90%) for prediction of functional recovery. However, the specificity was suboptimal (54%).[40] In comparison, ^{18}F-FDG PET scanning had relatively lower sensitivity but had the best diagnostic accuracy. Similar findings were shown by Schinkel et al. in yet another meta-analysis.[228] The lower specificity of nuclear imaging for predicting myocardial functional recovery may be related to the variable extent of subendocardial scarring. The areas of subendocardial scar show evidence of viability on nuclear imaging because of the preserved perfusion in the subepicardial and midmyocardial regions but their contractility is unlikely to improve after revascularization due to the scarred subendocardial region.

Sympathetic innervation in heart failure

Sympathetic nervous system activation is well known to be a key determinant of adverse cardiac remodeling in advanced HF.[234] Indeed, contemporary medical management of HF largely involves blocking the neurohormonal cascade that is mediated by the sympathetic nervous system. In patients with HF, several abnormalities of sympathetic innervation of the myocardium have been documented. These abnormalities are characterized by downregulation, desensitization, or dysfunction of the pre- and postsynaptic β-adrenoreceptors and an excess of norepinephrine release. As will be discussed, assessing the activity of myocardial sympathetic innervation in the failing heart has been shown to be a powerful predictor of outcome, further expanding the important role of nuclear imaging in the management of such patients.

For imaging sympathetic innervation, SPECT primarily employs ^{123}I-metaiodobenzylguanidine (MIBG), a noradrenaline analog. ^{123}I-MIBG is taken up by the sympathetic nerve terminals but is not catabolized and has no biologic effects. After ^{123}I-MIBG injection, early (15–30 minutes) and late (up to 4 hours) images are taken to calculate the heart-to-mediastinum ratio (HMR) of radionuclide uptake, as well as the rate of washout between the early and late images (Figure 7.29). The HMR is a highly reproducible index of myocardial ^{123}I-MIBG uptake, while the washout rate is a proxy for level of cardiac sympathetic activation.[235] Impaired sympathetic innervation as measured by ^{123}I-MIBG uptake is a strong predictor of cardiac morbidity and mortality in HF and may be a more powerful predictor than age and New York Heart Association (NYHA) class.[236] The ADMIRE-HF (AdreView Myocardial Imaging for Risk Evaluation in Heart Failure) prospective study in 961 patients demonstrated that an HMR less than 1.6 was associated with a greater than 11% risk of cardiac death, compared to less than 2% for an HMR of 1.6 or more.[237] In addition, ^{123}I-MIBG uptake has been shown to be an independent predictor of sudden death, regardless of LVEF.[238] The ^{123}I-MIBG washout rate is also a strong independent predictor of sudden cardiac death in systolic HF with a rate of 27% or more associated with a greater than sixfold risk of sudden death.[239] As a majority of severe HF patients with a primary prevention indication for an ICD never actually use their device, ^{123}I-MIBG imaging may become a valuable tool to help identify those patients at the highest risk of sudden cardiac death who are the most likely to benefit from such therapies.

In addition to prediction of cardiac morbidity and mortality, ^{123}I-MIBG imaging has also been shown to assess response to drug therapy. Angiotensin converting enzyme inhibitors and angiotensin receptor blockers improve cardiac sympathetic activity as measured by increased ^{123}I-MIBG uptake in patients with HF.[240,241] The use of β-blockers and aldosterone blockers has also been demonstrated to improve ^{123}I-MIBG uptake in HF patients.[242,243,244]

Advanced nuclear imaging in heart failure

The molecular mechanisms underlying adverse cardiac remodeling are an intense area of research. Advances in nuclear imaging have facilitated better understanding of these mechanisms through the use of radiolabeled ligands. One such application has been in imaging matrix metalloproteinases (MMP), which are extracellular degradative enzymes that have been shown to be crucial in the development of HF. Activated by catecholamines, angiotensin, and endothelin, MMPs have been shown to be upregulated in animal models of ischemic cardiomyopathy. Using ^{111}In-RP782, a radiolabeled MMP ligand, investigators have shown increased MMP activity not only in infarcted myocardium (increased fivefold) but also in noninfarcted remote myocardium (twofold increase).[245] Thus, localizing and tracking MMP activity by radiotracer imaging may aid in better assessing postinfarction ventricular remodeling. Other potential targets include integrins—the proteins involved in cell proliferation and angiogenesis—that can be tracked by binding with the PET ligand ^{18}F-fluoro-galacto-RGD. Preclinical studies demonstrate upregulation of integrin expression after myocardial infarction that persists until 6 months after reperfusion. These studies imply a role for radionuclide ligand imaging in monitoring angiogenesis in the process of myocardial remodeling and repair.[246]

Transplantation of human bone marrow cells has been shown in animal postinfarct models to improve contractile function.[247,248] However, trials of bone marrow cell therapy in patients with advanced ischemic HF have demonstrated mixed results, with absolute increases in LVEF of only about 3% in two studies[249,250] and no improvement in a third study.[251] Among the perceived limitations of bone marrow cell therapy is the variability in successful delivery and engrafting of implanted cells in the areas of damaged myocardium. Nuclear imaging is emerging as a noninvasive approach for labeling and tracking cells to gain an understanding into rate and mechanisms of cell engraftment. In a human study using ^{18}F-FDG labeling of unselected bone marrow or CD34-enriched cells infused in patients with acute coronary syndrome, PET imaging demonstrated 1.3–2.6% and 14–39% cell detection rates in infarcted myocardium, respectively.[252] Radiolabeled cell tracking may also aid researchers in developing new methods for cell delivery by allowing better understanding of the mechanisms involved in bone marrow cell homing and biodistribution to target tissue.

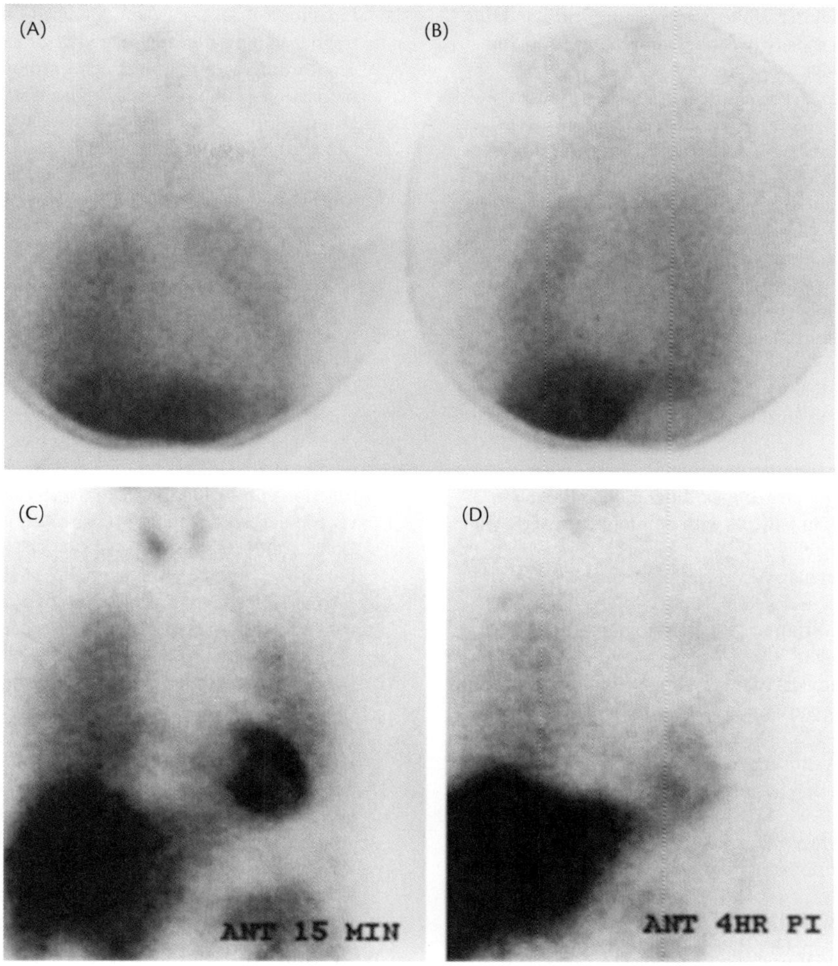

Fig. 7.29 MIBG planar images of a patient with a dilated cardiomyopathy (A) and (B) demonstrating a very low heart:mediastinum uptake suggesting poor sympathetic innervation. MIBG planar images at initial injection (C) and 4 hours later (D) demonstrating rapid washout of tracer.

Nuclear imaging after cardiac transplantation

Cardiac allograft vasculopathy (CAV) is a common occurrence after heart transplantation, seen in greater than 50% of heart transplant recipients by angiography at 10 years, and associated with increased mortality.[253] Coronary angiography has traditionally been the primary screening tool for detection of CAV. However, as angiography provides only an assessment of the coronary luminal diameter, diffuse or mild intimal disease may be missed. Furthermore, serial coronary angiography, as may be required to assess progression of CAV, exposes the patient to the risks of repeated invasive procedures. Nuclear imaging techniques, being noninvasive in nature, can be particularly attractive in this setting. In a study of 78 heart transplant patients who underwent both invasive angiogram and nuclear stress imaging within 48 hours of each other, SPECT imaging demonstrated a sensitivity of 92% and specificity of 86% for detection of significant CAV.[254] The presence of CAV by SPECT was also predictive of future cardiac events, with a relative risk of 4.1. Other similar studies have also confirmed the high specificity and sensitivity of nuclear imaging for predicting CAV and cardiac events.[255,256] In addition, abnormal myocardial perfusion by PET has also been shown to correlate with intravascular ultrasound measures of coronary plaque burden in heart transplant recipients, proposing a role for this modality as well in the evaluation of CAV.[257]

References

1. Badgett RG, Lucey CR, Mulrow CD. Can the clinical examination diagnose left-sided heart failure in adults? JAMA 1997;277:1712–19.
2. Capomolla S, Ceresa M, Pinna G, et al. Echo-Doppler and clinical evaluations to define hemodynamic profile in patients with chronic heart failure: Accuracy and influence on therapeutic management. Eur J Heart Fail 2005;7:624–30.
3. Shah MR, Hasselblad V, Stevenson LW, et al. Impact of the pulmonary artery catheter in critically ill patients: Meta-analysis of randomized clinical trials. JAMA 2005;294:1664–70.
4. Wheeler AP, Bernard GR, Thompson BT, et al. Pulmonary-artery versus central venous catheter to guide treatment of acute lung injury. N Engl J Med 2006;354:2213–24.
5. Shure D. Pulmonary-artery catheters—peace at last? N Engl J Med 2006;354:2273–74.
6. Oh JK. Echocardiography as a noninvasive Swan-Ganz catheter. Circulation 2005;111:3192–4.
7. Quinones MA, Otto CM, Stoddard M, et al. Recommendations for quantification of Doppler echocardiography: A report from the

Doppler quantification task force of the nomenclature and standards committee of the american society of echocardiography. J Am Soc Echocardiogr 2002;15:167–84.
8. Rudski LG, Lai WW, Afilalo J, et al. Guidelines for the echocardiographic assessment of the right heart in adults: A report from the American Society of Echocardiography endorsed by the European Association of Echocardiography, a registered branch of the European Society of Cardiology, and the Canadian Society of Echocardiography. J Am Soc Echocardiogr 2010;23:685–713; quiz 786–88.
9. Ristow B, Ali S, Ren X, et al. Elevated pulmonary artery pressure by Doppler echocardiography predicts hospitalization for heart failure and mortality in ambulatory stable coronary artery disease: The heart and soul study. J Am Coll Cardiol 2007;49:43–9.
10. Himelman RB, Stulbarg M, Kircher B, et al. Noninvasive evaluation of pulmonary artery pressure during exercise by saline-enhanced Doppler echocardiography in chronic pulmonary disease. Circulation 1989;79:863–71.
11. Giardini A. Limitations inherent to the simplified Bernoulli equation explain the inaccuracy of Doppler echocardiographic estimates of pulmonary artery pressures in patients with pulmonary hypertension. Chest 2011;140:270; author reply 270–1.
12. Yared K, Noseworthy P, Weyman AE, et al. Pulmonary artery acceleration time provides an accurate estimate of systolic pulmonary arterial pressure during transthoracic echocardiography. J Am Soc Echocardiogr 2011;24:687–92.
13. Chemla D, Castelain V, Humbert M, et al. New formula for predicting mean pulmonary artery pressure using systolic pulmonary artery pressure. Chest 2004;126:1313–17.
14. Friedberg MK, Feinstein JA, Rosenthal DN. A novel echocardiographic Doppler method for estimation of pulmonary arterial pressures. J Am Soc Echocardiogr 2006;19:559–62.
15. Abbas AE, Fortuin FD, Schiller NB, et al. Echocardiographic determination of mean pulmonary artery pressure. Am J Cardiol 2003;92:1373–6.
16. Mahan G, Dabestani A, Gardin JM, et al. Estimation of pulmonary artery pressure by pulsed Doppler echocardiography. Circulation 1983;68:367.
17. Dabestani A, Mahan G, Gardin JM, et al. Evaluation of pulmonary artery pressure and resistance by pulsed Doppler echocardiography. Am J Cardiol 1987;59:662–8.
18. Kitabatake A, Inoue M, Asao M, et al. Noninvasive evaluation of pulmonary hypertension by a pulsed Doppler technique. Circulation 1983;68:302–9.
19. Aduen JF, Castello R, Lozano MM, et al. An alternative echocardiographic method to estimate mean pulmonary artery pressure: Diagnostic and clinical implications. J Am Soc Echocardiogr 2009;22:814–19.
20. Nagueh SF, Appleton CP, Gillebert TC, et al. Recommendations for the evaluation of left ventricular diastolic function by echocardiography. J Am Soc Echocardiogr 2009;22:107–33.
21. Nagueh SF, Bhatt R, Vivo RP, et al. Echocardiographic evaluation of hemodynamics in patients with decompensated systolic heart failure. Circ Cardiovasc Imaging 2011;4:220–7.
22. Ritzema JL, Richards AM, Crozier IG, et al. Serial Doppler echocardiography and tissue Doppler imaging in the detection of elevated directly measured left atrial pressure in ambulant subjects with chronic heart failure. JACC Cardiovasc Imaging 2011;4:927–34.
23. Rohde LE, Palombini DV, Polanczyk CA, et al. A hemodynamically oriented echocardiography-based strategy in the treatment of congestive heart failure. J Card Fail 2007;13:618–25.
24. Grayburn PA, Appleton CP, DeMaria AN, et al. Echocardiographic predictors of morbidity and mortality in patients with advanced heart failure: The beta-blocker evaluation of survival trial (BEST). J Am Coll Cardiol 2005;45:1064–71.
25. Xie GY, Berk MR, Smith MD, et al. Prognostic value of Doppler transmitral flow patterns in patients with congestive heart failure. J Am Coll Cardiol 1994;24:132–9.
26. Pinamonti B, Di Lenarda A, Sinagra G, Camerini F. Restrictive left ventricular filling pattern in dilated cardiomyopathy assessed by Doppler echocardiography: Clinical, echocardiographic and hemodynamic correlations and prognostic implications. Heart muscle disease study group. J Am Coll Cardiol 1993;22:808–15.
27. Cintron G, Johnson G, Francis G, et al. Prognostic significance of serial changes in left ventricular ejection fraction in patients with congestive heart failure. The V-HEFT VA cooperative studies group. Circulation 1993;87:17–23.
28. Wong M, Staszewsky L, Latini R, et al. Severity of left ventricular remodeling defines outcomes and response to therapy in heart failure: Valsartan heart failure trial (VAL-HEFT) echocardiographic data. J Am Coll Cardiol 2004;43:2022–7.
29. Wong M, Staszewsky L, Latini R, et al. Valsartan benefits left ventricular structure and function in heart failure: VAL-HEFT echocardiographic study. J Am Coll Cardiol 2002;40:970–5.
30. Quinones MA, Greenberg BH, Kopelen HA, et al. Echocardiographic predictors of clinical outcome in patients with left ventricular dysfunction enrolled in the solvd registry and trials: Significance of left ventricular hypertrophy. Studies of left ventricular dysfunction. J Am Coll Cardiol 2000;35:1237–44.
31. Edner M, Bonarjee VV, Nilsen DW, et al. Effect of enalapril initiated early after acute myocardial infarction on heart failure parameters, with reference to clinical class and echocardiographic determinants. Consensus ii multi-echo study group. Clin Cardiol 1996;19:543–8.
32. Randomised, placebo-controlled trial of carvedilol in patients with congestive heart failure due to ischaemic heart disease. Australia/New Zealand Heart Failure Research Collaborative Group. Lancet 1997;349:375–80.
33. Lang RM, Bierig M, Devereux RB, et al. Recommendations for chamber quantification: A report from the American Society of Echocardiography's guidelines and standards committee and the Chamber Quantification Writing Group, developed in conjunction with the European Association of Echocardiography, a branch of the European Society of Cardiology. J Am Soc Echocardiogr 2005;18:1440–63.
34. Gudmundsson P, Rydberg E, Winter R, Willenheimer R. Visually estimated left ventricular ejection fraction by echocardiography is closely correlated with formal quantitative methods. Int J Cardiol 2005;101:209–12.
35. Senior R, Kaul S, Lahiri A. Myocardial viability on echocardiography predicts long-term survival after revascularization in patients with ischemic congestive heart failure. J Am Coll Cardiol 1999;33:1848–54.
36. Allman KC, Shaw LJ, Hachamovitch R, Udelson JE. Myocardial viability testing and impact of revascularization on prognosis in patients with coronary artery disease and left ventricular dysfunction: A meta-analysis. J Am Coll Cardiol 2002;39:1151–8.
37. Afridi I, Grayburn PA, Panza JA, et al. Myocardial viability during dobutamine echocardiography predicts survival in patients with coronary artery disease and severe left ventricular systolic dysfunction. J Am Coll Cardiol 1998;32:921–6.
38. Cwajg JM, Cwajg E, Nagueh SF, et al. End-diastolic wall thickness as a predictor of recovery of function in myocardial hibernation: Relation to rest-redistribution T1-201 tomography and dobutamine stress echocardiography. J Am Coll Cardiol 2000;35:1152–61.
39. Afridi I, Kleiman NS, Raizner AE, Zoghbi WA. Dobutamine echocardiography in myocardial hibernation. Optimal dose and accuracy in predicting recovery of ventricular function after coronary angioplasty. Circulation 1995;91:663–70.
40. Bax JJ, Wijns W, Cornel JH, et al. Accuracy of currently available techniques for prediction of functional recovery after revascularization in patients with left ventricular dysfunction due to chronic coronary artery disease: Comparison of pooled data. J Am Coll Cardiol 1997;30:1451–60.
41. Picano E, Lattanzi F, Orlandini A, et al. Stress echocardiography and the human factor: The importance of being expert. J Am Coll Cardiol 1991;17:666–9.

42. Hoffmann R, Lethen H, Marwick T, et al. Analysis of interinstitutional observer agreement in interpretation of dobutamine stress echocardiograms. J Am Coll Cardiol 1996;27:330–6.
43. Bonow RO, Carabello BA, Chatterjee K, et al. 2008 focused update incorporated into the ACC/AHA 2006 guidelines for the management of patients with valvular heart disease: A report of the American College of Cardiology/American Heart Association Task Force on Practice Guidelines (Writing Committee to Revise the 1998 Guidelines for the Management of Patients with Valvular Heart Disease). Endorsed by the Society of Cardiovascular Anesthesiologists, Society for Cardiovascular Angiography and Interventions, and Society of Thoracic Surgeons. J Am Coll Cardiol 2008;52:e1–142.
44. Baumgartner H, Hung J, Bermejo J, et al. Echocardiographic assessment of valve stenosis: Eae/ase recommendations for clinical practice. J Am Soc Echocardiogr 2009;22:1–23; quiz 101–2.
45. Zoghbi WA, Enriquez-Sarano M, Foster E, et al. Recommendations for evaluation of the severity of native valvular regurgitation with two-dimensional and Doppler echocardiography. J Am Soc Echocardiogr 2003;16:777–802.
46. Lancellotti P, Tribouilloy C, Hagendorff A, et al. European Association of Echocardiography recommendations for the assessment of valvular regurgitation. Part 1: Aortic and pulmonary regurgitation (native valve disease). Eur J Echocardiogr 2010;11:223–44.
47. Lancellotti P, Moura L, Pierard LA, et al. European association of echocardiography recommendations for the assessment of valvular regurgitation. Part 2: Mitral and tricuspid regurgitation (native valve disease). Eur J Echocardiogr 2010;11:307–32.
48. Zamorano JL, Badano LP, Bruce C, et al. EAE/ASE recommendations for the use of echocardiography in new transcatheter interventions for valvular heart disease. J Am Soc Echocardiogr 2011;24:937–65.
49. Reeves ST, Finley AC, Skubas NJ, et al. Basic perioperative transesophageal echocardiography examination: A consensus statement of the American Society of Echocardiography and the Society of Cardiovascular Anesthesiologists. J Am Soc Echocardiogr 2013;26:443–56.
50. Yiu SF, Enriquez-Sarano M, Tribouilloy C, et al. Determinants of the degree of functional mitral regurgitation in patients with systolic left ventricular dysfunction: A quantitative clinical study. Circulation 2000;102:1400–6.
51. Iung B. Management of ischaemic mitral regurgitation. Heart 2003;89:459–64.
52. Pino PG, Galati A, Terranova A. Functional mitral regurgitation in heart failure. J Cardiovasc Med (Hagerstown) 2006;7:514–23.
53. Levine RA, Schwammenthal E. Ischemic mitral regurgitation on the threshold of a solution: From paradoxes to unifying concepts. Circulation 2005;112:745–58.
54. Trichon BH, Felker GM, Shaw LK, et al. Relation of frequency and severity of mitral regurgitation to survival among patients with left ventricular systolic dysfunction and heart failure. Am J Cardiol 2003;91:538–43.
55. Tcheng JE, Jackman JD, Jr., Nelson CL, et al. Outcome of patients sustaining acute ischemic mitral regurgitation during myocardial infarction. Ann Intern Med 1992;117:18–24.
56. Lamas GA, Mitchell GF, Flaker GC, et al. Clinical significance of mitral regurgitation after acute myocardial infarction. Survival and ventricular enlargement investigators. Circulation 1997;96:827–33.
57. Borger MA, Alam A, Murphy PM, et al. Chronic ischemic mitral regurgitation: Repair, replace or rethink? Ann Thorac Surg 2006;81:1153–61.
58. Aklog L, Filsoufi F, Flores KQ, et al. Does coronary artery bypass grafting alone correct moderate ischemic mitral regurgitation? Circulation 2001;104:I68–75.
59. Rogers JH, Franzen O. Percutaneous edge-to-edge mitraclip therapy in the management of mitral regurgitation. Eur Heart J 2011;32:2350–7.
60. Gummert JF, Rahmel A, Bucerius J, et al. Mitral valve repair in patients with end stage cardiomyopathy: Who benefits? Eur J Cardiothorac Surg 2003;23:1017–22; discussion 1022.
61. Grigioni F, Enriquez-Sarano M, Zehr KJ, et al. Ischemic mitral regurgitation: Long-term outcome and prognostic implications with quantitative Doppler assessment. Circulation 2001;103:1759–64.
62. Calafiore AM, Gallina S, Di Mauro M, et al. Mitral valve procedure in dilated cardiomyopathy: Repair or replacement? Ann Thorac Surg 2001;71:1146–52; discussion 1152–3.
63. Kongsaerepong V, Shiota M, Gillinov AM, et al. Echocardiographic predictors of successful versus unsuccessful mitral valve repair in ischemic mitral regurgitation. Am J Cardiol 2006;98:504–8.
64. Lancellotti P, Gerard PL, Pierard LA. Long-term outcome of patients with heart failure and dynamic functional mitral regurgitation. Eur Heart J 2005;26:1528–32.
65. Shamim W, Francis DP, Yousufuddin M, et al. Intraventricular conduction delay: A prognostic marker in chronic heart failure. Int J Cardiol 1999;70:171–8.
66. Xiao HB, Brecker SJ, Gibson DG. Effects of abnormal activation on the time course of the left ventricular pressure pulse in dilated cardiomyopathy. Br Heart J 1992;68:403–7.
67. Xiao HB, Roy C, Fujimoto S, Gibson DG. Natural history of abnormal conduction and its relation to prognosis in patients with dilated cardiomyopathy. Int J Cardiol 1996;53:163–70.
68. Littmann L, Symanski JD. Hemodynamic implications of left bundle branch block. J Electrocardiol 2000;33(Suppl):115–21.
69. Aaronson KD, Schwartz JS, Chen TM, et al. Development and prospective validation of a clinical index to predict survival in ambulatory patients referred for cardiac transplant evaluation. Circulation 1997;95:2660–7.
70. Cleland JG, Daubert JC, Erdmann E, et al. The effect of cardiac resynchronization on morbidity and mortality in heart failure. N Engl J Med 2005;352:1539–49.
71. Bristow MR, Saxon LA, Boehmer J, et al. Cardiac-resynchronization therapy with or without an implantable defibrillator in advanced chronic heart failure. N Engl J Med 2004;350:2140–50.
72. Abraham WT, Fisher WG, Smith AL, et al. Cardiac resynchronization in chronic heart failure. N Engl J Med 2002;346:1845–53.
73. Hunt SA, Abraham WT, Chin MH, et al. 2009 focused update incorporated into the ACC/AHA 2005 guidelines for the diagnosis and management of heart failure in adults: a report of the American College Of Cardiology Foundation/American Heart Association Task Force on Practice Guidelines developed in collaboration with the International Society for Heart and Lung Transplantation. J Am Coll Cardiol 2009;53:e1–90.
74. Leclercq C, Faris O, Tunin R, et al. Systolic improvement and mechanical resynchronization does not require electrical synchrony in the dilated failing heart with left bundle-branch block. Circulation 2002;106:1760–3.
75. Ghio S, Constantin C, Klersy C, et al. Interventricular and intraventricular dyssynchrony are common in heart failure patients, regardless of qrs duration. Eur Heart J 2004;25:571–8.
76. Yu CM, Lin H, Zhang Q, Sanderson JE. High prevalence of left ventricular systolic and diastolic asynchrony in patients with congestive heart failure and normal qrs duration. Heart 2003;89:54–60.
77. Gorcsan J, 3rd, Abraham T, Agler DA, et al. Echocardiography for cardiac resynchronization therapy: Recommendations for performance and reporting—a report from the American Society Of Echocardiography Dyssynchrony Writing Group endorsed by the Heart Rhythm Society. J Am Soc Echocardiogr 2008;21:191–213.
78. Pitzalis MV, Iacoviello M, Romito R, et al. Ventricular asynchrony predicts a better outcome in patients with chronic heart failure receiving cardiac resynchronization therapy. J Am Coll Cardiol 2005;45:65–9.
79. Pitzalis MV, Iacoviello M, Romito R, et al. Cardiac resynchronization therapy tailored by echocardiographic evaluation of ventricular asynchrony. J Am Coll Cardiol 2002;40:1615–22.
80. Bax JJ, Marwick TH, Molhoek SG, et al. Left ventricular dyssynchrony predicts benefit of cardiac resynchronization therapy in patients with end-stage heart failure before pacemaker implantation. Am J Cardiol 2003;92:1238–40.

81. Bax JJ, Bleeker GB, Marwick TH, et al. Left ventricular dyssynchrony predicts response and prognosis after cardiac resynchronization therapy. J Am Coll Cardiol 2004;44:1834–40.
82. Gorcsan J, Kanzaki H, Bazaz R, et al. Usefulness of echocardiographic tissue synchronization imaging to predict acute response to cardiac resynchronization therapy. Am J Cardiol 2004;93:1178–81.
83. Notabartolo D, Merlino JD, Smith AL, et al. Usefulness of the peak velocity difference by tissue Doppler imaging technique as an effective predictor of response to cardiac resynchronization therapy. Am J Cardiol 2004;94:817–20.
84. Yu C-M, Fung JW-H, Zhang Q, et al. Tissue Doppler imaging is superior to strain rate imaging and postsystolic shortening on the prediction of reverse remodeling in both ischemic and nonischemic heart failure after cardiac resynchronization therapy. Circulation 2004;110:66–73.
85. Yu C-M, Fung W-H, Lin H, et al. Predictors of left ventricular reverse remodeling after cardiac resynchronization therapy for heart failure secondary to idiopathic dilated or ischemic cardiomyopathy. Am J Cardiol 2003;91:684–8.
86. Vieira MLC, Cury AF, Naccarato G, et al. Analysis of left ventricular regional dyssynchrony: Comparison between real time 3d echocardiography and tissue Doppler imaging. Echocardiography 2009;26:675–83.
87. Takeuchi M, Jacobs A, Sugeng L, et al. Assessment of left ventricular dyssynchrony with real-time 3-dimensional echocardiography: Comparison with Doppler tissue imaging. J Am Soc Echocardiogr 2007;20:1321–9.
88. Chung ES, Leon AR, Tavazzi L, et al. Results of the Predictors of Response to CRT (PROSPECT) trial. Circulation 2008;117:2608–16.
89. Bax JJ, Gorcsan J, 3rd. Echocardiography and noninvasive imaging in cardiac resynchronization therapy: Results of the PROSPECT (Predictors Of Response To Cardiac Resynchronization Therapy) study in perspective. J Am Coll Cardiol 2009;53:1933–43.
90. Suffoletto MS, Dohi K, Cannesson M, et al. Novel speckle-tracking radial strain from routine black-and-white echocardiographic images to quantify dyssynchrony and predict response to cardiac resynchronization therapy. Circulation 2006;113:960–8.
91. Tanaka H, Nesser HJ, Buck T, et al. Dyssynchrony by speckle-tracking echocardiography and response to cardiac resynchronization therapy: Results of the Speckle Tracking and Resynchronization (STAR) study. Eur Heart J 2010;31:1690–700.
92. Delgado V, van Bommel RJ, Bertini M, et al. Relative merits of left ventricular dyssynchrony, left ventricular lead position, and myocardial scar to predict long-term survival of ischemic heart failure patients undergoing cardiac resynchronization therapy. Circulation 2011;123:70–8.
93. Gorcsan J, 3rd. Finding pieces of the puzzle of nonresponse to cardiac resynchronization therapy. Circulation 2011;123:10–12.
94. Khan FZ, Virdee MS, Palmer CR, et al. Targeted left ventricular lead placement to guide cardiac resynchronization therapy: The target study: A randomized, controlled trial. J Am Coll Cardiol 2012;59:1509–18.
95. Stanton T, Hawkins NM, Hogg KJ, et al. How should we optimize cardiac resynchronization therapy? Eur Heart J 2008;29:2458–72.
96. Oz MC, Rose EA, Levin HR. Selection criteria for placement of left ventricular assist devices. Am Heart J 1995;129:173–7.
97. Rao V, Slater JP, Edwards NM, et al. Surgical management of valvular disease in patients requiring left ventricular assist device support. Ann Thorac Surg 2001;71:1448–53.
98. Shapiro GC, Leibowitz DW, Oz MC, et al. Diagnosis of patent foramen ovale with transesophageal echocardiography in a patient supported with a left ventricular assist device. J Heart Lung Transplant 1995;14:594–7.
99. Potapov EV, Stepanenko A, Dandel M, et al. Tricuspid incompetence and geometry of the right ventricle as predictors of right ventricular function after implantation of a left ventricular assist device. J Heart Lung Transplant 2008;27:1275–81.
100. Dang NC, Topkara VK, Mercando M, et al. Right heart failure after left ventricular assist device implantation in patients with chronic congestive heart failure. J Heart Lung Transplant 2006;25:1–6.
101. Nakatani S, Thomas JD, Savage RM, et al. Prediction of right ventricular dysfunction after left ventricular assist device implantation. Circulation 1996;94:216–21.
102. Grant AD, Smedira NG, Starling RC, Marwick TH. Independent and incremental role of quantitative right ventricular evaluation for the prediction of right ventricular failure after left ventricular assist device implantation. J Am Coll Cardiol 2012;60:521–8.
103. Fitzpatrick JR, Frederick JR, Hiesinger W, et al. Early planned institution of biventricular mechanical circulatory support results in improved outcomes compared with delayed conversion of a left ventricular assist device to a biventricular assist device. J Thorac Cardiovasc Surg 2009;137:971–7.
104. Ammar KA, Umland MM, Kramer C, et al. The ABCs of left ventricular assist device echocardiography: A systematic approach. Eur Heart J Cardiovasc Imaging 2012;13:885–99.
105. McCarthy PM, Nakatani S, Vargo R, et al. Structural and left ventricular histologic changes after implantable lvad insertion. Ann Thorac Surg 1995;59:609–13.
106. Xydas S, Rosen RS, Ng C, et al. Mechanical unloading leads to echocardiographic, electrocardiographic, neurohormonal, and histologic recovery. J Heart Lung Transplant 2006;25:7–15.
107. Levin HR, Oz MC, Chen JM, et al. Reversal of chronic ventricular dilation in patients with end-stage cardiomyopathy by prolonged mechanical unloading. Circulation 1995;91:2717–20.
108. Timek TA, Lai DT, Tibayan F, et al. Annular versus subvalvular approaches to acute ischemic mitral regurgitation. Circulation 2002;106:I27–I32.
109. Lam KM-T, Ennis S, O'Driscoll G, et al. Observations from non-invasive measures of right heart hemodynamics in left ventricular assist device patients. J Am Soc Echocardiogr 2009;22:1055–62.
110. Frogel J, Vodur S, Horak J. Transesophageal echocardiography diagnosis of extracardiac left ventricular assist device inflow cannula obstruction in a patient with Thoratec intracorporeal ventricular assist device biventricular support. J Am Soc Echocardiogr 2008;21:5–6.
111. Geyer H, Caracciolo G, Abe H, et al. Assessment of myocardial mechanics using speckle tracking echocardiography: Fundamentals and clinical applications. J Am Soc Echocardiogr 2010;23:351–69.
112. Feigenbaum H, Mastouri R, Sawada S. A practical approach to using strain echocardiography to evaluate the left ventricle. Circ J 2012;76:1550–5.
113. Mor-Avi V, Lang RM, Badano LP, et al. Current and evolving echocardiographic techniques for the quantitative evaluation of cardiac mechanics: ASE/EAE consensus statement on methodology and indications endorsed by the Japanese Society of Echocardiography. J Am Soc Echocardiogr 2011;24:277–313.
114. Bansal M, Kasliwal RR. How do I do it? Speckle-tracking echocardiography. Indian Heart J 2013;65:117–23.
115. Bansal M, Sengupta PP. Longitudinal and circumferential strain in patients with regional LV dysfunction. Curr Cardiol Rep 2013;15:339.
116. Brown J, Jenkins C, Marwick TH. Use of myocardial strain to assess global left ventricular function: A comparison with cardiac magnetic resonance and 3-dimensional echocardiography. Am Heart J 2009;157:102 e101–5.
117. Mistry N, Beitnes JO, Halvorsen S, et al. Assessment of left ventricular function in st-elevation myocardial infarction by global longitudinal strain: A comparison with ejection fraction, infarct size, and wall motion score index measured by non-invasive imaging modalities. Eur J Echocardiogr 2011;12:678–83.
118. Ingul CB, Stoylen A, Slordahl SA, et al. Automated analysis of myocardial deformation at dobutamine stress echocardiography: An angiographic validation. J Am Coll Cardiol 2007;49:1651–9.
119. Stanton T, Leano R, Marwick TH. Prediction of all-cause mortality from global longitudinal speckle strain: Comparison with

ejection fraction and wall motion scoring. Circ Cardiovasc Imaging 2009;2:356–64.
120. Bansal M, Chan J, Leano R, et al. Effects of perhexiline on myocardial deformation in patients with ischaemic left ventricular dysfunction. Int J Cardiol 2010;139:107–12.
121. Chan J, Hanekom L, Wong C, et al. Differentiation of subendocardial and transmural infarction using two-dimensional strain rate imaging to assess short-axis and long-axis myocardial function. J Am Coll Cardiol 2006;48:2026–33.
122. Kansal MM, Panse PM, Abe H, et al. Relationship of contrast-enhanced magnetic resonance imaging-derived intramural scar distribution and speckle tracking echocardiography-derived left ventricular two-dimensional strains. Eur Heart J Cardiovasc Imaging 2012;13:152–8.
123. Mollema SA, Delgado V, Bertini M, et al. Viability assessment with global left ventricular longitudinal strain predicts recovery of left ventricular function after acute myocardial infarction. Circ Cardiovasc Imaging 2010;3:15–23.
124. Antoni ML, Mollema SA, Atary JZ, et al. Time course of global left ventricular strain after acute myocardial infarction. Eur Heart J 2010;31:2006–13.
125. D'Andrea A, Cocchia R, Caso P, et al. Global longitudinal speckle-tracking strain is predictive of left ventricular remodeling after coronary angioplasty in patients with recent non-st elevation myocardial infarction. Int J Cardiol 2011;153:185–91.
126. Bochenek T, Wita K, Tabor Z, et al. Value of speckle-tracking echocardiography for prediction of left ventricular remodeling in patients with ST-elevation myocardial infarction treated by primary percutaneous intervention. J Am Soc Echocardiogr 2011;24:1342–8.
127. Zaliaduonyte-Peksiene D, Vaskelyte JJ, Mizariene V, et al. Does longitudinal strain predict left ventricular remodeling after myocardial infarction? Echocardiography 2012;29:419–27.
128. Hanekom L, Jenkins C, Jeffries L, et al. Incremental value of strain rate analysis as an adjunct to wall-motion scoring for assessment of myocardial viability by dobutamine echocardiography: A follow-up study after revascularization. Circulation 2005;112:3892–900.
129. Bansal M, Jeffriess L, Leano R, Mundy J, Marwick TH. Assessment of myocardial viability at dobutamine echocardiography by deformation analysis using tissue velocity and speckle-tracking. JACC Cardiovasc Imaging 2010;3:121–31.
130. Cho GY, Marwick TH, Kim HS, et al. Global 2-dimensional strain as a new prognosticator in patients with heart failure. J Am Coll Cardiol 2009;54:618–24.
131. Bertini M, Ng AC, Antoni ML, et al. Global longitudinal strain predicts long-term survival in patients with chronic ischemic cardiomyopathy. Circ Cardiovasc Imaging 2012;5:383–91.
132. Jasaityte R, Dandel M, Lehmkuhl H, Hetzer R. Prediction of short-term outcomes in patients with idiopathic dilated cardiomyopathy referred for transplantation using standard echocardiography and strain imaging. Transplant Proc 2009;41:277–80.
133. Bertini M, Ng AC, Borleffs CJ, et al. Longitudinal mechanics of the periinfarct zone and ventricular tachycardia inducibility in patients with chronic ischemic cardiomyopathy. Am Heart J 2010;160:729–36.
134. Haugaa KH, Smedsrud MK, Steen T, et al. Mechanical dispersion assessed by myocardial strain in patients after myocardial infarction for risk prediction of ventricular arrhythmia. JACC Cardiovasc Imaging 2010;3:247–56.
135. Haugaa KH, Goebel B, Dahlslett T, et al. Risk assessment of ventricular arrhythmias in patients with nonischemic dilated cardiomyopathy by strain echocardiography. J Am Soc Echocardiogr 2012;25:667–73.
136. Mor-Avi V, Lang RM, Badano LP, et al. Current and evolving echocardiographic techniques for the quantitative evaluation of cardiac mechanics: ASE/EAE consensus statement on methodology and indications endorsed by the Japanese Society of Echocardiography. Eur J Echocardiogr 2011;12:167–205.
137. Jacobs LD, Salgo IS, Goonewardena S, et al. Rapid online quantification of left ventricular volume from real-time three-dimensional echocardiographic data. Eur Heart J 2006;27:460–8.
138. Caiani EG, Corsi C, Sugeng L, et al. Improved quantification of left ventricular mass based on endocardial and epicardial surface detection with real time three dimensional echocardiography. Heart 2006;92:213–19.
139. Sapin PM, Schroeder KD, Smith MD, et al. Three-dimensional echocardiographic measurement of left ventricular volume in vitro: Comparison with two-dimensional echocardiography and cineventriculography. J Am Coll Cardiol 1993;22:1530–7.
140. van der Zwaan HB, Geleijnse ML, McGhie JS, et al. Right ventricular quantification in clinical practice: Two-dimensional vs. Three-dimensional echocardiography compared with cardiac magnetic resonance imaging. Eur J Echocardiogr 2011;12:656–64.
141. Burgess MI, Jenkins C, Chan J, Marwick TH. Measurement of left ventricular dyssynchrony in patients with ischaemic cardiomyopathy: A comparison of real-time three-dimensional and tissue Doppler echocardiography. Heart 2007;93:1191–6.
142. Kleijn SA, van Dijk J, de Cock CC, et al. Assessment of intraventricular mechanical dyssynchrony and prediction of response to cardiac resynchronization therapy: Comparison between tissue Doppler imaging and real-time three-dimensional echocardiography. J Am Soc Echocardiogr 2009;22:1047–54.
143. Deplagne A, Lafitte S, Reuter S, et al. Absence of additional improvement in outcome of patients receiving cardiac resynchronization therapy paced at the most delayed left ventricular region. Arch Cardiovasc Dis 2009;102:641–9.
144. Saito K, Okura H, Watanabe N, et al. Comprehensive evaluation of left ventricular strain using speckle tracking echocardiography in normal adults: Comparison of three-dimensional and two-dimensional approaches. J Am Soc Echocardiogr 2009;22:1025–30.
145. Maffessanti F, Nesser HJ, Weinert L, et al. Quantitative evaluation of regional left ventricular function using three-dimensional speckle tracking echocardiography in patients with and without heart disease. Am J Cardiol 2009;104:1755–62.
146. Yodwut C, Weinert L, Klas B, et al. Effects of frame rate on three-dimensional speckle-tracking-based measurements of myocardial deformation. J Am Soc Echocardiogr 2012;25:978–85.
147. Sengupta PP, Pedrizzetti G, Kilner PJ, et al. Emerging trends in cv flow visualization. JACC Cardiovasc Imaging 2012;5:305–16.
148. Bolger AF, Heiberg E, Karlsson M, et al. Transit of blood flow through the human left ventricle mapped by cardiovascular magnetic resonance. J Cardiovasc Magn Reson 2007;9:741–7.
149. Pedrizzetti G, Domenichini F, Tonti G. On the left ventricular vortex reversal after mitral valve replacement. Ann Biomed Eng 2010;38:769–73.
150. Dyverfeldt P, Kvitting JP, Carlhall CJ, et al. Hemodynamic aspects of mitral regurgitation assessed by generalized phase-contrast mri. J Magn Reson Imaging 2011;33:582–8.
151. Lefebvre XP, Yoganathan AP, Levine RA. Insights from in-vitro flow visualization into the mechanism of systolic anterior motion of the mitral valve in hypertrophic cardiomyopathy under steady flow conditions. J Biomech Eng 1992;114:406–13.
152. Carlhall CJ, Bolger A. Passing strange: Flow in the failing ventricle. Circ Heart Fail 2010;3:326–31.
153. Markl M, Geiger J, Kilner PJ, et al. Time-resolved three-dimensional magnetic resonance velocity mapping of cardiovascular flow paths in volunteers and patients with Fontan circulation. Eur J Cardiothorac Surg 2011;39:206–12.
154. Fyrenius A, Wigstrom L, Ebbers T, et al. Three dimensional flow in the human left atrium. Heart 2001;86:448–55.
155. Hope MD, Meadows AK, Hope TA, et al. Clinical evaluation of aortic coarctation with 4D flow MR imaging. J Magn Reson Imaging 2010;31:711–18.
156. Markl M, Kilner PJ, Ebbers T. Comprehensive 4D velocity mapping of the heart and great vessels by cardiovascular magnetic resonance. J Cardiovasc Magn Reson 2011;13:7.

157. Lanzer P, Botvinick EH, Schiller NB, et al. Cardiac imaging using gated magnetic resonance. Radiology 1984;150:121–7.
158. Karamitsos TD, Hudsmith LE, Selvanayagam JB, et al. Operator induced variability in left ventricular measurements with cardiovascular magnetic resonance is improved after training. J Cardiovasc Magn Reson 2007;9:777–83.
159. Mandapaka S, Hundley WG. Dobutamine cardiovascular magnetic resonance: A review. J Magn Reson Imaging 2006;24:499–512.
160. Anderson JL, Horne BD, Pennell DJ. Atrial dimensions in health and left ventricular disease using cardiovascular magnetic resonance. J Cardiovasc Magn Reson 2005;7:671–5.
161. Reichek N. MRI myocardial tagging. J Magn Reson Imaging 1999;10:609–16.
162. Petersen SE, Jung BA, Wiesmann F, et al. Myocardial tissue phase mapping with cine phase-contrast mr imaging: Regional wall motion analysis in healthy volunteers. Radiology 2006;238:816–26.
163. Gerber BL, Raman SV, Nayak K, et al. Myocardial first-pass perfusion cardiovascular magnetic resonance: History, theory, and current state of the art. J Cardiovasc Magn Reson 2008;10:18.
164. Wagner A, Mahrholdt H, Holly TA, et al. Contrast-enhanced mri and routine single photon emission computed tomography (SPECT) perfusion imaging for detection of subendocardial myocardial infarcts: An imaging study. Lancet 2003;361:374–9.
165. Kwong RY, Sattar H, Wu H, et al. Incidence and prognostic implication of unrecognized myocardial scar characterized by cardiac magnetic resonance in diabetic patients without clinical evidence of myocardial infarction. Circulation 2008;118:1011–20.
166. Kwong RY, Chan AK, Brown KA, et al. Impact of unrecognized myocardial scar detected by cardiac magnetic resonance imaging on event-free survival in patients presenting with signs or symptoms of coronary artery disease. Circulation 2006;113:2733–43.
167. Abdel-Aty H, Cocker M, Meek C, et al. Edema as a very early marker for acute myocardial ischemia: A cardiovascular magnetic resonance study. J Am Coll Cardiol 2009;53:1194–201.
168. Aletras AH, Tilak GS, Natanzon A, et al. Retrospective determination of the area at risk for reperfused acute myocardial infarction with T2-weighted cardiac magnetic resonance imaging: Histopathological and displacement encoding with stimulated echoes (dense) functional validations. Circulation 2006;113:1865–70.
169. Selvanayagam JB, Kardos A, Francis JM, et al. Value of delayed-enhancement cardiovascular magnetic resonance imaging in predicting myocardial viability after surgical revascularization. Circulation 2004;110:1535–41.
170. Kim RJ, Wu E, Rafael A, Chen EL, et al. The use of contrast-enhanced magnetic resonance imaging to identify reversible myocardial dysfunction. N Engl J Med 2000;343:1445–53.
171. Kirschbaum SW, Rossi A, van Domburg RT, et al. Contractile reserve in segments with nontransmural infarction in chronic dysfunctional myocardium using low-dose dobutamine cmr. JACC Cardiovasc Imaging 2010;3:614–22.
172. Wellnhofer E, Olariu A, Klein C, et al. Magnetic resonance low-dose dobutamine test is superior to scar quantification for the prediction of functional recovery. Circulation 2004;109:2172–4.
173. Pegg TJ, Selvanayagam JB, Jennifer J, et al. Prediction of global left ventricular functional recovery in patients with heart failure undergoing surgical revascularisation, based on late gadolinium enhancement cardiovascular magnetic resonance. J Cardiovasc Magn Reson 2010;12:56.
174. Kwon DH, Halley CM, Carrigan TP, et al. Extent of left ventricular scar predicts outcomes in ischemic cardiomyopathy patients with significantly reduced systolic function: A delayed hyperenhancement cardiac magnetic resonance study. JACC Cardiovasc Imaging 2009;2:34–44.
175. Delfino JG, Fornwalt BK, Oshinski JN, Lerakis S. Role of MRI in patient selection for CRT. Echocardiography 2008;25:1176–85.
176. Westenberg JJM, Lamb HJ, van der Geest RJ, et al. Assessment of left ventricular dyssynchrony in patients with conduction delay and idiopathic dilated cardiomyopathy: Head-to-head comparison between tissue Doppler imaging and velocity-encoded magnetic resonance imaging. J Am Coll Cardiol 2006;47:2042–8.
177. Budge LP, Helms AS, Salerno M, et al. MR cine dense dyssynchrony parameters for the evaluation of heart failure: Comparison with myocardial tissue tagging. JACC Cardiovasc Imaging 2012;5:789–97.
178. White JA, Yee R, Yuan X, et al. Delayed enhancement magnetic resonance imaging predicts response to cardiac resynchronization therapy in patients with intraventricular dyssynchrony. J Am Coll Cardiol 2006;48:1953–60.
179. Ypenburg C, Roes SD, Bleeker GB, et al. Effect of total scar burden on contrast-enhanced magnetic resonance imaging on response to cardiac resynchronization therapy. Am J Cardiol 2007;99:657–60.
180. Bleeker GB, Kaandorp TAM, Lamb HJ, et al. Effect of posterolateral scar tissue on clinical and echocardiographic improvement after cardiac resynchronization therapy. Circulation 2006;113:969–76.
181. Chalil S, Stegemann B, Muhyaldeen SA, et al. Effect of posterolateral left ventricular scar on mortality and morbidity following cardiac resynchronization therapy. Pacing Clin Electrophysiol 2007;30:1201–9.
182. Casolo G, Minneci S, Manta R, et al. Identification of the ischemic etiology of heart failure by cardiovascular magnetic resonance imaging: Diagnostic accuracy of late gadolinium enhancement. Am Heart J 2006;151:101–8.
183. McCrohon JA, Moon JCC, Prasad SK, et al. Differentiation of heart failure related to dilated cardiomyopathy and coronary artery disease using gadolinium-enhanced cardiovascular magnetic resonance. Circulation 2003;108:54–9.
184. Kotani J-I, Mintz GS, Castagna MT, et al. Intravascular ultrasound analysis of infarct-related and non-infarct-related arteries in patients who presented with an acute myocardial infarction. Circulation 2003;107:2889–93.
185. Felker GM, Thompson RE, Hare JM, et al. Underlying causes and long-term survival in patients with initially unexplained cardiomyopathy. N Engl J Med 2000;342:1077–84.
186. Bohl S, Schulz-Menger J. Cardiovascular magnetic resonance imaging of non-ischaemic heart disease: Established and emerging applications. Heart Lung Circ 2010;19:117–32.
187. Iles L, Pfluger H, Phrommintikul A, et al. Evaluation of diffuse myocardial fibrosis in heart failure with cardiac magnetic resonance contrast-enhanced t1 mapping. J Am Coll Cardiol 2008;52:1574–80.
188. Assomull RG, Prasad SK, Lyne J, et al. Cardiovascular magnetic resonance, fibrosis, and prognosis in dilated cardiomyopathy. J Am Coll Cardiol 2006;48:1977–85.
189. Nazarian S, Bluemke DA, Lardo AC, et al. Magnetic resonance assessment of the substrate for inducible ventricular tachycardia in nonischemic cardiomyopathy. Circulation 2005;112:2821–5.
190. Gersh BJ, Maron BJ, Bonow RO, et al. 2011 ACCF/AHA guideline for the diagnosis and treatment of hypertrophic cardiomyopathy: A report of the American College of Cardiology Foundation/American Heart Association Task Force on Practice Guidelines. Circulation 2011;124:e783–831.
191. Rickers C, Wilke NM, Jerosch-Herold M, et al. Utility of cardiac magnetic resonance imaging in the diagnosis of hypertrophic cardiomyopathy. Circulation 2005;112:855–61.
192. Olivotto I, Maron MS, Autore C, et al. Assessment and significance of left ventricular mass by cardiovascular magnetic resonance in hypertrophic cardiomyopathy. J Am Coll Cardiol 2008;52:559–66.
193. Harrigan CJ, Appelbaum E, Maron BJ, et al. Significance of papillary muscle abnormalities identified by cardiovascular magnetic resonance in hypertrophic cardiomyopathy. Am J Cardiol 2008;101:668–73.
194. Kwon DH, Setser RM, Thamilarasan M, et al. Abnormal papillary muscle morphology is independently associated with increased left ventricular outflow tract obstruction in hypertrophic cardiomyopathy. Heart 2008;94:1295–301.
195. Austin BA, Kwon DH, Smedira NG, et al. Abnormally thickened papillary muscle resulting in dynamic left ventricular outflow tract

obstruction: An unusual presentation of hypertrophic cardiomyopathy. J Am Soc Echocardiogr 2009;22:105 e105–6.
196. Choudhury L, Mahrholdt H, Wagner A, et al. Myocardial scarring in asymptomatic or mildly symptomatic patients with hypertrophic cardiomyopathy. J Am Coll Cardiol 2002;40:2156–64.
197. Maron MS, Appelbaum E, Harrigan CJ, et al. Clinical profile and significance of delayed enhancement in hypertrophic cardiomyopathy. Circ Heart Fail 2008;1:184–91.
198. Rubinshtein R, Glockner JF, Ommen SR, et al. Characteristics and clinical significance of late gadolinium enhancement by contrast-enhanced magnetic resonance imaging in patients with hypertrophic cardiomyopathy. Circ Heart Fail 2010;3:51–8.
199. Adabag AS, Maron BJ, Appelbaum E, et al. Occurrence and frequency of arrhythmias in hypertrophic cardiomyopathy in relation to delayed enhancement on cardiovascular magnetic resonance. J Am Coll Cardiol 2008;51:1369–74.
200. Bruder O, Wagner A, Jensen CJ, et al. Myocardial scar visualized by cardiovascular magnetic resonance imaging predicts major adverse events in patients with hypertrophic cardiomyopathy. J Am Coll Cardiol 2010;56:875–87.
201. O'Hanlon R, Grasso A, Roughton M, et al. Prognostic significance of myocardial fibrosis in hypertrophic cardiomyopathy. J Am Coll Cardiol 2010;56:867–74.
202. Perugini E, Rapezzi C, Piva T, et al. Non-invasive evaluation of the myocardial substrate of cardiac amyloidosis by gadolinium cardiac magnetic resonance. Heart 2006;92:343–9.
203. Maceira AM, Joshi J, Prasad SK, et al. Cardiovascular magnetic resonance in cardiac amyloidosis. Circulation 2005;111:186–93.
204. Modell B, Khan M, Darlison M, et al. Improved survival of thalassaemia major in the uk and relation to t2* cardiovascular magnetic resonance. J Cardiovasc Magn Reson 2008;10:42.
205. Anderson LJ, Wonke B, Prescott E, et al. Comparison of effects of oral deferiprone and subcutaneous desferrioxamine on myocardial iron concentrations and ventricular function in beta-thalassaemia. Lancet 2002;360:516–20.
206. Anderson LJ, Westwood MA, Holden S, et al. Myocardial iron clearance during reversal of siderotic cardiomyopathy with intravenous desferrioxamine: A prospective study using T2* cardiovascular magnetic resonance. Br J Haematol 2004;127:348–55.
207. Moon JC, Sachdev B, Elkington AG, et al. Gadolinium enhanced cardiovascular magnetic resonance in anderson-fabry disease. Evidence for a disease specific abnormality of the myocardial interstitium. Eur Heart J 2003;24:2151–5.
208. Rudolph A, Abdel-Aty H, Bohl S, et al. Noninvasive detection of fibrosis applying contrast-enhanced cardiac magnetic resonance in different forms of left ventricular hypertrophy relation to remodeling. J Am Coll Cardiol 2009;53:284–91.
209. Bohl S, Wassmuth R, Abdel-Aty H, et al. Delayed enhancement cardiac magnetic resonance imaging reveals typical patterns of myocardial injury in patients with various forms of non-ischemic heart disease. Int J Cardiovasc Imaging 2008;24:597–607.
210. Imbriaco M, Spinelli L, Cuocolo A, et al. Mri characterization of myocardial tissue in patients with fabry's disease. AJR Am J Roentgenol 2007;188:850–3.
211. Mahrholdt H, Wagner A, Deluigi CC, et al. Presentation, patterns of myocardial damage, and clinical course of viral myocarditis. Circulation 2006;114:1581–90.
212. Laissy J-P, Hyafil F, Feldman LJ, et al. Differentiating acute myocardial infarction from myocarditis: Diagnostic value of early- and delayed-perfusion cardiac mr imaging. Radiology 2005;237:75–82.
213. Abdel-Aty H, Boye P, Zagrosek A, et al. Diagnostic performance of cardiovascular magnetic resonance in patients with suspected acute myocarditis: Comparison of different approaches. J Am Coll Cardiol 2005;45:1815–22.
214. Ingkanisorn WP, Paterson DI, Calvo KR, et al. Cardiac magnetic resonance appearance of myocarditis caused by high dose il-2: Similarities to community-acquired myocarditis. J Cardiovasc Magn Reson 2006;8:353–60.
215. Rieker O, Mohrs O, Oberholzer K, et al. [Cardiac MRI in suspected myocarditis]. Rofo 2002;174:1530–6.
216. Gutberlet M, Spors B, Thoma T, et al. Suspected chronic myocarditis at cardiac MR: Diagnostic accuracy and association with immunohistologically detected inflammation and viral persistence. Radiology 2008;246:401–9.
217. Yilmaz A, Mahrholdt H, Athanasiadis A, et al. Coronary vasospasm as the underlying cause for chest pain in patients with pvb19 myocarditis. Heart 2008;94:1456–63.
218. Yelgec NS, Dymarkowski S, Ganame J, Bogaert J. Value of mri in patients with a clinical suspicion of acute myocarditis. Eur Radiol 2007;17:2211–17.
219. Schulz-Menger J, Wassmuth R, Abdel-Aty H, et al. Patterns of myocardial inflammation and scarring in sarcoidosis as assessed by cardiovascular magnetic resonance. Heart 2006;92:399–400.
220. De Cobelli F, Pieroni M, Esposito A, et al. Delayed gadolinium-enhanced cardiac magnetic resonance in patients with chronic myocarditis presenting with heart failure or recurrent arrhythmias. J Am Coll Cardiol 2006;47:1649–54.
221. Vignaux O, Dhote R, Duboc D, et al. Clinical significance of myocardial magnetic resonance abnormalities in patients with sarcoidosis: A 1-year follow-up study. Chest 2002;122:1895–901.
222. Patel MR, Cawley PJ, Heitner JF, et al. Detection of myocardial damage in patients with sarcoidosis. Circulation 2009;120:1969–77.
223. Roberts WC, McAllister HA, Jr., Ferrans VJ. Sarcoidosis of the heart. A clinicopathologic study of 35 necropsy patients (group 1) and review of 78 previously described necropsy patients (group 11). Am J Med 1977;63:86–108.
224. Hendel RC, Berman DS, Di Carli MF, Heidenreich PA, Henkin RE, Pellikka PA, et al. ACCF/ASNC/ACR/AHA/ASE/SCCT/SCMR/SNM 2009 appropriate use criteria for cardiac radionuclide imaging: A report of the American College of Cardiology Foundation Appropriate Use Criteria Task Force, the American Society of Nuclear Cardiology, the American College of Radiology, the American Heart Association, the American Society of Echocardiography, the Society of Cardiovascular Computed Tomography, the Society for Cardiovascular Magnetic Resonance, and the Society of Nuclear Medicine. J Am Coll Cardiol 2009;53:2201–29.
225. Neglia D, Michelassi C, Trivieri MG, et al. Prognostic role of myocardial blood flow impairment in idiopathic left ventricular dysfunction. Circulation 2002;105:186–93.
226. Cecchi F, Olivotto I, Gistri R, et al. Coronary microvascular dysfunction and prognosis in hypertrophic cardiomyopathy. N Engl J Med 2003;349:1027–35.
227. Schneider CA, Voth E, Gawlich S, et al. Significance of rest technetium-99 m sestamibi imaging for the prediction of improvement of left ventricular dysfunction after q wave myocardial infarction: Importance of infarct location adjusted thresholds. J Am Coll Cardiol 1998;32:648–54.
228. Schinkel AFL, Poldermans D, Elhendy A, Bax JJ. Assessment of myocardial viability in patients with heart failure. J Nucl Med 2007;48:1135–46.
229. Inaba Y, Chen JA, Bergmann SR. Quantity of viable myocardium required to improve survival with revascularization in patients with ischemic cardiomyopathy: A meta-analysis. J Nucl Cardiol 2010;17:646–54.
230. Rizzello V, Poldermans D, Biagini E, et al. Prognosis of patients with ischaemic cardiomyopathy after coronary revascularisation: Relation to viability and improvement in left ventricular ejection fraction. Heart 2009;95:1273–7.
231. Mielniczuk LM, Beanlands RS. Does imaging-guided selection of patients with ischemic heart failure for high risk revascularization improve identification of those with the highest clinical benefit?: Imaging-guided selection of patients with ischemic heart failure for high-risk revascularization improves identification of those with the highest clinical benefit. Circ Cardiovasc Imaging 2012;5:262–70; discussion 270.

232. Schinkel AFL, Bax JJ, Poldermans D, et al. Hibernating myocardium: Diagnosis and patient outcomes. Curr Probl Cardiol 2007;32:375–410.
233. Samady H, Elefteriades JA, Abbott BG, et al. Failure to improve left ventricular function after coronary revascularization for ischemic cardiomyopathy is not associated with worse outcome. Circulation 1999;100:1298–304.
234. McMurray JJ, Pfeffer MA. Heart failure. Lancet 2005;365:1877–89.
235. Carrio I. Cardiac neurotransmission imaging. J Nucl Med 2001;42:1062–76.
236. Nakata T, Miyamoto K, Edoi A, et al. Cardiac death prediction and impaired cardiac sympathetic innervation assessed by mibg in patients with failing and nonfailing hearts. J Nucl Cardiol 1998;5:579–90.
237. Jacobson AF, Senior R, Cerqueira MD, et al. Myocardial iodine-123 meta-iodobenzylguanidine imaging and cardiac events in heart failure. Results of the prospective ADMIRE-HF (Adreview myocardial imaging for risk evaluation in heart failure) study. J Am Coll Cardiol 2010;55:2212–21.
238. Tamaki S, Yamada T, Okuyama Y, et al. Cardiac iodine-123 metaiodobenzylguanidine imaging predicts sudden cardiac death independently of left ventricular ejection fraction in patients with chronic heart failure and left ventricular systolic dysfunction: Results from a comparative study with signal-averaged electrocardiogram, heart rate variability, and qt dispersion. J Am Coll Cardiol 2009;53:426–35.
239. Kioka H, Yamada T, Mine T, et al. Prediction of sudden death in patients with mild-to-moderate chronic heart failure by using cardiac iodine-123 metaiodobenzylguanidine imaging. Heart 2007;93:1213–18.
240. Kasama S, Toyama T, Kumakura H, et al. Effects of candesartan on cardiac sympathetic nerve activity in patients with congestive heart failure and preserved left ventricular ejection fraction. J Am Coll Cardiol 2005;45:661–7.
241. Somsen GA, van Vlies B, de Milliano PA, et al. Increased myocardial [^{123}I]-metaiodobenzylguanidine uptake after enalapril treatment in patients with chronic heart failure. Heart 1996;76:218–22.
242. Fukuoka S, Hayashida K, Hirose Y, et al. Use of iodine-123 metaiodobenzylguanidine myocardial imaging to predict the effectiveness of beta-blocker therapy in patients with dilated cardiomyopathy. Eur J Nucl Med 1997;24:523–29.
243. Gerson MC, Craft LL, McGuire N, et al. Carvedilol improves left ventricular function in heart failure patients with idiopathic dilated cardiomyopathy and a wide range of sympathetic nervous system function as measured by iodine 123 metaiodobenzylguanidine. J Nucl Cardiol 2002;9:608–15.
244. Kasama S, Toyama T, Kumakura H, et al. Effect of spironolactone on cardiac sympathetic nerve activity and left ventricular remodeling in patients with dilated cardiomyopathy. J Am Coll Cardiol 2003;41:574–81.
245. Su H, Spinale FG, Dobrucki LW, et al. Noninvasive targeted imaging of matrix metalloproteinase activation in a murine model of postinfarction remodeling. Circulation 2005;112:3157–67.
246. Higuchi T, Bengel FM, Seidl S, et al. Assessment of alphavbeta3 integrin expression after myocardial infarction by positron emission tomography. Cardiovasc Res 2008;78:395–403.
247. Caspi O, Huber I, Kehat I, et al. Transplantation of human embryonic stem cell-derived cardiomyocytes improves myocardial performance in infarcted rat hearts. J Am Coll Cardiol 2007;50:1884–93.
248. Laflamme MA, Chen KY, Naumova AV, et al. Cardiomyocytes derived from human embryonic stem cells in pro-survival factors enhance function of infarcted rat hearts. Nat. Biotechnol 2007;25:1015–24.
249. Assmus B, Honold J, Schachinger V, et al. Transcoronary transplantation of progenitor cells after myocardial infarction. N Engl J Med 2006;355:1222–32.
250. Assmus B, Walter DH, Seeger FH, et al. Effect of shock wave-facilitated intracoronary cell therapy on LVEF in patients with chronic heart failure: The cellwave randomized clinical trial. JAMA 2013;309:1622–31.
251. Perin EC, Willerson JT, Pepine CJ, et al. Effect of transendocardial delivery of autologous bone marrow mononuclear cells on functional capacity, left ventricular function, and perfusion in chronic heart failure: The focus-cctrn trial. JAMA 2012;307:1717–26.
252. Hofmann M, Wollert KC, Meyer GP, et al. Monitoring of bone marrow cell homing into the infarcted human myocardium. Circulation 2005;111:2198–202.
253. Taylor DO, Stehlik J, Edwards LB, et al. Registry of the international society for heart and lung transplantation: Twenty-sixth official adult heart transplant report—2009. J Heart Lung Transplant 2009;28:1007–22.
254. Ciliberto GR, Ruffini L, Mangiavacchi M, et al. Resting echocardiography and quantitative dipyridamole technetium-99 m sestamibi tomography in the identification of cardiac allograft vasculopathy and the prediction of long-term prognosis after heart transplantation. Eur Heart J 2001;22:964–71.
255. Hacker M, Tausig A, Romuller B, et al. Dobutamine myocardial scintigraphy for the prediction of cardiac events after heart transplantation. Nucl Med Commun 2005;26:607–12.
256. Elhendy A, Sozzi FB, van Domburg RT, et al. Accuracy of dobutamine tetrofosmin myocardial perfusion imaging for the noninvasive diagnosis of transplant coronary artery stenosis. J Heart Lung Transplant 2000;19:360–6.
257. Wu Y-W, Chen Y-H, Wang S-S, et al. Pet assessment of myocardial perfusion reserve inversely correlates with intravascular ultrasound findings in angiographically normal cardiac transplant recipients. J Nucl Med 2010;51:906–12.

CHAPTER 8

Pharmacologic management of advanced heart failure

Akshay S. Desai MD MPH and Marc A. Pfeffer MD PhD

Introduction

Substantial progress in the development and application of evidence-based therapy has fueled measurable improvements in quality and quantity of life for heart failure (HF) patients, particularly those with reduced left ventricular ejection fraction (LVEF).[1] However, most therapies delay but do not reverse disease progression, and the prevalence of symptomatic HF in the aging population has steadily increased over time. HF currently affects 2.8% of the adult population and over 11% of the expanding elderly population (>80 years) in the United States. A projected 25% increase in HF prevalence by 2030 will vault HF-associated costs to more than $44 billion.[2,3]

As the overall burden of HF increases, so too will the proportion of patients surviving to reach the more advanced, symptomatic stages of their disease. The American Heart Association (AHA) defines patients with end-stage refractory HF as having stage D disease, reflecting symptom limitation during daily life despite usual recommended therapy, and a low likelihood of durable remission into less symptomatic disease.[4,5] While they constitute the minority of the community-dwelling HF population,[6] these patients in the final stage of the HF continuum comprise a population that consumes a disproportionate share of healthcare resources due to considerable HF-associated morbidity, high rates of readmission, and 1-year mortality rates exceeding 50% despite the application of maximal medical treatment. The optimal stepped therapy of patients with chronic symptomatic HF (ACC/AHA stage C) is well informed by randomized clinical trials and summarized in published professional guidelines (see Chapter 1),[7,8,9,10] but best practices for management of those in stage D are less clearly defined. Indeed, in this fragile population, therapies previously considered lifesaving may no longer be tolerated, forcing withdrawal or dose reduction of guideline-recommended therapies. Accordingly, in this chapter we seek to outline an approach to pharmacologic treatment of the advanced HF patient, identifying gaps in the current evidence base for treatment of this small but growing population. The rapidly evolving role of cardiac replacement therapies (mechanical circulatory support, cardiac transplantation) in the management of this challenging population is addressed in Chapters 14–16.

When is heart failure truly refractory?

For the minority of patients presenting with fulminant HF symptoms and progressive hemodynamic instability due to cardiogenic shock, the onset of refractory disease is readily apparent. For the rest, however, the progression of chronic symptomatic HF toward the end-stage is often subtle and underappreciated by treating clinicians. Risk prediction models including the Heart Failure Survival Score[11] and Seattle Heart Failure Model[12] may help to generate actuarial estimates of survival based on clinical factors, but it remains unclear how these scores should be leveraged to influence decision-making and treatment for individual HF patients. Some of the more powerful predictors of poor outcome are ongoing HF symptoms at rest or with minimal exertion limiting activities of daily living (New York Heart Association [NYHA] functional class III–IV), repeated hospitalizations for HF decompensation,[13] loss of lean body mass,[14] worsening renal function,[15] hyponatremia,[16] low blood pressure, and the need to withdraw neurohormonal antagonists due to intolerance.[17] In general, the onset of these sentinel events despite the application of "optimal" treatment heralds the onset of stage D and should trigger consideration of advanced HF therapies or palliative interventions. Patients in this category represent a heterogeneous group ranging from ambulatory patients who are symptom-limited with minimal exertion to hospitalized patients with cardiogenic shock on vasoactive therapy requiring emergent consideration of mechanical circulatory support. The Interagency Registry for Mechanically Assisted Circulatory Support (INTERMACS) profiles elaborate the clinical spectrum of these patients, and are increasingly useful in identifying patients who are most likely to benefit from durable mechanical support as either lifetime therapy or bridge to transplantation (Table 8.1).[18]

A key challenge in the identification of stage D patients is differentiating those patients who are truly treatment refractory from those who are suboptimally or incompletely treated. The vast majority of symptoms and recurrent hospitalizations in HF patients are related to congestive exacerbations;[19] accordingly, residual congestion, as estimated by the physical examination, cardiac biomarker levels, noninvasive testing, or invasive hemodynamic assessment, is a powerful predictor of subsequent morbidity and mortality. In the Acute Decompensated Heart Failure National Registry (ADHERE) experience, 21% of patients admitted with clinical evidence of decompensation/volume overload were discharged without weight loss or with a gain in weight despite administration of diuretics, suggesting that inadequate treatment (or response) may in large measure contribute to the risk of subsequent clinical events.[20] Beyond adequate management of volume status, there is ample data that the benefits of neurohormonal antagonists, including angiotensin converting enzyme (ACE) inhibitors,[21] angiotensin receptor blockers (ARBs),[22] and β-blockers[23,24] are proportional to the administered

Table 8.1 INTERMACS profiles of advanced heart failure

Profile	Shorthand	Definition
1	"Critical cardiogenic shock"	Patient has life-threatening hypotension and profound low cardiac output with rapidly escalating inotropic support
2	"Progressive decline"	Patient has been demonstrated "dependent" on inotropic support but nonetheless shows signs of continuing deterioration
3	"Stable but inotrope-dependent"	Patient is clinically stable on mild–moderate doses of intravenous inotropes, or has a temporary circulatory support device, after repeated documentation of failure to wean without symptoms
4	"Resting symptoms"	Patient is at home on oral therapy but frequently has symptoms of congestion at rest or with activities of daily living
5	"Exertion intolerant"	Patient is comfortable at rest but unable to engage in any activity, living predominantly within the home
6	"Exertion limited"	Patient is comfortable at rest without evidence of fluid overload, is able to do some mild activity
7	"Advanced NYHA class III"	Patient is clinically stable with a reasonable level of comfortable activity, despite history of previous decompensation

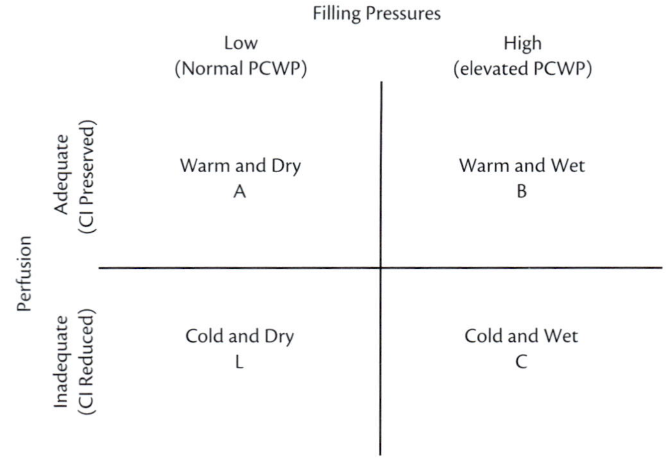

Fig. 8.1 Hemodynamic profiles in advanced heart failure. CI = Cardiac Index; PCWP = Pulmonary Capillary Wedge Pressure.

or maximally tolerated dose. Although guidelines recommend that physicians initiate and titrate these medications to the doses shown to prolong life in clinical trials, evidence suggests that these treatments are markedly underutilized in clinical practice.[25,26] A genuine effort to attempt dose titration is particularly important, since the inability to tolerate a dose considered maximally effective may be another distinguishing feature of stage D disease.[27]

Hemodynamic profiles to guide selection of therapy

The optimal approach to pharmacologic therapy in the advanced HF patient may vary according to the hemodynamic profile at the time of initial evaluation. According to the schema initially proposed by Stevenson et al.,[28] patients with advanced HF may be subclassified based on a bedside assessment into four groups based on the filling pressures that are high or low ("wet" or "dry") and perfusion that is adequate or critically limited ("warm" or "cold"). Key to the identification of elevated filling pressures are typical symptoms or physical examination findings of congestion including orthopnea, elevated jugular venous pressure, S3 gallop, worsening peripheral edema, ascites, and less commonly, rales. Poor perfusion is most accurately estimated by a narrow pulse pressure (<25% of the systolic blood pressure) or evidence of end-organ dysfunction (cool forearms and legs, worsening renal function, altered mental status). When available, invasive hemodynamic data may provide further refinement of this classification through direct measurement of the pulmonary capillary wedge pressure and cardiac output (Figure 8.1). For patients with adequate perfusion (profiles A and B), the primary goals are maintenance or correction of the volume status with judicious use of diuretics as well as titration of disease-modifying therapies to facilitate the more long-term favorable ventricular remodeling and slowing of disease progression. By contrast, for those with inadequate perfusion (profiles C and D), temporary or permanent withdrawal of neurohormonal antagonists or introduction of intravenous inotropic drugs or vasodilators may be necessary to facilitate acute hemodynamic stabilization. A subset of these patients may tolerate gradual reintroduction of an oral HF regimen after restoration of normal volume status and optimization of perfusion using intravenous drugs. Such therapy tailored to hemodynamic goals as measured by a pulmonary artery catheter, while not appropriate in routine application, may be particularly helpful in those profile C patients with low cardiac output and marked elevation in systemic vascular resistance who might be expected to recruit latent contractile reserve with effective vasodilator therapy.

The evidence base for pharmacologic treatment of "advanced" heart failure

The 2013 ACC/AHA guidelines for the management of chronic HF recommend that initial therapy in the stage D patient begin with conventional HF therapies appropriate for those in stage C.[29] While this strategy is intuitively appealing, few stage D patients have been enrolled in randomized clinical trials of these treatments (Figure 8.2). The vast majority of these trials selected patients for enrollment on the basis of ejection fraction and NYHA functional class, deliberately excluding those with the comorbidity profile and marginal hemodynamic status that characterizes those with truly end-stage disease. Of the major trials enrolling patients with more advanced HF symptoms (NYHA III–IV), few enrolled more than a handful of class IV patients (Table 8.2). The relatively low rates of control group mortality at 1 year in most of these studies (~10%) in comparison with the Evaluation Study of Congestive Heart Failure and Pulmonary Catheterization Effectiveness (ESCAPE) (38%)[30] and REMATCH (75%)[31] population of patients being considered for pulmonary artery catheter placement or LV assist device (LVAD) as destination therapy, respectively, highlights that those with the most advanced disease are largely underrepresented in clinical trials (Figure 8.3).[32]

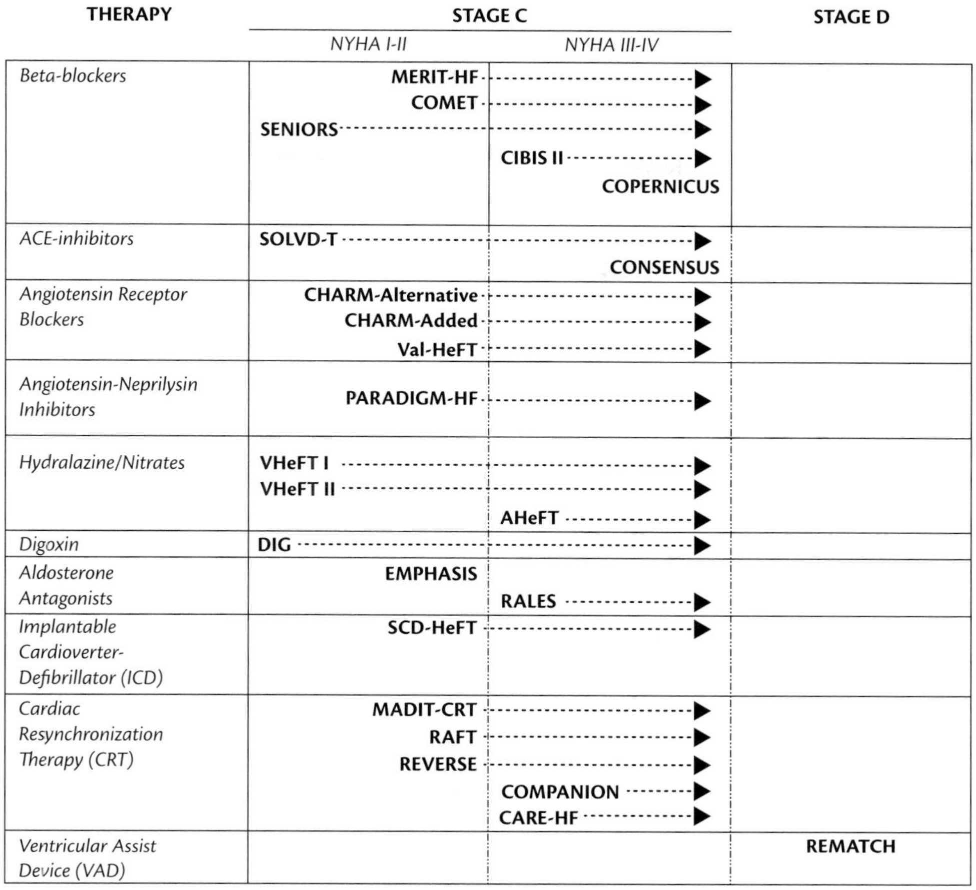

Fig. 8.2 Randomized trials of core heart failure therapies according to heart failure stage and severity.

Patients approaching end-stage disease may become increasingly intolerant of standard HF therapies, forcing dose reduction or even discontinuation of neurohormonal antagonists. Utilization of standard HF therapies in the most advanced HF populations being considered for LVAD or transplantation is therefore quite low compared with more stable ambulatory HF patients. Even at specialized HF centers, data from the INTERMACS registry suggests that by the time of VAD implantation, a minority of patients are still treated with β-blockers and ACE inhibitors (Table 8.3). The ability to successfully reintroduce these therapies after institution of mechanical circulatory support with an LVAD highlights that tolerability is largely a function of the acute hemodynamic state. Accordingly, used judiciously, these therapies may still be appropriate for many patients with highly symptomatic disease.

β-Blockers

Overall, β-adrenergic receptor blockers are now established as a cornerstone of therapy for patients with HF and reduced ejection fraction. Randomized trials have consistently demonstrated an approximate 30% incremental reduction in the rates of death across the HF spectrum with the addition of β-blockers to ACE inhibitors[33] Of the large scale trials of β-blocker treatment in chronic HF, only two included a substantive fraction of advanced HF patients. The Cardiac Insufficiency Bisoprolol Study-II (CIBIS-II)[34] randomized 2647 subjects with LVEF 35% or less and NYHA III–IV symptoms on standard therapy including diuretics and an ACE inhibitor to treatment with bisoprolol or placebo (target 10 mg/day). The trial was stopped early at a mean follow-up of 1.3 years due to a significant mortality advantage to those in the bisoprolol group (156 (11.8%) vs. 228 (17.3%) deaths, hazard ratio 0.66, 95% CI 0.54–0.81, $p <$ 0.0001). Subgroup analysis of the benefits in the 445 (17%) patients with NYHA IV symptoms suggested no variation in the benefits of bisoprolol treatment by HF severity. Similar findings were apparent in the subgroup of advanced HF patients with severe LV dysfunction enrolled in the Metoprolol CR/XL Randomized Intervention Trial in Heart Failure (MERIT-HF). In 795 subjects with NYHA III–IV symptoms (10% NYHA IV) and LVEF less than 25%, treatment with metoprolol succinate was associated with a 39% reduction in all-cause mortality (45 deaths [11.7% per patient year] vs. 72 deaths [19.1% per patient year], $p = 0.0086$), similar to the 34% mortality reduction observed in the population as a whole.[35]

The Carvedilol Prospective Randomized Cumulative Survival Study (COPERNICUS)[36] deliberately set out to test the benefits of β-blockade in a population with severe chronic HF. This trial randomized 2289 patients with LVEF less than 25%, symptoms of HF at rest or with minimal exertion, and clinical "euvolemia" to treatment with carvedilol (target 25 mg twice daily) or placebo. However, even here, what we now consider stage D patients with systolic blood pressure less than 85 mmHg, advanced chronic kidney disease (creatinine >2.8 mg/dl), and those requiring treatment with intravenous inotropic agents or vasodilators were excluded. Over a mean period of 10.4 months, during which standard treatment including diuretics and an ACE inhibitor or ARB was continued, those randomized to carvedilol experienced a 35% reduction in the risk of all-cause mortality (mortality rate 12.8% vs. 19.7% per patient year, $p = 0.0014$) and a 24% reduction in the combined disk

Table 8.2 Randomized trials of pharmacologic therapy in patients with advanced heart failure

Trial	N	% NYHA III–IV	Intervention (target dose)	Control group mortality at 1 year	Primary endpoint	Relative risk reduction
ACE inhibitors						
CONSENSUS I (1987)	253	IV: 100%	Enalapril 20 mg bid	52%	Death	40%
SOLVD-T (1991)	2569	III: 30% IV: 2%	Enalapril 20 mg bid	16%	Death	16%
Angiotensin receptor blockers						
Val-HeFT (2001)	5010	III: 36% IV: 2%	Valsartan 160 mg bid	9%	CV death or morbidity	13%
CHARM-Alternative (2003)	2028	III: 49% IV: 4%	Candesartan 32 mg daily	13%	CV death or HF hospitalization	23%
CHARM-Added (2003)	2548	III: 73% IV: 3%	Candesartan 32 mg daily	11%	CV death or HF hospitalization	15%
Angiotensin-neprilysin inhibitors						
PARADIGM-HF (2014)	8399	III: 24% IV: 0.7%	LCZ696 (sacubitril/valsartan) 200 mg bid	8.4%	CV death or HF hospitalization	20% (vs. enalapril)
Aldosterone receptor antagonists						
RALES (1999)	1663	III: 70% IV: 30%	Spironolactone 25–50 mg daily	24%	Death	30%
Hydralazine-ISDN						
VHeFT I (1986)	459	NR	Hydralazine 75 mg tid-qid, ISDN 40 mg qid	26%	Death	34%
A-HeFT (2004)	1050	III: 95% IV: 4%	Hydralazine 75 mg tid, ISDN 40 mg tid	~9%	Composite score (death, HF hospitalization, QOL)	43% (survival)
β-Blockers						
CIBIS-II (1999)	2647	III: 83% IV: 17%	Bisoprolol 10 mg daily	13%	Death	34%
MERIT-HF (1999)	3991	III: 55% IV: 4%	Metoprolol Succinate 200 mg daily	11%	Death	34%
COPERNICUS (2001)	2289	NR	Carvedilol 25 mg bid	20%	Death	35%
SENIORS (2005)	2128	III: 39% IV: 2%	Nebivolol 10 mg daily	10%	Death or CV hospitalization	14%
Digitalis glycosides						
DIG (1997)	6800	III: 30% IV: 2%	Digoxin	~10%	Death	0%
Ivabradine						
SHIFT (2010)	6558	III: 50% IV: 2%	Ivabradine 7.5 mg bid	~8%	CV death or HF hospitalization	18%
LVAD						
REMATCH (2001)	129	IV: 100%	LVAD (DT)	75%	Death	48%

bid, twice daily; CV, cardiovascular; HF, heart failure; LVAD, left ventricular assist device; qid, four times daily; QOL, quality of life; tide, three times daily. ; ISDN, Isosorbide dinitrate.

of death or HF hospitalization. Notably, despite the severity of their disease, 66% of patients assigned to carvedilol were successfully titrated to the target dose of 25 mg twice daily by 12 weeks, and 60% were maintained at this dose at study end. Fewer patients in the carvedilol group experienced adverse events requiring permanent discontinuation of study drug than in the placebo group. The benefits and tolerability were similar in all subgroups examined, including the 624 subjects at highest risk due to recent or recurrent HF decompensation or severely depressed cardiac function for whom treatment with carvedilol was associated with a 33% reduction

Table 8.3 Medical therapy in practice among patients with advanced heart failure

	REMATCH	Brigham and Women's Hospital	INTERMACS
	(*n* = 129)	(*n* = 61)	(*n* = 5407)
ACE inhibitor	57%	16%	31%
ARB	14%	13%	8%
β-Blocker	22%	31%	52%
Aldosterone antagonist	36%	52%	36%
Digoxin	86%	NR	NR
Loop diuretic	96%	93%	79%
Intravenous inotropic drugs	68%	84%	81%

Data for Brigham and Women's Hospital and INTERMACS drawn from INTERMACS Quarterly Quality Assurance Report December 2011 as reported to Brigham and Women's Hospital, and reflecting preimplant medications for implants from June 2006 through December 2011.

ACE, antiotensin converting enzyme; ARB, angiotensin receptor blocker.

in death or hospitalization for a cardiovascular reason (95% CI 13–49%, $p = 0.002$) (Figure 8.4). Notably, although low blood pressure is a potent marker of risk in advanced HF and a frequently cited reason for withholding β-blocker treatment, the relative benefits of carvedilol in COPERNICUS were similar in patients with low and preserved systolic blood pressure prior to treatment.[37]

Taken together, these data suggest potential benefits of β-blockers in stable patients with advanced HF comparable to those with less severe disease. Accordingly, guidelines recommend initiation of these agents in all patients with symptomatic HF, barring contraindications. Since the negative inotropic effects may initially be poorly tolerated in hospitalized patients with decompensated HF, β-blocker therapy should be initiated only after hemodynamic stabilization and restoration of normal volume status. As in the clinical trials, the starting doses should be low (e.g., 1.25 mg daily bisoprolol, 12.5–25 mg daily metoprolol succinate, 3.125 mg bid carvedilol) with gradual uptitration (e.g., every 2 weeks) toward the target or maximally tolerated doses. In patients who begin with low systolic blood pressure, α-adrenergic blockade may be poorly tolerated, and use of a β_1 selective agent such as metoprolol or bisoprolol may be preferable.

The development of worsening HF symptoms in patients treated with β-blockers should not automatically prompt dose reduction or discontinuation. While β-blockers may be justifiably withheld in patients with cardiogenic shock, this is not likely to be necessary for the vast majority of patients with acute decompensated HF who have adequate end-organ perfusion.[28] In the Organized Program to Initiate Lifesaving Treatment in Hospitalized Patients with Heart Failure (OPTIMIZE-HF), continuation of β-blockade was associated with lower postdischarge mortality.[38] Conversely, in the Carvedilol or Metoprolol European Trial, reduction in β-blockade during HF hospitalization was associated with higher risk of subsequent mortality.[39] Since the decision to reduce the dose was based on clinical judgment, this observation may be confounded by withdrawal in the sicker HF patients. For those in whom clinical hypoperfusion necessitates adjustment of the β-blocker dose, dose reduction is likely preferable to abrupt discontinuation. Rechallenge with β-blockers following hemodynamic stabilization and normalization of filling pressures should be considered; for those with particularly marginal cardiac output in whom tolerability is a particular concern, even more gradual dose titration (e.g., monthly, rather than biweekly titration) may facilitate introduction

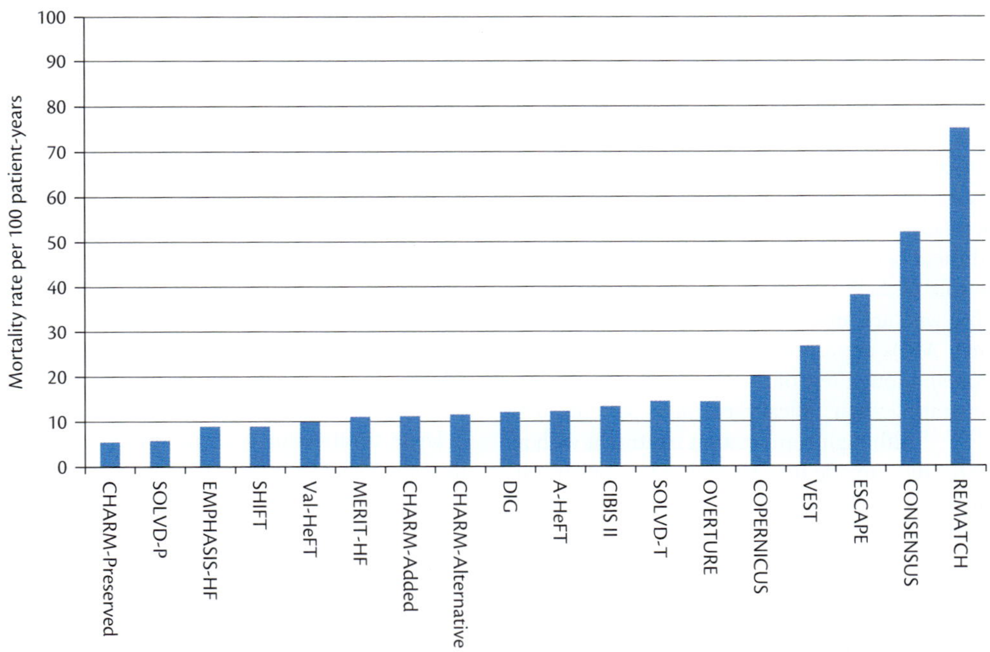

% NYHA III	38	0	0	50	36	55	73	49	30	95	83	30	48	–	85	–	0	0
% NYHA IV	2	0	0	2	2	4	3	4	2	4	17	2	2.1	–	14	–	100	100

Fig. 8.3 Placebo group mortality in selected randomized trials of heart failure patients.

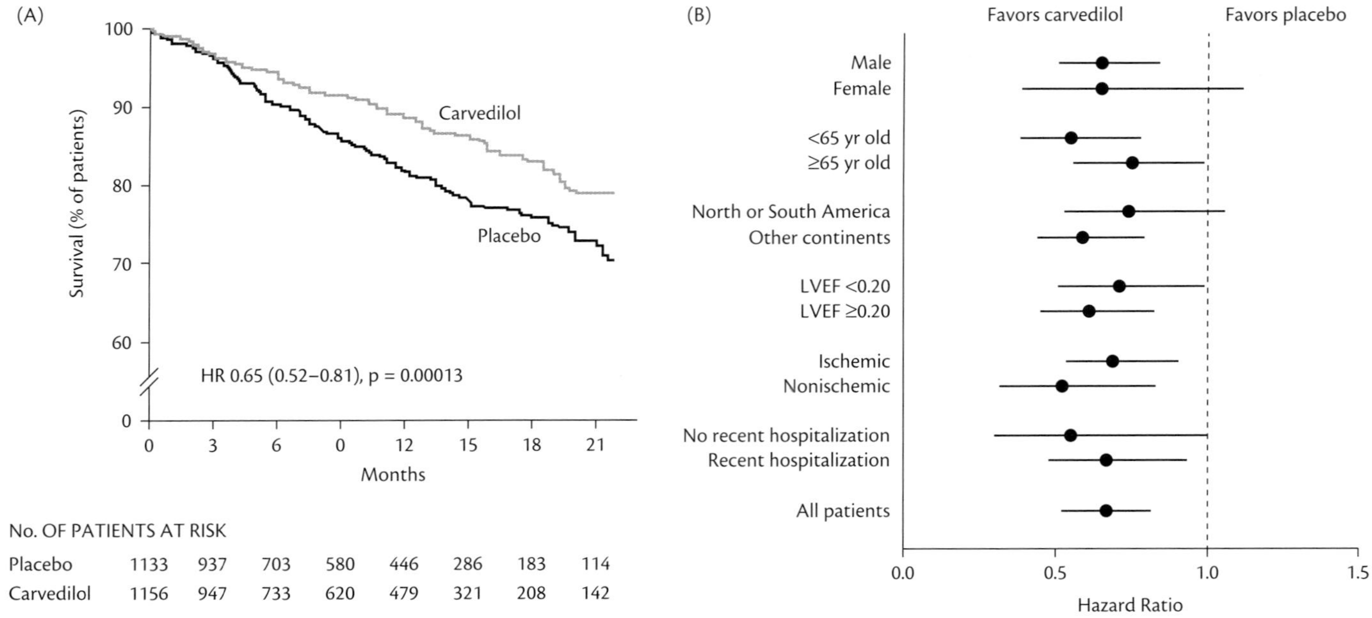

Fig. 8.4 COPERNICUS trial. (A) Kaplan–Meier analysis of time to death in placebo and carvedilol groups; (B) hazard ratios (and 95% confidence intervals) for death from any cause among key subgroups.

of low doses that may still be associated with substantive improvements in remodeling and clinical outcomes.[23]

ACE inhibitors, ARBs, and other oral vasodilators

Based on data from multiple large prospective randomized clinical trials enrolling patients across the spectrum of HF severity, current guidelines recommend consideration of ACE inhibitors in all patients with HF and LVEF 40% or less, including those with (stage C) and without (stage B) clinical symptoms.[29] The first large prospective trial of ACE inhibition in HF, the Cooperative North Scandinavian Enalapril Survival Study (CONSENSUS),[40] specifically targeted patients with advanced disease, and successfully enrolled a particularly high-risk population with a 1-year mortality of 52% in the placebo arm. Subjects randomized to enalapril experienced a 40% reduction in mortality at 6 months that was sustained out to at least 4 years, with a statistically measurable benefit enduring at 10-year follow-up in the open-label extension.[41] Subsequent trials (SOLVD, VHeFT II) extended these benefits to those with less advanced disease, solidifying the role of ACE inhibitors for patients across the HF spectrum. In those who are intolerant of ACE inhibitors due to cough or angioedema, ARBs are a proven alternative (when used at the appropriate doses), though few of the large randomized controlled trials demonstrating their efficacy enrolled patients with class IV symptoms.[22,42,43] Although combination treatment with an ACE inhibitor and ARB did provide incremental reductions in cardiovascular morbidity and mortality in the CHARM-Added study,[44] the higher rates of hypotension, renal dysfunction, and hyperkalemia associated with this combination frequently preclude use of this regimen in the advanced HF population.

With HF progression, the renin–angiotensin–aldosterone system (RAAS) may become indispensable for maintenance of blood pressure, renal perfusion, and glomerular filtration, making continued RAAS blockade challenging. Accordingly, 10–30% of patients with advanced HF are unable to tolerate ACE inhibitors due to hypotension or renal dysfunction, and these patients are also likely to be intolerant of ARBs.[17,45,46] Intolerance of ACE inhibitors due to circulatory–renal limitations is a poor prognostic sign, associated with a 2.5-fold increase in the risk of mortality.[17] For these patients, substitution of a combination of isordil and hydralazine may be an effective alternative.[47,48] In the Vasodilator Heart Failure Trial (VHeFT-1),[49] treatment with the isosorbide dinitrate/hydralazine combination was associated with significant reductions in mortality over 3-year follow-up compared with placebo, though subsequent data from VHeFT II suggests that this regimen may be less effective than enalapril.[47] This two-drug combination is occasionally better tolerated than ACE inhibitors in patients with marginal blood pressure who require vasodilation, and has been used to facilitate weaning from inotropic infusions in patients with advanced disease.[50] Only 3% of those enrolled in the African-American Heart Failure Trial (A-HeFT)[51] testing the isosorbide dinitrate/hydralazine combination as an add-on to standard HF treatment (including an ACE inhibitor or ARB in 87% and β-blocker in 74%) had NYHA class IV symptoms. Although this trial was terminated early for mortality benefit in the treatment arm, there is insufficient data to recommend routine use of this strategy in the advanced HF population where tolerability of add-on treatment is likely to be poor. However, clinical experience suggests that nitrates alone may be a useful adjunct to ACE inhibitors to help further reduce filling pressures and improve exercise tolerance in patients with advanced HF.[52,53]

Dose titration of ACE inhibitors and ARBs toward the target doses achieved in clinical trials is encouraged by the guidelines based on the results of dose-ranging trials suggesting incremental benefit at higher dose.[21,22] Although the evidence base is limited, comparable tolerability and efficacy of dose titration in the NYHA class IV patients who have been studied suggests that these results may broadly applicable to the population with more advanced HF.[54] Since the absolute reduction in clinical events with high-dose relative to lower-dose ACE inhibition appears to be small (<1%), maintenance of lower doses may be reasonable for those at particularly high risk for adverse events including hyperkalemia, worsening renal function, and hypotension during dose titration (such as elderly patients with borderline blood pressure). However, ACE inhibitor intolerance may be difficult to anticipate based on clinical factors, underscoring the clinical importance of an adequate trial of dose titration. In the Assessment of Lisinopril and Survival (ATLAS)[21] study, only 4.2% of ACE inhibitor naive patients could not be titrated to the medium doses of lisinopril (12.5–15 mg once daily) required for randomization; during the course of the trial, 27% of those assigned to high-dose (32.5–35.0 mg once daily) and 30.7% of those assigned to low-dose (2.5–5.0 mg once daily) lisinopril required study drug withdrawal, suggesting similar rates of adverse events in both arms.[54] Again, however, the representation of class IV patients was limited (225 of 3164 enrolled subjects, 7.1%). As with β-blockers, where clinical trial target doses are not tolerated, downtitration appears preferable to discontinuation.

Aldosterone antagonists

Suppression of aldosterone production by ACE inhibitors and ARBs in HF patients is transient and incomplete.[55,56,57] The central role of aldosterone in HF pathophysiology and the broad range of potentially deleterious cardiovascular and renal consequences of mineralocorticoid receptor activation in HF patients has fueled interest in combination blockade of the RAAS using aldosterone receptor antagonists in addition to ACE inhibitors. The Randomized Aldactone Evaluation Study (RALES)[58] randomized 1663 patients with severe HF (class IV symptoms within the 6 months prior to randomization, and class III or IV HF symptoms at the time of enrollment) and ejection fraction (EF) 35% or less already treated with an ACE inhibitor to treatment with spironolactone 25 mg daily or placebo. This trial, one of the few to deliberately target a population with advanced disease, was terminated early at mean follow-up of 24 months due to a dramatic 30% reduction in mortality among those treated with spironolactone (284 (35%) vs. 386 (46%) deaths, RR 0.70, 95% CI 0.60–0.82, $p < 0.001$). Understandably, since RALES was conducted before the major β-blocker mortality trials were completed, only 11% of those enrolled were treated with β-blockers. However, the favorable impact of aldosterone antagonists in the EPHESUS[59] trial of post-MI HF and the EMPHASIS-HF[60] trial of NYHA II HF confirm and extend the incremental benefits of aldosterone antagonism in HF patients treated with both ACE inhibitors and β-blockers.[60] Collectively, the data from these trials provides a compelling rationale for utilization of aldosterone antagonists as the "third drug" across the spectrum of patients with symptomatic HF and reduced EF.

The primary concern regarding utilization of aldosterone antagonists in patients with advanced HF is the risk of life-threatening hyperkalemia.[61] Hospitalizations and deaths associated with hyperkalemia were observed to increase dramatically following the publication of the RALES trial, underscoring the imperative for careful patient selection and longitudinal surveillance of potassium and renal function following initiation of these agents.[62] Patients with age 75 years, male gender, diabetes, creatinine 2.0 mg/dl or more, serum potassium 5.0 mmol/L or more, and those treated with more than one inhibitor of the RAAS appear to be at particularly high risk.[63] However, since those at high risk for hyperkalemia are also frequently those at highest risk for worsening HF, the net benefit of spironolactone or eplerenone prescription may still be favorable. In the RALES trial, those with eGFR less than 60 ml min^{-1} 1.73 m^{-2} derived greater absolute benefits from spironolactone treatment than those with preserved eGFR despite a more than twofold increase in risk of hyperkalemia prompting dose reduction or discontinuation.[64] Moreover, aldosterone antagonists are associated with lower risk of sudden death in the post-MI HF population,[65] perhaps in part because of the impact on reducing rates of hypokalemia.[66] Thus, while the risks of hyperkalemia must be considered, introduction of aldosterone antagonists should be considered in those with advanced HF in the context of careful laboratory monitoring. A suggested algorithm for initiation of aldosterone antagonists in advanced HF is provided in Box 8.1.

Box 8.1 Suggested algorithm for initiation of aldosterone antagonists in advanced heart failure

1. Optimize dosing of ACE/ARB and β-blocker
2. Check serum potassium prior to initation, avoid for K ≥ 5.0 mEq/L
3. Estimate glomerular filtration rate to assess specific risk of hyperkalemia
    - Creatinine may underestimate severity of renal dysfunction, particularly in elderly patients
    - Caution with eGFR <50 mL/min/1.73 m^2, avoid for eGFR <30 mL/min/1.73 m^2
4. Discontinue or reduce dosage of potassium supplements
5. Initiate at low dose (spironolactone 12.5 mg, eplerenone 25 mg)
6. Monitor potassium levels within 1 week of initiation or dose change, and at regular intervals thereafter (q3–6 months)
7. Reduce dose or discontinue for K^+ ≥5.5 mEq/L or Cr ≥ 2.5 mg/dL
8. Do not titrate beyond target doses (spironolactone 25 mg, eplerenone 50 mg)
9. Suspend treatment in setting of diarrhea or dehydration

ACE, antiotensin converting enzyme; ARB, angiotensin receptor blocker; eGFR, estimated glomerular filtration rate.

Angiotensin–neprilysin inhibitors

Although ACE inhibitors have long been considered first-line therapy for heart failure in patients with reduced ejection fraction, recent data has suggested the potential to improve outcomes in selected patients by substituting a new class of agents that simultaneously inhibit the angiotensin receptor and neprilysin, an enzyme that is important for the breakdown of a number of key endogenous vasodilators including natriuretic peptides.[135,136] The PARADIGM-HF (Prospective comparison of ARNi with ACEi to Determine Impact on Global Mortality and Morbidity in Heart Failure) trial was a prospective, double-blind, randomized, active-comparator trial of the angiotensin-receptor neprilysin inhibitor LCZ696 in comparison with enalapril in 8399 patients with NYHA II-IV heart failure and left ventricular ejection fraction ≤ 40% who were treated with guideline-directed medical therapy including an ACE-inhibitor or angiotensin-receptor blocker (dose equivalent to enalapril 10 mg daily). Prior to randomization, all patients completed a sequential run-in period to demonstrate tolerability of enalapril and LCZ696 at target doses (enalapril 10 mg twice daily, LCZ696 200 mg twice daily). Over median 27 months follow up, treatment with LCZ696 rather than enalapril in this population was associated with a 20% reduction in the primary composite outcome of cardiovascular death or heart failure hospitalization (HR 0.80; 95% CI 0.73 to 0.87; $p < 0.001$) as well as a 16% reduction in death from any cause (HR 0.84; 95% CI 0.76 to 0.93; $p < 0.001$).[137] Over 80% of the deaths in the trial were due to cardiovascular causes, and treatment with LCZ696 reduced both sudden cardiac death (HR 0.80; 95% CI 0.68 to 0.94; $p = 0.008$) and death due to worsening heart failure (HR 0.79; 95% CI 0.64-0.98; $p = 0.034$) compared with enalapril.[138] Although patients with advanced heart failure symptoms were eligible and comprised approximately 25% of the randomized population, patients intolerant of ACE-inhibitors or ARBs and those with systolic blood pressure < 100 mm Hg were excluded. Accordingly, the majority of subjects randomized were NYHA II or III, and only a handful of patients classified as NYHA IV (0.7%) successfully completed the run-in period. Even in this selected population, symptomatic hypotension was more common with LCZ696 than enalapril, suggesting that tolerability may be an issue for patients with more tenuous hemodynamics. Accordingly, while these data are provocative and may transform the therapy of many patients with heart failure and reduced ejection fraction, their relevance to the advanced heart failure population remains unclear.

Digitalis glycosides

Historically, the cardiac glycosides were the mainstay of HF therapy. With demonstration of the survival benefits of RAAS antagonists and β-blockers and the neutral impact of digoxin on mortality in the pivotal Digitalis Investigation Group (DIG) trial, the utilization of this effective agent has waned. Notably, however, digoxin treatment during that study was associated with significant reduction in HF hospitalizations, with an effect most pronounced in the highest risk subjects with severely reduced EF (<25%) or NYHA III/IV symptoms.[67] Although there are no recent trials, the more contemporary use of implantable defibrillators in the HF population may mitigate the concerns of the heightened risk for sudden death observed in the DIG trial.[67] The risk–benefit ratio of digoxin appeared most favorable in those with serum concentrations less than 1.0 ng/ml, with no incremental benefits at higher levels.[68] In this context, current treatment guidelines acknowledge that the judicious use of digoxin may improve functional capacity and reduce hospitalizations in patients with persistent HF symptoms despite optimal medical therapy with β-blockers, ACE inhibitors, and diuretics.[7] Accordingly, prescription of digoxin at low dose (0.125–0.25 mg daily) may be appropriate for many patients with advanced HF, excepting those with conduction system disease or advanced renal disease. Since data from two separate trials has suggested a significant rate of clinical deterioration following interruption of digoxin treatment in stable HF patients with reduced EF not treated with β-blockers, withdrawal of digoxin treatment is not recommended in the absence of concern for toxicity.[69,70]

Sinoatrial node inhibition

Ivabradine has recently received approval for use to reduce the risk of HF hospitalization in patients with LVEF 35% or less, sinus rhythm (heart rate ≥75), and symptomatic HF (NYHA class II–IV) despite treatment with β-blockers, ACE inhibitors (or ARBs), and mineralocorticoid blocker. Since relatively few class IV patients were included in the SHIFT[71] study which was the basis for this approval, information on use in advanced HF is currently rather limited. Although clearly not indicated as a substitute for β-blocker, the relative absence of a blood pressure lowering action or an increase in creatinine with this sinoatrial node inhibitor raises the potential for benefit in patients in whom tachycardia persists despite use of standard medications.

Anticoagulation

Although patients with HF and reduced EF are known to be at increased risk for thromboembolic events, the absolute risk of stroke or arterial embolism appears to be low (1–3% per year), even among those with severe left ventricular (LV) dysfunction.[72,73,74] Accordingly, it has been challenging to demonstrate a net benefit to routine anticoagulation with warfarin.[75,76,77] In the Warfarin versus Aspirin in Reduced Cardiac Ejection Fraction (WARCEF) trial, 2305 patients with sinus rhythm, no contraindication to warfarin anticoagulation, and LVEF 35% or less were randomized in double-blind, double-dummy fashion to treatment with warfarin (INR target 2.0–3.5) or aspirin (325 mg daily). The median EF among enrolled subjects was 24.7 ± 7.5%, with 680 subjects (29.7%) reporting NYHA III and only 18 subjects (1.2%) NYHA IV functional capacity. At mean follow-up of 3.5 ± 1.8 years, the incidence of the composite primary outcome of ischemic stroke, intracerebral hemorrhage, or death from any cause was no different between the two arms, but the rates of major hemorrhage were greater in those assigned to warfarin. Although data in advanced HF are limited, given this apparent increase in risk and lack of incremental benefit, use of warfarin anticoagulation in those without a specific indication (atrial fibrillation, known intracardiac thrombus, prior history of thromboembolism) is discouraged.[7] For those HF patients with atrial fibrillation who require anticoagulation, the novel anticoagulants such as dabigatran, rivaroxaban, and apixaban may be reasonable alternatives to warfarin,[78,79,80] since the relative efficacy with regard to prevention of stroke and systemic embolism appears to be similar, even among those with significantly reduced EF and more advanced (NYHA III–IV) symptoms.[81]

Antiarrhythmic drugs

While atrial and ventricular arrhythmias are common in patients with advanced HF and may contribute to morbidity and mortality, efforts at pharmacologic suppression with antiarrhythmic drugs have generally been associated with increased mortality.[82,83,84] The negative inotropic effects of many antiarrhythmic drugs as well as the associated risk of proarrhythmic side effects make them particularly challenging to use in the advanced HF population. Accordingly, there is no indication to use these agents to suppress the asymptomatic ventricular premature depolarizations or brief episodes of nonsustained ventricular tachycardia that may become more frequent as HF progresses. For most of these patients, continued titration of β-blocker therapy and correction of underlying electrolyte abnormalities (particularly hypokalemia) is adequate. For those HF patients with poorly tolerated atrial fibrillation, symptomatic ventricular arrhythmias, or recurrent defibrillator discharges who require antiarrhythmic drug treatment, amiodarone and dofetilide are the only agents associated with neutral effects on mortality in randomized trials and are therefore the preferred alternatives.[85,86]

Specific challenges in advanced heart failure

Refractory volume overload

Since sodium and fluid retention are responsible for the vast majority of congestive symptoms in patients with advanced HF, loop

Confirm Adherence
1) Taking medications as prescribed
2) Fluid In take restricted to <2L/day
3) Sodium Intake restricted to <2g/day

Optimize Loop Diuretic Dosing
1) BID or TID dosing to limit post-diuretic sodium retention
2) Torsemide or Bumetanide in preference to furosemide in patients with significant right sided symptoms, ascites, and edema
3) Dosing earlier in day to limit non adherence due to nocturia
4) Elevate lower extremities and lie supine for 30–60 minutes after diuretic administration

Consider Combination Diuretic Strategies
1) Addition of thiazide diuretics (e.g. hydrochlorothiazide 12.5–25 mg qd or metolazone 1.25–10 mg qd) 30 minutes prior to loop diuretic (caution with hypokalemia)
2) Addition of spironolactone (25–50 mg qd, caution with hyperkalemia)

Utilization of Intravenous Diuretics
1) Bolus Infusion in Adequate Dose (>= total daily oral dose, consider 2.5 x total maintenance oral dose in furosemid equivalents)
2) Continuous Infusion (reasonable to trial as an up front strategy or if bolus dosing fails)

Consider Alternative Strategies
1) Low dose dopamine (e.g. 2–3 mcg/kg/min)
2) Low dose nesiritide (0.005 mcg/kg/min, do not titrate, avoid if SBP<90 mm Hg)
3) Ultrafiltration (avoid in patients with severely impaired perfusion or shock)
4) Hemodynamic-guided Therapy (insertion of PA catheter)

Fig. 8.5 Management of refractory volume overload. BID = twice daily; TID = three times daily, PA = pulmonary artery.

diuretics remain a cornerstone of daily management. Loop diuretic requirements typically increase as HF progresses, and high maintenance doses (>200 mg daily furosemide or equivalent) may be necessary to maintain normal fluid balance. Resistance to diuretic therapy may occur in part due to enhanced tubular reabsorption of sodium and water in the face of progressive neurohormonal activation, but is further exacerbated by altered diuretic pharmacology in patients with more severe disease. Chronic administration of loop diuretics leads to changes within the distal nephron that enhance tubular sodium reabsorption and blunt natriuretic effects ("braking phenomenon"). Systemic absorption of oral diuretics may be delayed in the face of gut edema, and efficient transport of diuretics to their site of action within the tubular lumen of the nephron may be impaired, especially among those with comorbid renal dysfunction.[87,88,89] Compensatory sodium retention by the kidney as diuretic concentrations wane within the tubule may further attenuate natriuretic effect, particularly in patients with high dietary intake of sodium. Comorbid renal dysfunction in HF patients may further limit diuretic responsiveness; however, an elevated serum creatinine alone should not discourage attempts at diuresis in patients with obvious volume overload, since effective relief of venous congestion may actually improve renal perfusion and clearance.[90] These and other unexplained confounding factors may in part account for the observational data associating higher diuretic use with worse prognosis.[91,92,93,94,95,96]

For patients in whom even maximal doses of loop diuretics are associated with suboptimal response, several options are reasonable to consider (Figure 8.5). Restriction of dietary sodium intake to less than 2 g/day and more frequent diuretic dosing (e.g., two to three times daily rather than once daily) can limit the impact of post-diuretic sodium retention. Utilization of loop diuretics with greater oral bioavailability (e.g., bumetanide or torsemide) in place of furosemide may be associated with achievement of higher peak serum concentrations and greater natriuretic effect (Table 8.4). Sequential blockade of the nephron using different diuretic classes in combination may also facilitate a more effective diuretic response. While ineffective as monotherapy in HF patients, thiazide diuretics (e.g., hydrochlorothiazide, metolazone) may dramatically enhance diuresis when administered 30–60 minutes prior to a loop diuretic. Addition of spironolactone has also been associated with improved response in selected HF patients refractory to high-dose loop diuretics. Caution should be taken with such combination approaches due to enhanced risk for serious electrolyte abnormalities, particularly hypokalemia and hypomagnesemia.

Intravenous loop diuretics are administered to 90% of patients who are hospitalized with acute decompensated HF, and can be delivered by bolus or continuous infusion. Continuous infusion of loop diuretics offers the potential advantage of maintaining constant serum levels, delivering effective drug doses continuously to the urinary site of action, and minimizing the impact of rebound sodium retention that occurs with bolus dosing of diuretics that have a short serum half-life. This issue as well as the impact of loop diuretic dosing was critically evaluated in the Diuretic Optimization Strategies Evaluation (DOSE) Trial,[97] which enrolled 308 patients with acute exacerbations of chronic HF who had previously been treated with loop diuretics (80–240 mg furosemide daily or equivalent) and randomized them in 2 × 2 fashion to a low-dose (total intravenous furosemide dose equal to total daily oral loop diuretic dose in furosemide equivalents) or high-dose (total daily intravenous furosemide dose 2.5 times the daily total loop diuretic dose) strategy and to administration of furosemide either by intravenous bolus every 12 hours or by continuous intravenous infusion.

Table 8.4 Pharmacology of commonly used oral diuretics in heart failure

	Dosage[a] (mg/day)	Fractional sodium excretion(FeNA+, %)	Oral bioavailability	Half-life	Duration of action
Furosemide	20–600 mg	20–25%	~50%(highly variable)	1.5–2 h	6–8 h
Bumetanide	0.5–10 mg	20–25%	80–100%	1 h	4–6 h
Torsemide	10–400 mg	20–25%	80–100%	3–4 h	12–16 h
Ethacrynic acid	50–100 mg	20–25%	~100%	1 h	4–6 h
Metolazone	2.5–10 mg	5–8%	65%	8–14 h	12–24 h
Hydrochlorothiazide	25–100 mg	5–8%	60–70%	9–10 h	6–12 h
Chlorothiazide	250–1000 mg	5–8%	15–30%	1.5–2.5 h	6–12 h
Spironolactone	25–50 mg[b]	2%	~90%	1–2 h[c]	2–3 days
Amiloride	2.5–20 mg	2%	15–25%	6–9 h	24 h

[a] Higher dosages commonly divided twice daily.

[b] Higher dosages occasionally administered with careful monitoring of potassium and renal function.

[c] Canrenone, the active metabolite of spironolactone, has 13–24 hour half-life, which extends duration of effect.

Data adapted from Ernst and Moser[134] and Yancy, et al.[7]

Notably, there was no significant difference between the bolus and continuous infusion groups with regard to patient symptoms or renal function at 72 hours; however, the high-dose strategy was associated with greater urine output and a nonsignificant trend to greater improvement in patient symptoms. Overall, these data suggest that mode of intravenous diuretic administration is unlikely to have major impact on diuresis as long as the administered dose is sufficient. Nonetheless, local clinical experience suggests that some patients who fail to respond to high doses of bolus diuretics do seem to improve with transition to a continuous infusion.

Where volume overload and right ventricular (RV) dysfunction are sufficient to provoke ascites, increased intra-abdominal pressure and renal vein compression may further compromise the renal pressure gradient for filtration, exacerbating renal function.[98] In these patients, direct abdominal decompression through paracentesis may enhance renal blood flow and facilitate diuresis. An alternative approach to decongestion is the direct mechanical removal of salt and water through ultrafiltration. In patients with moderate congestive HF, venovenous ultrafiltration rapidly lowers right atrial and pulmonary capillary wedge pressures (PCWP) and results in sustained improvement in exercise tolerance.[99,100] Ultrafiltration may also reduce diuretic-induced neurohormonal activation, restore responsiveness to diuretics, and improve outcomes.[101] Although data from early randomized controlled trials suggest that use of ultrafiltration as up-front treatment in selected patients with acute decompensated HF was associated with enhanced weight loss and improved exercise capacity, hemodynamics, and hospitalizations relative to standard treatment with diuretics,[102,103] subsequent trials have failed to confirm these results. Most recently, the CARRESS trial suggested that a strategy of ultrafiltration in patients with acute decompensated HF complicated by cardiorenal syndrome was inferior to stepped pharmacologic therapy emphasizing loop diuretics, with similar weight loss and a higher rate of adverse events at 96 hours.[104]

Unfortunately, the current data supporting the use of ultrafiltration in the advanced HF population is limited. Patarroyo et al.[105] examined the value of slow continuous ultrafiltration in the management of a highly selected group of 63 patients with advanced HF, worsening renal function, and congestion refractory to intensive attempts at hemodynamically guided medical therapy using a pulmonary arterial catheter. The selection criteria defined an extremely ill population of patients at with LVEF 26 ± 15%, serum sodium of 133 ± 6 meq/L, baseline creatinine of 1.9 ± 0.8 mg/dl, mean central venous pressure of 20 mmHg, mean PCWP of 30 mmHg, and cardiac index of 1.8 L min^{-1} m^{-2} defining hemodynamics consistent with cardiogenic shock. At baseline, 18% were being treated with inotropic agents. After 48 hours of ultrafiltration, improvement in hemodynamics with reductions in filling pressures and increase in cardiac index was reported, but there was no significant improvement in blood urea nitrogen or serum creatinine. More concerning was that after initiation of ultrafiltration, 59% of these advanced HF patients required conversion to continuous dialysis during the hospital course, and 14% were dialysis dependent at discharge. Despite apparent effective decongestion, in this population with advanced disease refractory to conventional therapy, in-hospital mortality was high, with 19 of 63 (30%) patients dying before discharge and 6 additional patients discharged with terminal care in hospice. While this is a small patient sample from a single clinical center, these sobering data clearly highlight that ultrafiltration is of limited utility as salvage therapy for patients with worsening renal function in the setting of advanced, medically refractory HF.

Alternative therapies that have been explored as alternatives or adjuncts to loop diuretic therapy for volume removal in the acute HF setting include natriuretic peptides (nesiritide, ularitide), vasopressin antagonists (tolvaptan, conivaptan), and adenosine receptor antagonists (rolofylline). In randomized controlled trials, none of these agents has been effective in providing sustained improvements in clinical outcomes.[106,107,108] Initial enthusiasm for use of nesiritide to manage decompensated HF based on its acute hemodynamic effects[109] was tempered by meta-analyses suggesting increased risk of worsening renal function and mortality over longer-term follow-up.[110,111] Formal review of these data by the US Food and Drug Administration (FDA) culminated in the call for an adequately powered prospective randomized controlled trial to formally assess the balance of risk and benefit. The recently completed ASCEND-HF trial of 7141 patients with acute HF suggested a neutral effect of nesiritide relative to placebo on mortality, rehospitalizations, and renal function, arguing strongly against the routine use of nesiritide to manage HF in clinical practice.[106] Low-dose nesiritide (0.005 μg kg^{-1} min^{-1}) and low-dose dopamine (2–3 μg kg^{-1} min^{-1}) are currently being investigated as adjunctive therapy to facilitate diuresis in hospitalized HF patients as part of the ROSE trial (NCT01132846). Until these data are available, clinicians should reserve use of these agents for those patients without contraindications in whom adequate trials of combination diuretic therapy have failed to relieve substantive volume overload.

The novel peptide serelaxin, a recombinant version of the human relaxin-2 that regulates maternal adaptations to pregnancy, is associated with several potentially beneficial hemodynamic effects including increased cardiac output, improved renal blood flow, and reduced arterial compliance that might be useful in patients with acute HF. In the RELAX-AHF trial,[111a] among 1161 patients hospitalized with decompensated HF (including 329 with NYHA III and 135 with NYHA IV symptoms 30 days prior to randomization), a 48-hour infusion of serelaxin was associated with significant improvements in dyspnea, congestion, and hospital length of stay relative to placebo. Although there was no discernible impact of serelaxin treatment on cardiovascular death or readmissions, fewer deaths were observed at 180 days in serelaxin-treated patients. The role of this agent in the future management of the acute HF syndrome requires clarification in future randomized trials.

Impaired perfusion/cardiogenic shock

A particularly challenging subset of HF patients is those who present with volume overload and clinical evidence of end-organ hypoperfusion (hemodynamic profile C in the Stevenson classification). These patients with hypotension, resting tachycardia, narrow pulse pressure, pulsus alternans, cool extremities, obtundation or altered mental status, or worsening renal function often fail to respond to treatment with diuretics alone, and may require temporary or permanent withdrawal of neurohormonal antagonists and/or management with intravenous vasodilator or inotropic agents to improve systemic perfusion and increase renal blood flow. With minimal perfusion pressure and critical clinical status, intensive monitoring is required, and any pharmacologic intervention may have unintended adverse consequences in these fragile patients. Selection of appropriate pharmacologic treatment for these patients may be facilitated by direct ascertainment of hemodynamic parameters including filling pressures, cardiac output, and systemic vascular resistance. Notably, the Evaluation Study of Congestive Heart Failure and Pulmonary Artery Catheterization Effectiveness (ESCAPE) trial randomized 433 patients with advanced HF (6 month mortality 19%) and acute decompensation to management guided by a pulmonary artery catheter (PAC) or the clinical assessment alone and found no incremental benefit of PAC-guided treatment with regard to mortality or hospitalization during 6 month follow-up and a higher rate of adverse events.[30] While these data discourage routine use of a PAC to guide therapy of acute HF, they do not preclude a role in management of medically refractory HF patients or those with cardiogenic shock who were systematically excluded from the trial. Specific circumstances in which utilization of hemodynamic monitoring may be indicated to facilitate HF treatment are outlined in recent clinical guidelines[7] and summarized in Box 8.2.

Box 8.2 Indications for pulmonary artery catheterization in patients with heart failure

- Clinically indeterminate volume status, perfusion, systemic or pulmonary vascular resistance
- Clinically significant hypotension (e.g., symptomatic decline in blood pressure or systolic blood pressure <90 mmHg) or worsening renal function with empiric heart failure therapy
- Evaluation of candidacy for advanced therapies such as ventricular assist device or transplant (in particular assessment of pulmonary vascular resistance)
- Presumed cardiogenic shock requiring escalation of pressor support and consideration of mechanical circulatory support
- Severe clinical decompensation with uncertain relative contributions from elevated filling pressures, hypoperfusion, abnormal vascular tone
- Apparent inotrope dependence or severe symptoms that persist despite adjustment of recommended therapies

For patients with low cardiac output and high systemic vascular resistance, intravenous vasodilators are the preferred initial treatment strategy (Table 8.5). Dilation of the venous circulation reduces ventricular preload and filling pressures, while dilation of the systemic circulation reduces afterload and increases cardiac output, enhancing the response to intravenous diuretics. The best-studied intravenous vasodilator in advanced HF is sodium nitroprusside, which provides balanced arterial and venous vasodilation with rapid and marked dose-dependent reductions in systemic vascular resistance. Since empiric dosing of nitroprusside is associated with risks of hypotension, nitroprusside is typically administered under the guidance of invasive hemodynamic monitoring with a PAC. The dose is adjusted to "optimize" hemodynamics (typically a systemic

Table 8.5 Intravenous vasodilator drugs for advanced heart failure

	Half-life (min)	Cardiac output (CO)	Systemic vascular resistance (SVR)	Pulmonary vascular resistance (PVR)	Central venous pressure (CVP)	Mean arterial pressure (MAP)
Nitroglycerine	3	↑	↓	↓	↓↓↓	↓
Nitroprusside	1–2[a]	↑↑↑	↓↓↓	↓↓	↓	↓↓↓
Nesiritide	18	↑↑	↓↓	↓↓	↓↓	↓↓

[a]Thiocyanate metabolite has extended half-life of ~3 days.

Table 8.6 Inotropic drugs for advanced heart failure

	Half-Life (mins)	Cardiac Output (CO)	Systemic Vascular Resistance (SVR)	Pulmonary Vascular Resistance (PVR)	LV End Diastolic Pressure (LVEDP)	Mean Arterial Pressure (MAP)
Dobutamine	2.4	↑	↓	↔	↓	↓
Dopamine[a]	2	↑	↓	↔	↔	↑
2–10 μg/kg/min		↑ ↔	↑↑	↑	↑	↑↑
10–20 μg/kg/min						
Milrinone	150	↑	↓↓	↓↓	↓	↓↓
Levosimendan	60[b]	↑	↓	↓	↓	↓

[a]Hemodynamic effects vary according to dopamine dose: β-adrenergic receptor effects predominate at low dose, α-adrenergic effects at higher doses.

[b]Levosimendan has an active metabolite with an elimination half-life of 70–80 hours in heart failure patients.

vascular resistance of 1000–1200 dyne s cm^{-5} and cardiac index >2.1 ml min^{-1} m^{-2}) with concurrent titration of intravenous diuretics to normalize filling pressures. Once an optimal hemodynamic profile is achieved, maintenance is accomplished through weaning and substitution of the intravenous agent with oral vasodilator agents including ACE inhibitors, nitrates, and hydralazine.[112] Thiocyanate toxicity is a potential risk of nitroprusside exposure and is associated with dose, duration, and hepatic dysfunction. Nitroglyerine and nesiritide are reasonable alternatives to nitroprusside in this application and are frequently administered without hemodynamic monitoring, but provide less reduction in systemic vascular resistance at the doses commonly used in clinical practice.

For patients with low cardiac output and a marginal or low systemic vascular resistance, cardiac reserve may be limited, and use of inotropic drugs in preference to vasodilators is often necessary to improve symptoms and end-organ perfusion. The hemodynamic benefits of inotropic drugs in patients with advanced HF must be balanced against the established risks of morbidity and mortality in both short-term and long-term application. Routine administration of milrinone to hospitalized patients with acute decompensated HF in the OPTIME-CHF study was associated with a higher rate of tachyarrhythmias and hypotension in comparison with placebo.[113] As well, in the ESCAPE trial, in-hospital usage of inotropes was associated with a higher risk of death and rehospitalization at 6 months.[114] Despite the hope that levosimendan, a calcium sensitizer, might be a safer inotropic agent due to its lack of effect on intracellular calcium levels, data from Randomized Evaluations of Levosimendan (REVIVE-1 and REVIVE-2) studies suggests that this agent is similarly associated with higher risks of arrhythmias, hypotension, and all-cause mortality.[115]

Given these important limitations, inotropic drugs should be considered treatments of last resort, reserved for temporary stabilization of selected patients with rapidly progressive hemodynamic deterioration or treatment-refractory HF who are not candidates for vasodilator treatment. All agents carry appear to carry similar risks, and selection of the appropriate agent is conditioned in part based on the desired hemodynamic effects (Table 8.6). Milrinone is a more potent vasodilator than dobutamine, and is preferred for patients with significant pulmonary hypertension and RV failure due to greater impact on pulmonary vascular resistance. However, its prolonged half-life and greater impact on systemic blood pressure make it challenging to use in patients with marginal blood pressure or significant renal dysfunction. In this context, dobutamine or dopamine may be preferred first-line agents. Distinct from dobutamine, which is a pure β-agonist with inotropic and vasodilating properties, dopamine exhibits dose-dependent effects at a variety of dopaminergic and adrenergic receptors. Selective agonism of D1 receptors at by dopamine at low doses (2–3 μg kg^{-1} min^{-1}) may occasionally be exploited to facilitate renal vasodilation and enhanced urine output, while the inotropic (β-adrenergic) effects dominate at higher doses. With continued dose escalation, activation of α-adrenergic receptors by dopamine may result in vasoconstriction that may have deleterious consequences for HF patients. In patients who fail to respond to a single inotropic agent at adequate dose, the combination of a β-agonist and phosphodiesterase inhibitor may provide synergistic effects. The dosage of inotropes should be minimized and early efforts at rapid weaning encouraged to limit the duration of exposure and attendant adverse effects. Where successful weaning is not possible, recognition of end-stage disease and early consideration of more durable therapy such as mechanical circulatory support or cardiac transplantation is warranted, given considerably improved outcomes in comparative evaluation (see Chapters 14–16).[31] In some end-stage HF patients who are not candidates for advanced therapies, continuous outpatient support with inotropes is occasionally considered as a means to palliation of HF symptoms.[116] However, the expected survival of patients treated with such home infusions is less than 50% at 6 months, suggesting that the incremental quality of life gains for most patients may not balance out the added cost and complexity near the end of life.[31,117] This use to reduce the symptoms of severe refractory HF is recognized as not being administered to extend survival, but may help patients to successfully transition from the hospital to home or "bridge" to important life events.

Pulmonary hypertension/right ventricular failure

Pulmonary hypertension commonly complicates advanced HF and is associated with greater disability and reduced survival.[118] For many such patients with World Health Organization group 2 pulmonary hypertension, pulmonary vascular resistance is normal, and restoration of normal left heart filling pressures with standard HF treatments (afterload reduction and diuresis) is sufficient to reduce pulmonary pressures to the normal range. As the duration and severity of HF increases, however, mixed pulmonary hypertension, characterized by an elevated pulmonary vascular resistance and elevated PCWP, is more likely to be present.[119] Although intrinsic pulmonary vascular disease related to sleep-disordered breathing, parenchymal lung disease, or venous thromboembolism may contribute, this phenomenon is frequently related to chronic untreated passive pulmonary hypertension.[120] The RV is particularly sensitive to changes in afterload, and progressive development of RV dysfunction in patients with pulmonary hypertension is an additional marker of poor prognosis.[121,122]

The diagnostic evaluation and management of patients with pulmonary arterial hypertension and RV failure is reviewed in detail in Chapters 21 and 22. Among patients with pulmonary hypertension due to left HF, the primary therapeutic strategy is to minimize left heart filling pressures with vasodilators and diuretics in order to relieve the hydrostatic component of elevation in pulmonary venous pressures that contributes to pulmonary hypertension. For patients with mixed pulmonary hypertension and elevated pulmonary vascular resistance, the use of selective pulmonary vasodilators is frequently considered, but carries the potential for a substantial increase in transpulmonary flow that may overwhelm the compensatory capacity of the failing LV and precipitate pulmonary edema.[123] Despite acute hemodynamic benefits,[124] use of endothelin receptor antagonists to treat pulmonary hypertension in patients with HF and reduced EF has not been associated with consistent improvement in functional capacity or clinical outcomes in randomized trials.[125,126,127,128] The phosphodiesterase-5 (PDE-5) inhibitor sildenafil has been associated with improvement in symptoms and functional capacity in ambulatory patients with chronic HF, pulmonary hypertension, and HF with reduced LVEF,[129,130] but did not improve effort tolerance or clinical status in unselected patients with HF and preserved EF enrolled in the RELAX trial.[131] Definitive assessment of the role of PDE-5 inhibitors in HF patients awaits the completion of larger randomized trials powered to examine clinical outcomes. In the interim, for those with advanced HF and reduced EF in whom elevated filling pressure persist despite maximal medical therapy, maximal ventricular unloading with mechanical circulatory support using a LV assist device may be the most effective approach.[132,133]

Conclusion

While the pharmacologic management of patients with stage C HF is well defined by a large evidence base from randomized clinical trials, patients with stage D disease represent a population that has been largely excluded from systematic study to date and who are beyond the reach of guideline-directed medical therapy. While the design of clinical trials for this population is under way and will eventually support a more systematic approach, medical therapy of those with HF progression to stage D currently remains largely empiric, guided primarily by expert consensus and clinical judgment. Titration of standard HF therapies in this population must be undertaken cautiously and requires close surveillance with frequent reassessment to assess the appropriate balance of risk and benefit. The requirement for compassionate, team-based care and the need for close partnership between specialized clinicians and cardiac surgeons in selecting appropriate candidates for mechanical circulatory support and transplantation underscores that optimal management of these patients is increasingly the province of specialized centers with concentrated clinical expertise.

References

1. Cubbon RM, Gale CP, Kearney LC, et al. Changing characteristics and mode of death associated with chronic heart failure caused by left ventricular systolic dysfunction: a study across therapeutic eras. Circulation;4:396–403.
2. Roger VL, Go AS, Lloyd-Jones DM, et al. Heart disease and stroke statistics—2012 update: a report from the American Heart Association. Circulation 2012;125:e2–220.
3. Heidenreich PA, Trogdon JG, Khavjou OA, et al. Forecasting the future of cardiovascular disease in the United States: a policy statement from the American Heart Association. Circulation 2011;123:933–44.
4. Allen LA, Stevenson LW, Grady KL, et al. Decision making in advanced heart failure: a scientific statement from the American Heart Association. Circulation 2012;125:1928–52.
5. Hunt SA, Baker DW, Chin MH, et al. ACC/AHA Guidelines for the Evaluation and Management of Chronic Heart Failure in the Adult: Executive Summary A Report of the American College of Cardiology/American Heart Association Task Force on Practice Guidelines (Committee to Revise the 1995 Guidelines for the Evaluation and Management of Heart Failure): developed in collaboration with the International Society for Heart and Lung Transplantation; endorsed by the Heart Failure Society of America. Circulation 2001;104:2996–3007.
6. Ammar KA, Jacobsen SJ, Mahoney DW, et al. Prevalence and prognostic significance of heart failure stages: application of the American College of Cardiology/American Heart Association heart failure staging criteria in the community. Circulation 2007;115:1563–70.
7. Yancy CW, Jessup M, Bozkurt B, et al. 2013 ACCF/AHA Guideline for the Management of Heart Failure: A Report of the American College of Cardiology Foundation/American Heart Association Task Force on Practice Guidelines. Circulation 2013;128:e240–327.
8. McMurray JJ, Adamopoulos S, Anker SD, et al. ESC Guidelines for the diagnosis and treatment of acute and chronic heart failure 2012: The Task Force for the Diagnosis and Treatment of Acute and Chronic Heart Failure 2012 of the European Society of Cardiology. Developed in collaboration with the Heart Failure Association (HFA) of the ESC. Eur Heart J 2012;33:1787–847.
9. McKelvie RS, Moe GW, Ezekowitz JA, et al. The 2012 Canadian Cardiovascular Society heart failure management guidelines update: focus on acute and chronic heart failure. Can J Cardiol 2012;29:168–81.
10. Lindenfeld J, Albert NM, Boehmer JP, et al. HFSA 2010 Comprehensive heart failure practice guideline. J Card Fail 2010;16:e1–194.
11. Aaronson KD, Schwartz JS, Chen TM, et al. Development and prospective validation of a clinical index to predict survival in ambulatory patients referred for cardiac transplant evaluation. Circulation 1997;95:2660–7.
12. Levy WC, Mozaffarian D, Linker DT, et al. The Seattle Heart Failure Model: prediction of survival in heart failure. Circulation 2006;113:1424–33.
13. Setoguchi S, Stevenson LW, Schneeweiss S. Repeated hospitalizations predict mortality in the community population with heart failure. Am Heart J 2007;154:260–6.
14. Anker SD, Negassa A, Coats AJ, et al. Prognostic importance of weight loss in chronic heart failure and the effect of treatment with angiotensin-converting-enzyme inhibitors: an observational study. Lancet 2003;361:1077–83.
15. Hillege HL, Nitsch D, Pfeffer MA, et al. Renal function as a predictor of outcome in a broad spectrum of patients with heart failure. Circulation 2006;113:671–8.
16. Packer M, Lee WH, Kessler PD, et al. Role of neurohormonal mechanisms in determining survival in patients with severe chronic heart failure. Circulation 1987;75:IV80–92.
17. Kittleson M, Hurwitz S, Shah MR, et al. Development of circulatory-renal limitations to angiotensin-converting enzyme inhibitors identifies patients with severe heart failure and early mortality. J Am Coll Cardiol 2003;41:2029–35.
18. Boyle AJ, Ascheim DD, Russo MJ, et al. Clinical outcomes for continuous-flow left ventricular assist device patients stratified by pre-operative INTERMACS classification. J Heart Lung Transplant 2011;30:402–7.
19. Zile MR, Bennett TD, St John Sutton M, et al. Transition from chronic compensated to acute decompensated heart failure: pathophysiological insights obtained from continuous monitoring of intracardiac pressures. Circulation 2008;118:1433–41.
20. Gheorghiade M, Zannad F, Sopko G, et al. Acute heart failure syndromes: current state and framework for future research. Circulation 2005;112:3958–68.

21. Packer M, Poole-Wilson PA, Armstrong PW, et al. Comparative effects of low and high doses of the angiotensin-converting enzyme inhibitor, lisinopril, on morbidity and mortality in chronic heart failure. ATLAS Study Group. Circulation 1999;100:2312–18.
22. Konstam MA, Neaton JD, Dickstein K, et al. Effects of high-dose versus low-dose losartan on clinical outcomes in patients with heart failure (HEAAL study): a randomised, double-blind trial. Lancet 2009;374:1840–8.
23. Bristow MR, Gilbert EM, Abraham WT, et al. Carvedilol produces dose-related improvements in left ventricular function and survival in subjects with chronic heart failure. MOCHA Investigators. Circulation 1996;94:2807–16.
24. Fiuzat M, Wojdyla D, Kitzman D, et al. Relationship of beta-blocker dose with outcomes in ambulatory heart failure patients with systolic dysfunction: results from the HF-ACTION (Heart Failure: A Controlled Trial Investigating Outcomes of Exercise Training) trial. J Am Coll Cardiol 2012;60:208–15.
25. O'Connor CM, Stough WG, Gallup DS, et al. Demographics, clinical characteristics, and outcomes of patients hospitalized for decompensated heart failure: observations from the IMPACT-HF registry. J Card Fail 2005;11:200–5.
26. Dahlstrom U, Hakansson J, Swedberg K, Waldenstrom A. Adequacy of diagnosis and treatment of chronic heart failure in primary health care in Sweden. Eur J Heart Fail 2009;11:92–8.
27. Granger BB, Swedberg K, Ekman I, et al. Adherence to candesartan and placebo and outcomes in chronic heart failure in the CHARM programme: double-blind, randomised, controlled clinical trial. Lancet 2005;366:2005–11.
28. Nohria A, Lewis E, Stevenson LW. Medical management of advanced heart failure. JAMA 2002;287:628–40.
29. Hunt SA, Abraham WT, Chin MH, et al. 2009 focused update incorporated into the ACC/AHA 2005 Guidelines for the Diagnosis and Management of Heart Failure in Adults: a report of the American College of Cardiology Foundation/American Heart Association Task Force on Practice Guidelines: developed in collaboration with the International Society for Heart and Lung Transplantation. Circulation 2009;119:e391–479.
30. Binanay C, Califf RM, Hasselblad V, et al. Evaluation study of congestive heart failure and pulmonary artery catheterization effectiveness: the ESCAPE trial. JAMA 2005;294:1625–33.
31. Rose EA, Gelijns AC, Moskowitz AJ, et al. Long-term use of a left ventricular assist device for end-stage heart failure. N Engl J Med 2001;345:1435–43.
32. Skali H, Pfeffer MA, Lubsen J, Solomon SD. Variable impact of combining fatal and nonfatal end points in heart failure trials. Circulation 2006;114:2298–303.
33. Chatterjee S, Biondi-Zoccai G, Abbate A, et al. Benefits of beta blockers in patients with heart failure and reduced ejection fraction: network meta-analysis. BMJ 2013;346:f55.
34. The Cardiac Insufficiency Bisoprolol Study II (CIBIS-II): a randomised trial. Lancet 1999;353:9–13.
35. Goldstein S, Fagerberg B, Hjalmarson A, et al. Metoprolol controlled release/extended release in patients with severe heart failure: analysis of the experience in the MERIT-HF study. J Am Coll Cardiol 2001;38:932–8.
36. Packer M, Fowler MB, Roecker EB, et al. Effect of carvedilol on the morbidity of patients with severe chronic heart failure: results of the Carvedilol Prospective Randomized Cumulative Survival (COPERNICUS) study. Circulation 2002;106:2194–9.
37. Rouleau JL, Roecker EB, Tendera M, et al. Influence of pretreatment systolic blood pressure on the effect of carvedilol in patients with severe chronic heart failure: the Carvedilol Prospective Randomized Cumulative Survival (COPERNICUS) study. J Am Coll Cardiol 2004;43:1423–9.
38. Fonarow GC, Abraham WT, Albert NM, et al. Influence of beta-blocker continuation or withdrawal on outcomes in patients hospitalized with heart failure: findings from the OPTIMIZE-HF program. J Am Coll Cardiol 2008;52:190–9.
39. Metra M, Torp-Pedersen C, Cleland JG, et al. Should beta-blocker therapy be reduced or withdrawn after an episode of decompensated heart failure? Results from COMET. Eur J Heart Fail 2007;9:901–9.
40. Effects of enalapril on mortality in severe congestive heart failure. Results of the Cooperative North Scandinavian Enalapril Survival Study (CONSENSUS). The CONSENSUS Trial Study Group. N Engl J Med 1987;316:1429–35.
41. Swedberg K, Kjekshus J, Snapinn S. Long-term survival in severe heart failure in patients treated with enalapril. Ten year follow-up of CONSENSUS I. Eur Heart J 1999;20:136–9.
42. Granger CB, McMurray JJ, Yusuf S, et al. Effects of candesartan in patients with chronic heart failure and reduced left-ventricular systolic function intolerant to angiotensin-converting-enzyme inhibitors: the CHARM-Alternative trial. Lancet 2003;362:772–6.
43. Cohn JN, Tognoni G. A randomized trial of the angiotensin-receptor blocker valsartan in chronic heart failure. N Engl J Med 2001;345:1667–75.
44. McMurray JJ, Ostergren J, Swedberg K, et al. Effects of candesartan in patients with chronic heart failure and reduced left-ventricular systolic function taking angiotensin-converting-enzyme inhibitors: the CHARM-Added trial. Lancet 2003;362:767–71.
45. Bart BA, Ertl G, Held P, et al. Contemporary management of patients with left ventricular systolic dysfunction. Results from the Study of Patients Intolerant of Converting Enzyme Inhibitors (SPICE) Registry. Eur Heart J 1999;20:1182–90.
46. Kostis JB, Shelton B, Gosselin G, et al. Adverse effects of enalapril in the Studies of Left Ventricular Dysfunction (SOLVD). SOLVD Investigators. Am Heart J 1996;131:350–5.
47. Cohn JN, Johnson G, Ziesche S, et al. A comparison of enalapril with hydralazine-isosorbide dinitrate in the treatment of chronic congestive heart failure. N Engl J Med 1991;325:303–10.
48. Fonarow GC, Chelimsky-Fallick C, Stevenson LW, et al. Effect of direct vasodilation with hydralazine versus angiotensin-converting enzyme inhibition with captopril on mortality in advanced heart failure: the Hy-C trial. J Am Coll Cardiol 1992;19:842–50.
49. Cohn JN, Archibald DG, Ziesche S, et al. Effect of vasodilator therapy on mortality in chronic congestive heart failure. Results of a Veterans Administration Cooperative Study. N Engl J Med 1986;314:1547–52.
50. Binkley PF, Starling RC, Hammer DF, Leier CV. Usefulness of hydralazine to withdraw from dobutamine in severe congestive heart failure. Am J Cardiol 1991;68:1103–6.
51. Taylor AL, Ziesche S, Yancy C, et al. Combination of isosorbide dinitrate and hydralazine in blacks with heart failure. N Engl J Med 2004;351:2049–57.
52. Elkayam U, Johnson JV, Shotan A, et al. Double-blind, placebo-controlled study to evaluate the effect of organic nitrates in patients with chronic heart failure treated with angiotensin-converting enzyme inhibition. Circulation 1999;99:2652–7.
53. Johnson JB, Gross JF, Hale E. Effects of sublingual administration of nitroglycerin on pulmonary-artery pressure in patients with failure of the left ventricle. N Engl J Med 1957;257:1114–17.
54. Massie BM, Armstrong PW, Cleland JG, et al. Toleration of high doses of angiotensin-converting enzyme inhibitors in patients with chronic heart failure: results from the ATLAS trial. The Assessment of Treatment with Lisinopril and Survival. Arch Int Med 2001;161:165–71.
55. Borghi C, Boschi S, Ambrosioni E, Melandri G, Branzi A, Magnani B. Evidence of a partial escape of renin-angiotensin-aldosterone blockade in patients with acute myocardial infarction treated with ACE inhibitors. J Clin Pharmacol 1993;33:40–5.
56. Staessen J, Lijnen P, Fagard R, Verschueren LJ, Amery A. Rise of plasma aldosterone during long-term captopril treatment. N Engl J Med 1981;304:1110.
57. Swedberg K, Eneroth P, Kjekshus J, Snapinn S. Effects of enalapril and neuroendocrine activation on prognosis in severe congestive heart failure (follow-up of the CONSENSUS trial). CONSENSUS Trial Study Group. Am J Cardiol 1990;66:40D-4D; discussion 4D-5D.

58. Pitt B, Zannad F, Remme WJ, et al. The effect of spironolactone on morbidity and mortality in patients with severe heart failure. Randomized Aldactone Evaluation Study Investigators. N Engl J Med 1999;341:709–17.
59. Pitt B, Remme W, Zannad F, et al. Eplerenone, a selective aldosterone blocker, in patients with left ventricular dysfunction after myocardial infarction. N Engl J Med 2003;348:1309–21.
60. Zannad F, McMurray JJ, Krum H, et al. Eplerenone in patients with systolic heart failure and mild symptoms. N Engl J Med 2011;364:11–21.
61. Juurlink DN, Mamdani MM, Lee DS, et al. Rates of hyperkalemia after publication of the Randomized Aldactone Evaluation Study. N Engl J Med 2004;351:543–51.
62. McMurray JJ, O'Meara E. Treatment of heart failure with spironolactone—trial and tribulations. N Engl J Med 2004;351:526–8.
63. Desai A. Hyperkalemia associated with inhibitors of the renin-angiotensin-aldosterone system: balancing risk and benefit. Circulation 2008;118:1609–11.
64. Vardeny O, Wu DH, Desai A, et al. Influence of baseline and worsening renal function on efficacy of spironolactone in patients With severe heart failure: insights from RALES (Randomized Aldactone Evaluation Study). J Am Coll Cardiol 2012;60:2082–9.
65. Pitt B, White H, Nicolau J, et al. Eplerenone reduces mortality 30 days after randomization following acute myocardial infarction in patients with left ventricular systolic dysfunction and heart failure. J Am Coll Cardiol 2005;46:425–31.
66. Pitt B, Bakris G, Ruilope LM, et al. Serum potassium and clinical outcomes in the Eplerenone Post-Acute Myocardial Infarction Heart Failure Efficacy and Survival Study (EPHESUS). Circulation 2008;118:1643–50.
67. The effect of digoxin on mortality and morbidity in patients with heart failure. The Digitalis Investigation Group. N Engl J Med 1997;336:525–33.
68. Ahmed A, Rich MW, Love TE, et al. Digoxin and reduction in mortality and hospitalization in heart failure: a comprehensive post hoc analysis of the DIG trial. Eur Heart J 2006;27:178–86.
69. Packer M, Gheorghiade M, Young JB, et al. Withdrawal of digoxin from patients with chronic heart failure treated with angiotensin-converting-enzyme inhibitors. RADIANCE Study. N Engl J Med 1993;329:1–7.
70. Uretsky BF, Young JB, Shahidi FE, et al. Randomized study assessing the effect of digoxin withdrawal in patients with mild to moderate chronic congestive heart failure: results of the PROVED trial. PROVED Investigative Group. J Am Coll Cardiol 1993;22:955–62.
71. Swedberg K, Komajda M, Bohm M, et al. Ivabradine and outcomes in chronic heart failure (SHIFT): a randomised placebo-controlled study. Lancet 2010;376:875–85.
72. Dunkman WB. Thromboembolism and antithrombotic therapy in congestive heart failure. J Cardiovasc Risk 1995;2:107–17.
73. Dunkman WB, Johnson GR, Carson PE, Bhat G, Farrell L, Cohn JN. Incidence of thromboembolic events in congestive heart failure. The V-HeFT VA Cooperative Studies Group. Circulation 1993;87:VI94–101.
74. Katz SD. Left ventricular thrombus and the incidence of thromboembolism in patients with congestive heart failure: can clinical factors identify patients at increased risk? J Cardiovasc Risk 1995;2:97–102.
75. Cokkinos DV, Toutouzas PK. Antithrombotic therapy in heart failure: a randomized comparison of warfarin vs. aspirin (HELAS). Eur J Heart Fail 1999;1:419–23.
76. Cleland JG, Findlay I, Jafri S, et al. The Warfarin/Aspirin Study in Heart Failure (WASH): a randomized trial comparing antithrombotic strategies for patients with heart failure. Am Heart J 2004;148:157–64.
77. Massie BM, Collins JF, Ammon SE, et al. Randomized trial of warfarin, aspirin, and clopidogrel in patients with chronic heart failure: the Warfarin and Antiplatelet Therapy in Chronic Heart Failure (WATCH) trial. Circulation 2009;119:1616–24.
78. Granger CB, Alexander JH, McMurray JJ, et al. Apixaban versus warfarin in patients with atrial fibrillation. N Engl J Med 2011;365:981–92.
79. Connolly SJ, Ezekowitz MD, Yusuf S, et al. Dabigatran versus warfarin in patients with atrial fibrillation. N Engl J Med 2009;361:1139–51.
80. Patel MR, Mahaffey KW, Garg J, et al. Rivaroxaban versus warfarin in nonvalvular atrial fibrillation. N Engl J Med 2011;365:883–91.
81. van Diepen S, Hellkamp AS, Patel MR, et al. Efficacy and Safety of Rivaroxaban in Patients With Heart Failure and Nonvalvular Atrial Fibrillation: Insights From ROCKET AF. Circulation 2013;6:740–7.
82. Preliminary report: effect of encainide and flecainide on mortality in a randomized trial of arrhythmia suppression after myocardial infarction. The Cardiac Arrhythmia Suppression Trial (CAST) Investigators. N Engl J Med 1989;321:406–12.
83. Waldo AL, Camm AJ, deRuyter H, et al. Effect of d-sotalol on mortality in patients with left ventricular dysfunction after recent and remote myocardial infarction. The SWORD Investigators. Survival With Oral d-Sotalol. Lancet 1996;348:7–12.
84. Kober L, Torp-Pedersen C, McMurray JJ, et al. Increased mortality after dronedarone therapy for severe heart failure. N Engl J Med 2008;358:2678–87.
85. Torp-Pedersen C, Møller M, Bloch-Thomsen PE, et al. Dofetilide in patients with congestive heart failure and left ventricular dysfunction. Danish Investigations of Arrhythmia and Mortality on Dofetilide Study Group. N Engl J Med 1999;341:857–65.
86. Singh SN, Fletcher RD, Fisher SG, et al. Amiodarone in patients with congestive heart failure and asymptomatic ventricular arrhythmia. Survival Trial of Antiarrhythmic Therapy in Congestive Heart Failure. N Engl J Med 1995;333:77–82.
87. De Bruyne LK. Mechanisms and management of diuretic resistance in congestive heart failure. Postgrad Med J 2003;79:268–71.
88. Vasko MR, Cartwright DB, Knochel JP, Nixon JV, Brater DC. Furosemide absorption altered in decompensated congestive heart failure. Ann Intern Med 1985;102:314–18.
89. Vargo DL, Kramer WG, Black PK, Smith WB, Serpas T, Brater DC. Bioavailability, pharmacokinetics, and pharmacodynamics of torsemide and furosemide in patients with congestive heart failure. Clin Pharmacol Therapeut 1995;57:601–9.
90. Tang WH, Mullens W. Cardiorenal syndrome in decompensated heart failure. Heart 2010;96:255–60.
91. Cooper HA, Dries DL, Davis CE, et al. Diuretics and risk of arrhythmic death in patients with left ventricular dysfunction. Circulation 1999;100:1311–15.
92. Ahmed A, Husain A, Love TE, et al. Heart failure, chronic diuretic use, and increase in mortality and hospitalization: an observational study using propensity score methods. Eur Heart J 2006;27:1431–9.
93. Hasselblad V, Gattis Stough W, Shah MR, et al. Relation between dose of loop diuretics and outcomes in a heart failure population: results of the ESCAPE trial. Eur J Heart Fail 2007;9:1064–9.
94. Eshaghian S, Horwich TB, Fonarow GC. Relation of loop diuretic dose to mortality in advanced heart failure. Am J Cardiol 2006;97:1759–64.
95. Neuberg GW, Miller AB, O'Connor CM, et al. Diuretic resistance predicts mortality in patients with advanced heart failure. Am Heart J 2002;144:31–8.
96. Mielniczuk LM, Tsang SW, Desai AS, et al. The association between high-dose diuretics and clinical stability in ambulatory chronic heart failure patients. J Card Fail 2008;14:388–93.
97. Felker GM, Lee KL, Bull DA, et al. Diuretic strategies in patients with acute decompensated heart failure. N Engl J Med 2011;364:797–805.
98. Tang WH, Tong W, Jain A, et al. Evaluation and long-term prognosis of new-onset, transient, and persistent anemia in ambulatory patients with chronic heart failure. J Am Coll Cardiol 2008;51:569–76.
99. Agostoni PG, Marenzi GC, Pepi M, et al. Isolated ultrafiltration in moderate congestive heart failure. J Am Coll Cardiol 1993;21:424–31.
100. Agostoni P, Marenzi G, Lauri G, et al. Sustained improvement in functional capacity after removal of body fluid with isolated ultrafiltration in chronic cardiac insufficiency: failure of furosemide to provide the same result. Am J Med 1994;96:191–9.

101. Bart BA. Treatment of congestion in congestive heart failure: ultrafiltration is the only rational initial treatment of volume overload in decompensated heart failure. Circ Heart Fail 2009;2:499–504.
102. Bart BA, Boyle A, Bank AJ, et al. Ultrafiltration versus usual care for hospitalized patients with heart failure: the Relief for Acutely Fluid-Overloaded Patients With Decompensated Congestive Heart Failure (RAPID-CHF) trial. J Am Coll Cardiol 2005;46:2043–6.
103. Costanzo MR, Guglin ME, Saltzberg MT, et al. Ultrafiltration versus intravenous diuretics for patients hospitalized for acute decompensated heart failure. J Am Coll Cardiol 2007;49:675–83.
104. Bart BA, Hernandez AF. Ultrafiltration in heart failure with cardiorenal syndrome. N Engl J Med 2013;368:1159–60.
105. Patarroyo M, Wehbe E, Hanna M, et al. Cardiorenal outcomes following slow continuous ultrafiltration therapy in refractory patients with advanced decompensated heart failure. J Am Coll Cardiol 2012;60:1906–12.
106. O'Connor CM, Starling RC, Hernandez AF, et al. Effect of nesiritide in patients with acute decompensated heart failure. N Engl J Med 2011;365:32–43.
107. Massie BM, O'Connor CM, Metra M, et al. Rolofylline, an adenosine A1-receptor antagonist, in acute heart failure. N Engl J Med;363:1419–28.
108. Konstam MA, Gheorghiade M, Burnett JC, Jr., et al. Effects of oral tolvaptan in patients hospitalized for worsening heart failure: the EVEREST Outcome Trial. JAMA 2007;297:1319–31.
109. Colucci WS, Elkayam U, Horton DP, et al. Intravenous nesiritide, a natriuretic peptide, in the treatment of decompensated congestive heart failure. Nesiritide Study Group. N Engl J Med 2000;343:246–53.
110. Sackner-Bernstein JD, Skopicki HA, Aaronson KD. Risk of worsening renal function with nesiritide in patients with acutely decompensated heart failure. Circulation 2005;111:1487–91.
111. Sackner-Bernstein JD, Kowalski M, Fox M, Aaronson K. Short-term risk of death after treatment with nesiritide for decompensated heart failure: a pooled analysis of randomized controlled trials. JAMA 2005;293:1900–5.
111a. Teerlink JR1, Cotter G, Davison BA, et al. Serelaxin, recombinant human relaxin-2, for treatment of acute heart failure (RELAX-AHF): a randomised, placebo-controlled trial. Lancet 2013;381(9860):29–39.
112. Stevenson LW. Tailored therapy to hemodynamic goals for advanced heart failure. Eur J Heart Fail 1999;1:251–7.
113. Cuffe MS, Califf RM, Adams KF, Jr., et al. Short-term intravenous milrinone for acute exacerbation of chronic heart failure: a randomized controlled trial. JAMA 2002;287:1541–7.
114. Elkayam U, Tasissa G, Binanay C, et al. Use and impact of inotropes and vasodilator therapy in hospitalized patients with severe heart failure. Am Heart J 2007;153:98–104.
115. Packer M, Colucci WS, Fisher L, et al. Effect of levosimendan on the short-term clinical course of patients with acutely decompensated heart failure. JACC Heart Fail 2013;1:103–11.
116. Hershberger RE, Nauman D, Walker TL, et al. Care processes and clinical outcomes of continuous outpatient support with inotropes (COSI) in patients with refractory endstage heart failure. J Card Fail 2003;9:180–7.
117. Miller LW. Outpatient dobutamine for refractory congestive heart failure: advantages, techniques, and results. J Heart Lung Transplant 1991;10:482–7.
118. Butler J, Chomsky DB, Wilson JR. Pulmonary hypertension and exercise intolerance in patients with heart failure. J Am Coll Cardiol 1999;34:1802–6.
119. Khush KK, Tasissa G, Butler J, et al. Effect of pulmonary hypertension on clinical outcomes in advanced heart failure: analysis of the Evaluation Study of Congestive Heart Failure and Pulmonary Artery Catheterization Effectiveness (ESCAPE) database. Am Heart J 2009;157:1026–34.
120. Fang JC, DeMarco T, Givertz MM, et al. World Health Organization Pulmonary Hypertension group 2: pulmonary hypertension due to left heart disease in the adult—a summary statement from the Pulmonary Hypertension Council of the International Society for Heart and Lung Transplantation. J Heart Lung Transplant 2012;31:913–33.
121. Ghio S, Gavazzi A, Campana C, et al. Independent and additive prognostic value of right ventricular systolic function and pulmonary artery pressure in patients with chronic heart failure. J Am Coll Cardiol 2001;37:183–8.
122. Anavekar NS, Skali H, Bourgoun M, et al. Usefulness of right ventricular fractional area change to predict death, heart failure, and stroke following myocardial infarction (from the VALIANT ECHO Study). Am J Cardiol 2008;101:607–12.
123. Bocchi EA, Bacal F, Auler Junior JO, et al. Inhaled nitric oxide leading to pulmonary edema in stable severe heart failure. Am J Cardiol 1994;74:70–2.
124. Torre-Amione G, Young JB, Colucci WS, et al. Hemodynamic and clinical effects of tezosentan, an intravenous dual endothelin receptor antagonist, in patients hospitalized for acute decompensated heart failure. J Am Coll Cardiol 2003;42:140–7.
125. Coletta AP, Cleland JG. Clinical trials update: highlights of the scientific sessions of the XXIII Congress of the European Society of Cardiology—WARIS II, ESCAMI, PAFAC, RITZ-1 and TIME. Eur J Heart Fail 2001;3:747–50.
126. Louis A, Cleland JG, Crabbe S, et al. Clinical Trials Update: CAPRICORN, COPERNICUS, MIRACLE, STAF, RITZ-2, RECOVER and RENAISSANCE and cachexia and cholesterol in heart failure. Highlights of the Scientific Sessions of the American College of Cardiology 2001. Eur J Heart Fail 2001;3:381–7.
127. Kaluski E, Kobrin I, Zimlichman R, et al. RITZ-5: randomized intravenous TeZosentan (an endothelin-A/B antagonist) for the treatment of pulmonary edema: a prospective, multicenter, double-blind, placebo-controlled study. J Am Coll Cardiol 2003;41:204–10.
128. McMurray JJ, Teerlink JR, Cotter G, et al. Effects of tezosentan on symptoms and clinical outcomes in patients with acute heart failure: the VERITAS randomized controlled trials. JAMA 2007;298:2009–19.
129. Lewis GD, Shah R, Shahzad K, et al. Sildenafil improves exercise capacity and quality of life in patients with systolic heart failure and secondary pulmonary hypertension. Circulation 2007;116:1555–62.
130. Guazzi M, Vicenzi M, Arena R, Guazzi MD. PDE5 inhibition with sildenafil improves left ventricular diastolic function, cardiac geometry, and clinical status in patients with stable systolic heart failure: results of a 1-year, prospective, randomized, placebo-controlled study. Circ Heart Fail 2011;4:8–17.
131. Redfield MM, Chen HH, Borlaug BA, et al. Effect of phosphodiesterase-5 inhibition on exercise capacity and clinical status in heart failure with preserved ejection fraction: a randomized clinical trial. JAMA 2013;309:1268–77.
132. Zimpfer D, Zrunek P, Roethy W, et al. Left ventricular assist devices decrease fixed pulmonary hypertension in cardiac transplant candidates. J Thorac Cardiovasc Surg 2007;133:689–95.
133. Haft J, Armstrong W, Dyke DB, et al. Hemodynamic and exercise performance with pulsatile and continuous-flow left ventricular assist devices. Circulation 2007;116:I8–15.
134. Ernst ME, Moser M. Use of diuretics in patients with hypertension. N Engl J Med 2009;361:2153–64.
135. Braunwald EB. The Path to an Angiotensin Receptor Antagonist-Neprilysin Inhibitor in the Treatment of Heart Failure. J Am Coll Cardiol 2015;65(10):1029–41.
136. McMurray JJV. Neprilysin inhibition to treat heart failure: a tale of science, serendipity, and second chances. Eur J Heart Fail 2015;17:242–47.
137. Mcmurray JJV, Packer M, Desai AS, et al. Angiotensin–Neprilysin Inhibition versus Enalapril in Heart Failure. N Engl J Med 2014;371:993–1004.
138. Desai AS, McMurray JJ, Packer M, et al. Effect of the angiotensin-receptor-neprilysin inhibitor LCZ696 compared with enalapril on mode of death in heart failure patients. Eur Heart J 2015 Aug 7;36(30):1990–7.

CHAPTER 9

Arrhythmias in heart failure: The atrioventricular node and above

Steven Stevens MD, Kalyanam Shivkumar MD PhD, and Noel G. Boyle MD PhD

Atrial fibrillation

Atrial fibrillation (AF) and congestive heart failure (CHF) commonly occur together and each may exacerbate the other. The Framingham Heart Study demonstrated that each condition increases the risk for developing the other. There is a 15% 5-year incidence of new-onset CHF among patients with AF; the converse is also true, with a 25% 5-year incidence of new AF in patients with CHF.[1] The prevalence of AF progresses with worsening CHF: AF occurs in 10% of of patients in New York Heart Association (NYHA) class I and II, and in up to 50% in NYHA class IV.[2]

Pathophysiology

AF and CHF are interconnected in a complex interplay, in which each contributes to progression of the other. AF contributes to CHF via loss of atrioventricular (AV) synchrony which decreases cardiac output and leads to diastolic dysfunction. Irregular and rapid ventricular responses lead to variable filling cycles and inadequate handling of diastolic volume loading of the left ventricle. CHF leads to rising filling pressures which decrease left atrial (LA) compliance, and increase LA pressure, which stretches the tissues. There is activation of the renin–aldosterone–angiotensin system (RAAS) which promotes scarring and fibrosis of the LA, which leads to shortened refractoriness of the atrial tissues and conditions favorable for maintenance AF. The end result is LA enlargement, diastolic dysfunction, increased filling pressures with lower cardiac output, and predisposition for sustaining AF and progression of heart failure (Figure 9.1).[3]

Ionic and microscopic remodeling can be seen acutely in AF, with reductions in L-type calcium channels and potassium currents which occurs over 1–2 days, with structural remodeling of sarcoplasmic reticulum, changes in nuclear chromatin staining, and changes in connexin-40 sarcomere structures which occur over 1 week.[4] Sarcomere calcium handling is changed in the atrium with calcium overload and reduction in ryanodine receptor and calsequestrin expression, which lead to increased triggered activity. Furthermore, decreased atrial contractility results from decreases in phosphorylated protein kinase A and myosin-binding protein kinase C.[5]

Insights into the interplay of AF and heart failure have been demonstrated by Nattel and coworkers. In a canine model of ventricular tachypacing induced CHF (220–240 bpm for 5 weeks), ionic remodeling reversed within 4 weeks, but not structural remodeling.[6] Interestingly, in this study there was partial reversibility of structural remodeling with decreased fibrosis observed after treatment of angiotensin converting enzyme (ACE) inhibitors and also decreased angiotensin II levels.

Knowledge of the electrical mechanisms of AF activation and propagation remains limited. A landmark observation by Haïssaguerre et al. was that the pulmonary veins could be a source of ectopic rhythms which can trigger paroxysmal AF.[7] This is the foundation of modern AF ablation and pulmonary vein isolation. However, as AF persists and the atria remodel, reentrant circuits become predominant in the maintenance of the fibrillation. Two proposed theories are the *multiple wavelet theory*, which describes a diffuse process, and the *reentry rotors theory*, a more focal process, hence amendable to ablation.[8,9] Reentry rotors, first demonstrated in sheep hearts and recently successfully ablated in human hearts, may provide a mechanistic approach to ablation of more persistent AF.[10,11,12] Overall, AF likely has multiple mechanisms at play, but clearly there are ectopic triggers, and as well as a propensity for reentry to maintain AF (Figure 9.2).[13,14]

Although study of the mechanisms in the persistence of AF has been insightful in understanding the interplay with CHF, current treatment options are limited by lack of therapies to reverse this pathophysiology. Hence, current treatment approaches are targeted toward reduction in the frequency and duration of episodes, control of heart rate, and stroke reduction.

Clinical

AF is classified clinically as paroxysmal (self-terminating episodes lasting <7 days), persistent (non-self-terminating episodes lasting 7 days to 6 months), and permanent (AF for >6 months for which attempts at termination have failed or which is an accepted rhythm). Paroxysms of AF or runs of rapid ventricular response may instigate heart failure exacerbation or be caused by heart failure exacerbation. Therefore, treatment goals of heart failure must address AF.

Therapeutic approaches require risk stratification for stroke and assessment of need for anticoagulation, control of ventricular rate, and attempts to maintain sinus rhythm (when appropriate). AF treatment strategies can be divided into rate control and rhythm control. Fortunately, many of the same medications used to treat heart failure also treat AF: β-blockers and digoxin will

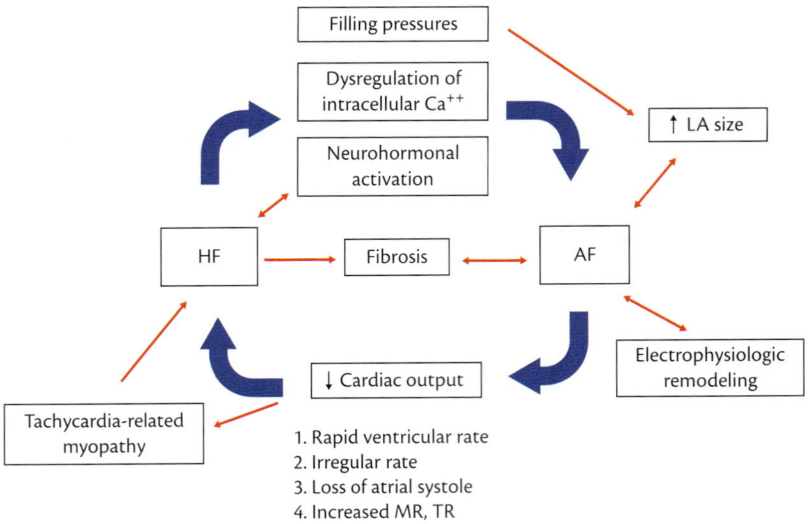

Fig. 9.1 Pathophysiological interactions of atrial fibrillation and heart failure. LA, left atrium; MR, mitral regurgitation, TR, tricuspid regurgitation.
Anter E, Jessup M, Callans DJ. Atrial Fibrillation and Heart Failure. Circulation 2009; 119: 2516–25.

help control heart rate, while ACE inhibitors may lead to reverse remodeling and reductions in AF burden. Antiarrhythmic drugs, on the other hand, do not have a primary role in the treatment of heart failure; hence the rhythm control strategy, although effective in treating AF, has not demonstrated a survival benefit in heart failure patients.[15] Except for amiodarone and dofetilide, most antiarrhythmics have been shown to increase mortality in patients with structural heart disease and heart failure.[16,17,18] Furthermore, risk stratification for stroke is central to the management of AF, especially in CHF which increases the risk of thromboembolism (Figure 9.3).[19]

Rate control

Rate control in the acute phase of heart failure can be achieved with intravenous calcium channel blockers or β-blockers.[20] These medications should be used with caution in the hypotensive or low normotensive patient, since hypotension may be exacerbated by negative inotropic medications. Infusions of short-acting medications such as esmolol may be useful to allow for a quickly reversible therapeutic trial, although such an approach is not evidence based. If rate control cannot be tolerated because of hypotension, then either inotropic blood pressure support and/or emergent cardioversion may be required.[21]

The strategy for long-term rate control has more evidence basis than acute treatment. β-Blockers serve a dual role in treating heart failure and controlling rate, whereas digoxin is beneficial as an adjunct and also reduces heart failure exacerbations. The combination therapy with carvedilol and digoxin has been found more effective than either alone.[22] The target for heart rate in the AF Follow-up Investigation of Rhythm Management (AFFIRM) trial was defined as less than 80 beats per minute at rest, and 110 beats per minute during a 6-minute walk test.[23] The Rate Control Efficacy (RACE-2) trial randomized patients to conventional strict control (<80 beats per minute at rest) or to a "lenient" approach (<110 beats per minute at rest) and found there to be no significant difference in mortality, NYHA class, and heart failure hospitalizations.[24]

Rhythm control

Maintenance of sinus rhythm with a strategy that may include a combination of rate control therapy, antiarrhythmic medication, cardioversion, and radiofrequency ablation can be especially challenging in the heart failure patient. Several factors make rhythm control more difficult to achieve in this patient population, including LA enlargement, comorbidities such as hypertension and obstructive sleep apnea, increased sympathetic tone, and lack of safe antiarrhythmic medications in structural heart disease. Nevertheless, despite lack of advantages over rate control in mortality, stroke reduction, or hospitalization, rhythm control has a vital role in treating symptomatic patients.

Acute rhythm control can be achieved with either pharmacotherapy or direct current (DC) cardioversion. Electrical cardioversion with 200 J biphasic energy with pads placed in the anterior-posterior position is over 94% effective (compared to 79% with monophasic energy), and there is little benefit and potential harm (from repeat cardioversion) in using lower energy levels.[21,25,26] Adverse events from cardioversion are rare, and include stroke, arrhythmia, and skin burns.[26,27] In the CHF patient, care must be taken to assess for hypokalemia and/or digoxin toxicity prior to cardioversion. Potassium repletion, especially if the patient is on digoxin, is important to reduce the risk of ventricular arrhythmias. The 7% risk of stroke without anticoagulation is the most serious complication, and this can be greatly reduced.[28] Comparison of strategies to reduce stroke associated with cardioversion have demonstrated equivalence of anticoagulation for 4 weeks followed by cardioversion and performing a transesophageal echocardiogram immediately before cardioversion to exclude appendage thrombus.[21,29] Important to remember is that the risk of stroke persists after cardioversion due to atrial stunning, and anticoagulation should be continued for a minimum of 4 weeks.[21] Patients in AF over 48 hours before cardioversion will have increased risk of thromboembolism formation in the LA appendage,[28,30] and should be managed similarly to those with AF of unknown duration, discussed above. Optimization of heart failure status before cardioversion is essential, as increased sympathetic

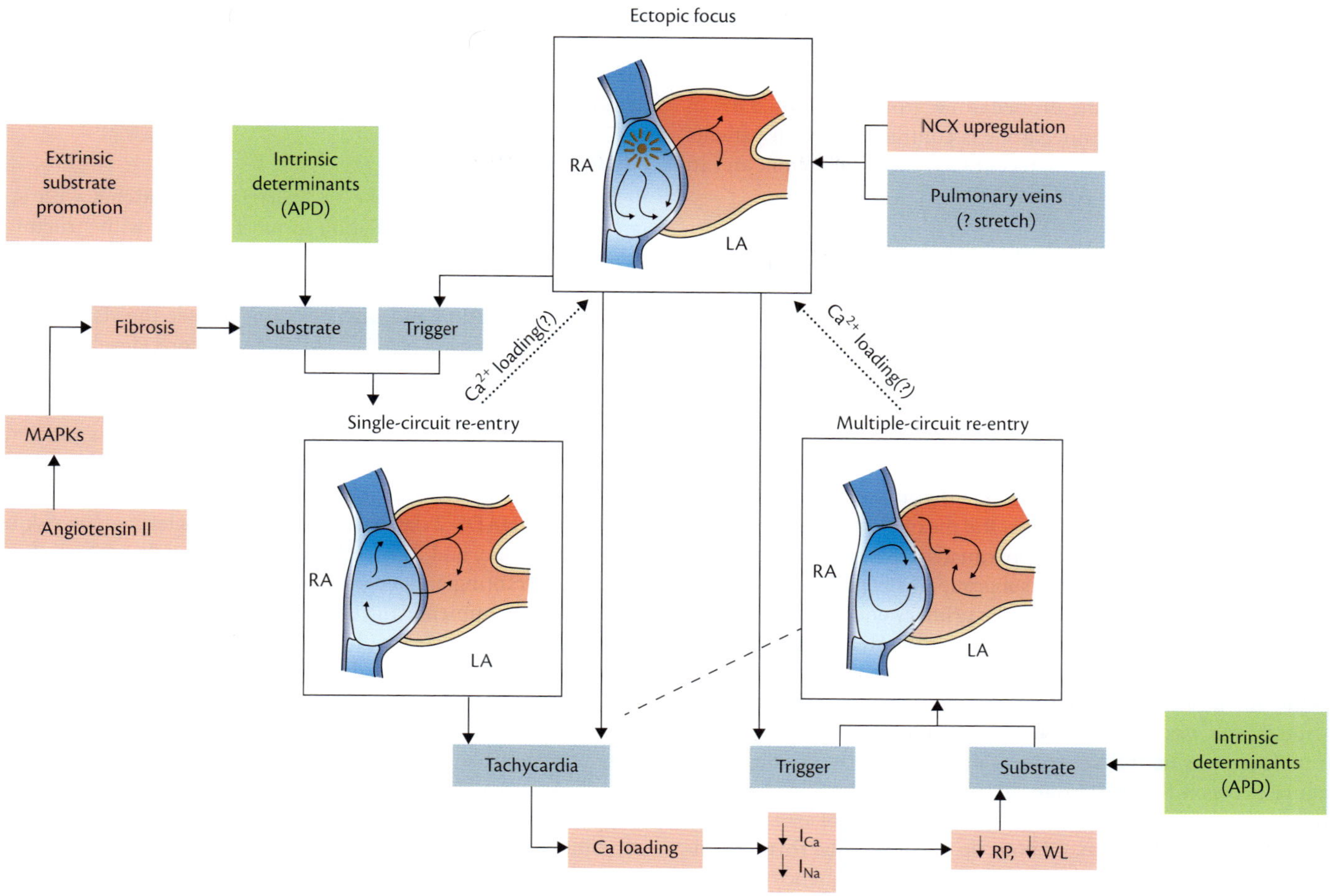

Fig. 9.2 Principal mechanisms that can produce atrial fibrillation (AF). Reentry involves a vulnerable substrate, which requires a trigger for reentry initiation. Ischemia, inflammation, and dilation make atria more vulnerable to AF. AF that results from any mechanism causes tachycardia-induced remodeling. Even if AF is initially maintained by ectopic activity or single-circuit reentry in a given patient, spatially heterogeneous refractoriness induced by atrial tachycardia remodeling (ATR) creates conditions favorable to multiple-circuit reentry, which may then become the AF-maintaining mechanism. Thus, multiple-circuit re-entry may be a final common pathway AF mechanism in many patients. LA, left atrium; PVs, pulmonary veins; RA, right atrium; RP, refractory period; WL, wavelength; APD, action potential duration; NCX, sodium calcium exchanger; MAPKs, mitogen-activated protein kinases.

Adapted from Nattel S. et al., (2008) Basic Science for the Clinical Electrophysiologist: Atrial Remodelling and Atrial Fibrillation, Circulation: Arrhythmia and Electrophysiology, 1, 62–68 and Nattel, S. (2002) New Ideas about Atrial Fibrillation 50 years on, Nature 415, 219–226.

tone in heart failure exacerbations will also predispose to early recurrence of AF.

Pharmacological cardioversion when done safely provides a less invasive option but a lower success rate with higher risk of adverse drug effects. Ibutilide is approximately 50% effective at cardioversion; however, the risk of torsades de pointes increases to 11.4% compared to 3.6% in non-heart-failure patients.[31,32] Class Ic agents flecainide and propafenone are contraindicated in structural heart disease because of proarrhythmia, and should not be used for chemical cardioversion.[33] Amiodarone remains an option for medical cardioversion; however, amiodarone given intravenously concomitantly with an oral load achieved sinus rhythm in 80% within 1 month (50% within 24 hours) compared to 40% of placebo patients.[34] However, a lower success rate would be expected in patients with structural heart disease, and the conversion rate is lower among patients with LA enlargement.[34]

Like acute management, drug therapy for maintenance of sinus rhythm in structural heart disease has only a few viable options. Several trials including the AFFIRM, the Sotalol-Amiodarone Atrial Fibrillation Efficacy Trial (SAFE-T), and Canadian Trial of Atrial Fibrillation(CTAF) have demonstrated amiodarone to be approximately 70% effective in maintaining sinus rhythm at 1 year, and more effective than sotalol or class I agents (40%).[15,35,36] More importantly, in the Grupo de Estudio de la Sobrevida en la Insuficienca Cardica en Argentina (GESICA trial), low-dose amiodarone (300 mg) proved to be safe in severe CHF (80% NYHA III–IV), with reduction in mortality (33% vs. 41%, $p = 0.024$ over 2 years).[37]

The only other antiarrhythmic medication that has demonstrated safety in heart failure in large randomized trial is dofetilide. Specifically, NYHA class II and III heart failure patients were studied in the Danish Investigators of Arrhythmia and Mortality on Dofetilide (Diamond HF) trial, where dofetilide maintained sinus rhythm in 75% of patients at 1 year. However, because of 3% risk of torsades, inpatient hospitalization to monitor for QT prolongation during initiation is mandatory.[38]

More recently, dronedarone initially showed promise as a novel class III agent similar to amiodarone, but without toxicity related to the iodine moiety. However, the ANDROMEDA study randomized 627 patients hospitalized for heart failure to dronedarone or placebo and found an early increase in death related to heart failure exacerbation in the dronedarone group, 8.1% vs. 3.8% at 2 months.[17] Currently dronedarone is contraindicated in patients with NYHA class IV CHF or recent CHF hospitalization, and in patients with permanent AF.[17,39,40]

Rate control versus rhythm control

The landmark study comparing rate control to rhythm control is the AFFIRM trial, reported in 2002.[41] In summary, there was no difference in mortality or thromboembolic events between the two groups with 5 years of follow-up. The mean age of patients in the trial was 69 years. Entry required AF, an additional risk factor for stroke, and controlled symptoms. Since the rhythm control strategy is generally used to control symptoms of AF, this trial was not designed to address the effectiveness of rhythm control for the indication of symptom relief. Of note, the mean ejection fraction (EF) in both groups was 55%, and approximately 23% of the patients had a history of heart failure. In the subgroup of 939 patients with heart failure there was no difference in the primary endpoint.

The Atrial Fibrillation and Congestive Heart Failure Trial (AF-CHF) compared rhythm control versus rate control in 1376 patients with EF less than 35% and clinical heart failure.[15] Amiodarone was used in 82% of patients in the rhythm control arm. There was no difference in death, stroke, or worsening heart failure between the two groups at 5 years of follow-up. Freedom from AF was achieved in just 20% in the rate control arm and 70% in the rhythm control arm. Of note, no patients in the rhythm control arm of this study were treated with radiofrequency ablation (Figure 9.4).

While rhythm control does not lead to decreased mortality or heart failure, it remains a preferred option in symptomatic patients. The restoration and maintenance of sinus rhythm is a good prognostic indicator, as evident in CHF-STAT trial and Diamond HF studies, each showing a reduction in mortality if sinus rhythm is restored.[42] In summary, the choice between a strategy of rhythm versus rate control should be guided by management of symptoms and patient preference, with no significant difference in mortality or stroke demonstrated in clinical trials.

Anticoagulation

Reduction in risk for stroke in heart failure patients with AF requires systemic anticoagulation in most patients with structural heart disease. Heart failure itself carries a 2.8% annual risk of stroke in the CHADS-2 validation study, and common comorbidities such as hypertension and diabetes can increase the risk to 5.8% per year.[19] The more recent CHADS-VASc score, developed in a Danish registry, offers a more refined risk stratification, by adding an extra point for female gender and vascular disease, and a two-tier point system for age: 1 point for age 65–75 years and 2 for age over 75 years. This results in reclassification of the lower-risk patients in the CHADS-2 system, with 39% of those deemed low risk by the CHADS-2 database reclassified as intermediate risk by CHA2DS2-VASc, and 21% reclassified as high risk, with all these patients warranting anticoagulation.[43,44] The European Society of Cardiology recommends the CHA2DS2-VASc score as first line in risk stratification for stroke (Table 9.1).[45]

Warfarin remains the gold standard for preventive treatment in AF patients at intermediate or high risk for stroke. A pooled meta-analysis of the five placebo controlled trials confirms a 68% reduction in stroke for patients taking warfarin compared to placebo.[46] Anti-platelet agents, aspirin and clopidogrel have been compared to warfarin and are much less efficacious, even when combined.[47] However, warfarin has many downsides, including requiring frequent INR testing, dietary consistency, and careful management to avoid drug interactions.

The availability of the newer anticoagulants made an immediate impact in the field of stroke prevention in AF. The novel anticoagulants include a direct thrombin inhibitor (dabigatran) and factor XA inhibitors (rivaroxaban, abixaban and edoxaban). The Randomized Evaluation of Long-term Anticoagulation (RELY)

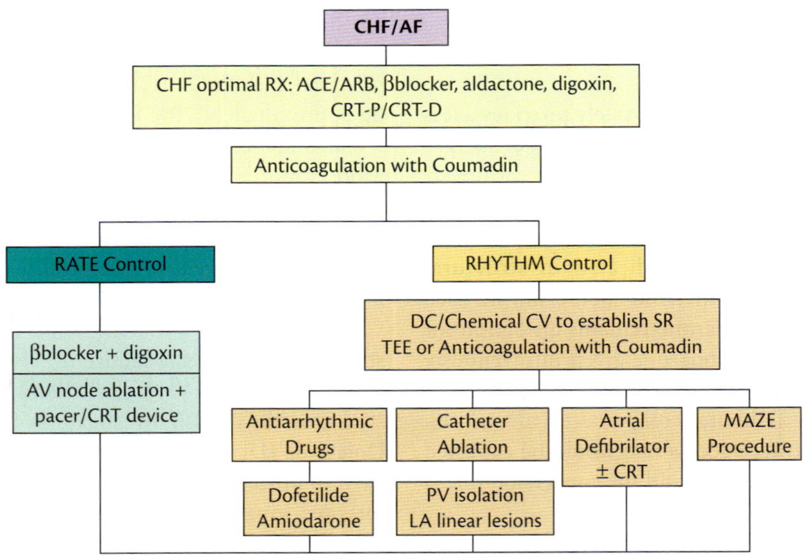

Fig. 9.3 Overview of the management of patients with atrial fibrillation and congestive heart failure.
Reprinted from Cardiology Clinics, 27(1), Boyle N, Shivkumar K, Atrial Fibrillation in Congestive Heart Failure, 79–93, copyright (2009) with permission from Elsevier.

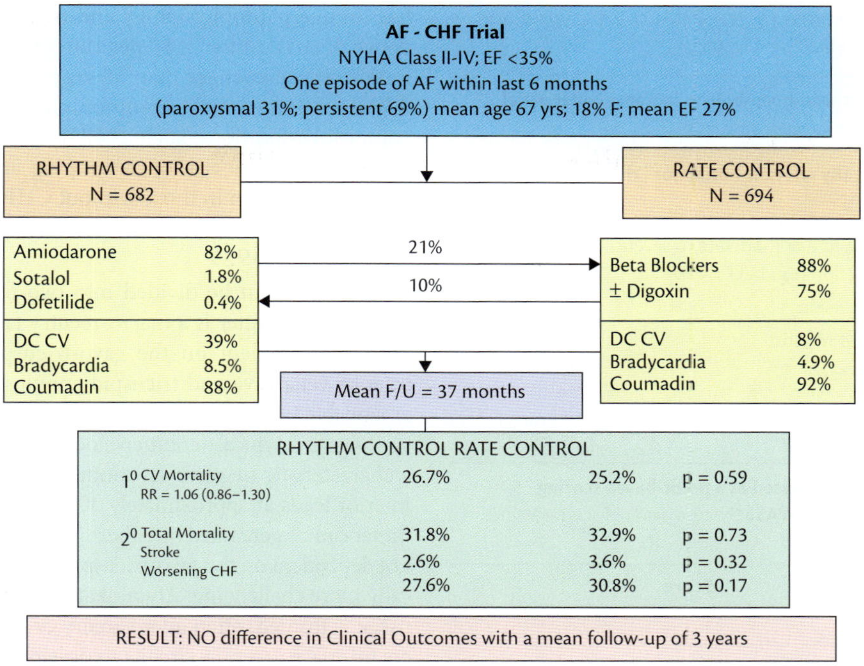

Fig. 9.4 Design and outcomes of the AF-CHF trial.

Reprinted from Cardiology Clinics, 27(1), Boyle N, Shivkumar K, Atrial Fibrillation in Congestive Heart Failure, 79–93, copyright (2009) with permission from Elsevier.

trial, reported in 2009, compared dabigatran to warfarin, and found that at 150 mg twice a day dosing dabigatran was superior for stroke reduction with equivalent bleeding risks. Rivaroxaban had similar results in a clinical trial in 2011, with the advantage of once a day dosing.[48] Apixiban also showed superiority over warfarin for stroke prevention, mortality, and bleeding in a randomized clinical trial reported in 2011.[49] A meta-analysis confirmed the superiority and increased safety of the three novel antithrombotics over warfarin. In the 44 563 patients analyzed there was a 22% relative reduction in stroke, 12% reduction in all-cause mortality, and 55% reduction in intracranial hemorrhage.[50] Disadvantages of the novel anticoagulants include gastrointestinal side effects, lack of monitoring to confirm compliance, and cost. Another concern is that 3 of the current 4 novel anticoagulants do not have a reversal agent available at present. For Dabigatran, a monoclonal antibody reversal agent, idarucizumab, was recently approved for clinical use.

It is estimated that up to 90% of intracardiac thrombi responsible for stroke in patients with AF originate in the LA appendage.[51] Invasive methods to prevent stroke in AF include surgical excision of the atrial appendage or percutaneous occlusion of the appendage ostium. The Watchman occlusion device was evaluated in a randomized trial, and had similar stroke rates as warfarin, though the procedural complication rate was too high to warrant approval by the US Food and Drug Administration (FDA).[52] Newer methods are under investigation, including the Lariat atrial occluder, which requires percutaneous pericardial access to tie off the appendage externally.[53] Lastly, surgical appendage closure at the time of other cardiac surgery may reduce stroke rates, though clinical data are lacking and thrombus is often seen on transesophageal echo even after attempted closure.[54] One problem with this approach is that approximately 35% of strokes that occur in AF occur from sources other than the appendage including the cerebral vasculature and the aorta.[46]

Catheter ablation

AF ablation with pulmonary vein isolation remains a viable treatment option for symptomatic AF that cannot be treated adequately with antiarrhythmic therapy.[55] Heart failure patients often have multiple comorbidities and LA enlargement, making them unfavorable ablation candidates. However, single-center studies have demonstrated similar efficacy in catheter ablation for AF in heart failure patients as compared with normal controls, with freedom of AF at 1 year around 70%.[56,57] Hsu et al. found that in the 86% of patients with inadequate rate control, a 20% increase in EF was achieved with AF ablation, which raises the possibility that tachycardia-related cardiomyopathy plays a larger role in heart failure with AF than generally appreciated.[56]

An intriguing study, the Pulmonary Vein Antrum Isolation versus AV Node Ablation with Biventricular Pacing for Treatment of Atrial Fibrillation in Patients with Congestive Heart Failure (PABA-CHF), demonstrated that pulmonary vein isolation resulted in improved 6-minute walk distance, increased EF, and improved symptoms compared to AV node ablation and pacing.[58] While pulmonary vein isolation can be valuable in reducing the frequency of AF in paroxysmal AF, the efficacy is much lower in patients with long-term persistent or permanent AF.[59] If rate control cannot be achieved medically, then AV node ablation with biventricular pacing remains a viable option. Data in the heart failure population is lacking, but a meta-analysis of 1181 patients who underwent AV node ablation and pacemaker implantation demonstrated improved outcomes in symptoms, NYHA functional class, EF, and hospitalizations compared to medical management.[60]

Atrial flutter

Atrial flutter often is grouped into the same category as AF, and while many of the clinical features remain common to both, each

Table 9.1 (a) Risk factors for stroke; (b) the CHADS-VASc score, and (c) adjusted stroke rates for CHADS-VASc scores

(a) Risk factors for stroke and thromboembolism in nonvalvular atrial fibrillation

"Major" risk factors	"Clinically relevant nonmajor" risk factors
Previous stroke, TIA, or systemic embolism	Heart failure or moderate to severe LV systolic dysfunction (e.g., LVEF £40%)
Age >75 years	Hypertension
	Diabetes mellitus
	Female sex
	Age 65–74 years
	Vascular disease[a]

(b) Risk factor-based approach expressed as a point-based scoring system, with the acronym CHA2DS2-VASc (Note: maximum score is 9 since age may contribute 0, 1, or 2 points)

Risk factor	Score
CHF/LV dysfunction	1
Hypertension	1
Age ≥75 years	2
Diabetes mellitus	1
Stroke/TIA/ thromboembolism	2
Vascular disease[a]	1
Age 65–74	1
Sex category (i.e., female sex)	1
Maximum score	9

(c) Adjusted stroke rate according to CHA_2D5_2-VASc score

CHA_2DS_2-VASc score	Patients (n = 7329)	Adjusted stroke rate (%/ year)[b]
0	1	0%
I	422	1.3%
2	1230	2.2%
3	1730	3.2%
4	1718	4.0%
5	1159	6.7%
6	679	9.8%
7	294	9.6%
8	82	6.7%
9	14	15.2%

CHF, congestive heart failure; LV, left ventricle; TIA, transient ischemic attack.

[a] Prior myocardial infarction, peripheral artery disease, aortic plaque. Actual rates of stroke in contemporary cohorts may vary from these estimates.

[b] Based on Lip et al.[43]

From ESC Guidelines on Atrial Fibrillation, European Heart Journal 2010; 31:2369–2429. With permission of Oxford University Press (UK) © European Society of Cardiology, www.escardio.org/guidelines.

has unique pathophysiology and treatment approaches. The incidence of atrial flutter is 88 per 100 000 person years, but is uncommon in those younger than 50 years, at only 5 per 100 000.[61] Like AF, atrial flutter most commonly occurs in patients with other comorbid conditions, such as CHF, or conditions leading to atrial enlargement. The risk of developing atrial flutter in CHF is 3.5 times greater than in those without CHF.[61]

Pathophysiology

Atrial flutter can be divided into two forms, typical and atypical. Typical atrial flutter is a macro-reentry tachyarrhythmia in the right atrium, dependent on the cavo-tricuspid isthmus (between the inferior vena cava and tricuspid annulus) conduction slowing, and amendable to catheter ablation at that isthmus. On a 12-lead electrocardiogram, typical (counter-clockwise) atrial flutter demonstrates a characteristic negative sawtooth pattern of the flutter waves in the inferior leads at approximately 300 beats per minute. Atypical atrial flutter can be generated by either right or LA reentrant circuits that are not dependent on the cavo-tricuspid isthmus, making ablation technically more challenging. Atypical atrial flutter usually occurs after scar tissue is formed, often after surgery or ablation, which creates barriers for macro-reentry circuits to develop. Early studies demonstrated that atrial flutter loops could be induced and mapped epicardially after applying crush injury to the right atria, and could be terminated by extending the lesion to the area between the AV groove and the inferior vena cava, which is currently the target for isthmus ablation.[62] Atrial flutter has been studied extensively and as a model for macro-reentry arrhythmias. Principles for mapping and catheter ablation for many arrhythmias come from the original work by Waldo et al. describing techniques for entraining reentry circuits of atrial flutter.[63]

Clinical

The effects of atrial flutter on heart failure are deleterious. In 1999, Alboni et al. took hemodynamic measurements of 23 consecutive patients in atrial flutter and sinus rhythm and demonstrated increased atrial pressures with a subsequent fall in systemic systolic pressure and rise in diastolic pressures.[64] Consequently, like AF, atrial flutter may lead to heart failure exacerbation. While AF has a wealth of clinical data to establish evidence-based treatment strategies in rate control, rhythm control, and anticoagulation, atrial flutter is less common and there is less evidence-based data. Therefore, treatment strategies for rate control and anticoagulation for atrial flutter are often grouped under the same approaches as for AF, and are similar to those discussed in the previous section. The risk of stroke in atrial flutter has been evaluated in retrospective analysis as well as a small prospective study, and ranges from 1.6% to 2.3%, slightly less than that of AF.[65,66] The most fundamental difference in atrial flutter, as compared to AF, is that it is a more organized rhythm, and more difficult to rate control adequately, and because of this, rhythm control is often the preferred strategy. Fortunately, in contrast to AF, catheter-based treatment for typical atrial flutter is highly effective, and often curative, and the guidelines reflect this by making initial catheter ablation for recurrent symptomatic typical atrial flutter a recommended treatment strategy.[67]

Catheter ablation

The majority of atrial flutter rhythms are right atrial and cavo-tricuspid isthmus dependent and therefore amendable to catheter ablation by creating a line of block along the isthmus between the inferior vena cava and tricuspid valve. In a randomized controlled trial, Natale et al. compared atrial flutter ablation to antiarrhythmic medication in 61 patients, and over 21 months of follow-up the radiofrequency ablation group was in sinus rhythm more often (80% vs. 36%, $p < 0.01$) and had higher quality of life and fewer hospitalizations.[68] Subsequently, a randomized multicenter trial compared atrial flutter ablation as first-line therapy to medical therapy with amiodarone. Of note, 62% of the patients in this study had structural heart disease. Over a mean of 13 months of follow-up, atrial flutter recurred in 3.8% in the ablation group and 29.5% in the amiodarone group ($p < 0.01$).[69] Among the various studies evaluating radiofrequency (RF) ablation of atrial flutter, the success rate for long-term freedom from recurrence of atrial flutter is consistently greater than 90%.[70] One caveat is that there is a high concordance of atrial flutter and AF, so that successful ablation of atrial flutter may not effect the later occurrence of AF. This was demonstrated in 59 patients who underwent atrial flutter ablation and followed for a mean of 13 months, with 9.4% having recurrent atrial flutter and 26.4% with recurrent AF.[71] Another relationship between AF and flutter is that when AF is treated with antiarrhythmics, the rhythm can organize to atrial flutter, which is often right sided and isthmus dependent, which may be effectively treated by ablation.[72] Overall the low complication rate coupled with a high success rate of isthmus-dependent atrial flutter catheter ablation has a class I indication as first-line treatment in both US and European guidelines.[67]

Atypical atrial flutter is less common and it is usually found in patients with atrial scarring such as congenital heart disease, after surgical scars in the right or left atrium, and after previous ablation. Catheter ablation for atypical flutter is technically more challenging and often less successful than for typical atrial flutter. If the rate cannot be controlled and ablation is unsuccessful, AV node ablation with biventricular pacing may be the only option in these challenging patients.

Supraventricular tachycardias

Supraventricular tachycardias (SVT), including AV nodal rentry, accessory pathway-mediated tachycardia, and atrial tachycardia occur in patients with and without structural heart disease. However, if left untreated any incessant tachycardia can lead to ventricular dysfunction and dilation, known as tachycardia-related cardiomyopathy. Therefore, this section discusses tachycardia-related cardiomyopathy as a consequence of SVT.

The three major categories of SVT include: (1) AV nodal reentry tachycardia, related to paroxysmal reentry tachycardia occurring within the slow and fast pathways in the AV node; (2) accessory pathway-mediated tachycardia, either in the form of (a) orthodromic, narrow complex tachycardia with reentry down the AV node and up the accessory pathway or (b) preexcited supraventricular tachycardia, with antegrade conduction over the accessory pathway and retrograde conduction over the AV node; (3) atrial tachycardia caused by a focal or microreentry rhythm initiating in the atrium. All of these SVT mechanisms can cause tachycardia-related cardiomyopathy, as can AF and atrial flutter, and controlling the rate is paramount to treatment of the resulting cardiomyopathy. Likewise, in patients with known structural heart disease, SVT can exacerbate heart failure and treatment of the tachycardia is clinically important.

Tachycardia-mediated cardiomyopathy

This was first demonstrated in an experiment by Whipple et al., who paced canine hearts at 330 beats per minute and demonstrated signs of CHF in the dogs.[73] Likewise, supraventricular tachycardia was demonstrated to cause cardiomyopathy in pigs through rapid atria pacing, with structural abnormalities seen at 1 week, and progressing to severe dilatation with biventricular failure by 3 weeks.[74] Cellular mechanisms of tachycardia-related cardiomyopathy include depletion of ATP reserves, oxidative stress, and ultimately fibrosis. This process can be limited by treatment with ACE inhibitors and antioxidants before rapid pacing.[75,76]

Often patients are diagnosed with initial presentation of heart failure and tachycardia, and it may be difficult to distinguish if the tachycardia is secondary to the cardiomyopathy or if it is causal. This may be especially true in nonischemic cardiomyopathy, which may follow the same clinical course of tachycardia-related cardiomyopathy, including improvement over time after initiation of treatment. One diagnostic dilemma is that other forms of cardiomyopathy do not exclude a comorbid tachycardia-related cardiomyopathy, and certainly tachycardia can make any form of structural heart disease acutely and chronically worse. Overall, the contribution of tachycardia-related cardiomyopathy to patients with systolic dysfunction may be underappreciated (Figure 9.5).[77] In a multicenter prospective cohort of AF patients with EF less than 45% who underwent AV nodal ablation, 25% of patients subsequently had improvement in EF to more than 45% over 12 months, hence tachycardia may have been contributing to the cardiomyopathy.[78] Tachycardia-related cardiomyopathy typically improves with treatment of the abnormal heart rate, though the heart may not completely normalize. This was demonstrated in a cohort of 24 patients with tachycardia-related cardiomyopathy (92% atrial arrhythmias) followed for 14 months, who had normalization of their EF (31.2 to 55%) but remained with dilated end-systolic volume compared to normal controls (33 vs. 22 ml/m^2, $p < 0.0001$).[79]

In the setting of SVT in patients with other forms of cardiomyopathy, there is increased myocardial work in tachycardia and treating the SVT expediently is necessary.

The usual methods of using adenosine infusion to break reentry tachycardia and suppressing tachycardia with β-blockers apply,

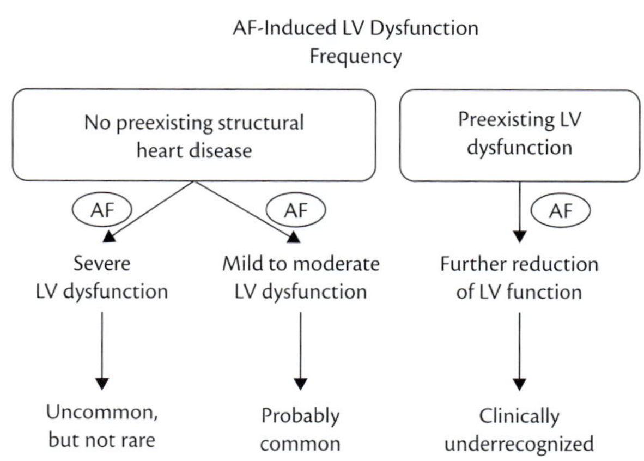

Fig. 9.5 Frequency of left ventricular dysfunction induced by atrial fibrillation. Cha YM, Redfield M, Shen WK, Gersh BJ, Atrial Fibrillation and Ventricular Dysfunction: A Vicious Electromechanical Cycle, Circulation 2004; 109: 2839–43.

though care must be taken to avoid precipitation of further left ventricular (LV) dysfunction with negative inotropes. Catheter ablation is ideal in SVT since this can be done safely with high success rates (typically >95%) and low complication rates.[59]

Supraventricular tachycardia contributes to CHF in a small subset of patients who may be amendable to dramatic improvement and even cure. Tachycardia-related cardiomyopathy is often a reversible process, although the diagnosis can be difficult to differentiate from other forms of cardiomyopathy and tachycardia secondary to decompensated heart failure. Treatment approaches include controlling the rate and catheter-based ablation, which for many SVT patients may be a definitive treatment.

Supraventricular arrhythmias post cardiac transplant

The transplanted heart does not have the same risks and frequencies of arrhythmias, and the differential diagnosis for underlying causes must be broadened.

Most transplants today are done with the bicaval method, so that the pulmonary veins and a patch of the posterior atrial wall of the recipient are sutured to the donor heart. This causes a form of bidirectional conduction block at the suture line, isolating the pulmonary veins, which is the goal of catheter-based AF ablation. This may be why there is a low incidence of AF in these patients. Additionally the transplanted hearts are denervated when initially transplanted, and become reinnervated heterogeneously over time so that sympathetic tone, which drives arrhythmias, may not have the same effects as in normal hearts.

The most comprehensive review of transplanted heart SVT comes from work of Vaseghi et al. in 2008, which reported on a cohort of 729 post-transplant recipients between 1994 and 2006 and characterized arrhythmias, including those that went on to have electrophysiology study for definitive diagnosis. AF only occurred in 7% of the recipients, and atrial flutter in 9%, with 57% of those arrhythmias occurring in the immediate postoperative period (Figure 9.6). Only those with transplant rejection or vasculopathy had AF or flutter after the postoperative period. Other SVT occurred in 7% of patients. Of the 24 patients who underwent electrophysiology study, atrial flutter was the most common rhythm found (58%) followed by scar-related atrial tachycardia (29%) (Figure 9.7).[80]

Treatment goals in the post-transplant patient with supraventricular arrhythmia needs special attention. Adenosine cannot be used without pacing back-up because the denervated heart may be extremely sensitive to it, leading to prolonged heart block.[81] β-Blockers should be use be used with caution as the transplant heart may be more sensitive to them. Verpamil and diltiazam may interact in the P-450 system with immunosuppression medications, and levels should be monitored closely. Amiodarone also interacts with immunosuppression (cyclosporine and tacrolimus) metabolism and may lead to transient bradycardia in the initial postoperative period after transplantation.[82] However, without further data, use of antiarrhythmics other than amiodarone is not proven safe in post-transplant patients, especially since QT prolongation post-transplant is associated with mortality, and QT prolongation from amiodarone has a lower incidence of torsades compared to other antiarrhythmics.[83] Care must be taken to rule out rejection and vasculopathy, as these are highly associated with AF and flutter.[84] As with all patients, typical atrial flutter, AV nodal reentry tachycardia, and accessory pathway-mediated tachycardia should be considered for ablation since this can be done safely and effectively.

Bradyarrhythmias in cardiomyopathy

Bradyarrhythmias are common in cardiomyopathy and may include sinus node dysfunction, tachy–brady syndrome, and

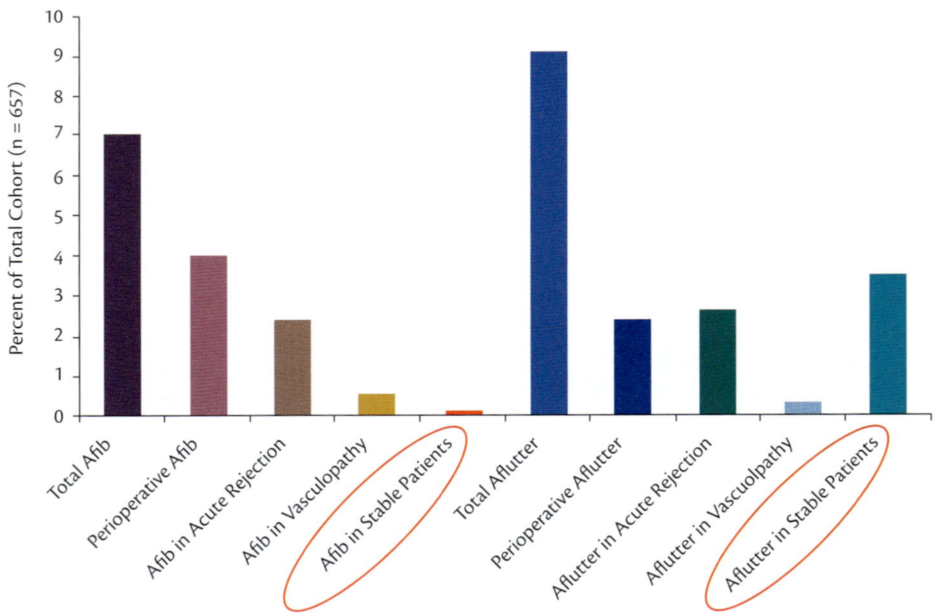

Fig. 9.6 Incidence of atrial flutter and atrial fibrillation after heart transplantation.

Reprinted from Journal of the American College of Cardiology, 51, Vaseghi M, Boyle N, Kedia R, et al. Supraventricular Tachycardia in Post-Orthotopic Heart Transplant Recipients, 2241–49, copyright (2008) with permission from Elsevier.

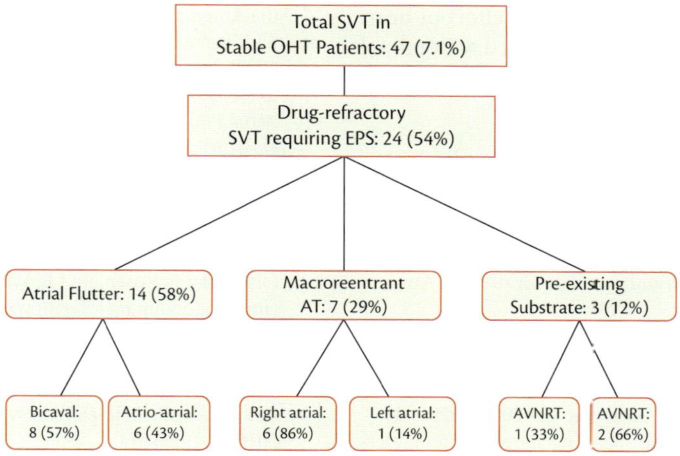

Fig. 9.7 Classification of supraventricular tachycardia in stable orthotopic heart transplant patients.
Reprinted from Journal of the American College of Cardiology, 51, Vaseghi M, Boyle N, Kedia R, et al. Supraventricular Tachycardia in Post-Orthotopic Heart Transplant Recipients, 2241–49, copyright (2008) with permission from Elsevier.

conduction disease. Treatment is usually permanent pacemaker implantation for symptomatic bradycardia, and biventricular pacing if there is left bundle branch block (LBBB) and EF is less than 35%. This section focuses on several specific cardiomyopathies and conduction disease that accompanies them, namely ischemic cardiomyopathy and the nonischemic cardiomyopathies secondary to specific conditions.

Ischemic cardiomyopathy

Conduction disease is common in ischemic heart disease both in the acute and chronic settings. In acute myocardial infarction, Mobitz I (Wenckebach) has an incidence of 4–10%, accounts for 90% of second-degree heart block, and is often transient, while Mobitz II occurs in large anterior myocardial infarctions, implies infrahisian block, and often occurs with fascicular or bundle branch block.[85,86] Complete heart block occurs in 6% of acute myocardial infarctions, and if associated with inferior myocardial infarctions, may be reversible and related to vagal tone; however, with anterior myocardial infarctions, complete heart block implies extensive infarction and is often irreversible.[86,87] Whether heart block occurs after anterior or inferior myocardial infarction, the prognosis is worse than in those without heart block.[88]

Infiltrative cardiomyopathies

Hemochromatosis is a hereditary disorder of iron overload with infiltrative cardiomyopathy known to cause significant conduction disease. Autopsy studies demonstrated significant infiltration of the sinoatrial (SA) and AV nodes with iron deposits.[89] The prevalence of hemochromatosis among patients with a conduction disorder is higher than one might expect, and a Swedish study of 232 unselected men treated with pacemakers found that 2% to had hemochromatosis.[90] Amyloid cardiomyopathy, a systemic infiltrative disease with amyloid deposits, from either monoclonal gammopathy or chronic inflammation, manifests with cardiac involvement in approximately 50% of cases, and heart failure, arrhythmias, and conduction disease are commonly present.[91] The Mayo Clinic published a cohort of 229 patients with AL-amyloid from 1970 through 1980, and heart failure and arrhythmia accounted for 40% of mortality in those patients.[92]

Inflammatory cardiomyopathies

Sarcoidosis is a systemic granulomatous inflammatory disease, with myocardial involvement in approximately 50% of patients, and in up to 5% of patients myocardial sarcoid is their only manifestation of the disease.[93] Myocardial involvement can lead to global or focal ventricular dysfunction and conduction disease.[93]

Chagas disease is a common form of idiopathic cardiomyopathy in Latin America, related to chronic infection with the *Trypanosoma cruzi* protozoan parasite, which may remain dormant in myocardial tissue. Conduction disease is usually manifested by hemiblock in early stages of the disease and eventually complete heart block. There is also a high incidence of ventricular arrhythmias in the setting of advanced Chagas cardiomyopathy.[94]

Lyme disease from *Borrelia* infection often presents with acute myocarditis and AV block that is transient and related to inflammation. In the chronic phase many years after initial infection, patients may present with dilated nonischemic cardiomyopathy, though in this stage conduction abnormalities are typically bundle branch block and hemiblock.[95] Giant cell myocarditis is an acute inflammatory condition with noncaseating granuloma formation in the myocardium. Both conduction disorders and ventricular tachycardia are common, and related to local myocardial inflammation.[96]

Conclusion

Arrhythmias above the AV node are common in heart failure, have a high morbidity, and may complicate management of the heart failure. AF is the most common arrhythmia in heart failure, with each condition promoting the other, and treatment of both conditions must be coordinated. Supraventricular tachycardias occur in structurally normal and failing hearts, and when present in the setting of CHF, tachycardia-related cardiomyopathy should be considered. Catheter ablation remains a highly effective and safe option for SVT and atrial flutter. Atrial arrhythmia in post-transplant patients is often an indication of rejection or transplant vasculopathy and further evaluation is required. Bradyarrhythmias in cardiomyopathy are common in ischemic cardiomyopathy, and when present in nonischemic cardiomyopathy may be associated with infiltrative or inflammatory cardiomyopathies. CHF and arrhythmias are frequent comorbid conditions, and a collaborative effort of heart failure specialists and electrophysiologists is required for optimal treatment of the heart failure patient.

References

1. Wang TJ, Larson MG, Levy D, et al. Temporal relations of atrial fibrillation and congestive heart failure and their joint influence on mortality: The Framingham Heart Study. Circulation 2003;107:2920–5.
2. Maisel WH, Stevenson LW. Atrial fibrillation in heart failure: Epidemiology, pathophysiology, and rationale for therapy. Am J Cardiol 2003;91:2D–8D.
3. Boyle NG, Shivkumar K. Atrial fibrillation in congestive heart failure: Current management. Cardiol Clin 2009;27:79–93, viii–ix.
4. Allessie M, Ausma J, Schotten U. Electrical, contractile and structural remodeling during atrial fibrillation. Cardiovasc Res 2002;54:230–46.
5. Yeh YH, Wakili R, Qi XY, et al. Calcium-handling abnormalities underlying atrial arrhythmogenesis and contractile dysfunction in dogs with congestive heart failure. Circ Arrhythm Electrophysiol 2008;1:93–102.
6. Li D, Shinagawa K, Pang L, et al. Effects of angiotensin-converting enzyme inhibition on the development of the atrial fibrillation substrate in dogs with ventricular tachypacing-induced congestive heart failure. Circulation 2001;104:2608–14.
7. Haissaguerre M, Jais P, Shah DC, et al. Spontaneous initiation of atrial fibrillation by ectopic beats originating in the pulmonary veins. N Engl J Med 1998;339:659–66.
8. Allessie MA, de Groot NM, Houben RP, et al. Electropathological substrate of long-standing persistent atrial fibrillation in patients with structural heart disease: Longitudinal dissociation. Circ Arrhythm Electrophysiol 2010;3:606–15.
9. Vaquero M, Calvo D, Jalife J. Cardiac fibrillation: From ion channels to rotors in the human heart. Heart Rhythm 2008;5:872–9.
10. Skanes AC, Mandapati R, Berenfeld O, et al. Spatiotemporal periodicity during atrial fibrillation in the isolated sheep heart. Circulation 1998;98:1236–48.
11. Jalife J, Berenfeld O, Skanes A, Mandapati R. Mechanisms of atrial fibrillation: Mother rotors or multiple daughter wavelets, or both? J Cardiovasc Electrophysiol 1998;9:S2–12.
12. Narayan SM, Krummen DE, Shivkumar K, et al. Treatment of atrial fibrillation by the ablation of localized sources: Confirm (conventional ablation for atrial fibrillation with or without focal impulse and rotor modulation) trial. J Am Coll Cardiol 2012;60:628–36.
13. Nattel S, Burstein B, Dobrev D. Atrial remodeling and atrial fibrillation: Mechanisms and implications. Circ Arrhythm Electrophysiol 2008;1:62–73.
14. Mittal S, Ayati S, Stein KM, Schwartzman D, et al. Transthoracic cardioversion of atrial fibrillation: Comparison of rectilinear biphasic versus damped sine wave monophasic shocks. Circulation 2000;101:1282–7.
15. Roy D, Talajic M, Nattel S, et al. Rhythm control versus rate control for atrial fibrillation and heart failure. N Engl J Med 2008;358:2667–77.
16. Reiffel JA, Correia J. Structural heart disease: Its importance in association with antiarrhythmic drug therapy. Clin Cardiol 1994;17:II3–6.
17. Kober L, Torp-Pedersen C, McMurray JJ, et al. Increased mortality after dronedarone therapy for severe heart failure. N Engl J Med 2008;358:2678–87.
18. Echt DS, Liebson PR, Mitchell LB, et al. Mortality and morbidity in patients receiving encainide, flecainide, or placebo. The cardiac arrhythmia suppression trial. N Engl J Med 1991;324:781–8.
19. Gage BF, Waterman AD, Shannon W, et al. Validation of clinical classification schemes for predicting stroke: Results from the national registry of atrial fibrillation. JAMA 2001;285:2864–70.
20. Demircan C, Cikriklar HI, Engindeniz Z, et al. Comparison of the effectiveness of intravenous diltiazem and metoprolol in the management of rapid ventricular rate in atrial fibrillation. Emerg Med J 2005;22:411–14.
21. Fuster V, Ryden LE, Cannom DS, et al. Acc/aha/esc 2006 guidelines for the management of patients with atrial fibrillation: A report of the American College Of Cardiology/American Heart Association Task Force on Practice Guidelines and the European Society of Cardiology Committee for Practice Guidelines (Writing Committee to Revise the 2001 Guidelines for the Management of Patients with Atrial Fibrillation): developed in collaboration with the European Heart Rhythm Association and the Heart Rhythm Society. Circulation 2006;114:e257–54.
22. Khand AU, Rankin AC, Martin W, et al. Carvedilol alone or in combination with digoxin for the management of atrial fibrillation in patients with heart failure? J Am Coll Cardiol 2003;42:1944–51.
23. Olshansky B, Rosenfeld LE, Warner AL, et al. The atrial fibrillation follow-up investigation of rhythm management (affirm) study: Approaches to control rate in atrial fibrillation. J Am Coll Cardiol 2004;43:1201–8.
24. Van Gelder IC, Groenveld HF, Crijns HJ, et al. Lenient versus strict rate control in patients with atrial fibrillation. N Engl J Med 2010;362:1363–73.
25. Botto GL, Politi A, Bonini W, et al. External cardioversion of atrial fibrillation: Role of paddle position on technical efficacy and energy requirements. Heart 1999;82:726–30.
26. Ricard P YK, Rinaldi JP,Bergonzi M, Saoudi N. Cardioversion of atrial fibrillation: How and when? Eur Heart J Suppl 2003: H40–44.
27. Rabbino MD, Likoff W, Dreifus LS. Complications and limitations of direct-current countershock. JAMA 1964;190:417–20.
28. Bjerkelund CJ, Orning OM. The efficacy of anticoagulant therapy in preventing embolism related to d.C. Electrical conversion of atrial fibrillation. Am J Cardiol 1969;23:208–16.
29. Klein AL, Grimm RA, Murray RD, et al. Use of transesophageal echocardiography to guide cardioversion in patients with atrial fibrillation. N Engl J Med 2001;344:1411–20.
30. Arnold AZ, Mick MJ, Mazurek RP, et al. Role of prophylactic anticoagulation for direct current cardioversion in patients with atrial fibrillation or atrial flutter. J Am Coll Cardiol 1992;19:851–5.
31. Volgman AS, Carberry PA, Stambler B, et al. Conversion efficacy and safety of intravenous ibutilide compared with intravenous procainamide in patients with atrial flutter or fibrillation. J Am Coll Cardiol 1998;31:1414–19.
32. Stambler BS, Wood MA, Ellenbogen KA, et al. Efficacy and safety of repeated intravenous doses of ibutilide for rapid conversion of atrial flutter or fibrillation. Ibutilide repeat dose study investigators. Circulation 1996;94:1613–21.
33. Camm AJ. Safety considerations in the pharmacological management of atrial fibrillation. Int J Cardiol 2008;127:299–306.
34. Vardas PE, Kochiadakis GE, Igoumenidis NE, et al. Amiodarone as a first-choice drug for restoring sinus rhythm in patients with atrial fibrillation: A randomized, controlled study. Chest 2000;117:1538–45.
35. Singh BN, Singh SN, Reda DJ, et al. Amiodarone versus sotalol for atrial fibrillation. N Engl J Med 2005;352:1861–72.
36. Roy D, Talajic M, Dorian P, et al. Amiodarone to prevent recurrence of atrial fibrillation. Canadian trial of atrial fibrillation investigators. N Engl J Med 2000;342:913–20.
37. Doval HC, Nul DR, Grancelli HO, et al. Randomised trial of low-dose amiodarone in severe congestive heart failure. Grupo de Estudio de la Sobrevida en la Insuficiencia Cardiaca en Argentina (GESICA). Lancet 1994;344:493–8.
38. Torp-Pedersen C, Moller M, Bloch-Thomsen PE, et al. Dofetilide in patients with congestive heart failure and left ventricular dysfunction. Danish investigations of arrhythmia and mortality on dofetilide study group. N Engl J Med 1999;341:857–65.
39. Camm AJ, Lip GY, De Caterina R, Savelieva I, et al. 2012 focused update of the esc guidelines for the management of atrial fibrillation: An update of the 2010 ESC guidelines for the management of atrial fibrillation developed with the special contribution of the European Heart Rhythm Association. Europace 2012;14:1385–413.
40. Connolly SJ, Camm AJ, Halperin JL, et al. Dronedarone in high-risk permanent atrial fibrillation. N Engl J Med 2011;365:2268–76.

41. Wyse DG, Waldo AL, DiMarco JP, et al. A comparison of rate control and rhythm control in patients with atrial fibrillation. N Engl J Med 2002;347:1825–33.
42. Deedwania PC, Singh BN, Ellenbogen K, et al. Spontaneous conversion and maintenance of sinus rhythm by amiodarone in patients with heart failure and atrial fibrillation: Observations from the Veterans Affairs Congestive Heart Failure Survival Trial of Antiarrhythmic Therapy (CHF-STAT). The Department Of Veterans Affairs CHF-STAT Investigators. Circulation 1998;98:2574–9.
43. Lip GY, Nieuwlaat R, Pisters R, et al. Refining clinical risk stratification for predicting stroke and thromboembolism in atrial fibrillation using a novel risk factor-based approach: The Euro Heart Survey on Atrial Fibrillation. Chest 2010;137:263–72.
44. Olesen JB, Lip GY, Hansen ML, et al.Validation of risk stratification schemes for predicting stroke and thromboembolism in patients with atrial fibrillation: Nationwide cohort study. BMJ 2011;342:d124.
45. Camm AJ, Lip GY, De Caterina R, et al. 2012 focused update of the ESC guidelines for the management of atrial fibrillation: An update of the 2010 ESC guidelines for the management of atrial fibrillation developed with the special contribution of the european heart rhythm association. Eur Heart J 2012;33:2719–47.
46. Hart RG, Halperin JL. Atrial fibrillation and stroke: Concepts and controversies. Stroke 2001;32:803–8.
47. Connolly S, Pogue J, Hart R, et al. Clopidogrel plus aspirin versus oral anticoagulation for atrial fibrillation in the Atrial Fibrillation Clopidogrel Trial With Irbesartan For Prevention Of Vascular Events (ACTIVE W): A randomised controlled trial. Lancet 2006;367:1903–12.
48. Patel MR, Mahaffey KW, Garg J, et al. Rivaroxaban versus warfarin in nonvalvular atrial fibrillation. N Engl J Med 2011;365:883–91.
49. Granger CB, Alexander JH, McMurray JJ, et al. Apixaban versus warfarin in patients with atrial fibrillation. N Engl J Med 2011;365:981–92.
50. Miller CS, Grandi SM, Shimony A, Filion KB, Eisenberg MJ. Meta-analysis of efficacy and safety of new oral anticoagulants (dabigatran, rivaroxaban, apixaban) versus warfarin in patients with atrial fibrillation. Am J Cardiol 2012;110:453–60.
51. Blackshear JL, Odell JA. Appendage obliteration to reduce stroke in cardiac surgical patients with atrial fibrillation. Ann Thorac Surg 1996;61:755–9.
52. Holmes DR, Reddy VY, Turi ZG, et al. Percutaneous closure of the left atrial appendage versus warfarin therapy for prevention of stroke in patients with atrial fibrillation: A randomised non-inferiority trial. Lancet 2009;374:534–42.
53. Bartus K, Bednarek J, Myc J, et al. Feasibility of closed-chest ligation of the left atrial appendage in humans. Heart Rhythm 2011;8:188–93.
54. Kanderian AS, Gillinov AM, Pettersson GB, et al. Success of surgical left atrial appendage closure: Assessment by transesophageal echocardiography. J Am Coll Cardiol 2008;52:924–9.
55. Wilber DJ, Pappone C, Neuzil P, et al. Comparison of antiarrhythmic drug therapy and radiofrequency catheter ablation in patients with paroxysmal atrial fibrillation: A randomized controlled trial. JAMA 2010;303:333–40.
56. Hsu LF, Jais P, Sanders P, Garrigue S, et al. Catheter ablation for atrial fibrillation in congestive heart failure. N Engl J Med 2004;351:2373–83.
57. Chen MS, Marrouche NF, Khaykin Y, et al. Pulmonary vein isolation for the treatment of atrial fibrillation in patients with impaired systolic function. J Am Coll Cardiol 2004;43:1004–9.
58. Khan MN, Jais P, Cummings J, et al. Pulmonary-vein isolation for atrial fibrillation in patients with heart failure. N Engl J Med 2008;359:1778–85.
59. Lee G, Sanders P, Kalman JM. Catheter ablation of atrial arrhythmias: State of the art. Lancet 2012;380:1509–19.
60. Wood MA, Brown-Mahoney C, Kay GN, Ellenbogen KA. Clinical outcomes after ablation and pacing therapy for atrial fibrillation: A meta-analysis. Circulation 2000;101:1138–44.
61. Granada J, Uribe W, Chyou PH, et al. Incidence and predictors of atrial flutter in the general population. J Am Coll Cardiol 2000;36:2242–46.
62. Rosenbleuth A, Garcia Ramos J. Studies on flutter and fibrillation II. The influence of artificial obstacles on experimental auricular flutter. Am Heart J 1947;33:677–84.
63. Waldo AL, MacLean WA, Karp RB, et al. Entrainment and interruption of atrial flutter with atrial pacing: Studies in man following open heart surgery. Circulation 1977;56:737–45.
64. Alboni P, Scarfo S, Fuca G, et al. Atrial and ventricular pressures in atrial flutter. Pacing Clin Electrophysiol 1999;22:600–4.
65. Biblo LA, Yuan Z, Quan KJ, et al. Risk of stroke in patients with atrial flutter. Am J Cardiol 2001;87:346–9, A349.
66. Seidl K, Hauer B, Schwick NG, et al. Risk of thromboembolic events in patients with atrial flutter. Am J Cardiol 1998;82:580–3.
67. Blomstrom-Lundqvist C, Scheinman MM, Aliot EM, et al. ACC/AHA/ESC guidelines for the management of patients with supraventricular arrhythmias—executive summary: A report of the American College of Cardiology/American Heart Association Task Force on Practice Guidelines and the European Society of Cardiology Committee for Practice Guidelines (Writing Committee to Develop Guidelines for the Management of Patients with Supraventricular Arrhythmias). Circulation 2003;108:1871–909.
68. Natale A, Newby KH, Pisano E, et al. Prospective randomized comparison of antiarrhythmic therapy versus first-line radiofrequency ablation in patients with atrial flutter. J Am Coll Cardiol 2000;35:1898–904.
69. Da Costa A, Thevenin J, Roche F, et al. Results from the Loire-Ardeche-Drome-Isere-Puy-de-Dome (LADIP) trial on atrial flutter, a multicentric prospective randomized study comparing amiodarone and radiofrequency ablation after the first episode of symptomatic atrial flutter. Circulation 2006;114:1676–81.
70. Lee KW, Yang Y, Scheinman MM. Atrial flutter: A review of its history, mechanisms, clinical features, and current therapy. Curr Probl Cardiol 2005;30:121–67.
71. Philippon F, Plumb VJ, Epstein AE, et al. The risk of atrial fibrillation following radiofrequency catheter ablation of atrial flutter. Circulation 1995;92:430–5.
72. Schumacher B, Jung W, Lewalter T, et al. Radiofrequency ablation of atrial flutter due to administration of class ic antiarrhythmic drugs for atrial fibrillation. Am J Cardiol 1999;83:710–13.
73. Whipple GH, Sheffield LT, Woodman EG, et al. Reversible congestive heart failure due to rapid stimulation of the normal heart. Proc N Engl Cardiovasc Soc 1962;20:39–40.
74. Spinale FG, Hendrick DA, Crawford FA, et al. Chronic supraventricular tachycardia causes ventricular dysfunction and subendocardial injury in swine. Am J Physiol 1990;259:H218–29.
75. Moe GW, Montgomery C, Howard RJ, et al. Left ventricular myocardial blood flow, metabolism, and effects of treatment with enalapril: Further insights into the mechanisms of canine experimental pacing-induced heart failure. J Lab Clin Med 1993;121:294–301.
76. Shite J, Qin F, Mao W, et al. Antioxidant vitamins attenuate oxidative stress and cardiac dysfunction in tachycardia-induced cardiomyopathy. J Am Coll Cardiol 2001;38:1734–40.
77. Cha YM, Redfield MM, Shen WK, Gersh BJ. Atrial fibrillation and ventricular dysfunction: A vicious electromechanical cycle. Circulation 2004;109:2839–43.
78. Redfield MM, Kay GN, Jenkins LS, et al. Tachycardia-related cardiomyopathy: A common cause of ventricular dysfunction in patients with atrial fibrillation referred for atrioventricular ablation. Mayo Clin Proc 2000;75:790–5.
79. Dandamudi G, Rampurwala AY, Mahenthiran J, et al. Persistent left ventricular dilatation in tachycardia-induced cardiomyopathy patients after appropriate treatment and normalization of ejection fraction. Heart Rhythm 2008;5:1111–14.
80. Vaseghi M, Boyle NG, Kedia R, et al. Supraventricular tachycardia after orthotopic cardiac transplantation. J Am Coll Cardiol 2008;51:2241–9.

81. Ellenbogen KA, Thames MD, DiMarco JP, et al. Electrophysiological effects of adenosine in the transplanted human heart. Evidence of supersensitivity. Circulation 1990;81:821–8.
82. Thajudeen A, Stecker EC, Shehata M, et al. Arrhythmias after heart transplantation: Mechanisms and management. J Am Heart Assoc 2012;1:e001461.
83. Vrtovec B, Radovancevic R, Thomas CD, et al. Prognostic value of the qtc interval after cardiac transplantation. J Heart Lung Transplant 2006;25:29–35.
84. Cui G, Tung T, Kobashigawa J, Laks H, Sen L. Increased incidence of atrial flutter associated with the rejection of heart transplantation. Am J Cardiol 2001;88:280–4.
85. Feigl D, Ashkenazy J, Kishon Y. Early and late atrioventricular block in acute inferior myocardial infarction. J Am Coll Cardiol 1984;4:35–8.
86. Simons GR, Sgarbossa E, Wagner G, et al. Atrioventricular and intraventricular conduction disorders in acute myocardial infarction: A reappraisal in the thrombolytic era. Pacing Clin Electrophysiol 1998;21:2651–63.
87. Lim CH, Toh CC, Low LP. Atrioventricular and associated intraventricular conduction disturbances in acute myocardial infarction. Br Heart J 1971;33:947–54.
88. Meine TJ, Al-Khatib SM, Alexander JH, et al. Incidence, predictors, and outcomes of high-degree atrioventricular block complicating acute myocardial infarction treated with thrombolytic therapy. Am Heart J 2005;149:670–4.
89. James TN. Pathology of the cardiac conduction system in hemochromatosis. N Engl J Med 1964;271:92–4.
90. Rosenqvist M, Hultcrantz R. Prevalence of a haemochromatosis among men with clinically significant bradyarrhythmias. Eur Heart J 1989;10:473–8.
91. Kyle RA. Amyloidosis. Circulation 1995;91:1269–71.
92. Kyle RA, Greipp PR. Amyloidosis (Al). Clinical and laboratory features in 229 cases. Mayo Clin Proc 1983;58:665–83.
93. Doughan AR, Williams BR. Cardiac sarcoidosis. Heart 2006;92:282–8.
94. Rassi A, Jr., Dias JC, Marin-Neto JA, Rassi A. Challenges and opportunities for primary, secondary, and tertiary prevention of chagas' disease. Heart 2009;95:524–34.
95. Cox J, Krajden M. Cardiovascular manifestations of Lyme disease. Am Heart J 1991;122:1449–55.
96. Lakdawala NK, Givertz MM. Dilated cardiomyopathy with conduction disease and arrhythmia. Circulation 2010;122:527–34.

CHAPTER 10

Ventricular arrhythmias in heart failure

John D. Ferguson MBChB MD
and John P. DiMarco MD PhD

Introduction

Ventricular arrhythmias (VA) and pump failure are the two most common causes of death in patients with heart failure (HF). HF specialists and electrophysiologists typically work together closely in managing these patients. Although antiarrhythmic drug therapy has remained static for many years, device therapy and catheter ablation strategies have evolved rapidly and now are the primary modalities of antiarrhythmic therapy for many patients.

Diagnosis of ventricular arrhythmia

The diagnosis of VA should include at minimum a history, physical examination, 12-lead ECG (Box 10.1), electrolytes, assessment of ventricular function, and screening for coronary artery disease. In patients with implantable cardioverter defibrillators (ICDs) and pacemakers, interrogation and analysis of the stored electrogram data often provide diagnostic information. Cardiac MRI (CMR) is increasingly helpful in the detection of myocardial scar and other myocardial abnormalities which may alter decisions regarding therapy. Invasive electrophysiological studies are used less frequently but may be crucial to distinguish supraventricular tachycardia (SVT) from ventricular tachycardia (VT) and may help to determine the efficacy of drug therapy. Noninvasive programmed stimulation (NIPS) via an ICD can be used to assess the inducibility of VT. Treadmill testing is useful for the assessment of exercise-induced VA.

Symptoms

Sustained VA usually results in symptoms but premature ventricular contractions (PVCs), nonsustained ventricular tachycardia (NSVT), slow sustained monomorphic ventricular tachycardia (SMVT), and short episodes of VT terminated by ICD anti-tachycardia pacing (ATP) may not cause any discernible symptoms.[1] Palpitations are a common symptom signaling arrhythmia and a careful history should be taken of the frequency and duration of episodes, associated symptoms, and precipitating factors. Lightheadedness, syncope, dyspnea, and chest pain may also occur. In patients with syncope and structural heart disease it is safer to initially presume that the syncope is related to ventricular tachyarrhythmia rather than other more benign etiologies. Admission for telemetry and urgent assessment is usually warranted in such patients.

Physical signs

In patients presenting with ongoing sustained VT, the primary objective is to determine whether there is hemodynamic instability. Physical signs of hemodynamic compromise are hypotension, cool extremities, rapid low-volume pulse, diaphoresis, pallor, raised venous pressure, pulmonary congestion, altered mental status, and ultimately loss of consciousness. In patients with significant instability, emergency cardioversion should be performed.

Ambulatory electrocardiogram recordings

Ambulatory ECG recordings are extremely useful in managing patients with ventricular arrhythmia. In patients who are suspected of ventricular arrhythmia and do not have a definitive diagnosis, the ambulatory ECG is useful for correlating symptoms with heart rhythm. This strategy should only be used in patients who are at relatively low risk. Most patients who are at increased risk of sudden death from VA (see Box 10.2) should be assessed more urgently as inpatients.

In patients who already have ECG documentation of VA, the ambulatory ECG is useful in guiding treatment strategy and subsequently assessing response to treatment. For instance, in patients with reduced left ventricular (LV) function and frequent PVCs on 12-lead ECG, a 24 hour ambulatory ECG is useful in quantifying the PVC burden. If PVCs account for more than 10% of heart beats during this period, a more aggressive strategy, including catheter ablation, should be considered to maximize the chance of recovery of LV function. Repeat assessment of PVC burden with ambulatory ECG following ablation is helpful in assessing the efficacy of therapy.

ICD electrograms

The proportion of HF patients who have either primary or secondary prevention ICDs has increased dramatically over the last decade. A thorough assessment of ICD stored data is an important tool in the management of episodes of VA. In fact, the ICD electrograms are increasingly the only record of VA, most episodes of which are promptly treated by the device. The ICD interrogation report provides important information for subsequent ablation.

Echocardiography and cardiac magnetic resonance imaging

Assessment of LV function is important in guiding both antiarrhythmic and ICD therapies, both of which are discussed later in the

Box 10.1 Practical tips for diagnosis of wide-complex tachycardias

There are multiple published criteria for distinguishing ventricular tachycardia (VT) from supraventricular tachycardia (SVT) using the 12-lead ECG. These criteria are difficult to remember and the sensitivity and specificity are suboptimal. This box includes both clinical features and ECG criteria to help diagnose wide-complex tachycardias.

- Favoring SVT
  - Irregularly, irregular intervals
  - "Classic" left or right bundle branch block (LBBB or RBBB) pattern
  - QRS unchanged or just wider than sinus QRS
  - Structural heart disease absent
  - History of SVT or WPW
- Favoring ventricular tachycardia
  - Structural heart disease present (prior MI, cardiomyopathy)
  - Regular except for fusion beats
  - AV dissociation (atrial capture, fusion beats)
  - QRS axis −60 to180°
  - QRS duration >140 ms for RBBB type V1 morphology; V1 >160 ms for LBBB type V1 morphology
  - Delayed activation during initial phase of the QRS complex:
    - LBBB pattern—R wave in V1, V2 >40 ms
    - RBBB pattern—onset of R wave to nadir of S >100 ms
- Concordance of all QRS complexes across the precordial leads

chapter. Patients with increasing ventricular arrhythmia may have a significant decline in LV function compared to prior assessment. It is important to consider the potential causes of this deterioration, particularly in patients with coronary artery disease. In patients presenting with VT storms (≥3 episodes in 24 hours), LV function is frequently depressed. This often reflects transient stunning related to repeated shocks, decompensated HF, and metabolic derangement.

In patients with sustained VT who are scheduled for catheter ablation, assessment of the location and extent of myocardial scar is helpful to guide the sites of ablation. Patients with severely depressed LV function or recent myocardial infarction should have mural thrombus excluded with echocardiography prior to instrumentation of the left ventricle. Cardiac MR with gadolinium late enhancement imaging can provide location of scar and assessment as to whether the scar is endocardial, epicardial or intramyocardial. A frequent limitation to cardiac MR is an implanted ICD. Cardiac MR has a small risk of damaging the ICD generator or causing heating of myocardium at the tip of the ICD lead which could require lead replacement. In addition, the generator and the lead may cause significant artifact degrading the images of the myocardium, especially of the anterior wall.

Coronary angiography

In patients presenting with ventricular fibrillation or polymorphic VT a low threshold for coronary angiography is appropriate to exclude critical ischemia. Episodes of ventricular arrhythmia with shock therapy are invariably associated with a rise in cardiac enzymes, especially troponins, and are often incorrectly labeled as myocardial infarction. In patients with sustained VT who do not

Box 10.2 Indications and contraindications for ICD therapy

I Indications for secondary prevention

A Documented episode of cardiac arrest due to ventricular fibrillation (VF), not due to a transient or reversible cause

B Documented sustained ventricular tachyarrhythmia (VT), either spontaneous or induced by an electrophysiology (EP) study (patients with syncope), not associated with an acute myocardial infarction (MI), and not due to a transient or reversible cause

II Indications for primary prevention

A Documented familial or inherited conditions with a high risk of life-threatening VT, such as long QT syndrome or hypertrophic cardiomyopathy

B Coronary artery disease with a documented prior MI, a measured left ventricular ejection fraction (LVEF) <35%, and inducible, sustained VT or VF at EP study. (The EP test must be performed more than 4 weeks after the qualifying MI.)

C Documented prior MI and a measured LVEF <30%

D Patients with ischemic dilated cardiomyopathy, documented prior MI, New York Heart Association (NYHA) class II and III heart failure, and measured LVEF <35%

E Patients with nonischemic dilated cardiomyopathy >3 (preferably 9) months, NYHA class II and III heart failure, and measured LVEF <35%

F Patients who meet all current Centers for Medicare & Medicaid Services coverage requirements for a cardiac resynchronization therapy (CRT) device and have NYHA class IV heart failure

III Exclusions

A NYHA classification IV without CRT

B Cardiogenic shock or symptomatic hypotension while in a stable baseline rhythm

C Had a coronary artery bypass graft or percutaneous transluminal coronary angioplasty within past 3 months

D Had an enzyme-positive MI within past 40 days

E Clinical symptoms or findings that would make them a candidate for coronary revascularization

F Any disease, other than cardiac disease (e.g., cancer, uremia, liver failure), associated with a likelihood of survival less than 1 year

G Patient must not have irreversible brain damage from preexisting cerebral disease

Modified from Pub 100-03 Medicare National Coverage Determinations. Chapter 1, Part 1, Section 20.4 (Rev. 29, 03-04-05).[37]

report a prior history of worsening chest pain, the yield of finding coronary stenoses during angiography is very low.

Electrophysiology study

Invasive electrophysiology (EP) study can be used to distinguish VT from SVT in patients who present with broad-complex tachycardia and a nondiagnostic ECG. It is also used in patients with undocumented palpitations or syncope and the presence of structural heart disease. The EP study is also used to assess the risk of sudden death, especially in those with reduced LV function. Patients with inducible sustained monomorphic VT are at increased risk of sudden death. Ventricular fibrillation can be induced in most patients if very aggressive pacing is used, but this may be a nonspecific finding and not a good predictor of sudden death. The EP study can also be performed to assess the efficacy of either drug or ablation therapy of sustained VT.

The use of the EP study to risk stratify patients with HF has fallen in the past decade. The sensitivity and specificity of predicting death from VA using the invasive EP study remains poor. Assessment of LV ejection fraction (LVEF) has become the primary measure for identifying patients at increased risk of sudden death from ventricular arrhythmia and candidates suitable for primary ICD therapy (see Box 10.2).

Noninvasive programmed stimulation

Noninvasive programmed stimulation (NIPS) is a relatively simple way to perform an EP study by using a previously implanted ICD or pacemaker. NIPS is useful in assessing the inducibility of VA after changes in drug therapy or ablation. For example, the introduction of amiodarone may partially suppress a VT but slow the cycle length. NIPS could help assess whether ICD detection and therapy programming is appropriate for the slower cycle length of VT.

Acute management of sustained ventricular tachycardia

The goal of acute therapy of sustained VT is to rapidly restore a stable rhythm with a physiologically appropriate rate and thereby prevent organ damage or further hemodynamic deterioration. Patients with severe hypotension, chest pain, or evidence for hypoperfusion of critical organs should be considered hemodynamically unstable, and direct current cardioversion is usually the most expeditious method for terminating the arrhythmia. In many patients, however, the tachycardia is not immediately life-threatening and the patient is conscious and not in severe distress. In such patients, pharmacologic cardioversion is the procedure of choice.[2,3]

Pharmacologic conversion of a sustained VT episode has not been studied in large controlled randomized trials. Observational and limited controlled trial data, however, indicate that intravenous procainamide is the most effective available agent.[4,5,6] Intravenous lidocaine and β-adrenergic blocking agents have very limited efficacy. There are patients with idiopathic sustained VT who may respond to either verapamil or adenosine. These patients usually have structurally normal hearts and they would not have a history of HF. Verapamil and diltiazem are contraindicated in wide-complex tachycardias of unknown mechanism in patients with structural heart disease.[2,3]

Adenosine may be used if there is a high likelihood that the arrhythmia is supraventricular in origin.[7] In many supraventricular arrhythmias, adenosine will either terminate the tachycardia or provide diagnostic information if atrioventricular (AV) or ventriculoatrial (VA) block occur.

Termination of an episode of VT with procainamide will depend on achievement of a transiently high plasma concentration which will usually gradually slow and then terminate the tachycardia. Infusion of 50–100 mg every minute up to a total dose of 15–17 mg/kg is most effective but blood pressure and QRS duration must be carefully followed before each increment is administered (Figure 10.1). Slower rates of infusion are likely to be less effective.[6]

Amiodarone and sotalol are also available for intravenous use but are not as effective as high dose procainamide infusions. However, intravenous amiodarone may be very useful in preventing early recurrence.[8,9,10] An oral formulation of procainamide is no longer available. Therefore, starting a patient on intravenous amiodarone, if VT returns after an initial pharmacologic or electrical conversion is the most reasonable alternative. Intravenous sotalol in patients with sustained venmtricular arrhythmias is used mostly as replacement in patients previously on oral therapy whose arrhythmias had been well controlled on sotalol.[11]

Some patients will have multiple episodes (≥3 within 24 hours) of VT or fibrillation requiring ICD therapies or external shocks. This syndrome has been referred to as "electrical storm."[12,13] In these patients, a search for and reversal of any contributing factors are critical to long-term success. β-Adrenergic blockers have been shown to be important adjuncts to other antiarrhythmics, usually amiodarone. In selected patients with drug-refractory VT in whom no reversible cause is identified, catheter ablation or left stellate ganglion blockade may be effective.

Nonsustained ventricular tachycardia

NSVT will be commonly detected during ECG monitoring in HF patients with both ischemic and nonischemic cardiomyopathies.[14] The frequency and complexity of ventricular ectopy are likely to increase during periods of worsening HF. A number of trials have tested the hypothesis that antiarrhythmic drug therapy, either empirically administered or when guided by arrhythmia suppression during serial ambulatory ECG monitoring, would improve survival and prevent sudden death. The drug most carefully evaluated has been amiodarone. In 1997, the Amiodarone Trials Meta-analysis Investigators reviewed 13 randomized controlled trials comparing amiodarone to placebo in patients with either recent myocardial infractions or congestive HF.[15] They estimated that prophylactic amiodarone would reduce arrhythmic/sudden death by 29% and total mortality by 13%. The studies included in this meta-analysis were completed before modern therapy for HF including aggressive revascularization, renin–angiotensin system and β-adrenergic blockade, and aldosterone antagonism was widely practiced. In the Sudden Cardiac Death—Heart Failure Trial (SCD-HeFT)[16] which was completed in 2004, empiric amiodarone had no advantage over placebo in patients with New York Heart Association (NYHA) class II symptoms and actually increased mortality in patients with class III symptoms. A more recent meta-analysis of 15 randomized trials showed that prophylactic amiodarone had no overall benefit on mortality.[17]

Drug therapy in ICD recipients

ICD therapy is now the primary option for prevention of sudden death and treatment of sustained VT in patients with congestive

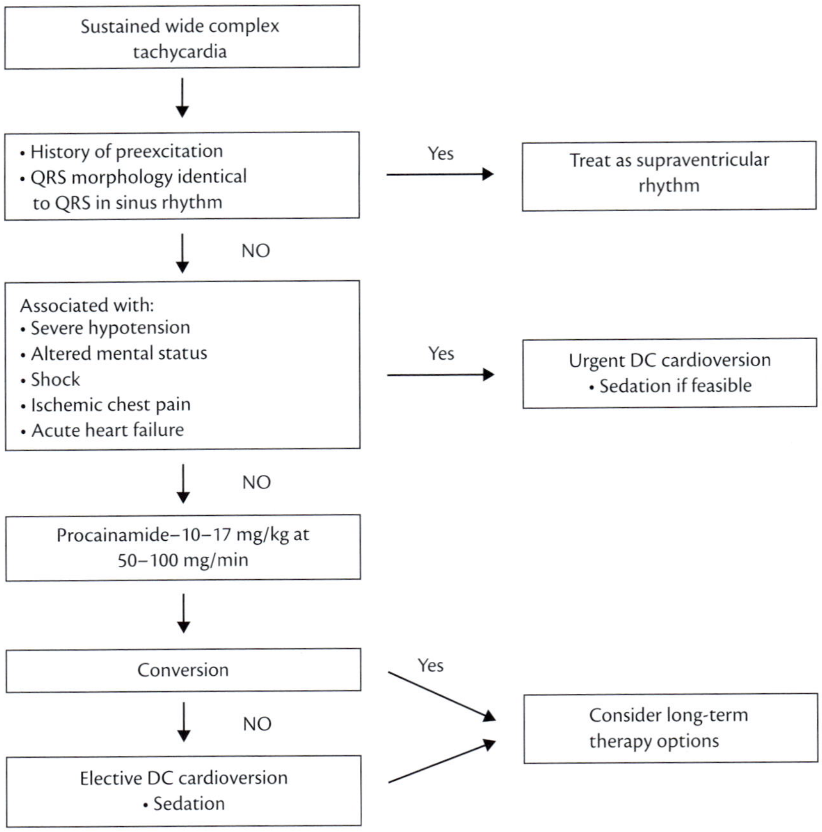

Fig. 10.1 Management of sustained wide-complex tachycardia.

HF and ventricular dysfunction. ICD shocks are, however, painful and may cause significant psychological distress. Antiarrhythmic drugs are therefore often prescribed in an effort to reduce shock frequency. In addition, atrial arrhythmias are common in HF ICD patients and antiarrhythmic drugs are often used to prevent atrial arrhythmias as well.

In addition to the known extracardiac side effects of antiarrhythmic drugs, the potential for drug–ICD interactions must be considered.[18,19] Antiarrhythmic drugs with sodium channel blocking properties (Vaughan Williams class I) may increase defibrillation threshold. Pure class III agents are unlikely to do so and may actually decrease defibrillation energy requirements. Pacing thresholds may rarely be affected. Antiarrhythmic drugs frequently prolong VT cycle lengths and may require changes in programmed detection zones. Antiarrhythmic drugs may result in sinus bradycardia or worsen AV conduction, increasing the need for atrial and/or ventricular pacing.

Amiodarone and sotalol are the drugs most commonly used as adjuncts to ICD therapy.[20,21,22] Pacifico et al.[20] randomized 302 patients with prior sustained arrhythmias and secondary prevention ICDs to either sotalol (160–320 mg daily) or placebo. Sotalol resulted in a 48% reduction of the primary endpoint of death from any cause or delivery of first shock for any cause. Overall shock frequency was significantly reduced to 1.43 ± 3.53 shocks per year in the sotalol group from 3.89 ± 10.65 shocks per year in the placebo group. In the Optimal Pharmacological Therapy in Cardioverter Defibrillator Patients Trial (OPTIC),[21] β-adrenergic blockade only, sotalol, and amiodarone plus β-blockade were compared. Sotalol, and to a greater degree, miodarone plus β-blockade, significantly decreased the frequency of shocks, both appropriate and inappropriate. There are, however, more recent data that suggest that antiarrhythmic drug therapy to prevent ICD shocks may not always be beneficial. Kowey et al.[23] reported a phase II dose-ranging study of celivarone, a noniodinated analog of amiodarone, in patients with ICDs. Celivarone had no significant effect on ICD shock frequency or mortality in this trial. However, the study included a small calibrator group treated with amiodarone. Although the amiodarone group had fewer ICD shocks, they also had a higher mortality. Until more definitive data on the value of adjunct antiarrhythmic therapy become available, it seems reasonable to restrict such therapy to patients with frequent, symptomatic episodes.

Implantable cardioverter defibrillators

The first published report on the use of a totally implanted defibrillator was in 1980.[24] In the ensuing years, the ICD has developed into the most important single therapy for preventing sudden death and treating sustained VT. In the United States over 130 000 ICDs are implanted annually with over three-fourths of the implants used for primary prevention of sudden cardiac death in patients with systolic HF.[25,26,27,28]

An ICD has two essential components: an ICD generator and a lead system for sensing, pacing, and shock delivery. The initial ICD generator was a bulky (230 g) device that required an abdominal implant and used epicardial lead patches. Over time, advances in technology have allowed the devices to become smaller and permitted the use of transvenous or subcutaneous lead systems. The ICD generator contains sensing circuits, memory storage, capacitors, voltage enhancers, a battery, a telemetry module, and a control microprocessor. The initial implanted defibrillator detected ventricular fibrillation (VF) using a probability density function analysis of the sensed ventricular electrogram. It was soon recognized that organized VT also needed to be a target of ICD therapy and sensed ventricular rate is now the basic measure used to detect arrhythmias. Current ICDs have programming options that include pacing for bradycardia, resynchronization therapy, biphasic defibrillation, advanced arrhythmia discrimination in slower zones, and remote monitoring.

After implant, the ICD is programmed with one or more VT or VF detection zones. In slower zones, discrimination algorithms may be used to identify supraventricular arrhythmias so that therapy may be withheld. Episodes of a tachycardia in a VT zone are often treated with several bursts of ATP first, followed by a shock, if necessary (Figures 10.2 and 10.3). In a VF zone, a single burst of ATP during high-voltage charging is often employed before shock delivery. Electrograms from each episode are stored and may be retrieved for subsequent analysis.

The ICD has been shown to be effective for preventing sudden cardiac death in a number of randomized clinical trials.[16,29,30,31,32,33,34,35,36,37] These trials are usually referred to as either secondary prevention trials in which patients had previously experienced a prior episode of cardiac arrest, VF, or VT, or primary prevention trials in which patients at high risk for sudden death but without known prior episodes were studied. The major clinical trials of ICD therapy are summarized in Table 10.1 and Figure 10.4.

The three most important secondary prevention ICD trials were the Antiarrhythmics Versus Implantable Defibrillators (AVID) Study,[29] the Canadian Implantable Defibrillator Study (CIDS),[30] and the Cardiac Arrest Study—Hamburg (CASH).[31] In AVID, 1016 cardiac arrest and unstable VT survivors were randomly assigned to either drug therapy (amiodarone, or infrequently sotalol) or an ICD. Other indicated therapies including β-adrenergic blockers, renin–angiotensin system inhibitors, and revascularization were permitted. The primary endpoint, total mortality, was decreased by 39%, 27%, and 31% at the 1, 2, and 3 year time points respectively. In CIDS, 696 patients with cardiac arrest, sustained VT, or syncope with induced VT were randomized between an ICD and amiodarone. ICD therapy resulted in a 19.7% lower mortality at the 2 year follow-up point. CASH included only cardiac arrest survivors (n = 346) and randomized them to either an ICD or drug therapy (amiodarone, metoprolol, or propafenone). The propafenone arm was terminated early due to excess mortality. At the 2 year time point, the mortality rate was 37% lower in the ICD group than in the combined amiodarone and metoprolol group.

Even in localities with skilled and efficient emergency medical care, most out-of-hospital cardiac arrest victims will not survive. Limiting ICD therapy to cardiac arrest survivors would therefore miss almost all potential sudden cardiac arrest victims. A number of ICD trials have been completed that demonstrated conclusively that ICD therapy is also often effective for primary prevention of sudden death in patients with both ischemic and nonischemic cardiomyopathies. The two largest primary prevention trails were the Multicenter Automatic Defibrillator Implantation Trial II (MADIT II)[33] and SCD-HeFT.[16] In MADIT II, patients had ischemic heart disease with prior myocardial infarction and a LVEF of 30% or less. ICD therapy compared to investigator-selected standard medical therapy resulted in a hazard ratio of 0.69. SCD-HeFT included patients with both ischemic and nonischemic cardiomyopathy, class II or class III HF symptoms, and a LVEF of 35% or less. Patients were randomized to either an ICD, amiodarone, or placebo. Overall, ICD therapy resulted in a hazard ratio of 0.77 with the benefit seen in the subgroup with class II HF.

Several studies of ICD therapy for primary prevention have not shown benefit.

The Coronary Artery Bypass Graft-Patch Trial (CABG-Patch)[34] randomized low ejection fraction in patients undergoing surgical coronary revascularization to either no therapy or an epicardial ICD system. Mortality was slightly higher in the ICD group. Two studies have looked at ICD therapy for primary prevention in high-risk patients early after myocardial infarction. In both the Defibrillator in Acute Myocardial Infarction Trial (DINAMIT)[36] and the Immediate Risk Stratification Improves Survival (IRIS) study,[37] no overall benefit was seen. In these two studies, a decrease in arrhythmic deaths in the ICD group was balanced by

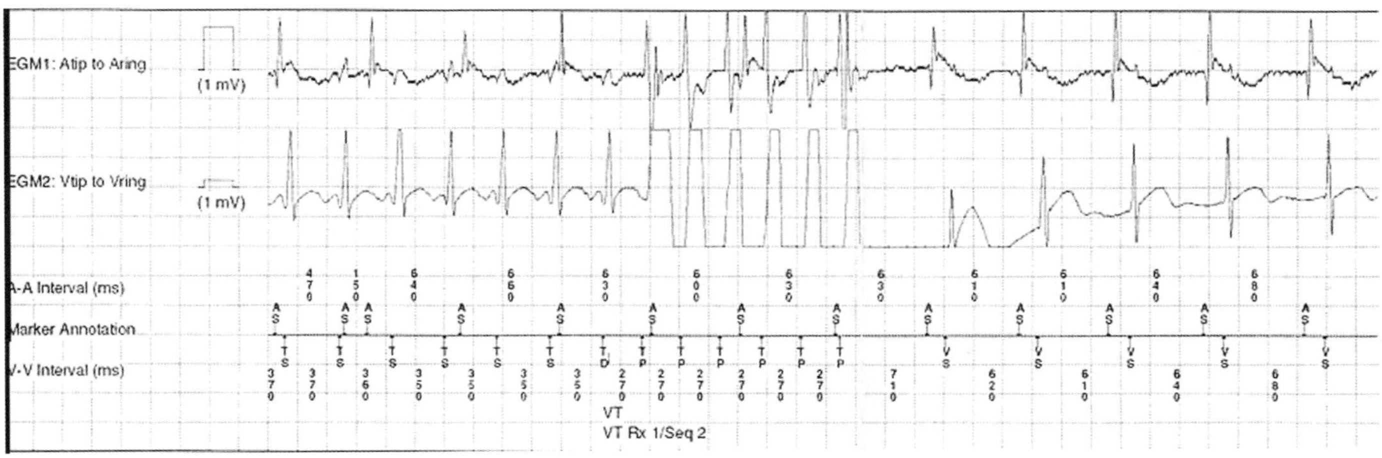

Fig. 10.2 Termination of ventricular tachycardia with ATP. The tracings shown are atrial and ventricular electrograms and an annotated marker channel. At the beginning of the tracing, the patient is in ventricular tachycardia with AV dissociation. A burst of anti-tachycardia pacing (TP) breaks the tachycardia and restores sinus rhythm.

Table 10.1 Major clinical trials of ICD therapy

Trial	Year	Patients (n)	LVEF	Additional study features	Hazard ratio	95% CI	p
Secondary prevention trials							
AVID	1997	1016	Prior cardiac arrest, VT	NA	0.62	(0.43–0.82)	<0.02
CIDS	2000	659	VT, prior cardiac arrest, syncope	NA	0.82	(0.60–1.1)	0.142
CASH	2000	191	Prior cardiac arrest	NA	0.766		0.081 (1-sided)
Primary prevention trials							
MADIT I	1996	196	≤35%	NSVT and EP+	0.46	(0.26–0.82)	0.009
MADIT II	2002	1232	≤30%	Prior MI	0.69	(0.51–0.93)	0.016
CABG-Patch	1997	900	≤36%	+SAECG and CABG	1.07	(0.81–1.42)	0.63
DEFINITE	2004	485	≤35%	NICM, PVCs, or NSVT	0.65	(0.40–1.06)	0.08
IRIS	2009	898	≤40%	Recent MI, HR >90 ± NSVT	1.04	(0.81–1.35)	0.78
DINAMIT	2004	674	≤35%	6–40 days post-MI and impaired HRV	1.08	(0.76–1.55)	0.66
SCD-HeFT	2006	1676	≤35%	Prior MI or NICM, class II or III CHF	0.77	(0.62–0.96)	0.007

AVID, Antiarrhythmics Versus Implantable Defibrillator; CABG-Patch, Coronary Artery Bypass Graft-Patch Trial; CASH, Cardiac Arrest Study Hamburg; CIDS, Canadian Implantable Defibrillator Study; CHF, congestive heart failure; DEFINITE, Defibrillators in Nonischemic Cardiomyopathy Treatment Evaluation; DINAMIT, The Defibrillator in Acute Myocardial Infarction Trial; HR, hazard ratio; HRV, heart rate variability; ICD, implantable cardioverter defibrillator; IRIS, Immediate Risk Stratification Improves Survival; LVEF, left ventricular ejection fraction; MADIT I and II, Multicenter Automatic Implantable Defibrillator Trials I and II; MI, myocardial infarction; NICM, nonischemic cardiomyopathy; NSVT, nonsustained ventricular tachycardia, SAECG, signal averaged ECG; SCD-HeFT, Sudden Cardiac Death in Heart Failure Trial; VT, ventricular tachycardia.

a corresponding increase in nonarrhythmic mortality. Based on these results, the Center for Medicare Services issued a National Coverage Decision[38] relating to ICD therapy in 2005 (see Box 10.2). These guidelines are in general agreement with recommendations from professional societies.

ICD therapy has evolved during a period in which pharmacologic management of patients with HF has improved dramatically. As a result, survival rates in HF patients during medical therapy are now much better than they were when the first ICD trials were reported. For this reason, there has been considerable interest in defining the "optimal" candidate for a primary prevention ICD. In an analysis of data from MADIT II,[39] the authors identified five factors which influenced ICD benefit: NYHA function class III, atrial fibrillation (AF), QRS duration greater than 120 ms, age over 70 years, and blood urea nitrogen (BUN) more than 26 mg/dl. Patients with no risk factors had no benefit from ICD therapy and benefit was markedly reduced in patients with two or more risk factors. Patient with one or two risk factors had the greatest change of benefit. In an analysis of the national Medicare ICD registry data, Bilchick et al.[40] identified seven predictors of mortality after ICD implant. These

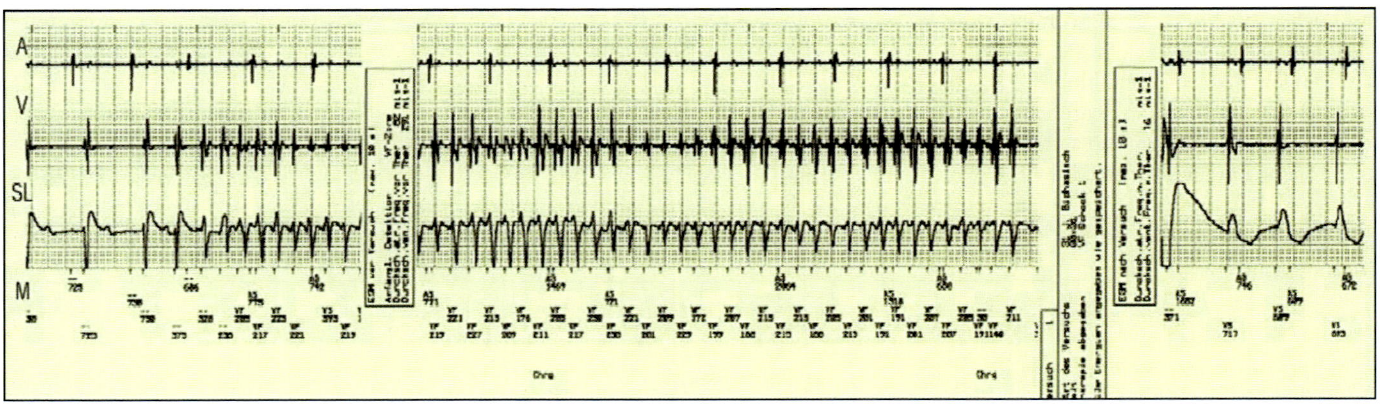

Fig. 10.3 ICD electrograms during rapid ventricular tachycardia. The tracings are stored electrograms from the atrial (A), right ventricular (V), and shock leads (SL) with a marker channel (M). The ventricular electrogram shows initiation of a rapid polymorphic ventricular tachycardia which is sensed by the ICD as ventricular fibrillation (VF). The device charges and shock delivery terminates the arrhythmia. With this device, the actual shocks are not shown.

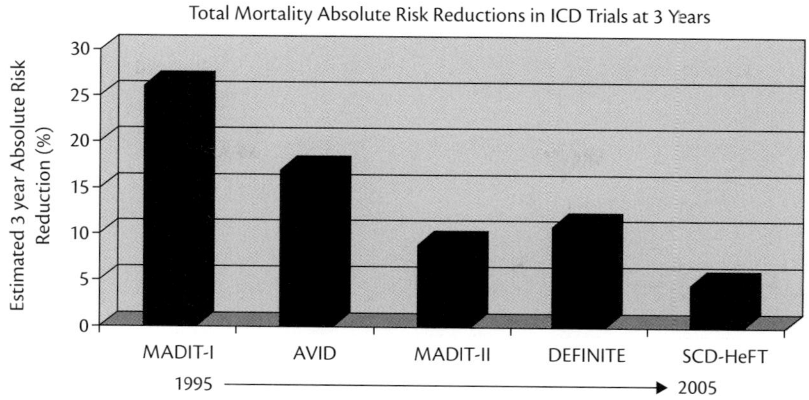

Fig. 10.4 Decreased ICD benefit over time. The graph shows how absolute reductions in total mortality have decreased over time in ICD studies. This decrease is attributable to several factors including better medical management of heart failure and ischemia, low event rates in the studies, and different entry criteria.

included age 75 years or over, class III HF, chronic lung disease, chronic kidney disease, AF, ejection fraction 20% or less, and diabetes. Points were assigned to each risk factor and nomograms relating survival to total point score were calculated. It must be remembered, however, that cardiac resynchronization has independent positive effects on mortality in addition to simply symptoms of HF.[41] At present, in the United States, over 40% of current primary prevention ICD recipients now receive a cardiac resynchronization device.

ICD follow-up and complications

All patients who received an ICD should have both periodic routine checks and urgent follow-up if problems arise.[42] With current ICD models, most follow-up device interrogations can be performed remotely, but virtually all ICD patients should still be seen in person by their cardiologist, HF specialist, or electrophysiologist at least once or twice annually.[43]

At each device interrogation the programmed parameters for bradycardia and tachycardia detection and therapy should be confirmed. Expected device longevity can be estimated based on battery voltage, device parameters, and therapy history. Sensing and capture thresholds and pacing impedance values for each active lead should be measured. All devices also include event logs and store electrograms from specified arrhythmic events. These electrograms should be examined to make sure that tachycardia identification is accurate and therapy effective. Pocket erosions and lead and pocket infections remain common clinical problems. Patients should be instructed to call if they note any change in their pocket or if they have unexplained bloodstream infections. At each clinic visit, the pocket should be carefully examined for signs of infection or inflammation. Pain in a chronic ICD pocket should always arouse suspicion for a chronic low-grade infection.

In-hospital complications

The most common in-hospital complications after ICD insertion are lead dislodgement or perforation, pocket hematoma, pneumothorax, arrhythmias, and if a LV lead is attempted, coronary sinus dissection.[44,45] Early complications are related to the experience and training of the operator, the type of device selected, and certain patient characteristics. Early ICD implants using epicardial patch systems that required a thoracotomy were associated with significant mortality (2–8%) but with transvenous systems, early mortality is much lower and usually due to recurrent arrhythmias. Procedural complications are more frequent with ICD generator changes particularly if a new lead is added.[46]

Late complications

Complications after hospital discharge are also unfortunately common during ICD therapy. The most frequent device-related adverse events are inappropriate shocks, infections, lead or device malfunction, and pacing or lead-related hemodynamic effects. Psychological well-being may also be affected in patients with multiple shocks, either inappropriate or appropriate.

Infections

Infections related to ICDs are a growing problem.[46,47,48] Superficial incisional infections that do not invade the pocket may be seen early after implant and can often be managed with antibiotics and good wound care. Late infections, either direct infection of the pocket or secondary infection of the leads from a remote site, are much more serious. Complete removal of the device and leads and antibiotic therapy are required to control the infection. Patients with evidence for associated valvular endocarditis will need a prolonged course of therapy.

Inappropriate shocks

A number of events can result in the delivery of inappropriate shocks in ICD recipients. Atrial tachyarrhythmias are the most common cause and antiarrhythmic drugs, β-adrenergic blocking agents, and electrogram discrimination algorithms are the most common approaches for prevention. Lead or device malfunctions leading to oversensing are also frequently encountered (Figure 10.5). Some ICD leads have experienced a higher than expected fracture rate. Newer ICD models have incorporated automatic checks of lead integrity to prevent inappropriate shocks due to lead fractures but these are not always effective.

Hemodynamic consequences

Congestive HF may be caused by lead-induced tricuspid valve dysfunction and by dyssynchrony caused by inappropriate right ventricular apical pacing. Loss of LV lead capture during cardiac resynchronization therapy (CRT) is another common cause of ICD-related HF worsening.

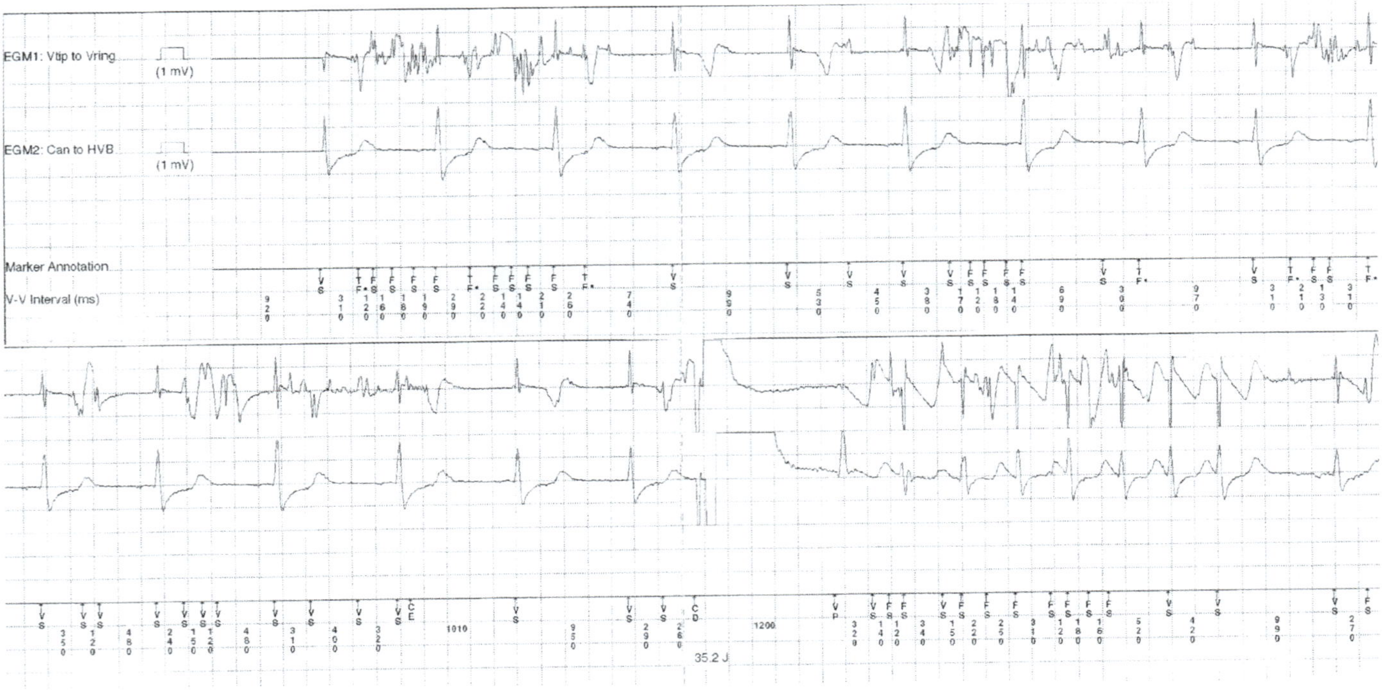

Fig. 10.5 Electrograms showing noise due to a lead fracture. The tracings are from a single-lead ICD. The rapid, high-amplitude spikes seen on the Vtip to Vring electrogram are due to intermittent contact caused by a lead fracture.

Psychological effects

Anxiety, depression, and post-traumatic stress disorder may be seen in ICD recipients. Rare or single shocks are well-tolerated by most but frequent shocks consistently will result in emotional distress and a reduced quality of life.

Ablation

Indications for catheter ablation

The 2009 European Heart Rhythm Association and Heart Rhythm Society's consensus document on catheter ablation of VA lists the current indications for this procedure as symptomatic sustained monomorphic VT that recurs despite therapy with antiarrhythmic drugs or in patients who do not desire or are intolerant of antiarrhythmic medications.[1] VT ablation is also indicated for control of incessant monomorphic VT or VT storm that is not due to a transient reversible cause, for patients with frequent PVCs, NSVT, or VT that results in myocardial dysfunction (due to tachycardia-related cardiomyopathy), for patients with VT from bundle branch reentry or intrafascicular VTs and, with recurrent sustained polymorphic VT or VF that is refractory to antiarrhythmic medications when there is a suspected trigger (single PVC morphology) that can be targeted for ablation. Catheter ablation is increasingly being used as a primary treatment for recurrent VT resulting in recurrent ICD shocks.[49,50] Recent data suggest the substrate-based ablation may reduce the incidence of ICD shocks in patients with a history of myocardial infarction who are undergoing an ICD placement for secondary prevention of sudden death.[51]

Principles of ablation

The majority of sustained VA arises from reentry around myocardial scar.[52,53] Reentrant circuits require areas of slow conduction which allow time for repolarization of the rest of the myocardial circuit thus allowing for perpetuation of the conduction around that circuit. Channels of slow conduction are found within scar tissue and their border zones. The exit site is the location where conduction exits the slow conduction zone to more rapidly conducting myocardium. Exit sites are prime targets for catheter ablation. Less commonly, VT may also arise from a single myocardial focus capable of abnormal automaticity. EP study and mapping techniques can now identify these substrates which can then be the targets for catheter ablation. Catheter ablation technology continues to evolve rapidly but the following concepts remain the cornerstones of ablation.

Access

Electrode catheters are usually advanced via the femoral veins to the high right atrium, the bundle of His, the coronary sinus, and the right ventricular apex. These catheters are used for the basic EP study. Access to the right ventricle is via the femoral veins. Access to the LV was traditionally via the retrograde aortic approach in which the ablation catheter is advanced through a femoral artery sheath, up the aorta, and then across the aortic valve to reach the left ventricle. There is now a growing trend to use the transseptal route for LV access. This has been helped by the increased experience in transseptal puncture from AF ablation procedures and the use of long deflectable sheaths to help direct the ablation catheter across the mitral valve into the LV. The advantage of this technique is that it helps to avoid a tortuous or diseased aorta in patients with peripheral vascular disease. Epicardial access can be obtained by percutaneous subxiphoid needlestick or by a surgical pericardial window.[54] A long sheath is inserted into the pericardial space through which a standard ablation catheter is passed and used for mapping and ablation. Rarely, an epicardial focus can be successfully mapped and ablated via the epicardial coronary veins, accessed via the coronary sinus emptying into the right atrium.[55] Surgical thoracotomy is used in a small number of patients who fail these catheter ablation techniques. In these patients, ablation can be performed under direct vision using surgical ablation that produces larger and deeper lesions or using resection of aneursymal scar.[56] Patients with an epicardial focus close to a coronary artery, those who have failed epicardial catheter ablation, or those who require epicardial mapping but have adhesions following bypass surgery may benefit from this open heart approach.

Programmed stimulation

The initial step to mapping of VT is induction of the VT using programmed stimulation. Ideally, the clinical tachycardia can be reliably induced prior to ablation but is noninducible after ablation. Typically this is done via pacing from the right ventricular apex. Programmed stimulation is performed with a drive train of eight beats using a single cycle length (S1) which is then followed by single or double extrastimuli (S2, S3). With successive drive trains, the coupled extrastimuli are progressively shortened, usually by 10 ms. This process is continued until VT is induced or the extrastimuli no longer capture (ventricular refractory period). Once sustained VT is induced, the QRS morphology and cycle length are analyzed and matched to ECGs of the clinical VT. Ideally the clinical VT is induced reliably several times prior to ablation. Once the VT has been analyzed it can be terminated, preferably using right ventricular pacing. If pacing fails then electrical cardioversion is required to restore sinus rhythm. The amount of programmed stimulation performed is largely governed by the hemodynamic instability of each episode. It is common to also induce nonclinical morphologies of VT, especially after initial ablation. Many of these nonclinical morphologies are also targeted for ablation. With sufficiently aggressive pacing, VF can be induced in most patients but this is nonspecific and not clinically useful.

Voltage and activation mapping

Three-dimensional (3D) electroanatomical mapping systems allow the operator to assign electrograms sensed from the tip of the mapping catheter to specific locations on a 3D computer model of the heart. These models can be created either by importing CT or MRI scans, using the myocardial contours traced from intracardiac ultrasound catheter, or by sweeping the mapping catheter around the inside of the chamber and assimilating the 3D points into a chamber geometry. Voltage maps are created by measuring the amplitude of the electrogram signal at multiple sites of chamber of interest using the mapping catheter. Scar produces low-amplitude signal compared to healthy myocardium. A threshold for endocardial scar is 1.5 mV (dense scar <0.5 mV, border zone 0.5–1.5 mV).[1] The low-voltage regions representing scar can then be displayed on a color map of the chamber of interest (Figures 10.6, 10.7, and 10.8). The VT circuits are commonly located within these regions of scar which serve as a good target for further mapping. Activation maps during VT are generated in a similar manner but the timing of the onset of the electrogram is compared to a timing reference, commonly the onset of the QRS of the VT/PVC. A color map of the activation times can then be displayed to help identify the location of the electrical circuit within the ventricle. Activation mapping is performed during sustained VT. It takes time to collect multiple activation points and so this technique can only be performed in sustained VT that is hemodynamically stable.

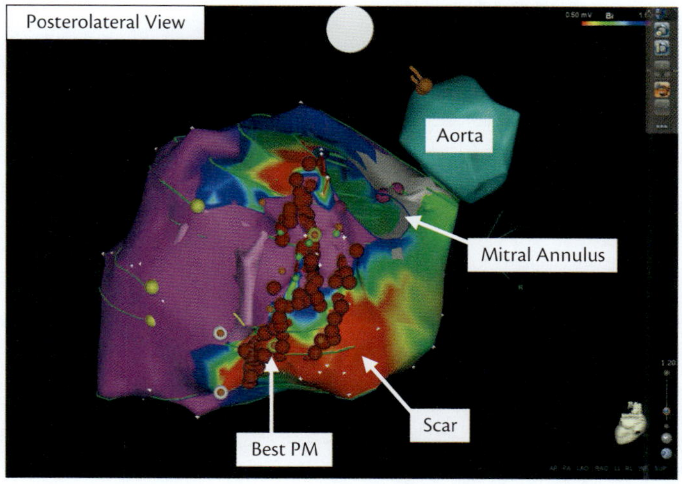

Fig. 10.6 Electroanatomical map of VT ablation. This is the posterolateral view of a Carto map of the left ventricle during ablation of sustained monomorphic VT in a patient with ischemic cardiomyopathy. The 3D geometry was traced from the endocardial contours of intracardiac ultrasound images. These contours are displayed as the green contours seen well overlying the purple lateral wall and these are collated to form a 3D image of the left ventricle and aortic root. The color range represents electrogram voltage. Red (<1.5 mV) represents dense myocardial scar. Purple (>2.5 mV) represents voltage of what is considered normal myocardium. The site of the best pace map are shown (Best PM). The sites of ablation along the edge of the scar are represented by the red dots.

Entrainment and pace mapping

Pacing from the mapping catheter at suspected sites of VT produces a unique QRS morphology at each pacing site. Comparing the paced 12-lead QRS morphology to the targeted VT helps to locate the exit site. Pacing at an exit site of should produce a perfect

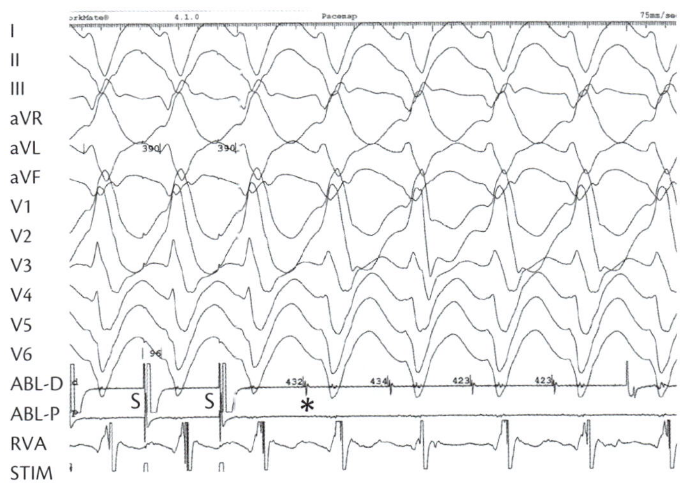

Fig. 10.7 Entrainment pacing during sustained ventricular tachycardia (VT). In this tracing the 12-lead ECG, right ventricular apex (RVA), and ablation distal and proximal (ABL D + P) electrograms are displayed during pacing (first 3 beats at 390 ms) and continuing ventricular tachycardia. The pacing is from the ABL D which is positioned at the Best PM site in Figure 10.7A. The 12-lead QRS morphology during pacing is very similar to that during sustained VT, making this a good pace map in 12 out of 12 leads. The time from the last paced beat (S) to the first electrogram of the continuing VT (*) is 432 ms. This is known as the postpacing interval and is very close to the cycle length of the VT (423 ms). A postpacing interval within 20 ms of the VT cycle length is an indicator that the ablation catheter is within the circuit of the VT.

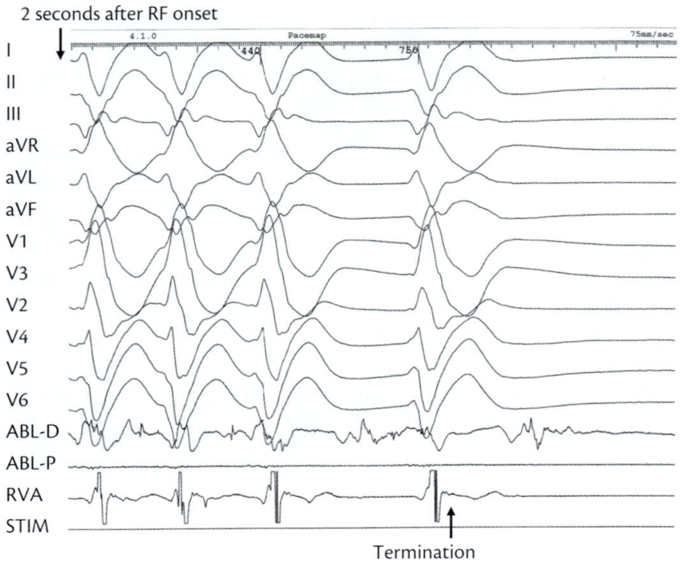

Fig. 10.8 Termination of ventricular tachycardia (VT). Radiofrequency ablation at the Best PM site (Figure 10.1A) which had a good pace map and a postpacing intervals close to the VT cycle length (Figure 10.7B) was successful in terminating the VT in less than 5 seconds after the onset of ablation.

match in all ECG leads (12/12 pace match). Pacing can be performed during sinus rhythm which is useful in patients who have hemodynamically unstable VT. More precise information can be obtained by pacing during stable VT using a process called entrainment. Entrainment pacing is done by pacing during sustained VT at a rate only a little faster than the VT for 20–30 seconds aiming to capture the ventricle but not terminate the VT. Again the paced 12-lead QRS is compared to the clinical VT to assess the proximity to the exit site. More precise information about the location of the pacing site can be obtained by measuring the time from stimulation to onset of the QRS and by measuring the postpacing intervals once VT has resumed. If available, this information can help accurately pinpoint the optimal sites for ablation. Unfortunately, pacing techniques are frequently limited by hemodynamic instability, lack of ventricular capture when pacing in scar, unintended termination of VT, or conversion of the VT to a different morphology during pacing.

Endocardial ablation

Once a successful site has been identified, catheter ablation is performed either with standard radiofrequency or increasingly, with addition of a saline-irrigated catheter tip which allows deeper myocardial lesions.[57] Judging how much ablation to perform at a particular site remains a challenge. Ablation lesions are generally 3–6 mm deep and wide. Transmural lesions are not possible in most ventricles with current technology and so mid or epicardial VT circuits may require additional epicardial ablation. In scar-related VT, it is common to successfully ablate the initial clinical VT but subsequently be able to induce other morphologies. Commonly multiple VTs (~3) need to be ablated.[1]

Ablation endpoints vary between patients. Ideally, the "clinical" arrhythmia is documented on 12-lead ECG and available at the time of the procedure. With the increasing use of ICD therapy, ECG documentation of the clinical VT is not always obtainable. ICDs will usually terminate VT before a 12-lead ECG can be obtained. In such cases the number of VTs, their individual cycle lengths, and electrogram morphologies can be compared with any VT induced at the time of the procedure. A careful note should be made of any changes in antiarrhythmic drugs that may alter the rate of a clinical VT at the time of subsequent ablation. In this situation, 12-lead ECG documentation of QRS morphology is a better indicator than simply using ICD electrogram rate of prior VTs.

Ablation endpoints include:

- Clinical VT noninducible after being reliably induced prior to ablation. This endpoint is associated with a lower risk (~37%) of VT recurrence compared to patients who have persistent inducibility of the clinical VT (~80% recurrence). In patients with a single clinical morphology, the persistent induction of different morphologies after successful ablation of the clinical VT has little effect on outcome.
- Modification of inducible VT. With the widespread use of ICDs, which make ECG documentation of the clinical VT more difficult, another endpoint is often used. Many centers aim to ablate all VTs with the same or longer cycle length than that recorded on ICD but not all of those with faster rates.
- No VT morphology inducible following ablation. This is the preferable endpoint but is not possible to achieve in all patients, especially those with very poor LV function or ischemia who may not tolerate repeated ventricular stimulation, episodes of VT, and shocks during the procedure. It is widely recommended that the minimum endpoint should be ablation of the clinical VT. There is less consensus on how many of residual, previously undocumented VTs should be ablated.[1,50]

Epicardial ablation

One reason for failure of endocardial ablation is a circuit that arises from the epicardium. Many of these circuits can now be ablated using an epicardial approach. This technique is more commonly required in patients with nonischemic cardiomyopathy but other diseases may also involve the epicardium. There is not yet consensus on the indications for epicardial ablation. The percutaneous subxiphoid puncture, developed in Brazil for the treatment of VT related to Chagas disease, is the technique most widely used.[1,50,54] A surgical subxiphoid window may be required and is preferable in patients with prior cardiac surgery who are likely to have adhesions. A flexible sheath is inserted into the pericardial space and a conventional ablation catheter is used for mapping, usually an irrigated tip catheter. The same principles for mapping of the endocardium are used in the epicardium with the additional caveats of avoiding coronary artery and left phrenic nerve damage, managing saline and blood accumulation in the pericardium, and avoiding introduction of air which may raise defibrillation thresholds.[58] Although most cases are being done as a separate procedure in patients who have failed a previous endocardial attempt, some high-volume centers are performing epicardial mapping de novo in patients suspected of an epicardial focus. In a series of patients with and without structural heart disease who had failed prior endocardial ablation, 59 patients underwent epicardial mapping.[59]An epicardial circuit was mapped and successfully ablated in three-quarters of patients. Although the epicardial approach does carry significant risk, the procedure appears to offer success in patients who may not be ablated using conventional endocardial techniques.

Surgical approach

The advances in catheter ablation and widespread use of ICDs has reduced the need for surgical ablation. Nevertheless, surgical aneurysectomy or resection of scar remains an option for some patients with ischemic cardiomyopathy and VT refractory to other therapies.[60] In other patients who have epicardial mapping showing a VT site too close to a coronary artery, surgical ablation under direct vision during thoracotomy can be effective. In patients with a history of VT undergoing surgical LV assist device (LVAD) insertion, both endocardial and epicardial surgical ablation can be performed concomitantly to minimize subsequent ventricular arrhythmia.

Premature ventricular complex ablation

PVCs are common in patients with HF and structural heart disease.[61] PVCs may also be accompanied by short runs of NSVT. It is well documented that frequent PVCs may be the cause of a reversible cardiomyopathy.[1,62,63] It is usually difficult to distinguish whether the PVCs are the primary problem or secondary to the cardiomyopathy. Cases in which PVCs represent more than 10% of heart beats on 24 hour ECG with most PVCs of the same QRS morphology are more likely to be PVC-induced cardiomyopathy. PVC ablation in these patients may result in significant recovery of their LV function.[64] Patients with multiple PVC morphologies are not good ablation candidates. Catheter ablation is usually preferred to antiarrhythmic drugs, which are often contraindicated in patients with structural heart disease. Idiopathic PVCs commonly arise from the right ventricular outflow tract but may also arise from the LV outflow tract, aortic cusps, or pulmonary artery.

Ablation in ischemic cardiomyopathy

The mechanism of VT in patients with prior myocardial infarction is usually reentry around myocardial scar but focal mechanisms can occur in 5–10% of patients.[53] Early reperfusion strategies have resulted in smaller infarcts and less aneurysm formation but in patients with chronic ischemic cardiomyopathy the risk of arrhythmia still remains significant. Ventricular tachycardia occurs at an annual rate of 1–2% of patients after myocardial infarction.[1] Although programmed stimulation can induce VT in almost 90% of patients with ischemic cardiomyopathy and clinical sustained VT, the rate and morphology often differs from that of spontaneous occurring VT. Many of these VTs are hemodynamically unstable. These factors have led to increasing utilization of substrate-based ablation which uses voltage and pace mapping during sinus rhythm to identify targets for ablation.[1,49,50,52] This minimizes the episodes of unstable VT during the procedure and is better tolerated by patients with reduced LV function. Most VT can be ablated from the endocardial approach but some VT, more commonly prior inferior infarction, may require an epicardial approach.[49,59] Outcomes of ablation vary considerably depending on the study population. Successful ablation of all clinical VTs is achieved in 38–72% with a procedural mortality of 0.5–8%.[1,50] Over 12 months follow-up 50–88% of patients will remain free of VT, most continuing on previously ineffective antiarrhythmic drugs.

Ablation in nonischemic cardiomyopathy

Sustained monomorphic VT is less common in nonischemic cardiomyopathy (NICM) but the mechanism is usually also reentry.[1,50,65] Areas of scar in NICM tend to be smaller, often close to the valve annulus and more often located in the mid-myocardium or epicardial layers. It is common to induce multiple morphologies of VT in this patient group and endocardial ablation alone is less successful. Mapping and ablating epicardial sits increases the success in this patient group,[59] but the optimal timing of epicardial ablation is yet to be determined.

Bundle branch reentry

Bundle branch reentry should be suspected in patients who have existing His–Purkinje disease (bundle branch block or significant intraventricular conduction delay). In this form of tachycardia, the circuit conducts retrograde up one bundle, most commonly the left bundle, and anterograde down the other bundle.[1,50] Most commonly this produces typical left bundle branch block pattern on ECG, often with heart rates of more than 200 bpm. Bundle branch reentry can usually be successfully treated by ablation of the right bundle branch, distal to the His signal. This does not often result in heart block although subsequent pacing for bradycadia is common in patients with His–Purkinje system disease. Antiarrhythmic drugs tend to be ineffective and ablation is first-line treatment with a success rate of close to 100%.

Polymorphic VT and ventricular fibrillation

Patients with polymorphic VT/VF usually present with a storm, receiving multiple shocks within 24 hours. Initial therapy with antiarrhythmic drugs, β-blockers, anesthesia, and hemodynamic support may fail to suppress these arrhythmia. Catheter ablation should be considered when polymorphic VT/VF is repeatedly initiated by a single PVC focus.[1,49,50,66] Mapping and ablation of these PVCs needs to be done during the acute storm and small series have reported successful control of the arrhythmia. Sympathectomy may play a role in patients with polymorphic VT/VF refractory to other therapies.[67]

Mechanical support for VT ablation

In patients with VT storms mechanical support can both help to maintain hemodynamic status and also reduce the number of episodes of VT. Intra-aortic balloon pumps have been used for a number of years for this indication but more recently percutaneous LVAD insertion has shown promise. In addition, mechanical support has also been used to support patients during VT ablation procedures, allowing for hemodynamic stability during long periods of sustained VT. This approach allows for prolonged and more detailed mapping of VTs that would otherwise have had to be terminated because of hypotension.

Risks of ablation

Ablation of VT in structurally normal hearts is relatively safe and only rarely results in complications. In patients with significant structural heart disease and multiple comorbidities the complication rate is significant. In a multicenter study of VT ablation in patients with advanced structural disease the complication rate approached 8% with a mortality of 3%.[68] More recently, ablation in a post-infarct population resulted in complications in less than 5%.[51] Most of the data on complications comes from experienced centers and may underestimate the risk in other populations.

Significant complications include vascular injury, thromboembolism, air embolism, cardiac tamponade, damage to the heart valves, the conduction system or the coronary arteries, myocardial ischemia, HF, and radiation exposure.[1,50]

Epicardial ablation carries additional risk. Specific risks include bleeding, injury to the coronary arteries or the left phrenic nerve, altered defibrillation thresholds, and pericarditis.[1] A study of 136 epicardial procedures in 3 experienced centers reported an acute complication rate of 5% and late complications 2% but no deaths.[69] Some degree of pericardial bleeding occurs in almost 30% of patients.[70] Although most bleeding is minor and stops shortly after pericardial access is achieved, occasionally surgical intervention is required. Subdiaphragmatic bleeding including hepatic laceration is rare but important to recognize. Damage to coronary arteries is an important concern and documentation of the location of the major epicardial vessels to the tip of the ablation catheter is usually required prior to ablation. A distance of more than 5 mm from the coronary artery is considered safe. Pericarditis occurs in around 30% of patients and is minimized by the injection of steroids following ablation.

LVAD and transplantation as treatments for refractory ventricular tachycardia

Mechanical support devices are sometimes necessary to bridge patients with refractory arrhythmia to heart transplantation. Farrar et al. used biventricular support devices. Others have shown that LV support alone may be sufficient to bridge patients to transplant. Occasionally, VADs may increase VT. Surgical VT endocardial cryoablation at the time of LVAD placement is possible and may decrease VT episode frequency. Catheter ablation following LVAD placement can be successful if care is taken to avoid the LVAD cannula. ICD back-up is still required for most LVAD patients since right ventricular output may fall during VT.

Transplantation for refractory VT is thought to represent less than 1% of all heart transplants performed in the United States each year. The United Network of Organ Sharing, the governing body for transplant allocation in the United States, has strict criteria to list patients for this indication and requires that the arrhythmia be symptomatic, recurring, life-threatening, and refractory to all therapy, or have prolonged, documented periods of electromechanical dissociation following electrical cardioversion. Listing for this criterion requires special exemption status (1Ae) that necessitates a regional conference call for clinical justification and approval.

References

1. Aliot EM, Stevenson WG, Almendral-Garrote JM, et al. EHRA/HRS Expert Consensus on Catheter Ablation of Ventricular Arrhythmias: developed in a partnership with the European Heart Rhythm Association (EHRA), a Registered Branch of the European Society of Cardiology (ESC), and the Heart Rhythm Society (HRS); in collaboration with the American College of Cardiology (ACC) and the American Heart Association (AHA). Europace 2009;11:771–817.
2. Neumar RW, Otto CW, Link MS, et al. Part 8: adult advanced cardiovascular life support: 2010 American Heart Association Guidelines for Cardiopulmonary Resuscitation and Emergency Cardiovascular Care. Circulation 2010;122: S729–67.
3. Zipes DP, Camm AJ, Borggrefe M, et al. ACC/AHA/ESC 2006 guidelines for management of patients with ventricular arrhythmias and the prevention of sudden cardiac death: a report of the American College of Cardiology/American Heart Association Task Force and the European Society of Cardiology Committee for Practice Guidelines (Writing Committee to Develop Guidelines for Management of Patients With Ventricular Arrhythmias and the Prevention of Sudden Cardiac Death). J Am Coll Cardiol 2006;48: e247–346.
4. Gorgels AP, van den Dool A, Hofs A, et al. Comparison of procainamide and lidocaine in terminating sustained monomorphic ventricular tachycardia. Am J Cardiol 1996;78:43–46.
5. Marill KA, deSouza IS, Nishijima DK, et al. Amiodarone is poorly effective for the acute termination of ventricular tachycardia. Ann Emerg Med 2006;47:217–24.
6. Marill KA, deSouza IS, Nishijima DK, et al. Amiodarone or procainamide for the termination of sustained stable ventricular tachycardia: an historical multicenter comparison. Acad Emerg Med 2010;17:297–306.
7. Marill KA, Wolfram S, Desouza IS, et al. Adenosine for wide-complex tachycardia: efficacy and safety. Crit Care Med 2009;37:2512–18.
8. Levine JH, Massumi A, Scheinman MM, et al. Intravenous amiodarone for recurrent sustained hypotensive ventricular tachyarrhythmias. Intravenous Amiodarone Multicenter Trial Group. J Am Coll Cardiol 1996;27:67–75.
9. Scheinman MM, Levine JH, Cannom DS, et al. Dose-ranging study of intravenous amiodarone in patients with life-threatening ventricular tachyarrhythmias. The Intravenous Amiodarone Multicenter Investigators Group. Circulation 1995;92:3264–72.
10. Kowey PR, Levine JH, Herre JM, et al. Randomized, double-blind comparison of intravenous amiodarone and bretylium in the treatment of patients with recurrent, hemodynamically destabilizing ventricular tachycardia or fibrillation. The Intravenous Amiodarone Multicenter Investigators Group. Circulation 1995;92:3255–63.
11. Ho DS, Zecchin RP, Richards DA, et al. Double-blind trial of lignocaine versus sotalol for acute termination of spontaneous sustained ventricular tachycardia. Lancet 1994;344:18–23.
12. Huang DT, Traub D. Recurrent ventricular arrhythmia storms in the age of implantable cardioverter defibrillator therapy: a comprehensive review. Prog Cardiovasc Dis 2008;51:229–36.
13. Eifling M, Razavi M, Massumi A. The evaluation and management of electrical storm. Texas Heart Inst J 2011;38:111–21.
14. Katritsis DG, Zareba W, Camm AJ. Nonsustained ventricular tachycardia. J Am Coll Cardiol 2012;60:1993–2004.
15. Amiodarone Trials Meta-Analysis Investigators. Effect of prophylactic amiodarone on mortality after acute myocardial infarction and in congestive heart failure: meta-analysis of individual data from 6500 patients in randomised trials. Lancet 1997;350:1417–24.
16. Bardy GH, Lee KL, Mark DB, et al.; Sudden Cardiac Death in Heart Failure Trial (SCD-HeFT) Investigators. Amiodarone or an implantable cardioverter-defibrillator for congestive heart failure. N Engl J Med 2005;352:225–37.
17. Piccini JP, Berger JS, O'Connor CM. Amiodarone for the prevention of sudden cardiac death: a meta-analysis of randomized controlled trials. Eur Heart J 2009;30:1245–53.
18. Bollmann A, Husser D, Cannom DS. Antiarrhythmic drugs in patients with implantable cardioverter-defibrillators. Am J Cardiovasc Drugs 2005;5:371–8.
19. Beadle R, Williams L, Lim HS. Drug-implantable cardioverter-defibrillator interactions. Expert Rev Cardiovasc Ther 2010;8:1267–73.
20. Pacifico A, Hohnloser SH, Williams JH, et al. Prevention of implantable-defibrillator shocks by treatment with sotalol. d,l-Sotalol Implantable Cardioverter-Defibrillator Study Group. N Engl J Med 1999;340:1855–62.
21. Connolly SJ, Dorian P, Roberts RS, et al. Optimal Pharmacological Therapy in Cardioverter Defibrillator Patients (OPTIC) Investigators. Comparison of beta-blockers, amiodarone plus beta-blockers, or sotalol for prevention of shocks from implantable cardioverter defibrillators: the OPTIC Study: a randomized trial. JAMA 2006;295:165–71.
22. Ferreira-Gonzalez I, Dos-Subira L, Guyatt GH. Adjunctive antiarrhythmic drug therapy in patients with implantable cardioverter defibrillators: a systematic review. Eur Heart J 2007;28:469–77.
23. Kowey PR, Crijns HJ, Aliot EM, et al. ALPHEE Study I. Efficacy and safety of celivarone, with amiodarone as calibrator, in patients with an implantable cardioverter-defibrillator for prevention of implantable

cardioverter-defibrillator interventions or death: the ALPHEE study. Circulation 2011;124:2649–60.

24. Mirowski M, Reid PR, Mower MM, et al. Termination of malignant ventricular arrhythmias with an implanted automatic defibrillator in human beings. N Engl J Med 1980;303:322–4.
25. Hammill SC, Kremers MS, Stevenson LW, et al. Review of the registry's fourth year, incorporating lead data and pediatric ICD procedures, and use as a national performance measure. Heart Rhythm 2010;7:1340–5.
26. DiMarco JP. Implantable cardioverter-defibrillators. N Engl J Med 2003;349:1836–47.
27. Epstein AE, Dimarco JP, Ellenbogen KA, et al. American College of Cardiology/American Heart Association Task Force on Practice. American Association for Thoracic Surgery. Society of Thoracic Surgeons. ACC/AHA/HRS 2008 guidelines for device-based therapy of cardiac rhythm abnormalities: executive summary. Heart Rhythm 2008;5:934–55.
28. Tracy CM, Epstein AE, Darbar D, et al. 2012 ACCF/AHA/HRS focused update incorporated into the ACCF/AHA/HRS 2008 guidelines for device-based therapy of cardiac rhythm abnormalities: a report of the American College of Cardiology Foundation/American Heart Association Task Force on Practice Guidelines and the Heart Rhythm Society. J Am Coll Cardiol 2013;61: e6–75.
29. The Antiarrhythmics Versus Implantable Defibrillators (AVID) Investigators. A comparison of antiarrhythmic-drug therapy with implantable defibrillators in patients resuscitated from near-fatal ventricular arrhythmias. N Engl J Med 1997;337:1576–83.
30. Connolly SJ, Gent M, Roberts RS, et al. Canadian implantable defibrillator study (CIDS): a randomized trial of the implantable cardioverter defibrillator against amiodarone. Circulation 2000;101:1297–302.
31. Kuck KH, Cappato R, Siebels J, Ruppel R. Randomized comparison of antiarrhythmic drug therapy with implantable defibrillators in patients resuscitated from cardiac arrest: the Cardiac Arrest Study Hamburg (CASH). Circulation 2000;102:748–54.
32. Moss AJ, Hall WJ, Cannom DS, et al. Improved survival with an implanted defibrillator in patients with coronary disease at high risk for ventricular arrhythmia. Multicenter Automatic Defibrillator Implantation Trial Investigators. N Engl J Med 1996;335:1933–40.
33. Moss AJ, Zareba W, Hall WJ, et al. Multicenter Automatic Defibrillator Implantation Trial II Investigators. Prophylactic implantation of a defibrillator in patients with myocardial infarction and reduced ejection fraction. N Engl J Med 2002;346:877–83.
34. Bigger JT,Jr. Prophylactic use of implanted cardiac defibrillators in patients at high risk for ventricular arrhythmias after coronary-artery bypass graft surgery. Coronary Artery Bypass Graft (CABG) Patch Trial Investigators. N Engl J Med 1997;337:1569–75.
35. Kadish A, Dyer A, Daubert JP, et al. Defibrillators in Non-Ischemic Cardiomyopathy Treatment Evaluation (DEFINITE) Investigators. Prophylactic defibrillator implantation in patients with nonischemic dilated cardiomyopathy. N Engl J Med 2004;350:2151–8.
36. Hohnloser SH, Kuck KH, Dorian P, et al. DINAMIT I. Prophylactic use of an implantable cardioverter-defibrillator after acute myocardial infarction. N Engl J Med 2004;351:2481–8.
37. Steinbeck G, Andresen D, Seidl K, et al. IRIS I. Defibrillator implantation early after myocardial infarction. N Engl J Med 2009;361:1427–36.
38. Center for Medicare Services. Pub. 100-03 Medicare National Coverage Determinations Available at: <http://www.cms.gov/transmittals/downloads/R29NCD.pdf>.
39. Goldenberg I, Vyas AK, Hall WJ, et al., MADIT-II. I. Risk stratification for primary implantation of a cardioverter-defibrillator in patients with ischemic left ventricular dysfunction. J Am Coll Cardiol 2008;51:288–96.
40. Bilchick KC, Stukenborg GJ, Kamath S, Cheng A. Prediction of mortality in clinical practice for Medicare patients undergoing defibrillator implantation for primary prevention of sudden cardiac death. J Am Coll Cardiol 2012;60:1647–55.
41. Cleland JG, Daubert JC, Erdmann E, et al. Cardiac Resynchronization-Heart Failure (CARE-HF) Study Investigators. The effect of cardiac resynchronization on morbidity and mortality in heart failure. N Engl J Med 2005;352:1539–49.
42. Chugh SS, Wood MA. ICD follow up and troubleshooting. In: Ellenbogen K, Wood M, ed., Cardiac Pacing and ICDs. Blackwell, Oxford; 2008; p. 463.
43. Varma N, Epstein AE, Irimpen A, et al., TRUST I. Efficacy and safety of automatic remote monitoring for implantable cardioverter-defibrillator follow-up: the Lumos-T Safely Reduces Routine Office Device Follow-up (TRUST) trial. Circulation 2010;122:325–32.
44. Freeman JV, Wang Y, Curtis JP, et al. The relation between hospital procedure volume and complications of cardioverter-defibrillator implantation from the implantable cardioverter-defibrillator registry. J Am Coll Cardiol 2010;56:1133–9.
45. van Rees JB, de Bie MK, Thijssen J, et al. Implantation-related complications of implantable cardioverter-defibrillators and cardiac resynchronization therapy devices: a systematic review of randomized clinical trials. J Am Coll Cardiol 2011;58:995–1000.
46. Poole JE, Gleva MJ, Mela T, et al., REPLACE Registry I. Complication rates associated with pacemaker or implantable cardioverter-defibrillator generator replacements and upgrade procedures: results from the REPLACE registry. Circulation 2010;122:1553–61.
47. Baddour LM, Cha YM, Wilson WR. Clinical practice. Infections of cardiovascular implantable electronic devices. N Engl J Med 2012;367:842–9.
48. Baddour LM, Epstein AE, Erickson CC, et al. American Heart Association Rheumatic Fever, Endocarditis, and Kawasaki Disease Committee.Council on Cardiovascular Disease in Young, Council on Cardiovascular Surgery and Anesthesia, Council on Cardiovascular Nursing.Council on Clinical Cardiology.Interdisciplinary Council on Quality of Care, American Heart Association. Update on cardiovascular implantable electronic device infections and their management: a scientific statement from the American Heart Association. Circulation 2010;121:458–77.
49. Yamada T, Kay GN. Optimal ablation strategies for different types of ventricular tachycardias. Nat Rev Cardiol 2012;9:512–25.
50. Natale A, Raviele A, Al-Ahmad A, et al. Venice Chart International Consensus document on ventricular tachycardia/ventricular fibrillation ablation. J Cardiovasc Electrophysiol 2010;21:339–79.
51. Reddy VY, Reynolds MR, Neuzil P, et al. Prophylactic catheter ablation for the prevention of defibrillator therapy. N Engl J Med 2007;357:2657–65.
52. Stevenson WG, Soejima K. Catheter ablation for ventricular tachycardia. Circulation 2007;115:2750–60.
53. Crawford T, Cowger J, Desjardins B, et al. Determinants of postinfarction ventricular tachycardia. Circ Arrhythm Electrophysiol 2010;3:624–31.
54. Sosa E, Scanavacca M. Epicardial mapping and ablation techniques to control ventricular tachycardia. J Cardiovasc Electrophysiol 2005;16:449–52.
55. Baman TS, Ilg KJ, Gupta SK, et al. Mapping and ablation of epicardial idiopathic ventricular arrhythmias from within the coronary venous system. Circ Arrhythm Electrophysiol 2010;3:274–9.
56. Lee R, Mitchell JD, Garan H, et al. Operation for recurrent ventricular tachycardia. Predictors of short- and long-term efficacy. J Thorac Cardiovasc Surg 1994;107:732–42.
57. Stevenson WG, Wilber DJ, Natale A, et al.; Multicenter Thermocool VT Ablation Trial Investigators. Irrigated radiofrequency catheter ablation guided by electroanatomic mapping for recurrent ventricular tachycardia after myocardial infarction: the multicenter thermocool ventricular tachycardia ablation trial. Circulation 2008;118:2773–82.
58. Tedrow U, Stevenson WG. Strategies for epicardial mapping and ablation of ventricular tachycardia. J Cardiovasc Electrophysiol 2009;20:710–13.
59. Schmidt B, Chun KR, Baensch D, et al. Catheter ablation for ventricular tachycardia after failed endocardial ablation: epicardial substrate or inappropriate endocardial ablation?. Heart Rhythm 2010;7:1746–52.
60. Raja SG, Salehi S, Bahrami TT. Impact of technique of left ventricular aneurysm repair on clinical outcomes: current best available evidence. J Card Surg 2009;24:319–24.

61. Maskin CS, Siskind SJ, LeJemtel TH. High prevalence of nonsustained ventricular tachycardia in severe congestive heart failure. Am Heart J 1984;107:896–901.
62. Baman TS, Lange DC, Ilg KJ, et al. Relationship between burden of premature ventricular complexes and left ventricular function. Heart Rhythm 2010;7:865–9.
63. Kanei Y, Friedman M, Ogawa N, et al. Frequent premature ventricular complexes originating from the right ventricular outflow tract are associated with left ventricular dysfunction. Ann Noninvasive Electrocardiol 2008;13:81–5.
64. Bogun F, Crawford T, Reich S, et al. Radiofrequency ablation of frequent, idiopathic premature ventricular complexes: comparison with a control group without intervention. Heart Rhythm 2007;4:863–7.
65. Mathuria N, Tung R, Shivkumar K. Advances in ablation of ventricular tachycardia in nonischemic cardiomyopathy. Curr Cardiol Rep 2012;14:577–83.
66. Pogwizd SM, McKenzie JP, Cain ME. Mechanisms underlying spontaneous and induced ventricular arrhythmias in patients with idiopathic dilated cardiomyopathy. Circulation 1998;98:2404–14.
67. Vaseghi M, Shivkumar K. Neuraxial modulation for ventricular arrhythmias: a new hope. Heart Rhythm 2012;9:1888–9.
68. Calkins H, Epstein A, Packer D, et al. Catheter ablation of ventricular tachycardia in patients with structural heart disease using cooled radiofrequency energy: results of a prospective multicenter study. Cooled RF Multi Center Investigators Group. J Am Coll Cardiol 2000;35:1905–14.
69. Sacher F, Roberts-Thomson K, Maury P, et al. Epicardial ventricular tachycardia ablation a multicenter safety study. J Am Coll Cardiol 2010;55:2366–72.
70. d'Avila A. Epicardial catheter ablation of ventricular tachycardia. Heart Rhythm 2008;5: S73–5.

CHAPTER 11

Cardiac resynchronization

James P. Daubert MD, Brett Atwater MD, and Kevin Jackson MD

Patient selection for cardiac resynchronization therapy

Cardiac resynchronization therapy (CRT) provides hemodynamic and clinical benefits for patients with heart failure (HF). CRT has been associated with a 30–50% reduction in all-cause mortality or HF hospitalization among thousands of carefully selected patients enrolled in clinical trials.[1,2,3,4] Cost-effectiveness analyses have repeatedly demonstrated the attractiveness of CRT for eligible patients.[5] Unfortunately the risk–benefit ratio is highly variable among patients with HF. Up to 30% of patients implanted with current-generation CRT devices fail to demonstrate clinical benefit with CRT therapy and up to 50% of patients fail to demonstrate echocardiographic response.[6,7] This chapter aims to review the current state of the art for identification of patients likely to benefit from CRT.

Mechanism of action of cardiac resynchronization therapy

Ventricular conduction delay is common among patients with HF and results in decreased stroke volume, worsening mitral regurgitation, and increased ventricular wall stress.[8] Conduction delay is frequently manifest on surface electrocardiogram (ECG) as prolongation of the QRS interval in left bundle branch block (LBBB), right bundle branch block (RBBB), or nonspecific intraventricular conduction delay (IVCD) patterns. Prolongation of the QRS interval independently predicts HF hospitalization and death among patients with systolic HF.[9,10] The objective of CRT is to approximate normal ventricular conduction to deliver near simultaneous mechanical contraction of the right ventricle (RV), interventricular septum, and left ventricular (LV) free wall. In selected patients CRT improves a variety of cardiac hemodynamics, including cardiac output, systolic pressure, mitral regurgitation, and left atrial pressure.[11,12]

Methods for identifying ventricular dyssynchrony

Because CRT is meant to restore ventricular synchrony it stands to reason that methods that characterize and identify significant dyssynchrony could improve our ability to select patients who will benefit from CRT. A variety of methods have been developed to identify and quantify ventricular dyssynchrony.

Electrocardiogram QRS duration

To date the only recommended method for identifying patients with dyssynchrony is QRS prolongation on surface ECG. Clinical trials of CRT enrolled subjects with a minimum QRS duration of 120–150 ms but the mean QRS in each study was substantially higher (Table 11.1).[1,13,14,15,16] Post-hoc analyses of the REVERSE and MADIT-CRT studies demonstrated that the clinical response to CRT was directly correlated to the baseline QRS duration.[17] Similar studies performed in large single-center analyses have shown no significant correlation between QRS duration and clinical or echocardiographic outcomes.[18] A meta-analysis including 5813 patients enrolled in 5 clinical trials showed that patients with a QRS duration of 150 ms or more derived a significant reduction in clinical adverse events (risk ratio = 0.6, $p < 0.001$) while patients with a QRS duration less than 150 ms derived no reduction in clinical adverse events (risk ratio = 0.95, $p = 0.49$).[19]

More recently, Sweeney and colleagues described new electrocardiographic analytic methods to obtain detailed information about LV myocardial scar location, baseline and biventricular-paced electrical vectors, and the activation times of the RV and LV.[20] Baseline electrocardiographic characteristics associated with echocardiographic response to CRT included LV scar burden as measured by the Selvester score and LV activation time. Biventricular-paced electrocardiographic characteristics associated with response to CRT included increasing R-wave amplitude in V1 to V2, and an axis shift from the left axis deviation to right axis deviation. The predicted probability of reverse remodeling ranged from less than 20% for patients with adverse predictors to 99% for patients with positive predictors.

Echocardiographic methods for identification of dyssynchrony

Prolongation of the QRS interval and mechanical dyssynchrony may not always be concordant. Leclercq and colleagues compared mechanical dyssynchrony and electrical dispersion during RA pacing, LV-only pacing, and biventricular pacing in dogs with tachycardia-induced cardiomyopathy and a LBBB electrocardiographic pattern.[21] Using tagged-MRI they found that mechanical dyssynchrony was reduced during both LV-only pacing and biventricular pacing while electrical dispersion was reduced only during biventricular pacing. Bleeker and colleagues reported that up to 30% of HF patients with QRS duration less than 120 ms have significant mechanical dyssynchrony by echocardiographic tissue Doppler imaging and 20–30% of HF patients with QRS duration greather than 120 ms may not have mechanical dyssynchrony.[22] Taken together, these data suggest that an imaging-based assessment of mechanical dyssynchrony may provide additional useful information when selecting patients for CRT.

Early single-center studies evaluating echocardiography for identification and quantitation of ventricular dyssynchrony used tissue Doppler imaging techniques to assess septal and lateral LV wall motion.[23,24] Septal to lateral wall delay of more than 65 ms, or standard deviation of time to peak systolic velocity of 12 segments greater than 33 ms, predicted clinical improvement

Table 11.1 Inclusion/exclusion criteria and key baseline subject characteristics of major CRT trials

	MUSTIC (n = 67)	PATH-CHF (n = 36)	MIRACLE (n = 453)	MIRACLE-ICD (n = 369)	CONTAK (n = 490)	COMPANION (n = 1520)	MADIT-CRT (n = 1820)	RAFT (n = 1798)	REVERSE (n = 610)
Cardiac rhythm	SR	SR	SR	SR	SR	SR	SR	SR	SR
NYHA class	III	III, IV	III, IV	III, IV	II, III, IV	III, IV	I, II	II, III	I, II
NYHA class distribution (%)	100	86/14	91/9	89/9	33/59/8	85/15	15/85	80/20	18/82
Minimum QRS (ms)	≥150	≥120	≥130	≥130	≥120	≥120	≥130	≥120	≥120
Mean ± SD QRS (ms)	176 ± 19	175 ± 32	166 ± 20	164 ± 22	158 ± 26	160	159	158 ± 24	154 ± 24
LVEF (%)	≤35	≤35	≤35	≤35	≤35	≤35	≤30	≤30	≤40
Mean ± SD LVEF (%)	23 ± 7	21 ± 7	22 ± 6	24 ± 1	21 ± 7	22	24 ± 5	23 ± 6	27 ± 7

LVEF, left ventricular ejection fraction; NYHA, New York Heart Association; SR, sinus rhythm.

or echocardiographic response to CRT. Further, these small studies suggested these cut-off values predicted CRT response better than ECG QRS duration. Newer methods using myocardial deformation analysis based on ultrasonic pixel "speckle" tracking can identify areas of transmural scar in addition to dyssynchrony information, potentially allowing the implanting physician to target the LV lead to viable myocardium.[25]

Echocardiographic assessment of mechanical dyssynchrony: clinical trials

The Predictors of Response to CRT (PROSPECT) study enrolled 498 patients from 53 international centers with LV ejection fraction (LVEF) 35% or less, QRS duration 130 ms or more, and NYHA class III or IV HF and evaluated 12 echocardiographic parameters as possible predictors of a positive response to CRT.[26] Clinical outcomes were improved in 69% of patients, whereas LV end-systolic volume decreased more than 15% in 56% of patients. The core echocardiographic lab found high variability in the measurement of each echocardiographic parameter arising from technical and interpretative factors at the enrolling centers. No single echocardiographic dyssynchrony parameter predicted clinical or echocardiographic response to CRT and it remains unclear whether this was related to the variability in parameter measurement.

The Resynchronization Therapy in Narrow QRS Study (ReThinQ) enrolled 250 patients at 34 centers with LVEF 35% or less, QRS duration 130 ms or more, and NYHA class III or IV HF with echocardiographic evidence of mechanical dyssynchrony.[27] Mechanical dyssynchrony was defined as a delay 65 ms or more in opposing wall delay by tissue Doppler imaging or a delay of 130 ms or more in septal to posterior wall QRS onset-to-peak displacement by M-mode echo in the parasternal long axis view. Overall the study showed no significant difference in clinical or echocardiographic outcomes between those patients randomized to CRT-on and those patients randomized to CRT-off. In a prespecified subgroup analysis, patients with QRS greater than120 ms showed significant improvements in NYHA class and peak oxygen consumption while those patients with a QRS duration less than 120 ms showed no improvements.

Delgado and colleagues evaluated speckle tracking among 397 patients with ischemic cardiomyopathy.[28] They found that two-dimensional speckle tracking radial strain analysis was feasible in 98% of patients. After 3 years of CRT, the survival rate of patients with LV radial dyssynchrony on baseline echocardiogram analysis (defined as a time delay between the anteroseptal and posterior segments of 130 ms or more) was 82% compared with 65% for patients without substantial dyssynchrony ($p < 0.001$). Further, they found that patients with leads placed in the area of latest mechanical contraction and in areas without speckle tracking-defined scar had better survival than patients with leads placed in areas with scar or in areas with early baseline mechanical contraction.

In summary, the use of echocardiography to identify patients who are suitable for CRT implantation is experimental and is not currently recommended to replace or supplement QRS interval. The ongoing Echocardiography Guided Cardiac Resynchronization Therapy (ECHO-CRT) study plans to enroll over 2300 patients with QRS duration 130 ms or more, and echocardiographic evidence of mechanical dyssynchrony. This study may offer more insight into the usefulness of newer echocardiographic methods, including speckle tracking, for the identification of dyssynchrony and prediction of clinical response to CRT.

MRI methods for assessment of mechanical dyssynchrony

Contrast-enhanced MRI offers excellent spatial resolution and is able to assess scar tissue noninvasively while offering the ability to assess mechanical dyssynchrony in three dimensions.[29] Bleeker and colleagues evaluated whether MRI findings could predict clinical and echocardiographic CRT response in 40 patients with NYHA class III or IV HF, LVEF 35% or less, QRS duration 120 ms or more, LBBB, and chronic coronary artery disease.[30] Patients with transmural posterolateral scar tissue showed a low response rate compared to patients without posterolateral scar (14% vs. 81%; $p < 0.05$). Patients without posterolateral scar tissue on MRI and evidence of severe baseline dyssynchrony on tissue Doppler echocardiographic imaging (>65 ms delay between septal and lateral walls) had a response rate of 95% compared to a response rate of 11% among patients with a posterolateral scar and/or absent LV dyssynchrony on tissue Doppler imaging. Leyva and colleagues evaluated the use of preprocedure contrast-enhanced MRI for prediction of clinical outcomes in 559 consecutive patients who received CRT for existing clinical indications between 2000 and 2009.[31] At follow-up, patients with the LV lead placed in an area of scar ($n = 43$) or who did not have a preprocedure MRI ($n = 350$) had significantly higher risk of cardiovascular death or hospitalization, higher clinical composite score, and more advanced NYHA class than patients who had the LV lead placed in an area without scar on preprocedure MRI ($n = 166$).

In the RESPOND study, investigators studied whether MRI-guided LV lead placement could improve clinical and echocardiographic outcomes in patients with LVEF 35% or less, NYHA class III or IV HF, and QRS duration 120 ms or less.[32] A total of 60 patients were randomly assigned to optimal medical therapy or CRT-D implantation. At 6 month follow-up, the 6 minute walk distance increased significantly in the CRT group (146.3 m to 249.0 m),but not in the medical therapy group (120 m to 90 m); $p < 0.0001$). Significant improvements were also found in the clinical composite score, NYHA class, and quality of life score in the patients randomly assigned to receive CRT but not patients with assigned to medical therapy. In summary, MRI may allow identification of patients with QRS less than 120 ms who have significant mechanical dyssynchrony and may benefit from CRT; however, these findings are experimental and the use of MRI for identification of CRT candidates has not received the recommendation of guidelines committees.

Characteristics of CRT "super-responders"

Between 15% and 25% of CRT recipients obtain dramatic improvement in EF and/or LV volumes and are called "super-responders". No consistent definition has been applied across studies of CRT super-response but in general super-responders obtain more than 15% improvement in EF or more than 20% reduction in LV end-systolic volume. These patients enjoy dramatic improvements in HF symptoms and HF hospitalizations. Among patients enrolled in MADIT-CRT with mildly symptomatic HF, QRS greater than 130 ms, and LVEF 30% or less, the cumulative probability of HF or all-cause death at 2 years was 4% in super-responders, 11% in responders, and 26% in hyporesponders ($p < 0.001$).[33] Single-center studies identified underlying LBBB, female sex, lower baseline BNP,[34] and shorter duration of HF symptoms[35] as predictors of CRT super-response. Characteristics of patients enrolled in MADIT-CRT who obtained CRT super-response included female sex (odds ratio [OR] 1.96; $p = 0.001$), no prior myocardial infarction (OR 1.80; $p = 0.005$), QRS duration 150 ms or more (OR 1.79; $p = 0.007$), LBBB (OR 2.05; $p = 0.006$), body mass index morer than 30 kg/m^2 (OR 1.51; $p = 0.035$), and smaller baseline left atrial volume index (OR 1.47; $p < 0.001$).

Characteristics of CRT nonresponders

Much effort has been spent identifying patient characteristics that reduce the likelihood of CRT response. In addition to male sex, and ischemic cause of underlying cardiomyopathy, atrial fibrillation (AF), conduction block patterns other than LBBB, chronic underlying RV apical pacing preceding CRT implantation, and a high baseline premature ventricular contraction (PVC) burden have been associated with reduced likelihood of CRT response.

Atrial fibrillation

Data on the use of CRT in patients with AF and HF are limited because patients with AF were excluded from most of the major trials of CRT. A meta-analysis of data from 5 prospective studies of CRT in patients with AF and HF compared responses in 797 patients with sinus rhythm and 367 patients with AF. The majority (56%) of patients with AF had atrioventricular (AV) nodal ablation.[36] The NYHA class improved similarly in patients with sinus rhythm and AF but the improvements in 6 minute walk distance and the Minnesota Living With Heart Failure Questionnaire quality of life scores improved more in patients with sinus rhythm than AF.

AF likely reduces the benefit of CRT by eliminating the ability of the CRT device to restore both AV synchrony and intra- and interventricular synchrony. The irregularity of ventricular response and frequent episodes of rapid AV nodal conduction during AF reduce the percentage of biventricular pacing. Among patients with standard CRT implantation criteria and a history of atrial arrhythmia, the percentage biventricular pacing is a strong predictor of HF hospitalization and all-cause mortality (Figure 11.1).[37] Patients

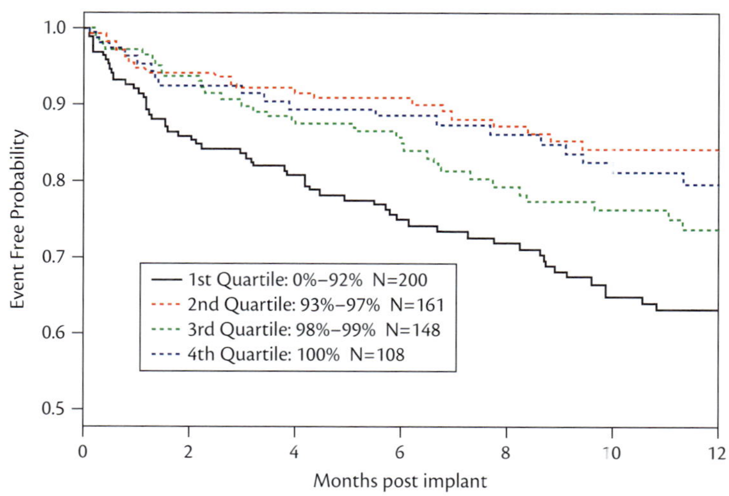

Fig. 11.1 Survival free from heart failure hospitalization and all-cause mortality in patients with a history of atrial arrhythmia. Q2 to Q4 versus Q1, HR 0.44, $p < 0.00001$; Q2 versus Q1, HR 0.34, $p < 0.001$.

Reprinted from the Journal of the American College of Cardiology, 53(4), Koplan BA et al., Heart Failure Decompensation and All-Cause Mortality in Relation to Percent Biventricular Pacing in Patients With Heart Failurels a Goal of 100% Biventricular Pacing Necessary?, 355–60, copyright (2009) with permission from Elsevier.

in this study with more than 92% biventricular pacing had a 66% reduction in HF hospitalization or all-cause mortality compared to patients with less than 92% biventricular pacing ($p < 0.00001$). The optimal percentage of biventricular pacing remains a matter of debate. Hayes and colleagues used data obtained from a large cohort of 36 935 patients enrolled in the LATTITUDE™ remote monitoring network to evaluate the relationship between percent biventricular pacing and all-cause mortality.[38] They found that patients with more than 99.6% biventricular pacing had a 24% reduction in all-cause mortality compared to patients with less than 99.6% biventricular pacing. Slowing AV nodal conduction either medically or with AV nodal ablation or restoring sinus rhythm using either antiarrhythmic drugs or ablation procedures can improve the percentage of biventricular pacing.

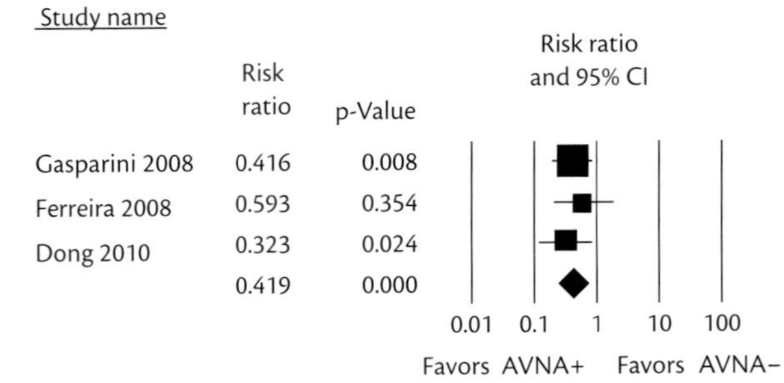

Fig. 11.2 Risk ratios for all-cause mortality in CRT patients with atrial fibrillation undergoing AV node ablation versus medical therapy with rate-controlling drugs. Reprinted from Journal of the American College of Cardiology, 59(8), Ganesan AN et al., Role of AV Nodal Ablation in Cardiac Resynchronization in Patients With Coexistent Atrial Fibrillation and Heart Failure: A Systematic Review, 719-26, copyright (2012) with permission from Elsevier.

Role of AV nodal ablation in CRT therapy for patients with atrial fibrillation

The use of AV nodal ablation in combination with CRT in patients with AF and HF was evaluated in an observational study of 673 patients with EF 35% or less, QRS 120 ms or more, and NYHA class II–IV HF.[39] Of the 162 patients in the cohort with chronic AF, 48 were given medical therapy for rate control to achieve more than 85% biventricular pacing and 114 underwent AV node ablation. Overall, patients with either chronic AF or sinus rhythm had clinical and echocardiographic response to CRT; however, among the patients with chronic AF, only those who had AV nodal ablation showed a significant increase in LVEF ($p < 0.001$), reverse remodeling effect ($p < 0.001$), and improved exercise tolerance ($p < 0.001$). A second, larger observational study was performed in 1285 consecutive patients with LVEF 35% or less, QRS 120 ms or more, and NYHA class II–IV HF.[40] Among the patients with chronic AF, 118 had AV nodal ablation and 55 received medical therapy to slow AV nodal conduction enough to achieve over 85% biventricular pacing. During 34 months median follow-up, mortality was significantly lower in patients treated with AV node ablation (4.3 vs. 15.2% in patients treated with drugs for rate control, adjusted hazard ratio 0.26 for all-cause mortality and 0.15 for HF mortality). In a systematic review investigators identified 6 studies reporting outcomes after AV nodal ablation in patients with AF undergoing CRT for symptomatic HF and LV dyssynchrony, including 768 CRT-AF patients, 339 of whom underwent AV nodal ablation and 429 were treated with medical therapy aimed at rate control alone.[41] Compared to patients who had CRT with medical therapy for rate control, patients who had CRT with AV nodal ablation had significant reductions in all-cause mortality (risk ratio 0.42), cardiovascular mortality (risk ratio 0.44), and improvement in mean NYHA functional class (risk ratio −0.52) (Figure 11.2).

Role of atrial fibrillation ablation in patients with CRT

One small study has compared a rhythm control approach of AF ablation by pulmonary vein isolation to AV nodal ablation to achieve 100% biventricular pacing.[42] Patients with symptomatic drug-resistant AF, an EF of 40% or less, and NYHA class II or III HF were randomly assigned to undergo either pulmonary vein isolation or AV node ablation with biventricular pacing. In all, 41 patients underwent pulmonary vein isolation, and 40 underwent AV node ablation with biventricular pacing. At 6 month follow-up patients randomized to pulmonary vein isolation had a better Minnesota Living With Heart Failure Questionnaire quality of life score (60 vs. 82, lower scores indicating better quality of life; $p < 0.001$), a longer 6 minute walk distance (340 m vs. 297 m, $p < 0.001$), and a higher LVEF (35% vs. 28%, $p < 0.001$) than patients randomized to AV node ablation and CRT.

Baseline RBBB or IVCD

The majority of patients enrolled in clinical trials of CRT had a baseline LBBB ECG pattern. Retrospective subgroup analyses of these studies show that patients with RBBB or IVCD derived less clinical and echocardiographic benefit than patients with LBBB.[43,44] The largest report of the use of CRT in patients with RBBB was a retrospective subgroup analysis of the MADIT-CRT trial.[45] Among 1817 patients, 1281 (70%) had baseline LBBB, 228 (13%) had RBBB, and 308 (17%) had nonspecific IVCD. Patients with LBBB had significantly reduced risk of death or HF event,ventricular tachycardia,and improved echocardiogram parameters with CRT-D versus implantable cardioverter defibrillator (ICD) alone. Patients with RBBB or IVCD had no significant reduction in death, HF events, or ventricular tachycardia. The study was underpowered to detect differences in this subgroup. Although non-LBBB patients did not obtain statistically significant differences in clinical endpoints, non-LBBB patients treated with CRT-D did have significant improvement in LV volumes compared with non-LBBB patients treated with ICD only ($p < 0.001$) for all parameters. These reductions were present in both RBBB and IVCD patients. It remains unclear whether clinical outcomes of CRT with RBBB and IVCD are worse because of the higher rate of comorbid adverse predictors and disease severity or decreased efficacy of CRT. Extensive LV conduction delay is frequently present in patients with RBBB and left axis deviation referred for CRT.[46] In a severely diseased conduction system, delay may be present in both the right and left bundle branches, with the manifest ECG pattern determined by the bundle with the slowest conduction. The PACE-RBBB study is currently randomizing 75 subjects with LVEF of 35% or less, NYHA class III or IV HF, and RBBB to ventricular back-up pacing (VVI), right ventricular (RV) dual-chamber pacing, or biventricular pacing using echocardiographic optimization. Prospectively collected data from this trial should help determine if CRT offers clinical and echocardiographic advantages over ICD therapy in patients with RBBB.

Chronic underlying right ventricular apical pacing

The Dual-Chamber and VVI Implantable Defibrillator (DAVID) study showed that chronic RV apical pacing can cause LV dilation, reduced LVEF, and increases HF hospitalizations and death in patients with baseline HF.[47] Less is known about the effect of chronic RV apical pacing in patients with normal baseline LVEF. The PACE trial investigators randomized 177 patients with normal baseline LVEF in whom a biventricular pacemaker had been successfully implanted to receive biventricular pacing (89 patients) or RV apical pacing (88 patients).48 At 12 months, the mean LVEF was significantly lower in the RV-pacing group than in the biventricular pacing group (54% vs. 62%, p <0.001), whereas the LV end-systolic volume was significantly higher in the RV pacing group than in the biventricular-pacing group (35.7 ml vs. 27.6 ml, p <0.001), with a relative difference between the groups in the change from baseline of 25% (p <0.001). Despite worsening EF, patients randomized to RV pacing had no significant increase in HF hospitalizations or death. The PREVENT-HF study investigators randomized 108 patients undergoing pacemaker implantation for high-grade AV block to RV-only pacing (n = 58) or biventricular pacing (n = 50).[49] At 12 months follow-up they found no significant differences in LV volume or EF measurements. The BLOCK-HF study evaluated patients with AV block destined to receive ventricular pacing who had an LVEF of 50% or less and randomized them to receive CRT or conventional dual-chamber RV pacing.[50] In results presented in preliminary fashion at the 2012 American Heart Association (AHA) meeting the investigators found a 26% reduction in the composite endpoint of mortality, HF hospitalization, or increase in the LV end-systolic volume of 15% or more. At this time it remains unclear whether patients with preserved LV function and no evidence of HF benefit from biventricular pacing compared to RV-only pacing. In contrast, patients with underlying HF and depressed LVEF who are expected to receive more than 40% ventricular pacing appear to benefit from biventricular rather than RV-only pacing.

Baseline premature ventricular contraction burden

Similar to AF, frequent PVCs are suspected to reduce the effectiveness of CRT by reducing the percentage of biventricular-paced beats and by causing fusion of some additional percentage of paced beats. In the MADIT-CRT trial, 15% of enrolled subjects had more than 5000 PVCs on preimplant 24-hour Holter monitoring. Among patients with nonischemic cardiomyopathy the RV outflow tract was the most common origin for PVCs. Although a high burden of PVCs is relatively common in CRT recipients, little work has been done investigating the role of PVC burden in predicting response to CRT therapy or the role of PVC suppression after CRT implantation to improve outcomes. One prospective multicenter nonrandomized observational study has assessed the effect of PVC ablation in CRT nonresponders.[51] Subjects were enrolled if they if they had less than 5% improvement in the LVEF and/or LV end-systolic volume of less than 10% with no associated improvement in clinical status 1 year after CRT implantation and had more than 10 000 PVCs/day on Holter monitoring. A total of 65 subjects were enrolled. Follow-up echocardiography 6 months after ablation revealed CRT response with improvements in mean LVEF (26.2% to 32.7%, p <0.001), LV end-systolic volume (178 ml to 145 ml, p <0.001) and median NYHA class (3.0 to 2.0, p <0.001). LVEF improved when the percentage of preablation PVC burden was greater than 14.3%. Of the 65 patients enrolled, 22 did not show significant improvement in LVEF after PVC ablation. These patients had a lower burden of PVCs and a higher percentage of biventricular pacing before ablation than patients who responded.

Summary of current guidelines for CRT patient selection

In 2012 the American College of Cardiology (ACC), the American Heart Assocation (AHA), and the Heart Rhythm Society (HRS) provided an update to their joint guidelines for device-based therapies of cardiac rhythm abnormalities.[52] This update incorporated new data for the use of CRT in patients with NYHA class II HF derived from the RAFT and MADIT-CRT studies. A summary of the guideline recommendations is presented in Table 11.2.

Device implantation

Evolution of biventricular pacing

The first fully implantable pacemaker was designed by Rune Elmqvist and placed by Dr. Ake Senning in 1958 at the Karolinska Institute in Solna, Sweden.[53] The patient, who suffered from complete heart block, required 26 device change-outs during his life, but ultimately survived an additional 43 years, outliving both the inventor and the surgeon. Dramatic improvements in component technology have occurred over the years and modern pacemakers now last a decade or longer before requiring battery replacement.

While early, single-chamber pacemakers provided life-saving therapy for patients with severe bradyarrhythmias, the atrioventricular dyssynchrony induced by RV-only pacing often led to deterioration of cardiac function and symptoms of congestive HF. In the early 1980s, techniques were developed for inserting transvenous leads into both the right atrium (RA) and ventricle for use with pacemakers capable of dual-chamber sensing and pacing (DDD).[54] By matching the ventricular pacing rate to the intrinsic sinus rate, these devices are able to restore AV synchrony and thereby mimic normal cardiac physiology.

In the early 1990s, several small case series were published suggesting a benefit for dual-chamber pacing in patients with severe cardiomyopathy but without a typical bradycardia indication for device implantation.[55,56] In the short term, the authors reported an improvement in LVEF and reduction in NYHA class HF symptoms with DDD pacing. It was hypothesized that the optimization of AV timing in these patients resulted in a reduction in mitral valve regurgitation with a further reduction in preload, thereby improving overall cardiac dynamics.

Despite enthusiasm over these early successes, subsequent trials of dual-chamber pacing for treatment of HF failed to prove long-term benefit. In a small prospective trial of 12 patients, Gold and colleagues found that in patients with HF, DDD pacing had a significant increase in the primary outcome of HF hospitalization or death.[57] The benefit of AV synchrony on diastolic filling time was likely outweighed by the deleterious effects of RV apical pacing on overall cardiac performance. RV apical pacing results in a reversal of the normal electrical activation pattern from apex to base. A decrease in LVEF, thought to be a consequence of abnormal septal motion and loss of mechanical–electrical coupling, results in inefficient myocardial performance. The deleterious consequence of RV pacing was subsequently confirmed in the DAVID trial, where RV pacing greater than 40% conferred a more than fivefold increase

Table 11.2 Indications for CRT

Indication	Level of evidence	Notes
Class I		
1. CRT is indicated for patients who have LVEF £35%, sinus rhythm, LBBB with a QRS duration ≥150 ms, and NYHA class II, III, or ambulatory IV symptoms on GDMT	A for NYHA class III/IV B for NYHA class II	Modified recommendation (specifying CRT in patients with LBBB of ≥150 ms; expanded to include those with NYHA class II symptoms)
Class IIa		
1. CRT can be useful for patients who have LVEF £35%, sinus rhythm, LBBB with a QRS duration 120–149 ms, and NYHA class II, III, or ambulatory IV symptoms on GDMT[16,17,18,20,21,22]	B	New recommendation
2. CRT can be useful for patients who have LVEF £35%, sinus rhythm, a non-LBBB pattern with a QRS duration ≥150 ms, and NYHA class III/ambulatory class IV symptoms on GDMT[16,17,18,21]	A	New recommendation
3. CRT can be useful in patients with atrial fibrillation and LVEF £35% on GDMT if (a) the patient requires ventricular pacing or otherwise meets CRT criteria and (b) AV nodal ablation or pharmacologic rate control will allow near 100% ventricular pacing with CRT[23,24,25,26,48]	B	Modified recommendation (wording changed to indicate benefit based on ejection fraction rather than NYHA class; level of evidence changed from C to B)
4. CRT can be useful for patients on GDMT who have LVEF £35% and are undergoing new or replacement device placement with anticipated requirement for significant (>40%) ventricular pacing[25,27,28,29]	C	Modified recommendation (wording changed to indicate benefit based on ejection fraction and need for pacing rather than NYHA class); class changed from IIb to IIa)
Class IIb		
1. CRT may be considered for patients who have LVEF£30%, ischemic etiology of heart failure, sinus rhythm, LBBB with a QRS duration of ≥150 ms, and NYHA class I symptoms on GDMT[20,21]	C	New recommendation
2. CRT may be considered for patients who have LVEF £35%, sinus rhythm, a non-LBBB pattern with QRS duration 120–149 ms, and NYHA class III/ambulatory class IV on GDMT[21,30]	B	New recommendation
3. CRT may be considered for patients who have LVEF £35%, sinus rhythm, a non-LBBB pattern with a QRS duration ≥150 ms, and NYHA class II symptoms on GDMT[20,21]	B	New recommendation
Class III: No benefit		
1. CRT is not recommended for patients with NYHA class I or II symptoms and non-LBBB pattern with QRS duration <150 ms[20,21,30]	B	New recommendation
2. CRT is not indicated for patients whose comorbidities and/or frailty limit survival with good functional capacity to <1 year[19]	C	Modified recommendation (wording changed to include cardiac as well as noncardiac comorbidities)

in death or hospitalization for CHF.[58] Thus further efforts to treat symptomatic CHF with dual-chamber pacing were abandoned.

In 1994, Cazeau and colleagues published the first case report of dedicated biventricular pacing for the treatment of congestive HF.[59] Using an epicardial lead placed on the LV free wall via thoracotomy and endocardial leads placed in the RA and left atrium (LA) via the coronary sinus (CS) and RV, they demonstrated a decrease in pulmonary capillary wedge pressure (PCWP) and an increase in cardiac output with temporary four-chamber pacing. Based upon these acute results, the investigators implanted a permanent pacing system, using Y-adaptors to provide simultaneous RV and LV pacing. After 6 weeks of biventricular pacing, the patient lost 17 pounds (~8 kg) and had symptomatic improvement to NYHA functional class II.

Two years later, this same group reported the results of biventricular pacing in their first eight patients.[60] Patients were "screened" for acute hemodynamic response with temporary pacing prior to insertion of a permanent system. At follow-up, half of the patients showed remarkable clinical improvement, confirming the results from their first patient. Based upon these results, enthusiasm grew for the application of CRT as a novel therapy for severe, drug-refractory CHF. In 1998, Daubert et al. published their series of the first, fully endocardially-placed CRT systems with LV leads inserted via the CS.[61] The widespread application of CRT thus began in earnest.

Anatomy of the coronary sinus

Early implanters discovered quickly that a major limitation of effective biventricular pacing was the ability to insert and locate the LV lead in an appropriate branch of the CS. Despite improvements in implant techniques and tools, failure rates for placement of LV leads via the CS still range between 7.5% and 10% in major clinical trials.[4,62] Most of

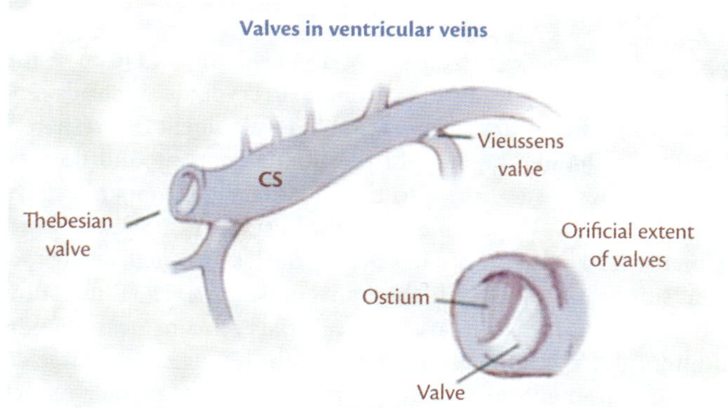

Fig. 11.3 Valves of the coronary sinus.
Habib A, Lachman N, Christensen KN, Asirvatham SJ. The anatomy of the coronary sinus venous system for the cardiac electrophysiologist. Europace (2009) 11 Suppl 5:v15–21, by permission of Oxford University Press.

these implant failures are due to difficulty accessing the CS ostium or advancing the pacing lead into an adequately stable position.

The CS runs in the posterior coronary groove between the LA and LV and the ostium opens into the postero-septal region of the RA near the tricuspid valve. The ostium itself is 5–15 mm in diameter and is partially covered by a Thebesian valve in approximately 60% of patients.[63] In a small subset of patients, the ostium is completely enclosed by the valve with only small fenestrations allowing venous drainage, thereby presenting a major impediment to CS access. In addition, RA dilation may lead to an abnormally high insertion of the CS ostium, making intubation with a fixed-shape catheter or wire difficult.

The body of the CS is made up of muscle fibers that are continuous with the LA, thus encircling the CS proper in a muscular sleeve. A second valve (the valve of Vieussens) located at the junction of the great cardiac vein and the vein of Marshall is present in about 8% of patients and may present a further obstacle for LV lead advancement (Figure 11.3).[64] This valve may also divert a wire into the diminutive vein of Marshall and care must be taken to confirm proper wire positioning in the main CS prior to catheter advancement or venogram balloon inflation. Inadvertent catheter advancement into the vein of Marshall can lead to venous dissection and hemopericardium.

Gross anatomic studies have shown a median number of six LV veins draining into the CS.[63] The nearest branch to the CS ostium is the middle cardiac vein (MCV) which may be covered by a small valve or originate with a separate ostium. The MCV runs in the interventricular groove toward the ventricular apex and is usually not a suitable target for LV lead placement. Three distinct veins drain the lateral wall of the LV. The posterolateral branch, the most prominent and consistent of these veins, usually enters the CS within 1 cm of the ostium. The lateral marginal vein and lateral branches off the anterior interventricular vein (AIV) are variably present (Figure 11.4). In patients with prior myocardial infarction, first-order branches to the lateral wall off the CS are often diminutive or absent.[65] For CRT implantation, where mid-lateral LV wall lead placement is generally preferred, this region was accessible from at least two CS tributaries (posterolateral and AIV) in greater than 85% of patients. In approximately 20% of patients, the mid-lateral LV wall was also accessible from branches off the MCV.

Imaging of the cardiac venous system to target LV lead placement is a critical part of the implant procedure. In most cases, this is accomplished after CS access via occlusive venography with a balloon-tipped catheter. Rotational venography may provide a more complete assessment of the CS branches and their takeoff, which can be difficult to appreciate in one or two-view venograms. Multislice computed tomography (MSCT) has been used preprocedure to assess the cardiac vasculature prior to the implant procedure and correlates well with occlusive venograms.[66] In addition, MSCT may reveal a high CS ostium takeoff and aid in catheter selection for successful CS access.[67]

Preprocedure dyssynchrony and scar analysis

Based upon the historic inclusion criteria from the major trials of CRT, the original guidelines for implantation included evidence of electrical dyssynchrony on ECG with a QRS duration greater than 120 ms. In their 2012 update, however, both the AHA and the ACC refined this recommendation to patients with LBBB and a QRS duration greater than 150 ms (class I indication). Those with a QRS duration between 120 and 150 ms were given a class IIa indication due to combined evidence from multiple trials showing marginal benefit from CRT in this population.[68] The decision to "downgrade" the indication in these patients is not without

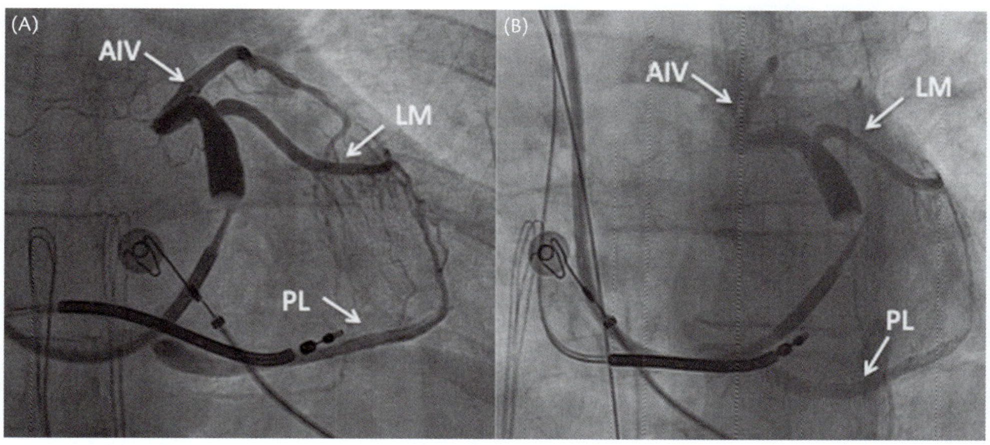

Fig. 11.4 Anatomy and branches of the coronary sinus. (A) The anteroposterior (AP) view demonstrates the posterolateral (PL), lateral marginal (LM), and anterior interventricular vein (AIV). (B) In the left anterior oblique (LAO) view, note the apparent absence of lateral branches from the AIV.

controversy, however, as it is based upon subgroup analysis and has the potential of withholding a beneficial therapy in a large cohort of patients with HF.

In patients with marginal electrical dyssynchrony (QRS 120–150 ms), there is growing evidence that echocardiographic measures of LV mechanical dyssynchrony may help to identify patients likely to respond to CRT. Mechanical dyssynchrony is defined as discordant contraction between the RV and LV (interventricular) or within the LV itself (intraventricular) and can be measured by transthoracic echocardiography using M-mode, tissue Doppler, or speckle tracking strain analysis. It has been shown that significant delay between the septal and posterior LV walls predicts response to CRT regardless of degree of electrical delay or type of bundle branch block.[69]

In addition to assisting in proper patient selection, echocardiographic dyssynchrony analysis can be used to effectively target the LV lead and improve the response rate to CRT. In the Targeted Left Ventricular Lead Placement to Guide Cardiac Resynchronization Therapy (TARGET) study, 220 patients were randomized to either standard LV lead placement or targeted placement based on the latest wall of activation on echocardiographic speckle tracking analysis. More patients with an LV lead placed on or near the wall with latest activation on speckle tracking strain analysis had LV reverse remodeling CRT than those with unguided LV lead placement (70% vs. 55%, $p = 0.031$).[70] Similarly, the Speckle Tracking Assisted Resynchronization Therapy for Electrode Region (STARTER) trial presented at the 2012 HRS meeting found reduced HF hospitalization in patients with guided LV lead placement versus those without (11% vs. 22%, $p = 0.031$).

The location and extent of transmural LV scar by contrast-enhanced MRI has been shown to predict poor response to CRT. In addition, placement of the LV lead on a region of dense LV infarct is independently associated with worse cardiovascular outcomes and survival.[71] Therefore, in patients with ischemic cardiomyopathy undergoing CRT implantation, preprocedure assessment of LV scar via MRI may help guide lead localization (Figure 11.5).

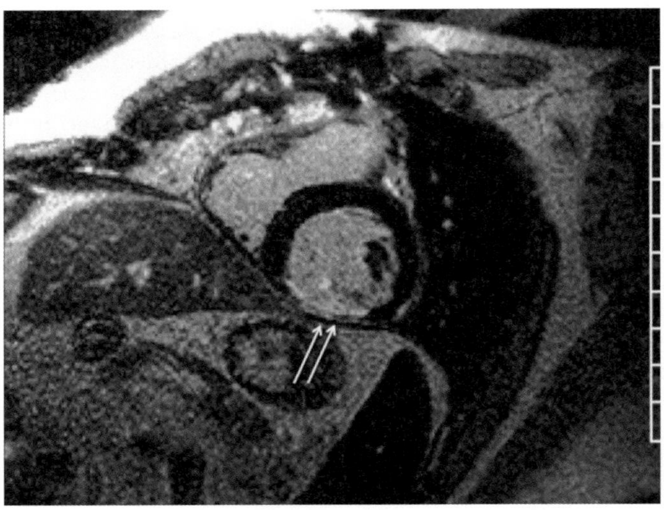

Fig. 11.5 Contrast-enhanced cardiac MRI demonstrating near transmural scarring of the posterolateral wall of the left ventricle (double arrow).

Implantation techniques

Compared to the earliest days of LV lead implantation using stylet-driven pacing leads, the current delivery tools and leads represent a significant improvement. The development of preshaped sheaths that follow the curvature of the lateral wall and floor of the RA allows easier access to the CS.[72] Device companies have improved LV lead design and shapes with smaller tip sizes and isodiametric lead bodies to aid in tracking the lead through small, tortuous side branches. Despite these advances, however, failure of LV lead placement in recent large clinical trials remains near 10%. In addition, given the growing evidence for the importance of targeted LV lead placement, tools and techniques deserve further refinement to improve the response rate to CRT.

During the procedure, the implanting physician may be presented with limited options for LV lead placement. In 70% of patients, at least three suitable CS side branches are available; however, in patients with ischemic cardiomyopathy and extensive lateral transmural scar, options may be more limited.[65] In addition, women tend to have a smaller diameter of both the main CS and side branches, independent of LV end-diastolic diameter. Even when a posterior or lateral CS branch is present, anatomic characteristics such as a steep takeoff angle, a small ostial diameter, and vessel tortuosity may make lead implantation difficult or impossible.

Standard techniques for implantation of the LV lead involve probing for the CS ostium with a wire through a preformed sheath followed by advancement of the pacing lead into the target branch over an angioplasty wire. A steep takeoff or tortuous anatomy may make traditional advancement of the LV lead over an angioplasty wire difficult or impossible. New catheter-based techniques using contrast injection to localize the CS ostium and telescoping delivery systems which allow direct advancement of the sheath into the target branch may allow more efficient, targeted LV lead placement.[73] These systems utilize inner directional catheters and guide sheaths to allow direct lead delivery into the target branch (Figure 11.6). Nonrandomized data have shown that CRT implant procedures using contrast injection through telescoping catheter delivery systems result in fewer failed LV leads (1.9% vs. 8.1%, $p = 0.02$), improved targeted lead placement, and reduced fluoroscopic times compared to standard over-the-wire techniques.[74]

Procedural complications

Acute complications related to the CRT implantation procedure are rare. In an analysis of over 2000 implants from two large randomized trials of CRT, the incidence of procedure-related death was 0.4%.[15] In actual clinical practice, however, in-hospital mortality was substantially higher after CRT implantation at 1.1%, although it was only slightly higher than for non-CRT ICD implantation (0.9%).[75]

CS dissection or perforation was observed in an average of 2.0% of 4512 implants in 6 CRT trials, with a declining incidence in more recently reported trials.[76] In nearly half of these patients, CRT was still successfully implanted and only a minority required inotropic support or drainage for hemopericardium. Recognition of CS dissection raises concern for the occurrence of cardiac tamponade, although fortunately most CS dissections do not progress to tamponade.[76] It is felt that the low pressure within the cardiac venous system as well as the adipose tissue that encases the CS help to limit pericardial bleeding in the majority of cases.

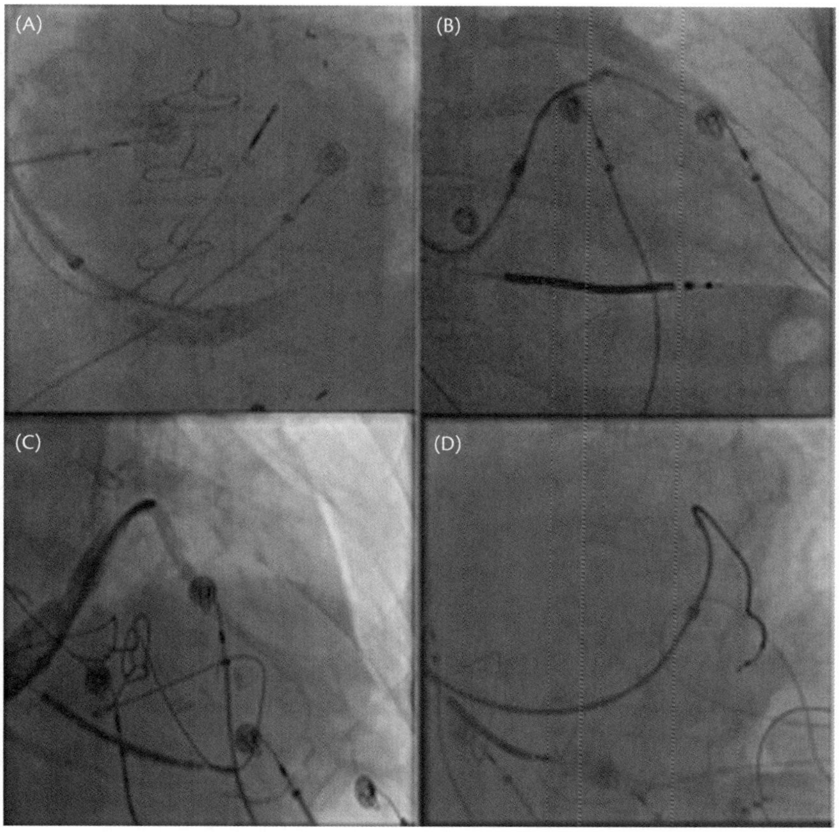

Fig. 11.6 Steps in left ventricular lead implantation using a telescoping catheter-based system. (A) The coronary sulcus (CS) is identified with contrast puffed through CS guide attached to the contrast injection system. The outer sheath is then advanced over the CS guide. (B) Once the outer sheath is in place in the mid-CS, the CS guide is removed. The vein selector is attached to the contrast injection system and inserted into the delivery guide. Both vein selector and deliver guide are advanced through the outer sheath. The target vein is identified with contrast injection through the vein selector. (C) The delivery guide is advanced over the vein selector into the target branch. (D) LAO view of LV lead advanced through delivery guide into final position.

Troubleshooting lead implantation

The most common reasons for failed LV lead implantation include inability to access the CS ostium, inability to advance the lead into the target branch, and acute lead dislodgement or instability. Several techniques have been reported to overcome these obstacles.

The CS ostium is located in the postero-septal region of the RA and is accessed by withdrawing the CS guide catheter across the tricuspid valve with counterclockwise torque. With significant RA enlargement, however, the ostium may enter more superiorly, making localization using this technique difficult. Rarely, the CS ostium may enter the atrium in an anomalous fashion. When initial attempts at CS cannulation fail, a selective coronary angiogram with cine-fluoroscopy of the venous phase may help locate a high or unusual ostial insertion (Figure 11.7).

Once the ostium is located, advancement of the catheter into the main body of the CS may be hindered by a prominent Thebesian valve or a steep takeoff due to atrial enlargement. When a wire can be placed into the main CS but there is resistance to catheter advancement, an occlusive balloon can be used as an anchor, allowing sufficient straightening of the ostium for successful catheter placement.[77] With this technique, a compliant venography or coronary artery balloon is advanced over a wire into the main CS or AIV. Once inflated, back-traction is applied to the balloon to effectively straighten the CS ostium allowing catheter advancement. This balloon-traction technique can also be used to "trap" a wire in a tortuous target vessel to prevent prolapse during lead advancement (Figure 11.8).

Invasive angioplasty techniques have been adopted by electrophysiologists to open partially occluded target branches in the CS.[78] A small-diameter (2.5 or 3.0 mm) coronary balloon can be advanced over a 0.014 inch (0.36 mm) angioplasty wire across a lesion with inflation to rated burst pressure in order to open the stenosis and allow lead passage. When tortuous branch anatomy allows passage of the wire but not the LV lead, additional techniques may be necessary for successful lead implantation. Balloon occlusion of the main CS superior to the branch takeoff can deflect the advancing force more directly into the target branch and thereby prevent wire and lead prolapse. Alternatively, if the wire can be advanced into the branch and back into the main CS via a collateral, a gooseneck snare can be used to capture the distal end of the wire. This end of the wire is then withdrawn through the access sheath and the lead can be advanced either antegrade or retrograde into the target location.

Advancements in left ventricular lead technology

Improving the response rates to CRT relies on multiple factors including proper patient selection, targeted lead placement, arrhythmia management, and device optimization. Placing the

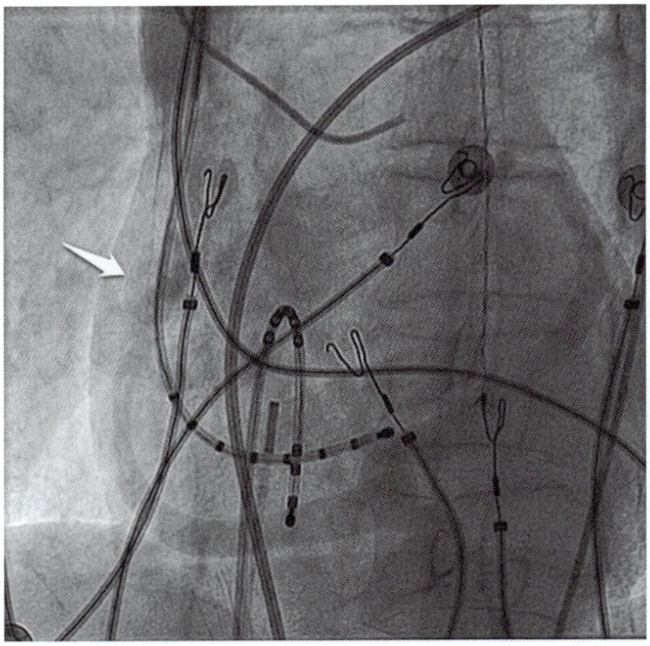

Fig. 11.7 Anomalous coronary sinus identified during venous phase of coronary angiography. The ostium drains into the high posterolateral right atrium (single arrow).

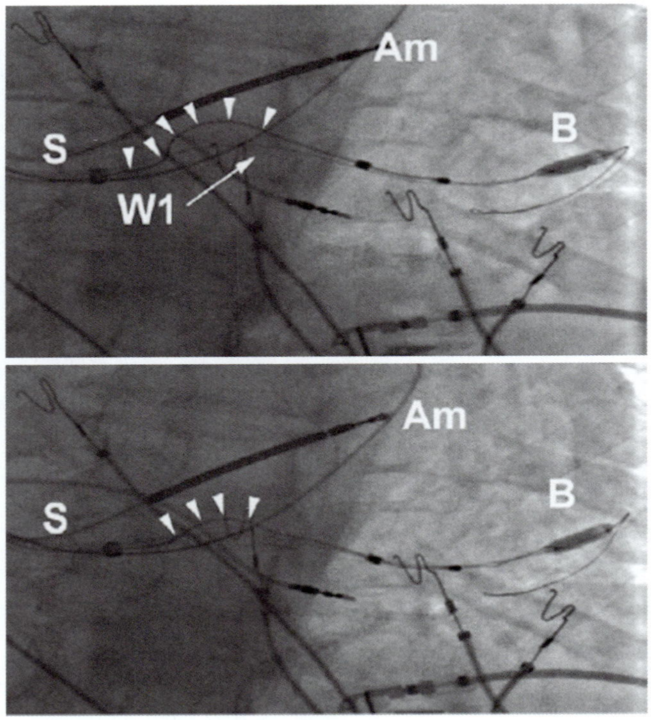

Fig. 11.8 Straightening of a tortuous coronary sinus ostium with anchoring balloon to facilitate left ventricular lead advancement. In the top panel, the coronary balloon is inflated to pin the wire advanced through the tip of the left ventricular lead. In the bottom panel, traction is applied to the ballon and the tortuous branch is straightened allowing lead advancement (arrows).
from reference (77)).

lead in the target branch requires the proper tools, technique, and pacing leads capable of tracking tortuous anatomy and remaining stably positioned once deployed.

Recent advancements in CRT lead technology have improved stability and lead tracking into difficult target vessels. Early LV leads were straight and unipolar and dislodgement rates were high. Current leads with angled or coiled distal tips allow "passive fixation" into the target vessel with lower rates of lead dislodgement. A new "active fixation" lead utilizing an expandable mesh on the lead coating which anchors the lead into the vessel may further reduce lead dislodgment.[79] Another recent advance has been the development of a quadripolar LV pacing lead, allowing multiple pacing vector configurations to overcome inadvertent phrenic nerve stimulation.[80] Further advances in lead fixation and multi-electrode pacing are in development.

Postimplantation follow-up

Early postoperative follow-up

In addition to careful routine clinical examination patients should undergo radiographic, ECG, and device interrogation early postoperatively. Chest radiography (CXR) should be performed to exclude pneumothorax and hemothorax, confirm lead position, and exclude dislodgement (Figure 11.9). The lateral view CXR is critical for confirming that the LV lead overlies the left lateral wall and is relatively posterior. Nomenclature for LV lead position based on CXR has been published and correlated with outcome.[81]

Continuous telemetry should be performed with attention to AF or other arrhythmias, VT, or VF which may in some cases be triggered by CRT, and for loss of LV capture. Atrial arrhythmias are a concern due to the risk of thromboembolism and possible need to initiate or reinitiate anticoagulation, but also due to the loss of CRT related to intrinsically conducted impulses. New onset of recurrent VT or VF may necessitate temporary discontinuation of CRT. Device interrogation is advised within 72 hours of implantation.[82] This can confirm lead function (sensing, thresholds, impedance), help to exclude lead dislodgement, verify that set-screws connecting the leads with the device header are tight, ensure that biventricular pacing is occurring, and evaluate for phrenic nerve or diaphragmatic stimulation (Table 11.3).

Postdischarge follow-up

After hospital discharge, follow-up should focus on detection of HF exacerbations, pocket hematoma, erosion or infection, lead dislodgement or fracture, extracardiac stimulation, arrhythmias, and loss of biventricular pacing. Owing to advanced HF, frequent follow-up is warranted. Medications such as β-blockers may be uptitrated due to improved systolic blood pressure and diuretics may need downtitration. Various CRT devices and their monitoring systems provide diagnostics such as thoracic impedance, heart rate variability, patient activity, atrial or ventricular arrhythmias, patient weight, or blood pressure and this may help provide advanced warning of impending HF.[83] Pocket complications cluster in the first few weeks, and consequently early follow-up is important. Erosion or infection can occur at any time; thus at least yearly follow-up is advised, [82] but patient education is important too. Arrhythmia, device, and lead follow-up is transitioning to being predominantly done remotely, at least in the United States.[84]

Complications of CRT therapy

Life-threatening complications are infrequent in the postdischarge phase after CRT device implantation but they may occur, and a

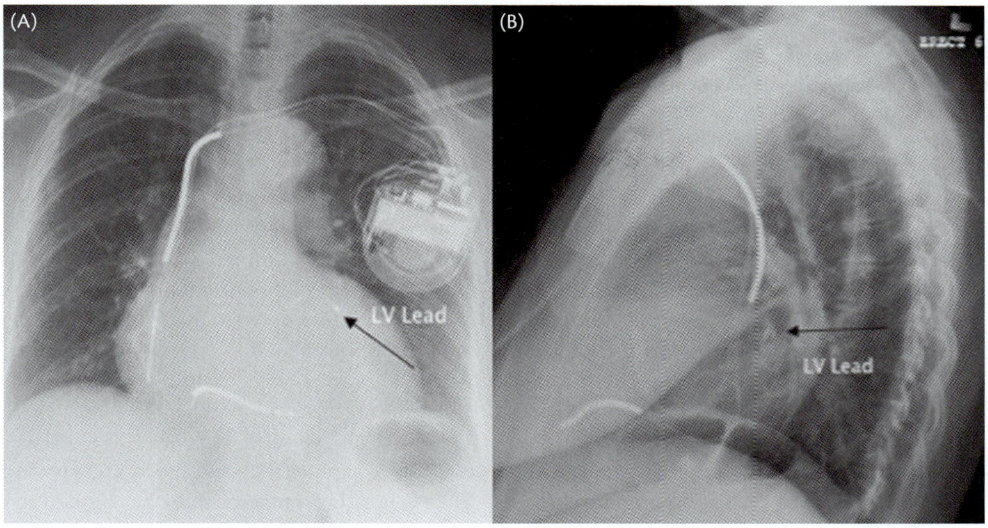

Fig. 11.9 (A) shows a PA chest radiograph and (B) a lateral view after placement of a CRT-D device. The lead is in the anterolateral branch in a basal position.

Table 11.3 Critical CRT-D device data and interpretation

Device data	Use and interpretation
% Ventricular pacing (VP)	Should be close to 100%
Biventricular (BiVP), right (RVP), and left ventricular pacing (LVP)	Some devices provide breakdown on % pacing in each chamber to further explore insufficient resynchronization
% Atrial pacing (AP)	Ideally near 0% or in case of severe sinus node dysfunction near 100%; AV delay for AS versus AP difficult to predict and may differ enormously[137]
Premature ventricular complexes (PVCs)	Total number and percent ideally very low; may be cause for loss of CRT Could represent atrial undersensing with intrinsic conduction or oversensing T-waves or double counting R-waves Consider antiarrhythmic or ablation if >10–20%
Mode switch, atrial high rate episodes, AT/AF episodes	Confirm with electrogram to exclude atrial oversensing (far-field R-waves) Frequent cause of failure to respond to CRT
BiVP via resynchronization algorithm	Counter for LVP after RV sensing (e.g., PVC); unlikely to provide optimal CRT
Ventricular sensing (VS)	Estimate of the percentage of sensed ventricular events should be close to 0% VS episodes (continuous ventricular sensing) may indicate intrinsic AV conduction (programmed AV delay too long or too low upper rate[99]) or atrial undersensing with intrinsic AV conduction
VT/VF	Correlation with HF status and AF Adjust detection, therapy (ATP or shock), antiarrhythmic agent or ablation as in conventional ICD

AF, atrial fibrillation; AS, atrial sensing; AT, atrial tachycardia; HF, heart failure; ICD, implantable cardioverter defibrillator.

Fung JW, Yu CM. Current Heart Failure Reports. 2008;5(1):44–50, Springer.

careful systematic approach is needed to detect and manage them. Cardiac tamponade related to LV or other lead insertion can present after hospital discharge and was reported in 0.17% of device implants when limiting the definition to 30 days or longer postimplant.[85] Most did not require lead extraction. Some cases of hemopericardium are clinically occult but important if lead extraction or manipulation is under consideration.[86] Symptoms and signs can include pain, dyspnea, presyncope, hypotension, pulsus paradoxus; echocardiography and sometimes CT scanning can be diagnostic.

Proarrhythmia related to left or biventricular pacing[87] is another life-threatening complication that classically occurs before hospital discharge,[88] but may occur later. In a small published series of eight patients, the mean time from CRT implantation to the onset of VT storm was 16 days.[89] Shukla and colleagues reported on five proarrhythmia cases all occurring within 1 week.[87] Both monomorphic VT and polymorphic VT have been described; the former perhaps due to preferential access to a reentry circuit the latter possibly related to QT prolongation induced by epicardial rather than endocardial stimulation.[89,90,91] While antiarrhythmic drugs and ablation have been used, deactivation of CRT is often immediately effective, although the long-term prognosis has been poor in some series. While the incidence of CRT-induced proarrhythmia is difficult to ascertain due to difficulty separating it from the inherent risk of arrhythmia in advanced congestive HF patients, in the series by Nayak and colleagues, as many as 4% of CRT patients were identified as exhibiting it.[89]

A similar controversy surrounds whether a reduction in VT/VF has been universally noted in CRT trials, including the MIRACLE-ICD trial.[92] The CARE-HF trial also showed a reduced rate of total and of sudden cardiac death in the CRT pacemaker arm compared to the medical therapy arm.[93] In the smaller REVERSE study an overall nonsignificant reduction in VT/VF was observed, but the reduction did reach statistical significance in the responder group.[94] On the other hand, results from the MADIT-CRT trial provides solid evidence that resynchronization therapy had antiarrhythmic benefit with an overall 29% reduction in the incidence of VT or VF in the CRT arm, although the benefit was confined to patients with native LBBB.[95]

LV lead-related problems including dislodgement, phrenic nerve capture with diaphragmatic stimulation, or loss of LV capture are the most common subacute complications of cardiac resynchronization, reported in 7–8% of patients in a compilation of several early multicenter CRT trials.[96] Problems with the LV lead far outnumber those with RA or RV leads. Unlike some other studies, patients in the MADIT-CRT trial randomized to the non-CRT arm did not receive an LV lead or CRT device, providing an opportunity to compare the incremental complications associated with the greater complexity of the CRT system. Complications were classified as serious if they were life threatening or required operative intervention. Acute (0–30 day) complications were more common in the CRT arm than the ICD arm, including both serious (5% vs. 3%) as well as nonserious (23% vs. 9%). Beyond 30 days, serious complications were equally prevalent in the two arms (2%), whereas nonserious complications remained more frequent in the CRT patients (20% vs. 11%). Higher rates of pneumothorax or hemothorax, infections needing operation, tamponade and especially CS dissection accounted for the serious complication differential between arms. The nonserious complications in the CRT arm were predominantly related to LV lead, many of which were ameliorated with programming.[97]

In a systematic review of 6 CRT trials including 3095 system implantations, the overall lead dislodgement rate was 5.7%, varying from 2.8% to 10.6%.[76] In the RAFT trial, lead dislodgement occurred in 2.2% of patients in the ICD arm and 6.9% of the CRT arm.[62] Interestingly the highest dislodgement rate was found in the REVERSE trial which reported such events out to 12 months, suggesting that LV lead dislodgements may continue to accrue beyond the early postoperative period, necessitating careful ongoing follow-up. Specifically, the rate of LV lead dislodgement between 1 and 12 months after implantation was 3.4% (9 of 262 systems).[98] The lack of definitive fixation for (most) LV leads probably accounts for the small ongoing dislodgement rate at least over the first 6–12 months compared to RA or RV leads.

Loss of biventricular pacing

Although telemetry may be helpful in monitoring for LV capture, 12-lead ECG is essential (Table 11.4). A baseline for future comparison should be established intraoperatively or at device follow-up when capture is confirmed by device interrogation. Figure 11.10 shows an example of 12-lead ECGs recorded pre- and post-CRT implant. Figure 11.10A shows a LBBB-like configuration in a patient with underlying AV block necessitating continuous RV pacing. Moreover, the QRS morphology is dramatically different. Note the negativity in lead I and the R-wave in lead V1 reflecting activation away from the lateral wall of the LV and from LV toward RV (or posterior to anterior) respectively. An R-wave in V1 simulating a RBBB-type of conduction pattern is also seen in about 10% of conventional RV-paced patients.[99] However, the appearance of such a RBBB-type pattern should raise suspicion of inadvertent lead location in the LV or CS. Elimination of the R-wave after moving electrodes V1 and V2 down to the 5th intercostal space, in combination with disappearance of the dominant R-wave in V3–6 is consistent with RV apical pacing.[99] One algorithm reported by Ammann and colleagues utilizes the presence of either an R/S ratio greater than 1 in V1 or an R/S ratio less than 1 in lead I as confirming the presence of LV capture with sensitivity and specificity of nearly 95%.[100] Their algorithm proved somewhat limited in a follow-up analysis by Ploux and colleagues, which examined different LV lead locations while restricting RV lead position to the RV apex.[101] In this series, an R/S ratio less than 1 was observed in EGG lead I in 12 patients (24%) during RV pacing. On the other hand,during biventricular pacing,particularly from an inferior or posterior LV lead location, the R/S ratio of less than 1 was absent in a significant proportion (24–36%). Adding to the complexity is the pattern with an RV outflow tract lead in which case bona fide biventricular capture may demonstrate a mostly negative QRS complex in V1 with a right inferior frontal plane axis.[99]

Table 11.4 Frontal plane axis in uni- and biventricular pacing

Univentricular pacing		**Biventricular pacing (LV free wall plus RV)**
Pacing site	**Frontal axis**	**Frontal axis**
LV free wall	+180	n/a
RV apex	−60 to −120	−90 to −180
RV outflow	+30 to +120	+120 to +180

Modified from Daubert JC, Saxon L, Adamson PB, Auricchio A, Berger RD, Beshai JF, et al. 2012 EHRA/HRS expert consensus statement on cardiac resynchronization therapy in heart failure: implant and follow-up recommendations and management. Heart Rhythm. 2012;9(9):1524–76; Porciani MC, Rao CM, Mochi M, Cappelli F, Bongiorno G, Perini AP, et al. A real-time three-dimensional echocardiographic validation of an intracardiac electrogram-based method for optimizing cardiac resynchronization therapy. Pacing Clin Electrophysiol. 2008;31(1):56–63, Wiley.

Figure 11.11A shows the 12-lead ECG from a patient who reports improved energy level 3 months post-CRT implant. Notably, it fails to demonstrate definitive LV capture according to the algorithm of Ammann and colleagues. All leads had excellent pacing thresholds and adequate safety margin. Figure 11.11B shows the intrinsic rhythm with native LBBB; note the similar PR interval to Figure 11.11A, suggesting near pseudofusion (with slight fusion). Panels C and D of Figure 11.11 show RV and LV (univentricular) pacing respectively (both in VVI mode to avoid fusion with native conduction). Finally, Figure 11.11E shows biventricular pacing with the AV interval reduced to 40 ms (to avoid any fusion) and then 100 ms in Figure 11.11F (as compared to the original setting of 140 ms in Figure 11.11A). The benefit of evaluating the baseline ECG and native conduction (when present) as a point of comparison to the biventricular-paced ECG is well illustrated by this example.

Upper rate behavior of biventricular devices differs from standard antibradycardia pacemakers due to the goal of having 100% (bi-)ventricular pacing.[102] The occurrence of sinus tachycardia due to exercise, emotion, or HF exacerbation can lead to loss of biventricular pacing when the P-P interval during sinus tachycardia becomes less than the total atrial refractory period (TARP), that is when the maximal tracking rate is reached. However, a hysteresis phenomenon exists for exit from upper rate behavior. In order to exit from the upper rate response and reestablish biventricular pacing, the conducted AV interval (AS-VS) which is longer than the programmed AV interval (AS-VP) plus the PVARP, must become longer than the upper rate interval.[102] PVCs can also initiate an upper rate-type of response if the spontaneous P-wave falls in the PVARP and is untracked with the intrinsic PR interval plus the PVARP exceeding the URL.[102]

As discussed earlier, AF is a common cause of failure to deliver effective biventricular pacing and of nonresponse to CRT. CRT

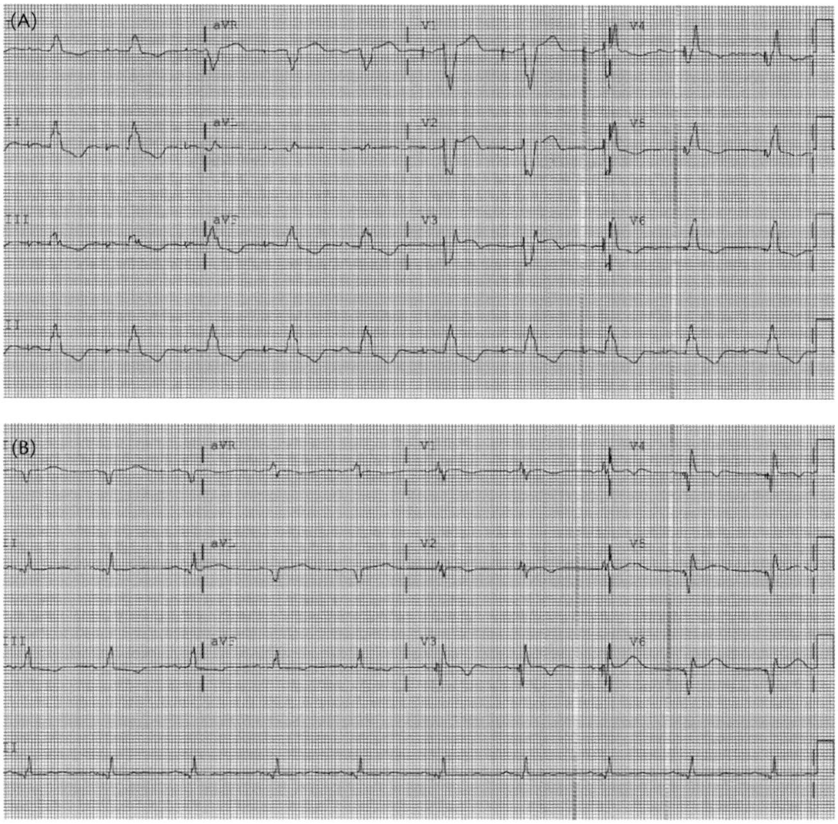

Fig. 11.10 12-lead ECGs recorded before (A) and after (B) a CRT implant. (A) A LBBB-like configuration in a patient with underlying AV block who had received continuous RV pacing. (B) Note that post-CRT the PR and the QRS duration are both shorter and the QRS is negative in lead 1 and has a prominent R-wave in V1.

devices have several algorithms to try to mitigate the loss of biventricular pacing. These include algorithms that deliver biventricular pacing upon sensing an intrinsic activation, increase the lower pacing rate temporarily when sensed beats occur during AF, or seek to minimize the variation in R-R intervals.[103] Counts of biventricular pacing may overestimate fully paced complexes due to unrecognized fusion beats during AF. Examining multiple ECG leads via a 12-lead Holter has been reported to be beneficial in detecting underdelivery of biventricular pacing (Figure 11.12).[104]

An obvious cause that biventricular pacing could be "lost" is failure to capture. On the other hand, necessity to pace at an excessively high output will deplete the battery and subject the patient to the risks of generator change.[105] Confirming LV capture was potentially challenging in the early generation, Y-connected RV-LV pacing systems where it was unknown which lead might lose capture first.[102] In dedicated CRT devices, the threshold can be checked for each channel (LV or RV) individually. Confusing capture with intrinsic conduction is still possible and therefore setting the pacing mode to VVI (above the intrinsic rate) or programming of a nonphysiologic short AV interval should be used. Anodal capture represents an additional confounder. LV pacing may be configured in bipolar mode (provided the LV lead is bipolar or even quadripolar) or unipolar using an RV lead (or generator can in some CRT devices). At a sufficient output with a unipolar LV lead in the LV to RV configuration, capture may occur at both the cathode (LV) and anode (RV). When RV (anodal) capture is lost as the output is reduced, the change in morphology on the surface and intracardiac electrograms could be misinterpreted as loss of LV capture resulting in programming an excessively high output.[102] Automated algorithms are now available to ensure consistent LV capture without excessive output. The automated capture methodology utilizes the conducted response from the LV to the RV and the timing of it to differentiate an LV-generated impulse versus an intrinsically conducted beat or a PVC.[106] In an analysis of 134 patients, the automated LV capture threshold was found to be safe and effective and uncovered a 1.5 V or greater variation in threshold in 15% of patients. Another algorithm using the evoked response on an independent (nonpacing) LV electrode has been reported also.[107]

Nonresponders

A number of different definitions of response have been used in clinical trials and in clinical practice. Using a randomized double-blind design comparing cardiac resynchronization with only back-up VVI pacing at 30 bpm in the MIRACLE study, 34% of patients felt moderately or markedly improved in the control arm as compared with 60% in the CRT arm.[15] Improvements in the three coprimary endpoints of NYHA functional class, 6 minute hall walk, and HF quality of life, were all superior in the CRT arm but improvement also occurred in these subjective measures in the "placebo" arm. For some of the more objective secondary objectives, such as maximal oxygen consumption (peak VO_2) or reduction in LV end-systolic dimension by echocardiography, the mean improvement in the control arm was negligible. In the MADIT-CRT trial, the non-CRT group who received only back-up ventricular pacing nevertheless had a mean reduction in LV echocardiographic end-systolic volume of 18 ml, though it was far less than the CRT arm which remodeled by 57 ml at 1 year as compared

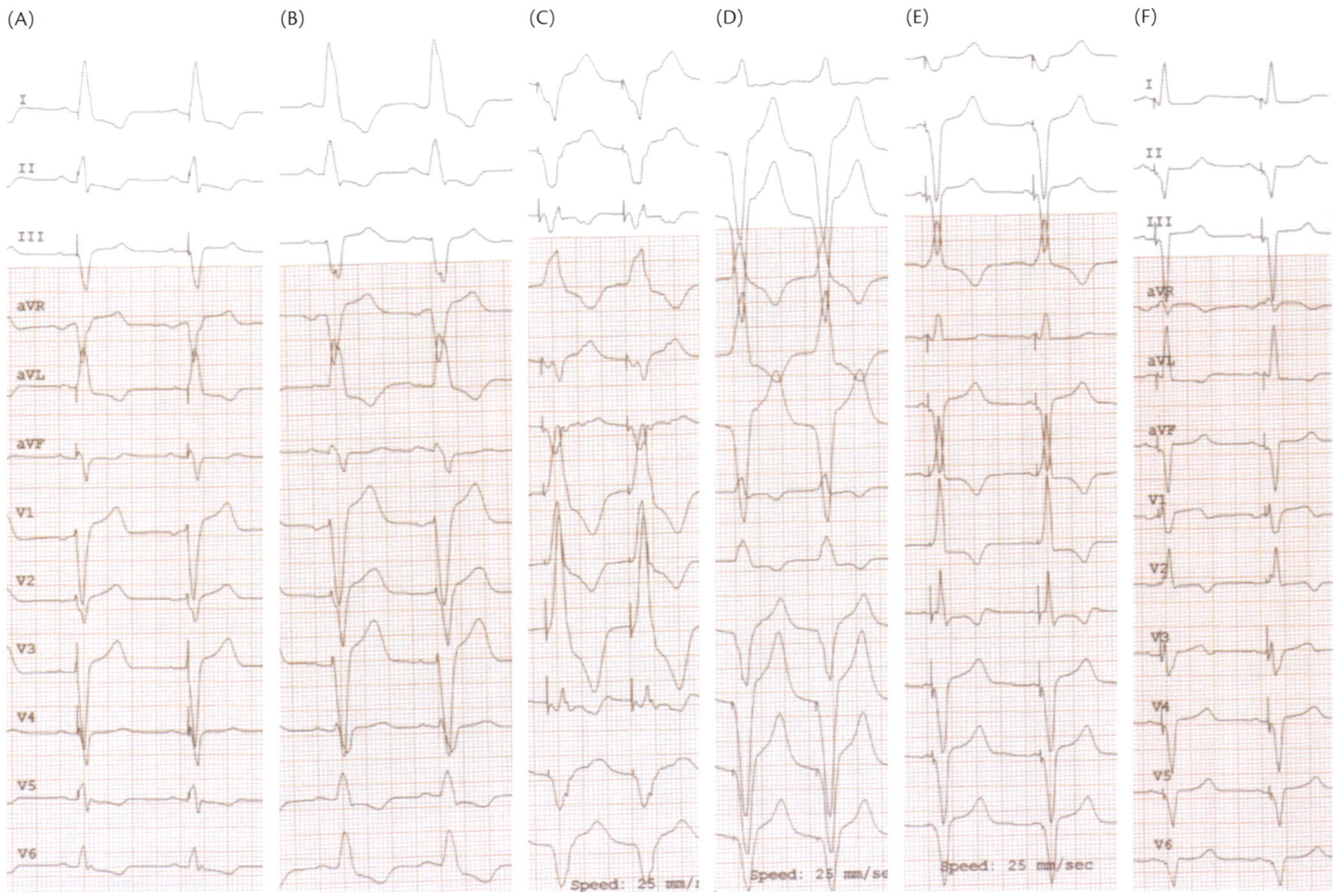

Fig. 11.11 12-lead rhythm strip with leads as shown in (A) for each panel. See text for details.

to the baseline echo.[4] The percentage nonresponse to CRT varies from about 20–30% for subjective measures to 35–50% for echocardiographic measures (Figure 11.13).[84]

With these limitations in defining and addressing the issue of nonresponders, Mullens and colleagues showed that a number of factors can contribute to the lack of improvement after CRT, which they defined as persistent advanced HF symptoms (i.e., NYHA III or IV) and/or lack of ventricular remodeling. They observed suboptimal AV intervals, arrhythmias (especially PVCs or AF), poor lead position, anemia, less than 90% biventricular pacing, inadequate medical therapy, and lack of underlying wide QRS as contributors.[108] In this small nonrandomized study, patients who were deemed to have had a favorable intervention (such as AV interval optimization) had improved survival. Cheng and colleagues queried the Medtronic Carelink database for the relative frequency of various possible reasons for loss of CRT therapy.[109] Prior studies have shown that CRT needs to be delivered nearly 100% to have an optimal response. Overall, 40% of patients had less than 98% biventricular pacing and 11% had less than 90% pacing. Atrial arrhythmias caused the most CRT loss overall, but in patients with less than 90% biventricular pacing too long an AV interval (resulting in ventricular sensing) became the dominant cause (Box 11.1).

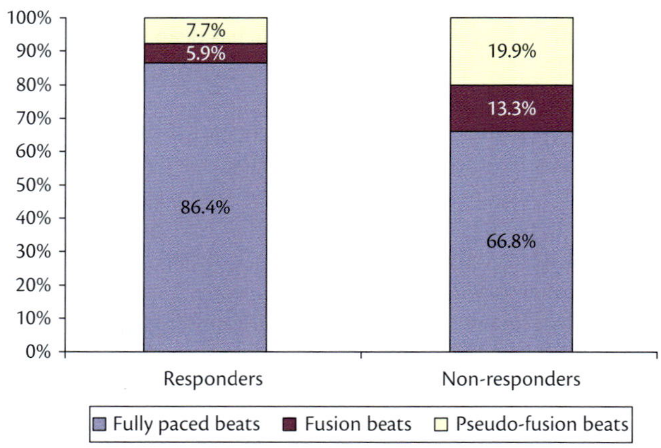

Fig. 11.12 Data from 12-lead Holter monitoring of CRT patients with atrial fibrillation to determine accurate biventricular pacing versus fusion and pseudofusion counts and correlation with response to CRT.

Reprinted from Journal of the American College of Cardiology, 60(16), Lakkireddy D, Di Biase L, Ryschon K, Biria M, Swarup V, Reddy YM, et al. Radiofrequency Ablation of Premature Ventricular Ectopy Improves the Efficacy of Cardiac Resynchronization Therapy in Nonresponders. 1531–9, copyright (2012) with permission from Elsevier.

AV interval optimization

Proper AV interval programming is unquestionably important in CRT, and a number of methodologies have been proposed (Table 11.5). It has been repeatedly demonstrated that the optimal AV delay can vary both between patients. Figure 11.14 shows a schematic representation of (left-sided) atrial and ventricular systolic and diastolic events from a mechanical perspective. It is well appreciated that too short an AV or PR interval as in the case of AV nodal reentrant tachycardia or too long as in extreme first

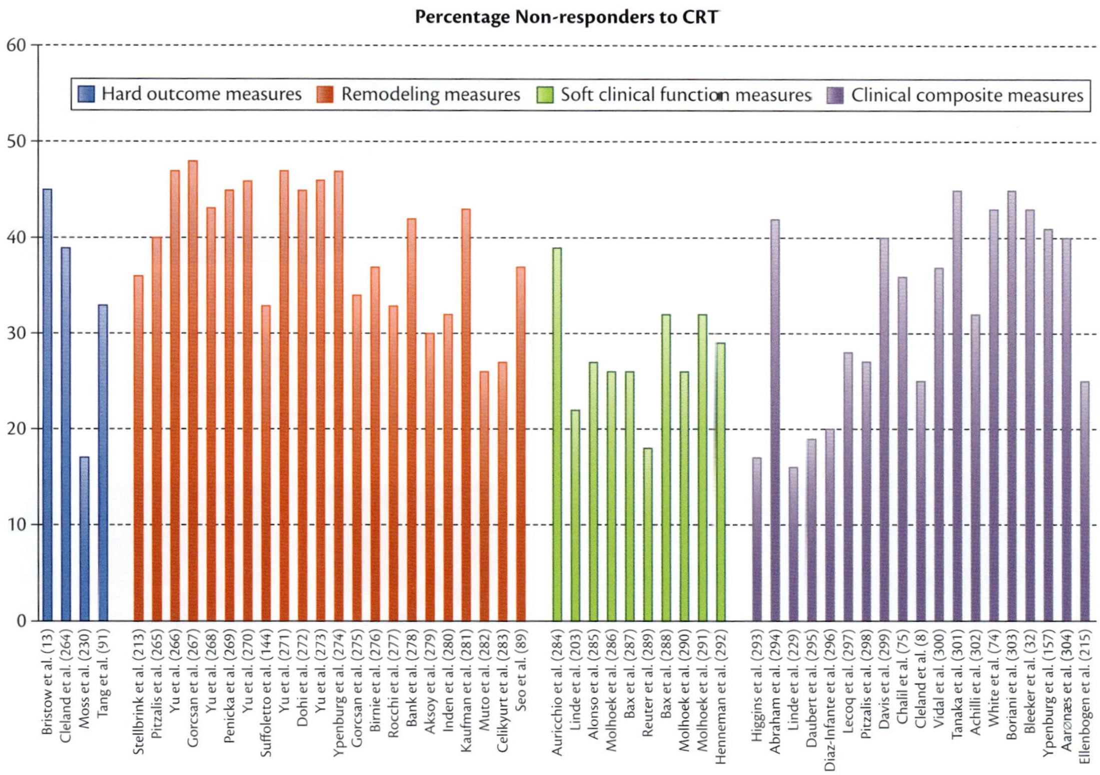

Fig. 11.13 Percent nonresponder is plotted by study and type of endpoint. See text. Note that more patients are characterized as nonresponders with left ventricular remodeling as the definition.

Reprinted from HeartRhythm, 9(9), Daubert JC, Saxon L, Adamson PB, Auricchio A, Berger RD, Beshai JF, et al. 2012 EHRA/HRS expert consensus statement on cardiac resynchronization therapy in heart failure: implant and follow-up recommendations and management, 1524–76, copyright (2012) with permission from Elsevier.

degree AV block can lead to symptomatic hemodynamic deterioration. In CRT, the AV interval must be short enough that pacing is uniformly delivered, yet not so short that atrial, especially LA, contraction is preempted (lower left panel, Figure 11.14). Phillipe Ritter developed a method for selecting the optimal AV interval; notably this was developed in patients with complete AV block, normal LV function, and for a standard (right ventricular-only) DDD pacemaker.[110,111,112] The first step is to determine the longest AV interval still providing ventricular capture; this will result in fusion of E and A waves since the E wave is delayed (lower right panel, Figure 11.14). Next the AV interval is shortened until the longest AV interval producing truncation of the A-wave is found (lower middle panel, Figure 11.14). The optimal AV delay can be calculated algebraically, however due to the complexities of this approach many centers use iterative adjustments of the AV interval with analysis of the mitral inflow waveforms to achieve distinct E and A waves (top panel, Figure 11.14).

Box 11.1 Causes of nonresponse to CRT (and loss of CRT)

- Insufficient CRT
  - Atrial fibrillation
  - Ventricular ectopic beats
  - Upper rate behavior
- Suboptimal lead position
- Myocardial scar
- Latency
- AV interval programming
  - Fusion or pseudofusion or pacing inhibition due to short PR interval
  - Interatrial conduction delay
  - Latency and delayed LV conduction
  - Paced AV delay versus sensed delay
- Lack of electrical dyssynchrony
- Echocardiographic response without clinical response

An alternative (or complementary) echocardiographic approach to AV interval optimization looks at LV ejection rather than filling, comparing the aortic velocity–time integral (VTI) with different programmed AV intervals. Insert illustrates measurement of the aortic VTI to optimize the AV interval. The VTI method is relatively quicker than the mitral inflow analysis, particularly in its algebraic format. Like any method there are limitations in accuracy. One study found beat-to-beat variability less than 3 cm (~15%) and since multiple beats were averaged, a standard error of the mean was 1 cm (~5%).[113] The aortic VTI method was compared in a small, randomized study (n = 40) to an empiric setting of 120 ms. Interestingly the mean "optimal" AV delay was 119 ms but the range of optimal delays was 60–200 ms. By clinical criteria (NYHA functional class and QOL score) the optimized group fared better and there were trends toward more improvement in echocardiographic remodeling.[113,114] In a small randomized comparison of the aortic VTI method with the mitral inflow method, the optimal

Table 11.5 Methods of programming the AV delay

Fixed AVD	100–130 ms for AS-BVP Offset for AP-BVP usually 30–60 ms: may substantially underestimate difference
Mitral inflow methodologies	
Ritter algebraic method	The optimal AVD is calculated using the formula V_S-MVC SAVD – VS-MVCLAVD + SAVD, where SAVD and LAVD are short and long AVDs, respectively, and V_S-MVC is the time interval between the ventricular sensing (V_S) and MVC[118]
Iterative approach	Set AVD to avoid truncation of A (at short AVD)or fusion of E and A (at long AVD)
Mitral VTI	Adjust AVD to achieve highest mitral VTI
Aortic VTI	
Invasive hemodynamic	Maximize LV *dp/dt* or pulse pressure while adjusting AV delay
Noninvasive hemodynamic (finger plythysmography)	Maximize systolic pressure while adjusting AV delay
Electrogram	
Aurricchio	Aurricchio IAVD × 0.7 -55 (if QRS >150)[116]
Expert Ease for HF	SAVD = K1 × QRS + K2 × SAVI + K3 where K1 = –0.728, K2 = 0.757 and K3 = 71.3 for biventricular pacing with free wall LV lead[118]
QuickOpt (St. Jude, Sylmar, CA, USA)	APD (intracardiac electrogram) + 60 if APD <100 or +30 if APD >100[119,120]
PEA	RV lead-based hemodynamic sensor measures intensity of S1 event (start of isovolumetric contraction) at range of V-V and AVDs; V-V selected then AVD chosen from inflection point of PEA versus AVD curve[111,127]

APD, atrial depolarization duration; AVD, AV delay; PEA, peak endocardial acceleration.

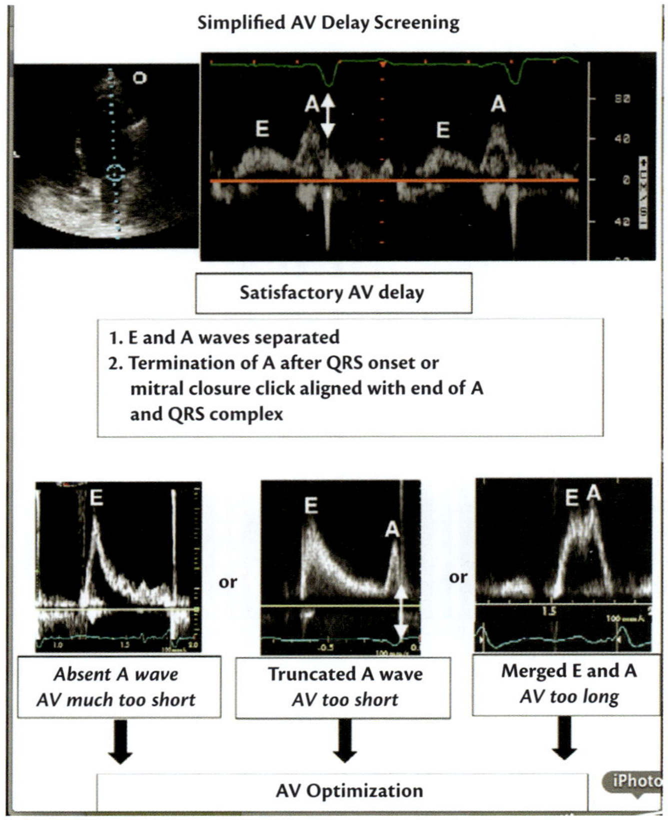

Fig. 11.14 Schematic representation of (left-sided) atrial and ventricular systolic and diastolic events from a mechanical perspective.

Reprinted from Journal of the American Society of Echocardiography, 21(3), Gorcsan J, 3rd, Abraham T, Agler DA, Bax JJ, Derumeaux G, Grimm RA, et al. Echocardiography for cardiac resynchronization therapy: recommendations for performance and reporting--a report from the American Society of Echocardiography Dyssynchrony Writing Group endorsed by the Heart Rhythm Society, 191–213, copyright (2008) with permission from Elsevier.

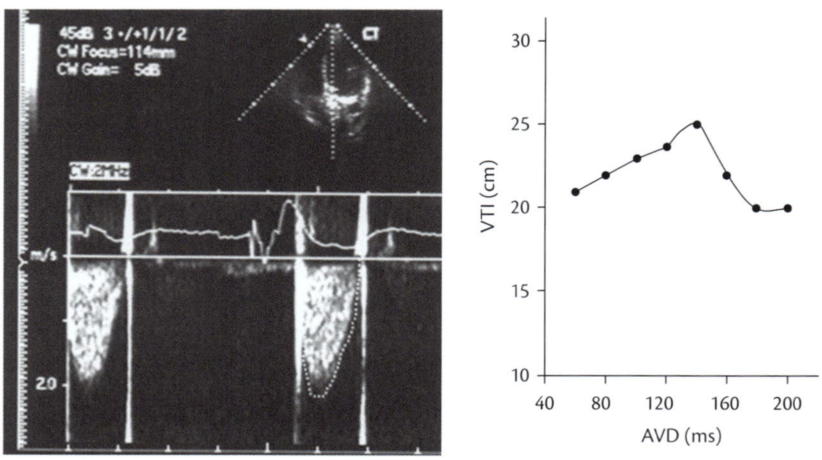

Fig. 11.15 Method of measuring the aortic velocity–time integral to optimize the atrioventricular interval.

Reprinted from HeartRhythm, 3(2), Kerlan JE, Sawhney NS, Waggoner AD, Chawla MK, Garhwal S, Osborn JL, et al. Prospective comparison of echocardiographic atrioventricular delay optimization methods for cardiac resynchronization therapy, 148–54, copyright (2006) with permission from Elsevier.

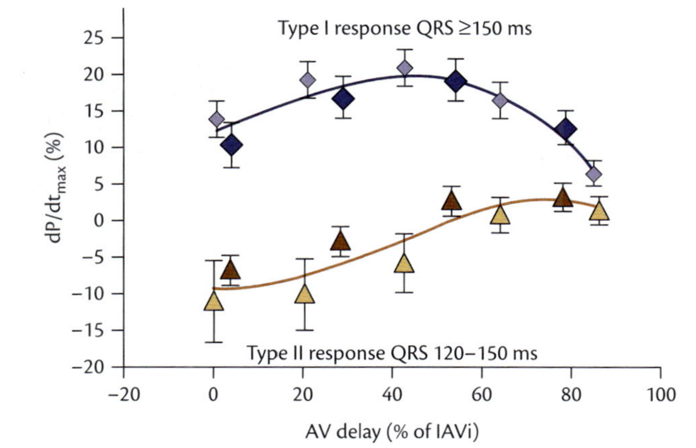

Fig. 11.16 The optimal atrioventricular delay (by LV *dp/dt*) could be predicted on the basis of the intrinsic QRS and PR intervals.

Auricchio A, Stellbrink C, Block M, Sack S, Vogt J, Bakker P, et al. Effect of pacing chamber and atrioventricular delay on acute systolic function of paced patients with congestive heart failure. The Pacing Therapies for Congestive Heart Failure Study Group. The Guidant Congestive Heart Failure Research Group. Circulation. 1999;99(23):2993–3001.

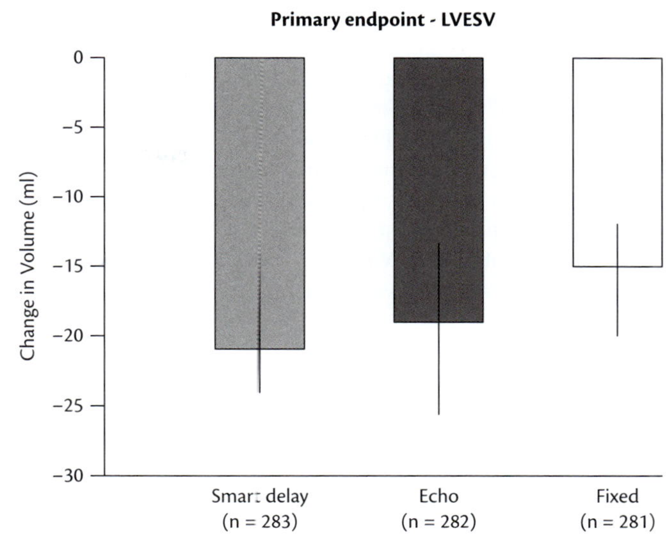

Fig. 11.17 Primary endpoint of the SMART-AV trial comparing the electrogram-based Smart Delay against echocardiographic mitral method and a fixed atrioventricular delay of 120 ms. See text for details.

Ellenbogen KA, Gold MR, Meyer TE, Fernndez Lozano I, Mittal S, Waggoner AD, et al. Primary results from the SmartDelay determined AV optimization: a comparison to other AV delay methods used in cardiac resynchronization therapy (SMART-AV) trial: a randomized trial comparing empirical, echocardiography-guided, and algorithmic atrioventricular delay programming in cardiac resynchronization therapy. Circulation. 2010;122(25):2660–8.

AV delay was longer with the VTI approach (119 ± 34 ms vs. 95 ± 24 ms, $p \leq 0.001$) and the aortic VTI improved more at the optimal setting than at the optimal inflow setting, which is not especially surprising; long-term outcomes were not evaluated.[114] In another comparison study, the VTI of mitral inflow was found to be superior to either aortic VTI, diastolic filling time, or the Ritter method of mitral inflow optimization when compared to invasive LV *dp/dt* after CRT implant.[115]

Nonechocardiographic approaches to device optimization have been described as well. Auricchio and colleagues noticed early on that the AV delay could be predicted relatively sufficiently on the basis of the intrinsic AV interval and the QRS duration (Figure 11.16).[116] This methodology or modifications of it has been used in several clinical trials (see Table 11.4 and Box 11.1).

Recently, the large SmartDelay Determined AV Optimization: A Comparison to Other AV Delay Methods Used in Cardiac Resynchronization Therapy (SMART-AV) trial[117] compared a fixed AV delay of 120 ms with an echo-based mitral inflow iterative approach and a modified electrogram approach[118] derived from Auricchio's method;[116] the patients (n = 1014) were randomized 1:1:1. The modified electrogram approach had been validated against LV *dp/dt* and was found to outperform the Ritter method, aortic VTI, and several fixed delays.[118] Interestingly, no significant differences were found in the primary endpoint (LV end-systolic volume 6 months after implant) or other echocardiographic or clinical secondary outcomes in the SMART-AV trial (Figure 11.17).

Another electrogram approach[119,120] measures duration of atrial depolarization from intracardiac electrograms in an effort

Table 11.6 AV interval programming and/or optimization in CRT trials

Trial	Programming	Echocardiographic optimization
MIRACLE[15]	By echo optimization	Mitral inflow optimization at predischarge, 3, 6 months
CARE-HF[93]	By echo optimization	Mitral inflow optimization at predischarge "to provide the maximum left ventricular filling time"
COMPANION[138,116]	Proprietary algorithm based on measures of the intrinsic PR interval, the QRS interval, and the intracardiac atrioventricular interval at the time of implantation[116]	No echocardiographic optimization
MADIT-CRT[4]	Expert Ease[116,138] Algorithm based on native PR, QRS and intrinsic device electrogram intervals	At investigator discretion based on mitral inflow optimization if algorithm interval unacceptable to investigator
RAFT[62]	Sensed AV 100 ms Paced AV 130 ms	None
REVERSE (Linde, 2006)	By echo optimization	Mitral inflow optimization predischarge "to provide the maximum left ventricular filling time" without A-wave truncation

to account for delayed LA activation in some patients; the programmed AV delay is adjusted up by either 60 or 30 ms depending upon whether the atrial depolarization is under or over 100 ms respectively.[119,120] This approach, (QuickOpt™, St. Jude Medical, Sylmar, CA, USA) adds an LV-RV sequential programming based on the intrinsic activation timing and conduction to the contralateral ventricle with paced stimuli. Sogaard and colleagues had demonstrated that optimized sequential biventricular pacing, with preactivation of either the LV or the RV, could further augment the response of simultaneous biventricular pacing.[121] The device-based V-V algorithm was validated in a prior study.[122] The FREEDOM trial compared the device-based A-V and V-V optimization performed every 3 months with a control group receiving CRT with a fixed AV interval (or one-time echocardiographic-based optimization at investigator discretion) in 1647 patients.[123] As presented in a late-breaking clinical trial at the HRS meeting in 2010, the primary endpoint was not significantly different although there was a trend toward a higher clinical response rate with frequent optimization; echocardiographic outcomes were not assessed.

An important and often overlooked aspect of AV interval optimization relates to whether the atrium is tracked or paced. The fundamental problem is that the more important chamber to "optimize" is the left, yet for the most part sensing is from the RA and RV and atrial pacing when employed is from the RA. The location of the RA lead can have a significant impact on when the intrinsic P-wave is sensed. Pacing from the RA free wall or appendage can augment the delay between the activation time at the RA lead and LA mechanical events. Atrial pacing during CRT has been found to be significantly less effective than atrial tracking using a VDD mode,[124] a mode used in several early CRT trials.[15]

The American Society of Echocardiography recommends routine echocardiographic assessment after CRT implantation and consideration of optimization depending upon diastolic filling patterns.[125] Most of the historic, randomized controlled trials establishing the benefit of CRT have used echocardiographic or interval-based optimization (Table 11.6) However, even before the "negative" findings of SMART-AV[117] and FREEDOM[123] were available, most CRT implants were not optimized to adjust AV (or VV) intervals according to the two different registry samples.[122,126,127] The tedious and time-consuming nature of the echocardiographic approach and the variation in algorithms and settings between different manufacturers may stifle these activities as well. The SMART AV

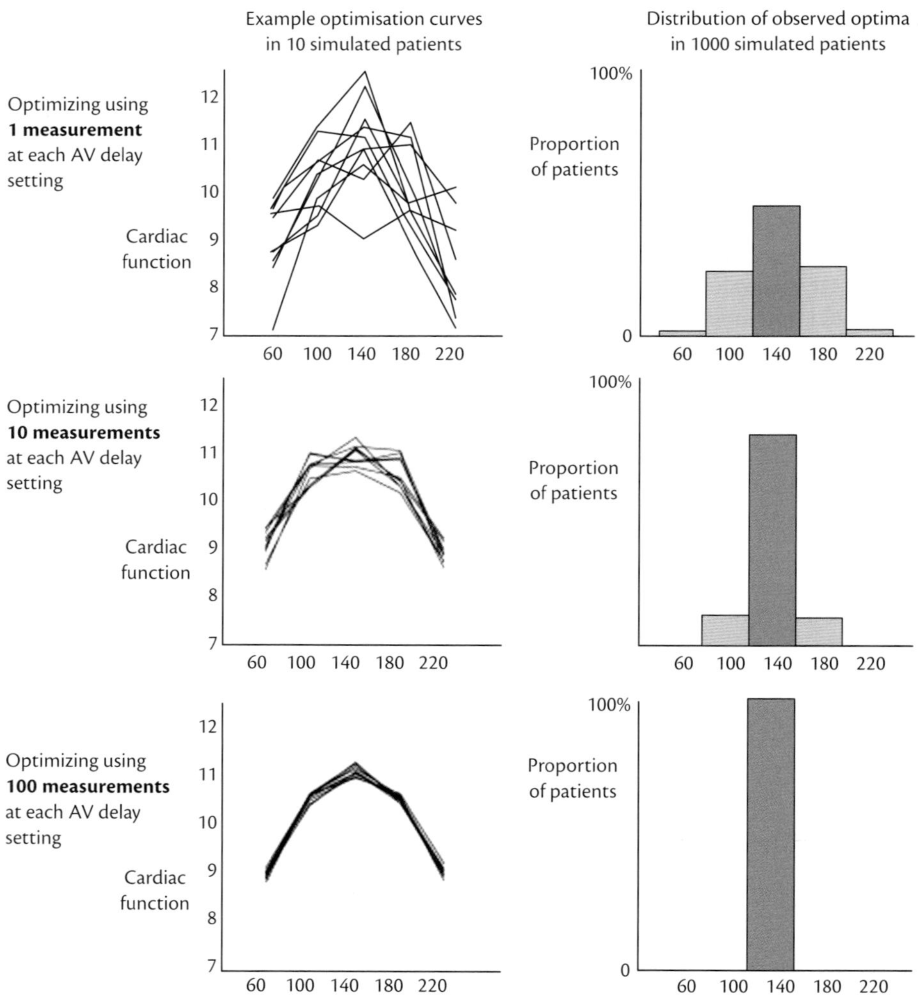

Fig. 11.18 Variation in aortic velocity–time integral is illustrated and inaccuracy of optimization with limited number of samples.
Pabari PA, Willson K, Stegemann B, van Geldorp IE, Kyriacou A, Moraldo M, et al. Heart Failure Reviews, When is an optimization not an optimization? Evaluation of clinical implications of information content (signal-to-noise ratio) in optimization of cardiac resynchronization therapy, and how to measure and maximize it. 2011;16(3):277–90, Springer.

and FREEDOM investigators suggested that routine optimization may not be warranted on the basis of their data but that selected patients, such as nonresponders to CRT, might benefit from tweaking of the programming. A better understanding of the lack of benefit in these two large studies is needed in the wake of numerous smaller studies showing improved outcomes or measurements with optimization of one sort or another.

Pabari and colleagues blame the lack of reproducibility and errors in measurements for the failure of echocardiographic optimization techniques. For instance, taking a single aortic VTI measurement gave an optimal AV delay of 40 ms, 80 ms, and 160 ms on different determinations; however, averaging 100 beats at a given setting produced a single clear optimal interval of 140 ms (Figure 11.18).[128] Another study casting some doubt on attempts to optimize device function acutely found that baseline LV *dp/dt* predicted outcome, but improvement of *dp/dt* with CRT was not predictive of survival.[129] This study did not evaluate LV remodeling. Could other acute measures, such as echocardiographic volume or dyssynchrony, blood pressure, or other measures be applicable to predict improved outcome if *dp/dt* is not capable? It seems that routine optimization is not beneficial but the study by Bogaard and colleagues suggests we may need a randomized trial of interventions in nonresponders to see if long-term benefit is derived.[117,123]

End-of-life issues

CRT is a major advance in the treatment of patients with advanced HF and has demonstrated reduction in both morbidity and mortality.[4,15,16,62,130,131] While recent studies have expanded our knowledge of the use of this therapy in patients with less symptomatic but structurally advanced ventricular dysfunction, only limited evidence exists for understanding the benefit and limitations of CRT in NYHA class IV patients.[132] Only anecdotal evidence and small case series are available exploring the use of CRT in nonambulatory or inotrope-dependent NYHA class IV patients.[133,134] More data is needed but other options such as heart transplantation, ventricular assist device, or palliative care should be considered.

In patients already receiving CRT we have seen that many are categorized as nonresponders.[84] In rare cases deactivation of CRT may lead to improvement, especially in narrower QRS or non-LBBB patients.[108] Case series have demonstrated programming or operative interventions that may be beneficial and possibly improve outcome.[16,108] Nevertheless, refractory progression of HF or other comorbidities may warrant consideration of withdrawal of CRT, ICD, or even bradycardia pacing and has been summarized in a recent HRS consensus statement.[135]

References

1. Higgins SL, Hummel JD, Niazi IK, et al. Cardiac resynchronization therapy for the treatment of heart failure in patients with intraventricular conduction delay and malignant ventricular tachyarrhythmias. J Am Coll Cardiol 2003;42(8):1454–9.
2. Abraham WT, Young JB, Leon AR, et al. Effects of cardiac resynchronization on disease progression in patients with left ventricular systolic dysfunction, an indication for an implantable cardioverter-defibrillator, and mildly symptomatic chronic heart failure. Circulation 2004;110(18):2864–8.
3. Linde C, Abraham WT, Gold MR, et al. Randomized trial of cardiac resynchronization in mildly symptomatic heart failure patients and in asymptomatic patients with left ventricular dysfunction and previous heart failure symptoms. J Am Coll Cardiol 2008;52(23):1834–43.
4. Moss AJ, Hall WJ, Cannom DS, et al. Cardiac-resynchronization therapy for the prevention of heart-failure events. N Engl J Med 2009;361(14):1329–38.
5. Linde C, Mealing S, Hawkins N, et al. Cost-effectiveness of cardiac resynchronization therapy in patients with asymptomatic to mild heart failure: insights from the European cohort of the REVERSE (Resynchronization Reverses remodeling in Systolic Left Ventricular Dysfunction). Eur Heart J 2011;32(13):1631–9.
6. Pires LA, Abraham WT, Young JB, Johnson KM. Clinical predictors and timing of New York Heart Association class improvement with cardiac resynchronization therapy in patients with advanced chronic heart failure: results from the Multicenter InSync Randomized Clinical Evaluation (MIRACLE) and Multicenter InSync ICD Randomized Clinical Evaluation (MIRACLE-ICD) trials. Am Heart J 2006;151(4):837–43.
7. van Bommel RJ, Bax JJ, Abraham WT, et al. Characteristics of heart failure patients associated with good and poor response to cardiac resynchronization therapy: a PROSPECT (Predictors of Response to CRT) sub-analysis. Eur Heart J 2009;30(20):2470–7.
8. Strickberger SA, Conti J, Daoud EG, et al. Patient selection for cardiac resynchronization therapy: from the Council on Clinical Cardiology Subcommittee on Electrocardiography and Arrhythmias and the Quality of Care and Outcomes Research Interdisciplinary Working Group, in collaboration with the Heart Rhythm Society. Circulation 2005;111(16) 2146–50.
9. Aaronson KD, Schwartz JS, Chen TM, et al. Development and prospective validation of a clinical index to predict survival in ambulatory patients referred for cardiac transplant evaluation. Circulation 1997;95(12):2660–7.
10. Baldasseroni S, Opasich C, Gorini M, et al. Left bundle-branch block is associated with increased 1-year sudden and total mortality rate in 5517 outpatients with congestive heart failure: a report from the Italian network on congestive heart failure. Am Heart J 2002;143(3):398–405.
11. Nelson GS, Berger RD, Fetics BJ, et al. Left ventricular or biventricular pacing improves cardiac function at diminished energy cost in patients with dilated cardiomyopathy and left bundle-branch block. Circulation 2000;102(25):3053–9.
12. Nelson GS, Curry CW, Wyman BT, et al. Predictors of systolic augmentation from left ventricular preexcitation in patients with dilated cardiomyopathy and intraventricular conduction delay. Circulation 2000;101(23):2703–9.
13. Cazeau S, Leclercq C, Lavergne T, et al. Effects of multisite biventricular pacing in patients with heart failure and intraventricular conduction delay. N Engl J Med 2001;344(12):873–80.
14. Young JB, Abraham WT, Smith AL, et al. Combined cardiac resynchronization and implantable cardioversion defibrillation in advanced chronic heart failure: the MIRACLE ICD Trial. JAMA 2003;289(20):2685–94.
15. Abraham WT, Fisher WG, Smith AL, et al. Cardiac resynchronization in chronic heart failure. N Engl J Med 2002;346(24):1845–53.
16. Bristow MR, Saxon LA, Boehmer J, et al. Cardiac-resynchronization therapy with or without an implantable defibrillator in advanced chronic heart failure. N Engl J Med 2004;350(21):2140–50.
17. Gold MR, Thébault C, Linde C, et al. Effect of QRS duration and morphology on cardiac resynchronization therapy outcomes in mild heart failure/clinical perspective. Circulation 2012;126(7):822–9.
18. Mollema SA, Bleeker GB, van der Wall EE, et al. Usefulness of QRS duration to predict response to cardiac resynchronization therapy in patients with end-stage heart failure. Am J Cardiol 2007;100(11):1665–70.
19. Sipahi I Carrigan TP, Rowland DY, et al. Impact of QRS duration on clinical event reduction with cardiac resynchronization therapy: Meta-analysis of randomized controlled trials. Arch Intern Med 2011;171(16):1454–62.
20. Sweeney MO, van Bommel RJ, Schalij MJ, et al. Analysis of ventricular activation using surface electrocardiography to predict left ventricular reverse volumetric remodeling during cardiac resynchronization therapy. Circulation 2010;121(5):626–34.

21. Leclercq C, Faris O, Tunin R, et al. Systolic improvement and mechanical resynchronization does not require electrical synchrony in the dilated failing heart with left bundle-branch block. Circulation 2002;106(14):1760–3.
22. Bleeker GB, Schalij MJ, Molhoek SG, et al. Relationship between QRS duration and left ventricular dyssynchrony in patients with end-stage heart failure. J Cardiovasc Electrophysiol 2004;15(5):544–9.
23. Gorcsan J, 3rd, Kanzaki H, Bazaz R, et al. Usefulness of echocardiographic tissue synchronization imaging to predict acute response to cardiac resynchronization therapy. Am J Cardiol 2004;93(9):1178–81.
24. Yu C-M, Fung JW-H, Zhang Q, et al. Tissue Doppler imaging is superior to strain rate imaging and postsystolic shortening on the prediction of reverse remodeling in both ischemic and nonischemic heart failure after cardiac resynchronization therapy. Circulation 2004;110(1):66–73.
25. Becker M, Hoffmann R, Kuhl HP, et al. Analysis of myocardial deformation based on ultrasonic pixel tracking to determine transmurality in chronic myocardial infarction. Eur Heart J 2006;27(21):2560–6.
26. Chung ES, Leon AR, Tavazzi L, et al. Results of the Predictors of Response to CRT (PROSPECT) Trial. Circulation 2008;117(20):2608–16.
27. Beshai JF, Grimm RA, Nagueh SF, et al. Cardiac-resynchronization therapy in heart failure with narrow QRS complexes. N Engl J Med 2007;357(24):2461–71.
28. Delgado V, van Bommel RJ, Bertini M, et al. Relative merits of left ventricular dyssynchrony, left ventricular lead position, and myocardial scar to predict long-term survival of ischemic heart failure patients undergoing cardiac resynchronization therapy/clinical perspective. Circulation 2011;123(1):70–8.
29. Kim RJ, Fieno DS, Parrish TB, et al. Relationship of MRI delayed contrast enhancement to irreversible injury, infarct age, and contractile function. Circulation 1999;100(19):1992–2002.
30. Bleeker GB, Kaandorp TAM, Lamb HJ, et al. Effect of posterolateral scar tissue on clinical and echocardiographic improvement after cardiac resynchronization therapy. Circulation 2006;113(7):969–76.
31. Leyva F, Foley PW, Chalil S, et al. Cardiac resynchronization therapy guided by late gadolinium-enhancement cardiovascular magnetic resonance. J Cardiovasc Magn Reson 2011;13:29.
32. Foley PWX, Patel K, Irwin N, et al. Cardiac resynchronisation therapy in patients with heart failure and a normal QRS duration: the RESPOND study. Heart 2011;97(13):1041–7.
33. Hsu JC, Solomon SD, Bourgoun M, et al. Predictors of super-response to cardiac resynchronization therapy and associated improvement in clinical outcome: the MADIT-CRT (multicenter automatic defibrillator implantation trial with cardiac resynchronization therapy) study. J Am Coll Cardiol 2012;59(25):2366–73.
34. Rickard J, Kumbhani DJ, Popovic Z, et al. Characterization of super-response to cardiac resynchronization therapy. Heart Rhythm 2010;7(7):885–9.
35. Steffel J, Milosevic G, Hürlimann A, et al. Characteristics and long-term outcome of echocardiographic super-responders to cardiac resynchronisation therapy: "real world" experience from a single tertiary care centre. Heart 2011;97(20):1668–74.
36. Upadhyay GA, Choudhry NK, Auricchio A, et al. Cardiac resynchronization in patients with atrial fibrillation: a meta-analysis of prospective cohort studies. J Am Coll Cardiol 2008;52(15):1239–46.
37. Koplan BA, Kaplan AJ, Weiner S, et al. Heart failure decompensation and all-cause mortality in relation to percent biventricular pacing in patients with heart failure. Is a goal of 100% biventricular pacing necessary? J Am Coll Cardiol 2009;53(4):355–60.
38. Hayes DL, Boehmer JP, Day JD, et al. Cardiac resynchronization therapy and the relationship of percent biventricular pacing to symptoms and survival. Heart Rhythm 2011;8(9):1469–75.
39. Gasparini M, Auricchio A, Regoli F, et al. Four-year efficacy of cardiac resynchronization therapy on exercise tolerance and disease progression: the importance of performing atrioventricular junction ablation in patients with atrial fibrillation. J Am Coll Cardiol 2006;48(4):734–43.
40. Gasparini M, Auricchio A, Metra M, et al. Long-term survival in patients undergoing cardiac resynchronization therapy: the importance of performing atrio-ventricular junction ablation in patients with permanent atrial fibrillation. Eur Heart J 2008;29(13):1644–52.
41. Ganesan AN, Brooks AG, Roberts-Thomson KC, et al. Role of AV nodal ablation in cardiac resynchronization in patients with coexistent atrial fibrillation and heart failure: a systematic review. J Am Coll Cardiol 2012;59(8):719–26.
42. Khan MN, Jais P, Cummings J, et al. Pulmonary-vein isolation for atrial fibrillation in patients with heart failure. N Engl J Med 2008;359(17):1778–85.
43. Aranda JM, Jr., Conti JB, Johnson JW, et al. Cardiac resynchronization therapy in patients with heart failure and conduction abnormalities other than left bundle-branch block: analysis of the Multicenter InSync Randomized Clinical Evaluation (MIRACLE). Clin Cardiol 2004;27(12):678–82.
44. Egoavil CA, Ho RT, Greenspon AJ, Pavri BB. Cardiac resynchronization therapy in patients with right bundle branch block: analysis of pooled data from the MIRACLE and Contak CD trials. Heart Rhythm 2005;2(6):611–15.
45. Zareba W, Klein H, Cygankiewicz I, et al. Effectiveness of cardiac resynchronization therapy by QRS morphology in the Multicenter Automatic Defibrillator Implantation Trial–Cardiac Resynchronization Therapy (MADIT-CRT): clinical perspective. Circulation 2011;123(10):1061–72.
46. Fantoni C, Kawabata M, Massaro R, et al. Right and left ventricular activation sequence in patients with heart failure and right bundle branch block: a detailed analysis using three-dimensional non-fluoroscopic electroanatomic mapping system. J Cardiovasc Electrophysiol 2005;16(2):112–9; discussion 20–1.
47. Wilkoff BL, Cook JR, Epstein AE, et al.; Dual Chamber and VVI Implantable Defibrillator Trial Investigators. Dual-chamber pacing or ventricular backup pacing in patients with an implantable defibrillator: The Dual Chamber And VVI Implantable Defibrillator (DAVID) trial. JAMA 2002;288(24):3115–23.
48. Yu C-M, Chan JY-S, Zhang Q, et al. Biventricular pacing in patients with bradycardia and normal ejection fraction. N Engl J Med 2009;361(22):2123–34.
49. Stockburger M, Gómez-Doblas JJ, Lamas G, et al. Preventing ventricular dysfunction in pacemaker patients without advanced heart failure: results from a multicentre international randomized trial (PREVENT-HF). Eur J Heart Fail 2011;13(6):633–41.
50. Curtis AB, Adamson PB, Chung E, et al. Biventricular versus right ventricular pacing in patients with AV block (BLOCK HF): clinical study design and rationale. J Cardiovasc Electrophysiol 2007;18(9):965–71.
51. Lakkireddy D, Di Biase L, Ryschon K, et al. Radiofrequency ablation of premature ventricular ectopy improves the efficacy of cardiac resynchronization therapy in nonresponders. J Am Coll Cardiol 2012;60(16):1531–9.
52. Tracy CM, Epstein AE, Darbar D, et al. 2012 ACCF/AHA/HRS focused update of the 2008 guidelines for device-based therapy of cardiac rhythm abnormalities. Circulation 2012;126(14):1784–800.
53. Elmqvist R. Review of early pacemaker development. Pacing Clin Electrophysiol 1978;1(4):535–6.
54. Parsonnet V, Werres R, Atherley T, Littleford PO. Transvenous insertion of double sets of permanent electrodes. Atraumatic technique for atrial synchronous and atrioventricular sequential pacemakers. JAMA 1980;243(1):62–4.
55. Hochleitner M, Hortnagl H, Ng CK, et al. Usefulness of physiologic dual-chamber pacing in drug-resistant idiopathic dilated cardiomyopathy. Am J Cardiol 1990;66(2):198–202.
56. Auricchio A, Sommariva L, Salo RW, et al. Improvement of cardiac function in patients with severe congestive heart failure and coronary artery disease by dual chamber pacing with shortened AV delay. Pacing Clin Electrophysiol 1993;16(10):2034–43.
57. Gold MR, Feliciano Z, Gottlieb SS, Fisher ML. Dual-chamber pacing with a short atrioventricular delay in congestive heart failure: a randomized study. J Am Coll Cardiol 1995;26(4):967–73.

58. Sharma AD, Rizo-Patron C, Hallstrom AP, et al. Percent right ventricular pacing predicts outcomes in the DAVID trial. Heart Rhythm 2005;2(8):830–4.
59. Cazeau S, Ritter P, Bakdach S, et al. Four chamber pacing in dilated cardiomyopathy. Pacing Clin Electrophysiol 1994;17(11 Pt 2):1974–9.
60. Cazeau S, Ritter P, Lazarus A, et al. Multisite pacing for end-stage heart failure: early experience. Pacing Clin Electrophysiol 1996;19(11 Pt 2):1748–57.
61. Daubert JC, Ritter P, Le Breton H, , et al. Permanent left ventricular pacing with transvenous leads inserted into the coronary veins. Pacing Clin Electrophysiol 1998;21(1 Pt 2):239–45.
62. Tang AS, Wells GA, Talajic M, et al. Cardiac-resynchronization therapy for mild-to-moderate heart failure. N Engl J Med 2010;363(25):2385–95.
63. Noheria A, Desimone CV, Lachman N, et al. Anatomy of the coronary sinus and epicardial coronary venous system in 620 hearts: an electrophysiology perspective. J Cardiovasc Electrophysiol 2013;24(1):1–6.
64. Habib A, Lachman N, Christensen KN, Asirvatham SJ. The anatomy of the coronary sinus venous system for the cardiac electrophysiologist. Europace 2009;11 Suppl 5:v15–21.
65. Blendea D, Shah RV, Auricchio A, et al. Variability of coronary venous anatomy in patients undergoing cardiac resynchronization therapy: a high-speed rotational venography study. Heart Rhythm 2007;4(9):1155–62.
66. Van de Veire NR, Schuijf JD, Bleeker GB, et al. Magnetic resonance imaging and computed tomography in assessing cardiac veins and scar tissue. Europace 2008;10 Suppl 3:iii110–13.
67. Da Costa A, Gate-Martinet A, Rouffiange P, et al. Anatomical factors involved in difficult cardiac resynchronization therapy procedure: a non-invasive study using dual-source 64-multi-slice computed tomography. Europace 2012;14(6):833–40.
68. Sipahi I, Carrigan TP, Rowland DY, et al. Impact of QRS duration on clinical event reduction with cardiac resynchronization therapy: meta-analysis of randomized controlled trials. Arch Intern Med 2011;171(16):1454–62.
69. Hara H, Oyenuga OA, Tanaka H, et al. The relationship of QRS morphology and mechanical dyssynchrony to long-term outcome following cardiac resynchronization therapy. Eur Heart J 2012;33(21):2680–91.
70. Khan FZ, Virdee MS, Palmer CR, et al. Targeted left ventricular lead placement to guide cardiac resynchronization therapy: the TARGET study: a randomized, controlled trial. J Am Coll Cardiol 2012;59(17):1509–18.
71. Delgado V, van Bommel RJ, Bertini M, et al. Relative merits of left ventricular dyssynchrony, left ventricular lead position, and myocardial scar to predict long-term survival of ischemic heart failure patients undergoing cardiac resynchronization therapy. Circulation 2011;123(1):70–8.
72. Butter C, Gras D, Ritter P, et al. Comparative prospective randomized efficacy testing of different guiding catheters for coronary sinus cannulation in heart failure patients. J Interv Card Electrophysiol 2003;9(3):343–51.
73. Worley SJ. CRT delivery systems based on guide support for LV lead placement. Heart Rhythm 2009;6(9):1383–7.
74. Jackson KP, Hegland DD, Frazier MC, et al. Impact of using a telescoping-support catheter system for left ventricular lead placement on implant success and procedure time of cardiac resynchronization therapy. Pacing Clin Electrophysiol 2013;36(5):553–8.
75. Reynolds MR, Cohen DJ, Kugelmass AD, et al. The frequency and incremental cost of major complications among medicare beneficiaries receiving implantable cardioverter-defibrillators. J Am Coll Cardiol 2006;47(12):2493–7.
76. van Rees JB, de Bie MK, Thijssen J, et al. Implantation-related complications of implantable cardioverter-defibrillators and cardiac resynchronization therapy devices: a systematic review of randomized clinical trials. J Am Coll Cardiol 2011;58(10):995–1000.
77. Worley SJ. How to use balloons as anchors to facilitate cannulation of the coronary sinus left ventricular lead placement and to regain lost coronary sinus or target vein access. Heart Rhythm 2009;6(8):1242–6.
78. Worley SJ. Implant venoplasty: dilation of subclavian and coronary veins to facilitate device implantation: indications, frequency, methods, and complications. J Cardiovasc Electrophysiol 2008;19(9):1004–7.
79. Crossley GH, Exner D, Mead RH, et al. Chronic performance of an active fixation coronary sinus lead. Heart Rhythm 2010;7(4):472–8.
80. Forleo GB, Mantica M, Di Biase L, et al. Clinical and procedural outcome of patients implanted with a quadripolar left ventricular lead: early results of a prospective multicenter study. Heart Rhythm 2012;9(11):1822–8.
81. Singh JP, Klein HU, Huang DT, et al. Left ventricular lead position and clinical outcome in the multicenter automatic defibrillator implantation trial-cardiac resynchronization therapy (MADIT-CRT) trial. Circulation 2011;123(11):1159–66.
82. Wilkoff BL, Auricchio A, Brugada J, et al. HRS/EHRA Expert Consensus on the Monitoring of Cardiovascular Implantable Electronic Devices (CIEDs): Description of techniques, indications, personnel, frequency and ethical considerations: developed in partnership with the Heart Rhythm Society (HRS) and the European Heart Rhythm Association (EHRA); and in collaboration with the American College of Cardiology (ACC), the American Heart Association (AHA), the European Society of Cardiology (ESC), the Heart Failure Association of ESC (HFA), and the Heart Failure Society of America (HFSA). Endorsed by the Heart Rhythm Society, the European Heart Rhythm Association (a registered branch of the ESC), the American College of Cardiology, the American Heart Association. Heart Rhythm 2008;5(6):907–25.
83. Fung JW, Yu CM. Leveraging cardiac resynchronization therapy devices to monitor patients with heart failure. Curr Heart Fail Rep 2008;5(1):44–50.
84. Daubert JC, Saxon L, Adamson PB, et al. 2012 EHRA/HRS expert consensus statement on cardiac resynchronization therapy in heart failure: implant and follow-up recommendations and management. Heart Rhythm 2012;9(9):1524–76.
85. Polin GM, Zado E, Nayak H, et al. Proper management of pericardial tamponade as a late complication of implantable cardiac device placement. Am J Cardiol 2006;98(2):223–5.
86. Hirschl DA, Jain VR, Spindola-Franco H, et al. Prevalence and characterization of asymptomatic pacemaker and ICD lead perforation on CT. Pacing Clin Electrophysiol 2007;30(1):28–32.
87. Shukla G, Chaudhry GM, Orlov M, et al. Potential proarrhythmic effect of biventricular pacing: fact or myth? Heart Rhythm 2005;2(9):951–6.
88. Mykytsey A, Maheshwari P, Dhar G, et al. Ventricular tachycardia induced by biventricular pacing in patient with severe ischemic cardiomyopathy. J Cardiovasc Electrophysiol 2005;16(6):655–8.
89. Nayak HM, Verdino RJ, Russo AM, et al. Ventricular tachycardia storm after initiation of biventricular pacing: incidence, clinical characteristics, management, and outcome. J Cardiovasc Electrophysiol 2008;19(7):708–15.
90. Fish JM, Brugada J, Antzelevitch C. Potential proarrhythmic effects of biventricular pacing. J Am Coll Cardiol 2005;46(12):2340–7.
91. Medina-Ravell VA, Lankipalli RS, Yan GX, et al. Effect of epicardial or biventricular pacing to prolong QT interval and increase transmural dispersion of repolarization: does resynchronization therapy pose a risk for patients predisposed to long QT or torsade de pointes? Circulation 2003;107(5):740–6.
92. Young JB, Abraham WT, Smith AL, et al. Combined cardiac resynchronization and implantable cardioversion defibrillation in advanced chronic heart failure: The MIRACLE ICD trial. JAMA 2003;289(20):2685–94.
93. Cleland JGF, Daubert J-C, Erdmann E, et al. The effect of cardiac resynchronization on morbidity and mortality in heart failure. N Engl J Med 2005;352(15):1539–49.
94. Gold MR, Linde C, Abraham WT, et al. The impact of cardiac resynchronization therapy on the incidence of ventricular arrhythmias in mild heart failure. Heart Rhythm 2011;8(5):679–84.

95. Ouellet G, Huang DT, Moss AJ, et al. Effect of cardiac resynchronization therapy on the risk of first and recurrent ventricular tachyarrhythmic events in MADIT-CRT. J Am Coll Cardiol 2012;60(18):1809–16.
96. Leon AR, Abraham WT, Curtis AB, et al. Safety of transvenous cardiac resynchronization system implantation in patients with chronic heart failure: combined results of over 2,000 patients from a multicenter study program. J Am Coll Cardiol 2005;46(12):2348–56.
97. Daubert JP, Hranitzky PM, McNitt S, et al. MADIT-CRT: Resynchronization patients experience more complications than ICD-only patients but outcomes are not significantly impacted. Circulation 2011;124:A9364.
98. Daubert C, Gold MR, Abraham WT, et al. Prevention of disease progression by cardiac resynchronization therapy in patients with asymptomatic or mildly symptomatic left ventricular dysfunction: insights from the European cohort of the REVERSE (Resynchronization Reverses Remodeling in Systolic Left Ventricular Dysfunction) trial. J Am Coll Cardiol 2009;54(20):1837–46.
99. Barold SS, Herweg B, Giudici M. Electrocardiographic follow-up of biventricular pacemakers. Ann Noninvasive Electrocardiol 2005;10(2):231–55.
100. Ammann P, Sticherling C, Kalusche D, et al. An electrocardiogram-based algorithm to detect loss of left ventricular capture during cardiac resynchronization therapy. Ann Intern Med 2005;142(12 Pt 1):968–73.
101. Ploux S, Bordachar P, Deplagne A, et al. Electrocardiogram-based algorithm to predict the left ventricular lead position in recipients of cardiac resynchronization systems. Pacing Clinical Electrophysiol 2009;32:S2–7.
102. Barold SS, Herweg B. Upper rate response of biventricular pacing devices. J Intervent Card Electrophysiol 2005;12(2):129–36.
103. Aktas MK, Jeevanantham V, Sherazi S, et al. Effect of biventricular pacing during a ventricular sensed event. Am J Cardiol 2009;103(12):1741–5.
104. Kamath G, Cotiga D, Koneru J, et al. The utility of 12-lead Holter monitoring in patients with permanent atrial fibrillation for the identification of nonresponders after cardiac resynchronization therapy. J Am Coll Cardiol 2009;53:1050–5.
105. Poole JE, Gleva MJ, Mela T, et al. Complication rates associated with pacemaker or implantable cardioverter-defibrillator generator replacements and upgrade procedures: results from the REPLACE registry. Circulation 2010;122(16):1553–61.
106. Crossley GH, Mead H, Kleckner K, et al. Automated left ventricular capture management. Pacing Clin Electrophysiol 2007;30(10):1190–200.
107. Kalahasty G, Giudici M, Lobban J, et al. Acute clinical evaluation of a left ventricular automatic threshold determination algorithm based on evoked response sensing. Pacing Clin Electrophysiol 2012;35(3):348–56.
108. Mullens W, Grimm RA, Verga T, et al. Insights from a cardiac resynchronization optimization clinic as part of a heart failure disease management program. J Am Coll Cardiol 2009;53(9):765–73.
109. Cheng A, Landman SR, Stadler RW. Reasons for loss of cardiac resynchronization therapy pacing/clinical perspective. Circ Arrhythm Electrophysiol 2012;5(5):884–8.
110. Dupuis J-M, Kobeissi A, Vitali L, et al. Programming optimal atrioventricular delay in dual chamber pacing using peak endocardial acceleration: comparison with a standard echocardiographic procedure. Pacing Clin Electrophysiol 2003;26(1 Pt 2):210–13.
111. Ritter P, Padeletti L, Gillio-Meina L, Gaggini G. Determination of the optimal atrioventricular delay in DDD pacing. Comparison between echo and peak endocardial acceleration measurements. Europace 1999;1(2):126–30.
112. Ritter P, Dib J, Lelievre T. Quick determination of the opti- mal AV delay at rest in patients paced in DDD mode for complete AV block (abstract). Eur J Cardiac Pacing Electrophysiol 1994;4:A163.
113. Kerlan JE, Sawhney NS, Waggoner AD, et al. Prospective comparison of echocardiographic atrioventricular delay optimization methods for cardiac resynchronization therapy. Heart Rhythm 2006;3(2):148–54.
114. Sawhney NS, Waggoner AD, Garhwal S, et al. Randomized prospective trial of atrioventricular delay programming for cardiac resynchronization therapy. Heart Rhythm 2004;1(5):562–7.
115. Jansen AH, Bracke FA, van Dantzig JM, et al. Correlation of echo-Doppler optimization of atrioventricular delay in cardiac resynchronization therapy with invasive hemodynamics in patients with heart failure secondary to ischemic or idiopathic dilated cardiomyopathy. Am J Cardiol 2006;97(4):552–7.
116. Auricchio A, Stellbrink C, Block M, et al. Effect of pacing chamber and atrioventricular delay on acute systolic function of paced patients with congestive heart failure. The Pacing Therapies for Congestive Heart Failure Study Group. The Guidant Congestive Heart Failure Research Group. Circulation 1999;99(23):2993–3001.
117. Ellenbogen KA, Gold MR, Meyer TE, et al. Primary results from the SmartDelay determined AV optimization: a comparison to other AV delay methods used in cardiac resynchronization therapy (SMART-AV) trial: a randomized trial comparing empirical, echocardiography-guided, and algorithmic atrioventricular delay programming in cardiac resynchronization therapy. Circulation 2010;122(25):2660–8.
118. Gold MR, Niazi I, Giudici M, et al. A prospective comparison of AV delay programming methods for hemodynamic optimization during cardiac resynchronization therapy. J Cardiovasc Electrophysiol 2007;18(5):490–6.
119. Meine M, Min X, Kordmann M, et al. IEGM based method for estimating optimal AV delay in cardiac resynchronization therapy. J Card Fail 2004;10(4,Suppl):S74.
120. Porciani MC, Rao CM, Mochi M, et al. A real-time three-dimensional echocardiographic validation of an intracardiac electrogram-based method for optimizing cardiac resynchronization therapy. Pacing Clin Electrophysiol 2008;31(1):56–63.
121. Sogaard P, Egeblad H, Pedersen AK, et al. Sequential versus simultaneous biventricular resynchronization for severe heart failure: evaluation by tissue Doppler imaging. Circulation 2002;106(16):2078–84.
122. Baker JH, 2nd, McKenzie J, 3rd, Beau S, et al. Acute evaluation of programmer-guided AV/PV and VV delay optimization comparing an IEGM method and echocardiogram for cardiac resynchronization therapy in heart failure patients and dual-chamber ICD implants. J Cardiovasc Electrophysiol 2007;18(2):185–91.
123. Abraham WT, Gras D, Yu CM, et al.; FREEDOM Steering Committee. Rationale and design of a randomized clinical trial to assess the safety and efficacy of frequent optimization of cardiac resynchronization therapy: the Frequent Optimization Study Using the QuickOpt Method (FREEDOM) trial. Am Heart J 2010;159(6):944–8.
124. Bernheim A, Ammann P, Sticherling C, et al. Right atrial pacing impairs cardiac function during resynchronization therapy: acute effects of DDD pacing compared to VDD pacing. J Am Coll Cardiol 2005;45(9):1482–7.
125. Gorcsan J, 3rd, Abraham T, Agler DA, et al. Echocardiography for cardiac resynchronization therapy: recommendations for performance and reporting—a report from the American Society of Echocardiography Dyssynchrony Writing Group endorsed by the Heart Rhythm Society. J Am Soc Echocardiogr 2008;21(3):191–213.
126. Deering TF, Epstein AE, Goldman D, Greenberg S. Hype, hope or help: optimization of AV/PV and VV timing in the CRT-D population—Experience from the ACT registry (abstract). Europace 2006;8(Suppl 1):186.
127. Gras D, Gupta MS, Boulogne E, et al. Optimization of AV and VV delays in the real-world CRT patient population: an international survey on current clinical practice. Pacing Clin Electrophysiol 2009;32(Suppl 1):S236–9.

128. Pabari PA, Willson K, Stegemann B, et al. When is an optimization not an optimization? Evaluation of clinical implications of information content (signal-to-noise ratio) in optimization of cardiac resynchronization therapy, and how to measure and maximize it. Heart Fail Rev 2011;16(3):277–90.
129. Bogaard MD, Houthuizen P, Bracke FA, et al. Baseline left ventricular dP/dtmax rather than the acute improvement in dP/dtmax predicts clinical outcome in patients with cardiac resynchronization therapy. Eur J Heart Fail 2011;13(10):1126–32.
130. Cleland JG, Daubert JC, Erdmann E, et al. The effect of cardiac resynchronization on morbidity and mortality in heart failure. N Engl J Med 2005;352(15):1539–49.
131. Linde C, Abraham WT, Gold MR, et al. Randomized trial of cardiac resynchronization in mildly symptomatic heart failure patients and in asymptomatic patients with left ventricular dysfunction and previous heart failure symptoms. J Am Coll Cardiol 2008;52(23):1834–43.
132. Lindenfeld J, Feldman AM, Saxon L, et al. Effects of cardiac resynchronization therapy with or without a defibrillator on survival and hospitalizations in patients with New York Heart Association class IV heart failure. Circulation 2007;115(2):204–12.
133. Braunschweig F, Hauptman PJ. Cardiac resynchronization therapy in the intensive care setting; the promise and peril of using implantable devices off label. Eur J Heart Fail 2008;10(3):220–1.
134. Herweg B, Barold SS. When is it too late for cardiac resynchronization therapy? Pacing Clin Electrophysiol 2008;31(5):525–8.
135. Lampert R, Hayes DL, Annas GJ, et al. HRS Expert Consensus Statement on the Management of Cardiovascular Implantable Electronic Devices (CIEDs) in patients nearing end of life or requesting withdrawal of therapyThis document was developed in collaboration and endorsed by the American College of Cardiology (ACC), the American Geriatrics Society (AGS), the American Academy of Hospice and Palliative Medicine (AAHPM); the American Heart Association (AHA), the European Heart Rhythm Association (EHRA), and the Hospice and Palliative Nurses Association (HPNA). Heart Rhythm 2010;7(7):1008–26.
136. Lakkireddy D, Di Biase L, Ryschon K, et al. Radiofrequency ablation of premature ventricular ectopy improves the efficacy of cardiac resynchronization therapy in nonresponders. J Am Coll Cardiol 2012;60(16):1531–9.
137. Daubert JC, Pavin D, Jauvert G, Mabo P. Intra- and interatrial conduction delay: implications for cardiac pacing. Pacing Clin Electrophysiol 2004;27(4):507–25.
138. Auricchio A, Ding J, Spinelli JC, et al. Cardiac resynchronization therapy restores optimal atrioventricular mechanical timing in heart failure patients with ventricular conduction delay. J Am Coll Cardiol 2002;39(7):1163–9.

CHAPTER 12

Advanced heart failure in valvular heart disease

Blase A. Carabello MD

Introduction

Each valvular heart disease imparts a unique hemodynamic burden on the left ventricle (LV) and/or the right ventricle (RV). If this burden is severe and prolonged it results eventually in myocardial damage, heart failure (HF), and death. The following is an examination of how each lesion causes HF and how HF may be prevented or reversed.

Aortic stenosis: the quintessential pressure overload

Pathophysiology

The normal aortic orifice area is about 3.0 cm^2. Narrowing from aortic stenosis (AS) to half that aperture causes little hemodynamic disturbance (Table 12.1). However, further narrowing leads to progressively higher pressure gradients between the LV and the aorta. The extra pressure required to force blood through the compromised aortic orifice represents the pressure overload of AS. In multiple ways this overload leads to HF. Mechanisms include maladaptive remodeling, impaired diastolic filling, abnormalities in coronary blood flow, and intrinsic LV injury with impaired myocardial contractility.

Afterload mismatch

Left ventricular ejection fraction (LVEF), and to some degree stroke volume, is inversely related to afterload, a property often quantified as systolic wall stress (σ):

$$(\sigma) = P \times r \,/\, 2th$$

where P is LV pressure, r is LV radius, and th is wall thickness. As LV pressure in the numerator of this equation increases, it can be offset by increased wall thickness (concentric hypertrophy, LVH) in the denominator. Thus in some cases afterload (stress) remains normal, helping to maintain ejection fraction (EF).[1] However in other cases LVH is inadequate to normalize stress, increased afterload impairs LV ejection, and HF ensues (Figure 12.1).[1,2] HF due to afterload mismatch in AS is probably the most easily treated. Aortic valve replacement (AVR) affords an immediate reduction in afterload, ejection performance improves almost instantaneously, and HF improves dramatically.[3]

Diastolic dysfunction

Unfortunately LVH in AS is a doubled-edged sword. While it helps to maintain ejection performance it also has pathologic consequences, one of which is to impair LV diastolic function.[4,5] Diastole is conventionally divided into two parts, active relaxation followed by passive diastolic filling. Pathologic LVH affects both of these phases. Active relaxation, which is characterized by the rate of descent of LV pressure decline, is delayed such that mitral valve opening is also delayed, shortening the time for LV filling.[5] Increased LV thickness compounded by increased extracellular collagen increases LV stiffness. Thus higher filling pressure is required to fill the LV to a given volume (Figure 12.2). Increased diastolic pressure in turn leads to lung congestion and the symptom of dyspnea.

In some patients the LV in AS remodels such that both compliance and end-diastolic volume are reduced so that although EF is normal, stroke volume is reduced.[6] Thus the key elements of HF, pulmonary congestion, and reduced cardiac output are present despite a normal EF. The syndrome of HF with normal EF in AS may be misleading to the clinician.[7,8] Reduced stroke volume also reduces the transvalvular gradient, causing the uninitiated to underestimate AS severity. However, if all of the other indicators of severe AS (valve area, heavy calcification, and reduced leaflet motion) are present, such patients benefit from AVR and fare poorly with medical therapy.[7,8,9]

Systolic dysfunction

In the majority of patients with AS and reduced EF, afterload is increased because increased LV systolic pressure is not offset by adequate concentric hypertrophy.[1] However, prolonged severe LV pressure overload also leads to myocardial damage as another cause of systolic dysfunction that compounds the syndrome of HF.

Table 12.1 Aortic valve area and mean aortic gradient

Aortic valve area (cm^2)	Gradient (mmHg)
3.0	3
2.0	8
1.0	30
0.8	47
0.7	62
0.6	84
0.5	121

Assumes a cardiac output of 5.5 L/min; heart rate of 75 bpm.

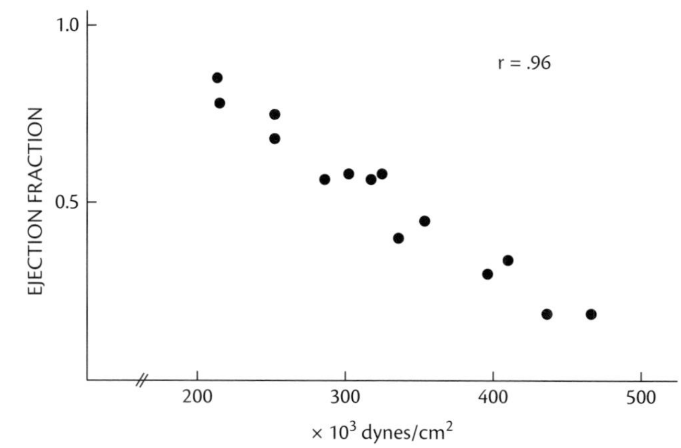

Fig. 12.1 The relationship between afterload (wall stress) and ejection is inverse. Thus afterload mismatch is a cause for reduced ejection fraction in patients with aortic stenosis.

Gunther S, Grossman W. Determinants of ventricular function in pressure-overload hypertrophy in man. Circulation 1979;59:679–88.

Multiple mechanisms exist to explain the myocardial dysfunction of AS. First, coronary blood flow reserve is impaired in AS potentiating subendocardial ischemia especially during exercise and the symptom of angina indicating episodic ischemia is common in AS.[10,11] It is known that increased levels of serum troponin correlate with HF and LV function and it is likely that repeated bouts of ischemia cause subtle LV damage that contributes to LV systolic dysfunction.[12,13] Second, abnormal calcium handling reduces inotropic state, in turn reducing LV function.[14] Apoptosis, microtubular excess, and genetic reprogramming also contribute to LV dysfunction in AS patients.[15,16,17,18] The foregoing mechanisms act in concert, leading to myocardial fibrosis[19,20] and end-stage HF defined as a syndrome of low EF, low gradient (low afterload), and low cardiac output (Figure 12.3).[21] Unlike the hemodynamics of afterload mismatch, low EF in this syndrome is due to severe myocardial damage and dysfunction and accordingly has a worse prognosis.[22]

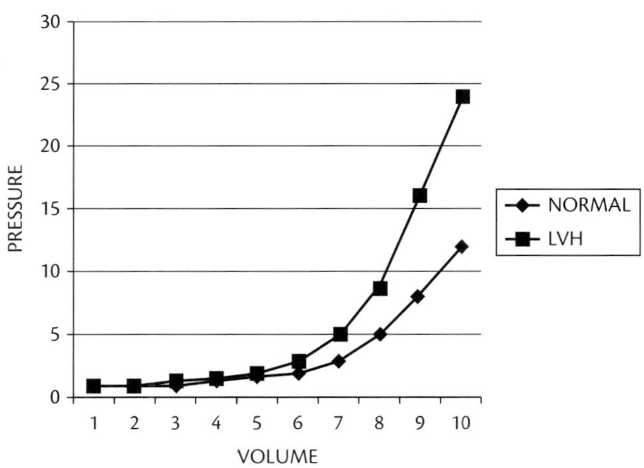

Fig. 12.2 Representative left ventricular (LV) pressure–volume curves for a normal subject and one with concentric left ventricular hypertrophy (LVH) typical of AS are shown. With LVH, greater pressure is required to fill the LV to a given volume.

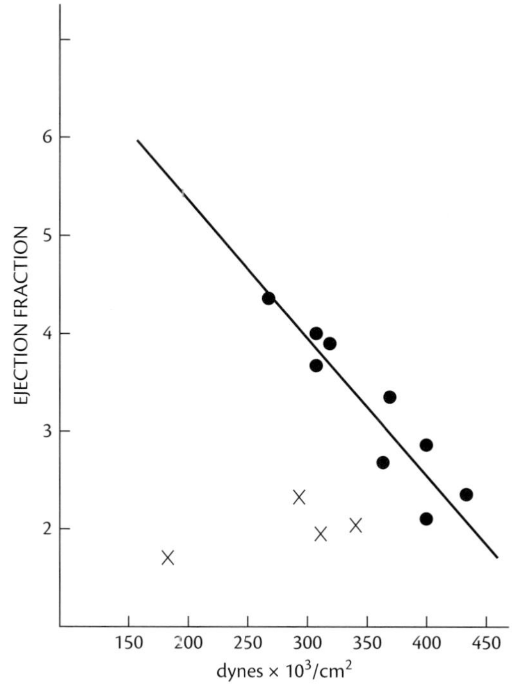

Fig. 12.3 The two mechanisms of left ventricular dysfunction are demonstrated by relating afterload (wall stress) to ejection fraction (EF). In some patients (circles) EF is reduced linearly with afterload so that afterload excess is the major cause of reduced EF. In other patients EF is reduced out of proportion to afterload excess (×). Thus intrinsic myocardial dysfunction is a primary cause of the reduced EF and also of a poor outcome.

Carabello BA, Green LH, Grossman W, Cohn LH, Koster JK, Collins JJ Jr. Hemodynamic determinants of prognosis of aortic valve replacement in critical aortic stenosis and advanced congestive heart failure. Circulation 1980;62:42–48.

Aortic stenosis versus pseudo aortic stenosis

Aortic valve area (AVA) is a key index used to judge AS severity. However, at low cardiac output AVA may be underestimated, in turn overestimating AS severity.[23] Aortic valve area is flow dependent, varying directly with cardiac output, especially at outputs of less than 5 L/min. In truly severe AS increasing output causes a concomitant increase in gradient and AVA increases only slightly. However, in pseudo aortic stenosis the AVA is small at baseline, suggesting severe AS, but as output increases (usually with infusion of a positive inotrope such as dobutamine) gradient increases only slightly leading to a large increase in calculated AVA.[24,25] It is likely that increased ventricular force and cardiac output open a mildly but not severely stenotic valve to a greater aperture. Patients with pseudo AS are managed reasonably well with standard HF therapy as opposed to AVR.[26]

Therapy for advanced heart failure in aortic stenosis

AS is a mechanical problem of LV outflow obstruction and the only effective solution to this mechanical obstruction is mechanical relief with AVR. Diuretics can temporarily relieve the symptom of dyspnea. Angiotensin converting enzyme (ACE) inhibitors useful in the therapy of other causes of HF may be used to treat hypertension if present but there is no evidence that these agents effectively treat HF in AS. For patients with a mean transvalvular gradient greater than 40 mmHg, afterload excess is the primary driver in causing reduced EF and in HF. In such patients AVR affords

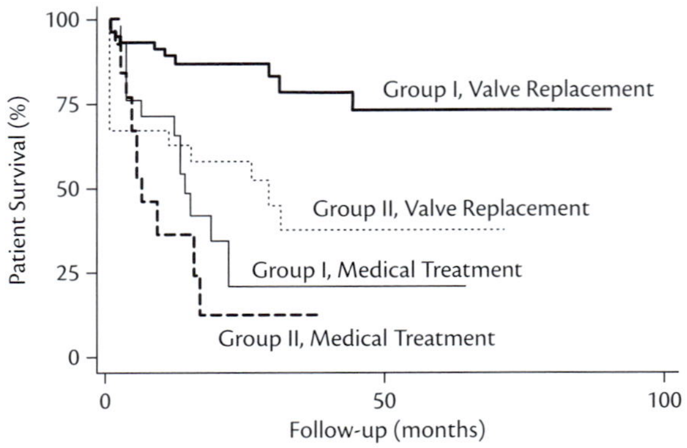

Fig. 12.4 Survival for aortic stenosis patients with advanced left ventricular dysfunction is depicted according to inotropic response and therapy. Group I patients had a positive response to dobutamine infusion with a greater than 20% increase in stroke volume while group II patients failed to have inotropic reserve. The best outcome was seen in a group I patient who underwent aortic valve replacement.

Monin JL, Quere JP, Monchi M, et al. Low-gradient aortic stenosis: operative risk stratification and predictors for long-term outcome: a multicenter study using dobutamine stress hemodynamics. Circulation 2003;108:319–24.

dramatic improvement in EF and in HF.[3] However, the mortality of AVR, which is about 2.5% for the general AS population and less than 1% for asymptomatic patients with normal LV function, ranges from 10 to 40% in the group of patients with low-gradient low EF.[22,27,28,29,30] Patients at the better end of this high mortality range include those with inotropic reserve (Figure 12.4),[30] those able to muster a gradient greater than 20 mmHg, and those without extensive myocardial infarction as the cause of their LV dysfunction.[28] Some low-gradient low-EF patients may benefit from transcatheter valve replacement (TAVR) that avoids the stress of surgery,[31] while some benefit from standard surgical AVR.[27] Which patients are beyond benefit from either form of AVR remains to be elucidated.

Aortic balloon valvotomy (BAV), in which a large balloon is inflated in the aortic orifice, offers temporary partial relief from AS in some low-gradient low-EF patients. Occasionally there is substantial improvement in HF following BAV, in which case the procedure is used as a bridge to definitive AVR.[32]

Low-gradient normal ejection fraction

Some patients with AS have reduced cardiac output (and thus HF) despite also having a normal EF. Such patients have concentric remodeling with increased wall thickness and decreased LV volume and thus a normal EF from a small LV volume yields a reduced stroke volume. If it is clear from valve area and valve morphology that AS is the cause of reduced stroke volume and the patients have symptoms consistent with low output and HF, AVR improves survival over medical therapy.[7,9]

Mitral stenosis

Most cases of mitral stenosis (MS) are caused by rheumatic heart disease. Women are affected about threefold greater than men. In some older patients, mitral annular calcification may significantly restrict the mitral orifice despite fairly normal leaflet motion. As the mitral orifice narrows, a pressure gradient develops between left atrium (LA) and LV, increasing LA pressure (Figure 12.5).[33] Concomitantly MS restricts LV inflow, reducing preload, LV diastolic volume, and cardiac output. The typical patient complains of dyspnea on exertion, orthopnea, and paroxysmal nocturnal dyspnea (PND). In developed nations EF and/or other ejection indexes of cardiac function are reduced in about one-third of patients yet myocardial contractility is usually normal. In such cases increased afterload caused by reflexive vasoconstriction in response to decreased cardiac output together with preload restriction reduce EF despite normal contractility (Figure 12.6).[34] In developing countries where the rheumatic process is more aggressive, myocardial damage may add a "myocardial factor", i.e., myocardial damage in addition to altered loading in causing LV dysfunction.[35] As MS worsens and LA pressure increases, pulmonary pressure (PAP) rises in concert as mean PAP must exceed LA pressure in order for there to be forward blood flow. Pulmonary vasoconstriction adds to PAP and severe pulmonary hypertension may ensue, placing a pressure overload on the RV, and right HF may develop as a result. In addition increased LA pressure in conjunction with the inflammatory changes from the rheumatic process engenders atrial fibrillation (AF). Failure to control the ventricular response in AF reduces LV filling time, further increasing left atrial pressure (LAP) and reducing cardiac output, worsening HF.

As noted earlier, most patients with MS are women and some develop significant stenosis during childbearing age. In patients with MS, HF may develop for the first time during pregnancy or be exacerbated by it. Typically cardiac output increases by about 70% during the second trimester. Since gradient increases by the square of the output, this increase in output would increase a 5 mmHg gradient to about 14 mmHg, potentially leading to pulmonary congestion.

Therapy for heart failure in mitral stenosis

Heart rate control

As heart rate increases diastole is shortened, reducing the time available for transfer of blood across the stenotic mitral orifice. Thus it makes empiric sense to control heart rate especially at the extremes seen in rapid AF. However, most trials of heart rate control either in patients in sinus rhythm or with more modest AF rates have not produced symptomatic improvement.[36,37] In general, agents that control heart rate (β-blockers and rate-controlling calcium channel blockers) are also negative inotropes that tend to reduce cardiac output and increase LV filling pressure, potentially negating the effects of rate control.

Diuretics

Most of the HF symptoms of MS stem from elevated LA pressure resulting from the transmitral pressure gradient. As such diuretics may be useful in controlling modest LA hypertension and the symptoms that accrue from it. Unfortunately transmitral flow is also dependent upon the transmitral gradient so that excessive reduction in filling pressure will also reduce cardiac output, leading to fatigue and prerenal azotemia.

Pulmonary vasodilators

Increased LA pressure leads to increased pulmonary artery (PA) pressure, both passively as more pressure is required from the RV to fill the LV, and actively due to pulmonary vasoconstriction. In some cases of MS the PA pressure is extraordinarily high, leading to right HF and the symptoms of ascites and edema. In addition,

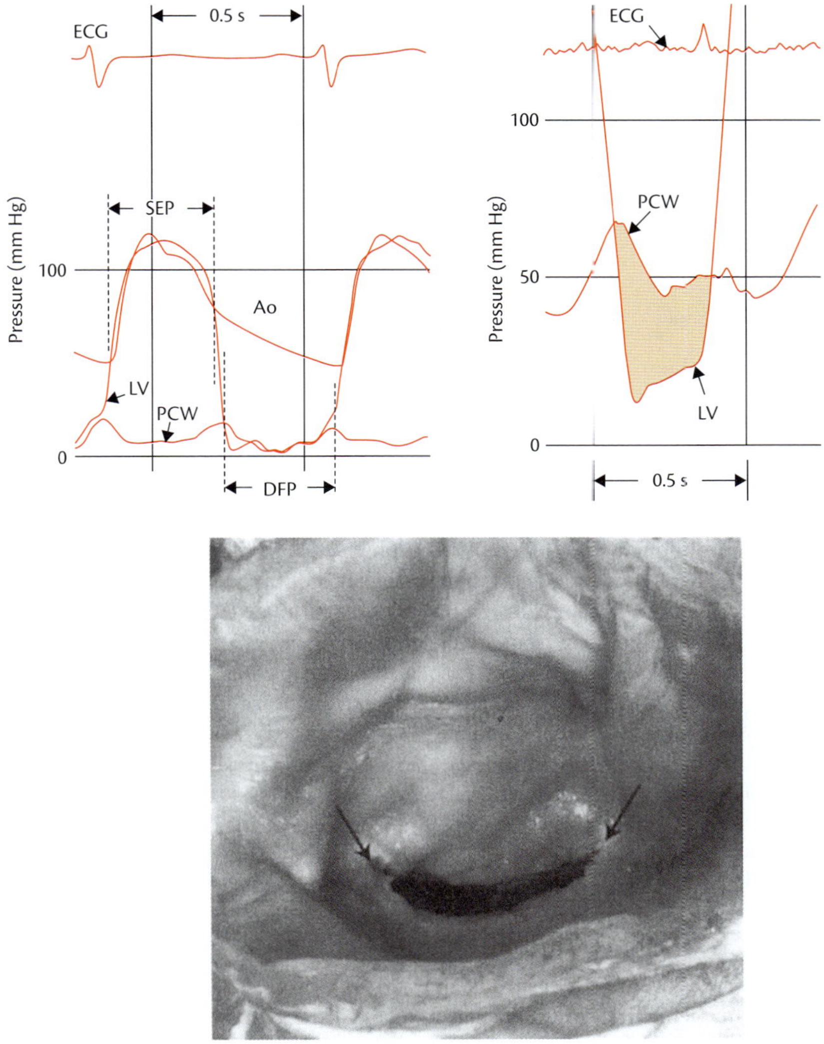

Fig. 12.5 A rheumatic mitral valve (left) and the subsequent pressure tracings characteristic of mitral stenosis (right).
Carabello BA. Mitral Stenosis. In: Hurst's: The Heart, 13th ed, Vol 2., Chapter 78, pp 1738–44. 2011.

during exercise the transmitral gradient and thus the PA pressure increases by the square of the cardiac output generating severe left atrial and pulmonary hypertension. Such high pressures can lead to rupture of dilated bronchial veins causing hemoptysis. It is known that a variety of agents can be used to reduce pulmonary vasoconstriction and thus reduce PAP. These include prostacycline analogs, endothelin antagonists, and phosodiesterase type 5 inhibitors. Whether these agents would be of any value in treating uncorrected MS is unknown. While decreasing pulmonary vasoconstriction might improve right HF, in theory these agents might increase cardiac output, hence increasing the transmitral gradient and, as such, increase the LA pressure leading to pulmonary edema.

Mechanical relief of rheumatic mitral stenosis

MS is a mechanical obstruction to LV inflow and the only effective treatment for HF due to MS is relief of that obstruction. Balloon mitral valvotomy (BMV) is the standard therapy used in most cases of rheumatic MS. Unlike in AS where leaflet motion is restricted by dozens of calcified nodular plaques, rendering BAV only partially effective in increasing orifice area, in MS obstruction comes from leaflet fusion at the valve commissures. Inflation of a large balloon placed into the mitral orifice transseptally fractures the commissural adhesions and restores valve opening.[38,39,40] If valve anatomy is unfavorable for BMV due to heavy calcification, leaflet scarring, or extensive disease of the subvalvular apparatus, mitral valve replacement (MVR) is done instead. Relief of mitral obstruction lowers LA and pulmonary artery pressure and increases cardiac output. Ideally MS should be corrected before more than mild symptoms develop and before more than mild pulmonary hypertension has occurred. However, even if far-advanced left- and or right-sided HF has ensued, most patients respond well to BMV or MVR. After the procedure PAP usually rapidly falls toward normal but occasionally it remains elevated; in this case persistent pulmonary hypertension and right HF can be treated with sildenafil.[41] In cases where there has been myocardial damage and there is HF beyond valvular obstruction, standard therapy for HF due to systolic dysfunction should be employed.

As nonrheumatic populations age, mitral annular calcification (MAC) is becoming a more common cause of MS and a more challenging one to correct. In patients with MAC the valve leaflets are

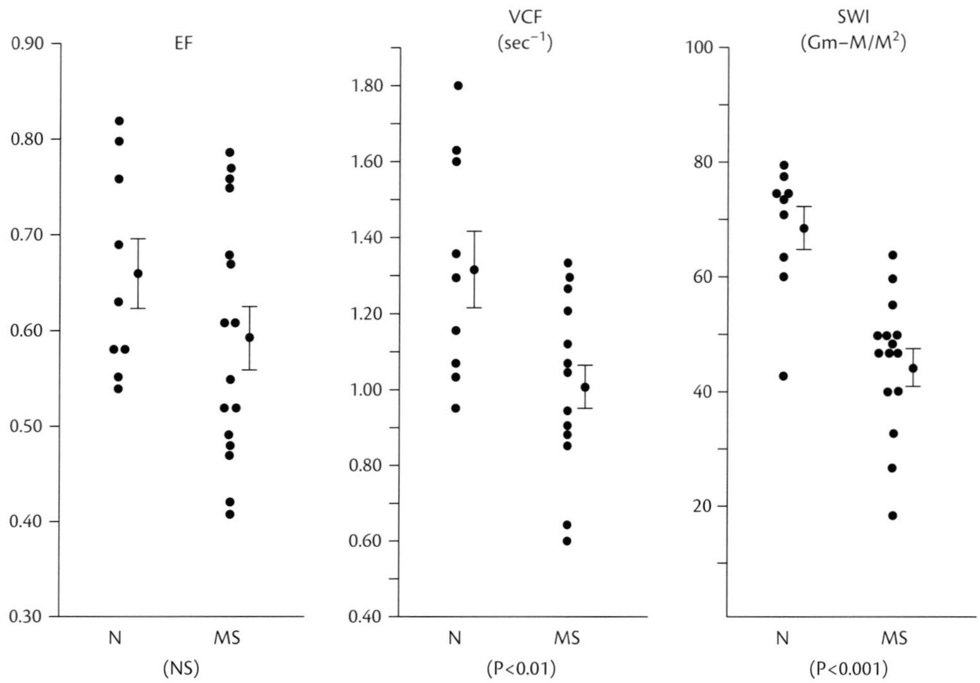

Fig. 12.6 Ejection fraction (EF), mean velocity of circumferential fiber shortening (VCF), and stroke work index (SWI) are shown for normal subjects (N) and those with mitral stenosis (MS). Although MS is viewed as a lesion that "protects" the left ventricle, about one-third of MS patients have reduced ejection performance due to abnormal loading conditions.

Gash AK, Carabello BA, Cepin D, Spann JF. Left ventricular ejection performance and systolic muscle function in patients with mitral stenosis. Circulation 1983 Jan;67(1):148–54.

relatively normal while impingement on the annulus from calcification reduces orifice area. MBV is ineffective in dilating the constricted orifice and MVR requires extensive debridement of the annulus.

Mitral regurgitation

Classification

In addressing mitral regurgitation (MR), primary MR (PMR) must be distinguished from secondary or functional MR (SMR). Primary MR occurs when pathology of one or more of the mitral valve components: the leaflets, the chordae tendineae, the papillary muscles, and/or the mitral annulus cause the valve to leak. When severe, PMR exerts a hemodynamic overload on the LV, eventually causing myocardial damage, HF, and death. Correction of PMR removes the overload and if corrected in a timely manner, allows myocardial repair and a normal lifespan.[42] Conversely SMR is almost an entirely different disease. In SMR the valve itself is usually normal but severe myocardial damage caused by myocardial infarction or idiopathic dilated cardiomyopathy leads to papillary muscle displacement, wall motion abnormalities, and annular dilatation, preventing the valve from coapting. Thus in SMR severe myocardial damage already exists and causes the MR, so it is much less clear that correcting the MR is beneficial to the patient.[43]

Pathophysiology of heart failure in primary mitral regurgitation

Acute primary mitral regurgitation

In severe acute MR, as might occur in chordal rupture, there is a sudden volume overload on the small and unprepared LV and LA. Increased preload from the volume overload and decreased afterload afforded by the extra pathway for LV ejection increase LVEF. However, because more than 50% of total LV stroke volume is ejected backward into the LA, forward stroke volume and cardiac output are reduced (Figure 12.7).[44] Simultaneously the volume overload on the LA increases LA pressure leading to pulmonary congestion. Thus there is HF despite normal LV function. Arterial vasodilators such as sodium nitroprusside may be used to reduce aortic impedance in an effort to increase forward flow while simultaneously decreasing MR.[45] However, the frequent coexistence of hypotension may contraindicate the use of vasodilators in favor of intra-aortic balloon counterpulsation (IAPB).[46] Balloon counterpulsation decreases afterload while supporting mean arterial pressure thereby increasing forward flow while decreasing MR. Most cases of severe acute MR require surgical repair of the mitral valve as definitive therapy.

Chronic primary severe mitral regurgitation

If MR develops gradually over time, severe compensated MR may develop, wherein the patient is asymptomatic, myocardial function is normal, and EF is enhanced (Figure 12.7). Compensation is afforded by enlargement of the LA so that it can accept the regurgitant volume at lower pressure and also by LV eccentric hypertrophy wherein sarcomeres are laid down in series, increasing myocyte length and chamber volume enabling increased total and forward stroke volume.[47] Unlike almost all other LV volume overloads (e.g., aortic regurgitation, complete heart block, anemia) MR is a pure volume overload.[48] In most other volume overloads the extra volume is pumped into the aorta where it increases pulse pressure and systolic blood pressure and thus are actually combined pressure and volume overloads. In MR systolic pressure

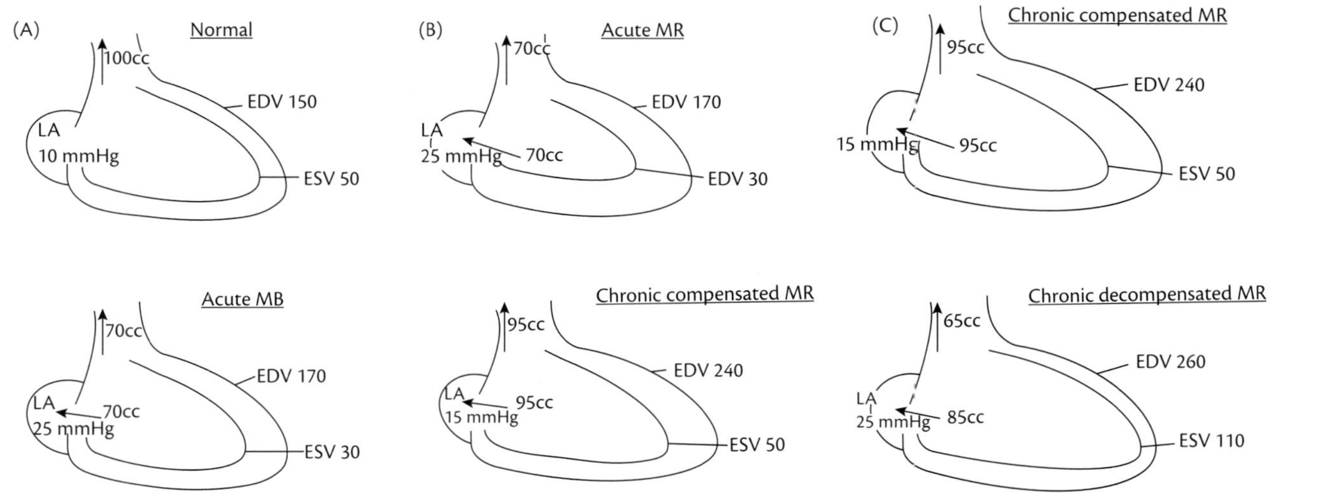

	Preload SL μ	Afterload E$$ Kdyne/cm²	CF	EF	RF	FSV CC's
N	2.07	90	N	−67	0	100
AMR	2.25	60	N	−82	−50	70

	Preload SL μ	Afterload E$$ Kdyne/cm²	CF	EF	RF	FSV CC's
AMR	2.25	60	N	−82	−5	70
CCMH	2.19	90	N	−79	−5	95

	Preload SL μ	Afterload E$$ Kdyne/cm²	CF	EF	RF	FSV CC's
CCMH	2.19	90	N	−79	−50	95
COLOR	2.19	120	↓	−58	−57	65

Fig. 12.7 The pathophysiologic stages of mitral regurgitation (MR). (A) Normal physiology is compared to that of acute MR. The acute volume overload of MR maximizes preload (sarcomere length, SL) and increases end-diastolic volume (EDV) modestly. The extra pathway for ejection into the left atrium (LA) reduces afterload (end-systolic stress, ESS) thereby further enhancing left ventricular (LV) ejection, reducing end-systolic volume (ESV). Contractility is normal (N) or enhanced. These factors act in concert to increase ejection fraction (EF) and total stroke volume. However regurgitation reduces forward stroke volume (FSV). The portion of total stroke volume regurgitated is referred to as the regurgitant fraction (RF). (B) Acute MR is compared to chronic compensated MR. Eccentric cardiac hypertrophy has intervened in chronic compensated MR, increasing EDV and both total and FSV. Increased LV size increases its radius and also ESS, in turn increasing ESV so that EF falls slightly. Note afterload is reduced only in acute MR. Increased LA size accommodates the RF at substantially lower filling pressure. (C) Chronic compensated MR is compared to chronic decompensated MR. In this stage LV contractile dysfunction has ensued causing a large increase in ESV and a fall in stroke volume and EF, although EF may still be maintained in the "normal" range by increased preload. Increased LV radius increases ESS leading to a further decline in LV function and further cardiac dilatation in turn increasing the RF.

Carabello BA: Mitral regurgitation: Basic pathophysiologic principles. Part I. Mod Concepts Cardiovasc Dis 57:53–58, 1988.

tends to low normal and the resultant LV remodeling reflects this, leading to a thin-walled dilated chamber.[49] This chamber geometry facilitates diastolic filling but also tends to increase LV afterload.[50,51,52] It is often held (wrongly) that MR reduces afterload due to the unloading of the LV by the extra-low-impedance pathway for LV ejection into the low pressure LA. While the concept is correct it is offset by the chamber geometry that develops: wall stress $(\sigma) = P \times r / 2th$, as discussed earlier in the chapter. The thin-walled, enlarged LV in MR leads to a large radius/thickness ratio, tending to increase wall stress. While afterload is reduced in acute MR it returns to normal in the chronic phase and actually is excessive in decompensated MR.[52]

The patient with severe MR may remain compensated for several years but, with time, persistent severe volume overload leads to LV dysfunction (see Figure 12.7). Such dysfunction may be heralded by the onset of symptoms but in some patients it is not. It also must be recognized that increased preload in MR may maintain EF in the "normal" range, falsely reassuring the clinician that the myocardium is still healthy. In fact the "normal" EF for the patient with severe MR is around 70% so that by the time it declines to less than 60% (or even 64%) LV damage has ensued.[53,54] Myocardial impairment in MR accrues from loss of contractile elements and also from abnormalities in calcium handling that leads to abnormal excitation-contraction.[55,56] Initially dysfunction appears reversible both by mitral valve repair and also in part by β-adrenergic blockade in animal models of MR and also in human patients (Figure 12.8A and B).[57,58] It is likely that MR leads to reduced forward cardiac output, in turn causing a reflexive increase in damaging catecholamines.[59,60,61] The goal of MR management is to intervene when or before even the mildest of symptoms develop[62,63] and/or before there is evidence of LV and/or RV dysfunction. Yearly examination that includes echocardiography surveils for a change in exercise tolerance and a change in LV function. Surgery is performed when early symptoms develop or when EF approaches 60% or when LV end-systolic dimension approaches 40 mm or if there is evidence that PAP is increasing.[53,54,64,65,66,67]

If the patient presents after these thresholds have been reached, prognosis is reduced but most patients still benefit from surgery. While unproven it is probably advisable for patients to undergo a course of standard HF therapy for 3 months prior to operation to help improve LV function prior to surgery.

Mitral valve repair versus mitral valve replacement

The mitral valve apparatus prevents LV to LA regurgitation during systole but this is only one of its functions. The mitral valve is an integral part of the LV, helps maintain LV shape, and aids in LV contraction.[68,69] Its destruction during MVR impairs LV function and leads to both increased operative and late mortality.[42,70,71,72,73,74,75] It is often believed that the fall in EF that is sometimes observed following mitral surgery is due to increased afterload imposed on the

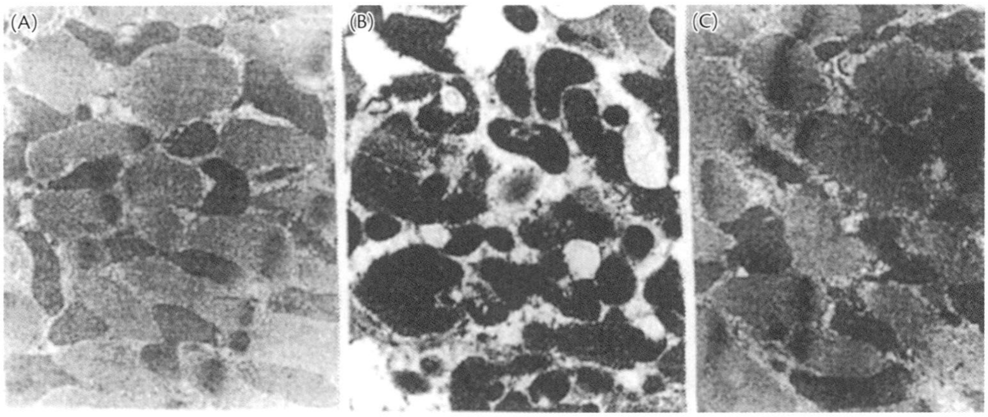

Fig. 12.8 (A) Histopathology of the myocardium from a normal dog (left), a dog with LV dysfunction from chronic MR (middle), and a dog 3 months after correction of the MR (right). During MR there is loss of contractile elements that recovers following surgery. (B) End-systolic elastance (EES) and EES corrected for volume, two measures of LV contractility, are shown before and after surgical correction of MR in patients. In many cases contractility improves, recapitulating the canine histology shown in (A).

(A) Reprinted from Journal of Thoracic Cardiovascular Surgery, 106(6), Spinale FG, Ishihara K, Zile M, DeFryte G, Crawford FA, Carabello BA, Structural basis for changes in left ventricular function and geometry because of chronic mitral regurgitation and after correction of volume overload, 1147–57. Copyright (1993) with permission from Elsevier. (B) Starling MR. Effects of valve surgery on left ventricular contractile function in patients with long-term mitral regurgitation. Circulation 199592(4):811–18.

LV by removal of the low-impedance pathway for ejection into the LA. In fact reduced postoperative EF is more related to destruction of the mitral valve apparatus than changes in load, as evidenced by the large fall in EF when the apparatus is destroyed versus only a small fall in EF when the valve is repaired.[71,72,73,74] If the valve cannot be repaired, replacement in which the native leaflets and their chordal attachments to the papillary muscles are maintained helps support LV function.[74] Thus mitral valve repair is important in avoiding postoperative HF, especially if there is evidence of preoperative LV dysfunction.

HF in PMR is best prevented by performing corrective surgery before symptoms or asymptomatic LV dysfunction has developed and by employing mitral repair instead of MVR. If LV dysfunction has developed mitral valve repair can still be employed with the expectation that HF may persist after surgery albeit improved compared to before surgery. Indeed, with mitral repair there is almost no degree of LV dysfunction that renders the patient inoperable.

Secondary mitral regurgitation

The majority of patients with SMR have advanced LV dysfunction from either myocardial infarction or dilated cardiomyopathy. Occasionally a strategically placed wall motion abnormality causes SMR with preserved EF but in most cases of SMR the EF is depressed. As such the majority of patients with SMR should undergo standard HF therapy with β-blockers, ACE inhibitors or angiotensin receptor blockers (ARBs), and aldosterone antagonists. Conduction abnormalities are common in patients with SMR and frequently contribute to the wall motion abnormalities responsible for SMR. In some cases cardiac resynchronization may dramatically reduce SMR and thus should be considered in SMR patients with widened QRS.[76,77]

Surgery for secondary mitral regurgitation

For PMR the concept is straightforward: MR causes the hemodynamic overload responsible for the eventual poor outcome, and correction of PMR by mitral repair resolves the problem. For SMR the issue is much more complicated. Correction of the MR only resolves the volume overload but does not recover infracted myocardium or reverse dilated cardiomyopathy. While it seems clear that the presence of SMR in HF worsens prognosis,[78,79] it has been difficult to show that surgical correction of SMR improves prognosis or even symptoms in some cases, despite the fact the valve surgery leads to reverse LV remodeling,[43,80,81,82] although a recent report is more encouraging.[83] It may be that while SMR has ill effects on the patient and their LV, the consequences of myocardial disease overwhelm the SMR in importance so that any benefit from MR surgery is not apparent. Further, while mitral repair is clearly the preferred method of correcting PMR, it is not clear if either repair or replacement is superior for treating SMR.[84]

Recently percutaneous approaches to MR have been investigated. One of these (MitraClip) clips the two mitral leaflets together in their mid-portions, reducing MR. The device leads to reverse LV remodeling[85,86,87] and randomized trials are under way examining if it has an effect on mortality in SMR.

Aortic regurgitation

Acute aortic regurgitation

In acute severe aortic regurgitation (AR) as might occur in infective endocarditis there is a sudden volume overload on a small, unprepared LV. Overfilling of the LV increases LV and LA diastolic pressure, leading to pulmonary congestion while forward cardiac output is reduced. Increased LV diastolic pressure may cause preclosure of the mitral valve, protecting the lungs from extremes in increased filling pressure; but preclosure also limits forward flow, reducing cardiac output further. Reduced output and backward diastolic flow into the LV reduce aortic systolic and diastolic pressure (Figure 12.9).[88] Reduced aortic diastolic pressure and increased LV diastolic pressure greatly reduce the gradient across the myocardium necessary to propel coronary blood flow that occurs nearly entirely during diastole. It is likely this combination of events causes myocardial ischemia and leads to a dire outcome when even mild HF complicates acute AR especially when there is echocardiographic evidence of mitral valve preclosure.[89] This

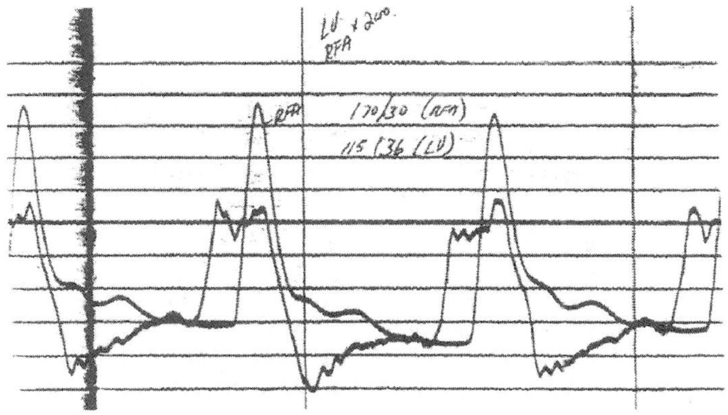

Fig. 12.9 Left ventricular (LV) and femoral artery (RFA) pressure tracings for a patient with acute aortic regurgitation (AR). Rapid equalization of pressures results in little gradient for driving coronary blood flow.

Reprinted from Cardiology Pearls, Carabello BA, Ballard WL, Gazes PC, Hanley & Belfus, Inc., (1994), with permission from Elsevier.

outcome likely is worsened by delay in diagnosis fostered by the subtle nature of the illness especially with regard to the physical examination. The rapid rise in LV pressure together with the rapid decline in aortic pressure reduces the aortic-to-LV gradient driving AR. Thus the murmur of acute AR is often unimpressive and limited to early diastole. Mitral preclosure causes S1 to be soft, so that the physical examination is quietly understated. Gradually increasing heart rate and subtle changes in respiratory rate or even mild dyspnea may presage cardiovascular collapse.

Acute severe AR accompanied by HF is a surgical emergency.[90] While no large randomized trials exist, mortality is about 75% with medical therapy versus about 25% with surgery. Attempts at medical therapy are fraught. Most pressor agents used to maintain blood pressure cause vasoconstriction and worsen AR. Vasodilators used to reduce filling pressure usually worsen hypotension and lower organ perfusion. Fears that a prosthetic valve may become infected are usually unfounded as the infection rate is less than 5% within even 48 hours of the last positive blood culture.[91]

Chronic aortic regurgitation

Pathophysiology

In patients with chronic AR the extra volume needed to compensate that lost to regurgitation is pumped into the aorta where it widens pulse pressure and increases systolic pressure.[48] Thus, unlike MR, AR is a combined volume and pressure overload and the LV in chronic AR remodels accordingly with both increased volume and thickness compared to normal.[92] Unlike MR, patients with compensated AR may remain so for many years.[93] Indeed, the average patient with MR develops an indication for intervention at a rate of 8% per year versus 4% per year for patients with chronic severe AR (Figure 12.10). However, eventually LV dysfunction and HF supervene. LV dysfunction in AR is caused both by afterload excess and also by myocardial damage and impaired contractility.[94,95,96] Although AR is often viewed as a lesion of volume overload (which it is), it is also a lesion that causes excessive afterload.[48,96] The increased systolic LV pressure and large LV radius increase wall stress (afterload) dramatically inhibiting LV ejection. The combined pressure and volume overload also cause myocardial damage characterized by an exuberance of extracellular matrix that replaces contractile elements and impairs contractile function.[94] Because AR is a disease of afterload, it was natural that there were pharmacologic attempts to reduce afterload in an effort to forestall disease progression. However, these efforts have met with highly variable results, so that no firm recommendation can be made about the use of vasodilators in treating chronic severe asymptomatic AR.[97,98] AVR (or occasionally valve repair) is the only effective way to prevent these permanent sequelae from occurring. Valve replacement should be timed before LV dysfunction affects prognosis. This threshold is approached when symptoms develop or when EF falls toward 0.55 or when end-systolic dimension approaches 50–55 mm.[99,100]

Advanced left ventricular dysfunction and heart failure

In cases where surgical correction of AR is delayed and severe LV dysfunction and HF have ensued, prognosis is reduced (Figure 12.11).[101] Standard medical therapy for HF is less straightforward in patients with AR than in other etiologies of HF. β-Blockers are problematic because by slowing heart rate they may increase AR by increasing diastolic length and thus the time period for retrograde flow. However, one recent study suggests safety of β-blocker use in AR patients with HF and relatively rapid heart rates.[102] The use of ACE inhibitors in AR has also been a cause of

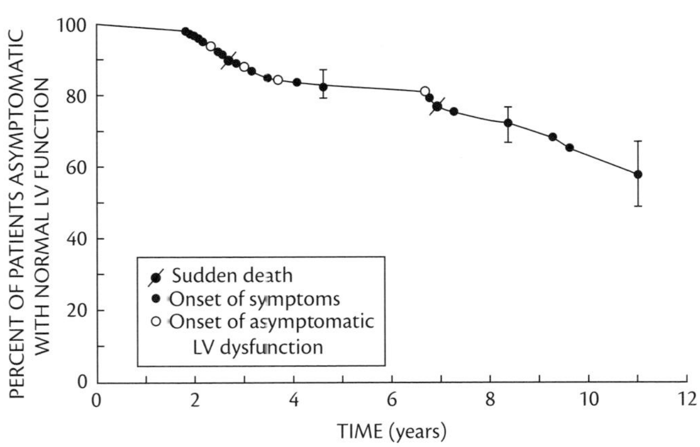

Fig. 12.10 Natural history of patients with severe aortic regurgitation. Endpoints including symptom onset, asymptomatic left ventricular dysfunction, or sudden death are reached slowly, at a rate of about 4% per year.

Bonow RO, Lakatos E, Maron BJ, Epstein SE. Serial long-term assessment of the natural history of asymptomatic patients with chronic aortic regurgitation and normal left ventricular systolic function. Circulation 1991;84(4):1625–35.

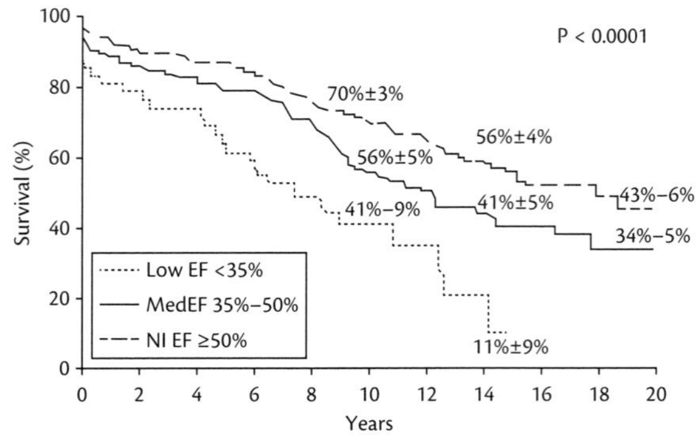

Low (EF <35%)	43	35	31	21	15	8	6	3			
MedEF (35%–50%)	134	115	104	55	78	50	34	30	19	9	2
NI (EF ≥50%)	373	245	238	134	141	112	35	40	32	17	1

Fig. 12.11 Postoperative survival for patients with aortic regurgitation, plotted according to preoperative ejection fraction (EF). As EF declines, prognosis worsens.
Chaliki HP, Mohty D, Avierinos JF, Scott CG, Schaff HV, Tajik AJ, Enriquez-Sarano M. Outcomes after aortic valve replacement in patients with severe aortic regurgitation and markedly reduced left ventricular function. Circulation 2002, 106(21):2687–93.

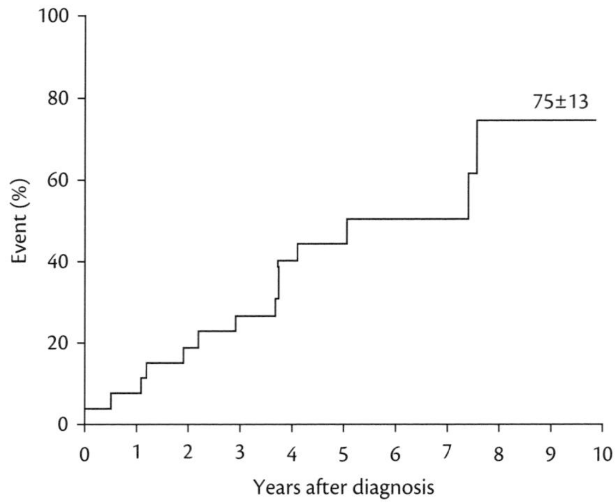

Fig. 12.12 Natural history of primary tricuspid regurgitation.
Reprinted from Journal of Thoracic Cardiovascular Surgery, 128(2), Messika-Zeitoun D et al., Medical and surgical outcome of tricuspid regurgitation caused by flail leaflet, 296–302, copyright (2004) with permission from Elsevier.

concern because by potentially disrupting extracellular matrix they might impair the coupling of myocyte contraction with the myocardial skeleton.[103] However, most studies demonstrate apparent safety of ACE inhibitor administration in AR.[104] Ultimately AVR is the definitive therapy for even decompensated AR, although once EF is depressed outcome is impaired compared to when AVR is done in a timely manner.

Tricuspid regurgitation

Primary tricuspid regurgitation

While most tricuspid regurgitation (TR) is secondary to other lesions that cause either pressure or volume overload on the RV, primary TR does occur rarely. In developed countries blunt chest trauma, often from a motor vehicle accident, damages the tricuspid valve owing to its relatively anterior location. Rheumatic heart disease, carcinoid disease, Ebstein's anomaly, and serotonergic drugs may cause deformity, scarring, and retraction of the tricuspid leaflets and subsequent TR. It is clear that severe TR causes RV volume overload and right-sided HF, eventually impairing survival (Figure 12.12).[105] However there may be a prolonged time period before this impact occurs and severe TR and even tricuspid valve removal in cases of infective endocarditis can be well tolerated at least initially.[106] RV dysfunction may occur in the presence of normal myocyte function[107] because distorted chamber geometry and severe TR increase right-sided filling pressure and reduce cardiac output. Management of primary TR is fraught especially when the underlying cause is incurable as in carcinoid disease. Unlike in MR where objective guidelines exist that trigger surgery, such triggers have not been defined for TR. In patients with advanced symptoms and valve anatomy that lends itself to repair, surgical repair should be performed because mortality following tricuspid valve replacement is quite high, approximately 20% in some series.[108,109] Indications for the choice of valve prosthesis are poorly defined. Many patients with primary TR are younger, militating toward mechanical valve replacement, and yet relatively low tricuspid flow velocity increases the risk of valve thrombosis in the tricuspid position. Further, tricuspid valve replacement in isolation is an uncommon procedure for which there are little outcome data compounding the uncertainty of the best therapy to employ.

Secondary tricuspid regurgitation

Most TR occurs secondary to pressure or volume overload placed upon the RV by other conditions that cause RV dilatation and tricuspid annular enlargement. Because the RV must generate much of the force needed to fill the LV, conditions that increase LV filling pressure overload the RV. Thus right HF and TR often accompany LV systolic and diastolic dysfunction and left-sided valvular heart disease, especially mitral disease. LV enlargement in mitral disease alters septal function thereby impeding RV performance both by mechanical distortion of the septum and also possibly by reducing RV contractility.[110,111] These conditions are often accompanied by pulmonary vasoconstriction, adding to the RV burden. Lung disease that distorts the pulmonary vasculature increases pulmonary vascular resistance and causes RV pressure overload, intensified when hypercapnia caused by advanced lung disease intensifies pulmonary vasoconstriction, worsening RV failure, and TR. Pulmonary vascular disease caused by acute or chronic pulmonary embolism or by primary pulmonary hypertension is an additional cause of pulmonary hypertension and secondary TR.

Right-sided volume overload, as occurs with atrial septal defect and other left-to-right shunts or by pulmonic regurgitation following repair of congenital heart disease, causes RV enlargement and secondary TR.

The basic approach to secondary TR is to improve its primary cause. Thus treatment of LV failure or of severe lung disease acts to reduce RV pressure overload with subsequent improvement of TR. Pulmonary vasodilators may improve symptoms but have not been shown to prolong life.

Tricuspid valve surgery during left-sided valve surgery

It may be reasoned that correction of left-sided valve disease will in turn improve RV function by reducing RV pressure and improving RV septal function. Unfortunately postoperative improvement in TR following left-sided valve surgery is unpredictable, with

TR sometimes worsening instead of improving. It may be that increased left-side cardiac output afforded by improved LV function volume overloads the RV, worsening TR. Failure to address the TR at the time of left-sided surgery is attended by increased mortality especially if a second operation is required to address the TR.[112,113] Therefore it is advisable to address even mild TR surgically at the time of left-sided valve operations.

Pulmonic insufficiency

Pulmonic insufficiency (PI) is the most common cause for reoperation in patients who have had previous surgery to correct congenital heart disease.[114] Postprocedure PI leads to right heart volume overload and RV failure, impacting quality of life and probably reducing survival. Balloon valvotomy for congenital pulmonary stenosis and surgical correction of tetralogy of Fallot (TOF) and failure of RV to PA conduits used in TOF surgery are the most common PI causes. Native valve failure is usually treated by percutaneous implantation of a bioprosthetic valve[115] while conduit failure is treated by a percutaneous valve implantation system.[116]

Summary

Each valvular lesion imposes a unique hemodynamic burden of the LV and/or RV. When these lesions are severe they eventually lead to HF and death if not appropriately corrected, and indeed the goal of therapy is to time mechanical intervention so as to prevent HF. The onset of symptoms presages a downhill course in all valve lesions and thus symptoms are an indication for mechanical valve intervention. In the absence of symptoms, asymptomatic LV dysfunction is a sign of deterioration that also requires mechanical correction; thus close echocardiographic surveillance for LV dysfunction is mandatory in following the patient with valve disease. If HF has already ensued, in most cases standard HF therapy is appropriate, to be followed by mechanical intervention. Mechanical intervention itself is consistently changing as surgical mortality and morbidity constantly improve. The advent of transcatheter techniques for valve replacement and repair already offer less invasive therapy to patients that would have been considered inoperable or at very high risk. It is likely that these techniques will become progressively easier and safer to employ opening the gateway to patients with valvular heart disease who, in the past, would have been relegated to develop HF and to die from it.

References

1. Huber D, Grimm J, Koch R, Krayenbuehl HP. Determinants of ejection performance in aortic stenosis. Circulation 1981;64:126–34.
2. Gunther S, Grossman W. Determinants of ventricular function in pressure-overload hypertrophy in man. Circulation 1979;59:679–88.
3. Carabello BA, Williams H, Gash AK, et al. Hemodynamic predictors of outcome in patients undergoing valve replacement. Circulation 1986;74(6):1309–16.
4. Hess OM, Ritter M, Schneider J, et al. Diastolic stiffness and myocardial structure in aortic valve disease before and after valve replacement. Circulation 1984;69:855–65.
5. Zile MR, Brutsaert DL. New concepts in diastolic dysfunction and diastolic heart failure: part II-causal mechanisms and treatment. Circulation 2002;105:1503–8.
6. Kupari M, Turto H, Lommi J. Left ventricular hypertrophy in aortic valve stenosis: preventive or promotive of systolic dysfunction and heart failure? Eur Heart J 2005;26:1790–96.
7. Hachicha Z, Dumensnil JG, Bogaty P, Pibarot P. Paradoxical low flow, low gradient severe aortic stenosis despite preserved ejection fraction is associated with higher afterload and reduced survival. Circulation 2007;115:2856–64.
8. Dumesnil JG, Pibarot P, Carabello BA. Paradoxical low flow and/or low gradient severe aortic stenosis despite preserved left ventricular ejection fraction: implications for diagnosis and treatment. Eur Heart J 2010;31:281–9.
9. Clavel MA, Dumesnil JG, Capoulade R, et al. Outcome of patients with aortic stenosis, small valve area and low-flow, low-gradient despite preserved left ventricular ejection fraction. J Am Coll Cardiol 2012;60:1259–67.
10. Marcus ML, Doty DB, Hiratzka LF, et al. Decreased coronary reserve: a mechanism for angina pectoris in patients with aortic stenosis and normal coronary arteries. N Engl J Med 1982;307:1362–66.
11. Nakano K, Corin WJ, Spann JF Jr, et al. Abnormal subendocardial blood flow in pressure overload hypertrophy is associated with pacing-induced subendocardial dysfunction. Circ Res 1989;65:1555–64.
12. Kupari M, Eriksson S, Turto H, et al. Leakage of cardiac troponin I in aortic valve stenosis. J Intern Med 2005;258(3):231–7.
13. Rosjo H, Andreassen J, Edvardsen T, Omland T. Prognostic usefulness of circulating high-sensitivity troponin T in aortic stenosis and relation to echocardiographic indexes of cardiac function and anatomy. Am J Cardiol 2011;108:88–91.
14. Ito K, Yan X, Feng X, et al. Transgenic expression of sarcoplasmic reticulum Ca^{2+} ATPase modifies the transition from hypertrophy to early heart failure. Circ Res 2001;89:422–29.
15. Olivetti G, Abbi R, Quaini F, et al. Apoptosis in the failing human heart. N Engl J Med 1997;336:1131–41.
16. Hein S, Arnon E, Kostin S, et al. Progression from compensated hypertrophy to failure in the pressure-overloaded human heart: structural deterioration and compensatory mechanisms. Circulation 2003;107:984–89.
17. Communal C, Singh K, Pimental DR, Colucci WS. Norepinephrine stimulates apoptosis in adult rat ventricular myocytes by activation of the β-adrenergic pathway. Circulation 1998;98:1329–34.
18. Tsutsui H, Oshihara K, Cooper GT. Cytoskeletal role in the contractile dysfunction of hypertrophied myocardium. Science 1993;260:682–87.
19. Weidemann F, Herrmann S, Stork S, et al. Impact of myocardial fibrosis in patients with symptomatic severe aortic stenosis. Circulation 2009;120:577–84.
20. Herrmann S, Stork S, Niemann M, et al. Low-gradient aortic valve stenosis: myocardial fibrosis and its influence on function and outcome. J Am Coll Cardiol 2011;58:402–12.
21. Carabello BA, Green LH, Grossman W, et al. Hemodynamic determinants of prognosis of aortic valve replacement in critical aortic stenosis and advanced congestive heart failure. Circulation 2980;62:42–48.
22. Connolly HM, Oh JK, Schaff HV, et al. Severe aortic stenosis with low transvalvular gradient and severe left ventricular dysfunction: result of aortic valve replacement in 52 patients. Circulation 2000;101:1940–46.
23. Blais C, Burwash JG, Mundigler G, et al. Projected valve area at normal flow rate improves the assessment of stenosis severity in patients with low flow, low-gradient aortic stenosis: the multicenter TOPAS (Truly or Psuedo Severe Aortic Stenosis) study. Circulation 2006;113:711–21.
24. Carabello BA, Ballard WL, Gazes PC, et al. Cardiology Pearls. Philadelphia: Hanley and Belfus; 1994.
25. Nishimura RA, Grantham JA, Connolly HM, et al. Low-output, low-gradient aortic stenosis in patients with depressed left ventricular systolic function: the clinical utility of the dobutamine challenge in the catheterization laboratory. Circulation 2002;106:809–13.
26. Fougeres E, Tribouilloy C, Monchi M, et al. Outcomes of pseudo-severe aortic stenosis under conservative treatment. Eur Heart J 2012;33(19):2426–33.
27. Brogan WC, Grayburn PA, Lange RA, Hillis LD. Prognosis after valve replacement in patients with severe aortic stenosis and a low transvalvular pressure gradient. J Am Coll Cardiol 1993;21:1657–60.

28. Levy F, Laurent M, Monin JL, et al. Aortic valve replacement for low-flow/low gradient aortic stenosis: operative risk stratification and long-term outcome: a European multicenter study. J Am Coll Cardiol 2008;51:1466–72.
29. Tribouilloy C, Levy F, Rusinaru D, et al. Outcome after aortic valve replacement for low-flow/low-gradient aortic stenosis without contractile reserve on dobutamine stress echocardiography. J Am Coll Cardiol 2009;53:1865–73.
30. Monin JL, Quere JP, Monchi M, et al. Low-gradient aortic stenosis: operative risk stratification and predictors for long-term outcome: a multicenter study using dobutamine stress hemodynamics. Circulation 2003;108:319–24.
31. Clavel MA, Webb JG, Rodes-Cabau J, et al. Comparison between transcatheter and surgical prosthetic valve implantation in patients with severe aortic stenosis and reduced left ventricular ejection fraction. Circulation 2010;122:1928–36.
32. Tissot CM, Attias D, Himbert D, et al. Reappraisal of percutaneous aortic balloon valvuloplasty as a preliminary treatment strategy in the transcatheter aortic valve implantation era. Euro Intervention 2011;7(1):49–56.
33. Carabello BA. Mitral stenosis. In: Walash R, Fang J, ed., Hurst's The Heart: Manual of Cardiology, 13th edn, Vol 2, Chapter 78. New York: McGraw-Hill; 2011, pp. 1738–44.
34. Gash AK, Carabello BA, Cepin D, Spann JF. Left ventricular ejection performance and systolic muscle function in patients with mitral stenosis. Circulation 1983;67(1):148–54.
35. Mohan JC, Khalilullah M, Arora R. Left ventricular intrinsic contractility in pure rheumatic mitral stenosis. Am J Cardiol 1989;64:240.
36. Stoll BC, Ashcom TL, Johns JP, et al. Effects of atenolol on rest and exercise hemodynamics in patients with mitral stenosis. Am J Cardiol 1995;75:482–4.
37. Monmeneu Menadas JV, Marin Ortuno F, Reyes Gomis F, et al. Beta-blockade and exercise capacity in patients with mitral stenosis in sinus rhythm. J Heart Valve Dis 2001;11:199–203.
38. Turi ZG, Reyes VP, Raju BS, et al. Percutaneous balloon versus surgical closed commissurotomy for mitral stenosis. A prospective, randomized trial. Circulation 1991;83:1179–85.
39. Reyes VP, Raju BS, Wynne J, et al. Percutaneous balloon valvuloplasty compared with open surgical commissurotomy for mitral stenosis. N Engl J Med 1994;331:961–67.
40. Ben Farhat M, Ayari M, Maatouk F, et al. Percutaneous balloon versus surgical closed and open mitral commissurotomy: seven-year follow-up results of a randomized trial. Circulation 1998;97:245–50.
41. Trachte AL, Lobato EB, Urdaneta F, et al. Oral sildenafil reduces pulmonary hypertension after cardiac surgery. Ann Thorac Surg 2005;79(1):194–7. Discussion 194–7.
42. Enriquez-Sarano M, Schaff HV, Orszulak TA, et al. Valve repair improves the outcome of surgery for mitral regurgitation: a multivariate analysis. Circulation 1995;91(4):1022–8.
43. Benedetto U, Melina G, Roscitano A, et al. Does combined mitral valve surgery improve survival when compared to revascularization alone in patients with ischemic mitral regurgitation? A meta-analysis on 2479 patients. J Cardiovasc Med (Hagerstown) 2009;10(2):109–14.
44. Carabello BA. Mitral regurgitation: Basic pathophysiologic principles. Part I. Mod Concepts Cardiovasc Dis 1988;57:53–8.
45. Yoran C, Yelin EL, Becker RM, et al. Mechanism of reduction of mitral regurgitation with vasodilator therapy. Am J Cardiol 1979;43(4):773–7.
46. Horstkotte D, Schulte HD, Niehues R, et al. Diagnostic and therapeutic considerations in acute, severe mitral regurgitation: experience in 42 consecutive patients entering the intensive care unit with pulmonary edema. J Heart Valve Dis 1993;2(5):512–22.
47. Spinale FG, Ishihara K, Zile M, et al. Structural basis for changes in left ventricular function and geometry because of chronic mitral regurgitation and after correction of volume overload. J Thorac Cardiovasc Surg 1993;106(6):1147–57.
48. Wisenbaugh T, Spann JF, Carabello BA. Differences in myocardial performance and load between patients with similar amounts of chronic aortic versus chronic mitral regurgitation. J Am Coll Cardiol 1984;3:916–23.
49. Carabello BA. The relationship of left ventricular geometry and hypertrophy to left ventricular function in valvular heart disease. J Heart Valve Dis 1995;4(Suppl 2):S132–8;discussion S138–9.
50. Zile MR, Tomita M, Nakano K, et al. Effects of left ventricular volume overload produced by mitral regurgitation on diastolic function. Am J Physiol 1991;261(5 Pt 2):H1471–80.
51. Corin WJ, Murakami T, Monrad ES, et al. Left ventricular passive diastolic properties in chronic mitral regurgitation. Circulation 1991;83(3):797–807.
52. Corin WJ, Monrad ES, Murakami T, et al. The relationship of afterload to ejection performance in chronic mitral regurgitation. Circulation 1987;76:59–67.
53. Enriquez-Sarano M, Tajik AJ, Schaff HV, et al. Echocardiographic prediction of survival after surgical correction of organic mitral regurgitation. Circulation 1994;90:830–7.
54. Tribouilloy C, Rusinaru D, Szymanski C, et al. Predicting left ventricular dysfunction after valve repair for mitral regurgitation due to leaflet prolapse: additive value of left ventricular end-systolic dimension to ejection fraction. Eur J Echocardiogr 2011;12(9):702–10.
55. Urabe Y, Mann DL, Kent RL, et al. Cellular and ventricular contractile dysfunction in experimental canine mitral regurgitation. Circ Res 1992;70(1):131–47.
56. Mulieri LA, Leavitt BJ, Martin BJ, et al. Myocardial force-frequency defect in mitral regurgitation heart failure is reversed by forskolin. Circulation 1993;88(6):2700–4.
57. Nakano K, Swindle MM, Spinale F, et al. Depressed contractile function due to canine mitral regurgitation improves after correction of the volume overload. J Clin Invest 1991;88(2):723.
58. Starling MR. Effects of valve surgery on left ventricular contractile function in patients with long-term mitral regurgitation. Circulation 1995;92(4):811–18.
59. Nagatsu M, Zile MR, Tsutsui H, et al. Native beta-adrenergic support of left ventricular dysfunction in experimental mitral regurgitation normalizes indexes of pump and contractile function. Circulation 1994;89(2):818–26.
60. Mehta RH, Supiano M, Oral H, et al. Relation of systemic sympathetic nervous system activation to echocardiographic left ventricular size and performance and its implications in patients with mitral regurgitation. Am J Cardiol 2000;86(11):1193–7.
61. Tsutsui H, Spinale FG, Nagatsu M, et al. Effects of chronic β-adrenergic blockade on the left ventricular and cardiocyte abnormalities of chronic canine mitral regurgitation. J Clin Invest 1994;93(6):2639–48.
62. Tribouilloy CM, Enriquez-Sarano M, Schaff HV, et al. Impact of preoperative symptoms on survival after surgical correction of organic mitral regurgitation: rationale for optimizing surgical indications. Circulation 1999;99(3):400–5.
63. Gillinov AM, Mihaljevic T, Blackstone EH, et al. Should patients with severe degenerative mitral regurgitation delay surgery until symptoms develop? Ann Thorac Surg;90(2):481–8.
64. Tribouilloy C, Grigioni F, Avierinos JF, et al.; MIDA Investigators. Survival implication of left ventricular end-systolic diameter in mitral regurgitation due to fall leaflets: a long-term follow-up multicenter study. J Am Coll Cardiol 2009;54:1961–68.
65. Bonow RO, Carabello BA, Kanu C, et al.; ACC/AHA Task Force on Practice Guidelines; ACC/AHA 2006 guidelines for the management of patients with valvular heart disease: a report of the American College of Cardiology/American Heart Association Task Force on Practice Guidelines. Circulation 2006;114(5):e84.231.
66. Crawford MD, Souchek J, Oprian CA, et al. Determinants of survival and left ventricular performance after mitral valve replacement: Department of Veterans Affairs Cooperative Study on Valvular Heart Disease. Circulation 1990;81(4):1173–81.
67. Ghoreishi M, Evans CF, DeFillippi CR, et al. Pulmonary hypertension adversely affects short-and long term survival after mitral valve

operation for mitral regurgitation: implications for timing of surgery. J Thorac Cardiovasc Surg 2011;142(6):1439–52.
68. Rushmer RF. Initial phase of ventricular systole: asynchronous contraction. Am J Physiol 1956;184(1):188.
69. Hansen DE, Sarris GE, Niczyporuk MA, et al. Physiologic role of the mitral apparatus in left ventricular regional mechanics, contraction synergy and global systolic performance. J Thorac Cardiovasc Surg 1989;97(4):521–33.
70. Sarris GE, Cahill PD, Hansen DE, et al. Restoration of left ventricular systolic performance after reattachment of the mitral chordate tendineae. The importance of valvular-ventricular interaction. J Thorac Cardiovasc Surg 1988;95(6):969–79.
71. Rozich JD, Carabello BA, Usher BW, et al. Mitral valve replacement with and without chordal preservation in patients with chronic mitral regurgitation: mechanisms for differences in postoperative ejection performance. Circulation 1992;86(6):1718–26.
72. Goldman ME, Mora F, Guarino T, et al. Mitral valvuloplasty is superior to valve replacement for preservation of left ventricular function: an intraoperative two-dimensional echocardiographic study. J Am Coll Cardiol 1987;10(3):568–75.
73. Horskotte D, Schulte HD, Bircks W, Strauer BE. The effect of chordal preservation on late outcomes after mitral replacement: a randomized study. J Heart Valve Dis 1993;2(2):150–8.
74. David TE, Burns RJ, Bacchus CM, Druck MN. Mitral valve replacement for mitral regurgitation with and without preservation of chordate tendineae. J Thorac Cardiovasc Surg 1984;88 (5, Pt 1):718–25.
75. Oline STS risk calculator: Available at: <http://riskcalc.sts.org/STSWebRiskCalc273/de.aspx>.
76. St John Sutton MG, Plappert T, Abraham WT, et al.; Multicenter InSync Randomized Clinical Evaluation (MIRACLE) Study Group. Effect of cardiac resynchronization therapy on left ventricular size and function in chronic heart failure. Circulation 2003;107(15):1985–90.
77. van Bommel RJ, Marsan NA, Delgado V, et al. Cardiac resynchronization therapy as a therapeutic option in patients with moderate-sever functional mitral regurgitation and high operative risk. Circulation 2011;124(8):912–19.
78. Trichon BH, Felker GM, Shaw LK, et al. Relation of frequency and severity of mitral regurgitation to survival among patients with left ventricular systolic dysfunction and heart failure. Am J Cardiol 2003;91(5):538–43.
79. Rossi A, Dini FL, Faggiano P, et al. Independent prognostic value of functional mitral regurgitation in patients with heart failure. A quantitative analysis of 1256 patients with ischemic and non-ischemic dilated cardiomyopathy. Heart 2011;97(20):1675–80.
80. Fattouch K, Guccione F, Sampognaro S, et al. Efficacy of adding mitral valve restrictive annuloplasty to coronary artery bypass grafting in patients with moderate ischemic mitral valve regurgitation: a randomized trial. J Thorac Cardiovasc Surg 2009;138(2):278–85.
81. Milhaljevic T, Lam BK, Rajeswaran JK, et al. Impact of mitral valve annuloplasty combined with revascularization in patients with functional ischemic mitral regurgitation. J Am Coll Cardiol 2007;49(22):2191–201.
82. Wu AH, Aaronson KD, Bolling SF, et al. Impact of mitral valve annuloplasty on mortality risk in patients with mitral regurgitation and left ventricle systolic dysfunction. J Am Coll Cardiol 2005;45(3):381–7.
83. Deja MA, Grayburn PA, Sun B, et al. Influence of mitral regurgitation repair on survival in the surgical treatment for ischemic heart failure trial. Circulation 2012;125(21):2639–48.
84. Cohn LH, Rizzo RJ, Adams DH, et al. The effect of pathophysiology on the surgical treatment of ischemic mitral regurgitation: operative and late risks of repair versus replacement. Eur J Cardiothorac Surg 1995;9(10):568–74.
85. Pleger ST, Schulz-Schonhagen M, Geis N, et al. One year clinical efficacy and reverse cardiac remodeling in patients with severe mitral regurgitation and reduced ejection fraction after MitraClip implantation. Eur J Heart Fail 2013;15(8):919–27.
86. Whitlow PL, Feldman T, Pedersen WR, et al.; EVEREST II Investigators. Acute and 12-month results with catheter-based mitral valve leaflet repair: the EVEREST II (Endovascular Valve Edge-to-Edge Repair) High Risk Study. J Am Coll Cardiol 2012;59(2):130–9.
87. Rudolph V, Lubos E, Schluter M, et al. Aetiology of mitral regurgitation differentially affects 2-year adverse outcomes after MitraClip therapy in high-risk patients. Eur J Heart Fail 2013;15(7):796–807.
88. Carabello BA, Ballard WL, Gazes PC. Cardiology Pearls. Philadelphia: Hanley & Belfus; 1994.
89. Sareli P, Klein HO, Schamroth CL, et al. Contribution of echocardiography and immediate surgery to the management of severe aortic regurgitation from active infective endocarditis. Am J Cardiol 1986;57(6):413–18.
90. Mokadam NA, Stout KK, Verrier ED. Management of acute regurgitation in left-sided cardiac valves. Tex Heart Inst J 2011;38(1):9–19.
91. al Jubair K, al Fagih MR, Ashmeg A, et al. Cardiac operations during active endocarditis. J Thorac Cardiovasc Surg 1992;104:487–490.
92. Feiring AJ, Rumberger JA. Ultrafast computer tomography analysis of regional radius-to-wall thickness ratios in normal and volume-overloaded human left ventricle. Circulation 1992;85(4):1423–32.
93. Bonow RO, Lakatos E, Maron BJ, Epsstein SE. Serial long-term assessment of the natural history of asymptomatic patients with chronic aortic regurgitation and normal left ventricular systolic function. Circulation 1991;84(4):1625–35.
94. Schwarz F, Flameng W, Schaper J, et al. Myocardial structure and function in patients with aortic valve disease and their relation to postoperative results. Am J Cardiol 1978;41(4):661–9.
95. Krayenbuehl HP, Hess OM, Monrad ES, et al. Left ventricle myocardial structure in aortic valve disease before, intermediate, and late after aortic valve replacement. Circulation 1989;79(4):744–55.
96. Taniguchi K, Nakano S, Kawashima Y, et al. Left ventricular ejection performance, wall stress, and contractile state in aortic regurgitation before and after aortic valve replacement. Circulation 1990;82:798–807.
97. Scognamiglio R, Rahimtoola SH, Faoli G, et al. Nifedipine in asymptomatic patients with severe aortic regurgitation and normal left ventricular function. N Engl J Med 1994;331:689–94.
98. Evangelista A, Tornos P, Samola A, et al. Long-term vasodilator therapy in patients with severe aortic regurgitation. N Engl J Med 2005;353:1342–9.
99. Henry WL, Bonow RO, Borer JS, et al. Observations on the optimum time for operative intervention for aortic regurgitation. I. Evaluation of the results of aortic valve replacement in symptomatic patients. Circulation 1980;61(3):471–83.
100. Klodas E, Enriquez-Sarano M, Tajik AJ, et al. Surgery for aortic regurgitation in women: contrasting indications and outcomes compared with men. Circulation 1996;94:2472–8.
101. Chaliki HP, Mohty D, Avierinos JF, et al. Outcomes after aortic valve replacement in patients with severe aortic regurgitation and markedly reduced left ventricular function. Circulation 2002;106(21):2687–93.
102. Sampat U, Varadarajan P, Turk R, et al. Effect of beta-blocker therapy on survival in patients with severe aortic regurgitation. J Am Coll Cardiol 2009;54(5):452–7.
103. Supino PG, Borer JS, Herrold EM, et al. Prognostic impact of systolic hypertension on asymptomatic patients with chronic severe aortic regurgitation and initially normal left ventricular performance at rest. Am J Cardiol;96(7):964–70.
104. Elder DH, Wei L, Szwejkowski BR, et al. The impact of renin-angiotensin-aldosterone system blockade on heart failure outcomes and mortality in patients identified to have aortic regurgitation: a large population cohort study. J Am Coll Cardiol 2011;58(20):2084–91.
105. Messika-Zeitoun D, Thomson H, Bellamy M, et al. Medical and surgical outcome of tricuspid regurgitation caused by flail leaflets. J Thorac Cardiovasc Surg 2004;128(2):296–302.

106. Arbulu A, Asfaw I. Management of infective endocarditis: seventeen years' experience. Ann Thorac Surg 1987;43(2):144–9.
107. Ishibashi Y, Rembert JC, Carabello BA, et al.Normal myocardial function in severe right ventricular volume overload hypertrophy. Am J Physiol Heart Circ Physiol 2001;280(1):H11–16.
108. Chang BC, Lim SH, Yi G, et al. Long-term clinical results of tricuspid valve replacement. Ann Thorac Surg 2006;81(4):1317–23, discussion 1323–4.
109. Filsoufi F, Anyanwu AC, Salzberg SP, et al. Long-term outcomes of tricuspid valve replacement in the current era. Ann Thorac Surg 2005;80:845–50.
110. Le Tourneau T, Deswarte G, Lablin N, et al. Right ventricular systolic function in organic mitral regurgitation: impact of biventricular impairment. Circulation 2013;127:1597–608.
111. Carabello BA. The myocardium in mitral regurgitation: a tale of 2 ventricles. Circulation 2013;127(15):1567–8.
112. Nath J, Foster E, Heidenreich PA. Impact of tricuspid regurgitation on long-term survival. J Am Coll Cardiol 2004;43(3):405–9.
113. Shiran A, Sagie A. Tricuspid regurgitation in mitral valve disease incidence, prognostic implications, mechanism, and management. J Am Coll Cardiol 2009;53(5):401–8.
114. Giamberti, A, Chessa M, Abella R, et al. Morbidity and mortality risk factors in adults with congenital heart disease undergoing cardiac reoperation. Ann Thorac Surg 2009;88:1284–9.
115. Giamberti A, Chessa M, Reali M, et al. Porcine bioprosthetic valve in the pulmonary position: mid-term results in the right ventricular outflow tract reconstruction. Pediatr Cardiol 2013;34:1190–3.
116. Butera G, Milanesi O, Spandoni I, et al. Melody transcatheter pulmonary valve implantation. Results from the registry of the Italian society of pediatric cardiology. Catheter Cardiovasc Interv 2013;81(2):310–16.

CHAPTER 13

High-risk heart failure surgery: Strategies for coronary artery bypass grafting and valve surgery in patients with reduced ejection fraction

Marzia Leacche MD, Garrick C. Stewart MD, and John G. Byrne MD

Introduction

Heart failure (HF) is a progressive disease marked by continuous remodeling of the ventricle in the wake of insults such as coronary artery disease (CAD) or valvular abnormalities. Medical therapies have been proven in randomized trials to reduce the risk of death from systolic HF, yet the prevalence of patients with refractory symptoms is on the rise. For patients with severely reduced systolic function, mechanical circulatory support devices have been developed but remain expensive and have a high incidence of adverse events. Meanwhile cardiac transplantation remains reserved for highly select patients with few comorbidities. These advanced therapies are insufficient to meet the needs of most patients with severe ventricular dysfunction.

HF surgery has a central role in the treatment of patients with refractory symptoms. When thoughtfully deployed, surgery can halt or even reverse the deleterious effects of pathological remodeling. Optimal management of chronic HF combines surgical and medical expertise in a multidisciplinary team approach. Successful surgery in patients with reduced left ventricular (LV) function relies on careful patient selection, thoughtful use of noninvasive imaging, and application of pioneering operative techniques. This chapter explores strategies for coronary revascularization in ischemic heart disease and surgery for left-sided valvular lesions in high-risk patients with HF.

Coronary artery disease and heart failure

The prevalence of CAD continues to increase, even as survival has improved dramatically after the initial presentation.[1] Breakthroughs in medical and percutaneous therapies have transformed CAD from an acute, often fatal, condition to one marked by chronic, debilitating symptoms frequently accompanied by impaired contractile function.[2] CAD is now recognized as the most important risk factor for the development of HF.[3] Ischemic cardiomyopathy has worse outcomes than many other forms of HF, in part due to the presence of comorbid conditions.[4] The high mortality rates of patients with ischemic HF coupled with a poor quality of life and frequent hospitalizations have stimulated efforts to identify patients with ischemic cardiomyopathy who may have reversible myocardial dysfunction.

Mechanisms of contractile dysfunction in the setting of CAD are heterogeneous. After myocardial infarction, fibrosis and loss of functional myocardium can lead to neurohormonal activation and ventricular remodeling of the remaining noninfarcted myocardium.[5] Survivors of infarction frequently have significant stenoses in coronaries outside the infarct-related arteries, thus jeopardizing myocardium that may be supplied by a stenotic vessel.[6] Residual CAD can also produce acute or chronic episodes of ischemia contributing to further deterioration of myocardium function, recurrent infarct, or sudden death. Chronic ischemia can contribute to progressive ventricular dysfunction due to apoptosis even in the absence of a clear acute ischemic event or myonecrosis.[7] Episodes of transient ischemia can lead to myocardial stunning that persists even after the ischemic insult has resolved, while recurrent episodes can produce significant myocardial dysfunction. Myocardial contractile elements may also undergo programmed disassembly in response to repeated bouts of reversible ischemia in chronic CAD, producing a condition known as myocardial hibernation.[8] Long-term prognosis is determined by the angiographic extent and severity of CAD, leading to interest in revascularizing patients with LV systolic dysfunction.[9]

Up to half of patients with CAD and reduced ejection fraction (EF) have significant areas of dysfunctional but viable myocardium (Figure 13.1).[10] Regions of viable hibernating tissue can be identified by noninvasive imaging techniques. The different imaging modalities can evaluate perfusion and cell membrane integrity

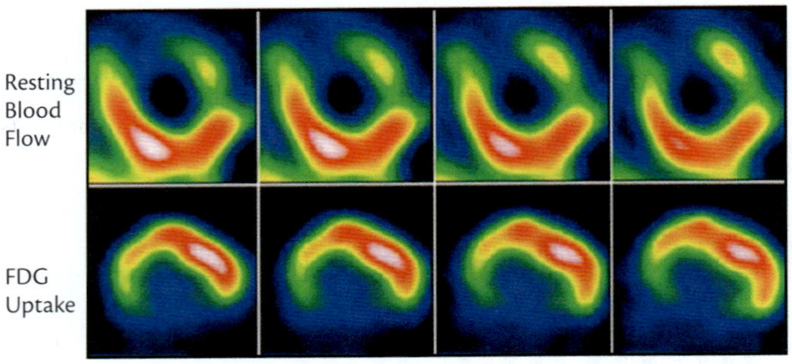

Fig. 13.1 Midventricular short axis images of resting blood flow (upper panel) and fluorodeoxyglucose (FDG) uptake on positron emission tomography (PET) (lower panel) in a patient with recent LAD occlusion and LV dysfunction. There is extensive reduction in resting blood flow in the anterior wall with enhanced FDG uptake (flow/metabolism mismatch). Data has emerged to suggest greater survival benefit as the degree of FDG PET mismatch increases, corresponding to regions of hibernating myocardium. The patient had improvement in ventricular function following CABG.

Allman KC. Journal of Nuclear Cardiology (2013) 20(4):621, Springer.

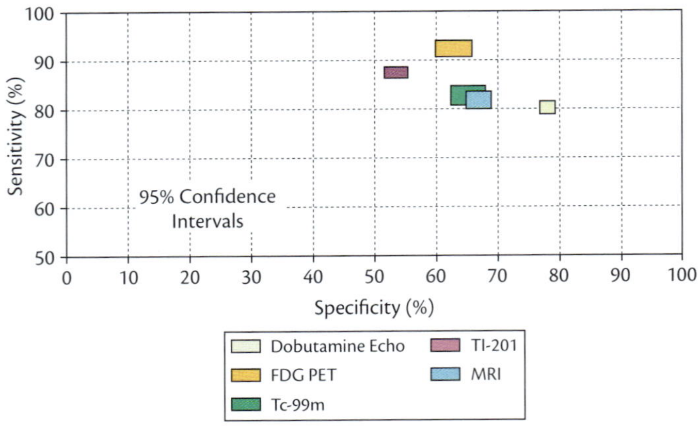

Fig. 13.2 Comparison of sensitivities and specificities (with 95% confidence intervals) of the various forms of viability testing used to predict recovery of regional myocardial function after revascularization. FDG, fluorodeoxyglucose; MRI, magnetic resonance imaging; PET, positron emission tomography; Tc, technetium, Tl, thallium.

Reprinted from Current Problems in Cardiology, 32, Schinkel et al., Hibernating Myocardium: Diagnosis and Patient Outcomes, 375–410, copyright (2007) with permission from Elsevier.

(thallium-201, technetium-99-sestamibi, and tetrofosmin), metabolic activity (^{18}F-FDG positron emission tomography [PET], ^{11}C-acetate), contractile reserve (dobutamine stress echocardiography), or the extent of infarcted myocardium (cardiac MRI). The diagnostic accuracy of cardiac magnetic resonance (CMR) can be enhanced by integrating end-diastolic wall thickness, low-dose dobutamine infusion, and delayed gadolinium contrast enhancement.[11] Selection of an appropriate viability modality is often guided by local availability and expertise (Figure 13.2). When there is moderate LV dysfunction (EF 30–50%), the available data clearly demonstrates the clinical utility of the imaging modalities listed above.[12] However, when there is more severe LV dysfunction (EF <30%) with dilatation, then PET scanning and CMR are more advantageous. There is even interest in combining the high sensitivity of PET with the high specificity of CMR to guide management of patients with indeterminate degrees of scarring and viability.[13] Moreover, the integrated noninvasive assessment of myocardial viability in tandem with stress perfusion imaging can identify normal, scarred, viable, or ischemic myocardium, providing incremental prognostic information for patients with suspected CAD.[14]

Coronary artery bypass surgery

Triage to coronary artery bypass surgery

Widespread use of viability testing in the 1990s led to data suggesting that outcomes after coronary revascularization depend on the predominant state of the dysfunctional heart muscle. Large areas of viable myocardium identify patients most likely to have a survival benefit from coronary revascularization.[15] In a meta-analysis of 2088 patients, among patients with viable myocardium, there was an 80% reduction in the annual cardiac death rate with revascularization compared to medical therapy.[15] The seminal studies of coronary artery bypass grafting (CABG) surgery compared to medical therapy demonstrated greater benefit of CABG in patients with mild-to-moderate LV dysfunction.[16,17,18,19] However, each of these trials excluded patients with severely reduced EF (<35%) since they were felt to be too high risk for surgery. In the subsequent decades, contemporary medical therapy for systolic HF has improved dramatically such that the incremental benefits of surgical intervention may be attenuated. Uncertainty arose about what to do in patients with both CAD and HF and led to the development of the Surgical Treatment for Ischemic Heart Failure (STICH) trial. STICH randomized 1212 patients to medical therapy alone or medical therapy plus CABG.[20] Participants had a LVEFlerss than 35% and CAD amenable to CABG surgery. Patients with left main stenosis greater than 50% were excluded, as were patients with Canadian Cardiovascular Society Class III or IV angina.

Recipients of contemporary medical therapy in STICH had an all-cause mortality that was similar to those patients randomized to CABG. CABG did, however, reduce the rates of cardiovascular death (relative risk reduction 19%) and cardiovascular hospitalization or death from any cause (relative risk reduction 26%) (Figure 13.3). During the trial, 11% of the patients randomized to medical therapy underwent CABG surgery and 9% of patients randomized for surgery received medical therapy alone.[21] Patients assigned to medical management who then underwent CABG surgery had lower 5-year mortality than those who received medicines alone (25% vs.42%), while those assigned to CABG who crossed over to medical therapy alone had higher 5-year mortality compared to those treated with CABG per protocol (59% vs. 33%). Clinician judgment still plays an important role in triage to CABG over medical therapy.

The primary outcome of STICH—that CABG added to medical therapy for ischemic cardiomyopathy failed to reduce all-cause mortality—must be interpreted in the light of several important limitations. Testing for the extent and degree of myocardial ischemia was not part of the entry criteria. The presence and magnitude of inducible myocardial ischemia has been consistently shown to predict future cardiovascular events as well as benefit from revascularization.[22] Patients with moderate or severe angina were also excluded as most clinicians believe there is at a minimum a quality of life, if not survival, benefit in such patients undergoing revascularization. Given the slow enrollment in STICH (two participants per site per year), it has been suggested that trial participants did not reflect usual practice with HF patients demonstrating

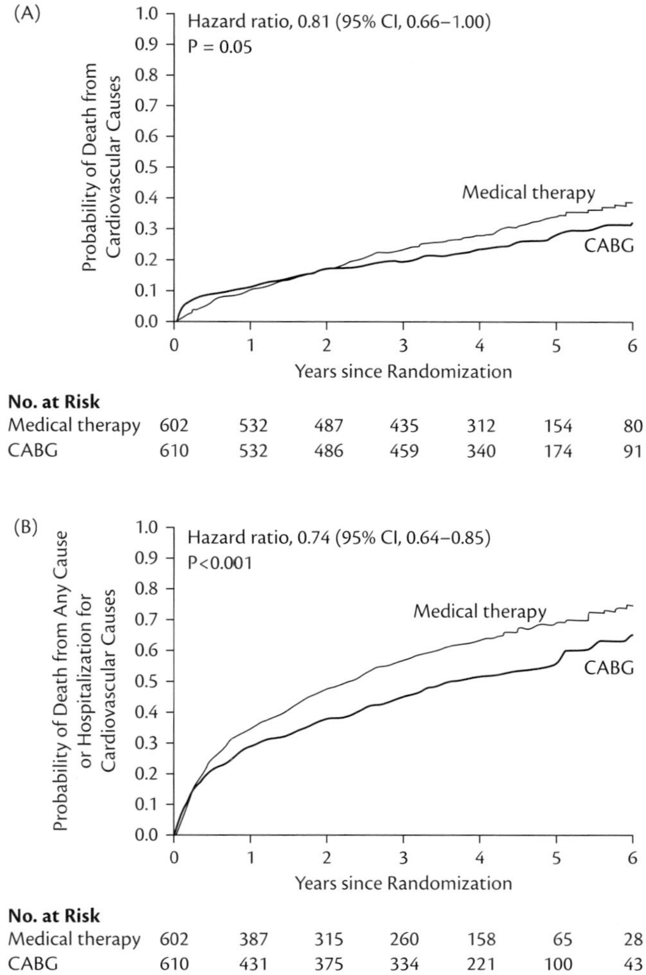

Fig. 13.3 Results from the Surgical Treatment for Ischemic Heart Failure (STICH) trial, which randomized 1212 patients to medical therapy alone or medical therapy plus coronary artery bypass grafting (CABG). Kaplan–Meier curves for the probability of death from cardiovascular causes (A) and death from any cause or hospitalization from cardiovascular causes (B).

From New England Journal of Medicine, Velasquez EJ, et al, Coronary-Artery Bypass Surgery in Patients with Left Ventricular Dysfunction, 364:1607–16, copyright © (2011) Massachusetts Medical Society. Reprinted with permission from Massachusetts Medical Society.

angina or reversible ischemia being triaged to revascularization before study entry. Moreover, it was hard to quantify how many viable territories each patients had as well as the quality of the targets. Both the inability to achieve complete anatomic revascularization and stress-induced ischemia after bypass surgery have been linked to an increased risk of death after CABG.

The impact of myocardial viability on outcomes after medical or surgical therapy was further evaluated in a substudy of STICH, the first study in which prerandomization viability test results did not influence the choice of subsequent treatment. Among the 601 (49.6%) of STICH participants with viability testing, mortality was significantly reduced in patients with viable compared to nonviable myocardium (37% vs. 51%, p = 0.003) over a median follow-up of 5.1 years.[23] Following on the primary STICH trial results which were negative for survival in CABG versus medical therapy, the presence of myocardial viability also failed to impact all-cause mortality after adjustment for other baseline variables. Myocardial viability indicated the likelihood of improved outcomes with either surgical or medical therapy, but did not identify patients with greater survival benefit from revascularization(Figure 13.4A).[23]

Revascularization is still the treatment of choice for patients with LVEF less than 35% and multivessel coronary disease when there is (1) left main disease or left main equivalent, (2) significant angina and/or inducible ischemia, (3) anterior wall viability, and (4) suitable grafting targets (Figure 13.4B).[24,25] The left internal mammary artery (LIMA) to left anterior descending (LAD) is the only graft that makes a difference in long-term survival.[26,27] This graft has superior long-term patency and confers the survival benefit observed in CABG patients. The LIMA to LAD has a patency rate of 90% at 10 years versus about 50% for saphenous vein grafts.[28,29] While patients with multivessel CAD benefit from a LIMA-LAD graft, surgical revascularization with conduits other than LIMA are less clear. Indeed, there is a high risk of early saphenous vein graft failure (6–30% at 12 months).[29,30] The superiority of the LIMA graft is also reflected in the lack of survival benefit in reoperative CABG surgery when the LIMA is already patent.[31] Whether non-LAD vessels should be grafted or stented needs to be determined. Further bypass surgery should not be offered to a patient who already had CABG surgery with an existing patent LIMA to the LAD. Alternatively, there should be consideration of redo CABG in a patient who has had only a saphenous vein graft to the LAD with a jeopardized blood supply to the anterior wall.[32] Multivessel percutaneous coronary interventions (PCI) may also be considered as an alternative in high-risk surgical patients who are expected to benefit from revascularization, though PCI is more often used for anginal relief rather than recovery of myocardial function.

In general, a greater number of viable myocardial segments translates into a greater likelihood of benefit from surgical revascularization.[33] In particular, the presence of extensive viability and/or ischemia may bolster the recommendation for surgical revascularization even in patients with a significant burden of extracardiac comorbidities. If ischemia is not present, viability alone should not trigger immediate revascularization until other concurrent causes of ventricular dysfunction (e.g., heavy alcohol use, tachycardia-mediated cardiomyopathy) are ruled out by careful history and physical examination.[34] Finally, the issue of how to evaluate the quality of the bypass targets remains controversial. In general small, heavily calcified vessels will not have the same run-off as a large-caliber noncalcified vessel. An individual approach to correlating viability testing to coronary angiography is required to determine if there is sufficient viable myocardium supplied by stenotic vessels with good distal bypass targets in order to develop a road map for targeted revascularization. If no viability or angina is present, there is no role for revascularization to treat systolic HF.

Preoperative considerations for high-risk CABG

Even though a high relative risk exists for patients with EF less than 35% triaged to CABG, for appropriately selected patients surgery can still be the preferred therapeutic strategy provided it is performed in an experienced center using a multidisciplinary team approach. Once a patient with HF and CAD has demonstrated appropriate myocardial viability and suitable bypass targets, an integrated preoperative risk assessment is mandatory. This should include care adjudication of extracardiac comorbid conditions as well as cardiac factors contributing to surgical risk. The Society of

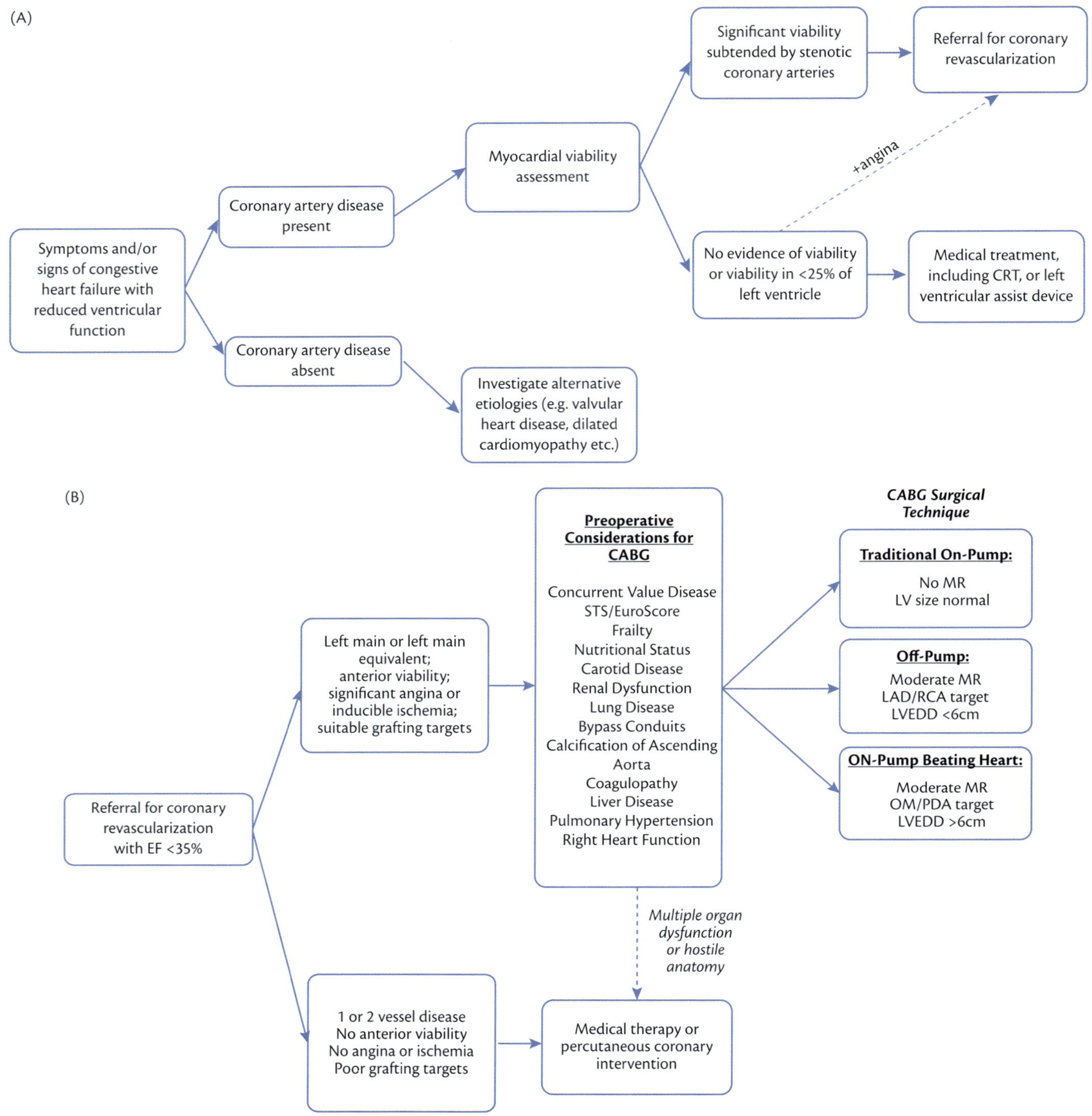

Fig. 13.4 (A) Algorithm for selecting appropriate coronary revascularization candidates with symptomatic heart failure and reduced ejection. (B) Integrative preoperative assessment of patients referred for coronary artery bypass grafting with reduced ejection fraction. EF, ejection fraction; LAD, left anterior descending; LV, left ventricle; LVEDD, left ventricular end-diastolic dimension; MR, mitral regurgitation; OM, obtuse marginal; PDA, posterior descending artery; RCA, right coronary artery; STS, Society of Thoracic Surgeons.

(A) Modified from Camici et al,. Contemporary Reviews in Cardiovascular Medicine Stunning, Hibernation, and Assessment of Myocardial Viability, Circulation, 117, 103–114.

Thoracic Surgeons (STS) Score and European System for Cardiac Operative Risk Evaluation (EuroSCORE) are the two most widely used risk stratification algorithms and may be employed to assess operative risk and guide discussion with patients and their families.[35,36] The presence of ventricular dysfunction and clinical HF are among the most important independent predictors of 30-day post-CABG mortality in both scoring systems. The following sections outline special preoperative considerations, many of which are excluded from current risk scores yet play a critical role in high-risk patient selection and management.

Frailty

Frailty assessment offers a powerful way to integrate the myriad subclinical physiologic insults across multiple organ systems that lead to a heightened vulnerability to stress. It may be particularly relevant for elderly patients and those undergoing cardiac surgery.[37] Commonly used bedside tools to assess frailty, which is mainly manifest as sarcopenia, include a simple handshake (grip strength) to seeing how fast the patient can walk (gait speed), or simply an "eyeball test".[38] Frailty as measured by gait speed has been shown to be an incremental predictor beyond STS score of morbidity and mortality in elderly patients undergoing cardiac surgery.[39] Since frailty manifests clinically as a deficit in functional capacity, it can be challenging to assess in patients with ischemic cardiomyopathy since HF patients may have a reduction in gait speed and strength. In general, patients with cognitive impairment, slow gait, and poor ambulation or who require assistance to complete basic daily tasks will do poorly with cardiac surgery.[40]

Nutritional status

Another important concept linked to frailty is nutrition status. Cardiac cachexia has been consistently associated with increased mortality in HF.[41] Low body mass index, recent unintentional weight loss, and hypoalbuminemia increase the risk for adverse events after surgery due to poor malnutrition status.[42] Patients should have comprehensive assessment of their nutritional status in advance of surgery, including assessment of caloric needs. Those patients exhibiting significant malnourishment should be considered for supplemental enteric feeding if surgery can be delayed long enough to bolster nutritional status.

Carotid disease

Severe extracranial carotid artery disease increases the risk of adverse neurologic outcomes after cardiac surgery. While carotid endarterectomy (CEA) has been shown to have favorable outcomes, the combination of CEA and CABG surgery increases the overall patient risk. The optimal surgical approach and timing of correcting concomitant carotid disease and CAD is still debatable. In the past few years, carotid stenting (CAS) has emerged as an effective alternative treatment to CEA. A recent meta-analysis of eight trials comparing CAS and CEA has shown that CEA and carotid stenting have equivalent risk of stroke or death.[43] In a cardiac population both carotid stenting and CEA have shown comparable adverse events (death, stroke, or myocardial infarction) equivalent results.[44] In order to minimize the overall length of the operation, carotid stenting is preferred over combined cardiac surgery and carotid endarterectomy. Carotid stenting can be performed without general anesthesia in the vascular or catheterization laboratory, so that potential neurologic changes can be monitored immediately. The patient usually is loaded with clopidogrel and will require it for 1 month, often precluding immediate CABG. If surgery is more urgent, the patient should be monitored in the intensive care unit (ICU) for at least 2 days after carotid stenting since vagal hypotension can sometimes occur after resolution of carotid stenosis.

Renal dysfunction

Renal impairment has been consistently shown to be an adverse prognostic marker in patients undergoing revascularization of viable myocardium.[45,46] It is not known how best to balance remaining kidney function with the degree of viability in the selecting candidates for high-risk revascularization. Patients with chronic kidney disease will definitively do better than those who can have off-pump coronary artery bypass (OPCAB) surgery compared to those who will need on-pump surgery.[47] Later-stage renal dysfunction (estimated glomerular filtration rate <30 ml/min) is not a contraindication to CABG surgery but renal replacement therapy may be necessary after surgery on either a temporary or permanent basis.

Lung disease

Many patients awaiting CABG will not have pulmonary function tests (PFTs) prior to admission for CABG. Initial assessment can include bedside spirometry and an arterial blood gas. If bedside spirometry is markedly abnormal (vital capacity <1 L, and FEV_1 between 50% and 25% of predicted), full PFTs should be obtained along with a noncontrast chest CT. If full PFTs confirm severe pulmonary dysfunction, the noncontrast chest CT is informative. In general, patients with severe pulmonary dysfunction but not grossly abnormality of chest CT will still do fine with surgery. If the patient has a severe restrictive ventilatory defect or diffuse pulmonary infiltrates on the chest CT, they most likely will not do well after surgery and will often need a tracheostomy in order to be safely weaned off the ventilator. In patients with severe pulmonary dysfunction, avoiding volume overload during and after the surgery is fundamental to achieving a good outcome and off-pump surgery is the preferred surgical approach. There should be particular attention during surgery to avoid damage to the lungs (creating air leaks) and to keep both pleural spaces closed.

Limited bypass conduits

Complete revascularization is the key to success in CABG surgery for ischemic cardiomyopathy. Sources for vascular conduits, in order of importance, are: LIMA, right internal mammary artery (RIMA), radial artery, greater saphenous vein, then lesser saphenous vein. Any combination of conduits may be ultimately used although the patient should have a LIMA to harvest or at least a RIMA which could be used as a free graft to the LAD.

Calcified ascending aorta

Patients with severe peripheral vascular disease or those on hemodialysis often have atherosclerotic plaque in the ascending aorta. If a patient has severe peripheral vascular disease or is on hemodialysis, a chest CT without intravenous contrast should be performed to assess the degree of calcification in the ascending aorta. Instrumentation of a calcified aorta can significantly increase the risk of stroke. If a patient is suitable to an off-pump approach, a proximal anastomotic device can be used for the proximal anastomoses thereby avoiding the application of the ascending aorta cross-clamp side-biter. If the patient is not suitable for off-pump surgery and needs to have an on-pump beating-heart approach, there has to be enough space to cannulate the ascending aorta safely and apply an anastomotic device.

Hematologic abnormalities

Heparin-induced thrombocytopenia (HIT) is a major hematologic contraindication to CABG surgery.[48] In patients with low or dropping platelet count, presence of an anti-platelet factor 4/heparin antibody should be confirmed with a serotonin release assay to avoid a false positive result. Patients with confirmed HIT require an alternative nonheparin anticoagulation during the surgery and immediately thereafter. Unlike heparin, alternative anticoagulants (e.g., direct thrombin inhibitors) cannot be easily reversed. Perioperative plasma exchange to remove the heparin antibodies is expensive, logistically challenging, and of uncertain benefit. The need for different anticoagulation strategies coupled with the risk of significant bleeding and transfusions weigh heavily against surgical intervention in HIT patients with multivessel coronary disease and HF.

Liver disease

Liver dysfunction can range from mild fatty liver disease to frank cirrhosis. Several scoring systems have been developed to assess surgical risk with concurrent liver disease. The Child–Pugh score classification is commonly used to assess degree of liver dysfunction depending upon serum bilirubin, creatinine levels, international normalized ratio (INR), hepatic encephalopathy, and ascites. The Model for End-Stage Liver Disease (MELD) score is now being used to assess prognosis in HF and risk for cardiac surgery.[49] The MELD score is derived from a linear regression model based on serum bilirubin, creatinine levels, and the INR. The mortality of patients increases with increasing score.[50] A MELD score greater than 13 and a Child–Pugh score B or C is a substantial contraindication for surgery in ischemic cardiomyopathy. If all variables are not available to measure the scores, an elevated INR without any sort of anticoagulation would warrant further evaluation before proceeding, including liver ultrasound, assessment of synthetic function (e.g., albumin) or even liver biopsy is there is a high index of suspicion for frank cirrhosis.

Pulmonary hypertension and right heart failure

Severe pulmonary hypertension without valve disease is a contraindication to surgical revascularization. With off-pump surgery it will not be possible to lift the heart to perform an obtuse marginal or a posterior descending artery graft if there is marked pulmonary hypertension. Such a patient would need on-pump beating-heart surgery. With severe pulmonary hypertension (not reversible with inhaled nitric oxide), the right ventricle will not perform well after surgery. A severely dilated right ventricle on echocardiography is a contraindication to surgical revascularization on-pump with a beating heart. Off-pump surgery is not contraindicated provided that there is viability in the right coronary territory and a good target (right coronary or posterior descending artery).

Patient preparation

Once a HF patient has been triaged to CABG, preoperative medical optimization is mandatory. In elective and semi-elective cases, the patient's volume status and hemodynamics should be optimized after admission with diuresis, judicious afterload reduction, and rhythm control. In select patients a pulmonary artery catheter may be required to ensure adequate hemodynamic preparation for bypass surgery. Patients who are euvolemic going into surgery will have a shorter length of stay and may be less likely to suffer hemodynamic embarrassment in the perioperative period.

Patients with severely reduced EF (<20–25%) should also undergo preliminary evaluation for mechanical circulatory support as a potential bailout strategy.[51] Options for LV support beyond a balloon pump should be considered in advance of surgery in case a patient cannot be weaned off cardiopulmonary bypass. Percutaneous or surgically implanted ventricular assist devices (VADs) are now available for the treatment of postsurgical shock. The degree of right HF must be adjudicated in case right ventricular (RV) support is warranted, since long-term dual ventricular support is currently available only to those eligible for cardiac transplantation. Important indices of right heart function include right atrial pressure, the appearance of the RV on echocardiography (e.g., RV to LV size ratio or tricuspid annular plane excursion), RV stroke work index, and evidence of congestion of the abdominal visceral with abnormal renal and hepatic function. Mechanical support can be used either as a bridge to recovery or transplantation or as permanent cardiac assist therapy. Patients ineligible for long-term mechanical support should be clearly identified in advance of high-risk CABG.

Thoughtful informed consent is the final, and perhaps most important, step of patient preparation. Candid estimates of perioperative morbidity and mortality, postoperative recovery time, and the potential for temporary or lasting mechanical support should be given to both the patient and their family before embarking on high-risk surgery. Expectations surrounding high-risk surgery must be carefully calibrated and any preoperative discussion should include the option of ongoing medical therapy or even targeted PCI. Given the complexity of decision-making, the attendant perioperative risks, and likelihood of a prolonged hospitalization, a social worker and other nonclinical members of the multidisciplinary team should be engaged early in the surgical hospitalization to maximize the available support.

Surgical technique

Several different approaches have been used to perform CABG surgery in patients with severe LV dysfunction. The two techniques of choice are off-pump CABG or on-pump beating-heart surgery. The advantage of both techniques is the absence of ischemic myocardial cardioplegic arrest. In patients who also present with right ventricular dysfunction, there is even a greater incentive to avoid cross-clamping and then needing to wean the patient from cardiopulmonary bypass.

OPCAB surgery has been shown in several trials to have comparable results to on-pump CABG surgery when performed by experienced surgeons.[52,53] When surgeons perform low numbers of off-pump compared to on-pump procedures (<20% off-pump), the patency rate and percent with complete revascularization are lower than in on-pump CABG surgery.[54] In a large meta-analysis of 23 nonrandomized studies including 7759 patients with EF less than 40%, of whom 2822 received OPCAB and 4937 underwent on-pump surgery, the early mortality rate of OPCAB was lower than in the on-pump group (odds ratio 0.64, 95% CI 0.51–0.81).[55] Incomplete revascularization, however, occurred more often in the OPCAB group. In experienced off-pump programs, the long-term graft patency is similar to that of on-pump surgery.[56] An on-pump beating-heart approach has been shown to lead to significant improvement of LV function with lower mortality and morbidity than traditional on-pump cardioplegia.[57] When compared to off-pump, the beating-heart technique can provide more complete revascularization at the price of a modestly increased risk of morbidity, such as increased blood loss, ventricular arrhythmias, inotropic support, ICU, hospital stay, and blood transfusion.[58]

The key to successful CABG is complete revascularization of viable myocardial territories. Most patients receive a sheathless intra-aortic balloon counterpulsation pump (IABP) in the operating room for support during the surgery or immediately thereafter, unless severe abdominal aorta atherosclerosis, aortic regurgitation, or abdominal aneurysm is present. In patients with pulmonary hypertension and RV dysfunction, inhaled epoprostenol is administered in the operating room while we keep low tidal volume ventilation. If this is unable to decrease pulmonary hypertension and RV dysfunction, then inhaled nitric oxide is used. Generally the patient will not tolerate an inodilator such as milrinone at this stage so further hemodynamic support is provided by epinephrine or norepinephrine.

In patients who need posterior descending artery (PDA) and a LAD bypass OPCAB can be performed if there is mild mitral regurgitation (MR) and the ventricle is normal or upper normal in size. In patients with larger ventricle (LVEDD ≥6.0 cm) and/or moderate MR, on-pump surgery can be performed without cross-clamping. In patients who need bypass on the lateral wall, but have a normal size ventricle and minimal MR, we perform the operation off-pump. If a patient has a large ventricle and moderate MR, the surgery can be performed on-pump with the heart beating.

On-pump CABG technique

Heparin is administered to achieve an activated clotting time (ACT) about 300 seconds. The LIMA to LAD anastomosis is performed first. For positioning, a lap sponge is placed behind the heart and an Octopus stabilizer (Medtronic Inc., Minneapolis, MN, USA) is deployed. We open the vessel and always place an intracoronary shunt (we use Maquet shunts) to avoid ischemia before performing the anastomosis. Depending on the coronary anatomy we may perform next the most critical lesion either an obtuse marginal (OM) branch or a PDA. To position the OM we place patient head down and rotate the operative table toward the surgeon, we open the right pleural space to have the heart dropped in the right pleural space, then we use the Octopus and Starfish suction cup device (Medtronic Inc., Minneapolis, MN, USA) to position the heart and stabilize. To position for the right coronary artery (RCA), we use only the stabilizer and to position for the PDA we use both the Octopus and the Starfish.

The proximal connections are performed after applying the side-biter to the ascending aorta and placing the IABP on standby while keeping the systolic blood pressure below 100 mmHg. We routinely use the epi-aortic ultrasound to scan the ascending aorta for plaque. If the ascending aorta cannot be safely clamped with the side-biter, we use the Novare proximal device (Novare Surgical Systems, Inc., Cupertino, CA, USA).

On-pump beating-heart approach

The on-pump beating-heart technique is used in patients with dilated ventricles, relatively small targets, and in the presence of moderate MR. We give heparin to achieve an ACT of 400 seconds prior to cannulation of the ascending aorta and the right atrium in the standard fashion. Then we proceed to perform the distal and the proximal anastomoses after applying an ascending aorta side-biter clamp. The LIMA to LAD graft is performed last. We use the Octopus and Starfish and place intracoronary shunts while having the heart decompress on cardiopulmonary bypass. The shunt provides a clean field.

Perioperative anticoagulation strategy

During the OPCAB procedure we reverse half-dose heparinization at the end of the procedure, while for on-pump beating-heart surgery we completely reverse the heparin. In patients with an IABP, if they are not bleeding within 6 hours we routinely start heparin infusion at a fixed rate (500 or 600 units) without titration. We also start aspirin and clopidogrel that same day, as the majority of these patients will have diffuse CAD. We continue a combination of clopidogrel and aspirin for 3 months unless they have coronary stents, which may mandate long-term dual anti-platelet therapy.

Post-CABG care

Bypass surgery can translate into remarkable improvements in angina, New York Heart Association (NYHA) class, and peak oxygen consumption on cardiopulmonary exercise testing.[59] Recovery of contractile functional can take days or weeks after restoration of normal blood flow to hibernating myocardium. Reverse remodeling can then improve diastolic function, reduce ventricular chamber size and restore the conical shape of the ventricle.[60] Optimization of ventricular performance after revascularization is predicated on careful postoperative management and timely reintroduction of medical therapy.

As the patient transitions from the surgical care unit to the step-down setting, slow weaning of inotropes is encouraged. Net volume status increases in the perioperative setting as patients receive colloid and crystalloid resuscitation. Euvolemia should be gradually restored with loop diuretic administration, with close monitoring of renal function and electrolyte loss. Patients should be euvolemic at discharge so that out-of-hospital rehabilitation can proceed without the danger of ongoing fluid shifts. Oral HF medications, including β-blockers and angiotensin converting enzyme (ACE) inhibitors (or angiotensin receptor blockers), should be reinstated as blood pressure and renal function allow. β-Blockers in particular have been shown to improve the performance of segments of hibernating myocardium.[61] Institution of guideline-based HF therapies may reduce the likelihood of early readmission while improving long-term survival.[62] Early postdischarge follow-up with a multidisciplinary team of both surgical and medical specialists can go a long way toward ensuring appropriate institution of longitudinal pharmacotherapy and guaranteeing maximal recovery following surgery.

Ventricular reconstruction for ischemic cardiomyopathy

Progressive remodeling of the ventricle after myocardial infarction can produce striking changes in the geometry and performance of the heart. Areas of transmural myocardial infarction may be thin-walled and dyskinetic or even aneurysmal, increasing the workload of the remaining viable myocardium.[63] Surgical attempts to restore the shape of the heart have focused on excising areas of densely infarcted tissue. Traditional surgical reconstruction has involved a linear repair involving the free wall, also known as the Dor procedure (or endoventricular circular patch plasty), though more modern techniques have evolved to include reconstruction of nonaneurysmal myocardium.[64,65] Myocardial segments eligible for reconstruction represent scar and thus should not have evidence viability on noninvasive testing. Despite promising case series, the prospective, randomized STICH trial failed to demonstrate a benefit when surgical ventricular reconstruction was performed with CABG.[66] Nevertheless, surgical ventricular reconstruction may be used by experienced surgeons in highly select cases, such as when thrombus is present within aneurysmal segments of the heart. Once a patient with reduced EF and a densely scarred myocardium has reached the point of inotrope dependence or stage D HF, mechanical circulatory support is indicated rather than surgical reconstruction of an end-stage ventricle.

Valve surgery for heart failure

Mitral regurgitation in patients with left ventricular dysfunction

MR can be caused by abnormalities of any component of the mitral valve apparatus: annulus, valve leaflets, chordae tendineae, papillary muscles, and adjacent LV free wall. In patients with LV systolic dysfunction and HF, MR can be classified according to whether or not ischemic heart disease is present. The distinction between ischemic and nonischemic MR has major implications for surgical therapy, with very different treatment decisions based on the nature of the valvular dysfunction. Patients with systolic dysfunction and significant chronic MR should only be referred for mitral surgery if they have refractory symptoms despite a background of guideline-based medical and resynchronization therapies.

All patients with MR and systolic dysfunction should receive neurohormonal antagonists with an attempt to titrate to target doses. For patients with a wide QRS complex on the surface electrocardiogram and LVEF less than 35%, particularly those with left bundle branch block and QRS duration greater than 150 ms, consideration should be given to cardiac resynchronization therapy.[67] Biventricular pacing has been shown to reduce the degree of MR and produce substantial reverse remodeling in patients with moderate-to-severe functional MR and high operative risk.[68,69] HF patients who are nonresponders to cardiac resynchronization pacing may be appropriate for referral for surgical correction of residual MR.

Ischemic mitral regurgitation

The most important mechanism of ischemic MR is mitral valve leaflet tethering due to chronic postinfarction remodeling, resulting in apical and lateral displacement of the papillary muscles (Figure 13.5). This shape change occurs after an inferior or posterior transmural myocardial infarction leads to displacement of the posteromedial papillary muscle.[70] The presence of MR can augment postinfarction remodeling and further exacerbate the degree of functional MR.[71] In addition, dynamic MR can occur during episodes of transient ischemia involving the papillary muscles.[72] Annular dilatation may also be present with chronic ventricular enlargement, though is always associated with concurrent leaflet tethering.

Transthoracic echocardiography (TEE) is the most important study for patients with suspected MR and can define regurgitant severity and operative risk. In patients with functional MR not due to primary leaflet pathology, LV remodeling may be evident along with annular dilatation, papillary muscle displacement, and leaflet tethering. Semiquantitative assessment of MR severity can be performed with color flow and continuous wave Doppler interrogation.[73] MR severity correlates with left atrial jet width area, pulmonary vein systolic flow reversal, effective regurgitant orifice area, and regurgitant fraction and volume.[74,75] Adverse outcomes with surgery for MR have been associated with an estimated regurgitant orifice larger than 20 mm^2, regurgitant volume 30 ml or more, and vena contracta width 4 mm or more.[76] Hemodynamic catheterization is only required if there is a discrepancy in clinical findings and noninvasive imaging or when estimated pulmonary artery systolic pressures are out of proportion to the degree of MR. In addition, coronary angiography should be performed before any consideration for mitral valve surgery, especially in patients with traditional coronary risk factors or in those with suspected postinfarct papillary muscle dysfunction or dynamic ischemic MR.

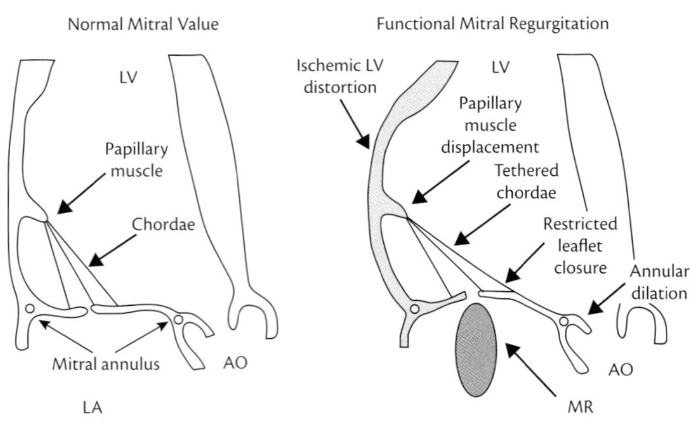

Fig. 13.5 Schematic of the normal mitral valve and functional mitral regurgitation. Ao, aorta; LA, left atrium; LV left ventricle; MR, mitral regurgitation.
Reprinted from Journal of the American College of Cardiology, 42, Levine et al., Ischemic mitral regurgitation, the dynamic lesion: clues to the cure, 1929–32, copyright (2003) with permission from Elsevier.

Two primary clinical decisions points arise in the treatment of ischemic MR: (1) whether or not to address the MR at the time of CABG surgery; and (2) if valve surgery is needed, whether the valve should be repaired or replaced (Figure 13.6).

Mitral surgery at time of CABG

Fundamentally, ischemic MR is a ventricular problem and not a valve problem. Valve interventions (annuloplasty ring, ring plus adjunct procedure, or replacement) have not been shown to improve survival, since survival has been linked to the degree of underlying ventricular dysfunction.[77,78] Thus, mitral valve intervention at the time of CABG is intended to improve symptoms and prevent late complications, such as worsening congestive HF, hospital readmission, and deteriorating quality of life.[79]

In a subgroup analysis of the STICH trial, patients with LVEF 35% or less and CAD amenable to CABG were assessed based upon their degree of MR. The decision to address the mitral valve during the CABG surgery was left to the surgeon. Among 1212 patients enrolled in STICH, 15% had moderate MR and 3% had severe MR. The question of whether or not to address the mitral valve in this setting primarily arises when the degree of MR is moderate. In the medical arm of STICH, the risk of death was strongly correlated to the degree of MR (moderate–severe MR had HR 2.01, 95% CI 1.42–2.85) In the CABG group, there was a trend toward better survival within the CABG plus mitral repair group versus CABG only (HR 0.62, 95% CI 0.35–1.08). If the degree of MR is severe and CABG is planned, most operators recommend addressing the mitral valve at the time of bypass surgery.

In one randomized trial, 73 patients referred for CABG with moderate ischemic MR and EF 30% or more were randomized to receive CABG with or without mitral valve repair (MVR). The study was stopped early since at 1 year there was a greater improvement in peak oxygen consumption (the primary endpoint) with CABG plus MVR.[80] The group undergoing concurrent MVR also had reduction in MR severity, improvement in LV remodeling, and lower natriuretic peptide levels, though the study was not powered to assess mortality differences. The study provided further support that moderate ischemic MR should be addressed at the time of CABG when there is moderately reduced systolic dysfunction.

The decision to address the mitral valve should be made before CABG surgery in the office or at the bedside and not by TEE in the operating room.[81] The TEE is mandatory but should not be the main source of information to determine whether surgical repair of

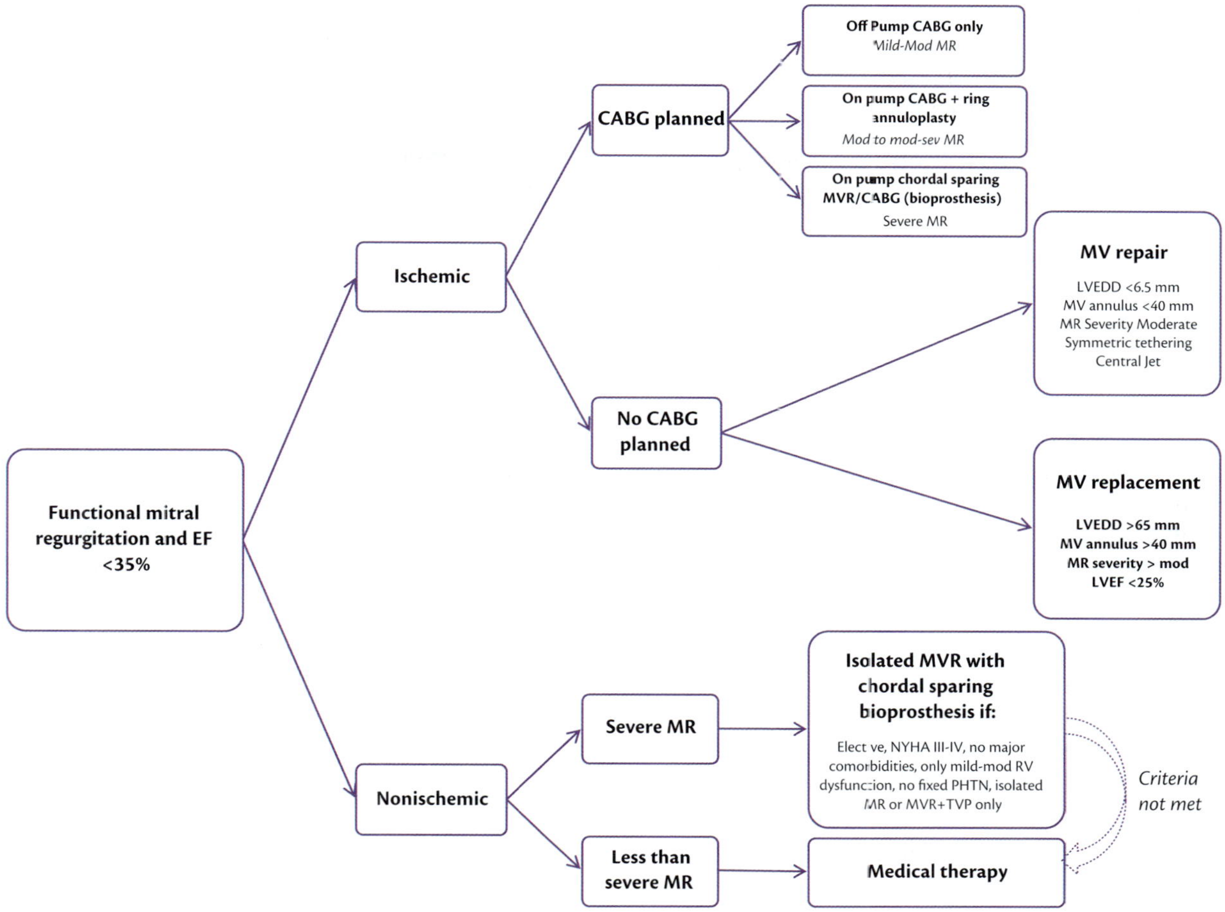

Fig. 13.6 Management strategy for patients with functional mitral regurgitation and reduced left ventricular function (EF <35%). CABG, coronary artery bypass grafting; LVEDD, left ventricular end-diastolic diameter; NYHA, New York Heart Association; PHTN, pulmonary hypertension; TVP, tricuspid valvuloplasty.

the mitral valve should be undertaken at the time of CABG. At the extremes, the decisions are fairly straightforward: if mild MR or less then leave the valve alone, if more than moderate–severe MR then operate on the valve. If moderate MR is present along with severe systolic dysfunction (EF <30%) the decision is more controversial. At that point, the choice is between CABG alone (on- or off-pump) and on-pump CABG with mitral valve surgery. The deciding factor between these two options is whether viable myocardium is present. If there is a large extent (≥5 segments) of viable myocardium, there can be a significant improvement in the degree of ischemic MR with CABG alone, particularly if there is viability in the inferior or lateral walls near the papillary muscles.[82]

Mitral valve ring annuloplasty alone with CABG will be sufficient if the ventricle is not too dilated (LV end-diastolic dimension <65 mm), the mitral annulus is not too dilated (<40 mm), the degree of MR is not too bad (moderate), there is a lower tethering area (<2 cm^2), there is symmetric tethering, and there is a central jet.[70,83,84] Predictors of recurrent mitral regurgitation after annuloplasty alone are a tenting height of 1 cm^2 or more, mitral annular dimension greater than 3.7 cm, MR grade greater than 3.5 with a central or complex jet, LV end-systolic volume greater than 145 ml, systolic sphericity index 0.7 or more, and a restrictive diastolic filling pattern.[85] Significant distortions of the ventricle or mitral valve apparatus will thwart the ability of ring annuplasty alone to address ischemic MR.

Mitral valve replacement versus repair

Based on the above echocardiographic criteria, if there is a low likelihood that ring annuloplasty alone will abolish MR, then adjunctive valve procedures are often considered to reconstruct the native mitral apparatus. In such cases, the valve should simply be replaced with a low-profile modern biological prosthesis using full chordal sparing technique. Once again, none of these adjunctive procedures have been proven to make a difference in long-term survival when compared to mitral valve replacement. If repair is undertaken, the patient must leave the operating room with a nearly perfect result or at most trivial residual MR. An inadequate repair is far worse than a valve replacement. If mild residual MR is present (coaptation <8 mm) then there is continuous adverse ventricular remodeling due to greater loading perpetuating a vicious positive feedback cycle whereby MR begets further MR.[76] There is no indication for mechanical valve replacement in ischemic MR, as the vast majority of patients will not live long enough to experience the extended durability of a mechanical prosthesis.

The key to successful mitral valve replacement is chordal sparing for both the anterior and posterior chordae.[86] Repair is superior to replacement when feasible and when the patient can leave the operating room with little MR. However, in the most complex settings, such as multiple regurgitant jets, the survival rates between repair and replacement are similar.[87,88] For extremely high-risk patients, mitral valve replacement is often safer and faster than attempting a complex and potentially lengthy MVR. Sicker or older patients with multiple comorbidities in most cases will not outlive biological mitral valve prostheses for ischemic MR.

Nonischemic mitral regurgitation

Patients with a nonischemic dilated cardiomyopathy will often have leaflet tethering, an apically displaced coaption point, and mitral annular dilatation leading to severe MR. The presence of MR in patients with severe LV systolic dysfunction is a predictor of poor survival.[89] The surgical criteria for nonischemic MR are not the same as for ischemic MR (discussed above). In patients with dilated cardiomyopathy, we tend to favor replacement over repair. Preservation of both the anterior and posterior chordal support (anterolateral papillary muscle and posteromedial papillary muscle, respectively) is the key to successful replacement. While it is common practice among surgeons to make an effort to preserve the posterior chordal support, the anterior chordal support is often neglected. Reattachment of the anterior chordae close to their anatomical positions preserves annular symmetry and allows natural chordal tension with more physiologic systolic and diastolic function of the left ventricle.[86] Standard posterior leaflet preservation can be achieved by plication of the leaflet tissue in the valve sutures. For the anterior leaflet the mid-portion of the leaflet is excised and the separate anterior and posterior segments are reattached to their respective commissures to preserve anatomical position.

Isolated mitral valve surgery: preferred surgical approach

In patients with isolated mitral valve disease and poor LV systolic function, two general surgical approaches can be used: median sternotomy with ischemic cardioplegic arrest or right thoractomy with fibrillatory arrest. Modified techniques use a combination of both (e.g., minimally invasive right thoracotomy with cardioplegic arrest). Our preferred approach is minimally invasive right thoracotomy with fibrillatory arrest (Figure 13.7).

Minimally invasive mitral valve surgery avoids full sternotomy and has been shown to produce less postoperative discomfort and enable earlier mobilization and hospital discharge compared to conventional sternotomy.[90] This approach is referred to as "minimally invasive" because of a reduction in surgical trauma and implies similar reductions in postoperative pain and length of rehabilitation. Whether or not such "minimally invasive" procedures are really less invasive in this expanded sense remains unproven, as there is no general agreement on the definition and no standard approach to the measurements of outcomes covered by the term.

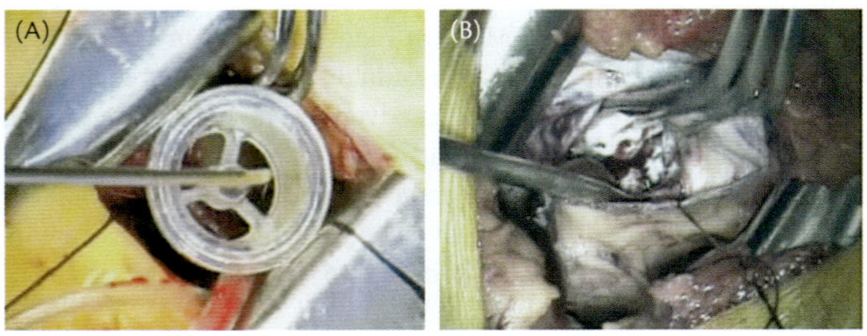

Fig. 13.7 Approach to minimally invasive mitral valve surgery. (A) Right anterolateral thoracotomy (5 cm) with a prosthetic valve held up next to thoracotomy to demonstrate the size of incision. (B) Operative exposure of the mitral valve using an atrial retractor.[118]

Reprinted from Annals of Thoracic Surgery, 85, Umakanthan et al., Safety of Minimally Invasive Mitral Valve Surgery Without Aortic Cross-Clamp, 1544–1550, copyright (2008) with permission from Elsevier.

The true value of minimally invasive mitral valve surgery through a right thoracotomy without aortic cross-clamping with the heart beating (cold fibrillatory arrest) is not the small lateral incision with its cosmetic advantages, faster recovery, and the ability to avoid retrosternal adhesions in reoperative settings. The true advantage lies in the avoidance of ischemic cardioplegic arrest while keeping the fibrillating heart cold and empty. In patients with LV systolic dysfunction requiring mitral valve (MV) surgery this mimics the benefit of off-pump beating-heart surgery for CABG. This technique has been described in a series of 504 consecutive patients undergoing minimally invasive mitral valve surgery. Of this cohort, 16% had an EF of 35% or less. Among these patients with systolic dysfunction undergoing minimally invasive MVR, 30-day mortality of the entire cohort was only 4%, substantially lower than the aggregate predicted STS mortality of 20%.[91]

One common theme of minimally invasive approaches to mitral valve surgery is the continued need for aortic cross-clamping and a cardioplegia delivery system. In our approach, myocardial protection is accomplished by keeping the heart decompressed, cooling to 28 °C to decrease myocardial oxygen consumption, and then perfusing the coronaries against an intact aortic valve with cold oxygenated blood. In a series of 66 consecutive patients with EF 35% or less who underwent MVR with the above technique, two-thirds of whom had ischemic MR, mortality was only 4.5% compared to the expected 6.5% according to the STS score, providing indirect evidence for the safety of minimally invasive mitral valve replacement without aortic cross-clamp in patients with severe cardiomyopathy.[92]

Surgery is indicated for functional MR in dilated cardiomyopathy provided severe MR is confirmed by transthoracic echocardiography (TTE), the surgery is elective, there is no more than mild-to-moderate RV dysfunction, and no major comorbid conditions. In contrast to decisions surrounding CABG, patient substrate must be largely limited to isolated mitral valve disease without significant cardiac or extracardiac comorbidity.

Aortic stenosis

Aortic stenosis (AS) is a disease for which there is no medical treatment. Characterizing the severity of stenosis is critical for determining the timing of surgical intervention and requires careful history, physical examination, and initial imaging with TTE.[93] AS accounts for over one-quarter of chronic valvular heart disease, with approximately 80% of symptomatic cases occurring in adult males. Age-related degenerative calcification is the most common cause in the United States, with other etiologies including congenitally bicuspid aortic valve and rheumatic heart disease. In addition to older age and male sex, smoking, diabetes, hypertension, and chronic kidney disease are risk factors for calcific AS, leading to a population with symptomatic disease often saddled with a heavy burden of comorbid conditions. The cardinal symptoms of AS are dyspnea, angina, and syncope.[94] There is typically a long latent phase during which progressive stenosis develops with variable rates of progression. Symptoms are rare until the valve orifice has narrowed to less than 1 cm^2. The onset of symptoms is a critical turning point in the natural history of the disease and heralds the need for surgical evaluation and treatment.

Obstruction to LV outflow produces a pressure gradient between the aorta the ventricular cavity. Initially the LV will compensate for the increased wall stress with concentric hypertrophy. Compensatory hypertrophy may accommodate a large pressure gradient for years before it becomes maladaptive and LV function declines, with chamber dilatation and reduced cardiac output. Moreover coronary flow reserve may be reduced because of increased oxygen demand of the hypertrophied LV and increased transmural pressure gradient along the longer distance blood must travel to reach the subendocardial layer. Subendocardial ischemia ensues even in the absence of coronary disease and the myocardium begins to be replaced by collagen and undergo fibrotic changes, eventually leading to combined systolic and diastolic dysfunction of the ventricle.[95] When there is underlying LV systolic dysfunction, severe AS may be present despite low transaortic velocity and mean gradient. It is estimated that 5–10% of all patients with AS have low-flow, low-gradient AS in the setting of LV dysfunction.[96] Such patients are at particularly high risk for complications and require further evaluation to determine if true valvular AS is present or whether the reduced estimated valve area on echocardiography relates to underlying cardiomyopathy.

The evaluation and management of patients with AS and a depressed EF can be vexing. Patients with anatomically severe AS and reduced EF (<40%) often have a relatively low pressure gradient (<30 mmHg) due to a weakened ventricle and afterload mismatch. The true severity of AS can be difficult to determine when the cardiac output and transvalvular gradient are low. If the ventricle itself is diseased and unable to generate sufficient systolic force to open the leaflets adequately, a reduced aortic valve area may be present at rest, overestimating AS severity. This conditions is known as pseudo-severe AS.[97] In such cases, LV dysfunction is the predominant pathology and may be caused by prior myocardial infarction or a primary cardiomyopathy. Patients with either true severe AS and a reduced EF or pseudo-severe AS have a low-flow state with low transaortic gradients contributing to an estimated aortic valve area of less than 1 cm^2. Pseudo-severe AS patients must be distinguished from those with true severe AS since patients with true severe AS and contractile reserve will usually benefit from valve surgery, whereas patients with pseudo-severe AS are not operative candidates for aortic valve replacement (AVR).[98,99,100]

Dobutamine stress echocardiography has a well-defined diagnostic role in patient with suspected AS and low EF.[101] The inotropic effects of low-dose dobutamine will increase transvalvular flow in patients with a contractile reserve.[102] Contractile reserve is defined as an increase in stroke volume with inotropic infusion of more than 20%. Dobutamine infusion, particularly at doses 20 $\mu g\ kg^{-1}\ min^{-1}$ or less, is generally well tolerated but should only be performed in experienced centers with a cardiologist in attendance. In patients with true severe AS and LV dysfunction dobutamine will increase cardiac output and mean transvalvular gradient, but the calculated aortic valve area will remain low (<1 cm^2) Patients with pseudo-severe AS will have an increase in aortic valve area into a range no longer considered severe (>1.2 cm^2) with little change in transvalvular gradient. Some patients will not show contractile reserve to dobutamine, signaling a poor prognosis (Figure 13.8).[103]

Surgery is indicated in true severe AS with contractile reserve after dobutamine challenge, and generally contraindicated for patients with pseudo-severe AS or those without contractile reserve.[104,105] Candidates for AVR for severe AS with reduced LV function are those who can undergo elective surgery and do not have multivalvular disease. Patients who require multiple valve replacements when there is severe EF are not appropriate candidates given the dramatic increase in ischemic clamp time. Other markers of increase risk with AVR include advanced age, frailty, renal failure requiring hemodialysis, and a small aortic annulus. Patients with low-gradient AS undergoing AVR have a significantly higher perioperative and long-term mortality if multivessel CAD is present.[100,106]

The absence of an LV contractile reserve is not an absolute contraindication to AVR, but it is a strong negative predictor of survival, particularly in those with severe AS with a mean gradient of less than 20 mmHg with dobutamine infusion. In a study of 81 patients with low-flow AS without contractile reserve, 5-year survival was higher in the surgical AVR patients compared to those medically managed (54% vs. 13%, $p < 0.001$) despite a higher operative mortality in the AVR group (22%).[107] In patients without contractile reserve, surgery can still be offered provided the following criteria are met: the mean gradient is greater than 30 mmHg, the aortic annulus is of adequate size for body surface area of the patient, there is no CAD, few major comorbitidies, age is less than 75 years, there is isolated AS only, and LVAD therapy is available as a back-up if there is ongoing hemodynamic compromise after AVR.

Aortic valve replacement

For patients with reduced EF and symptomatic severe AS, AVR is performed using the standard technique with cardiopulmonary bypass. The key to success in these patients is short ischemic cardioplegic arrest and avoidance of patient–prosthesis mismatch. In general, an attempt is made to place the largest aortic prosthesis that the annulus can accommodate. A small prosthesis is an independent risk factor for perioperative mortality in this group.[108] Patients with LV dysfunction are more sensitive to residual AS and its attendant afterload compared to patients with preserved LV function. In recipients with patient–prosthesis mismatch, survival is reduced threefold while freedom from congestive HF is reduced fourfold compared to those patients without residual patient–prosthesis mismatch.[109] The choice of valve prosthesis depends on patient age, anticipated lifespan, and preference for and tolerance of anticoagulation.

Transcatheter aortic valve replacement (TAVR) is an emerging option for patients thought to be inoperable or at extremely high risk for operative replacement. The Placement of Aortic Transcatheter Valves (PARTNER) trial randomized patients with severe AS to medical management versus TAVR (inoperable cohort) and surgical AVR versus TAVR (high-risk cohort). Inoperable patients had significant reduced rates of death at 1 year (HR 0.55, 95% CI 0.40–0.74) while high-risk patients had similar one-year survival, with a trend toward higher risk of stroke in the TAVR group.[110,111] It is important to note that patients were excluded from the trial if they had severe LV dysfunction (EF < 20%). In a substudy of the PARTNER trial, TAVR performed better than medical therapy in inoperable patients with EF less than 55%.[112] There will be an expanding role for TAVR in the treatment of patients with AS and LV dysfunction as higher-risk patients present for consideration of aortic valve surgery. The clinical complexities surrounding the menu of choices for valve replacement has contributed to the development of multidisciplinary heart teams so that patients can be evaluated and managed by a cohesive group of valvular disease specialists.[113]

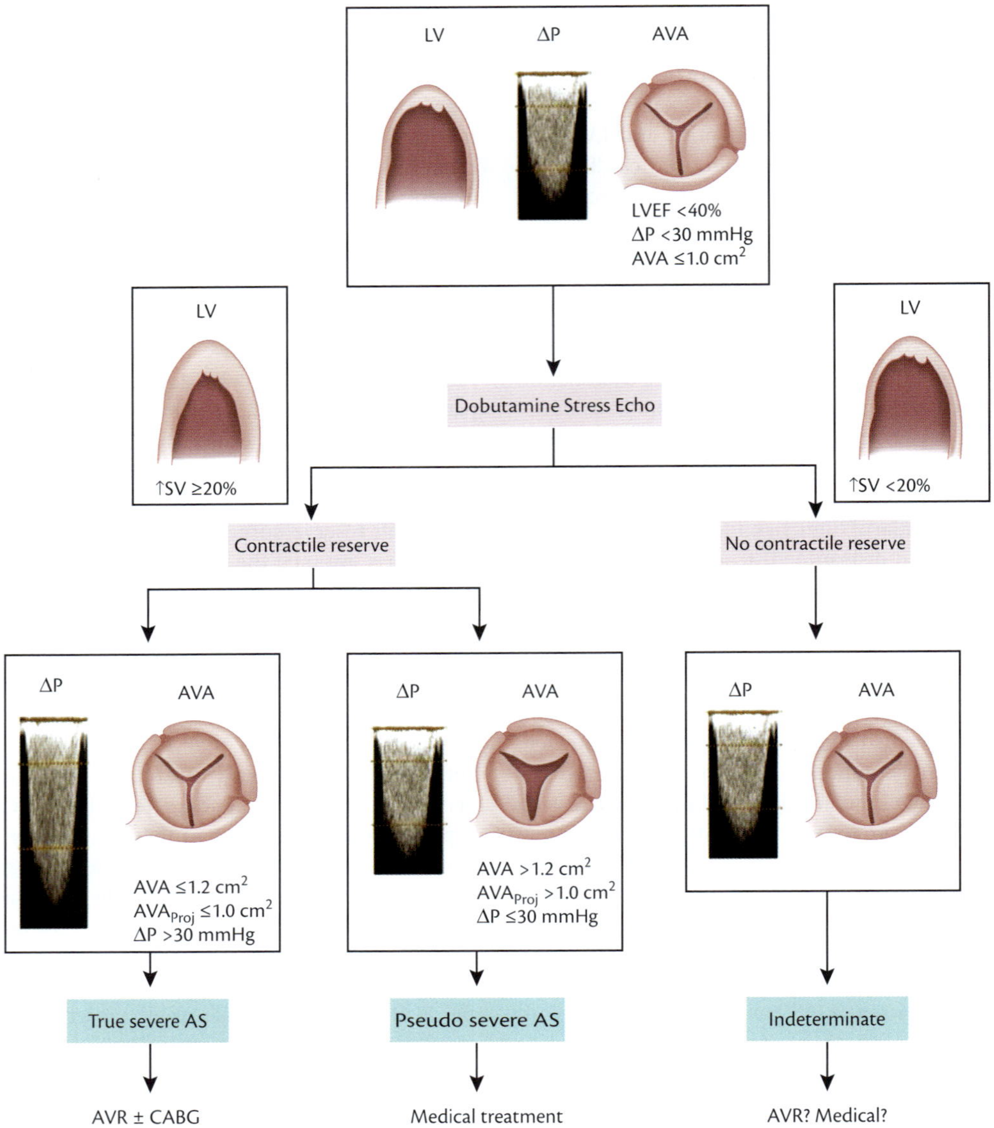

Fig. 13.8 Algorithm for decision-making in low-flow, low-gradient aortic stenosis (AS). AVA, aortic valve area; CABG, coronary artery bypass grafting; LV, left ventricle; LVEF, left ventricular ejection fraction; ΔP, transaortic pressure gradient; SV, stroke volume.

Reprinted from Journal of the American College of Cardiology, 54, Picano, E et al., The Emerging Role of Exercise Testing and Stress Echocardiography in Valvular Heart Disease, 2251–60, copyright (2009) with permission from Elsevier.

Aortic regurgitation

Valvular aortic regurgitation is commonly caused by valve leaflet abnormalities (endocarditis, congenital bicuspid valve) or aortic root dilatation. The prognosis of patients with chronic aortic regurgitation (AR) is determined by symptom status and LV size and function. An LV end-systolic volume more than 60 ml/m^2, an end-systolic dimension of more than 50 mm, or an EF less than 50% indicates a severely dysfunctional ventricle in the face of the chronic preload and afterload imposed by severe AR. Patients who are symptomatic or have these early signs of LV dysfunction should be referred for AVR. Surgical correction of severe AR usually results in some symptomatic improvement, regardless of the functional status of the ventricle.[114] The decision to refer for surgical therapy for AR becomes more challenging when severe LV systolic dysfunction is present since there are few data available and a questionable role for contractile reserve, in contrast to AS with reduced EF.[115] Dobutamine may accentuate the differences in ventricular size and function that are more prevalent in those who eventually recover following valve surgery.

AVR for AR is still recommended for those patients with NYHA class II–IV symptoms and EF 25–50%, understanding that they have a higher operative mortality (>10%) compared to those patients with preserved EF undergoing AVR. For those who survive, there is a significant improvement in LV performance and long-term survival compared to patients receiving medical management.[116] Although earlier studies with less sophisticated myocardial protection and valves with higher residual gradients demonstrated poor results for AVR for AR with severe LV impairment, more recent data suggests survival after AVR may be similar to those patient with better LV function.[103] For patients with EF less than 25% there is a limited role for AVR for severe AR. Surgery can still be offered if only isolated AVR is to be performed in an elective setting, if the patient is younger (<70 years old), without significant comorbidities, and if they are a candidate for LV assist device (LVAD) back-up. Contractile reserve demonstrated by dobutamine stress echocardiography can give some reassurance to proceed with surgery. Surgical technique is similar to that of AVR for AS; however, bioprostheses should be used in view of the potential need for LVAD and the risk of thrombosis with mechanical aortic valves with continuous flow mechanical support.

References

1. Roger VL, Go AS, Lloyd-Jones DM, et al. Heart disease and stroke statistics—2012 update: a report from the American Heart Association. Circulation 2012;125:e2–220.
2. Torabi A, Cleland JG, Khan NK, et al. The timing of development and subsequent clinical course of heart failure after a myocardial infarction. Eur Heart J 2008;29:859–70.
3. Fox KF, Cowie MR, Wood DA, et al. Coronary artery disease as the cause of incident heart failure in the population. Eur Heart J 2001;22:228–36.
4. Felker GM, Shaw LK, O'Connor CM. A standardized definition of ischemic cardiomyopathy for use in clinical research. J Am Coll Cardiol 2002;39:210–18.
5. Sutton MG, Sharpe N. Left ventricular remodeling after myocardial infarction: pathophysiology and therapy. Circulation 2000;101:2981–8.
6. Goldstein JA, Demetriou D, Grines CL, et al. Multiple complex coronary plaques in patients with acute myocardial infarction. N Engl J Med 2000;343:915–22.
7. Scarabelli T, Stephanou A, Rayment N, et al. Apoptosis of endothelial cells precedes myocyte cell apoptosis in ischemia/reperfusion injury. Circulation 2001;104:253–6.
8. Thijssen VL, Borgers M, Lenders MH, et al. Temporal and spatial variations in structural protein expression during the progression from stunned to hibernating myocardium. Circulation 2004;110:3313–21.
9. Bart BA, Shaw LK, McCants CB, Jr., et al. Clinical determinants of mortality in patients with angiographically diagnosed ischemic or nonischemic cardiomyopathy. J Am Coll Cardiol 1997;30:1002–8.
10. al-Mohammad A, Mahy IR, Norton MY, et al. Prevalence of hibernating myocardium in patients with severely impaired ischaemic left ventricles. Heart 1998;80:559–64.
11. Romero J, Xue X, Gonzalez W, Garcia MJ. CMR imaging assessing viability in patients with chronic ventricular dysfunction due to coronary artery disease: a meta-analysis of prospective trials. JACC Cardiovasc Imaging 2013;5:494–508.
12. Camici PG, Prasad SK, Rimoldi OE. Stunning, hibernation, and assessment of myocardial viability. Circulation 2008;117:103–14.
13. Allman KC. Noninvasive assessment myocardial viability: current status and future directions. J Nucl Cardiol 2013;20:618–37; quiz 38–9.
14. Bingham SE, Hachamovitch R. Incremental prognostic significance of combined cardiac magnetic resonance imaging, adenosine stress perfusion, delayed enhancement, and left ventricular function over preimaging information for the prediction of adverse events. Circulation 2011;123:1509–18.
15. Allman KC, Shaw LJ, Hachamovitch R, Udelson JE. Myocardial viability testing and impact of revascularization on prognosis in patients with coronary artery disease and left ventricular dysfunction: a meta-analysis. J Am Coll Cardiol 2002;39:1151–8.
16. Coronary artery surgery study (CASS): a randomized trial of coronary artery bypass surgery. Survival data. Circulation 1983;68:939–50.
17. Veterans Administration Coronary Artery Bypass Surgery Cooperative Study Group. Eleven-year survival in the Veterans Administration randomized trial of coronary bypass surgery for stable angina. N Engl J Med 1984;311:1333–9.
18. Yusuf S, Zucker D, Peduzzi P, et al. Effect of coronary artery bypass graft surgery on survival: overview of 10-year results from randomised trials by the Coronary Artery Bypass Graft Surgery Trialists Collaboration. Lancet 1994;344:563–70.
19. Varnauskas E. Twelve-year follow-up of survival in the randomized European Coronary Surgery Study. N Engl J Med 1988;319:332–7.
20. Velazquez EJ, Lee KL, Deja MA, et al. Coronary-artery bypass surgery in patients with left ventricular dysfunction. N Engl J Med 2011;364:1607–16.
21. Doenst T, Cleland JG, Rouleau JL, et al. Influence of crossover on mortality in a randomized study of revascularization in patients with systolic heart failure and coronary artery disease. Circ Heart Fail 2013;6:443–50.
22. Shaw LJ, Berman DS, Maron DJ, et al. Optimal medical therapy with or without percutaneous coronary intervention to reduce ischemic burden: results from the Clinical Outcomes Utilizing Revascularization and Aggressive Drug Evaluation (COURAGE) trial nuclear substudy. Circulation 2008;117:1283–91.
23. Bonow RO, Maurer G, Lee KL, et al. Myocardial viability and survival in ischemic left ventricular dysfunction. N Engl J Med 2011;364:1617–25.
24. Wijns W, Kolh P, Danchin N, et al. Guidelines on myocardial revascularization. Eur Heart J 2010;31:2501–55.
25. Fihn SD, Gardin JM, Abrams J, et al. 2012 ACCF/AHA/ACP/AATS/PCNA/SCAI/STS guideline for the diagnosis and management of patients with stable ischemic heart disease: a report of the American College of Cardiology Foundation/American Heart Association task force on practice guidelines, and the American College of Physicians, American Association for Thoracic Surgery, Preventive Cardiovascular Nurses Association, Society for Cardiovascular Angiography and Interventions, and Society of Thoracic Surgeons. Circulation 2012;126:e354–471.
26. Caracciolo EA, Davis KB, Sopko G, et al. Comparison of surgical and medical group survival in patients with left main coronary artery disease. Long-term CASS experience. Circulation 1995;91:2325–34.
27. Caracciolo EA, Davis KB, Sopko G, et al. Comparison of surgical and medical group survival in patients with left main equivalent coronary artery disease. Long-term CASS experience. Circulation 1995;91:2335–44.
28. Tatoulis J, Buxton BF, Fuller JA. Patencies of 2127 arterial to coronary conduits over 15 years. Ann Thorac Surg 2004;77:93–101.
29. Balacumaraswami L, Taggart DP. Intraoperative imaging techniques to assess coronary artery bypass graft patency. Ann Thorac Surg 2007;83:2251–7.
30. Alexander JH, Hafley G, Harrington RA, et al. Efficacy and safety of edifoligide, an E2F transcription factor decoy, for prevention of vein graft failure following coronary artery bypass graft surgery: PREVENT IV: a randomized controlled trial. JAMA 2005;294:2446–54.
31. Lytle BW, Loop FD, Taylor PC, et al. The effect of coronary reoperation on the survival of patients with stenoses in saphenous vein bypass grafts to coronary arteries. J Thorac Cardiovasc Surg 1993;105:605–12; discussion 12–14.
32. Comparison of coronary bypass surgery with angioplasty in patients with multivessel disease. The Bypass Angioplasty Revascularization Investigation (BARI) Investigators. N Engl J Med 1996;335:217–25.
33. D'Egidio G, Nichol G, Williams KA, et al. Increasing benefit from revascularization is associated with increasing amounts of myocardial hibernation: a substudy of the PARR-2 trial. JACC Cardiovasc Imaging 2009;2:1060–8.
34. Schinkel AF, Poldermans D, Rizzello V, et al. Why do patients with ischemic cardiomyopathy and a substantial amount of viable myocardium not always recover in function after revascularization? J Thorac Cardiovasc Surg 2004;127:385–90.
35. Hattler BG, Madia C, Johnson C, et al. Risk stratification using the Society of Thoracic Surgeons Program. Ann Thorac Surg 1994;58:1348–52.

36. Nashef SA, Roques F, Hammill BG, et al. Validation of European System for Cardiac Operative Risk Evaluation (EuroSCORE) in North American cardiac surgery. Eur J Cardiothorac Surg 2002;22:101–5.
37. Lee DH, Buth KJ, Martin BJ, et al. Frail patients are at increased risk for mortality and prolonged institutional care after cardiac surgery. Circulation 2010;121:973–8.
38. Studenski S, Perera S, Patel K, et al. Gait speed and survival in older adults. JAMA 2011;305:50–8.
39. Afilalo J, Eisenberg MJ, Morin JF, et al. Gait speed as an incremental predictor of mortality and major morbidity in elderly patients undergoing cardiac surgery. J Am Coll Cardiol 2010;56:1668–76.
40. Bagnall NM, Faiz O, Darzi A, Athanasiou T. What is the utility of preoperative frailty assessment for risk stratification in cardiac surgery? Interact Cardiovasc Thorac Surg 2013;17:398–402.
41. Anker SD, Ponikowski P, Varney S, et al. Wasting as independent risk factor for mortality in chronic heart failure. Lancet 1997;349:1050–3.
42. Engelman DT, Adams DH, Byrne JG, et al. Impact of body mass index and albumin on morbidity and mortality after cardiac surgery. J Thorac Cardiovasc Surg 1999;118:866–73.
43. Liu Z, Shi Z, Wang Y, et al. Carotid artery stenting versus carotid endarterectomy: systematic review and meta-analysis. World J Surg 2009;33:586–96.
44. Ziada KM, Yadav JS, Mukherjee D, et al. Comparison of results of carotid stenting followed by open heart surgery versus combined carotid endarterectomy and open heart surgery (coronary bypass with or without another procedure). Am J Cardiol 2005;96:519–23.
45. Cooper WA, O'Brien SM, Thourani VH, et al. Impact of renal dysfunction on outcomes of coronary artery bypass surgery: results from the Society of Thoracic Surgeons National Adult Cardiac Database. Circulation 2006;113:1063–70.
46. Hillis GS, Zehr KJ, Williams AW, et al. Outcome of patients with low ejection fraction undergoing coronary artery bypass grafting: renal function and mortality after 3.8 years. Circulation 2006;114:I414–19.
47. Boulton BJ, Kilgo P, Guyton RA, et al. Impact of preoperative renal dysfunction in patients undergoing off-pump versus on-pump coronary artery bypass. Ann Thorac Surg 2011;92:595–601; discussion 2.
48. Linkins LA, Dans AL, Moores LK, et al. Treatment and prevention of heparin-induced thrombocytopenia: Antithrombotic Therapy and Prevention of Thrombosis, 9th ed: American College of Chest Physicians Evidence-Based Clinical Practice Guidelines. Chest 2012;141:e495S–530S.
49. Kim MS, Kato TS, Farr M, et al. Hepatic dysfunction in ambulatory patients with heart failure: application of the MELD scoring system for outcome prediction. J Am Coll Cardiol 2013;61:2253–61.
50. Thielmann M, Mechmet A, Neuhauser M, et al. Risk prediction and outcomes in patients with liver cirrhosis undergoing open-heart surgery. Eur J Cardiothorac Surg 2010;38:592–9.
51. Wilson SR, Mudge GH, Jr., Stewart GC, Givertz MM. Evaluation for a ventricular assist device: selecting the appropriate candidate. Circulation 2009;119:2225–32.
52. Lamy A, Devereaux PJ, Prabhakaran D, et al. Off-pump or on-pump coronary-artery bypass grafting at 30 days. N Engl J Med 2012;366:1489–97.
53. Lamy A, Devereaux PJ, Prabhakaran D, et al. Effects of off-pump and on-pump coronary-artery bypass grafting at 1 year. N Engl J Med 2013;368:1179–88.
54. Khan NE, De Souza A, Mister R, et al. A randomized comparison of off-pump and on-pump multivessel coronary-artery bypass surgery. N Engl J Med 2004;350:21–8.
55. Jarral OA, Saso S, Athanasiou T. Off-pump coronary artery bypass in patients with left ventricular dysfunction: a meta-analysis. Ann Thorac Surg 2011;92:1686–94.
56. Fukui T, Tabata M, Morita S, Takanashi S. Early and long-term outcomes of coronary artery bypass grafting in patients with acute coronary syndrome versus stable angina pectoris. J Thorac Cardiovasc Surg 2013;145:1577–83, 83 e1.
57. Letsou GV, Wu YX, Grunkemeier G, et al. Off-pump coronary artery bypass and avoidance of hypothermic cardiac arrest improves early left ventricular function in patients with systolic dysfunction. Eur J Cardiothorac Surg 2011;40:227–32.
58. Darwazah AK, Bader V, Isleem I, Helwa K. Myocardial revascularization using on-pump beating heart among patients with left ventricular dysfunction. J Cardiothorac Surg 2010;5:109.
59. Carluccio E, Biagioli P, Alunni G, et al. Patients with hibernating myocardium show altered left ventricular volumes and shape, which revert after revascularization: evidence that dyssynergy might directly induce cardiac remodeling. J Am Coll Cardiol 2006;47:969–77.
60. Carluccio E, Biagioli P, Alunni G, et al. Effect of revascularizing viable myocardium on left ventricular diastolic function in patients with ischaemic cardiomyopathy. Eur Heart J 2009;30:1501–9.
61. Cleland JG, Pennell DJ, Ray SG, et al. Myocardial viability as a determinant of the ejection fraction response to carvedilol in patients with heart failure (CHRISTMAS trial): randomised controlled trial. Lancet 2003;362:14–21.
62. Yancy CW, Jessup M, Bozkurt B, et al. 2013 ACCF/AHA Guideline for the Management of Heart Failure: A Report of the American College of Cardiology Foundation/American Heart Association Task Force on Practice Guidelines. Circulation 2013;62(16):e147–239.
63. Di Donato M, Toso A, Dor V, et al. Surgical ventricular restoration improves mechanical intraventricular dyssynchrony in ischemic cardiomyopathy. Circulation 2004;109:2536–43.
64. Dor V. Left ventricular reconstruction: the aim and the reality after twenty years. J Thorac Cardiovasc Surg 2004;128:17–20.
65. Shapira OM, Davidoff R, Hilkert RJ, et al. Repair of left ventricular aneurysm: long-term results of linear repair versus endoaneurysmorrhaphy. Ann Thorac Surg 1997;63:701–5.
66. Jones RH, Velazquez EJ, Michler RE, et al. Coronary bypass surgery with or without surgical ventricular reconstruction. N Engl J Med 2009;360:1705–17.
67. Epstein AE, DiMarco JP, Ellenbogen KA, et al. 2012 ACCF/AHA/HRS focused update incorporated into the ACCF/AHA/HRS 2008 guidelines for device-based therapy of cardiac rhythm abnormalities: a report of the American College of Cardiology Foundation/American Heart Association Task Force on Practice Guidelines and the Heart Rhythm Society. Circulation 2013;127:e283–352.
68. Di Biase L, Auricchio A, Mohanty P, et al. Impact of cardiac resynchronization therapy on the severity of mitral regurgitation. Europace 2011;13:829–38.
69. van Bommel RJ, Marsan NA, Delgado V, et al. Cardiac resynchronization therapy as a therapeutic option in patients with moderate-severe functional mitral regurgitation and high operative risk. Circulation 2011;124:912–19.
70. Levine RA, Schwammenthal E. Ischemic mitral regurgitation on the threshold of a solution: from paradoxes to unifying concepts. Circulation 2005;112:745–58.
71. Beeri R, Yosefy C, Guerrero JL, et al. Mitral regurgitation augments post-myocardial infarction remodeling failure of hypertrophic compensation. J Am Coll Cardiol 2008;51:476–86.
72. Kaul S, Spotnitz WD, Glasheen WP, Touchstone DA. Mechanism of ischemic mitral regurgitation. An experimental evaluation. Circulation 1991;84:2167–80.
73. Zoghbi WA, Enriquez-Sarano M, Foster E, et al. Recommendations for evaluation of the severity of native valvular regurgitation with two-dimensional and Doppler echocardiography. J Am Soc Echocardiogr 2003;16:777–802.
74. Enriquez-Sarano M, Sinak LJ, Tajik AJ, et al. Changes in effective regurgitant orifice throughout systole in patients with mitral valve prolapse. A clinical study using the proximal isovelocity surface area method. Circulation 1995;92:2951–8.
75. Enriquez-Sarano M, Dujardin KS, Tribouilloy CM, et al. Determinants of pulmonary venous flow reversal in mitral regurgitation and its usefulness in determining the severity of regurgitation. Am J Cardiol 1999;83:535–41.

76. Bouma W, van der Horst IC, Wijdh-den Hamer IJ, et al. Chronic ischaemic mitral regurgitation. Current treatment results and new mechanism-based surgical approaches. Eur J Cardiothorac Surg 2010;37:170–85.
77. Mihaljevic T, Lam BK, Rajeswaran J, et al. Impact of mitral valve annuloplasty combined with revascularization in patients with functional ischemic mitral regurgitation. J Am Coll Cardiol 2007;49:2191–201.
78. Magne J, Girerd N, Senechal M, et al. Mitral repair versus replacement for ischemic mitral regurgitation: comparison of short-term and long-term survival. Circulation 2009;120:S104–11.
79. Deja MA, Grayburn PA, Sun B, et al. Influence of mitral regurgitation repair on survival in the surgical treatment for ischemic heart failure trial. Circulation 2012;125:2639–48.
80. Chan KM, Punjabi PP, Flather M, et al. Coronary artery bypass surgery with or without mitral valve annuloplasty in moderate functional ischemic mitral regurgitation: final results of the Randomized Ischemic Mitral Evaluation (RIME) trial. Circulation 2012;126:2502–10.
81. Byrne JG, Aklog L, Adams DH. Assessment and management of functional or ischaemic mitral regurgitation. Lancet 2000;355:1743–4.
82. Penicka M, Linkova H, Lang O, et al. Predictors of improvement of unrepaired moderate ischemic mitral regurgitation in patients undergoing elective isolated coronary artery bypass graft surgery. Circulation 2009;120:1474–81.
83. McGee EC, Gillinov AM, Blackstone EH, et al. Recurrent mitral regurgitation after annuloplasty for functional ischemic mitral regurgitation. J Thorac Cardiovasc Surg 2004;128:916–24.
84. Murphy MO, Ahmed K, Athanasiou T. Surgery for chronic ischemic mitral regurgitation—which mitral intervention? Expert review of cardiovascular therapy 2011;9:587–97.
85. Silbiger JJ. Mechanistic insights into ischemic mitral regurgitation: echocardiographic and surgical implications. J Am Soc Echocardiogr 2011;24:707–19.
86. Athanasiou T, Chow A, Rao C, et al. Preservation of the mitral valve apparatus: evidence synthesis and critical reappraisal of surgical techniques. Eur J Cardiothorac Surg 2008;33:391–401.
87. Vassileva CM, Boley T, Markwell S, Hazelrigg S. Meta-analysis of short-term and long-term survival following repair versus replacement for ischemic mitral regurgitation. Eur J Cardiothorac Surg 2011;39:295–303.
88. Gillinov AM, Wierup PN, Blackstone EH, et al. Is repair preferable to replacement for ischemic mitral regurgitation? J Thorac Cardiovasc Surg 2001;122:1125–41.
89. Agricola E, Ielasi A, Oppizzi M, et al. Long-term prognosis of medically treated patients with functional mitral regurgitation and left ventricular dysfunction. Eur J Heart Fail 2009;11:581–7.
90. Svensson LG, Atik FA, Cosgrove DM, et al. Minimally invasive versus conventional mitral valve surgery: a propensity-matched comparison. J Thorac Cardiovasc Surg 2010;139:926–32 e1–2.
91. Petracek MR, Leacche M, Solenkova N, et al. Minimally invasive mitral valve surgery expands the surgical options for high-risks patients. Ann Surg 2011;254:606–11.
92. Brittain EL, Goyal S, Leacche M, et al. Minimally-invasive mitral valve replacement without aortic cross-clamp is safe in patients with severe cardiomyopathy. J Am Coll Cardiol 2012;59:E1996.
93. Stewart GC, O'Gara PT. Valvular heart disease. In Irwin and Rippe's Intensive Care Medicine, 7th edition, Chapter 34. Philadelphia: Lippincott, Williams and Wilkins; 2012: pp. 328–46.
94. Ross J, Jr., Braunwald E. Aortic stenosis. Circulation 1968;38:61–7.
95. Carabello BA. Aortic stenosis: from pressure overload to heart failure. Heart Fail Clin 2006;2:435–42.
96. Mookadam F, Moustafa SE, Khandheria B. Management of aortic valve disease in the presence of left ventricular dysfunction. Expert Rev Cardiovasc Ther 2010;8:259–68.
97. Carabello BA. Clinical practice. Aortic stenosis. N Engl J Med 2002;346:677–82.
98. Quere JP, Monin JL, Levy F, et al. Influence of preoperative left ventricular contractile reserve on postoperative ejection fraction in low-gradient aortic stenosis. Circulation 2006;113:1738–44.
99. Tribouilloy C, Levy F, Rusinaru D, et al. Outcome after aortic valve replacement for low-flow/low-gradient aortic stenosis without contractile reserve on dobutamine stress echocardiography. J Am Coll Cardiol 2009;53:1865–73.
100. Clavel MA, Fuchs C, Burwash IG, et al. Predictors of outcomes in low-flow, low-gradient aortic stenosis: results of the multicenter TOPAS Study. Circulation 2008;118:S234–42.
101. Picano E, Pibarot P, Lancellotti P, et al. The emerging role of exercise testing and stress echocardiography in valvular heart disease. J Am Coll Cardiol 2009;54:2251–60.
102. Grayburn PA. Assessment of low-gradient aortic stenosis with dobutamine. Circulation 2006;113:604–6.
103. Carabello BA. Is it ever too late to operate on the patient with valvular heart disease? J Am Coll Cardiol 2004;44:376–83.
104. Bonow RO, Carabello BA, Chatterjee K, et al. 2008 Focused update incorporated into the ACC/AHA 2006 guidelines for the management of patients with valvular heart disease: a report of the American College of Cardiology/American Heart Association Task Force on Practice Guidelines (Writing Committee to Revise the 1998 Guidelines for the Management of Patients With Valvular Heart Disease): endorsed by the Society of Cardiovascular Anesthesiologists, Society for Cardiovascular Angiography and Interventions, and Society of Thoracic Surgeons. Circulation 2008;118:e523–661.
105. George TJ, Arnaoutakis GJ, Shah AS. Surgical treatment of advanced heart failure: alternatives to heart transplantation and mechanical circulatory assist devices. Prog Cardiovasc Dis 2011;54:115–31.
106. Levy F, Laurent M, Monin JL, et al. Aortic valve replacement for low-flow/low-gradient aortic stenosis operative risk stratification and long-term outcome: a European multicenter study. J Am Coll Cardiol 2008;51:1466–72.
107. Monin JL, Quere JP, Monchi M, et al. Low-gradient aortic stenosis: operative risk stratification and predictors for long-term outcome: a multicenter study using dobutamine stress hemodynamics. Circulation 2003;108:319–24.
108. Connolly HM, Oh JK, Schaff HV, et al. Severe aortic stenosis with low transvalvular gradient and severe left ventricular dysfunction:result of aortic valve replacement in 52 patients. Circulation 2000;101:1940–6.
109. Kulik A, Burwash IG, Kapila V, et al. Long-term outcomes after valve replacement for low-gradient aortic stenosis: impact of prosthesis-patient mismatch. Circulation 2006;114:I553–8.
110. Smith CR, Leon MB, Mack MJ, et al. Transcatheter versus surgical aortic-valve replacement in high-risk patients. N Engl J Med 2012;364:2187–98.
111. Leon MB, Smith CR, Mack M, et al. Transcatheter aortic-valve implantation for aortic stenosis in patients who cannot undergo surgery. N Engl J Med 2012;363:1597–607.
112. Kodali SK, Williams MR, Smith CR, et al. Two-year outcomes after transcatheter or surgical aortic-valve replacement. N Engl J Med 2012;366:1686–95.
113. Holmes DR, Jr., Rich JB, Zoghbi WA, Mack MJ. The heart team of cardiovascular care. J Am Coll Cardiol 2013;61:903–7.
114. Chaliki HP, Mohty D, Avierinos JF, et al. Outcomes after aortic valve replacement in patients with severe aortic regurgitation and markedly reduced left ventricular function. Circulation 2002;106:2687–93.
115. Tam JW, Antecol D, Kim HH, et al. Low dose dobutamine echocardiography in the assessment of contractile reserve to predict the outcome of valve replacement for chronic aortic regurgitation. Can J Cardiol 1999;15:73–9.
116. Bonow RO, Carabello BA, Chatterjee K, et al. 2008 focused update incorporated into the ACC/AHA 2006 guidelines for the management of patients with valvular heart disease: a report of the American College of Cardiology/American Heart Association Task Force on Practice Guidelines (Writing Committee to revise the 1998 guidelines for the management of patients with valvular heart disease). Endorsed by the Society of Cardiovascular Anesthesiologists, Society

for Cardiovascular Angiography and Interventions, and Society of Thoracic Surgeons. J Am Coll Cardiol 2008;52:e1–142.

117. Schinkel AF, Bax JJ, Poldermans D, et al. Hibernating myocardium: diagnosis and patient outcomes. Curr Probl Cardiol 2007;32:375–410.

118. Umakanthan R, Leacche M, Petracek MR, et al. Safety of minimally invasive mitral valve surgery without aortic cross-clamp. Ann Thorac Surg 2008;85:1544–9; discussion 49–50.

CHAPTER 14

Mechanical circulatory support: Patient selection, optimization, and in-patient management of the patient with a left ventricular assist device

Michael J. Domanski MD and Mandeep R. Mehra MD

A perspective on mechanical circulatory support

Though data are limited, about 2% of patients with clinical heart failure (HF) in the United States can be classified as refractory (stage D of the American College of Cardiology (ACC)/American Heart Association (AHA) ABCD classification) and have an approximately 80% 5-year mortality.[1,2] For the stage D patients who are appropriate candidates, heart transplantation, with a 1-year survival of 87% and a 10-year survival of 50%,[3] is the treatment that offers the best longevity and quality of life. However, only about 2200 donor hearts become available each year[4] in the US, making transplantation a treatment available to only a small minority of patients with advanced HF. Alternatives to allograft transplantation may include xenotransplantation, cellular therapy (stem cells, angiogenesis), or a mechanical total artificial heart (TAH). Current applicable science and engineering have not matured sufficiently at this time to establish any of these as effective, durable solutions.

In contrast, implantable left ventricular assist devices (LVADs) that support out-of-hospital ambulatory patients have been developed to the point of widespread and expanding clinical use and the technology continues to improve. Most of the rest of this chapter focuses on continuous-flow LVADs with the HeartMate II (Thoratec, Pleasanton, CA) and HeartWare HVAD (HeartWare, Inc., Framingham, MA) as the typical axial flow and centrifugal flow pump prototypes, understanding that the principles adduced apply to other LVAD systems of which many will be entering the marketplace.

Indications for LVAD implantation

Historically, the first use of LVADs was as a bridge to transplant; that is, to provide the hemodynamic support needed by highly selected patients to survive while awaiting transplant. However, the most frequent indication for LVAD placement now is as permanent support for patients who are not transplant candidates; that is, as "destination" devices. In this context, the indication is more aptly referred to as "lifetime therapy," indicating a durable device capable of prolonging lifespan with maintenance of a reasonable quality of life. Another indication is as a "bridge to decision" (in those currently ineligible for transplantation but with potentially reversible underlying relative contraindications such as renal insufficiency or pulmonary hypertension).

Indications for LVAD implantation in nontransplant candidates

In order to efficiently discuss the role of mechanical circulatory support (MCS), we introduce the INTERMACS classification scheme, put forth by Stevenson and her colleagues,[1] that classifies advanced HF according to level of dysfunction (Table 14.1). Patients in INTERMACS class 1 (IC1) are in cardiogenic shock, IC2 patients are deteriorating despite inotropic therapy, IC3 patients are stable but require inotropic therapy (or MCS or both), and the remaining profiles 4–7 imply varying stages of severity in ambulatory patients not on continuous inotropic therapy. The INTERMACS classification system is particularly valuable because prognosis is strongly related to the clinical attributes that determine the classification.

This discussion of LVAD indications proceeds with the assumption that rapidly reversible causes of HF are absent, that conventional medical therapies of HF have been attempted, and that the advanced HF state persists.

Placement of an LVAD is indicated when survival is considered to be improved compared to medical therapy. The REMATCH trial,[5] published in 2001, was the first randomized study, and demonstrated that survival of end-stage transplant-ineligible HF

Table 14.1 INTERMACS classification of limitation

INTERMACS profiles	Descriptions	Time frame for intervention
Profile 1: Critical cardiogenic shock	Patients with life-threatening hypotension despite rapidly escalating inotropic support, critical organ hypoperfusion, often confirmed by worsening acidosis and/or lactate levels *"Crash and burn"*	Definitive intervention needed within hours
Profile 2: Progressive decline	Patient with declining function despite IV inotropic support, may be manifest by worsening renal function, nutritional depletion, inability to restore volume balance *"Sliding on inotropes"* Also describes declining status in patients unable to tolerate inotropic therapy	Definitive intervention needed within a few days
Profile 3: Stable but inotrope dependent	Patient with stable blood pressure, organ function, nutrition, and symptoms on continuous intravenous inotropic support (or a temporary circulatory support device or both), but demonstrating repeated failure to wean from support due to recurrent symptomatic hypotension or renal dysfunction *"Dependent stability"*	Definitive intervention elective over a period of weeks to few months
Profile 4: Resting symptoms	Patient can be stabilized close to normal volume status but experiences daily symptoms of congestion at rest or during ADL. Doses of diuretics generally fluctuate at very high levels. More intensive management and surveillance strategies should be considered, which may in some cases reveal poor compliance that would compromise outcomes with any therapy. Some patients may shuttle between profiles 4 and 5	Definitive intervention elective over period of weeks to a few months
Profile 5: Exertion intolerant	Comfortable at rest and with ADL but unable to engage in any other activity, living predominantly within the house. Patients are comfortable at rest without congestive symptoms, but may have underlying refractory elevated volume status, often with renal dysfunction. If underlying nutritional status and organ function are marginal, patient may be more at risk than INTERMACS 4, and require definitive intervention	Variable urgency, depends upon maintenance of nutrition, organ function, and activity
Profile 6: Exertion limited	Patient without evidence of fluid overload is comfortable at rest, and with ADL and minor activities outside the home but fatigues after the first few minutes of any meaningful activity. Attribution to cardiac limitation requires careful measurement of peak oxygen consumption, in some cases with hemodynamic monitoring to confirm severity of cardiac impairment *"Walking wounded"*	Variable, depends on maintenance of nutrition, organ function, and activity level
Profile 7: Advanced NYHA III	A placeholder for more precise specification in future, this level includes patients who are without current or recent episodes of unstable fluid balance, living comfortably but with meaningful activity limited to mild physical exertion	Transplantation or circulatory support may not currently be indicated
Modifiers for profiles		Possible profiles to modify
TCS (temporary circulatory support)	Can modify only patients in hospital (other devices would be INTERMACS devices) Includes IABP, ECHO, TandemHeart, Levitronix, BVS 5000 or AB5000, Impella	Profiles 1, 2, 3 in hospital
A (arrhythmia)	Can modify any profile. Recurrent VTs that have recently contributed substantially to clinical compromise. This includes frequent ICD shock or requirement for external defibrillator, usually more than twice weekly	Any profile
FF (frequent flyer)	Can modify only outpatients, designating a patient requiring frequent emergency visits or hospitalizations for diuretics, ultrafiltration, or temporary IV vasoactive therapy.	Profile 3 if at home, 4, 5, 6. A frequent flyer would rarely be profile 7

ADL, activities of daily living; ICD, implantable cardioverter defibrillator; VT, ventricular tachyarrhythmia.

patients could be improved by implantation of an LVAD. Motivated by prolonged successful support of patients with LVADs placed as a bridge to transplant, REMATCH randomized 129 advanced HF patients who were not transplant candidates to optimal medical therapy or to optimal medical therapy and LVAD implantation with a first-generation pulsatile-flow device (Thoratec XVE). Entry criteria were a left ventricular ejection fraction (LVEF) 25% or less, peak VO_2 12 ml/kg/min or less, and NYHA functional class IV HF for at least 90 days despite treatment with diuretic, digitalis, and angiotensin converting enzyme (ACE) inhibitor; or the patient had to be inotrope dependent. The indications were later broadened to include patients who were in NYHA functional class III and IV HF for at least 28 days and who had received 14 days of intra-aortic balloon pump (IABP) therapy or were inotrope dependent despite weaning attempts with peak VO_2 14 ml/kg/min or less (only five patients were entered into the trial based on these criteria).

There was a highly significant 48% reduction in risk of all-cause mortality, the primary endpoint of the trial (Figure 14.1); 1-year survival was 52% in the device group and 25% in the medical therapy group. The 2-year survival was 23% in the device group

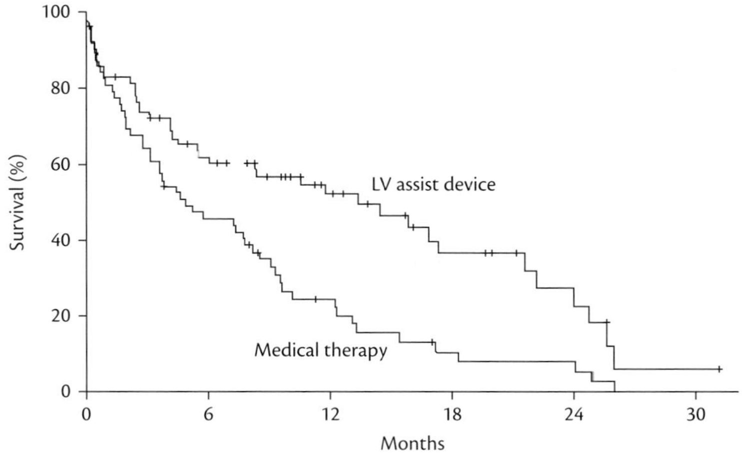

No. AT Risk						
LV assist device	68	38	22	11	5	1
Medical therapy	61	27	11	4	3	0

Fig. 14.1 REMATCH results.

From New England Journal of Medicine, Rose E, Gelljns A, Moskowitz A, et al. Long-term use of a left ventricular assist device for end-stage heart failure, 345; 1435–1443, copyright © (2001) Massachusetts Medical Society. Reprinted with permission from Massachusetts Medical Society.

and only 8% in the medical therapy group, confirming the tenuous prognosis of those meeting the eligibility criteria.

The central importance of the REMATCH trial is that this was the first demonstration that an LVAD could prolong a patient's life in the absence of a subsequent transplant. Also, the survival of medically treated patients with this severity of HF was well characterized in REMATCH and was dismal. This said, despite its superiority over medical therapy, survival in the LVAD group was also poor and the pulsatile LVADs did not achieve widespread clinical application as destination therapy.

The device used in the REMATCH trial was a large first-generation pulsatile device with limited durability. Pulsatile LVADs have now been essentially completely replaced by second-generation continuous-flow devices. These are small turbopumps that continuously pump blood from the left ventricle (LV) into the aorta. Current devices are quiet and allow tether-free movement using external battery packs, thus permitting many of the usual activities of daily living to continue.

The Thoratec HeartMate II continuous-flow LVAD has been studied in a randomized clinical trial comparing it to the pulsatile Thoratec XVE LVAD. Slaughter et al.[6] randomized 200 patients who had LVEF less than 25%, peak Vo_2 less than 14 ml kg^{-1} min^{-1} or less than 50% of predicted, were in NYHA functional class IIIb or IV for at least 45 of the 60 days preceding randomization, and were not considered candidates for cardiac transplantation. Alternatively, patients could be enrolled if they were IABP dependent for at least 7 days or inotrope dependent for 14 days prior to enrollment. The primary composite endpoint of the trial was survival free of disabling stroke or reoperation to repair or replace the LVAD.

The survival results are shown in Figure 14.2. Estimated 1-year and 2-year event-free survival for the continuous-flow LVAD was respectively 68% and 58% and for the pulsatile LVAD 55% and 24%: a dramatically better event-free survival with the continuous-flow device. While survival with the pulsatile device was marginally better than in the REMATCH trial, the reason was likely the 31% crossover rate to the continuous-flow LVAD. In fact, only 11% of the pulsatile-flow LVAD patients were alive with the pulsatile device still in place at 2 years.

There are comparatively limited data with medical therapy in the current era. In the INTrEPID study, Rogers et al.[7] compared matched patients with advanced HF treated with continuous-flow LVADs to patients treated with optimal medical therapy but no LVAD. Of importance is that patients treated medically had dismal survival (90% 1-year mortality) similar to the previously reported medically treated cohort in REMATCH. So, while the use of the continuous-flow LVAD materially improves survival compared to the pulastile devices, major strides have not occurred in medical therapy, giving us a stable estimate of survival without an LVAD. One reason for this is that as the HF transitions to late stages, the ability to tolerate disease-modifying neurohormonal therapy wanes significantly (see Chapter 8). Furthermore, no new therapy that can be applied in this progressive decline situation has become available and inotropic therapy remains the only supportive treatment. Inotropic therapy, however, is a double-edged sword that provides temporary support but with the potential to accelerate disease progression. Recently, published data from the INTERMACS Registry[8] suggest continued improvement in survival for LVAD-treated patients with a 2-year survival that now exceeds 70%, far better than could be expected with medical therapy.

The studies discussed so far are summarized in Figure 14.3. Patients entered into these studies correspond generally to classes IC1–IC4 and were not transplant candidates. However, the prognosis for patients in IC1 (cardiogenic shock; "crash and burn") even with an LVAD are much inferior to the results for patients in IC2–IC4 and IC1 patients should be stabilized with temporary LV or biventricular support devices (discussed below).

For some patients, the contraindications to transplant resolve following LVAD implantation. Pulmonary hypertension, hepatic dysfunction, and renal insufficiency may all improve in the hemodynamic milieu provided by the LVAD.[9,10,11] For these patients, the

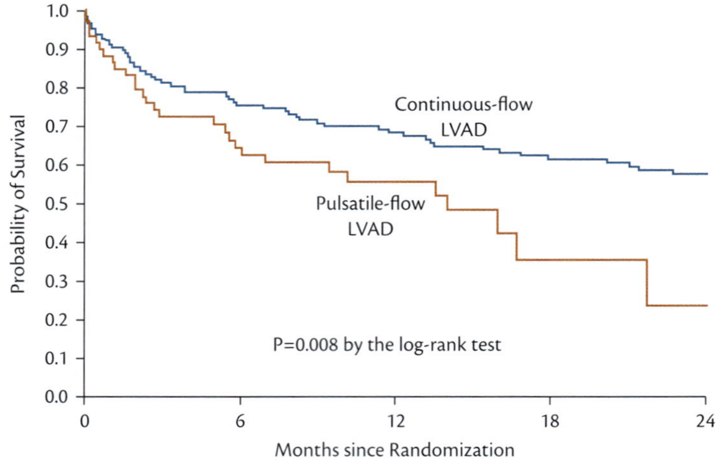

No. at Risk					
Continuous-flow LVAD	133	95	82	69	62
Pulsatile-flow LVAD	59	32	19	5	2

Fig. 14.2 Survival following continuous-flow left ventricular assist device (LVAD) versus pulsatile-flow LVAD.
From New England Journal of Medicine, Slaughter et al, Advanced Heart Failure Treated with Continuous-Flow Left Ventricular Assist Device,361:2241–2251, Copyright © (2001) Massachusetts Medical Society. Reprinted with permission from Massachusetts Medical Society.

LVAD, is, in effect, a "bridge" to transplant candidacy and to the improved prognosis that follows tranplantation.

From the above, a picture emerges of the patient who, in the absence of a transplant, has a better survival with an LVAD than without, many of whom may also be bridged to candidacy. Generally, the patients in these trials fit into the IC2–IC4 category and do not have an unacceptable comorbidity.

Using these data, the US Center for Medicare and Medicaid Services (CMS) defined the subset of nontransplant candidates for whom destination therapy improves survival and for whom they will reimburse device placement. To qualify, these patients must have the following characteristics:[12]

- NYHA class IV HF symptoms that have failed to respond to optimal medical management including dietary salt restriction, diuretics, digitalis, β-blockers, and ACE inhibitors (if tolerated) for at least 60 of the last 90 days
- LVEF) less than 25%

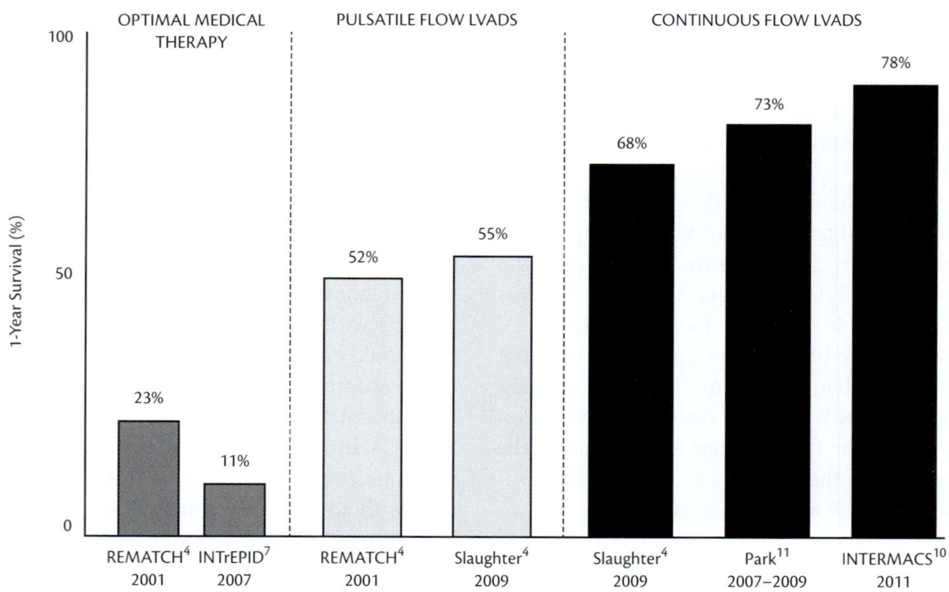

Fig. 14.3 Survival in advanced heart failure.
Mehra, Mandeep and Domanski, Michael, Should Left Ventricular Assist Device Should Be Standard of Care for Patients With Refractory Heart Failure Who Are Not Transplantation Candidates?: Left Ventricular Assist Devices Should Be Considered Standard of Care for Patients With Refractory Heart Failure Who Are Not Transplantation Candidates, Circulation, 126, 3081–3087.

- Functional limitation indicated by a peak oxygen consumption of less than 12 ml kg^{-1} min^{-1}; or the patient has a continued need for IV inotropic therapy owing to symptomatic hypotension, decreasing renal function, or worsening pulmonary congestion
- Adequate body size ($\geq$1.5 m^2) to support the LVAD implantation.

Bridge to transplantation

MCS is indicated in heart transplant candidates who are unable to maintain adequate organ perfusion to survive while awaiting transplant. In this setting the LVAD can materially improve long-term survival, not only by improving survival to transplant but also by presenting the patient for transplant in a hemodynamically compensated state with normal or improved renal, hepatic, and neurologic function.

Disadvantages of LVAD implantion include device-related complications, HLA sensitization, additional cardiovascular surgery with the risk of complications, and the additional complexity of the subsequent transplant procedure. Despite these concerns, available data suggest that survival following transplant in patients bridged to transplant is similar to the survival in transplanted patients not requiring MCS before transplant.[13,14]

To summarize, the available data show that:

- There exists a group of patients who have an extremely poor prognosis on medical therapy alone. These individuals generally correspond to IC1–IC4 patients. IC1 patients should be treated with temporary support, including biventricular as needed (see below). For this group of patients, survival is best for those who can be transplanted, worst for those who receive only optimal medical therapy, and intermediate for those receiving a destination continuous-flow LVAD (Figure 14.4).
- IC2–IC4 patients have improved survival following LVAD implantation compared to optimal medical therapy alone.
- Over time, survival of LVAD patients has improved but survival with optimal medical therapy in these patients remains similar to that seen in the REMATCH trial.
- Implicit in the decision-making is the understanding that survival with transplantation is superior to that currently available from LVAD placement for the small minority of patients for whom it becomes available and so the feasibility of transplantation should at least be considered in each of them.

Investigation of the role of the LVAD in "less sick" patients (those not yet requiring an inotrope) is ongoing in the REVIVE-IT trial.[15] This trial is a proof-of-concept study evaluating broadened indications for device use.

Patient selection and optimization

We have developed the indications for LVAD placement as they currently exist. However, patients meeting these indications vary substantially in their survival and functionality following implant, depending largely on the presence and severity of comorbidities (Table 14.2). A central task in the medical management of these patients is recognizing their prognosis-impacting attributes and incorporating these into the management plan. We turn now to issues of patient selection and optimization in individuals with nominal indications for MCS.

Right heart function

The role of the right heart is to provide sufficient oxygenated preload to the left heart to maintain perfusion and to do so with right-sided pressures low enough to avoid liver and kidney dysfunction. Inadequate right heart function following LVAD implantation is a frequent cause of morbidity (multiorgan system failure) and death following LVAD implantation as well as poorer outcomes after transplant.[16,17,18,19,20] For patients whose right ventricle (RV) fails and, as a result, require biventricular support, the hazard ratio for death is 3.27 compared to individuals receiving an LVAD and not requiring biventricular support (see Table 14.2). Hence, we need to assess the right heart function preoperatively to determine whether RV failure will occur post-LVAD implant. Parameters that portend a poor prognosis include low RV stroke work index (RVSWI), end-organ dysfunction, and moderate or

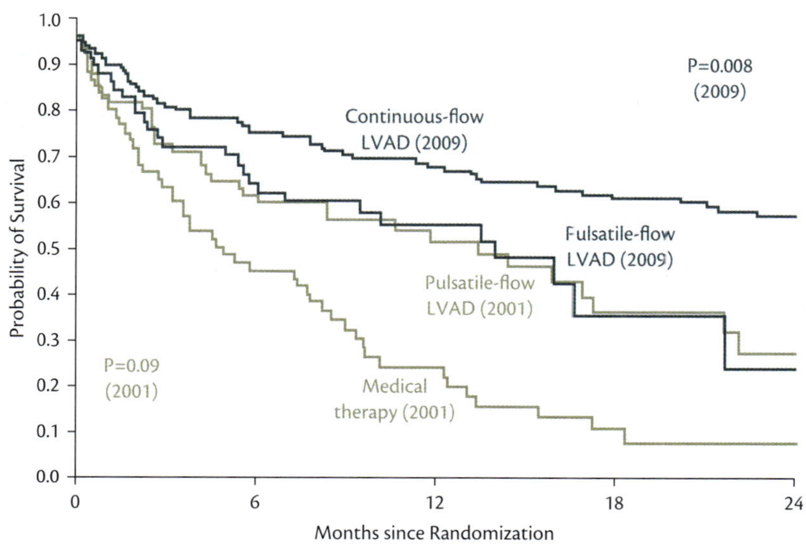

Fig. 14.4 Comparison of survival with transplantation, destination therapy with a continuous-flow left ventricular assist device (LVAD), and with a pulsatile LVAD.
From New England Journal of Medicine, Fang JC, Rise of the Machines—Left Ventricular Assist Devices as Permanent Therapy for Advanced Heart Failure;361:2282–2285, Copyright © (2009) Massachusetts Medical Society. Reprinted with permission from Massachusetts Medical Society.

Table 14.2 Preoperative risk factors for post-LVAD death in 43 666 primary implant patients, June 2006 to June 2011

	Early hazard		Constant hazard	
Risk factors	**HR**	***p*-value**	**HR**	***p*-value**
Age, older	1.54[a]	<0.0001	1.30[a]	0.0001
BSA, larger	1.48[b]	0.0006		
Female			1.36	0.01
History of				
CABG	1.84	<0.0001		
Valve surgery	1.81	0.0007		
CVA	1.74	0.005		
Bilirubin, higher	1.10[c]	<0.0001		
Creatinine, higher	1.16[d]	0.01		
BUN, higher			1.08[e]	0.001
RA pressure, higher	1.21[f]	0.0004		
Ascites	1.55	0.007		
Pulmonary hypertension			1.49	0.03
INTERMACS				
Level 1	2.87	<0.0001		
Level 2	1.84	0.001	1.35	0.01
Bridge to candidacy			1.38	0.009
Destination therapy			1.38	0.009
Pulsatile-flow LVAD			3.01	<0.0001
BiVAD	3.27	<0.0001		
Concomitant surgery	1.36	0.01		

BiVAD, biventricular assist device; BSA, body surface area; BUN, blood area nitrogen; CABG, coronary artery bypass grafting; CVA, cerebral vascular accident; HR, hazard ratio; INTERMACS, Interagency Registry for Mechanically Assisted Circulatory Support; LVAD, left ventricular assist device; RA, right atrial.

The hazard ratio denotes the increased risk: (a) from age 70 to 80; (b) of a 0.5-unit increase in BSA; (c) of a 1.0-unit increase in bilirubin; (d) of a 1.0-unit increase in creatinine; (e) of a 1.0-unit increase in BUN; and (f) of a 5.0-unit increase in RA pressure.

Reprinted from Journal of Heart and Lung Transplantation, 26, Radovancevic B et al., End-organ function in patients on long-term circulatory support with continuous-or pulsatile-flow assist devices, 815–818, copyright (2007) with permission from Elsevier. INTERMACS Registry data Reprinted from the American Journal of Cardiology, 53, Moreno F et al., Evaluation of size and dynamics of the inferior vena cava as an index of right sided cardiac function, 579–585, copyright (1984) with permission from Elsevier.

severe tricuspid regurgitation. Were it possible to provide an accurate preoperative prediction about whether a particular RV would fail following LVAD placement, management would be greatly simplified. Unfortunately, while some risk stratificaton is possible, precise prediction is not. For this reason continuing postoperative surveillance for the development of right-sided failure is essential to avoid organ system failure (kidneys, liver) including by placing a RV assist device if necessary.

Hemodynamic assessment

An initial question in a patient with a failing ciriculation in whom MCS is contemplated, is what type of durable MCS to apply, whether an LVAD or biventricular device. The device most commonly decided upon is the LVAD. Apart from loss of contractility caused by the underlying disease process, there are a number of stresses on the RV that attend the HF state and the placement of an LVAD.[21,22,23] Pulmonary vascular resistance (PVR) is frequently elevated in HF patients prior to surgery. Cardiopulmonary bypass challenges RV function by increasing PVR (increased RV afterload); causing major fluid shifts consequent upon administration of colloids and other fluids that increase RV load; and right coronary air embolism as a cardiopulmonary bypass-mediated inflammatory response can occur. Also, LVAD placement alters the geometry of the right (by leftward septal shift) and LV (remodeling), potentially compromising RV performance.

Reduced preoperative RV contractility increases the risk of RV failure. Contractile function can be inferred from the imaging workup (discussed below) but systolic (and diastolic) ventricular perfomance vary with different loading conditions as well as with contractility. Being able to estimate RV contractility independent of the loading conditions to the extent practical is important. The RVSWI is a measure of the capacity of the RV to add energy to the flow, and can be routinely estimated for clinical purposes as

$$\text{RVSWI} = \frac{(\text{PAM-RVEDP})\,\text{SV}}{\text{BSA}}$$

where BSA is body surface area, PAM is mean pulmonary artery pressure, RVEDP is RV end-diastolic pressure, and SV is stroke volume (cardiac output/heart rate).[24] In the intensive care unit (ICU) the central venous pressure (CVP) is generally substituted for RVEDP. There have been a number of studies of RVSWI as a predictor of postoperative right HF. Shenk et al.[25]showed an association between preoperative RVSWI and need for prolonged postimplant (>14 days) inotropic support (38% for <300 mmHg ml m^{-2}, 29% for 600–900 mmHg ml m^{-2} and 3% for RVSWI >900 mmHg ml m^{-2}). A RVSWI less than 300 mmHg ml m^{-2} has been associated with the need for insertion of a RV assist device (RVAD).[18,26]

Elevated PVR (particularly when >5 Wood units), though a relative contrainidcation to transplantation is not a barrier to MCS placement; indeed, PVR tends to fall after LVAD implant potentially bridging the patient to transplant candidacy.[16,18,27,28]

Additionally, more than moderate tricuspid regurgitation is a risk factor for right HF following LVAD implantation and should be corrected as part of the implant procedure.[6]

Scoring systems have been developed to assist in stratifying risk for RV failure after LVAD placement.[29,30] In general, poor hemodynamic indices, including elevated filling pressure, as well as evidence of end-organ dysfunction (kidney, liver) add risk. Each of the modeling schemes has a variety of limitations that reduce prediction accuracy.

Noninvasive assessment of the right ventricle

Noninvasive imaging can provide extensive characterization of the right heart and substantially extend the understanding available from invasive monitoring. Also, along with the physical examination, imaging is the only way to characterize the right heart structure and function outside the critical care setting.

Guidelines for the echo assessment of right heart function have been published by the American Society of Echocardiography (ASE)[31] and physicians specializing in advanced HF should be familiar with their application. Right atrial pressure can be

Table 14.3 Estimation of right heart pressure

Variable	Normal[a](0–5 [3] mmHg)	Intermediate[b](5–10 [8] mmHg)		High(15 mmHg)
IVC diameter	≤2.1 cm	≤2.1 cm	>2.1 cm	>2.1 cm
Collapse with sniff	>50%	<50%	>50%	<50%
Secondary indices of elevated RA pressure				Restrictive filling Tricuspid E/E′>6 Diastolic flow predominance in hepatic veins (systolic filling fraction <55%)

IVC, inferior vena cava; RA, right atrial.

[a] Ranges are provided for low and intermediate categories, but for simplicity, midrange values of 3 mmHg for normal and 8 mm Hg for intermediate are suggested.

[b] Intermediate (8 mmHg) RA pressures may be downgraded to normal (3 mmHg) if no secondary indices of elevated RA pressure are present, upgraded to high if minimal collapse with sniff (<35%) and secondary indices of elevated RA pressure are present, or left at 8 mmHg if uncertain.

estimated from echocardiographic investigation of the inferior vena cava (Table 14.3)[32] and used in calculations. Well-defined standards have been published for RV size and can be found in the ASE guidelines. Right ventricular systolic function can be estimated in a number of ways. For patients without an implanted device (including prior to LVAD placement), MRI can define RV structure and make a geometry-independent estimate of RV ejection fraction (normal ≥0.45). A geometry-independent estimate can also be made using a first-pass study with radionuclide ventriulograhy whether or not an implant is present. The geometry of the RV and difficulties with endocardial definition limit conventional echocardiography but the fractional area change can often be assessed, particularly with the use of an echocardiographic contrast material (normal ≥0.35). Tricuspid annular septal motion (TAPSE) is another measure of systolic function and is obtained using a two-dimensional guided M-mode cursuor positioned across the tricuspid annulus (normal ≥16 mm). By placing a tissue Doppler sample space at the tricuspid annulus assessment of tissue velocity (s') as a metric of systolic function (normal ≥10 cm/s), a variety of pressures can be estimated.

Right atrial pressure is used in a variety of calculations. Pressure gradients (in mmHg) across valves are estimated to be $4V^2$ where V is the speed (in meters/second) of the regurgitant jet, allowing RV systolic pressure to be estimated using the Doppler-derived velocity trace across the tricuspid valve and adding the right atrial pressure dervived from examination of the inferior vena cava (see Table 14.3). In the absence of pulmonic stenosis, this is also used to estimate pulmonary artery systolic pressure. Pulmonary artery diastolic pressure can be estimated if there is a pulmonary regurgitant jet using the estimated right atrial pressure as a measure of RV end-diastolic pressure. Also, a regression equation has been developed that makes use of the acceleration time of the pulmonary artery systolic velocity tralce to calculate mearn pulmonary artery pressure. Knowing the mean and systolic pressures in the pulmonary artery allows estimation of the pulmonary artery diastolic pressure.

Diastolic function of the RV can be assessed using tissue Doppler imaging of the tricuspid annulus (normal s' >6) and by assessing the E/A ratio in a manner analogous to assessing diastolic function of the LV (E/A <8 grade 1, >2.1 restrictive, and 0.8–2.1 with reduced s' grade 2). Right ventricular hypertrophy (free wall thickness >5 mm) can be diagnosed.

So, in summary, invasively and noninvasively, we can characterize the pre- and postoperative RV, estimate the preoperative liklihood that the RV will fail following implantation of an LVAD, and monitor for right heart dysfunction and failure following implantation. It is important to emphasize that there is no highly accurate method of preoperatively predicting RV failure post-LVAD. For this reason, early recognition of RV failure following LVAD implantation is essential to prevent multisystem organ failure (particularly kidneys and liver). The assessment of right heart function must take into account the right-sided hemodynamics, the structural and functional indices of the RV (size; severity of tricuspid regurgitation, TAPSE, and systolic function) and the presence or absence of hepatorenal comorbidity.

Treatment of right ventricular dysfunction

When right heart function is inadequate, treatment options include manipulation of RV preload and afterload, use of inotropic agents, and the placement of a a temporary or permanent RVAD. Additionally, a TAH or transplant can replace the right heart altogether.

Assuring adequate oxygenation and avoidance of hypercapnea and acidosis are imortant general measures in assuring appropriate right heart function. When right heart filling pressure is low (<10 mmHg) fluid loading to increase preload is indicated to increase right heart output.

Reduction of elevated afterload is essential to optimize output of the right heart. Nitric oxide acts by increasing cGMP in the pulmonary vasculature and is the most specific of the pulmonary vasodilators, causing essentially no systemic vasodilation and so avoding systemic hypotension.[33] Nitric oxide (5–40 ppm) is delivered by inhalation and so requires appropriate equipment. Standard nitrates are also effective pulmonary vasodilators but produce systemic vasodilation and the resulting systemic hypotension frequently limits the use of these drugs.[34,35] Prostaglandins (epoprostenol and iloprost) increase cGMP levels and result in nonspecific vasodilation, except perhaps in an inhaled form that may not have significant systemic effects.[36]

Milrinone is a phosphodiesteras inhibitor that increases cAMP level resulting in pulmonary and systemic vasodilation as well as increasing myocardial inotropy;[37] it may be considered as a vasodilator with inotropic properties. Dobutmine and isoproterenol also provide inotropic support to the RV and vasodilation. These three drugs, because they are nonselective vasodilators, can result in systemic hypotension. When right heart inotropic support is needed in a hypotensive patient epinephrine or norepinephrine should be considered because they are potent inotropes as well as pressors. When systemic vasoplegia complicates the clinical picture, resulting in systemic hypotension, vasopressin can be added as a pure vasoconstrictor. Digitalis is useful for long-term inotropic support of the chronically failing RV and sildenafil provides long-term pulmonary (and systemic) vasodilation.

Elevated right heart filling pressure, particularly exceeding about 15 mmHg, can result in kidney and liver failure. Diuresis is first line therapy. Nesiritide stimulates guanyl cyclase, raising cGMP levels causing diuresis; naturesis, and vasodilation;[38] reducing left heart filling pressure; and reducing systemic and PVR with an increase in cardiac output but not heart rate. However, the usefulness of this agent in right HF is less well established. Ultrafiltration is effective when pharmacologic agents do not produce the desired effect of volume reduction. None of these therapies have been shown to alter the long-term natural history of right HF and the scientific data available to guide the treatment of right HF are limited. In the current era, RV failure following continuous-flow LVAD implantation that is refractory to medical therapy has declined remarkably, occurring in only about 6% of cases.[39] Notable is the extremely poor prognosis that attends the need for biventricular support—43% 2-year survival (Figure 14.5),[39] underscoring the need for thoughtful patient selection and management.

When refractory RV dysfunction is recognized, MCS should be instituted promptly to avoid multiorgan system failure. In patients who require other than short-term biventricular support and who are transplant candidates, suppport with an implantable RVAD or a TAH is indicated. A key part of the decision regarding RV MCS is consideration of whether the right heart remains or would remain difficult to manage were it to be retained—for instance, if there were uncontrollable ventricular tachyarrhthmias, ventricular clots, or extensive ischemic damage. The CentriMag (Thoratex, Pleasanton, CA) temporary device is a reasonable choice for emergent support of a failing RV. If it is placed with cannulas compatible with the Thoratec PVAD, smooth conversion to long-term support is possible. However, destination therapy with these configurations is not practical and this biventricular support or TAH implantation should be limited to use as a bridge to transplant. It is essential that intraoperative management be instituted to focus on the right heart during LVAD placement. Right ventricular protection strategies include limitation of blood product transfusions, avoidance of right heart volume loading, protection of the right heart during cardiopulmonary bypass, and use of afterload reduction in the pulmonary circuit.

There is limited experience using two continuous-flow devices for biventricular support.

Decompensated heart failure and cardiogenic shock

Cardiogenic shock (IC1), is an important risk marker for death following LVAD implantation (see Table 14.2), with a hazard rato of 3.5 for IC1 patients.[39] This most likely indicates that with such extremely severe illness the major operative stress of LVAD placement is not tolerated. For this reason most centers now make use of effective temporary devices, some of which (e.g., the Impella; Abiomed, Inc., Danvers, MA) can be introduced percutaneously,[39] with the expectation that improved kidney and liver function will improve survival. Temporary LV or biventricular support is available and can incoporate an oxygenator in the circuit.

Renal function

Severe renal dysfunction preimplant predicts an adverse postimplant prognosis and the need for chronic dialysis is associated with a particularly poor prognosis and LVAD placement. Because of this, LVAD placement should generally be avoided in these patients.[40,41,42]

There are a number of mechanisms by which HF can be detrimental to renal function. Since the glomerular perfusion gradient is the difference between arterial and venous pressures across the kidneys, elevated right heart pressure (by increasing renal vein pressure) can reduce the GFR by reducing this pressure gradient. Where cardiac output is low, glomerular perfusion pressure and GFR are reduced and glomerular injury can result. Inotropic or mechanical support can improve renal perfusion by increasing cardiac output. High right-sided pressures can be lowered using diuretics. If diuretics are ineffective or result in the cardiorenal syndrome then mechanical fluid removal with ultrafiltration can

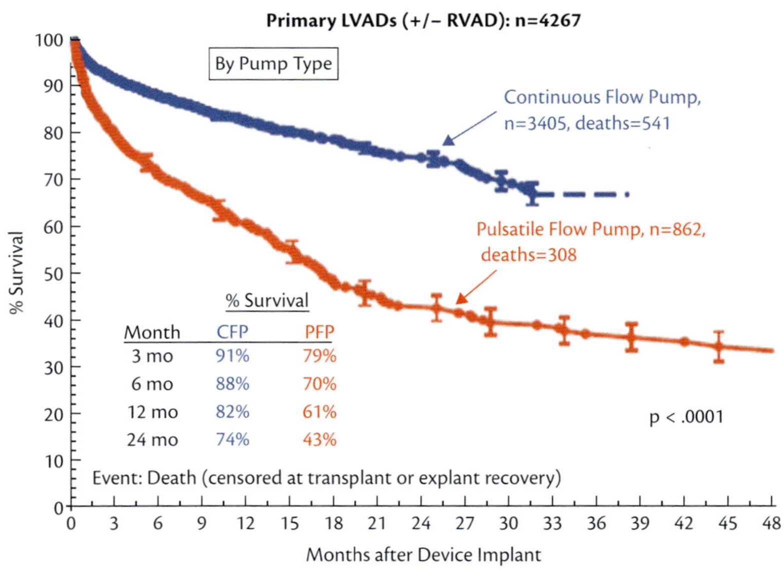

Fig. 14.5 Post-LVAD implant survival with and without biventricular assist.

Reprinted from Journal of Heart and Lung Transplantation, 31, Kirklin J, Naftel D, Kormos R, et al. The fourth INTERMACS annual report: 4,000 implants and counting, 117–126, copyright (2012) with permission from Elsevier.

Table 14.4 Risk assessment based on hepatic function

Child–Pugh score			
Measure	**1 point**	**2 points**	**3 points**
Bilirubin (mg/dl)	< 2.0	2.0–3.0	> 3.0
Albumin (mg/dl)	> 3.5	2.8–3.5	< 2.8
Ascites	Absent	Mild	Moderate
Encephalopathy	None	Suppressed with meds	Refractory to meds
INR	<1.7	1.7–2.3	> 2.3
Scores	**Class**		
5–6	A		
7–9	B		
10–15	C		
MELD score			
= [(0.957*ln(Cr mg/dl)) + (0.378*ln(bilirubin (mg/dl)) + (1.120*ln(INR))]*10 If patient was on HD at least twice in the past week then Cr = 4			
Score	**Postoperative 30-day mortality**		
0–5	3.2%		
6–10	8.6%		
11–15	21.9%		
16–20	44.0%		
21–25	55.6%		
26+	87.5%		

Teh, et al. MELD score. Gastroenterology 2007; 132: 1261–1269 and Child Pugh score calculator <http://prodruginfo.com/formulary/childpugh_score_calculator.htm> with permission from Elsevier.

be effectively combined, as necessary, with inotropic support of the right heart. Chronic neurohumoral activation is responsible for advancing damage to the kidneys[43] and many patients have significant intrinsic renal disease for this or other reasons. These patients should avoid nephrotoxic drugs.

Following LVAD implantation, a significant improvement in renal function can be expected depending on the amount of irreversible renal damage already present. It does not appear that continuous-flow devices have a different renal effect than pulsatile devices, but long-term renal outcomes have not been evaluated in the setting of continous-flow devices.

Hepatic function

Diminished hepatic function is associated with worse outcomes including bleeding, related generally to the severity of the dysfunction,[44] and patients with cirrhosis have poor outcomes. Two scoring systems, the MELD[45] and the Child–Pugh,[46] are used to assess the risk associated with hepatic dysfunction (Table 14.4). Hepatic decompensation risk following LVAD placement is predicted by the Child–Pugh score. Patients in Child–Pugh classes B and C are at markedly increased risk for postoperative hepatic failure. The MELD score derived from the INTERMACS database also incorporates renal dysfunction and predicts the the postoperative 30-day mortality.[47,48,49]

Patients with cirrhosis are at markedly increased risk for a poor outcome and LVAD placement should usually be avoided in such patients. On the other hand, patients with lesser degrees of hepatic damage generally experience improved or even normalized hepatic function following LVAD placement.[50]

Preoperative therapy is directed to improving hepatic function by improving perfusion with inotropic or MCS, as necessary, and reversal of the anticoagulated state with fresh frozen plasma. Right heart pressures are normalized using diuretics with mechanical fluid removal as necessary, and inotropic support of the left heart is used to increase cardiac output to assure adequate perfusion.

Hematologic function

As noted earlier, preoperative correction of INR is essential to risk reduction. When the platelet count is <150 000 or there has been a recent marked (>20%) decrease, heparin-induced thrombocytopenia (HIT) should be excluded using a serotonin release assay. If it is necessary to proceed in the presence of HIT, an alternative to heparin such as argatroban is necessary. If HIT antibodies become undetectable, heparin use is, once again, appropriate.[51] Thrombocytopenia represents an important risk marker for adverse outcome following LVAD implantation. The reasons remain speculative, but this is a marker for a more advanced inflammatory disease state, predicts need for higher blood product use, and is associated with right HF after LVAD insertion.

Pulmonary function

Patients with severe intrinsic lung disease are poor candidates for LVAD implantation. Indeed, when forced vital capacity (FVC), forced expiratory volume (FEV1), and diffusion capacity (DLCO) are less than 50% of predicted in the absence of pulmonary congestion, LVAD implantation should generally be avoided.[52] Patients requiring mechanical ventilatory support are at particularly high risk for poor outcome, and appropriate weaning prior to LVAD implant is advisable if feasible.[53] The preoperative workup should include chest radiograph, arterial blood gas, and spirometry for patients not in decompensated HF. Where anatomic abnormalities are suspected, prior thoracic surgery has occurred, or intersititial lung disease is suspected, a high-resolution CT scan should be considered.

Nutritional status

Obesity is not a contraindication to LVAD placement.[54] While poor nutritional status is associated with an increased risk of infection and poor outcome, there is little to suggest that prognosis is altered by nutritional intervention and so LVAD implant should not be delayed for the purpose of nutritional therapy. However, severe nutritional status portends an adverse prognosis and where feasible, improving nutrition as measured by prealbumin assessment may be wise.

Infection

Once an LVAD is infected bacteriologic cure is unlikely. In such cases, the combination of appropriate antibiotics followed by heart transplantation may effectively support the patient and allow cure of the infection. Immediate transplant is rarely feasible and is undertaken at increased risk in the presence of an active infection so that other approaches must be considered. If the patient can tolerate the absence of MCS for a period of time, perhaps with inotropic support, the LVAD can be removed, antibiotics administered to cure the infection, and then another LVAD implanted or transplant performed. This entails two major surgeries and carries substantial risk. A final option is chronic antibiotic suppression.

Even patients without a demonstrated active preoperative infection are at increased risk for a postoperative infection compared to their healthy contemporaries for a number of reasons, including the state of immunosuppression that accompanies HF, indwelling lines and, frequenly, hospitalizations that expose them to a variety of pathogens in addition to the presence of comorbities such as renal failure and malnutrition.[55,56,57,58]

In patients without active infection, preoperative antibiotic prophylaxis is indicated, with broad coverage of Gram-negative and Gram-positive organisms including MRSA (if hospitalized for >48 hours) and mupirocin ointment[59,60,61]to the nares. In special circumstances, antiviral or antifungal prophylaxis may be indicated.

Gastrointestinal bleeding

Continuous-flow LVADs appear to increase the risk of gastrointestinal (GI) bleeding. In one study there was a 22.8% rate of GI bleeding,[62] and GI bleeding is a frequent cause of readmission. A careful assessment should be undertaken prior to LVAD placement to exclude patients with lesions that would predispose to this complication.

Valvular heart disease

Valvular lesions vary in their impact on LVAD function. For some, no correction is needed while others interfere with effective circulatory support by the LVAD.

Mitral insufficiency

This generally does not require repair or replacement pre- or post-LVAD. Mitral regurgitation is reduced by the LVAD both directly by continuous pumping and by reduction in ventricular dilatation, which is a frequent cause of valve dysfunction in HF.[51] Additionally, for patients with a mechanical valve in place, the vigorous flow across the mitral valve serves to effectively wash the prosthesis so that thrombosis risk is reduced sufficiently for a mechanical valve to be placed or left in place.

Mitral stenosis

In contrast, mitral stenosis provides significant impedance to blood flow into the LV which increases the left atrial pressure and reduces pump flow. As a result, a stenotic mitral valve should be replaced at the time of LVAD placement.[51]

As noted above, mechanical or bioprosthetic valves are acceptable in the mitral position if already present. However, the disadvantage of a mechanical valve is the need for a greater degree of anticoagulation than would be required by the presence of the LVAD with a bioprosthetic valve and so if valve replacement is needed at the time of LVAD placement, a bioprosthetic device should be used.

Aortic stenosis

This does not require repair because the LVAD effectively bypasses the valve. However, the incidence of progressive disease, particularly insufficiency, may influence LVAD function in the long term. Importantly, if a mechanical prosthetic valve is already in position in the aortic location, most surgeons recommend conversion to a bioprosthesis or closure of the outflow. This is done to avoid thromboembolism risk due to reduced flow across the LV outflow when the LVAD is functioning at full capacity.

Aortic insufficiency

On the other hand, aortic insufficiency is a particular concern and tends to progress after implant, at least sometimes due to fusion of aortic valve leaflets.[51] Hence, if there is more than mild aortic insufficiency, aortic valve replacement should be performed When the aortic valve is replaced a bioprosthetic valve should be used to reduce the risk of thromboembolic complications. Alternatively, the aortic valve can be oversewn proximal to the takeoff of the coronaries. This prevents emboli from the heart proximal to the patch but results in immediate death if the LVAD fails.

Up to this point we have focused on appropriate patient selection and preoperative optimization. This chapter examines medical management of MCS patients and so the details of the intraoperative phase and routine ICU management (such as respirator management) are not within its scope.

Overall postimplant considerations

Hemodynamically, the goal of treatment is a mean arterial pressure of 70–90 mmHg with cardiac index greater than 2.2 L/min,[51,63,64] at a filling pressure in the left heart low enough to avoid lung congestion but sufficient to provide the preload needed to maintain these parameters. These hemodynamic parameters must be achieved without causing RV failure and at a right atrial (central venous) pressure that does not result in renal or hepatic dysfunction (generally ≤15 mmHg). Mean arterial pressure should remain below 90 mmHg to maximize flow (in continuous-flow devices, the afterload is crucial in detrmining LVAD outflow) and minimize bleeding risk. In addition to these basic hemodynamic requirements, other considerations modulate the final speed setting. For instance, where possible, LVAD flow is set so as to maintain opening of the aortic valve approxomately every third beat, which may help to reduce the risk of aortic thrombosis[65] and the progression of aortic insufficiency,[65,66,67] both of which have been associated with failure of the aortic valve to open. Another is reduction in the severity of mitral regurgitation. Postimplant management, then, focuses on (1) assuring that device speed is appropriately programmed; (2) that associated drug and ancillary device therapy (anticoagulation, neurohumoral antagonists, diuretics, ICD, etc.) are optimal; and (3) that problems with the device, patient, or patient–device interface are recognized.

Setting device speed

The specific design of the LVAD varies with the manufacturer. Here, we will attempt to state principles that are applicable to LVADs generally and not to a specific device. However, we use the Thoratec HeartMate II (HMII) (Figure 14.6) as the prototype example because a truly generic discussion is less informative and this device has accrued the most worldwide experience along with the HeartWare HVAD device.

One might begin by asking a simple question: "Why do people with advanced HF live longer with an LVAD?" A straightforward answer is that tissue perfusion is improved. This is easy to accept and probably, as a general statement, true. But, the next question is: "What represents optimal perfusion?" (which is what determines pump speed and drug treatment that impacts hemodynamics). At the present time, there is no precise answer to this question. There is a great deal that is just not known: What is the relationship between pump (plus heart) output and survival? Should we unload the heart as much as possible or not (i.e., does the degree of

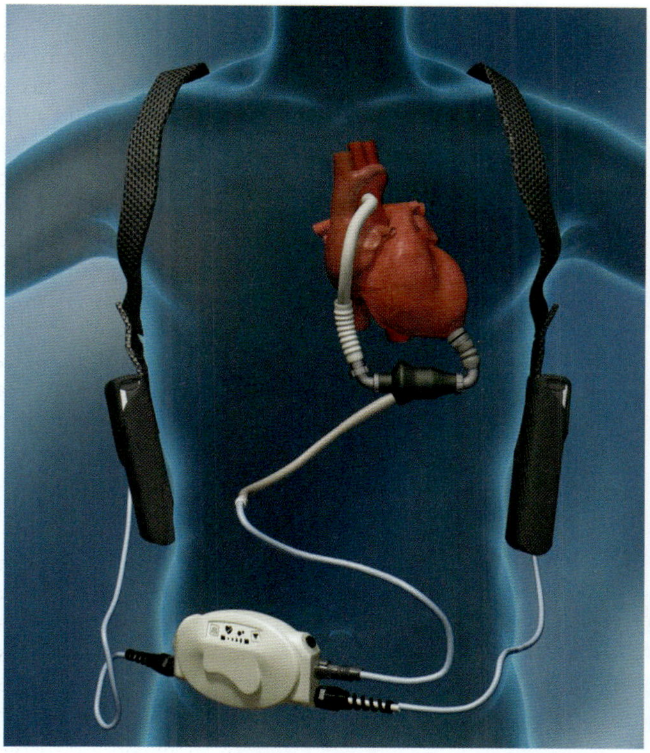

Fig. 14.6 The HeartMate II system.
Clinical management of continuous-flow left ventricular assist devices in advanced heart failure, Slaughter, Mark S., The Journal of Heart and Lung Transplantation (Elsevier).

unloading affect myocardial recovery)? How often, if at all, should the aortic valve open? The point here is that there is much to be learned about the patient/MCS interface. The approach described here is designed to allow safe operation with appropriate pressures but is based on the limited information that is available today.

Some LVAD systems are axial flow designs and others are centripetal with flow direction changed by the turbine. The HeartMate II is an axial flow device with an inlet cannula in the LV and outlet cannula in the proximal aorta (see Figure 14.6). The turbine continually pumps blood from the LV into the aorta, rotating at a speed set by the operator and powered via an electrical drive line that crosses the body wall to an external power source. The automatic control system electronics are also external.

Given the conceptual limitations of defining optimal speed discussed earlier, how can we provide an operational definition of the "optimal" speed setting? For the current purpose, the speed should be set to provide normal cardiac index, result in no rightward or leftward shift of the interventricular septum, and minimize mitral regurgitation. Additionally, we seek to set the speed so that the aortic valve opens occasionally, providing a pulse pressure of 10–15 mmHg, thus washing the proximal aorta to reduce the risk of thrombus formation.

Patients arrive from the operating room with the speed set. Because there are major postoperative volume changes, there is no advantage to adjusting the speed until later in the hospitalization unless there is evidence of inadequate hemodynamic support or the development of ventricular tachyarrhythmias suggesting a suckdown phenomenon. We describe an approach of optimizing speed using echocardiography closely following that described by Slaughter et al.[51]

Utilizing the echocardiographic four-chamber or short-axis view (Figure 14.7), the speed is decreased until the septum just begins to shift rightward into the RV. This is designated the lower rate limit. (With the HeartMate II the speed should not go below 8600 rpm during this procedure.) The aortic valve may or may not open, depending on the underlying contractile state of the myocardium. For some ventricles the aortic valve may be opening on every beat, for others the aortic valve may not be opening at all, depending on the inherent contractile function of the LV.

The rate is then increased until the septum just begins to bow into the LV. This is designated as the upper rate limit. The speed is then set to the midpoint between the upper and lower rate limit. With upper and lower rate limits defined, and starting with this midpoint, the speed can be changed to try to achieve specific goals. These might include minimizing mitral regurgitation and/or assuring that the aortic valve opens on every second or third beat, as discussed above. Generally, the attempt is to keep the set speed at least 400 rpm below the upper rate limit to avoid suckdown phenomena with the usual day-to-day changes in volume status.

Speed optimization should be undertaken before hospital discharge when the patient is stable, whenever there is a clinical suggestion of indadequte support at any time during the hospital stay or after discharge, and then occasionally as an outpatient.

Associated drug/device therapy

Anticoagulation is essential to prevent device clotting but is managed with the understanding that bleeding has been far more common than thrombosis, importantly due to an acquired von Willebrands syndrome that attends MCS.[68] The specific anticoagulation/antiplatelet regimen varies with the specific MCS device. Study of the HeartMate II[59] showed that an INR range of 1.5–2.0 minimizes thrombotic risk while limiting hemorragic events. For the HeartMate II aspirin 81–325 mg daily is also recommended although few data are available to support a specific recommendation. Coumadin is generally started on postoperative day 2 to day 5 without bridging with heparin because of the increased risk of hemorrhage. Exceptions are patients with devices or coagulation abnormalities who may require earlier, and perhaps more aggressive, anticoagulation.

Patients with an ICD should have the device turned on prior to discharge. Patients who do not have an ICD, such as those who presented with an acute myopathy, should have one placed before discharge because an ICD in this setting has been associated with improved survival.[70] Similarly, cardiac resynchronzation therapy should be continued.

While there is no evidence on which to base a recommendation regarding neurohumoral antagonists, the use of ACE inhibitors, β-blockers, and aldosterone antagonists is reasonable post-LVAD placement on theoretical grounds to help prevent continuing deterioration of ventricular function. For this reason, these agents may be particularly appropriate choices where blood pressure control (mean arterial pressure <90 mmHg) is needed.

LVAD system fundamentals and troubleshooting

In this section we discuss use of the LVAD data display to deduce patient physiology and LVAD function and troubleshooting of the LVAD.

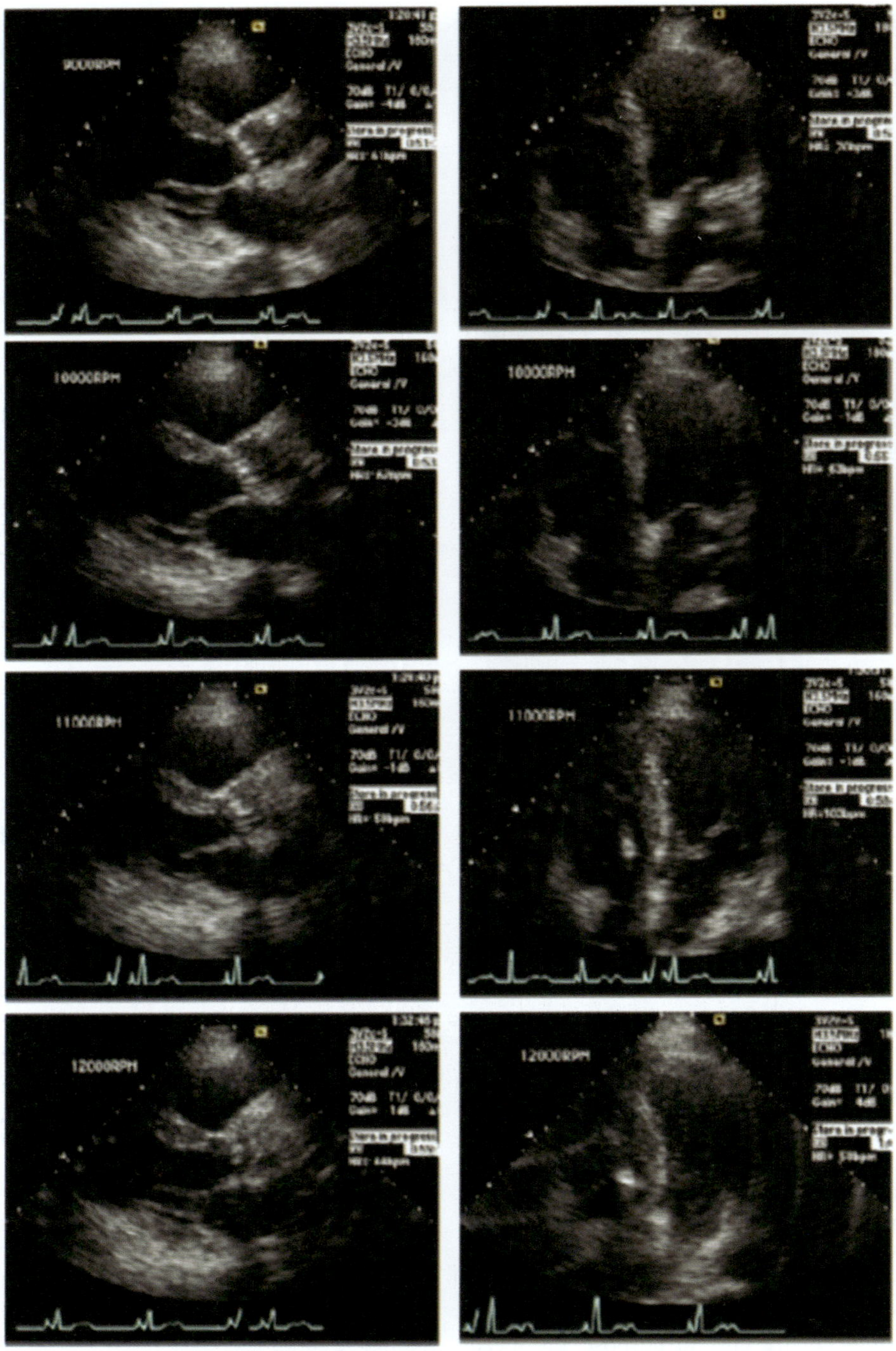

Fig. 14.7 Example of using echocardiography to set the speed of the left ventricular assist device.
Reprinted from Journal of Heart and Lung Transplantation, 29, Slaughter M, Pagani F, Rogers J, et al. Clinical management of continuous-flow left ventricular assist devices in advanced heart failure, S1–S39, copyright (2010) with permission from Elsevier.

Figure 14.8 shows the display for the HeartMate II. In the center of the console is the programmed turbine speed. The speed is set by the operator and the LVAD then delivers the power necessary to maintain the set speed. The speed and the power seen on the lower right of the display are the only parmeters that are actually measured. The flow, shown on the upper left side of the display panel, is estimated using an algorithm that incorporates pump power and pump speed. When the speed exceeds the expected speed range "+++" is displayed on the flow gauge and "– – –" is displayed when the speed falls below the expected range. Pulsatility index, displayed in the upper right, is also a calculated parameter and is discussed below.

One goal of this chapter is to provide a basis for understanding the LVAD well enough to troubleshoot (i.e., to recognize and correct a problem). A small investment in gaining a qualitative understanding of the energy economy of the device makes deducing the physiological state of the patient and the operating status of the LVAD relatively simple and obviates the need to memorize

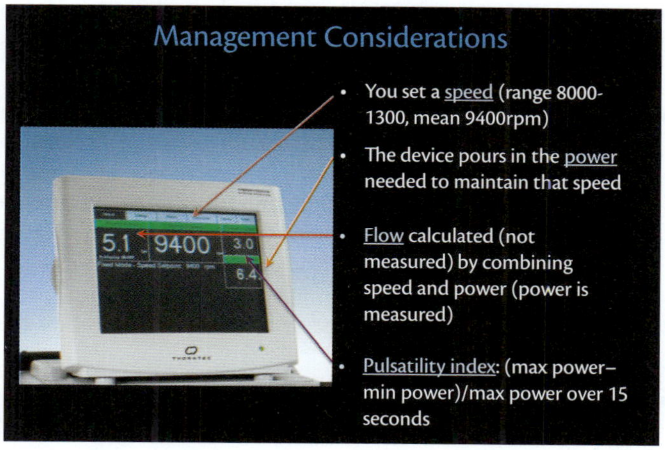

Fig. 14.8 Thoratech Heartmate II display.

the parameters expected from a multitude of possible physiological states. The qualitative nature of the following material must be emphasized. Were numerically accurate pressures and flows needed, a far more complex model that incorporates the complex, time-varying pressures, flows, and coupling of the device and patient would be required.

In order for blood to flow from the LV into the aorta, the rotor must add sufficient energy (quantified as an injection of total pressure, P_I) to the blood to overcome the pressure gradient between the LV and the aorta. Energy imparted by the rotor in excess of this manifests as flow velocity. In general, the more the energy injected by the rotor the greater the flow so long as the LV (acting as a reservoir) has sufficient volume (when it does not, tissue can be drawn against the inflow cannula in a suckdown phenomenon). Now, if there is obstruction to flow anywhere in the pump, there is a loss of energy that would otherwise have been available to cause flow. So, the volume of flow pumped will be diminished by obstruction(s) anywhere along the flow path (proximal or distal to the rotor). Now we can write a qualitative relationship that will be useful in understanding the impact of various situations on pump flow. Doing so is simplified by assuming that the flow is of a perfect fluid steadily flowing in a rigid tube without energy loss due to friction, the presence of a boundary layer, or any jets. As a result the expression is not quantitatively accurate but does allow the physician to deduce physiological state from the readings on the LVAD or, conversely, the readings expected from a given physiological state.

Referring to Figure 14.9, the total pressure in the flow as it exits into the aorta is composed of the sum of the total pressure in the LV and the total pressure added to the flow by the turbine, using

$$P_{LV} + P_I = P_{SAO} + {}^{1/2}\rho V^2$$

where P_I is total pressure added by the turbine, P_{LV} is the total pressure contributed by the LV, ρ is the density of the blood, P_{SAO} is the static pressure at the conduit exit, and V is the velocity at which the blood exits into the aorta from the LVAD conduit area, A.
Solving for V and multiplying by the conduit area gives the following expression for volume flow, Q:

$$Q = VA = A\left\{2/\rho\left[P_I - \left(P_{SAO} - P_{LV}\right)\right]\right\}^{1/2}$$

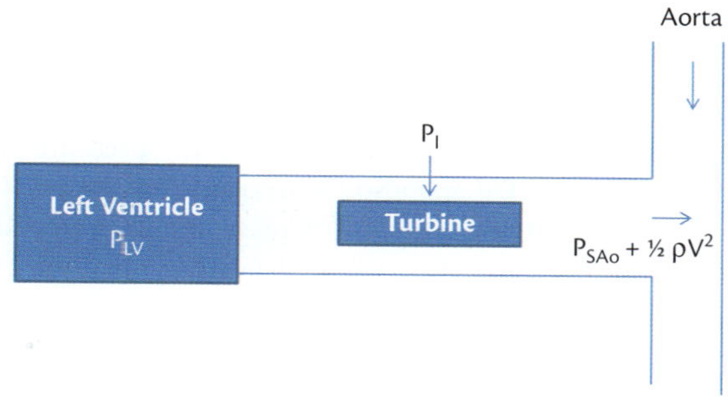

Fig. 14.9 Schematic of implanted left ventricular assist device (LVAD). P_{SAO}, static pressure in the aorta; P_{LV}, total pressure in the left ventricle; P_I, total pressure injected by the LVAD.

Because of the assumptions, this is written as proportional to ($\propto$) rather than equal:

$$Q \propto A\left\{2/\rho\left[P_I - \left(P_{SAO} - P_{LV}\right)\right]\right\}^{1/2} \qquad (1)$$

For the purpose of analysis, it is important to understand that power used by the LVAD to maintain the speed set by the operator is proportional to the flow, so that

$$\text{Power} \propto Q \qquad (2)$$

Now, we consider pulsatility index and then we will be in a position to relate pressures to flow and to power and conversely to interpret the telemetry data returned by the LVAD.

When the ventricle contracts, pressure is generated, resulting in increased flow into the LVAD (that may also open and cause flow through the aortic valve). The greater the flow through the LVAD, the greater the power the device injects to maintain speed. Hence, we can turn this around and use the fluctuation in power to quantify the ability of the heart to contract. This is the pulsatility index which is just the peak power over a 15-second interval minus the minimum power divided by the average power. Thus, the pulsatility index is a metric of the contractile function of the LV. The machine updates every second so the parameter is a running function of the preceding 15 seconds.

Now we are ready to consider what the console readings would be in a few examples of physiological states:

- **Outflow or inflow obstruction (not involving the rotor).** Whether inflow or outflow, there is a pressure drop across the obstruction(s). Hence, there is a nonzero P_{OB}. As a result some of the total energy (P_I) injected by the rotor is expended overcoming the gradient across the obstruction and the flow, Q, is reduced. As a result, the flow and thus the power (see equation 2) is reduced. So, in the setting of obstruction inside the pump and pump tubing (but not on the rotor) power will decrease. CT scan can be used to look for kinking of the inflow or outflow cannula and for clot. The CT scan does not, of course, provide visualization inside of the radio-opaque portions of the pump.
- **Sepsis.** The vasodilation attending sepsis would be expected to reduce the absolute aortic pressure far more than the absolute reduction in LV pressure and so with a decrease in LV-to-aorta gradient, the flow term (see equation 1) would increase and therefore so would the power (see equation 2).

- **Hypertension.** Elevated aortic pressure would increase the aorta-to-LV gradient and so reduce flow (equation 1) and, as a result, power would decline as well.
- **Hypovolemia/inadequate preload.** The LV pressure would decrease (both LVEDP and also the developed pressure) so that the aorta-to-LV gradient would increase resulting in reduced flow (equation 1) and thus reduced power (equation 2). An echocardiogram is useful to look for pericardial effusion (tamponade) or RV failure.
- **Suction events.** As discussed above, the LV serves as reservoir of blood to be pumped by the LVAD. If the flow into the LV is insufficient to replace the sum of the blood flowing out through the LVAD and the blood exiting through the aortic valve, cardiac structures will be pulled toward the inflow conduit of the LVAD. This can result in ventricular arrhythmias and markedly reduced flow. The HeartMate II monitors pulsatility index (PI) for sudden changes which are interpreted as suction events. If a difference of 45% per second or more from the average PI occurs, a suction event is diagnosed and the LVAD then executes a protocol in which it reduces speed to the low limit setting (or to a default of 9000 rpm) and then increases the rate by 100 rpm/s to the prior set rate. A suction event indicates that the pump is operating at a speed (and therefore a flow rate) faster than that ventricle can fill or that the inflow cannula is malpositioned. The differential diagnosis includes any entity that can impede filling of the left heart. These include hypovolemia, tamponade, right HF (including due to arrhythmias), and pulmonary embolus. Inflow cannula malposition can also result in suction events and can be assessed with chest radiograph and also with transesophageal echocardiography.
- **Clot on the rotor.** A final, but important special case, relates to the development of clot on the rotor. Flow is not directly measured by the HeartMate II. Rather, it is, as discussed before, approximated using the speed and the power. So, if the power goes up at a set speed, the device will register a greater flow. This is frequently the case. However, if the power needed to turn the rotor at a particular speed is increased, for instance by added drag resulting from the formation of a clot on the rotor, then the calculated flow would increase without an increase in the actual flow. Indeed, when one sees an otherwise unexplained gradual increase in power a clot needs to be in the differential diagnosis.

The above examples illustrate that making use of two simple relationships, one can deduce the behavior of the device and also work backward from the device readings to the physiological state.

Other management points

A number of practical details of management are covered here.

- **Blood pressure.** The ideal target for mean arterial blood pressure is 70–80 mmHg and should be kept to less than 90 mmHg as measured with an arterial line in place. Without an arterial line, blood pressure measurement is effected using a sphygmomanometer and a Doppler device. This is less accurate, particularly when there is a substantial pulse pressure since this technique does not allow determination of where in the cardiac cycle measurement occurs.
- **Anemia.** Patients with LVADs in place have an acquired von Willebrand disease and frequently have GI bleeding. Hemolysis is also common (see below).
- **Hemolysis** can present, and is most often pump related (though not necessarily) but should be searched for as part of any anemia workup in these patients. Plasma free hemoglobin in excess of 40 mg/dl or LDH in excess of 1000 mg/dl (this, when present on two measurements within 24 hours, was the base for defining hemolysis in the HeartMate II bridge to transplant trial[70]). The presence of hemolysis may prompt a reduction in pump speed, which can reduce hemolysis and should raise suspicion for the possibility of a pump thrombus.
- **Ventricular tachyarrhythmias**[71] are undesirable because they lead to low flow and, if not recognized in the outpatient, may lead to failure of the right heart. The presence of sustained ventricular tachyarrhmias should prompt a search for a cause. Common culprits include suckdown events, electrolyte imbalance, hemodynamic instability,and the use of inotropic agents. Cardioversion does not interfere with LVAD function. ICDs should be left on after implantation, making sure that the ICD is one whose function is not adversely affected by the presence of an LVAD.
- **Right HF** and its treatment have been discussed earlier.
- **Atrial fibrillation/flutter** is treated in much the same manner as in patients without an LVAD; rate is controlled or the patient cardioverted, and patients are anticoagulated according to standard guidelines.

Unique considerations with the HeartWare device

Management of the HeartWare ventricular assist device is similar to the HeartMate II LVAD with a few exceptions. First, the target INR is recommended is 2–3; second, cerebral thomboembolism events appear to be higher than with the HeartMate II. As a result, assuring aspirin responsiveness is recommended and, in its absence, addition of clopidogrel or dipyridamole should be considered. Also recommended is keeping mobile phones at least 50 feet (15 meters) away from the controllers to prevent radio interference. It appears that the sintered surface of the current HeartWare device leads to a lower neurological complication rate than the earlier nonsintered version. The motor speed of the controller ranges from 1800 to 4000 rpm and the typical clinical recommended range is 2400 rpm (power 21.5 W, flow 3 L/min) to 3200 rpm (power 8.5 W, flow 8 L/min). An interesting difference between the HeartWare and HeartMate devices is that the HeartWare HVAD controller uses the entered value of the hematocrit to calculate pump flow. The default hematocrit entered is 30% and it is recommended that, for an accurate flow assessment, the most recent hematocrit be entered when a change of more than 5% has occurred. The principles by which this pump operates are similar to those set out above.

Total artificial heart

As described in the previous chapter, the SynCardia TAH is a pulsatile, implantable pump that consists of two polyurethane ventricles with pneumatically driven diaphragms and four Medtronic-Hall tilting disc valves. In clinical trials, the device was effective for bridging to transplant in 79% of patients with inotrope-refractory biventricular failure. Survival after heart transplant was 86% at 1 year and 64% at 5 years, similar to national registry standards, leading to regulatory approval in the US and elsewhere. Particularly attractive features of this device are the ability to employ it in situations of biventricular failure, severe HF with restrictive cardiomyopathy, or conditions of extensive myocardial infarction particularly with mechanical complications such as cardiac or septal rupture. Other unique clinical conditions where this device may be employed include incessant refractory ventricular arrhythmias, complex congenital heart disease, severe allograft failure after cardiac transplant, patients with multiple mechanical valves, or INTERMACS 1 cardiogenic shock states where the predicted outcomes with a LVAD are less optimal.

A disadvantage of the TAH is the elimination of any possibility of myocardial recovery. Technical considerations are important for feasibility since the patient size must meet certain criteria, e.g., body surface area ≥ 1.7 m^2, and a thoracic diameter (anterior vertebral body to sternum at 10th thoracic vertebra) of 10 cm or more. A smaller device that can be implanted in smaller patients is under active development.

The pump diaphragms are activated by movement of air from an external driver, allowing for a maximal stroke volume of 70 ml. Typical drive pressures for the right pump are between 60 mmHg and 90 mmHg and between 180 and 200 mmHg on the left side. The device rate is set at a rate greater than 120 ejections per minute, and the percentage of time the pump spends in "systole" is typically set to 45–55%. These parameters are configured to allow for full ejection of blood volume, to prevent stasis and clinically significant hemolysis. Systemic anticoagulation is required with an INR target of 2.5–3.5.

There are specific clinical issues that are unique to TAH management. This device operates on a steep physiological curve and has little adaptability to tolerate either systemic blood pressure changes or large shifts in blood volume. As such, attention must be focused on these areas. If renal insufficiency ensues, volume management becomes difficult and use of adjunctive drugs with natriuretic expression is advocated by some but not all centers. Indeed, as the ventricles are excised, early on, most patients exhibit a sharp decline in renal function due to the loss of natriuretic peptide expression by the myocardium. This is why many advocate use of low-dose nesiritide as an exogenous source of B-type natriuretic peptide (BNP) early postoperatively until other endogenous renal regulatory systems become upregulated as the HF state settles.

The TAH creates a heightened inflammatory milieu, causes hemolysis due to the four mechanical valves and high flow state, and also interferes with erythropoiesis. These effects lead to a severe anemia that requires close attention and may worsen circulating blood volume issues.

In some cases, postoperative mechanical ventilator autocycling with a flow trigger, and subsequent loss of autocycling after switching to a pressure trigger, have been observed with the TAH. This problem may be resolved by use of a pressure trigger rather than a flow trigger setting. Interestingly this is more commonly observed in those with markedly elevated CVPs.

The TAH requires a bulky and unwieldy driver and controller system during in-hospital use but a smaller portable driver, called the "freedom" driver, is now available for transition to home discharge while patients are awaiting a transplant.

A fully implantable TAH that is durable, quiet, and does not require transcutaneous connections is another possible solution. Total cardiac replacement is available but current devices are large, noisy, require large percutaneous connections, and have limited life cycles. They can be effective in bridging to transplant and have been used as destination therapy, meaning without the intent to transplant, but are not practical for widespread application when long-term support is indicated for patients who desire a return to a reasonably normal outpatient existence.

So, as is the case for the other modalities discussed in this chapter, a TAH practical for widespread use does not exist. However, in contrast to xenotransplantation or stem cell based treatment, there are no fundamental *scientific* barriers to developing a TAH. The necessary blood-compatible biomaterials, long a major roadblock, exist; pump pressures needed are, by engineering standards, modest; more complex control technology than is needed for the TAH is in everyday use; and power systems could be constructed. Nonetheless, while necessary fundamental understandings are in place, the engineering challenge of developing a TAH with the above characteristics is daunting—hugely expensive, requiring a development process lasting many years, and not assured of success in the time frame needed by most industrial concerns.

Update on current and ongoing key clinical trials and tribulations

Current trials and clinical experience supports the application of LVADs as a life-saving and life-sustaining therapy for appropriately selected patients with advanced HF in INTERMACS Profiles 1 to 4.[72, 73] In the Risk Assessment and Comparative Effectiveness of Left Ventricular Assist Device and Medical Management in Ambulatory Heart Failure Patients (ROADMAP) study, the safety, feasibility and quality of life extending benefits in the INTERMACS 4 profile population were aptly demonstrated.[73] Extending implants into a less sick advanced HF population (Profiles 5–7) will require both a better understanding of the natural history of ambulatory advanced HF and better devices with lower complication rates. Just as thrombosis is a complication of all current LVADs, so are bleeding, disabling stroke, and infection. Stroke risk appears to be significantly higher in HVAD than in the HM II, although more conclusive data comparing the devices will need to await the final publication of the Evaluate the Heart- Ware Ventricular Assist System (ENDURANCE) trial or until INTERMACS compares these outcomes directly between the two pumps.[74] In currently presented series from ENDURANCE, the two year outcomes with the HVAD pump were numerically inferior to the Heartmate II device, largely due to the excessively higher (threefold) rates of observed disabling strokes. Strategies for improving communication and enhancing patient-centered decisions are being actively explored in the ongoing Decision Support Intervention for Patients and Caregivers Offered Destination Therapy Heart Assist Device (DECIDE LVAD) trial.[75] Is there a glimmer of hope in reducing risk of pump thrombosis with newer devices? Promising preliminary data have emerged about the next-generation magnetically levitated centrifugal-flow HeartMate 3 from its Conformité Européene Mark Trial. In the first 50 HeartMate 3 recipients who received the device in 10 centers across six countries, there were no reported adverse events of pump malfunction, pump thrombosis, or significant intravascular hemolysis through six months of support, although a 12% incidence of stroke was observed.[76] The pivotal Multi-center Study of MagLev Technology in Patients Undergoing MCS Therapy With HeartMate 3 (MOMENTUM 3) trial of the HeartMate 3 pump is ongoing in the United States.[77] This trial will test the hypothesis that the engineering advances in the Heartmate 3 pump will provide greater hemocompatibility. The fully magnetically levitated pump rotor allows for a wide range of operations while maintaining pump stability, has an internally built in pulsatility algorithm designed for prevention of pump stasis and the pump housing has wider spaces for blood component movement without incurring shear stress. In addition, the pivotal trial is designed to include all comers to allow LVAD therapy to be a "therapy in the journey of heart failure" without the artificial designations of compartmentalization to bridge to transplant versus destination therapy.[78] A number of smaller profile devices with the potential for earlier application using fully contained systems that use transcutaneous energy transfer are under development.

References

1. Stevenson L, Pagani F, Young J, et al. INTERMACS profiles of advanced heart failure: the current picture. J Heart Lung Transplant 2009;28:535–41.
2. Ammar K, Jacobson S, Maloney D, et al. Prevalence and prognostic significance of heart failure stages: application of the American College of Cardiology/American Heart Association heart failure staging criteria in the community. Circulation 2007;115:1563–70.
3. Hertz M, Aurora P, Christie J. Registry of the Interrnational Society for Heart and Lung Transplantation: a quarter century of thoracic transplantation. J Heart Lung Transplant 2008;27:937–42.
4. National Heart, Lung, and Blood Institute (NHLBI) website: <http://www.nhlbi.nih.gov>.
5. Rose E, Gelljns A, Moskowitz A, et al. Long-term use of a left ventricular assist device for end-stage heart failure. N Engl J Med 2001;1435–43.
6. Slaughter M, Rogers J, Milano C, et al. for the HeartMate II Investigators. Advanced heart failure treated with continuous flow left ventricular assist devices. N Engl J Med 2009;361:2241–51.
7. Rogers J, Butler J, Lansman S, et al. Chronic mechanical circulatory support for inotrope dependent heart failure patients who are not transplant candidates: results of the INTrEPID Trial. J Am Coll Cardiol 2007;50(8):741–7.
8. Lund L, Matthews J, Aaronson K. Patient selection for left ventricular assist devices. Eur J Heart Fail 2010;12:434–43.
9. Guillermo, T, Southard R, Mathias M, et al. Reversal of secondary pulmonary hypertension by axial and pulsatile mechanical circulatory support. J Heart Lung Transplant 2010;29:195–200.
10. Radovancevic B, Vrtovec B, deKor E, et al. End-organ function in patients on long-term circulatory support with continuous- or pulsatile-flow assist devices. J Heart Lung Transplant 2007;26:815–18.
11. Hasin T, Topilsky Y, Schirger J, et al. Changes in renal function after implantation of continuous flow left ventricular assist devices. J Heart Lung Transplant 2012;59:26–36.
12. Centers for Medicare & Medicaid Services. Decision memo for ventricular assist devices as destination therapy (CAG-00119N). <http://www.cms.gov/medicare-coverage-database/details/nca-decision-memo.aspx>.
13. Alba A, McDonald M, Rao V, et al. The effect of ventricular assist devices on the long-term post-transplant outcomes: a systematic review of observational studies. Eur Heart J Fail 2011;785–95.
14. Pat J, Piacentino V, Cuevas A, et al. Impact of left assist device bridging on post-transplant outcomes. Ann Thoracic Surg 2009;88:1457–61.
15. Baldwin T, Mann D. NHLBI's for program VAD therapy for moderately advanced heart failure: the REVIVE-IT pilot trial. J Card Failure 2010;16:855–8.
16. Dang N, Topkara V, Mercando M, et al. Right heart failure after left assist device implantation in patients with chronic congestive heart failure. J Heart Lung Transplant 2006;25:1–6.
17. Kavarana M, Pessin-Minsley M, Urtecho J, et al. Right ventricular dysfunction and organ failure in left ventricular assist device recipients. Ann Thorac Surg 2002;73:745–50.
18. Ochiai Y, McCarthy P, Smedira G, et al. Predictors of severe right ventricular failure after implantable left ventricular device insertion: analysis of 245 pateents. Circulation 2002;106(12 Suppl 1):1198–202.
19. Morgan J, John R, Lee B, et al. Is severe right ventricular failure in left ventricular assist device recipients a risk factor for unsuccessful bridging to transplant and post-transplant mortality. Ann Thorac Surg 2004;77:859–863.
20. Deng M, El-Banayousy A, Gronda E, et al. Mechanical circulatory support for advanced heart failure: effect of patient selection on outcome. Circulation 2001:103:231–7.
21. Thunberg C, Gaitan B, Arabia F, et al. Ventricular assist devices today and tomorrow. J Cardiothoracic Vasc Anesth 2010;24:656–80.
22. Dickstein M, Mets B, Heath M. Anesthetic considerations during left ventricular assist device implantation. In: Goldstein D, Oz M, ed., Cardiac Assist Devices. Armonk, NY: Futura; 2000, pp. 63–74.
23. Boehmer J. The right prediction. J Am Coll Cardiol 2012;529–30.
24. Slaughter M, Pagani F, Rogers J, et al. Clinical management of continuous-flow left ventricular assist devices in advanced heart failure. J Heart Lung Transplant 2010;29:S1–39.
25. Schenk S, McCarthy P, Blackstone E, et al. Duration of inotropic support after left ventricular device implantation: risk factors and impact on outcome. J Thoracic Cardiovasc Surg 2006; I31:447–54.
26. Fukamachi K, McCarthy P, Smedira N, et al. Preoperative risk factors for right ventricular failure after implantable left ventricular assist device insertion. Ann Thorac Surg 1999;68:2181–4.
27. Morgan J, John R, Lee B, et al. Is severe right ventricular failure in left ventricular assist device recipients a risk factor for unsuccessful bridging to transplant and post-transplant mortality. Ann Thorac Surg 2004;77:859–63.
28. Santambrogio L, Bianchi T, Fuardo M, et al. Right ventricular failure after left ventricular assist device insertion: preoperative risk factors. Interact Cardiovasc Thorac Surg 2006;5:379–82.
29. Fitzpatrick J, Frederick J, Hsu V, et al. Risk score derived from pre-operative data analysis. predicts the need for biventricular mechanical circulatory support. J Heart Lung Transplant 2008;27:1286–92.
30. Matthews J, Koelling T, Pagani F, et al. The right ventricular risk score: pre-operative tool for assessing the risk of right ventricular failure in left ventricular assist device candidates. J Am Coll Cardiol 2008;51:2163–72.
31. Rudski LG, Lai WW, Afilalo J, et al. Guidelines for the echocardiographic assessment of the right heart in adults: a report from the American Society of Echocardiography endorsed by the European Association of Echocardiography, a registered branch of the European Society of Cardiology, and the Canadian Society of Echocardiography. J Am Soc Echocardiogr 2010;23:685–713.
32. Moreno F, Hagan A, Holmen J. Evaluation of size and dynamics of the inferior vena cava as an index of right sided cardiac function. Am J Cardiol 1984:53:579–85.
33. Ramakrishna H. Recent advances in pulmonary hypertension therapy. Recent Pat Cardiovasc Drug Discov 3:28–36.
34. Stoivierska-Dzierzck B, Michler, R. The evolving management of acute right-sided heart failure in cardiac transplant recipients. J Am Coll Cardiol 38:923–31.
35. Overgaard C, Dzavik V. Inotropes and vasopressors: review of physiology and clinical use in cardiovascular disease. Circulation 2008;118:1047–56.
36. Safdat Z. Treatment of pulmonary arterial hypertension: the role of prostacyclin and prostaglandin analogs. Resp Med 2011;106:818–27.
37. Zewail Q, Nawar M, Vrtovec M, et al. Intravenous milrinone in the treatement of advanced congestive heart failure. Texas Heart Inst J 2003;30(2):109–13.

38. Hobbs R, Mills R. Therapeutic potential of nesiritide (recombinant b-type natriuretic peptide) in the treatment of heart failure. Expert Opin Investig Drugs 1999;8:1063–72.
39. Kirklin J, Naftel D, Kormos R, et al. The fourth INTERMACS annual report: 4,000 implants and counting. J Heart Lung Transplant 2012;31:117–26.
40. Farrar D. Preoperative of survival in patients with Thoratec ventricular assist devices as a bridge to heart transplantation. J Heart Lung Transplant 1994;13:93–100.
41. Sander S, Zimpfer D, Zrunek P, et al. Renal function and outcome after continuous flow left ventricular device implantation. Ann Thorac Surg 2009;87:1072–8.
42. Ma L, Fujinmo Y, Matsumiya G, et al. Renal function with left ventricular assist devices: the poorer the preoperative renal function the long the recovery. Med Sci Monit 2008;14:CR621–7.
43. Braunwald E. Biomarkers in heart failure. N Engl J Med 2008;358:2148–59.
44. Reinhartz O, Farrar D, Hershon J, et al. Importance of preoperative liver function as a predictor of survival in patients supported with Thoratec left ventricular devices as a bridge.to transplantation. J Thorac Cardiovasc Surg 1998;116:633–40.
45. Teh SH, Nagorney DM, Stevens SR, et al. Risk Factors for mortality after surgery in patients with cirrhosis. Gastroenterology 2007;132:1261–1269.
46. Child Pugh score calculator. <http://prodruginfo.com/formulary/child-pugh_score_calculator.htm>
47. Matthews J, Pagani F, Haft J. Model for end-stage liver disease score predicts left ventricular assist device operative transfusion requirements, morbidity, and mortality. Circulation 2010;121:214–20.
48. Concha P, Mertz K. Perioperative risk among patients with cirrhosis, Rev Med Child 2010;138:1165–71.
49. Modi A, Volhra H, Barlow C. Do patients with liver cirrhosis undergoing cardiac surgery have acceptable outcomes? Ventricular assist system in patients awaiting heart transplantation, J Thorac Cardiovasc Surg Interact Cardiovasc Thorac Surg 2010;11:630–34.
50. Frazier O, Rose E, Oz M, et al. Multicenter clinical evaluation of the Heartmate vented electric left ve ventricular assist system in patients awaiting heart transplantation. J Thorac Cardiovasc Surg 2001;122:1186–95.
51. Slaughter M, Pagani F, Rogers J, et al. Clinical management of continuous-flow left ventricular assist devices in advanced heart failure. J Heart Lung Transplant 2010;29: S1–39.
52. Miller L, Russel S. Candidate selection for long-term left ventricular assist device therapy for advanced heart failure. In: Kormos R, Miller L, ed., Mechanical Circulatory Support. Philadelphia, PA: Elsevier; 2012, pp. 72–87.
53. Oz M, Goldstein D, Pepino P, et al, Screening scale predicts patients successfully receiving long- term implantable left ventricular assist devices. Circulation 1995;92: II-169–73.
54. Mano A, Fujita K, Uenomachi K, et al. Body mass index is a useful predictor of prognosis after left ventricular assist system implantation, J Heart Lung Transplant 2009;28:428–33.
55. Stofkaova A. Leptin and adiponectin: from energy and metabolic dysbalance to inflammation and autoimmunity. Endocr Regul 2009;43:158–68.
56. Nunez J, Minana G, Bodi V, et al. Low lymphocyte count and cardiovascular diseases. Current Med Chem 2011;18:3226–33.
57. Betjes M, Langerak A, van der Spek A, et al. Premature aging of circulating T cells in patients with end-stage renal disease. Kidney Int 2011;80:208–17.
58. Vardeny O, Moran J, Sweitzer N, et al. Decreased T-cell response to influenza vaccination in patients with heart failure. Pharmacotherapy 2010;30:10–16.
59. Acharya M, Som R, Tsui S, What is the optimum antibiotic prophylaxis in patients undergoing implantation of a left ventricular assist device? Interact Cardiovasc Thorac Surg 2012;14:209–14.
60. Holman W, Skinner J, Waites K, et al. Infection during circulatory support with ventricular assist devices. Ann Thorac Surg 1999;68:711–16.
61. Saito S, Matsumiya G, Sakaguchi T, et al. Long-term medical control of inflow cuff infection in a patient with a left ventricular assist system. J Artif Organs 2009;12:58–60.
62. Aggarwal A, Pant R, Kumar S, et al. Incidence and management of gastrointestinal bleeding. Ann Thorac Surg 2012;93:1534–40.
63. St Ande A, DelRossa A. Hemodynamic management of patients in the first 24 hours after cardiac surgery. Crit Care Med 2005;33:2082–93.
64. El-Banayosy A, Korfer R, Ansoglu I, et al. Device and patient management in a bridge-to-transplant setting. Ann Thorac Surg 2001;71(3 Suppl): S98–102.
65. Hatano M, Kinugawa K, Shiga T, et al. Less frequent opening of the aortic valve and a continuous flow pump are risk factors for postoperative onset of aortic insufficiency in patients with a left ventricular assist device. Circ J 2011;75:1147–55.
66. Toda K, Fujita T, Shimahara Y, et al. Late aortic insufficiency related to poor prognosis during left ventricular assist device support Ann Thorac Surg 2011;92:929–34.
67. Mudd J, Cuda J, Halushka M, et al. Fusion of aortic valve commissures in patiens supported by a continuous axial flow left ventricular assist device. J Heart Lung Transplant 2008;27:1269–74.
68. Task Force 5ISHLT guidelines on the outpatient management of mechanical circulatory support device recipient. <http://www.ishlt.org/ContentDocuments/TaskForce5-OutpatientManagement_2012-03-22.pdf>
69. Boyle A, Russell S, Teuteberg J, et al. Low thromboembolism and pump thrombosis with the HeartMate II left ventricular assist device: analysis of outpatient anticoagulation. J Heart Lung Transplant 2009;28:881–7.
70. Rafaat M, Tanaka T, Kormos R, et al. Survival benefit of implantable cardioverter-defibrillators in left ventricular assist-supported heart failure patients. J Card Failure 2012;18:140–5.
71. Miller L, Pagani F, Russell S, et al. Use of a continuous flow device in patients awaiting heart transplantation. N Engl J Med 2007;357:885–96.
72. Kirklin JK, Naftel DC, Pagani FD, et al. Seventh INTERMACS annual report: 15,000 patients and counting. J Heart Lung Transplant 2015;Oct 8:pii: S1053–2498(15)01450–3. doi: 10.1016/j.healun.2015.10.003. [Epub ahead of print]
73. Estep JD, Starling RC, Horstmanshof DA, et al. ROADMAP Study Investigators. Risk Assessment and Comparative Effectiveness of Left Ventricular Assist Device and Medical Management in Ambulatory Heart Failure Patients: Results From the ROADMAP Study. J Am Coll Cardiol 2015;Oct 20;66(16):1747–61.
74. Pagani FD, Milano CA, Tatooles AJ, et al. HeartWare HVAD for the treatment of patients with advanced heart failure ineligible for cardiac transplantation: results of the ENDURANCE Destination Therapy Trial. J Heart Lung Transplant 2014;34:S9.
75. CORI-1310-06998 Trial of a Decision Support Intervention for Patients and Caregivers Offered Destination Therapy Heart Assist Device((DECIDE-LVAD). Available at: https://clinicaltrials.gov/ct2/show/NCT02344576).
76. Netuka I, Sood P, Pya Y, et al. Fully magnetically levitated left ventricular assist system for treating advanced HF: a multicenter study. J Am Coll Cardiol 2015;66:2579–89.
77. MOMENTUM 3 IDE Clinical Study Protocol (HM3™). Available at: <https://clinicaltrials.gov/ct2/show/NCT02224755>
78. Uriel N, Adatya S, Mehra MR. Evolution in mechanical circulatory support: are we at the precipice of a disruptive innovation? J Am Coll Cardiol 2015;66:2590–3.

CHAPTER 15

Mechanical circulatory support: Outpatient management

Mandeep R. Mehra MD and Michael J. Domanski MD

Introduction

Once the patient is discharged from the hospital to ambulatory status, long-term success with mechanical circulatory support (MCS) devices is critically dependent upon diligent monitoring including attention to early detection of device-related complications. Follow-up of these patients is complex and includes optimal volume management, recognition and therapy of right heart failure, anticoagulation management, surveillance for arrhythmia, blood pressure management, and assessing for bleeding complications (especially gastrointestinal (GI) bleeding), as well as neurological events and device malfunction, particularly pump thrombosis.[1] Infections are common in this population and require early diagnosis and treatment. In this chapter, we specifically discuss continuous-flow axial or centrifugal devices since these are by far the most common forms of circulatory support in patients who are not hospitalized.

Optimal device function

Once the patient becomes ambulatory, optimizing device function is critical. The principles include (1) maintenance of adequate perfusion during rest and activity, (2) avoidance of right heart failure, (3) optimizing anticoagulation to avoid pump thrombosis while minimizing bleeding risk, and (4) effectively decompressing the left ventricular cavity. Continuous-flow left ventricular assist devices (LVADs) are valveless and flow of blood through these devices depends primarily upon the preload, pump speed and afterload. The mechanics of pump function were discussed in detail in Chapter 14, including principles for troubleshooting the device. In general, the pump speed should be set to minimize mitral regurgitation, while achieving a midline position of the interventricular septum and intermittent opening of the aortic valve (to avoid stagnation of flow in the aortic root). This is typically achieved by performing a ramp study, wherein the device parameters are adjusted upwards or downwards, to achieve proper septal geometry and intermittent aortic valve opening.

The frequency of follow-up should be most intense early after discharge from pump placement, with increasing time intervals between visits in patients with an uncomplicated outpatient course: for example, weekly for the first month, then twice monthly for 2 months and then every other month. Each visit should include a clinical evaluation for right heart function, blood pressure management, assessment of driveline site cleanliness, patient rehabilitation progress, and extent of physical activity. Device as well as equipment function must also be assessed. A scheme for evaluating device parameters and their potential pathophysiological correlates is shown in Table 15.1. Continuing education of patients should be offered regarding monitoring of device integrity, caring for the driveline and attending to care of ancillary equipment including the controllers and battery packs.[2]

Hypertension and hypotension

Ideally, the blood pressure should be measured in supine and standing positions and orthostasis identified if present. Blood pressure must be measured using a Doppler instrument and should be maintained in the 70–90 mmHg range.[3,4] The residual pulsatility consequent upon heart contraction (the pulse pressure is usually no more than 5–15 mmHg) results in variation of the measured pressure. Studies have shown a correlation between the risk of neurological events and higher blood pressures, particularly with a centrifugal continuous-flow device. This recommended range of blood pressure ensures adequate forward flow while minimizing poor perfusion. Experience has shown that traditional neurohormonal antagonist therapy drugs provide excellent blood pressure control; dihydropyridine calcium channel blockers are also used when needed.[5]

The differential diagnosis of hypotension in LVAD patients is extensive and includes bleeding, dehydration, right heart failure, tamponade, infection, and device-related complications, such as improper cannula positioning, inadequate pump speed, or pump malfunction. Orthostatic hypotension should be evaluated at each clinical visit, dynamic changes recorded, and treatments adjusted accordingly.

These recommendations are based on expert consensus derived from a limited evidence base. Expanding the evidence base is required to refine management strategies. Examples include determining the effectiveness of antihypertensive agents in preventing strokes and the usefulness of neurohormonal blockade in preventing worsening heart function in these patients.

Table 15.1 A general scheme for device optimization and troubleshooting

Interrogation parameter	Possible pathophysiology	Suggested intervention
Increased pump power (decreased ventricular unloading)	Increased drag on rotor (thrombus)	Investigate for hemolysis and pump thrombosis Augment anticoagulation Increase pump flow Consider pump exchange if established thrombosis
High flow–low blood pressure	Excess vasodilation due to medications or infection	Evaluate for device-related infection Reduce vasodilators
Decreased flow	Low preload (hypovolemia, bleeding, arrhythmias)	Investigate for arrhythmia Optimize fluid status Investigate for covert or overt bleeding source
Low pulsatility index	Increased pump speed Poor ventricular contraction Low preload	Optimize pump speed downwards Assess for myocardial reserve
High pulsatility index	Decreased pump speed or flow Intrinsic myocardial recovery	Assess device for malfunction or ventricle for recovery

Arrhythmias

Atrial and ventricular arrhythmias result in significant morbidity, primarily because of compromised right ventricular filling and function, leading to inadequate left ventricular filling, heart failure, hypotension, and device compromise. Left atrial distention from congestion or mitral regurgitation may be an inciting cause and adequate decompression of the left ventricle may decrease this risk.

Atrial fibrillation also complicates anticoagulation management by requiring the standard levels of anticoagulation needed for stroke prophylaxis. This becomes particularly hazardous in patient populations prone to bleeding, such those with prior GI bleeding, or in very elderly people. In patients with poorly tolerated arrhythmia amiodarone or dofetilide may be effective in restoring and maintaining sinus rhythm. Ablative therapy is generally reserved for refractory cases.

The incidence of ventricular arrhythmias after implantation of an MCS device has been reported to be as high as 20% to 50%.[1,6] Although electrolyte imbalance in the setting of a diseased right heart and underlying pathological substrate can cause such arrhythmias, "suction" events are common. These events are caused by excessive decompression of the left ventricle and/or cannula positioning that facilitates contact with the heart wall. Any hemodynamic change that would allow the inflow cannula to come into contact with myocardial structures, particularly the interventricular septum, can precipitate a ventricular tachyarrhythmia. Such circumstances include bleeding or hypovolemia due to other causes, increased LVAD speeds, and improper angulation of the inflow cannula. Another cause of ventricular tachyarrhythmias is new reentrant circuits around the inflow cannula in the left ventricular apex. Isolated episodes of ventricular arrhythmia may be well tolerated, at least initially, and can be terminated with either antitachycardia pacing from an implantable cardioverter defibrillator (ICD) or with cardioversion. Most patients will have an ICD implanted before MCS implantation or before discharge following LVAD placement.[7]

If a suction event is suspected, evidence of hypovolemia from excessive diuresis, bleeding, or dehydration should be sought and corrected if present. Consideration should also be given to reducing the LVAD speed under the guidance of transthoracic echocardiography.

Right heart failure

Right heart failure is associated with increased morbidity and mortality, longer hospitalization, a higher rate of renal insufficiency and, generally, in a failure to thrive.[8] The severity of right heart failure preoperatively is the strongest predictor of right heart failure after LVAD implantation. Although continuous-flow devices are associated with less frequent occurrence of right heart failure than older pulsatile LVADs, the frequency of right heart failure remains at least 5–15%.[9] Early after implant, the frequency of right heart failure is present is as many as one-third of patients but the frequency declines over the following the 2 weeks. The fifth INTERMACS annual report, covering 6 years and more than 6000 durable MCS implants, found that severe right-sided failure requiring mechanical right-sided support increased the early (1–2 months) mortality compared to moderate or mild right ventricular dysfunction.[10] Even when MCS is not needed, the duration of required inotropic support is correlated with morbidity and failure to survive to transplant.

In the ambulatory phase, failing to optimize LVAD speed may result in distortion of the geometry of the ventricular septum, thereby compromising right heart function.[11] Therefore, as the left ventricle decompresses, device optimization should include attention to the right heart and settings should not result in worsening tricuspid regurgitation or increased dilatation of the right ventricular cavity.

Infection

LVAD therapy is attended by comorbidities that predispose to infection. These include malnutrition, renal failure, diabetes mellitus, and chronic lung disease. Often, these patients are compromised by the severe debilitation consequent upon their heart failure, with significant frailty a common problem. Pump design factors, suboptimal surgical technique, and poor percutaneous driveline care can predispose patients to infection risk. Indeed, infection commonly complicates the post-LVAD course with 16% of all LVAD patient deaths caused by infection.[12]

The International Society for Heart and Lung Transplantation (ISHLT) working group has proposed standardized criteria to define infections in LVAD patients.[13] This group divided infections into three categories: (1) LVAD-specific (if involving the pump, cannula, pocket, or percutaneous driveline); (2) LVAD-related (including infective endocarditis, bloodstream infections with or without an indwelling central venous catheter and/or mediastinitis), and (3) non-LVAD-related (including lower respiratory tract infection, cholecystitis, and urinary tract infection).

The most common LVAD-specific infections are percutaneous driveline infections. The need for a driveline to exit the skin predisposes to infections due to breakdown of the skin as a barrier to infection and remains a fundamental limitation of all currently available durable MCS devices. A rate of 0.48 events/patient-year was observed for driveline infections in a trial of lifetime ("destination") therapy.[9] In contrast, younger patients with fewer comorbidities experience a lower infection rate. In the HeartWare HVAD bridge to transplant trial, driveline exit site infection remained one of the most common postoperative complications with an incidence of 0.29 events/patient-year.[14] In order to prevent percutaneous driveline and related device infections, protocols for optimal inpatient and outpatient driveline care have been established and involve immobilization of the driveline, to prevent friction and breakdown of the skin barrier, as one of the most important components. If infection develops, depending on its severity, increased frequency of dressing changes, hospitalization for intravenous antibiotics, surgical revision, wound vacuum therapy, or even pump exchange may be needed.

Pump-related infection involving the blood–device surface interface is a rare but serious complication of LVAD implantation, may be difficult to eradicate, and requires chronic antibiotic suppression therapy. For those with a bridge to transplant indication, device-related infection allows for an upgrade to urgent transplant priority. Excess vasodilation due to infections may lower blood pressure and result in an increased flow across the device. Secondary antibiotic prophylaxis for dental, respiratory, genitourinary, and gastrointestinal procedures has not been studied in the LVAD population. The most recent guidelines state that antibiotic prophylaxis would be "reasonable and remains at the discretion of the physician."[2]

Gastrointestinal bleeding

Although bleeding at any location can occur as a result of the demands of anticoagulation, GI bleeding in patients with continuous-flow devices is the most common. Occurring in one-fifth of all patients, GI bleeding accounts for recurrent hospitalizations in one-tenth of LVAD patients.[15,16,17] Bleeding can occur anywhere along the GI tract; however, mechanisms of bleeding unique to continuous-flow devices have been the subject of great interest. It is postulated that relatively high nonphysiologic shear stress is imparted to blood components as they move through the device, which promotes von Willebrand factor (vWF) proteolysis by the metalloprotease ADAMTS13, leading to a decrease in high molecular weight (functional) vWF multimers.[18] In addition to an observed acquired type IIa vWD, development of angiodysplasia or arteriovenous malformations (AVMs) is the cause of as many as one-third of the GI bleeding episodes. The reduced pulse pressure encountered with continuous-flow devices may lead to intestinal hypoperfusion, causing regional hypoxia, vascular dilation, and subsequent angiodysplasia. Focal ischemia may also increase the proclivity to GI bleeding.

As with management of any case of major GI bleeding, anticoagulation medication should be discontinued and the anticoagulated state reversed if clinically necessary. To prevent device-related thrombosis, the pump speed may need to be increased to facilitate adequate flow and improve heat dissipation through the device during such episodes. Patients must be supported hemodynamically with intravenous fluids but blood products should be used sparingly, especially in patients listed for transplantation, since transfusion increases the risk of sensitization and thus the probability of acquiring a histocompatible donor. The risk to the patient of an adverse outcome due to bleeding must be weighed against the risk of pump thrombosis consequent upon of reversing anticoagulation with vitamin K or fresh frozen plasma. Once stabilized, a patient with GI bleeding should be evaluated with upper and lower endoscopy in conjunction with consultation with a gastroenterologist. If standard endoscopy does not demonstrate a bleeding site, capsule endoscopy or balloon enteroscopy should be performed to assess the small bowel. In the setting of persistent bleeding and negative endoscopic evaluation, a tagged red blood scan or angiography can be considered.

When no bleeding site is identified, therapeutic options are limited. There are no substantial data demonstrating benefit of reducing pump speed to increase pulsatility and change the shear stress profile in order to facilitate resolution of AVMs.[19] The long-term benefits of octreotide in patients with refractory GI bleeding from small-bowel AVMs have been extrapolated for use in the LVAD population.[17] Further studies are needed to determine whether this strategy is effective.

Stroke

Disabling stroke is one of the most feared complications of durable LVAD therapy and the rate of stroke has not declined with the use of continuous-flow rather than pulsatile devices.[20] Previously, hemorhagic stroke was more prevalent than ischemic stroke. This has now changed, with ischemic strokes being more common, likely as a result of acceptance of lower anticoagulation targets. Initial data on the HeartWare HVAD as a bridge to transplant demonstrates a stroke risk similar to that of other LVADs. Stroke risk is importantly related to blood pressure and most advocate a Doppler pressure of no greater than 85 mmHg.[5,21] To reduce the risk of thrombotic events, both anticoagulation and antiplatelet therapy are recommended beginning in the postoperative period and continuing following discharge. Optimal levels of both therapies remain to be defined.

The current relaxed INR (1.5–2.0) practice is based on a study of 331 HeartMate II (Thoratec, Pleasanton, CA) outpatients followed for 6 months that reported a total thrombotic event rate of 3.3% which was dwarfed by a hemorrhagic event rate of 22%. In addition to acceptance of a lower INR, lower aspirin dose of 81–325 mg are the current practice.[22] In the case of LVAD-associated ischemic stroke or transient ischemic attack, aggressive anticoagulation is not recommended in the acute setting in order to avoid potential transformation to hemorrhagic stroke. More recently, aortic root and carotid bulb thromboses have been reported, leading to consideration of the potential usefulness of routine screening of carotid arteries and the aortic root both post-LVAD implant and following discharge in the chronic follow-up period.[23,24]

Pump thrombosis

The incidence of clinically relevant pump thrombosis requiring device exchange was observed infrequently in both the original HeartMate II trial (4% of destination therapy (DT) and 1.4% of bridge-to-transplantation (BTT) patients) and in a subsequent retrospective analysis of 331 BTT HeartMate II outpatients published around the same time ($n = 3$, 0.009%). However, since then, a significantly increased rate of pump thrombosis has been reported in clinical practice, and may be as high as 10%, particularly in the 2011–2012 time frame.[25] Possible reasons for this increased incidence include evolving demographics of the LVAD population (increasing age and comorbidities likely to be prothrombotic); growing concern over recurrent GI bleeding leading to diminished INR targets and/or discontinuation of antiplatelet therapy, and potentially technical evolution in the HeartMate II device. Thrombus may evolve from small deposits of fibrin within the pump and its components, or the pump may ingest clot originating in the cardiac chambers. Clinically, a patient with pump thrombosis may present with acute or subacute heart failure symptoms and a new neurological deficit, and/or with the consequences of hemolysis such as dark-colored urine. An lactate dehydrogenase (LDH) level in excess of 1000 or three times the previous level, hemoglobinuria, and/or significantly elevated plasma free hemoglobin should also raise suspicion of LVAD thrombosis even in the absence of symptoms. In the case of a HeartMate II, classically, a large thrombus in contact with the rotor leads to power elevations or "spikes" due to increased drag and resultant decreased pulsatility index. In the case of significant flow obstruction, normal unloading of the ventricle with increasing pump speed will not be seen on ramp study. Additionally, arterial pulse pressure will increase due to increased preload without an associated increase in arterial blood pressure; this may be apparent as a change on LVAD sounds on auscultation. Definitive treatment is pump replacement/exchange and is recommended in all patients in whom reoperation is appropriate; intravenous heparin infusion may be initiated initially to prevent progression of thrombus. The use of direct platelet directed therapy or thrombolysis (directed or systemic) has not had favorable results and should only be used with great caution in highly selected situations. A paradigm has been offered to guide therapy in the setting of pump thrombosis, as summarized in Box 15.1.[25]

Box 15.1 A general recommendation for prevention and management of pump thrombosis

A. Preimplant

Thrombophilia assessment in patients with prior thromboembolic events (e.g., pulmonary embolism, left ventricular clots, arterial thrombosis) is recommended. Consider assessment of heterozygous factor V Leiden mutation, anti-phospholipid antibodies, protein S deficiency, and heterozygous MTHFR C667T (hyperhomocysteinemia).

B. Bridging anticoagulation

Avoid use of unopposed warfarin or other vitamin K antagonists, such as phenprocoumon and acenocoumarol. Bridging with intravenous unfractionated or low molecular weight heparins should be used. When anticoagulation is interrupted for a surgical procedure, use an effective bridging strategy. Do not use direct thrombin inhibitors.

C. Monitoring for dynamic thrombosis risk

Close monitoring for development of de-novo arrhythmias, such as atrial fibrillation. Consider surveillance for de-novo thrombi in the aortic root or carotid bulb, early after implant. These entities are not likely to cause pump thrombosis but will inform on the net adequacy of anticoagulant and antiplatelet regimens.

D. Monitoring for hemolysis

Assays for lactate dehydrogenase (LDH) differ, and local reference ranges and actionable targets must be developed. Biweekly LDH must be monitored, especially in the early phase, and a 2- to 2.5-fold rise in the case of a HeartMate II or a 1.67-fold rise in the HVAD from the upper limit of normal must prompt a critical attentiveness to management. Typically, these levels represent a value of 600 IU/L and 400 IU/L, respectively. Those with low-grade persistent LDH elevations may require attention to mechanical factors or testing to assess adequacy of antiplatelet regimens if the INR is consistently in range. Exclude glucose-6-phosphate dehydrogenase (G6PD) deficiency.

E. Monitoring for mechanical factors

Change in angular acuity of the inflow cannula may require close monitoring by serial chest radiography (HeartMate II device only) in the early time frame. We recommend that serial radiographs need to be superimposed to evaluate an increase in apposition angles with progressive ventricular decompression. Such patients should be monitored very closely for possible pump thrombosis. Avoiding disruption in anticoagulation stability and low flow through the device might be a reasonable clinical stance.

F. Vigilance during and after infection

Heightened states of inflammation (increasing C-reactive protein levels) during infections, represent a particularly vulnerable period for thrombosis. In such situations, close attention to intensify anticoagulation and more frequent monitoring of LDH levels is needed until the clinical condition subsides.

G. Avoidance of delay in therapy

When the diagnosis of pump thrombosis is clear (e.g., hemodynamic compromise, sustained LDH >1000 IU/L, peripheral palpable pulse, noncompressible left ventricle, new-onset mitral regurgitation) and there is no overt lapse in maintaining anticoagulation, trials of medical therapy with thrombolytics or with IV antiplatelet glycoprotein IIb/IIIA inhibitors only delay definitive therapy and are not advised. A surgical option for pump exchange should be entertained immediately, unless there are clinical factors, such as surgical futility.

Specific intervention in critical care situations

Absence of a pulse in an LVAD patient may prompt the initiation of the Adult Cardiac Life Support (ACLS) protocol. However, it is particularly important in this population to assess the patient first before reacting to alarms on the display or on telemetry. Patients often tolerate episodes of ventricular tachycardia (VT) and ventricular fibrillation (VF) on an LVAD, and will not require cardioversion.

When assessing blood pressure, a Doppler machine must be used to obtain a mean arterial pressure (MAP) reading. If an arterial line is placed, it is likely to show a diminished pulse pressure of approximately 5–15 mmHg. A first step in patient assessment should be to auscultate the left upper abdomen for a continuous LVAD hum. If a continuous humming sound is not audible, device malfunction should be suspected and acted upon. If a patient is truly clinically unstable, standard ACLS protocols should be invoked, bearing in mind a pulse cannot be used to monitor status or to dictate appropriate medical therapy. Furthermore, cardiopulmonary resuscitation (CPR) should be avoided unless clearly necessary. Because of the location of the LVAD and its associated connections to myocardial structures, CPR may dislodge components of the device, resulting in fatal bleeding. All emergent situations should involve the urgent consultation of a cardiac surgeon, LVAD coordinator, and/or specialized cardiologist.[1]

Special ambulatory issues with the total artificial heart

The SynCardia total artificial heart (TAH; SynCardia Systems, Inc., Tucson, AZ, USA) is a pulsatile, implantable pump that consists of two polyurethane ventricles with pneumatically driven diaphragms and four Medtronic-Hall tilting disc valves. Using a special portable driver, patients can now be discharged to home and undergo rehabilitation on the TAH.[1] Issues unique to this device include renal insufficiency, due to loss of natriuretic peptide stimulation as a result of excision of the ventricular chambers, and also a characteristic anemia.[26,27] It has been observed that TAH patients have a persistent anemia with hemoglobin ranging between 6 and 8 g/dl, resulting from a combination of chronic hemolysis, ineffective erythropoiesis, and inflammation (predominant). These patients are noted to have markedly elevated lactate dehydrogenase levels, undetectable or low haptoglobin levels, and elevated plasma free hemoglobin, as well as elevated high-sensitivity C-reactive protein and reticulocyte production indices. Iron deficiency must be corrected diligently although ineffective iron utilization may also play a role in this anemia.

Mechanical circulatory support and myocardial recovery

Spontaneous recovery of myocardial dysfunction to the point of explantation is unusual except in patients with certain specific etiologies of their cardiomyopathy. Etiologies where recovery occurs frequently include acute myocarditis, peripartum cardiomyopathy, tachycardia-induced cardiomyopathy, and toxic cardiomyopathies. However, even in the absence of a specific reversible cause, patients exposed to neurohormonal or cardiac resynchronization therapy may exhibit reverse remodeling, sometimes with a marked improvement in cardiac structure and function ("super-responders"). The notion that heart failure refractory to medical therapy cannot return to a less advanced stage is not accurate. In 1999, Frazier and Myers[28] reported five patients with sufficient myocardial recovery to achieve device explantation. Of these four patients remained stable off left ventricular device support ranging from 2 months to 3 years. Although many other investigators reported similar findings in small case series, it was not until 2006 that a protocol designed to achieve recovery was prospectively evaluated. This protocol, referred to as the Harefield Strategy,[29] included a staged approach beginning with optimizing medical therapy using high doses of neurohormonal therapy and digoxin (25 mg of carvedilol 3 times daily, digoxin 0.125 mg/day, lisinopril 40 mg/day, losartan 150 mg/day, and spironolactone 25 mg/day). These patients were then followed for improvement in left ventricular dimensions, and only if normalization "on and off" (15 minutes with transient discontinuation) device support was noted, were they moved into the next stage. In this phase, the non-selective β-blocker was transitioned to a β_1 selective blocker so that clenbuterol, a selective β_2 agonist, could be added to the pharmacologic regimen in an effort to facilitate physiologic hypertrophy. In their series, 11 of 15 patients (73%) with nonischemic cardiomyopathy supported by a first-generation pulsatile HeartMate LVAD were able to undergo device explantation after an average support time of nearly a year. Freedom from recurrent heart failure at 1 and 4 years was 100% and 88.9%, respectively, in these 11 patients.

With the emergence of second-generation devices, the same group reported similar findings using this protocol with the continuous-flow HeartMate II device in 20 patients with a non-ischemic cardiomyopathy of whom 12 were successfully explanted.[30] In these 12 patients, freedom from death and recurrent heart failure was 83.3% at 1 and 3 years. After an average follow-up exceeding 1 year, surviving explants preserved their ejection fraction (58.1 ± 13.8%), modestly increased their left ventricular end-diastolic (59.0 ± 9.3 mm) dimension and maintained an excellent peak aerobic capacity $(Vo_2)_{max}$ of 22.6 ± 5.3 ml kg^{-1} min^{-1}. It should be noted that these were young patients with nonischemic cardiomyopathy and the majority (8/12) had heart failure symptoms of less than 6 months duration. These results were not replicated in the HARPS (HArefield Recovery Protocol Study) conducted in the US in which only 2/17 patients demonstrated sufficient recovery to undergo explantation. The US patients were older and had a longer duration of heart failure symptoms than the UK study.

An earlier effort from the LVAD working group examined 67 patients supported with a first-generation pulsatile LVAD and 9% were subsequently weaned to explant recovery.[31] While less relevant in today's era with continuous-flow devices, these investigators used a practical algorithm for weaning which can be easily clinically replicated. Patients were evaluated monthly after LVAD implantation and those with left ventricular ejection fraction (LVEF) greater than 40% at reduced device support underwent dobutamine echocardiography with simultaneous hemodynamic monitoring. Baseline hemodynamic and echocardiographic data were obtained with the LVAD and then with the LVAD weaned to the lowest tolerated flow. Dobutamine was infused in 5-minute dose increments from 5 to 20 μg kg^{-1} min^{-1} with ECG and echocardiographic monitoring. Infusion rate was increased to 40 μg kg^{-1} min^{-1} if 85% of predicted maximum heart rate was not achieved. Hemodynamic and echocardiographic data were recorded after 3 minutes at each infusion rate. Using this protocol to ascertain myocardial reserve, 34% of patients were found to have reached the threshold for stress evaluation and 6 were ultimately explanted.

Formica and colleagues[32] have described a three-step protocol to assess myocardial reserve during LVAD support (with the HeartMate II continuous-flow device). Following optimization of medical therapy, three modalities are used to evaluate cardiac reserve: echocardiography (ECHO), cardiopulmonary exercise testing (CPXT), and right heart catheterization (RHC). Each is performed at rest and peak exercise and with the LVAD at full support and when weaned to the lowest possible flow. Testing is done over 4 days as follows:

- Day 1, resting ECHO with full and weaned LVAD support
- Day 2, bicycle CPXT with full LVAD support
- Day 3, CPXT combined with exercise ECHO with LVAD weaned
- Day 4, RHC at rest with full and weaned LVAD support, followed by bicycle exercise RHC with LVAD weaned.

The HeartMate II LVAD can support a low speed of approximately 6000 rpm, at which point net forward flow is deemed to be zero under usual preload and afterload conditions. In this protocol, pump speed is decreased by 400 rpm each minute to 6200 rpm. At 8000 rpm, 5000 IU of heparin is given (if INR <2.5). Heparin 2000 IU is readministered every 15 minutes to maintain activated clotting time levels of 200–250 seconds. Weaning is discontinued if patients became symptomatic or Doppler blood pressure declines by 20%. In their selected series, three of six nonischemic patients with duration of heart failure ranging from 2 to 8 months underwent successful device explantation after 8–16 months of hemodynamic support. Importantly, all three patients demonstrated recovery of biventricular function. Recovery was not predicted by the peak aerobic capacity or peak exercise cardiac output. In a follow-up analysis, these investigators demonstrated that patients who recovered and were explanted remained free of heart failure for 4–6 years. Interestingly, those who recovered were distinguished by absence of coronary artery disease, a shorter duration heart failure, less myocardial fibrosis, and less myocyte hypertrophy, and were supported at higher LVAD speeds.

Upon mechanical unloading of the ventricle through LVAD therapy, significant reverse remodeling is detected, often with near-normalization of structural abnormalities. However, this phenomenon does not always correlate with myocardial function recovery. Gene-expression profiling studies have revealed that less than 5% of dysregulated genes revert to normal with LVAD therapy, despite overall structural improvements.[33] Drakos and colleagues[34] reported in a cohort of 80 consecutive patients with ischemic and nonischemic heart failure supported with continuous-flow devices. At 6 months, 34% of patients had a relative increase in LVEF of greater than 50%. This study showed that the improvements in cardiac function did not manifest until after 6 months of support, and that these improvements persisted at the 1-year follow-up evaluation.

The coronary circulation and myocardial lood flow may be important in predicting and assessing myocardial recovery. However, this is not been attended to in clinical investigations. Gupta and colleagues[35] systematically evaluated myocardial perfusion and strain imaging in 18 chronically supported LVAD patients. They found that the myocardial perfusion patterns were not homogenous and rendered the assessment of ischemic versus nonischemic etiology practically impossible. This suggests that the continuous-flow LVADs induce alterations in blood flow across the coronary circulation that may have importance in determining viability of myocardium and potential for recovery.

Although myocardial recovery is an infrequent clinical phenomenon, we believe that structured evaluations to facilitate recovery and remission should be pursued. In order to be successful, it is likely that implantation of cardiac support devices in earlier stages of disease using partial support, maintaining the cardiac architecture (by not destroying the apical fulcrum) and attention to myocardial blood flow may be important attributes to focus upon. We suggest that two groups of patients suitable for myocardial recovery can be identified upfront. These include those patients with a nonischemic reversible cardiomyopathy (toxic, tachycardic, inflammatory) or in selected cases of acute coronary syndromes presenting with cardiogenic shock where revascularization supported by MCS may allow for recovery within a reasonable time period. In others, those with less advanced age and heart failure of a nonischemic and shorter duration should currently be considered as potential candidates for myocardial recovery assessment.

Conflict of interest

Dr. Mehra reports consulting for Thoratec, Boston Scientific, Medtronic, St. Judes, Abbott Vascular, National Institute of Health, American Board of Internal Medicine and ISHLT; Dr. Domanski reports no relevant conflicts.

References

1. Lala A, Mehra MR. Durable mechanical circulatory support in advanced heart failure: a critical care cardiology perspective. Cardiol Clin 2013;31(4):581–93, viii-ix.
2. Feldman D, Pamboukian SV, Teuteberg JJ, et al. The 2013 Int ernational Society for Heart and Lung Transplantation Guidelines for mechanical circulatory support: executive summary. J Heart Lung Transplant 2013;32:157–87.
3. Bennett MK, Roberts CA, Dordunoo D, et al. Ideal methodology to assess systemic blood pressure in patients with continuous-flow left ventricular assist devices. J Heart Lung Transplant 2010;29(5):593–4.
4. Lanier GM, Orlanes K, Hayashi Y, et al. Validity and reliability of a novel slow cuff-deflation system for noninvasive blood pressure monitoring in patients with continuous-flow left ventricular assist device. Circ Heart Fail 2013;6(5):1005–12.
5. Lampert BC, Eckert C, Weaver S, et al. Blood pressure control in continuous flow left ventricular assist devices: efficacy and impact on adverse events. Ann Thorac Surg 2014;97(1):139–46.
6. Raasch H, Jensen BC, Chang PP, et al. Epidemiology, management, and outcomes of sustained ventricular arrhythmias after continuous-flow left ventricular assist device implantation. Am Heart J 2012;164(3):373–8.
7. Boilson BA, Friedman PA. Role of implantable cardioverter-defibrillators in patients with continuous flow ventricular assist devices. Circ Arrhythm Electrophysiol 2013;6(4):663–5.
8. Kavarana MN, Pessin-Minsley MS, Urtecho J, et al. Right ventricular dysfunction and organ failure in left ventricular assist device recipients: a continuing problem. Ann Thorac Surg 2002;73:745–50.
9. Slaughter MS, Rogers JG, Milano CA, et al. Advanced heart failure treated with continuous-flow left ventricular assist device. N Engl J Med 2009;361:2241–51.
10. Kirklin JK, Naftel DC, Kormos RL, et al. Fifth INTERMACS annual report: risk factor analysis from more than 6,000 mechanical circulatory support patients. J Heart Lung Transplant 2013;32:141–56.
11. Mehra MR, Park MH, Landzberg MJ, et al.; on behalf of the International Right Heart Failure Foundation Scientific Working Group. Right heart failure: Toward a common language. J Heart Lung Transplant 2014;33(2):123–6.
12. Holman WL, Pamboukian SV, McGiffin DC, et al. Device related infections: are we making progress? J Card Surg 2010;25:478–83.
13. Hannan MM, Husain S, Mattner F, , et al. Working formulation for the standardization of definitions of infections in patients using ventricular assist devices. J Heart Lung Transplant 2011;30:375–84.

14. Aaronson KD, Slaughter MS, Miller LW, et al. Use of an intrapericardial, continuous-flow, centrifugal pump in patients awaiting heart transplantation. Circulation 2012;125:3191–200.
15. Demirozu ZT, Radovancevic R, Hochman LF, et al. Arteriovenous malformation and gastrointestinal bleeding in patients with the HeartMate II left ventricular assist device. J Heart Lung Transplant 2011;30:849–53.
16. Aggarwal A, Pant R, Kumar S, et al. Incidence and management of gastrointestinal bleeding with continuous flow assist devices. Ann Thorac Surg 2012;93:1534–40.
17. Suarez J, Patel CB, Felker GM, et al. Mechanisms of bleeding and approach to patients with axial-flow left ventricular assist devices. Circ Heart Fail 2011;4:779–84.
18. Klovaite J, Gustafsson F, Mortensen SA, et al. Severely impaired von Willebrand factor-dependent platelet aggregation in patients with a continuous-flow left ventricular assist device (HeartMate II). J Am Coll Cardiol 2009;53:2162–7.
19. Wever-Pinzon O, Selzman CH, Drakos SG, et al. Pulsatility and the risk of nonsurgical bleeding in patients supported with the continuous-flow left ventricular assist device HeartMate II. Circ Heart Fail 2013;6:517–26.
20. Peura JL, Colvin-Adams M, Francis GS, et al. Recommendations for the use of mechanical circulatory support: device strategies and patient selection: a scientific statement from the American Heart Association. Circulation 2012;126:2648–67.
21. Slaughter MS, Pagani FD, McGee EC, et al.; HeartWare Bridge to Transplant ADVANCE Trial Investigators. HeartWare ventricular assist system for bridge to transplant: combined results of the bridge to transplant and continued access protocol trial. J Heart Lung Transplant 2013;32(7):675–83.
22. Boyle AJ, Russell SD, Teuteberg JJ, et al. Low thromboembolism and pump thrombosis with the HeartMate II left ventricular assist device: analysis of outpatient anti-coagulation. J Heart Lung Transplant 2009;28:881–7.
23. Reul JT, Reul GJ, Frazier OH. Carotid-bulb thrombus and continuous-flow left ventricular assist devices: A novel observation. J Heart Lung Transplant 2014;33(1):107–9.
24. Freed BH, Jeevanandam V, Jolly N. Aortic root and valve thrombosis after implantation of a left ventricular assist device. J Invasive Cardiol 2011;23(4):E63–5.
25. Mehra MR, Stewart GC, Uber PA. The vexing problem of thrombosis in long-term mechanical circulatory support. J Heart Lung Transplant 2014;33(1):1–11.
26. Shah KB, Tang DG, Kasirajan V, et al. Impact of low-dose B-type natriuretic peptide infusion on urine output after total artificial heart implantation. J Heart Lung Transplant 2012;31(6):670–2.
27. Mankad AK, Tang DG, Clark WB, et al. Persistent anemia after implantation of the total artificial heart. J Card Fail 2012;18(6):433–8.
28. Frazier OH, Myers TJ. Left ventricular assist system as a bridge to myocardial recovery. Ann Thorac Surg 1999;68(2):734–41.
29. Birks EJ, Tansley PD, Hardy J, et al. Left ventricular assist device and drug therapy for the reversal of heart failure. N Engl J Med 2006;355(18):1873–84.
30. Birks EJ, George RS, Hedger M, et al. Reversal of severe heart failure with a continuous-flow left ventricular assist device and pharmacological therapy: a prospective study. Circulation 2011;123(4):381–90.
31. Maybaum S, Mancini D, Xydas S, et al.; LVAD Working Group. Cardiac improvement during mechanical circulatory support: a prospective multicenter study of the LVAD Working Group. Circulation 2007;115(19):2497–505.
32. Formica P, Murthy S, Edwards P, et al. A structured 3-step approach to evaluate cardiac recovery with continuous flow circulatory support. J Heart Lung Transplant 2010;29(12):1440–2.
33. Mann DL, Barger PM, Burkhoff D. Myocardial recovery and the failing heart: myth, magic, or molecular target? J Am Coll Cardiol 2012;60(24):2465–72.
34. Drakos SG, Wever-Pinzon O, Selzman CH, et al. Magnitude and time course of changes induced by continuous-flow left ventricular assist device unloading in chronic heart failure: insights into cardiac recovery.Kfoury AG; UCAR (Utah Cardiac Recovery Program) Investigators. J Am Coll Cardiol 2013;61(19):1985–94.
35. Gupta DK, Skali H, Rivero J, et al. Assessment of myocardial viability and left ventricular function in patients supported by a left ventricular assist device. J Heart Lung Transplant 2014;33(4):372–81.

CHAPTER 16

Cardiac transplantation: Overview

Josef Stehlik MD, MPH and Joann Lindenfeld MD

Introduction

Heart transplantation as a potential treatment for advanced heart failure (HF) has been explored in experimental models since the beginning of the 20th century. This research addressed the technical aspects of transplantation, preservation of donor organs, immune mechanisms of rejection, and approaches to immune suppression. In the 1960s, doctors Norman Shumway and Richard Lower started a heart transplant research program at Stanford University (California, USA) aimed at bringing this therapy to clinical care. The first human heart transplant was performed by Dr. Christian Barnard in 1967, and was quickly followed by transplants performed in the United States and other countries. While heart transplantation was technically successful, the lack of efficient and safe immunosuppression resulted in unacceptably high post-transplantation mortality. With the development of the percutaneous endomyocardial biopsy technique and criteria for histopathologic grading of myocardial rejection, as well as the availability of improved immunosuppression in the form of cyclosporine, orthotopic heart transplantation became a relatively routine therapy for advanced HF. Currently, heart transplantation is an accepted and effective approach to extending longevity and improving quality of life in selected patients with advanced heart disease. This chapter reviews the contemporary approach to donor and recipient selection and the logistics of the transplant process, and summarizes post-transplant outcomes.

Heart transplant indications and outcome

Patients with advanced HF whose symptoms cannot be controlled despite optimal medical therapy, resynchronization therapy, or alternative surgical or percutaneous therapies should be evaluated for heart transplantation. In addition, patients with debilitating angina and refractory ventricular arrhythmias may also be considered for heart transplantation.[1] As the number of donor organs is limited, the goal is to select patients who will derive the most incremental benefit from transplantation for both survival and quality of life.

Approximately 5000–6000 heart transplant procedures are performed worldwide annually.[2] While heart transplantation volumes have remained stable for more than a decade in North America and western Europe, a significant increase in the use of heart transplantation for treatment of advanced heart disease has taken place in other regions, including South America and Asia.

The International Registry for Heart and Lung Transplantation (ISHLT) captures donor and recipient data as well as post-transplant outcomes for approximately two-thirds of all heart transplant procedures worldwide. The demographic and outcome data reviewed in this section are largely based on this data source.[3,4]

Heart transplant recipient demographics

More than one-half of adult heart transplant recipients (54%) carry the diagnosis of nonischemic cardiomyopathy, and approximately one-third (37%) have ischemic cardiomyopathy. The remaining patients are transplanted for cardiomyopathy resulting from congenital heart disease (3%) or valvular heart disease (3%), and approximately 3% of heart transplant procedures are retransplantations. Less than 1% of patients undergo heart transplantation for other types of heart diseases, such as restrictive cardiomyopathy, infiltrative heart disease, hypertrophic cardiomyopathy, refractory angina, or refractory life-threatening arrhythmias. Among pediatric patients, the majority undergo heart transplantation for nonischemic cardiomyopathy (59%), and patients with congenital heart disease are the second largest group (38%). Approximately 1% of patients undergo repeat transplantation and the remaining patients have heart diseases of less common etiology.

Baseline demographic characteristics and comorbidities for a recent cohort of adult recipients, transplanted between 2006 and 2011, are shown in Table 16.1. The average age of a heart transplant recipient is 54 years. Compared to previous eras, more patients in their sixties are being transplanted, and while this is still done rarely (<2%), a higher number of patients 70 years old and above are also receiving heart transplants. Comorbidities, especially diabetes mellitus, hypertension, or previous cardiac surgery, are common. A higher number of patients with previous malignancy are also being considered for heart transplantation (Table 16.1). Perhaps the most notable development in the profile of patients being transplanted in recent years is the increasing use of mechanical circulatory support as a bridge to transplant. In 2010, 36% of adult and 25% of pediatric heart transplant recipients were on circulatory support (not including intraaortic balloon counterpulsation) at the time of heart transplantation.[3,4]

Post-transplantation survival

Survival of patients after heart transplantation far exceeds the expected survival of patients with American Heart Association

Table 16.1 Characteristics recorded at the time of transplant in patients transplanted between 2006 and June 2011. Continuous variables expressed as median (5th–95th percentile)

	(*n* = 17 868)
Age (years)	54.0 (24.0–67.0)
Gender (% female)	23.7%
Weight (kg)	79.4 (53.1–110.2)
Height (cm)	175.0 (157.5–188.0)
Body mass index	26.0 (19.2–34.9)
Comorbidities:	
Diabetes mellitus	25.4%
Hypertension	44.1%
Peripheral vascular disease	2.9%
COPD	4.2%
Prior malignancy	6.4%
Prior cardiac surgery	45.4%
Serum creatinine (mg/dl)	1.2 (0.7–2.3)
Mechanical ventilation	2.9%
Preoperative inotropic and circulatory support	
Intravenous inotropes	42.6%
IABP	6.2%
LVAD	27.3%
RVAD	3.8%
TAH	0.9%
ECMO	1.0%

COPD, chronic obstructive pulmonary disease; ECMO, extracorporeal membrane oxygenation; IABP, intraaortic balloon pump; LVAD, left ventricular assist device; RVAD, right ventricular assist device; TAH, total artificial heart.

The Journal of Heart and Lung Transplantation, 31, Stehlik J, Edwards LB, Kucheryavaya AY, Benden C, Christie JD, et al. The registry of the International Society for Heart and Lung Transplantation: 29th official adult heart transplant report—2012, 1052–106, copyright (2012) with permission from Elsevier.

(AHA) class D HF treated with medical therapies.[5] Among a cohort of 96 273 patients who received heart transplants between 1982 and 2010, the median survival was 10 years. The greatest hazard for mortality is seen in the first post-transplantation year—approximately 10% of patients die in this period. For patients surviving past the first year, the median survival is 13 years. In the above-mentioned cohort, 22% were alive at 20 years after transplantation. There has been a continued gradual improvement in post-transplantation survival, with most of this improvement resulting from decrease in 1-year mortality (Figure 16.1).[4,6] The leading causes of mortality include acute rejection, infection, cardiac allograft vasculopathy, malignancy, and renal failure. There are distinct differences in the incidence of the specific causes of mortality at different time-points after transplantation (Figure 16.2). As many of the causes of death can be viewed as a result of either insufficient or excessive immunosuppression, attempts have been made to individualize the level of immunosuppression. Since the risk of acute rejection decreases with time following transplant, gradual protocol-driven reduction of immunosuppression has become a standard approach.

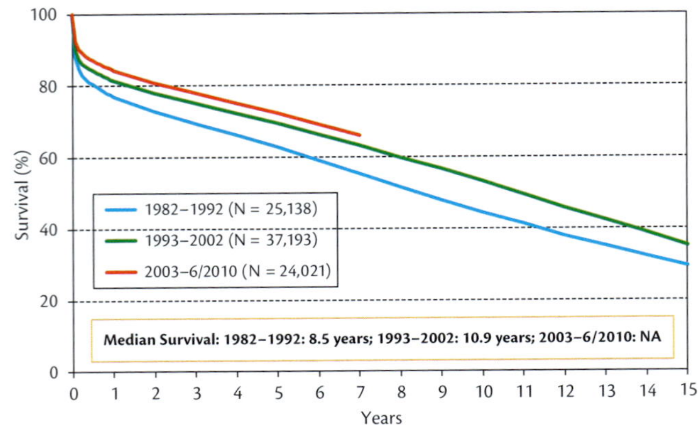

Fig. 16.1 Kaplan–Meier survival of adult heart transplant recipients transplanted between 1982 and 2010, by era. Survival rates were compared using the log-rank test statistic.

Journal of Heart and Lung Transplantation, 31, Stehlik J, Edwards LB, Kucheryavaya AY, Benden C, Christie JD, et al. The registry of the International Society for Heart and Lung Transplantation: 29th official adult heart transplant report—2012, 1052–106, copyright (2012) with permission from Elsevier.

Additional patient characteristics such as age, allosensitization, and previous history of rejection are often used to further tailor the level of immunosuppression. Recent investigations have examined whether changes in immunosuppression therapy informed by lymphocyte activity testing[7] or gene expression profiling[8] could lead to better results. In the absence of conclusive outcome studies, these approaches have not gained uniform acceptance. Therefore, changes in immunosuppression aimed at improving long-term survival are often made at a time when a post-transplantation complication associated with increased risk of mortality, such as cardiac allograft vasculopathy (CAV), renal dysfunction, or malignancy is identified. This is further explored in the section discussing post-transplantation morbidity.

Mortality risk factors

Knowledge of mortality risk factors is important for guiding decisions regarding candidacy of patients with advanced HF for heart

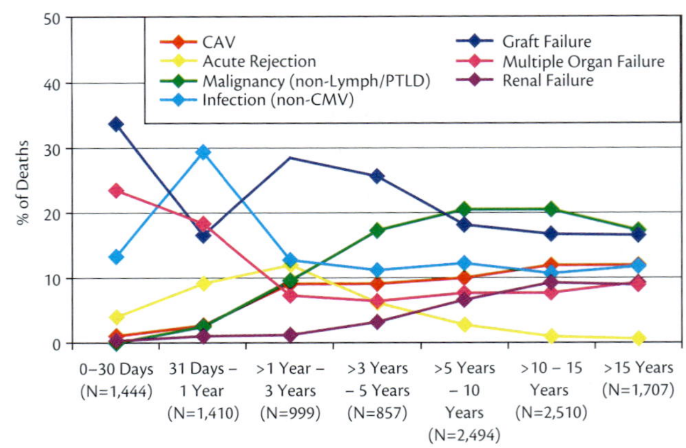

Fig. 16.2 Relative incidence of leading causes of death in patients dying between 2004 and June 2011.

Journal of Heart and Lung Transplantation, 31, Stehlik J, Edwards LB, Kucheryavaya AY, Benden C, Christie JD, et al. The registry of the International Society for Heart and Lung Transplantation: 29th official adult heart transplant report—2012, 1052–106, copyright (2012) with permission from Elsevier.

transplantation. Most adult patients are transplanted for either advanced idiopathic nonischemic cardiomyopathy or advanced ischemic cardiomyopathy. Compared to idiopathic cardiomyopathy patients, those with ischemic cardiomyopathy have a small excess in the relative risk of mortality—approximately 10–15%—that persists throughout their post-transplantation course. Patients transplanted for adult congenital heart disease have a twofold higher risk of mortality in the first post-transplantation year compared to nonischemic cardiomyopathy patients but better long-term survival, so that 10-year post-transplantation survival of these two groups is not different. Patients in need of retransplantation represent a group of patients at potentially high risk of post-transplantation mortality. A study from the Cardiac Transplant Research Database group reported that patients receiving retransplant within 1 year of their original transplant, and those receiving retransplant for acute rejection, had a risk of mortality that was several-fold higher than survival in primary heart transplant recipients.[9] As a result, the number of patients being retransplanted early has decreased significantly, and survival 1 year after retransplantation has improved from 55% for patients retransplanted in 1982–1992, to 82% in those retransplanted in 2003–2010. However, even in the current era, the risk of 1- and 5-year mortality after retransplantation exceeds that of a primary transplantation. Risk of transplantation in patients with less frequent causes of heart disease needs to be carefully evaluated at the time of assessment for transplant candidacy. An increasing number of patients with chemotherapy-induced cardiomyopathy are being treated for advanced HF and referred for transplantation evaluation.[10,11] It appears that in carefully selected patients with chemotherapy-induced cardiomyopathy, survival after transplantation is comparable to other patients, despite a higher risk of infection and malignancy post-transplantation.[12,13] Another challenging group is patients with AL amyloidosis. Survival of patients with cardiac AL amyloidosis can be improved with heart transplantation, when combined with preceding or subsequent chemotherapy aimed at inducing remission of the amyloidosis. However, recurrence of amyloidosis in the allograft is frequent, and post-transplantation survival is in general inferior compared to the typical transplant recipient. Therefore, heart transplantation as a treatment approach to cardiac AL amyloidosis remains controversial.[14,15,16,17]

The rapid rise of mechanical support use in patients awaiting heart transplantation also has implications for post-transplantation survival. The presence of temporary mechanical support such as extracorporeal membrane oxygenation (ECMO) or temporary pulsatile ventricular assist devices (VADs) at the time of transplant results in a two- to threefold increase in the risk of death at 1 and 5 years after transplantation.[4] The elevated risk of post-transplantation mortality, which used to be associated with permanent left ventricvular assist device (LVAD) use, appears to be very modest or absent altogether when the most recent cohorts of patients bridged with continuous-flow LVADs are examined.[18,19] The presence of biventricular support with biventricular assist devices or total artificial heart continues to be associated with increased risk of post-transplantation mortality.[4]

A number of additional donor and recipient characteristics have been identified as being associated with favorable or unfavorable outcome after transplantation. Donor characteristics are discussed in detail later in the chapter, but increasing age of adult donors is a strong and fairly linear predictor of both early and late mortality after adult heart transplantation. Similarly, recipient age is a strong predictor of early and late post-transplantation mortality, with a

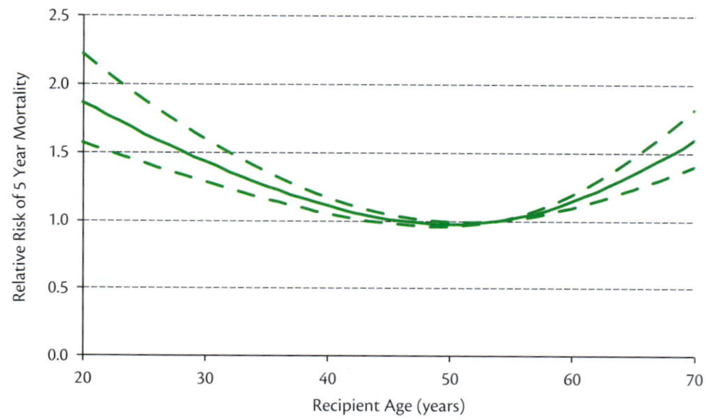

Fig. 16.3 Recipient age as a predictor of mortality 5 years after transplant.
Journal of Heart and Lung Transplantation, 31, Stehlik J, Edwards LB, Kucheryavaya AY, Benden C, Christie JD, et al. The registry of the International Society for Heart and Lung Transplantation: 29th official adult heart transplant report—2012, 1052–106, copyright (2012) with permission from Elsevier.

U-shaped relationship. Patients transplanted in their 40s and early 50s are at lowest risk while both younger and older recipients have a higher risk of mortality (Figure 16.3). The higher risk in younger patients is likely a result of a more responsive immune system resulting in a higher risk of rejection.[20,21] Higher rates of medication noncompliance may also play a role in higher mortality rates in younger recipients.[22] In contrast, the higher risk in older patients can be attributed to higher risk of malignancy and infection, as well as a higher comorbidity burden. A third perennial risk factor, which importance has changed little over the years, is allograft ischemic time. There is a small increase in mortality risk to approximately 240 minutes, but the risk increases sharply with further extension of the allograft ischemic time. Different myocardial cardioplegic preservation solutions have been formulated and their efficacy in reducing ischemic graft injury tested. Despite some promising experimental results, no consistent differences in outcome have been found among the commonly used cardioplegic solutions in clinical studies.[23,24,25] Ex-vivo machine perfusion of a beating heart allograft is a promising approach to reducing ischemic myocardial injury and extending the acceptable allograft ischemic time. Feasibility of this approach has been shown in experimental studies, initial clinical experience in lung transplantation has been described, and clinical trials using ex-vivo heart perfusion are ongoing.[26,27]

Significant recipient comorbidities, such as renal dysfunction, diabetes mellitus, obesity, infection preceding heart transplant, and ventilator support at the time of transplant, also increase the risk of post-transplantation mortality.[4,28,29,30,31,32] Recipient allosensitization (presence of anti-HLA antibodies in the recipient's serum) increases the risk of post-transplantation mortality.[33]

The risk associated with certain recipient characteristics is not always linear. Complex interactions between characteristics also mean that a sum of the individual relative risks may not provide an accurate quantification of the overall risk.[34] Unfortunately, reliable models that would allow for this quantification are not currently available.

Morbidity

Management of post-transplantation complications is described in detail in Chapter 19; in this section we review the incidence of the leading post-transplantation morbidities.

Acute graft rejection

The incidence of acute graft rejection is highest in the first several months after transplantation. In the 1990s, more than 40% of patients were hospitalized for rejection treatment in the first post-transplantation year. Introduction of the immunosuppressive induction agents, mycophenolate mofetil and tacrolimus has resulted in a steep decline of acute rejection incidence, with only 16% of patients transplanted in 2009 requiring treatment for acute rejection in the first post-transplantation year. The risk of acute rejection continues to decrease with time, now below 5%/year after the second post-transplantation year.[4]

A number of patient characteristics including younger age in the adult recipient population, African-American ethnicity, medication noncompliance, and recipient allosensitization increase the risk of rejection.[20,21,35] Patients who develop acute rejection in the first post-transplantation year remain at a higher risk of rejection later. It has been suggested that acute antibody-mediated rejection might have a higher impact on long-term survival compared to acute cellular rejection. This may be because we have a better understanding of the pathophysiology of acute cellular rejection, and therefore also more specific and efficient therapies, which is not the case for antibody-mediated rejection. When acute rejection is accompanied by hemodynamic compromise, the risk of subsequent death increases markedly, regardless of the rejection type.[36]

Cardiac allograft vasculopathy

CAV is a type of coronary artery disease characterized by diffuse intimal proliferation. CAV is characterized angiographically by diffuse narrowing of epicardial coronary arteries, with tapering of the distal segments and loss of small coronary branches. Approximately 25% of patients have angiographic evidence of CAV at 5 years after transplantation, and more than half have CAV at 10 years.[4] Intravascular coronary ultrasound studies have shown, however, that CAV starts early post-transplantation; coronary intimal thickness can be seen on intravascular ultrasound (IVUS) in many patients at 1 year after transplantation.[37,38] Risk factors for development of CAV include higher donor age, donor history of hypertension, cytomegalovirus (CMV)-positive donor allocation to a CMV-negative recipient, male donor sex, male recipient sex, and allograft rejection.[39,40] CAV represents a significant risk factor for mortality.[41] It appears that the incidence of CAV has decreased modestly in recent years.[4]

Infection

Infection is a relatively frequent complication following transplantation. The hazard is highest in the first year when the level of immunosuppression is high, but risk of significant infection continues throughout the post-transplantation period. Infection remains one of the leading causes of mortality after heart transplantation (Figure 16.4).

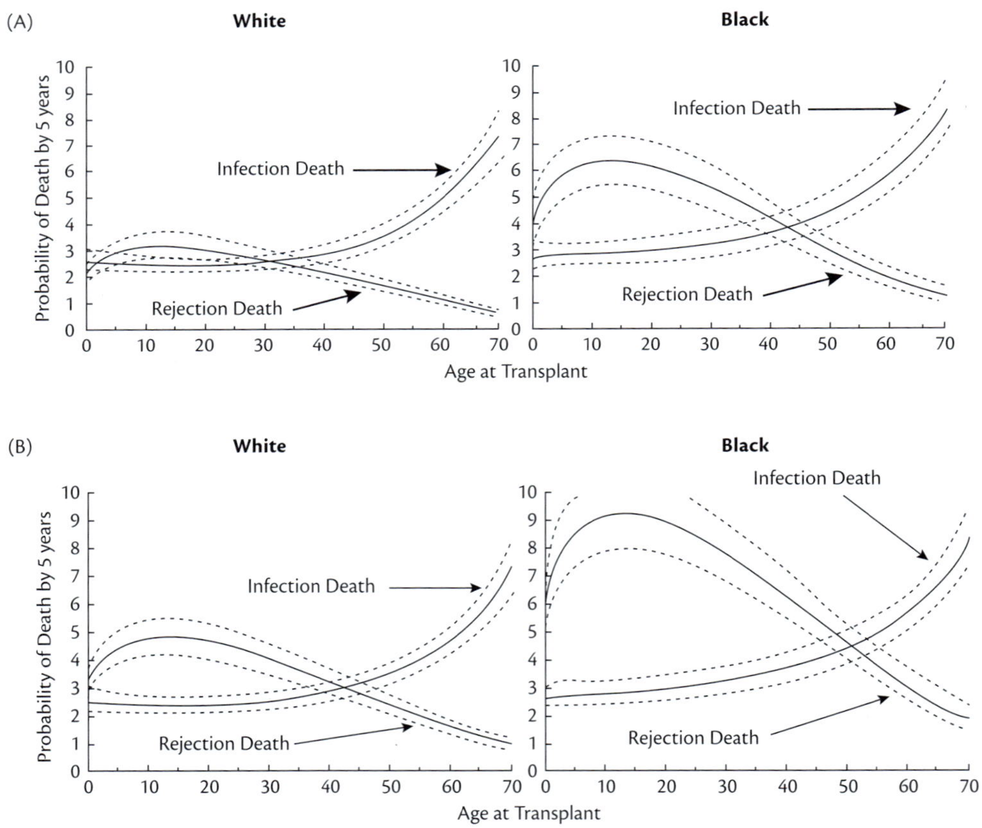

Fig. 16.4 Multivariate equations depicting the probability of death due to rejection or infection at 5 years after transplantation with respect to age at the time of transplantation in black or white (A) male and (B) female recipients transplanted in January 1, 2006.

Journal of Heart and Lung Transplantation, 30, George JF, Taylor DO, Blume ED, Kirklin JK, Naftel DC, Brown RN, Dipchand AI,McGiffin DC, Pamboukian SV, Tallaj JA. Minimizing infection and rejection death: clues acquired from 19 years of multi-institutional cardiac transplantation data, 151–7, copyright (2011) with permission from Elsevier.

Malignancy

The risk of malignancy is higher in transplant recipients compared to healthy individuals of similar age. The increase in the risk is believed to be associated with long-term exposure to immunosuppressive therapies, and the risk increases with time since transplantation. Skin cancer is the most frequent post-transplantation malignancy, seen in more than 20% of patients within 10 years of transplantation. In contrast to the general population, squamous cell cancer is much more frequent than basal cell carcinoma. Other malignancies which incidence is higher in solid organ transplant recipients include cervical carcinoma, hepatobiliary carcinoma, and renal carcinoma. In children, lymphoma is the most common malignancy. Post-transplantation lymphoproliferative disorder (PTLD) is a type of lymphoma seen after transplantation both in children and in adults. Risk factors for developing post-transplantation malignancy include older recipient age, higher cumulative exposure to immunosuppressive therapies, history of malignancy before transplantation, and sun exposure for skin cancer. Epstein–Barr virus (EBV) is believed to be responsible for development of PTLD, and EBV-negative recipients of EBV-positive donors are at a particularly high risk.[42]

Renal dysfunction

Renal dysfunction is a common problem after heart transplantation. Among patients transplanted in the United States between 1990 and 2000, 20% had a glomerular filtration rate less than 29 ml min^{-1} 1.73 m^{-2} or were receiving renal replacement therapy by 10 years after transplantation.[43] Severe renal dysfunction before or after transplantation is a predictor of mortality. Risk factors for post-transplantation development of renal dysfunction include recipient age, recipient history of kidney disease, and recipient history of diabetes mellitus. The incidence of severe renal dysfunction after heart transplant has been gradually decreasing over the past 20 years.

Donor management and evaluation

During the early days of heart transplantation, cardiac allografts were procured from donors after circulatory death. In the 1970s, clinical criteria for confirmation of brain death were established, which greatly facilitated the process of organ donation.[44,45] As a result, brain-dead donors have been used almost exclusively as source of allografts for cardiac transplantation. More recently, donation after circulatory death (DCD) has been used in lung and abdominal transplantation. Contemporary experience with this approach in heart transplantation has been limited, however, to a small number of programs.[46] While DCD may lead to an increase in the number of available donor allografts,[47] wider acceptance of this approach will require further examination of the logistical, legal, and bioethical aspects specific to heart transplantation.

Donor management is a term that describes activities that take place after establishment of the diagnosis of brain death in a prospective donor, and are directed at preserving and improving organ function for the purposes of organ donation and transplantation. Implementation of effective donor management is critical, as the process of brain death often results in hemodynamic instability. Initially, cerebral ischemia results in a potent sympathetic surge, mediated at the medullary level. In addition to hypertension and tachycardia seen at this stage, the sympathetic discharge can be detrimental to myocardial function; myocardial ischemia and injury results from calcium overload, depletion of high-energy phosphates, generation of oxygen free radicals, endothelial damage, and β-adrenoreceptor desensitization.[48,49,50,51] Later, at the time of herniation, ischemia of the spinal cord results in abrupt deactivation of the sympathetic nervous system, a drop in catecholamine levels, vasodilation, and hypotension. Endocrine changes resulting from brain death are believed to contribute to hemodynamic instability. Compromise of the hypothalamic–pituitary–adrenal axis can lead to depletion of thyroid hormone and cortisol levels, while diabetes insipidus can result in hypovolemia, hypernatremia, and further hypotension. All these events are occurring precisely at a time when clinical teams reduce the aggressiveness of medical care in a critically ill patient progressing to brain death. It is therefore important that processes are in place to allow for a seamless transition of care from the clinical teams in the intensive care unit to the personnel responsible for donor management. The initial hemodynamic goals of donor management will not differ significantly from the goals of the critical care team. Interventions should aim for normalization of systemic pressure, cardiac filling pressures, and cardiac output (general goals are: mean arterial pressure ≥60 mmHg, central venous pressure 6–10 mmHg, pulmonary capillary wedge pressure 8–12 mmHg, cardiac index >2.4 L $min^{-1}m^{-2}$). Crystalloids should be used to maintain normovolemia and hypotonic fluid may be necessary to prevent or treat hypernatremia in patients with diabetes insipidus. In patients with significant blood loss, transfusions should be used to achieve hematocrit greater than 30%, and normoglycemia should also be maintained. Respiratory management should be aggressive, including frequent suctioning and bronchoscopy, if needed; ventilator settings should be optimized to achieve normocapnia and prevent hypoxia. Hypothermia should be avoided.

Vasoactive agents are often needed for treatment of hypotension. While there are no conclusive data to assess efficacy of specific agents, low-dose vasopressors (vasopressin, norepinephrine, neosynephrine) should be used to treat the hypotension that is believed to result from peripheral vasodilation.[52] The need for agents with inotropic properties (dobutamine, epinephrine) should raise questions regarding abnormalities in myocardial contractility. Short-acting drugs such as sodium nitroprusside or esmolol should be used to treat hypertension. Invasive hemodynamic monitoring with a pulmonary artery catheter may be of benefit in donors where hemodynamic goals cannot be expeditiously achieved or maintained.[53] In patients with hemodynamic instability despite implementation of the above measures, hormonal supplementation with various combinations of corticosteroids, thyroid hormone, and insulin has been proposed to counteract the possible hormonal depletion resulting from brain death. While there is no consensus on the utility of this approach, some studies have shown benefit.[54,55,56]

With achievement of the hemodyamic goals, the *donor evaluation* process starts. From the cardiac transplant perspective, the goal is to exclude significant pre-existing heart disease, new myocardial dysfunction resulting from the critical condition leading to brain death, and the negative impact of the brain death process on myocardial function. Extracardiac factors are also carefully evaluated.

Extracardiac considerations

A careful medical, social, and travel history should be obtained. Donor mode of death has been linked with post-transplantation outcomes, but other donor characteristics appear to have a much stronger effect on survival.[57] When the donor cause of death is not clear, however, a cardiac cause of death has to be ruled out, as this would almost certainly prevent use of the heart for transplantation.

Donor age is considered very carefully as it has significant implications for graft survival. In the 1980s, allografts were sought predominantly from very young donors. Subsequently, it was shown that donor selection could be expanded to healthy donors of older age and median donor age has since increased.[4] Regional differences in the typical donor age also exist, influenced by variations in donor pool and local practice; for example, the median age of a heart donor in the United States is 34 years compared to 42 years in Europe. Post-transplantation mortality increases progressively with increasing donor age. When compared to a 30-year old donor, the relative risk of 1-year mortality is increased 50% in a 50-year-old donor and 100% in a 60-year-old donor. The negative impact of increasing donor age can be further potentiated by additional donor characteristics such as left ventricular (LV) hypertrophy or longer allograft ischemic time.[58] In North America, less than 10% of transplanted hearts come from donors 50 years of age or older.

The effects of donor and recipient height and weight are discussed in the section on donor–recipient matching.

Donor medical comorbidities also need to be considered during donor selection. Donor history of hypertension and diabetes mellitus have been associated with risk of recipient mortality. It is important to determine whether these comorbidities have resulted in development of coronary artery disease, myocardial hypertrophy, or myocardial dysfunction in the donor (see following section—Assessment of donor cardiac function).

Donor history of malignancy is usually considered a contraindication for heart transplantation, as donor malignancy can be transmitted to the recipient through the allograft.[59,60,61,62,63,64] A few notable exceptions where donation appears to be safe include donor history of noninvasive nonmelanoma skin tumors and history of primary low-grade brain tumors, as long as craniotomy or intracranial shunts have not been performed. Of note, brain tumors including glioblastoma multiforme, medulloblastoma, and astrocytoma should definitely be considered a contraindication to transplantation because of their tendency to metastasize.

Donors should be routinely screened for infectious diseases that could be transmitted to the recipient (Table 16.2). While a history of EBV, CMV, or toxoplasmosis is frequent and these do not represent contraindications to transplantation, the appropriate testing should be done as it will influence the selection and choice of antimicrobial prophylactic therapy after transplantation. Donor infection with HIV or syphilis represent an absolute contraindication to organ transplantation. Donors with hepatitis B (HBV) and hepatitis C (HBC) used to be considered as heart donors for recipients with the same viral disease; however, due to the risk of hepatitis reactivation in the recipient, most programs no longer use this approach.[65] Infection with human T-lymphotropic virus (HTLV) appears to be inconsequential, and donor screening for HTLV is no longer recommended in the United States. If the donor's social history, travel history, or medical history raise suspicion of any other potentially transmittable infection, appropriate testing should be completed before transplant. Reported donor-derived infections have included West Nile virus, rabies, Chagas disease, malaria, tuberculosis, measles, parvovirus, adenovirus, and enterovirus.[66]

Table 16.2 Recommended prospective donor screening tests for infectious diseases

Infectious agent	Screening test
Hepatitis B virus (HBV)	NAT If NAT not available: HBV surface antigen, core antibody, surface antibody
Hepatitis C virus (HCV)	NAT If NAT not available: HCV antibody
HIV	NAT If NAT not available: HIV antibody
Treponema pallidum	Treponemal antibody or TPHA and rapid plasma reagin (RPR)
Toxoplasma gondii	Toxoplasma antibody
Cytomegalovirus (CMV)	CMV antibody
Epstein–Barr virus (EBV)	EBV antibody panel
Herpes simplex virus (HSV)	HSV antibody
Bacterial infection	Blood and urine cultures
Fungal infection	Blood and urine cultures

NAT, nucleic acid testing; TPHA, *Treponema pallidum* particle agglutination assay,

Some donors may be diagnosed with bacterial or fungal infections. Some systemic infections, such as pneumonia or line-associated sepsis, do not necessarily represent a contraindication to transplantation, as long as the causative agent is identified, appropriate treatment is started, repeat blood cultures are sterile, and there is no evidence of endocarditis.[67] In contrast, use of organs from donors with severe systemic and possibly metastatic infections should be avoided, especially when the causative organism may be difficult to identify, as is the case, for example, in meningitis or encephalitis.[66]

Screening for infectious diseases is designed to minimize the risk of donor-derived infection. Some risk of disease transmission remains, even with screening, due to the lag between infection acquisition and initial test positivity. The period of false negativity is significantly reduced by implementation of nucleic acid testing (NAT). Compared to serology testing for antibodies, NAT decreases this period from more than 22 days to 10 days for HIV, from 50 days to 22 days for HBV, and from 94 days to 9 days for hepatitis C virus (HCV). The risk of contraction of an infectious disease in this window period should be assessed through careful social history. Recently updated criteria specific to organ transplantation identify donors at increased risk for HIV, HBV and HCV infection, and should be taken into consideration when making a decision to accept a donor.[68] The risk factors include history of the following in the preceding 12 months:

- new diagnosis or treatment of syphilis, gonorrhea, chlamydia, or genital ulcers
- sex with a person known or suspected to have HIV, HBV, or HCV infection
- men who have had sex with men (MSM)
- women who have had sex with a man with a history of MSM behavior

- sex in exchange for money or drugs
- sex with a person who had sex in exchange for money or drugs
- use of, or sex with a person who uses, illicit drugs by intravenous, intramuscular, or subcutaneous route
- jail, prison, juvenile correctional facility, or lock-up for more than 72 consecutive hours
- child who is less than 18 months of age and born to a mother known to be infected with, or at increased risk for, HIV, HBV, or HCV infection, or a child who has been breastfed within the preceding 12 months by a mother with these risks.

In the United States, recipients for whom an organ from a "high-risk" donor is being considered should be asked to sign an informed consent acknowledging this information.

Assessment of donor cardiac function

Echocardiography is now done routinely in most if not all potential heart donors. It provides assessment of myocardial structure, myocardial function, valvular function, and often also an estimate of pulmonary pressures. Some of the abnormalities that can be identified by echocardiography are discussed in this section.

Myocardial dysfunction

When myocardial dysfunction is present, it is imperative to determine its etiology. In donors without underlying heart disease, myocardial dysfunction is frequently a result of the sympathetic surge that accompanies brain death. The chamber size in this clinical scenario is normal and there is global systolic dysfunction, often with regional wall motion abnormalities typically in the anteroseptal region. Myocardial dysfunction caused by brain death is often reversible, and survival in recipients of hearts with initially depressed contractility is good.[69,70] When myocardial dysfunction is suspected to be a result of brain death, donor management should be extended, hemodynamics optimized, and the echocardiogram repeated in 6–12 hours if possible to assess for improvement of cardiac function. If significant myocardial dysfunction (LVEF<40%) or need for high-dose inotropic support persist despite optimization of preload and afterload, the heart should be considered not suitable for transplantation.

RV function should be assessed carefully in patients with chest trauma to rule out the possibility of myocardial contusion. This condition is often associated with increase in serum markers of myocardial injury. Myocardial dysfunction associated with ventricular remodeling (e.g., increase in ventricular size, evidence of myocardial scarring) suggests underlying heart disease and would be an indication to either decline the donor for heart transplantation, or to proceed with additional diagnostic testing.

Left ventricular hypertrophy

There is some disagreement regarding the extent to which donor LVH affects post-transplantation survival. Carefully selected donors with LVH appear to have favorable survival; however, donor history of hypertension has been identified as a risk factor for post-transplantation mortality,[4] and studies have shown that severe LVH (>13 mm) may compromise survival, especially if the allograft ischemic time is long or if the donor is older.[58,71,72] If hypertrophic cardiomyopathy is identified on echocardiography, the donor heart should not be used for transplantation.

Valvular dysfunction

Chest trauma can result in tricuspid valve injury, flail leaflet(s), and severe tricuspid regurgitation. If use of such a heart for transplantation is considered, the tricuspid valve must be repaired before transplantation. Any valvular regurgitation or stenosis of more than mild severity should trigger additional testing or refusal of the donor heart. Presence of a bicuspid aortic valve without more than mild stenosis, especially if the donor is young, does not represent a contraindication for transplantation, as the natural history of the disease is favorable. Bench repair of bicuspid valve before heart transplantation has been described.[73]

Congenital heart disease

In most instances, congenital heart disease in the donor represents a contraindication for transplantation. A heart with a small secundum atrial septal defect, without evidence of RV volume overload, can be considered for heart transplantation, with the defect surgically corrected at the time of transplantation. (Patent foramen ovale is inconsequential, and should also be closed at the time of transplant).

A 12-lead ECG should be obtained to rule our acute myocardial ischemia, chronic ischemic heart disease, arrhythmias, or other abnormalities.

Serum cardiac enzymes (troponin and CK-MB) are often elevated at the time of donor evaluation, and may reflect events surrounding cardiac resuscitation or brain death. In the absence of coronary artery disease or traumatic myocardial injury, elevation of cardiac enzymes, especially when transient, is not a contraindication to transplantation.[74]

Coronary angiography should be performed in most male donors 46 years of age or older and in female donors 55 years of age or older, to rule out the presence of significant coronary artery disease (CAD). In donors with history of cocaine use or three or more risk factors for CAD (hypertension, diabetes, tobacco use, dyslipidemia, premature coronary disease in the family), the age cutoff for angiography should be lower (35 years).[75] In situations where performing coronary angiography is not feasible, decisions regarding an acceptance of the donor should take into account the donor's likelihood of CAD, and the urgency of transplantation in the particular recipient should be determined. Allografts with mild nonobstructive lesions are often used, especially for older recipients. While surgical correction of obstructive donor CAD prior to transplantation has been reported, it is rarely done in clinical practice, and should be considered a contraindication to transplantation in most circumstances.[76]

Substance abuse

Use of cocaine causes vasoconstriction, endothelial dysfunction, and systemic hypertension, and promotes clotting. These effects are cardiotoxic; myocardial injury is likely, especially with intravenous cocaine use. The use of heart allografts from donors who use cocaine intravenously should be avoided, although hearts from donors with nonintravenous cocaine without evidence of myocardial dysfunction and LVH can be considered for transplantation.[67]

Ethanol is also a myocardial toxin and cardiac function in donors with history of heavy alcohol abuse should be examined carefully; a conservative approach to donor use in this clinical scenario seems appropriate.

Integrated information obtained through donor social and medical history, donor management, and donor diagnostic evaluation is used by clinical transplant teams to make decisions on organ suitability for transplantation, and the desirability of allocation to individual transplant candidates.

Contraindications to cardiac transplantation

Determining an individual's suitability for cardiac transplantation and transplantation-associated risk is a complex process, dependent upon a multitude of factors, including existing comorbidities, prior surgical history, and serum alloantibody status. Comorbidities may adversely affect both quality of life and survival following transplantation and, depending on their severity, may be either relative or absolute contraindications to transplantation. Conditions such as hypertension, diabetes, hyperlipidemia, obesity, chronic kidney disease, and vascular disease may be exacerbated by immunosuppressive medications.[77] Others, such as pulmonary hypertension or a history of prior cardiac surgery, increase perioperative risk. While exact criteria for individual contraindications vary among centers, the actual comorbidities and patient characteristics that are considered are fairly uniform. In the last several years both temporary and durable mechanical circulatory support (MCS) devices have been used as a "bridge to decision"—that is, to afford time to determine if conditions such as pulmonary hypertension or renal and hepatic dysfunction are reversible enough to allow successful transplantation. In some cases these devices provide the time and stability for important noncardiac surgery to be performed prior to transplantation or provide support during a period of observation following cancer therapy to assess the risk of recurrence. Table 16.3 lists contraindications for cardiac transplantation and indicates situations in which MCS might be used as a bridge to decision for transplantation and also indicates those problems often caused or exacerbated by immunosuppressive therapy.

Table 16.3 Contraindications to cardiac transplantation

Contraindications	Potentially modifiable with MCS	Comments on MCS support	Likely to be exacerbated or improved by immunosuppressive therapy
Absolute			
Any condition resulting in life expectancy <2 years, not modifiable by heart transplantation			
Relative			
Pulmonary			
Pulmonary hypertension	Yes	Data for risk/benefit ratio uncertain	
Pulmonary parenchymal disease	No		
Pulmonary infarction	Yes	May allow time for infarction to resolve	Exacerbated
Advanced age			
Chronic kidney disease	Yes	If due to cardiorenal syndrome	Exacerbated
Hepatic disease	Yes	If due to heart failure	
Vascular	Maybe	In some cases may allow surgical correction	Exacerbated
Cerebrovascular disease	No		
Peripheral arterial disease	No		
Abdominal aortic aneurysm	No		
Diabetes with neuropathy, nephropathy, or retinopathy	No		
Obesity	Unlikely		Exacerbated
Cachexia	Yes	May allow correction of cachexia but cachexia also increases risk of MCS surgery	
Resistant hypertension	No		Exacerbated
Active GI bleeding including peptic ulcer disease	No		Peptic ulcer disease exacerbated by steroids

(continued)

Table 16.3 Continued

Contraindications	Potentially modifiable with MCS	Comments on MCS support	Likely to be exacerbated or improved by immunosuppressive therapy
Active infection HIV Hepatitis B and C *Clostridium difficile* Active cholescystitis, diverticulitis Other serious infections	Active infection generally contraindicates MCS placement		Exacerbated
Systemic diseases:			
Severe progressive neurologic or neuromuscular disorders	No		
Active malignancy	In some cases	May allow time to be certain malignancy is unlikely to recur	Exacerbated
Autoimmune diseases	No		May improve
Sarcoidosis	No		May improve
Amyloidosis	No		
Unresolved tobacco abuse	Yes	May allow time for therapy and correction	
Inability to comply with pre- and post-transplant medical care Psychiatric disease Alcohol or drug abuse Nonadherence Inadequate social support	Maybe	May allow time for treatment of problems or mobilization of social support but all these factors also increase risk of MCS therapy	Complex medical regimen may make adherence more difficult
Surgical concerns Multiple sternotomies Radiation-induced heart disease Heparin-induced thrombocytopenia	No		

MCS, mechanical circulatory support.

Data from Mancini D, Lietz K. Selection of cardiac transplantation candidates in 2010. Circulation. 2010;122:173–83.

Any problem that limits life expectancy to less than 2 years despite a cardiac transplantation is an absolute contraindication to transplantation.[78,79] Examples include amyloidosis with multiorgan involvement or patients with HIV and multiple opportunistic infections. Severe irreversible pulmonary hypertension is also considered an absolute contraindication because of the risk of death due to right HF following transplantation.

Pulmonary issues

Pulmonary hypertension

Elevated pulmonary vascular resistance (PVR) is a risk factor for mortality following cardiac transplantation.[80] The excess mortality associated with elevated PVR is primarily due to RV failure, as the donor RV is usually not hypertrophied and may not be able to maintain a prolonged acute increase in systolic pressure in the face of increased PVR post-transplantation. Indeed, RV failure has been reported to be the cause of 20% of early heart transplant deaths.[81] The most recent ISHLT registry data, however, report only a modest incremental mortality risk associated with an elevated PVR of 3–5 Wood units or greater compared to less than 3 Wood units, but no difference between recipient PVR of 3–5 versus greater than 5 Wood units.[4] In a retrospective review of 405 cardiac transplants performed in a single center, 158 had pulmonary hypertension defined as PVR greater than 2.5 Wood units and (or) a transpulmonary gradient (TPG) greater than 12 mmHg.[82] Recipients with pulmonary hypertension were divided into tertiles by PVR (mild, PVR = 2.5–3 Wood units; moderate, PVR =3.1–4.5 Wood units; severe PVR ≥ 4.5 Wood units). There was no effect of PVR on 10-year mortality. Thus, some controversy exists about precise levels of PVR that contraindicate transplantation. Reversibility of an elevated PVR is considered to be associated with improved survival. The most common criteria for assessing the risk of right HF utilize PVR (mean pulmonary artery pressure minus mean pulmonary capillary wedge pressure divided by cardiac output) and the TPG (mean pulmonary artery pressure minus mean pulmonary capillary wedge pressure). The Stanford group reported that PVR greater than 2.5 Wood units, a TPGgreater than 15 mmHg, and a pulmonary artery systolic pressure greater than 50 mmHg all identified patients at high risk of mortality following cardiac transplantation.[83] Either a low baseline PVR (≤2.5 Wood units) or a PVR that could be reduced to 2.5 Wood units or less without symptomatic hypotension (systolic blood pressure ≤85 mmHg) best predicted a low 90-day mortality without RV failure. Other studies have confirmed that the reversibility of elevated PVR predicts a low postoperative mortality.[84,85] Nitroglycerine, nitroprusside, dobutamine, inhaled nitric oxide, and inhaled and intravenous prostaglandins have all been used to assess reversibility of pulmonary hypertension.[83,86,87]

Other potential therapies have been suggested for patients with high PVR. The 2012 ISHLT registry reported that in recipients with a PVR greater than 5 Wood units, a donor:recipient body weight ratio of 1.1–1.2 resulted in improved mortality compared to lower ratios.[4] When PVR is high and "fixed," oral sildenafil therapy may be considered.[88] Implantation of a LVAD to allow time for the PVR to decrease before cardiac transplantation is another option.[89] However, the risk of RV failure may be considerable in these patients and the excess morbidity and mortality of the LVAD procedure must be considered. In addition, sensitization to HLA antigens resulting from the LVAD procedure and the associated blood product transfusions may make finding a donor heart more difficult.[89] Liden et al. in a retrospective evaluation of 405 cardiac transplants (158 with pulmonary hypertension) matched 11 recipients with pulmonary hypertension (PVR >2.5 Wood units and/or a TPG >12 mmHg) who underwent pretransplantation LVAD placement with 22 recipients with pulmonary hypertension who did not have an LVAD prior to transplantation.[82] Mortality was not different between the two groups and 3 of the 11 LVAD subjects required post-transplantation MCS versus only 1 of the 22 without an LVAD, suggesting that there may not be an overall benefit of an LVAD if implanted solely to reduce pulmonary hypertension.

RV failure following transplantation may be affected by factors other than elevated pretransplant PVR including donor size, quality of the donor heart, and the presence of increased pulmonary resistance due to the lung edema and injury that occurs during cardiopulmonary bypass.

As a result, specific criteria for the level of pulmonary hypertension that are considered a contraindication to transplantation and for the determination of pulmonary hypertension reversibility vary between transplant centers. The most current guidelines suggest that "fixed pulmonary hypertension," as defined by a pulmonary artery systolic pressure greater than 60 mmHg, a mean TPG greater than 15 mmHg, and a PVR greater than 6 Wood units represent absolute contraindications to cardiac transplantation.[79]

Pulmonary parenchymal disease

Patients with severe pulmonary parenchymal diseases such as chronic bronchitis, emphysema, or interstitial lung disease are poor candidates for cardiac transplantation, as these problems affect operative and long-term mortality and substantially limit post-transplantation quality of life. In general, a forced expiratory volume in one second (FEV_1) of less than 1 L or 40% of predicted, that is not reversible with treatment of HF, is considered a contraindication to cardiac transplantation.[78,79]

Pulmonary infarction

Pulmonary emboli may lead to pulmonary hypertension, increasing the risk of right HF post-transplantation.[90] The development of a recent pulmonary infarction has been considered a contraindication to transplantation due to the risk of lung abscess, empyema, bronchopleural fistula, and systemic sepsis following transplantation.[90]

Age

Advanced recipient age is a risk factor for post-transplantation morbidity and mortality, even after accounting for associated comorbidities. While not all studies agree, the largest studies suggest that age is a factor in post-transplantation survival.[4,78,91] In a review of the United Network for Organ Sharing (UNOS) database of 14 441 first-time heart recipients transplanted between 1999 and 2006, Weiss et al. reported slightly better survival of patients younger than 60 years compared to patients 60 years or older.[92] Thirty-day, 1-year, and 5-year survival were 94%, 87%, and 75% in the younger group compared to 93%, 84%, and 69% in the older group (p <0.001).[92] Older patients had more infections but less rejection. Half of the excess mortality in the older group was seen in the first year post-transplantation. Although incremental age was determined to be a risk factor, the authors pointed out that older recipients received higher-risk donor hearts, which could explain part or all of the excess mortality attributed to age. Despite favorable results in carefully selected elderly recipients, many transplant programs continue to have an upper age limit, and a recent review suggests age greater than 72 years should be a relative contraindication.[79]

Chronic kidney disease

Renal dysfunction is common in patients with end-stage HF and it is often difficult to determine how much of it is due to chronic underlying kidney disease and how much is due to *cardiorenal syndrome*. Renal dysfunction due to the cardiorenal syndrome is likely to reverse with successful transplantation, while underlying chronic kidney disease may be exacerbated by calcineurin inhibitors. Careful evaluation of renal function pretransplantation is important as glomerular filtration rate (GFR) declines more rapidly with age in transplant recipients than in the general population.[93,94] The fall in GFR is likely to be due primarily to calcineurin inhibitor toxicity but may also be due to diabetes, hypertension, and vascular disease, all of which may be caused or exacerbated by immunsuppressive therapy, particularly calcineurin inhibitors and corticosteroids, following transplantation.[77] Unless the patient is a candidate for combined heart–kidney transplantation, severe irreversible chronic kidney disease (GFR <25–30 ml min^{-1} 1.73 m^{-2}) that is unrelated to HF is a relative contraindication to transplantation.[79] Both increasing age and diabetes increase the risk for the development of stage 5 chronic kidney disease (GFR <15 ml min^{-1} 1.73 m^{-2}) post-transplantation.[94]

Severe hepatic disease

Patients with severe underlying liver disease have an increased risk of anesthetic and surgical complications and mortality following cardiac surgery.[95,96] The Child classification (and its modifications) has been predictive of poor outcomes following cardiac surgery but it is uncertain whether this score outperforms the Standard Model for End-Stage Liver Disease (MELD) score.[96,97] The Child score uses encephalopathy, ascites, total bilirubin, albumin, and the INR or the prothrombin time while the MELD score uses total bilirubin, albumin, and INR. As most potential transplant recipients do not have encephalopathy or ascites, and many are taking oral anticoagulants, rendering the INR poorly predictive, variations of the Child score and the MELD score are imperfect tools for this group. Recently a modified MELD score (with albumin replacing INR to eliminate the confounding effects of anticoagulation) was found to be highly predictive of mortality following cardiac transplantation. Patients with a modified MELD score less than 14 had a 5-year survival of 82.2% compared to 55.1% in those with a modified MELD score greater than 20.[98] The precise criteria for excluding a candidate for cardiac transplantation because of underlying liver disease remain uncertain and vary between centers, although a recent review suggested that a total bilirubin greater than 2.5 mg/dl, serum transaminases more than three times normal, or an INR off warfarin greater than 1.5 should represent relative contraindications.[79]

Vascular disease

Vascular disease, including carotid, aortic, and peripheral arterial disease (PAD) are all predictors of cardiovascular mortality. Immunosuppressive therapy following transplantation causes and exacerbates known cardiac risk factors for vascular disease such as hypertension, diabetes, hyperlipidemia, and obesity.[77] Thus, symptomatic vascular disease has been considered a contraindication to transplantation because of the concern for vascular complications and acceleration of the underlying vascular disease.[78,79] In a prospective study of 239 transplant recipients without vascular disease prior to transplantation who underwent routine post-transplantation surveillance for vascular disease, 24 (10%) developed significant vascular disease, including carotid stenosis, femoral-popliteal and aortoiliac disease, and abdominal aortic aneurysms at a mean of 3.2 years post-transplantation.[99] In another cohort that did not undergo routine surveillance studies other than history and physical examination, vascular disease increased in prevalence from 6% at time of transplant evaluation to 17% at 10 years post-transplantation.[100] The authors noted that much of the vascular disease was due to medical interventions and suggested that transplant recipients with vascular disease pretransplantation were at increased risk for vascular injuries.

Pre-existing vascular disease has also been shown to have a deleterious effect on survival post-transplantation. In the largest study to date (1634 heart transplant recipients), Rogers et al. reported that vascular disease was a significant predictor of 30-day mortality.[101] Likewise, in a retrospective evaluation of 264 combined heart–kidney transplant recipients, pre-existing vascular disease was the strongest predictor of mortality.[102] In another retrospective study of 402 heart transplant recipients, there was a trend for higher mortality (hazard ratio = 1.5) in recipients with pre-existing vascular disease, and a significantly increased risk of post-transplantation cerebrovascular accident (CVA) (16.7% vs. 3.1%, $p = 0.001$) as well as development of new PAD (33% vs. 7%). The development of new abdominal aortic aneurysms was noted in all of these studies.[100,101,102,103]

Symptomatic cerebrovascular disease, defined as a previous transient ischemic attack or CVA, is associated with an increased post-transplantation risk of stroke and functional decline.[104] However, probably due to careful recipient selection, the absolute risk of stroke and functional decline in this study were low. Many HF patients suffer embolic transient ischemic attacks or strokes due to emboli caused by atrial fibrillation or LV thrombus, and those patients seem likely to have a lower risk of post-transplantation CVA than those with obstructive cerebrovascular disease, as the intracardiac source of emboli is removed.

These data support the recent suggestions that PAD not amenable to surgical or percutaneous therapy, symptomatic carotid stenosis, an ankle–brachial index less than 0.7, and uncorrected abdominal aneurysms larger than 6 cm be considered relative contraindications to transplantation.[79]

Diabetes

Diabetes is a particularly concerning comorbidity in cardiac transplant recipients because it causes chronic kidney disease and because immunosuppressive agents may cause direct renal injury and exacerbate diabetes and hypertension, further affecting renal function.[77] The presence of significant end-organ damage (e.g., neuropathy or nephropathy, but not retinopathy), has been considered a relative contraindication to heart transplantation.[78] Using the UNOS database, Russo et al. evaluated 20 412 first-time heart transplant recipients who underwent transplantation between January of 1995 and December of 2005. Diabetes was classified by the number of diabetes-related complications, which included a pretransplantation history of renal failure (serum creatinine ≥2.5 mg/dl), history of CVA, PAD, or severe obesity as defined by a body mass index (BMI) greater than 35 kg/m^2.[105] Patients with diabetes and no diabetes-related complications had a survival nearly equal to nondiabetic recipients. However, in those with diabetes-related complications, survival worsened progressively as the number of complications increased. Median survival was 10.1 years in transplant recipients without diabetes and 9 years ($p = 0.08$) in those with diabetes and no diabetes-related complications, as compared to 6.7 years in recipients with one diabetes-related complication and 3.6 years in recipients with two or more complications.[105] Death due to renal failure, CVA, and infection were increased as the number of diabetes-related complications increased. Functional status, as measured by the ability to independently perform activities of daily living, was reduced in diabetic recipients without complications, and each diabetes-related complication was associated with a further reduction in functional capacity.[105] Almuti et al. reported that the absolute decrease in GFR at 3 years following heart transplantation was the same in diabetic subjects as in their nondiabetic counterparts, despite a lower starting GFR in the diabetic patients.[106] However, more patients in the diabetic group developed end-stage renal disease because of the lower pretransplantation GFR.

Obesity and cachexia

In nontransplantation cardiac surgery patients, obesity is consistently associated with an increased risk of sternal wound infection, and variable reports of more pulmonary complications, thromboembolic disease, and nonsternal infection.[107,108] In a retrospective evaluation of 4515 heart transplant recipients from the Cardiac Transplant Research Database, pretransplantation obesity (>140% of ideal body weight) was associated with increased 4-year mortality in men and a similar, though nonsignificant, result in women.[28] Infection rates were increased in obese versus nonobese recipients. However, the most recent ISHLT registry did not identify obesity as a mortality risk.[4] Obese candidates wait longer for a donor heart and are less likely to receive a heart transplant than their nonobese counterparts, presumably due to the requirement for larger donor hearts.[109] In general, a BMI of 35 kg/m^2 or more or greater than 140% of ideal body weight is considered a relative contraindication for cardiac transplantation.[79]

A BMI less than 20 kg/m^2 or less than 80% of ideal body weight have both been associated with increased post-transplantation mortality.[111] However, a low BMI was not found to be a risk in another study.[111] Despite the conflicting data, cachexia (BMI <18–20 kg/m^2) is currently considered a relative contraindication for transplantation.[78,79]

Active infection

Active bacterial tissue infection is a contraindication to transplantation. *Clostridium difficile* infection, common in potential cardiac transplant recipients because of their frequent hospitalizations, is a contraindication to transplantation as it is more fulminant in the face of immunosuppression and may result in toxic megacolon.[112] Active cholecystitis and diverticulitis are also considered relative contraindications.[78,79]

Few data exist about cardiac transplantation in HIV-positive recipients. One study reported 100% 5-year survival in 7 patients with HIV, 5 of whom had HIV diagnosed pretransplantation and two who had seroconverted post-transplantation.[113] These patients had a mean CD4 count of 554±169/μl and undetectable antigen loads. Further data are needed to determine the long-term outcomes in these patients.

Overall, the results of cardiac transplantation in selected hepatitis B and C positive recipients are similar to those in noninfected recipients.[114,115,116] However, the incidence of liver disease appears to be higher in hepatitis B-positive recipients and thus they are less often considered for transplantation than hepatitis C positive recipients.[116] Potential recipients with either hepatitis B or hepatitis C should be evaluated for viral load and for the presence of significant liver disease, usually with a liver biopsy.

Resistant systemic hypertension

Hypertension refractory to multiple drug therapy is a relative contraindication to cardiac transplantation as both corticosteroids and calcineurin inhibitors may exacerbate hypertension.[77]

Active gastrointestinal bleeding

Any gastrointestinal bleeding that cannot be adequately controlled is a contraindication to cardiac transplantation because of the high levels of anticoagulation required during cardiopulmonary bypass. Active peptic ulcer disease is particularly problematic as corticosteroids may exacerbate the underlying disease.

Severe progressive neurologic or neuromuscular disorders

Muscular dystrophies represent an array of inherited mutations that affect the cytoskeleton and/or nuclear proteins, resulting in skeletal muscle myopathy. Many afflicted patients also develop a dilated cardiomyopathy that results in either sudden cardiac death or death due to progressive HF. Muscular dystrophy has been considered a relative contraindication to cardiac transplantation because progression of the skeletal myopathy limits the benefits of transplantation on both quality of life and survival. However, a recent study comparing the clinical outcomes following cardiac transplantation of 29 muscular dystrophy patients with 275 non-muscular dystrophy matched controls reported that survival at 1 and 5 years, infection rates, and the incidence of rejection and CAV were not significantly different in the two groups.[117] While it is likely that the transplanted muscular dystrophy patients were highly selected, the study suggests that selected patients can be considered for cardiac transplantation.

Systemic diseases

Malignancy

The incidence of cancer is increased in recipients of solid organ transplantation compared to the general population, and immunosuppression also enhances progression of the malignant disease.[118,119] Thus, active nondermatologic malignancy is felt to be a contraindication to cardiac transplantation and guidelines recommend at least a 2-year cancer-free period prior to transplantation. In a report of 232 cardiac transplant recipients who had chemotherapy-induced cardiomyopathy, 1-, 3- and 5-year survival were not different than those of contemporaneous recipients with other causes of HF, although the subjects in this study were younger and had fewer comorbidities than the average recipient.[120] Post-transplantation infection was increased in the cancer survivors (22% vs. 14%, $p = 0.0040$) as were post-transplantation malignancies, but the absolute increase in malignancy was modest (5% vs. 2%, $p = 0.006$). Conversely, recipients with chemotherapy-induced cardiomyopathy were more likely to be free of rejection than recipients who had had no previous malignancy (72% vs. 62%, $p = 0.03$).

Sarcoidosis, amyloidosis, autoimmune disease

Systemic diseases such as sarcoidosis and amyloidosis present considerable risk as they may recur in the transplanted heart and may cause substantial disease in other organs following transplantation. Although small single-center studies suggest a modest decrement in survival for heart transplant recipients with cardiac sarcoidosis, a retrospective review of the UNOS database reported that 65 cardiac transplant recipients with cardiac sarcoidosis actually had a slightly better 1-year survival than contemporaneous recipients with all other diagnoses.[121,122] Without transplantation, patients with HF due to cardiac amyloidosis have a poor prognosis. Combined heart–liver transplant has been reported to be successful for patients with transthyretin amyloidosis, where misfolding of the mutated transthyretin results in its deposition and damage in organs.[123] In patients with immunoglobulin light-chain (AL or primary systemic) amyloidosis, heart transplantation, followed by chemotherapy and/or stem cell transplantation, has been modestly successful,[124,125,126] but results are poor if neither chemotherapy or stem cell transplantation is possible.[124] Transplantation in patients with restrictive heart disease due to amyloidosis or radiation-induced cardiac disease is associated with poorer survival compared to other forms of restrictive cardiomyopathy.[127] Patients with systemic amyloidosis and multiple myeloma with more than two organs involved and autonomic dysfunction are generally excluded from cardiac transplantation.[79]

Autoimmune diseases such as systemic lupus erythematous and rheumatoid arthritis present relative contraindications due to the risk of recurrent disease in the transplanted heart and disease development in other organs. However, these patients may benefit from post-transplantation immunosuppression and thus should be considered on a case by case basis.

Unresolved tobacco abuse

Resumption of smoking post-transplantation occurs in 10–40% of pretransplant smokers and significantly increases the post-transplantation risk for CAV and cancer.[78,128,129,130,131] Indeed, after correcting for smoking pretransplantation, post-transplantation smoking remained a significant determinant of overall mortality in a multivariate analysis.[130] Most programs recommend 6 months of documented smoking abstinence. Urinary cotinine, a nicotine metabolite with a longer half-life than nicotine (19 vs. 2 hours), is most often utilized to monitor smoking recidivism as it is widely available, inexpensive, and easy to use.[131] Levels of urinary cotinine become undetectable after approximately 4 days.

Inability to comply with pre- and post-transplantation medical care

Psychiatric and psychosocial factors

Guidelines suggest that a careful psychosocial evaluation be performed pretransplantation, but specific tools are not well defined.[78,132] Instruments designed to predict a good psychosocial outcome following transplantation have been developed but are not yet validated.[133,134] Psychosocial evaluation should include an assessment of substance abuse, nonadherence, and measures of quality of life.

Substance abuse (alcohol and illicit drugs)

Active alcohol or substance abuse has been considered an absolute contraindication for transplantation.[78,79] Substance abuse and nonadherence have both been associated with poor outcomes in the general population (see below). Most programs require documentation of abstinence and participation in some form of a follow-up program to prevent recidivism.[78,135]

Nonadherence

In the general population as well as in transplant recipients, nonadherence is common and associated with poor outcomes. The rate of nonadherence with immunosuppressant medications in adult solid organ transplant populations has been estimated to average 23 per 100 cases and is associated with an increased risk of clinical events, including graft loss.[136,137,138] It has been difficult to determine demographic and transplant-related health history characteristics that predict post-transplantation nonadherence, but poor social support and poorer self-perceived health are important, as is history of nonadherence pretransplantation.[136,139,140] In one prospective study of 141 heart, liver, and lung recipients, self-reported pretransplant nonadherence was associated with an eightfold increase in post-transplantation nonadherence, which, in turn, was associated with an increase in acute rejection.[137]

Inadequate social support

Some degree of social support is necessary for transplant recipients for assistance with daily activities, especially in the first few weeks following transplantation, as well as for travel to scheduled appointments, emotional support, and coordination of a complex medical regimen. A social work evaluation is important as it will detect areas of lack of support that might preclude adherence to the complex medical care required following transplantation.[78]

Miscellaneous issues

Previous sternotomy

Previous sternotomy increases the operative risk for cardiac transplantation, but it is uncertain if there is an absolute number of prior surgeries that would preclude transplantation.[85,141]

Radiation-induced heart disease

Mediastinal radiotherapy for malignancy may result in valvular, coronary, and pericardial disease along with myocardial and pulmonary fibrosis and may also impact surgical outcomes.[142] Patients with previous chest radiation who have undergone subsequent sternotomy have a high rate of pulmonary complications following cardiac transplantation, prolonged ischemic times due to abnormal thoracic anatomy, and impaired wound healing due to radiation damage to tissues.[143,144] Patients with restrictive cardiomyopathy due to previous chemotherapy and radiation therapy or amyloidosis have a substantially increased mortality following cardiac transplantation compared to those with other forms of restrictive disease.[127]

Heparin-induced thrombocytopenia

Heparin-induced thrombocytopenia (HIT) is relatively common in potential transplant recipients due to the multiple exposures many of these patients have had to heparin. Once heparin is cleared from the circulation, no further anti-heparin antibody is produced, but antibody often persists for up to 100 days.[145] While transplantation should generally be delayed until the anti-heparin antibody is undetectable by enzyme-linked immunosorbent assay (ELISA) as there is inadequate data for the use of agents other than heparin during cardiopulmonary bypass, in urgent situations cardiac transplantation in these patients has been undertaken either with short exposure to heparin during the cardiopulmonary bypass, or with the use of nonheparin anticoagulants.[146,147] In nontransplantation cardiac surgery, plasmapheresis has been used successfully to prevent HIT during cardiopulmonary bypass in patients with heparin antibody; however, data in support of this approach for transplant surgery are lacking.[148] It has been suggested that immunosuppression may decrease the risk of HIT following cardiac transplantation.[149]

Donor–recipient matching

Recipients are matched to donors using both nonimmunologic factors (primarily body size) and immunologic factors (ABO blood type and human leukocyte antigens).

Nonimmunologic aspects of matching

Nonimmunologic matching of donor to recipient is done primarily by body weight and height. Typically, transplant candidates are listed on the UNOS transplant waiting list with a provision for the range of weight and height that will be accepted. Body weight is used as a rough surrogate for heart size and a donor/recipient body weight ratio of more than 0.8 is a frequently used criterion of acceptable size match, especially in cases of recipients with pulmonary hypertension. However, there are limited data to support this practice unless the recipient has severe pulmonary hypertension. Patel et al. evaluated the effect of donor/recipient weight ratios of less than 0.8, 0.8–1.2, and greater than 1.2 on 5-year mortality in 15 284 cardiac transplant recipients and found that the donor/recipient weight ratio did not predict mortality.[150] The most recent report of the ISHLT registry confirms these findings.[4] However, in recipients with a PVR greater than 5 Wood units, a donor/recipient body weight ratio of 1.1 to 1.2, compared to lower ratios, resulted in improved survival.[4]

While both age and sex of the donor may affect transplant outcomes, matching by age and sex is not routine. Male recipients have been reported to have a 10–15% improved mortality when they receive a male donor heart compared to a female donor heart.[151,152,153] A recent analysis of the largest cohort to date of over 60 000 heart transplant recipients confirmed a 10% increased mortality in male recipients of female donor hearts compared to male donor hearts and a 10% reduced mortality when female recipients receive hearts from female donors compared to male donors.[153] These results were not explained by either differences in body weight or the incidence of cellular or antibody-mediated rejection. Thus, sex mismatching does not appear to be inconsequential, but sex matching is not routinely done because of the other constraints of donor–recipient allocation.

Advanced donor age is a risk factor for mortality. One-year mortality progressively worsens as donor age increases above 30 years: the 1-year mortality risk is nearly twofold with a 60-year old donor compared to a 30-year old donor.[4] Older donor hearts are often used for older donors, but matching by age is influenced by many other factors, such as the urgency of the recipient's medical condition.

Immunologic aspects of matching

The cardiac donor is matched to recipient by ABO blood group and by avoidance of specific human leukocyte antigens (HLA) in allosensitized recipients. Recipient antibodies against donor ABO and HLA antigens, present at the time of transplantation, may result in hyperacute rejection or acute antibody-mediated rejection (AMR). Donor-specific anti-HLA antibodies that persist or develop de novo have also been associated with higher mortality and higher risk of late AMR with less consistent associations with CAV.[155,156,157] Recipient antibodies to other non-ABO, non-HLA antigens have been variably reported to be associated with poor outcomes but evidence is not yet adequate to mandate routine monitoring for these antibodies.[158,159]

ABO blood group matching

Although 29 blood group systems have been identified, it is the ABO system that is important in solid organ transplantation.[160] The ABO blood group in humans is defined by the type of blood group glycoprotein antigens present on the surface of the red blood cell.[161] Blood group antigens are also present on lymphocytes, platelets, and epithelial and endothelial cells. The four major ABO blood types in humans are O, A, B, and AB. Type A cells express type A antigen, type B cells express type B antigen, type AB cells express both A and B antigens, and type O cells express neither A or B antigens. Anti-A and anti-B antibodies do not form in the presence of either type A or B antigens, respectively, but do form when their respective antigen is absent. Accordingly, type O donors are said to be "universal donors" as they lack both A and B antigens while type AB recipients are "universal recipients" as they lack both anti-A and anti-B antibodies. If an ABO-incompatible donor organ (has either A or B antigen against which the recipient has antibodies) is transplanted, there will often be acute and severe AMR (hyperacute rejection) resulting in early graft loss.[162] Thus careful ABO matching has been important for successful cardiac transplantation. Due to the shortage of organ donors, ABO-incompatible cardiac transplantation was studied in infants as they do not generally develop antibodies against A and B blood group antigens until about 4–8 months of age, until the gastrointestinal tract is colonized with bacteria that have antigens similar to the A and B blood group antigens.[163,164,165] These bacterial antigens stimulate the formation of antibodies that cross-react with A and B blood group antigens expressed in the heart. ABO-incompatible cardiac transplantation in infants has been shown to result in survival comparable to ABO-compatible heart transplantation and to reduce wait times, and is now a standard practice in many countries.[163,166] ABO-incompatible transplantation has also been performed successfully in adults, primarily in kidney recipients, and rarely in heart recipients.[166,167,168]

Allosensitization

The HLA system is synonymous with the human major histocompatibility (MHC) locus and is an important effector for the rejection of tissue grafts in HLA-unmatched individuals. The function of MHC molecules is to present antigen peptides to T lymphocytes to help initiate the immune response. There are three HLA classes (I, II, and III) defined by their structure, location, and product function.[169] HLA class I consists of A, B, and Cw antigens, which are expressed constitutively on all nucleated cells of the body. HLA class II antigens include DR, DQ, and DP antigens, which are expressed on antigen-presenting cells, B lymphocytes, and activated microvascular endothelial cells.[170] Many other cells of the body, including T lymphocytes, will express HLA class II antigens in the presence of inflammation.[171] HLA class III encodes for a number of other proteins involved in immune function, but matching is not generally performed for HLA class III molecules.

Sensitization to HLA antigens is defined by the development of anti-HLA antibodies, which may occur with exposure to cells that express "nonself" HLA antigens. Common situations leading to sensitization include blood transfusion, pregnancy, and organ transplantation. Antibodies to the individual HLA antigens of the donor are termed "donor-specific antibodies" (DSA). Recipient sensitization to donor HLA antigens is of particular relevance in transplantation as preformed anti-HLA DSA may result in acute AMR and graft loss.[172] The de-novo development of DSA following transplantation is also associated with poor outcomes, although less acutely.[173,174]

Detection of anti-HLA antigens

The reported prevalence of anti-HLA antibodies depends upon the sensitivity of the specific method of detection. Over the last several decades, techniques for the measurement of anti-HLA antibodies have evolved significantly, from cell- or membrane-based methods to solid-phase assays that use solubilized and recombinant HLA molecules.[175,176] Individual HLA antibodies can now be detected with great sensitivity but the specificity of these antibodies in relation to cytotoxicity and rejection risk remains incompletely understood.[175]

The classic cell-based assay is the complement-dependent cytotoxicity (CDC) assay. In this assay lymphocytes are obtained from 20–40 random donors with both common and rare HLA antigens.[176,177] Lymphocytes from these individual donors are placed in wells, and serum from the recipient is added to each well, along with complement and a vital dye. When an anti-HLA antibody binds to the HLA antigen on the cell surface and activates complement, a membrane attack complex (MAC) forms and inserts into the cell membrane, resulting in cell death and subsequent cellular uptake of the vital dye. Dead cells can then be identified by confocal microscopy.[177] The panel reactive antibody (PRA) level is defined as the percentage of wells in which the recipient's serum resulted in donor lymphocyte cell lysis. If cell lysis occurs in 20 of the 40 wells, the PRA is 50%. The CDC assay can not distinguish cell lysis due to anti-HLA antibodies from that due to non-HLA antibodies.

Solid-phase immunoassays (SPI) are of two types—the ELISA and the bead assays (e.g., Luminex).[176,177] In SPI, solubilized or recombinant HLA molecules are used, eliminating any reaction with non-HLA antibodies. HLA molecules are bound to a microfilter plate in the ELISA assay and to polystyrene beads in the bead assays. Anti-HLA antibodies are enzyme conjugated (ELISA) or conjugated with fluorescent dye (Luminex) and bind to the solid matrix. In ELISA, the results are expressed in optical density ratios compared to a negative control. In the microbead (Luminex) assay, the assessment is expressed as molecules of equivalent soluble fluorochrome (MESF), or mean fluorescent index (MFI), or as standard fluorescent intensity (SFI) units. The results provide a semiquantitative assessment of antibody binding but do not reflect the amount of antibody.

Advantages and disadvantages of the cell-based versus the solid-phase methods of detecting HLA antibodies are summarized in Table 16.4. Although an increasing number of centers base acceptance of a donor organ on solid-phase assays, controversy and questions still exist.[175,176,177,178,179] The cell-based methods are significantly less sensitive than the solid-phase assays and do not identify individual HLA antigens. While they only identify antibodies that fix complement, some complement-fixing antibodies may be either non-HLA antibodies or may not be donor-specific. SPI identify individual specificities of the antibodies; however, they typically do not provide information on whether these antibodies are capable of binding complement. Non-complement-fixing antibodies would not be as likely to result in AMR, but might exclude a donor organ if a virtual crossmatch is done using information from the solid-phase immunoassay. A promising method for the determination of complement fixation uses antibody against C1q, a component of complement, to determine whether recipient anti-HLA antibodies bound on Luminex single-antigen beads are capable of fixing complement.[180] The C1q assay was used by Chin et al. in a study of 18 pediatric cardiac transplant recipients, of whom 13 were sensitized (PRA >20%) and 5 developed AMR. The investigators reported that the C1q assay was positive only in the five patients with DSA who developed AMR.[181]

Table 16.4 Comparison of cell-based and solid-phase methods of detecting anti-HLA antibodies

	Cell-based	Solid-phase
Sensitivity of method	Less sensitive	More sensitive
HLA antigens	Does not detect individual HLA antibodies	Does detect individual HLA antibodies
False-positive reactions	Non-HLA antibodies	May detect cryptic antigens on denatured DNA
Detection of complement fixation	Yes	No, but newer techniques may (C1q assay requires further validation)
Clear data to determine whether to decline donor	Criteria vary between centers	Criteria vary between centers
Reproducibility between centers	Yes	Not yet certain
Virtual crossmatch possible	No	Yes
Detection of post-transplant de-novo anti-HLA antibodies	No	Yes

Zeevi A, Girnita A, Duquesnoy R. Immunologic Research (2006), 255–64, Springer.

Many centers started to use SPI and the individual MFI (or MESF or SFI) for each specific anti-HLA antibody to make decisions regarding accepting or declining a donor with known HLA typing (virtual crossmatch). However, test result variability among individual laboratories makes consensus on what absolute MFI value should make an antigen "unacceptable" difficult. More data correlating MFI values with outcomes such as AMR would be valuable. Very high MFI values, however, do appear to predict antibody that will fix complement and lead to AMR.[181] In summary, SPI have supplanted the use of cell-based assays in many centers as they make it possible to perform a virtual crossmatch and to monitor for the ongoing presence and de-novo appearance of DSA.

SPI have also allowed the development of the calculated PRA (cPRA). The cPRA compares a recipient's individual HLA antibodies to the individual HLA antigen frequencies determined from 12 000 kidney donors in the United States between the years 2003 and 2005.[182] The cPRA represents the proportion of organ donors in the United States that would likely have one or more of the unacceptable HLA antigens for the individual recipient. The cPRA is helpful in determining how likely it is for a sensitized recipient to be offered a compatible donor match. The cPRA can be calculated on the UNOS website.[183]

Causes and prevalence of HLA sensitization

Major causes of HLA sensitization include transfusion, pregnancy, transplantation, and implantation of MCS devices. Allogeneic cryopreserved heart valves result in sensitization as well.[184,185] While inflammatory events alone do not appear to cause HLA sensitization, they do appear to enhance anti-HLA antibodies in previously sensitized individuals.[171,186]

Over 18% of patients transplanted between 2005 and 2011 had a PRA of 10% or greater.[4] This percentage of sensitized recipients is likely to increase as there is increased adoption of more sensitive antibody detection techniques and as more MCS devices are placed prior to transplantation.

Transfusion

All cellular components of blood can elicit sensitization to HLA antigens. HLA antigens are most densely expressed on lymphocytes and platelets and less so on other white blood cells.[187] Red blood cells (RBC) also express HLA antigens, although at a much lower density than other cells.[187] The sensitization response to a RBC transfusion depends on the patient's previous exposure to HLA antigens as well as the type of transfusion and number of units transfused. Most packed RBC have platelets routinely removed and are "leukoreduced" by filters or other techniques. However, leukoreduction leaves a small number of residual leukocytes permitting sensitization. In subjects with no previous pregnancies, RBCs rarely provoke sensitization. In a study of nulliparous females and males, sensitization was 1% in those with no previous transfusions and 1.7% in those who had a previous transfusion.[188] When antibodies do develop, they tend to be of low titer and usually disappear after a few months. Sensitization is most common in the young and decreases with age.[189] Transfusions result in HLA antibody induction more frequently and in higher titer in previously sensitized subjects.[189,190]

Pregnancy

During pregnancy the mother is exposed to the HLA antigens of the fetus, some of which are "foreign" as they are inherited from the father. Even in previously nontransfused subjects, HLA sensitization during pregnancy is quite common. Using a lymphocytotoxicity assay, one study reported a sensitization rate of 32% at the time of delivery.[191] Antibodies were not detected until the 28th week of gestation and declined following delivery, but some sensitization was detectable up to 30 years postpartum. In blood donors with previous pregnancies, antibodies were present in 5% using a cytotoxicity assay (Konoeda) and in 24–33% using a solid-phase immunoassay.[188] The prevalence of sensitization increased with the number of pregnancies.[188]

Organ transplantation

Transplantation of any organ may result in the formation of DSA. Ho et al. reported that 36% of 950 consecutive first heart transplant recipients developed new anti-HLA antibodies following transplantation. This study used the relatively insensitive CDC assay and did not determine donor specificity.[173] Using a more sensitive Luminex solid-phase technique in 243 cardiac transplant recipients, Smith et al. reported the development of de-novo anti-HLA antibodies in 58% of recipients and 5% of all recipients developed de-novo DSA.[173] The appearance of nondonor HLA antibodies as well as DSA was cumulative over time but did appear to occur less frequently after 8–9 years post transplantation in both studies.[173,174]

MCS devices

HLA sensitization with MCS devices is an important problem as 36% of all 2010 cardiac transplant recipients had some form of MCS, primarily LVADs, at the time of transplantation.[4,193] Sensitization is thought to be largely due to the administration of blood products, including RBC, plasma, and platelets during and following LVAD implantation.[193] While RBCs undergo leukofiltration prior to transfusion, some leukocytes remain to stimulate sensitization. Even in the absence of RBC transfusions, platelets and/or plasma transfusions appear to stimulate sensitization.[193] Sensitization increases as the total number of blood products transfused increases and as the duration of LVAD support increases.[85,193] Some studies report sensitization even when no cellular blood products are transfused and it has been postulated that the interaction of LVAD biomaterials with blood stimulates antibody production.[85,195] If true, one would suspect that second-generation continuous-flow LVADs would be less sensitizing than the first-generation pulsatile-flow devices since the the newer generations of devices have no valves and have significantly less device surface area exposed to blood. Studies are conflicting, however, on whether the types of devices differ in the rate of sensitization and whether rejection following transplantation (due to the presence of anti-HLA antibodies) differs between patients with the two types of devices.[193,196] It is important to remember that this is a complex comparison as the transfusion of blood products may be different between the types of LVADs both acutely and chronically and many anti-HLA antibodies formed may not be directed at the donor or may not be complement fixing and thus would not be expected to result in AMR.[197]

Cryopreserved allograft heart valves

Patients implanted with cryopreserved pulmonary and aortic valves should be considered to be at higher risk for HLA sensitization with any sensitizing event as these valves may have resulted in previous sensitization. Decellularized allografts appear to substantially reduce the frequency of HLA sensitization.[184,185]

Methods to avoid HLA sensitization

Avoiding or minimizing transfusion of blood products is key, particularly in previously sensitized patients, as their risk of sensitization is increased and, if sensitization occurs, it is likely to be prolonged.[85] Careful attention to minimizing blood draws and treating iron deficiency will reduce the need for RBC transfusions. Leukoreduction of blood products is standard and appears to help reduce sensitization, although not all studies agree.[189] There are other potential options for preventing desenstization. HLA matching for blood donations reduces sensitization, but there are significant logistic problems in both identifying HLA-matched donors and transporting blood products to the recipient rapidly.[189] Some preliminary studies using immunosuppression to reduce sensitization have been promising.[189] Also, the use of intravenous immunoglobulin (IVIg) during transfusion or other sensitizing event to reduce sensitization is an intriguing strategy. A recent study shows that sensitization to HLA antigens following pregnancy is lower in Rh-negative women who have received Rh immunoglobulin.[198]

Matching a donor to an allosensitized recipient

Direct crossmatch

The donor–recipient direct crossmatch is done with the CDC assay described previously, except that only the donor's T lymphocytes and the recipient's serum are used. The assay can be enhanced with anti-human globulin (AHG) and is then called AHG-CDC crossmatch. AHG is a complement-fixing antibody to anti-human immunoglobulin.[177] When added as an additional step the AHG binds to DSA already present on the lymphocyte surface, which helps activate the complement and improves the sensitivity of the CDC assay. If donor cells are killed, the direct crossmatch is considered positive. A positive AHG-CDC crossmatch is generally considered a contraindication to transplantation unless steps are taken to either desensitize the recipient prior to transplantation or to remove antibodies immediately prior or during the transplant procedure. The direct crossmatch adds several hours to the allocation process and the additional time required to transport donor cells may preclude acceptance of the donor heart, especially from more distant locations. Most transplant centers have now adopted the "virtual crossmatch" for sensitized recipients.

Virtual crossmatch

The "virtual" crossmatch involves comparing the individual HLA antigens of the prospective donor with the anti-HLA antibodies of the recipient, identified with solid-phase techniques. A positive virtual crossmatch is present if the recipient has anti-HLA antibodies directed against donor HLA antigens. A negative virtual crossmatch does predict the absence of acute AMR with reasonable accuracy. Stehlik et al. compared the AHG-CDC crossmatch to a virtual crossmatch using the Luminex assay.[199] An MFI of more than 2000 was defined as unacceptable for an individual antibody. The two methods were compared retrospectively in 181 sensitized cardiac transplant recipients and then prospectively in 28 sensitized recipients. The positive predictive value of the virtual crossmatch was 79% and the negative predictive value was 92%. Subsequently, 14 sensitized patients received allografts after a compatible virtual crossmatch with donors from distant locations. Their outcomes were compared with 14 sensitized patients who received organs after compatible prospective serologic crossmatch, and similar rejection rates and survival were found. The virtual crossmatch allowed acceptance of donors for sensitized recipients for whom an AHG-CDC crossmatch was not possible. While use of the virtual crossmatch has become accepted, a number of uncertainties remain. The MFI for an anti-HLA antibody that predicts AMR is not well defined and criteria for acceptability vary between centers. The higher the MFI value used, the lower the sensitivity of the approach and the greater the risk for rejection after transplant, but also the higher the likelihood of finding a donor heart. Furthermore, it is not certain that all antibodies detected by solid-phase techniques would bind complement and lead to rejection. Thus some donor hearts that would have resulted in an excellent outcome might be declined. In the face of a positive virtual crossmatch, a negative AHG-CDC assay would predict a good outcome but there is often not sufficient time to obtain donor tissue or to perform the assay prospectively. A C1q assay was recently developed for the Luminex platform and, as discussed previously, may predict the ability of anti-HLA antibodies to bind complement.[180]

The wait for acceptable donor hearts continues to increase and sensitized recipients wait longest.[200] As the waiting time increases for potential recipients, there is more likelihood that the patient will deteriorate and need an LVAD as a bridge to transplantation. Sensitization is likely to be enhanced by the need for blood product transfusions and the inflammatory milieu of the LVAD surgery. Furthermore, one significant and common complication of the current continuous-flow LVADs is bleeding. If transfusion is necessary in an already sensitized patient, sensitization is likely to be exacerbated.

Desensitization

In the past, if a sensitized potential recipient needed a prospective crossmatch a local donor was required so that tissue from the donor could be obtained rapidly in order to do a direct prospective crossmatch. The use of the virtual crossmatch has allowed matching to recipients from a much larger geographic area. However, many patients are highly sensitized, making a compatible virtual crossmatch unlikely. Desensitization protocols may be used in these patients in an attempt to reduce the anti-HLA antibody burden and increase the likelihood of finding a compatible donor. While protocols for desensitization vary widely between transplant centers, two general types of regimens utilizing IVIg are the most common. The mechanism of IVIg in reducing antibody burden is complex and not entirely understood, but probably includes anti-T and anti-B cell activity, blockade of complement activation, cytokine inhibition, as well as blockade of antibody binding sites.[201] A high- dose IVIg protocol utilizes monthly IVIg at a dose of 2 g/kg until antibodies (or antibody binding) are reduced enough to allow a compatible crossmatch.[202] If IVIg alone does not result in adequate desensitization, the anti-CD20 (anti-B cell) chimeric monoclonal antibody rituximab may be added.[203] The second commonly used protocol consists of plasmapheresis followed by hyperimmune anti-cytomegalovirus IVIg at a dose of 100 mg/kg, each given every other day.[204] Because of the potential for rebound in anti-HLA antibodies following plasmapheresis, an immunomodulating agent such as IVIg is generally combined with plasmapheresis. Cyclophosphamide has also been used successfully in some protocols.[200] More recently, bortezomib, a proteasome inhibitor approved for treatment of multiple myeloma, has been reported to reduce anti-HLA antibody burden by killing plasma cells.[205]

The wide variation in agents, doses and timing of densensitization protocols was outlined in a recent consensus conference publication.[206] With the recent development of SPI to define DSAs, as well as methods to assess complement fixation, randomized clinical trials evaluating specific desensitization protocols should be possible. It will be critical to determine if current desensitization protocols provide an acceptable long-term risk–benefit mortality ratio.

Outcomes in sensitized recipients

Several centers have reported a higher post-transplantation mortality in presensitized cardiac recipients compared to nonsensitized recipients.[207,208] However, from a multivariate analysis in a single-center study of 536 recipients, John et al. reported no effect of a PRA greater than 20% up to 5 years post transplantation.[209] The ISHLT registry reports a modest effect of PRA on survival at 1, 5 and 15 years post transplantation.[4] In a report utilizing UNOS data, Schaffer et al. reported that recipients with an initial PRA greate than 20% who had at least a 20% decline in PRA prior to transplant had a better 10-year survival than those with a PRA greater than 20% whose decline in PRA was less than 5% prior to transplantation (50% vs. 44%, $p = 0.007$).[210]

Development of de-novo DSA does appear to be associated with a higher mortality following transplantation. Using the CDC assay, Ho et al. reported that 36% of 950 consecutive first heart transplant recipients developed new anti-HLA antibodies following transplantation.[173] The 15-year graft survival was highest in patients who never developed alloantibodies (70%) or who displayed them only before transplantation (71%); graft survival in recipients who showed antibodies both before and after transplantation (56%), or only after transplantation (47%), was lower. Using a more sensitive solid-phase technique (Luminex) in 224 cardiac transplant recipients, Smith et al. retrospectively analyzed 224 cardiac transplant recipients without either DSA or "natural antibodies" prior to transplant.[174] The subjects had HLA antibody production determined every year after transplantation up to 13 years post transplantation. The development of de-novo and persistent DSA was strongly associated with poor patient survival (HR = 4.3, $p = 0.0001$).

Few data are available to address the long-term outcomes of sensitized cardiac transplant recipients who undergo desensitization. Kobashigawa et al. reported a single-center series of 95 patients with a PRA greater than 10%.[211] Twenty-one patients (mean PRA 70.5 ± 28.9%) underwent desensitization. They were compared to 74 sensitized recipients (PRA 18.8 ± 8.5%) and nonsensitized control recipients. Five-year survival and freedom from CAV were not different among the three groups but freedom from acute rejection in the first post-transplantation year was much lower in treated sensitized recipients (57.1%) than in either the untreated sensitized or the nonsensitized recipients (85.1% and 87.4%, respectively). The excess rejection in the treated subjects was primarily AMR. There was no difference in infection or other major adverse cardiovascular events in the three groups.

LVADs are increasingly used to bridge patients to transplantation and are associated with increased sensitization. For this and other reasons, it is possible that outcomes post transplantation are influenced by implantation of an LVAD. Arnaoutatus et al., using data from the UNOS registry for all HeartMate XVE and HeartMate II LVADs implanted between 2004 and 2009, reported that sensitized patients had 30-day and 1-year survival similar to survival in nonsensitized LVAD recipients.[212] Although PRA activity did not affect rejection in the year after cardiac transplantation for either device type, sensitization did prolong the time to transplantation and high class II alloantibody was associated with higher rates of primary graft dysfunction for both devices ($p < 0.05$).

The association of DSA with outcomes such as AMR, graft dysfunction, CAV, and mortality are likely to be clarified with current solid-phase assay methods that allow identification of antibodies to individual HLA antigens and antibody functionality with methods such as C1q assay.

Anatomy of the transplant process

The care of the transplant recipient over time is designed to optimize survival while limiting morbidity. The best possible outcomes would result by adjusting immunosuppression to achieve the lowest possible rates of both infection and rejection, thus incurring the fewest possible adverse effects of immunosuppressive therapies. However, there is currently no well-accepted test to determine the immunologic state of each individual and an individual's short- and long-term risk for cellular rejection, AMR, graft dysfunction, and CAV. Consequently, tapering of immunosuppression is done using frequent monitoring for rejection, including echocardiograms, myocardial biopsies, and gene expression profiling. Monitoring for CAV is done with coronary angiography and intracoronary ultrasound and monitoring for graft dysfunction is done primarily with echocardiograms. Some graft dysfunction is likely to be undiagnosed CAV but it is not clear if all graft dysfunction has an underlying immunologic cause. In the early days of transplantation, attention was focused on preventing rejection. However, immunosuppression has improved and a review of current causes of mortality and morbidity following transplantation suggests that the balance may currently be shifted to over-immunosuppression, but only if one assumes that the incidence of graft dysfunction and CAV would not be changed by reducing immunosuppression. Mortality is highest in the first year (and particularly the first 30 days) post transplantation with a 1-year mortality of about 10%. In the first 30 days, graft dysfunction accounts for 34% of deaths with 13% due to non-CMV infection and only 4% due to rejection (see Figure 16.2).[4] In the remainder of the first year, infection is responsible for 29% of deaths while graft dysfunction drops to 17% and rejection is responsible for 9%. For those who survive the first year following transplantation, there is a constant mortality rate of about 3–4% per year (see Figure 16.1). Graft dysfunction remains the most common single cause of death (24% of all deaths) until after 5 years, when malignancy increases to about 23% of all deaths and graft dysfunction drops to just under 20% (see Figure 16.2). After the first year, infection is a relative constant cause of death at 10–15%, CAV represents about 10–15%, while rejection is the cause of 12% of deaths at 1–3 years post transplantation and then drops to 5% or under. The prevalence of end-stage renal disease gradually increases over time and results in 9% of all deaths at 10 years following transplantation. It is quite likely that many of the cases of graft dysfunction are actually due to undiagnosed CAV.

Morbidity following transplantation is common, presumably due to the recipients' underlying diseases, aging, and complications of immunosuppressive therapy.[77] Recipients who survive 5 years following transplantation have a prevalence of hypertension of more than 90%, hyperlipidemia of 90%, diabetes of nearly 40%, and many have chronic renal dysfunction.[4] All of these comorbidities are caused or exacerbated by immunosuppressive therapy.[77] Rejection is more common in younger recipients while infection is a greater risk in older recipients, suggesting that enhanced immunosuppression might benefit the young and reduced immunosuppression might benefit the older recipient (see Figure 16.3).[213] Post-transplantation malignancy is also more common in elderly recipients, thus a reduction in immunosuppression in older recipients might also reduce this major cause of morbidity and mortality.

The risk of rejection is highest in the first year post-transplantation and decreases over time.[4] Thus, immunosuppression is typically prescribed at its high levels early post transplantation and then tapered over the first year, as long as rejection is absent. Induction therapy early post transplantation with polyclonal anti-lymphocyte globulins or interleukin-2 antagonists is currently utilized in about half of patients transplanted in the United States. While induction therapy reduces the risk of early rejection it does not prevent late rejection and does not appear to affect mortality.[4] Most programs use prednisone, a calcineurin inhibitor (tacrolimus or cyclosporine), and mycophenolate mofetil for chronic immunosuppression. Tacrolimus is now used much more commonly than cyclosporine as it appears that there is less early rejection, although it is not clear that long-term results are significantly different. While both calcineurin inhibitors may cause renal toxicity, cyclosporine appears to cause more hypertension and lipid abnormalities while tacrolimus has a more potent effect on exacerbation of diabetes.[77] It is standard to gradually taper immunosuppressive agents over the first year or two post-transplantation. Prednisone can be tapered off in more than half of patients with good long-term results.[214,215] Calcineurin inhibitor doses are decreased, though rarely discontinued, over time as well, but protocols vary widely. Myocardial biopsies are performed at frequent intervals for routine surveillance early post transplantation as immunosuppression is being tapered. After 6 months, many centers use gene expression monitoring as surveillance and myocardial biopsy only if gene expression studies are positive.[216,217] Late cellular rejection is unusual in the absence of early rejection, a marked reduction in immunosuppressive therapy, or concomitant infection. Thus, many centers discontinue routine surveillance myocardial biopsies once immunosuppressive therapy is no longer being tapered, especially in patients at low risk for rejection.[218] The risk of AMR was thought to be greatest early post transplantation due to preformed DSA, but DSA may appear de novo even years post transplantation and lead to poor outcomes primarily due to late AMR.[173,174] De-novo DSA appear in a modest percentage of recipients on a yearly basis and thus monitoring for DSA has been recommended after a potentially sensitizing event, as well as on a routine basis. However, it is not yet clear whether densensitization improves long-term outcomes.

CAV assumes increasing importance over time as a cause of death, and coronary angiography (with or without intracoronary ultrasound) is often performed yearly or every other year to detect early CAV. If CAV develops, therapies such as the addition of mammalian target of rapamycin (mTOR) inhibitors (sirolimus or everolimus) appear to significantly reduce the progression of CAV.[219,220]

Infection prophylaxis to prevent CMV, candida, and pneumocystis may often be discontinued as immunosuppression is tapered.

Routine screening for malignancy as recommended in the general population is warranted in transplant recipients, particularly in older subjects, and monitoring and treating skin cancers is critical at all ages. Cardiac transplant recipients require evaluation and therapy for comorbidities such as hypertension, hyperlipidemia, obesity, chronic kidney disease, and diabetes. In addition careful surveillance for the frequent drug–drug interactions that occur with immunosuppressive drugs is critical.[221]

On average, cardiac transplant recipients can expect to live 10 years following transplantation and many have much longer survival. Return to work, pregnancy, and physical activity are possible for recipients and most have a good quality of life. Malignancy, graft dysfunction, and CAV are major long-term problems that limit survival and quality of life. The development of tests to monitor the specific immunologic state of individual patients along with new immunosuppressive agents and improved understanding of the causes of graft dysfunction and CAV will significantly improve long-term outcomes for future cardiac transplant recipients.

References

1. Lindenfeld J, Albert NM, Boehmer JP, et al. HF SA 2010 Comprehensive Heart Failure Practice Guideline. J Card Fail 2010 16:e1–194.
2. <http://www.transplant-observatory.org/> (Accessed Nov 2012).
3. Kirk R, Dipchand AI, Edwards LB, et al. The registry of the international society for heart and lung transplantation: fifteenth pediatric heart transplantation report—2012. J Heart Lung Transplant 2012;31:1065–72.
4. Stehlik J, Edwards LB, Kucheryavaya AY, et al. The registry of the international society for heart and lung transplantation: 29th official adult heart transplant report—2012. J Heart Lung Transplant 2012;31:1052–64.
5. Hunt SA, Abraham WT, Chin MH, et al. 2009 focused update incorporated into the ACC/AHA 2005 Guidelines for the Diagnosis and Management of Heart Failure in Adults: a report of the American College of Cardiology Foundation/American Heart Association Task Force on Practice Guidelines: developed in collaboration with the International Society for Heart and Lung Transplantation. Circulation 2009;119: e391–479.
6. Johnson MR, Meyer KH, Haft J, et al. Heart transplantation in the United States, 1999–2008. Am J Transplant 2010;10:1035–46.
7. Kobashigawa JA, Kiyosaki KK, Patel JK, et al. Benefit of immune monitoring in heart transplant patients using ATP production in activated lymphocytes. J Heart Lung Transplant 2010;29:504–8.
8. Mehra MR, Kobashigawa JA, Deng MC, et al. Clinical implications and longitudinal alteration of peripheral blood transcriptional signals indicative of future cardiac allograft rejection. J Heart Lung Transplant 2008;27:297–301.
9. Radovancevic B, McGiffin DC, Kobashigawa JA, et al. Retransplantation in 7,290 primary transplant patients: a 10-year multi-institutional study. J Heart Lung Transplant 2003;22:862–8.
10. Eschenhagen T, Force T, Ewer MS, et al. Cardiovascular side effects of cancer therapies: a position statement from the Heart Failure Association of the European Society of Cardiology. Eur J Heart Fail 2011;13:1–10.
11. Cheng H, Force T. Molecular mechanisms of cardiovascular toxicity of targeted cancer therapeutics. Circ Res 2010;106:21–34.
12. Oliveira GH, Hardaway BW, Kucheryavaya AY, et al. Characteristics and survival of patients with chemotherapy-induced cardiomyopathy undergoing heart transplantation. J Heart Lung Transplant 2012;31:805–10.
13. Lenneman AJ, Wang L, Wigger M, et al. Heart transplant survival outcomes for adriamycin-dilated cardiomyopathy. Am J Cardiol 2013;111:609–12.
14. Sattianayagam PT, Gibbs SD, Pinney JH, et al. Solid organ transplantation in AL amyloidosis. Am J Transplant 2010;10:2124–31.
15. Dubrey SW, Burke MM, Hawkins PN, Banner NR. Cardiac transplantation for amyloid heart disease: the United Kingdom experience. J Heart Lung Transplant 2004;23:1142–53.
16. Roig E, Almenar L, Gonzalez-Vilchez F, et al. Outcomes of heart transplantation for cardiac amyloidosis: subanalysis of the spanish registry for heart transplantation. Am J Transplant 2009;9:1414–19.
17. Singh TP, Almond CS, Semigran MJ, et al. Risk prediction for early in-hospital mortality following heart transplantation in the United States. Circ Heart Fail 2012;5:259–66.
18. Nativi JN, Drakos SG, Kucheryavaya AY, et al. Changing outcomes in patients bridged to heart transplantation with continuous- versus pulsatile-flow ventricular assist devices: an analysis of the registry of the International Society for Heart and Lung Transplantation. J Heart Lung Transplant 2011;30:854–61.
19. Patlolla V, Patten RD, Denofrio D, et al. The effect of ventricular assist devices on post-transplant mortality an analysis of the United network for organ sharing thoracic registry. J Am Coll Cardiol 2009;53:264–71.
20. Kobashigawa JA, Kirklin JK, Naftel DC, et al. Pretransplantation risk factors for acute rejection after heart transplantation: a multiinstitutional study. The Transplant Cardiologists Research Database Group. J Heart Lung Transplant 1993;12:355–66.
21. Stehlik J, Starling RC, Movsesian MA, et al. Utility of long-term surveillance endomyocardial biopsy: a multi-institutional analysis. J Heart Lung Transplant 2006;25:1402–9.
22. McAllister S, Buckner EB, White-Williams C Medication adherence after heart transplantation: adolescents and their issues. Progr Transplant 2006;16:317–23.
23. George TJ, Arnaoutakis GJ, Baumgartner WA, et al. Organ storage with University of Wisconsin solution is associated with improved outcomes after orthotopic heart transplantation. J Heart Lung Transplant 2011;30:1033–43.
24. Lima ML, Fiorelli AI, Gomes OM, et al. Comparative analysis of the performance of various crystalloid cardioplegic solutions on myocardial protection after prolonged cold ischemia. Transplantat Proc 2011;43:80–3.
25. Cannata A, Botta L, Colombo T, et al. Does the cardioplegic solution have an effect on early outcomes following heart transplantation? Eur J Cardiothorac Surg 2012;41: e48–52; discussion e52–43.
26. Cypel M, Yeung JC, Machuca T, et al. Experience with the first 50 ex vivo lung perfusions in clinical transplantation. J Thorac Cardiovasc Surg 2012;144:1200–6.
27. Randomized Study of Organ Care System Cardiac for Preservation of Donated Hearts for Eventual Transplantation (PROCEEDII). Clinicaltrials.gov Identifier: NCT00855712.
28. Grady KL, White-Williams C, Naftel D, et al. Are preoperative obesity and cachexia risk factors for post heart transplant morbidity and mortality: a multi-institutional study of preoperative weight-height indices. Cardiac Transplant Research Database (CTRD) Group. J Heart Lung Transplant 1999;18:750–63.
29. Bourge RC, Naftel DC, Costanzo-Nordin MR, et al. Pretransplantation risk factors for death after heart transplantation: a multiinstitutional study. The Transplant Cardiologists Research Database Group. J Heart Lung Transplant 1993;12:549–62.
30. Kirklin JK, Naftel DC, Bourge RC, et al. Evolving trends in risk profiles and causes of death after heart transplantation: a ten-year multi-institutional study. J Thorac Cardiovasc Surg 2003;125:881–90.
31. Taylor DO, Stehlik J, Edwards LB, et al. Registry of the International Society for Heart and Lung Transplantation: Twenty-sixth Official Adult Heart Transplant Report—2009. J Heart Lung Transplant 2009;28:1007–22.
32. Weiss ES, Allen JG, Arnaoutakis GJ, et al. Creation of a quantitative recipient risk index for mortality prediction after cardiac transplantation (IMPACT). Ann Thorac Surg 2011;92:914–21; discussion 921–2.
33. Mehra MR, Uber PA, Uber WE, et al. Allosensitization in heart transplantation: implications and management strategies. Curr Opin Cardiol 2003;18:153–8.
34. Stehlik J, Feldman DS, Brown RN, et al. Interactions among donor characteristics influence post-transplant survival: a multi-institutional analysis. J Heart Lung Transplant 2010;29:291–8.
35. Kubo SH, Naftel DC, Mills RM, Jr., et al. Risk factors for late recurrent rejection after heart transplantation: a multiinstitutional, multivariable analysis. Cardiac Transplant Research Database Group. J Heart Lung Transplant 1995;14:409–18.

36. Mills RM, Naftel DC, Kirklin JK, et al. Heart transplant rejection with hemodynamic compromise: a multiinstitutional study of the role of endomyocardial cellular infiltrate. Cardiac Transplant Research Database. J Heart Lung Transplant 1997;16:813–21.
37. Kobashigawa JA, Tobis JM, Starling RC, et al. Multicenter intravascular ultrasound validation study among heart transplant recipients: outcomes after five years. J Am Coll Cardiol 2005;45:1532–37.
38. Mehra MR, Crespo-Leiro MG, Dipchand A, et al. International Society for Heart and Lung Transplantation working formulation of a standardized nomenclature for cardiac allograft vasculopathy—2010. J Heart Lung Transplant 2010;29:717–27.
39. Costanzo MR, Naftel DC, Pritzker MR, Heilman JK, 3rd, Boehmer JP, et al. Heart transplant coronary artery disease detected by coronary angiography: a multiinstitutional study of preoperative donor and recipient risk factors. Cardiac Transplant Research Database. J Heart Lung Transplant 1998;17:744–53.
40. McGiffin DC, Savunen T, Kirklin JK, et al. Cardiac transplant coronary artery disease. A multivariable analysis of pretransplantation risk factors for disease development and morbid events. J Thorac Cardiovasc Surg 1995;109:1081–8; discussion 1088–9.
41. Roussel JC, Baron O, Perigaud C, et al. Outcome of heart transplants 15 to 20 years ago: graft survival, post-transplant morbidity, and risk factors for mortality. J Heart Lung Transplant 2008;27:486–93.
42. Chinnock R, Webber SA, Dipchand AI, et al. A 16-year multi-institutional study of the role of age and EBV status on PTLD incidence among pediatric heart transplant recipients. Am J Transplant 2012;12(11):3061–8.
43. Ojo AO, Held PJ, Port FK, et al. Chronic renal failure after transplantation of a nonrenal organ. N Engl J Med 2003;349:931–40.
44. A definition of irreversible coma. Report of the Ad Hoc Committee of the Harvard Medical School to Examine the Definition of Brain Death. JAMA 1968;205:337–40.
45. Diagnosis of brain death. Statement issued by the honorary secretary of the Conference of Medical Royal Colleges and their Faculties in the United Kingdom on 11 October 1976. Br Med J 1976;ii:1187–8.
46. Boucek MM, Mashburn C, Dunn SM, et al. Pediatric heart transplantation after declaration of cardiocirculatory death. N Engl J Med 2008;359:709–14.
47. Noterdaeme T, Detry O, Hans MF, et al. What is the potential increase in the heart graft pool by cardiac donation after circulatory death? Transpl Int 2013;26(1):61–6.
48. Baroldi G, Di Pasquale G, Silver MD, et al. Type and extent of myocardial injury related to brain damage and its significance in heart transplantation: a morphometric study. J Heart Lung Transplant 1997;16:994–1000.
49. Shivalkar B, Van Loon J, Wieland W, et al. Variable effects of explosive or gradual increase of intracranial pressure on myocardial structure and function. Circulation 1993;87:230–9.
50. Kolin A, Norris JW. Myocardial damage from acute cerebral lesions. Stroke 1984;15:990–3.
51. Wood KE, Becker BN, McCartney JG, et al. Care of the potential organ donor. N Engl J Med 2004;351:2730–9.
52. Pennefather SH, Bullock RE, Mantle D, Dark JH. Use of low dose arginine vasopressin to support brain-dead organ donors. Transplantation 1995;59:58–62.
53. Potter CD, Wheeldon DR, Wallwork J. Functional assessment and management of heart donors: a rationale for characterization and a guide to therapy. J Heart Lung Transplant 1995;14:59–65.
54. Rosendale JD, Kauffman HM, McBride MA, et al. Aggressive pharmacologic donor management results in more transplanted organs. Transplantation 2003;75:482–7.
55. Salim A, Vassiliu P, Velmahos GC, et al. The role of thyroid hormone administration in potential organ donors. Arch Surg 2001;136:1377–80.
56. Wheeldon DR, Potter CD, Oduro A, et al. Transforming the "unacceptable" donor: outcomes from the adoption of a standardized donor management technique. J Heart Lung Transplant 1995;14:734–42.
57. Singhal AK, Sheng X, Drakos SG, Stehlik J. Impact of donor cause of death on transplant outcomes: UNOS registry analysis. Transpl Proc 2009;41:3539–44.
58. Wever Pinzon O, Stoddard G, Drakos SG, et al. Impact of donor left ventricular hypertrophy on survival after heart transplant. Am J Transplant 2011;11:2755–61.
59. Buell JF, Beebe TM, Gross TG, et al. United network for organ sharing publication on scientific registry of transplant recipients central nervous system donor cancer transmission data. Transplantation 2005;79:623.
60. Buell JF, Trofe J, Hanaway MJ, et al. Transmission of donor cancer into cardiothoracic transplant recipients. Surgery 2001;130:660–6; discussion 666–8.
61. Conlon PJ, Smith SR. Transmission of cancer with cadaveric donor organs. J Am Soc Nephrol 1995;6:54–60.
62. Penn I. Transmission of cancer with donor organs. Transplant Proc 1988;20:739–40.
63. Penn I. Malignant melanoma in organ allograft recipients. Transplantation 1996;61:274–8.
64. Kauffman HM, McBride MA, Cherikh WS, et al. Transplant tumor registry: donors with central nervous system tumors1. Transplantation 2002;73:579–82.
65. Shafii AE, Su JW, Smedira NG, et al. The effect of recipient hepatitis C virus infection on outcomes following heart transplantation. Transplant Proc 2010;42:1784–7.
66. Grossi PA, Fishman JA. Donor-derived infections in solid organ transplant recipients. Am J Transplant 2009;9(Suppl 4): S19–26.
67. Costanzo MR, Dipchand A, Starling R, et al. The International Society of Heart and Lung Transplantation Guidelines for the care of heart transplant recipients. J Heart Lung Transplant 2010;29:914–56.
68. Seem DL, Lee I, Umscheid CA, Kuehnert MJ. PHS Guideline for reducing human immunodeficiency virus, hepatitis B virus, and hepatitis C virus transmission through organ transplantation. Publ Health Rep 2013;128:247–343.
69. Zaroff JG, Babcock WD, Shiboski SC, et al. Temporal changes in left ventricular systolic function in heart donors: results of serial echocardiography. J Heart Lung Transplant 2003;22:383–8.
70. Kono T, Nishina T, Morita H, et al. Usefulness of low-dose dobutamine stress echocardiography for evaluating reversibility of brain death-induced myocardial dysfunction. Am J Cardiol 1999;84:578–82.
71. Kuppahally SS, Valantine HA, Weisshaar D, et al. Outcome in cardiac recipients of donor hearts with increased left ventricular wall thickness. Am J Transplant 2007;7:2388–95.
72. Zaroff JG, Rosengard BR, Armstrong WF, et al. Consensus conference report: maximizing use of organs recovered from the cadaver donor: cardiac recommendations, March 28–29, 2001, Crystal City, Va. Circulation 2002;106:836–41.
73. Navia JL, Atik FA, Marullo A, et al. Bench repair of donor aortic valve with minimal access orthotopic heart transplantation. Ann Thorac Surg 2005;80:313–15.
74. Khush KK, Menza RL, Babcock WD, Zaroff JG. Donor cardiac troponin I levels do not predict recipient survival after cardiac transplantation. J Heart Lung Transplant 2007;26:1048–53.
75. Zaroff JG, Rosengard BR, Armstrong WF, et al. Maximizing use of organs recovered from the cadaver donor: cardiac recommendations: March 28–29, 2001, Crystal City, Va. J Heart Lung Transplant 2002;21:1153–60.
76. Laks H, Scholl FG, Drinkwater DC, et al. The alternate recipient list for heart transplantation: does it work? J Heart Lung Transplant 1997;16:735–42.
77. Lindenfeld J, Page RL 2nd, Zolty R, et al. Drug therapy in the heart transplant recipient: Part III: common medical problems. Circulation 2005;111:113–17.
78. Mehra MR, Kobashigawa J, Starling R, et al. Listing criteria for heart transplantation: International Society for Heart and Lung Transplantation guidelines for the care of cardiac transplant candidates—2006. J Heart Lung Transplant 2006;25:1024–42.

79. Mancini D, Lietz K. Selection of cardiac transplantation candidates in 2010. Circulation 2010;122:173–83.
80. Kirklin JK, Naftel DC, Kirklin JW, et al. Pulmonary vascular resistance and the risk of heart transplantation. J Heart Transplant 1988;7(5):331–6.
81. Stobierska-Dzierzek B, Awad H, Michler RE. The evolving management of acute right-sided heart failure in cardiac transplant recipients. J Am Coll Cardiol 2001;38:923–31.
82. Liden H, Haraldsson A, Ricksten SE, et al. Does pretransplant left ventricular assist device therapy improve results after heart transplantation in patients with elevated pulmonary vascular resistance? Eur J Cardiothorac Surg 2009;35:1029–34.
83. Costard-Jäckle A, Fowler MB. Influence of preoperative pulmonary artery pressure on mortality after heart transplantation: testing of potential reversibility of pulmonary hypertension with nitroprusside is useful in defining a high risk group. J Am Coll Cardiol 1992;19:48–54.
84. Chen EP, Bittner HB, Davis RD, Van Trigt P. Pulmonary vascular impedance and recipient chronic pulmonary hypertension following cardiac transplantation. Chest 1997;112:1622–9.
85. Drakos SG, Kfoury AG, Gilbert EM, et al. Multivariate predictors of heart transplantation outcomes in the era of chronic mechanical circulatory support. Ann Thorac Surg 2007;83:62–7.
86. Givertz MM, Hare JM, Loh E, et al. Effect of bolus milrinone on hemodynamic variables and pulmonary vascular resistance in patients with severe left ventricular dysfunction: a rapid test for reversibility of pulmonary hypertension. J Am Coll Cardiol 1996;28:1775–80.
87. Stanek B, Sturm B, Frey B, et al. Bridging to heart transplantation: prostaglandin E1 versus prostacyclin versus dobutamine. J Heart Lung Transplant 1999;18:358–66.
88. Jabbour A, Keogh A, Hayward C, Macdonald P. Chronic sildenafil lowers transpulmonary gradient and improves cardiac output allowing successful heart transplantation. Eur J Heart Fail 2007;9:674–7.
89. Zimpfer D, Zrunek P, Roethy W, et al. Left ventricular assist devices decrease fixed pulmonary hypertension in cardiac transplant candidates. J Thorac Cardiovasc Surg 2007;133:689–95.
90. Young JN, Yazbeck J, Esposito G, et al. The influence of acute preoperative pulmonary infarction on the results of heart transplantation. J iHeart Transplant 1986;5:20–2.
91. Banner NR, Bonser RS, Clark AL, et al. UK guidelines for referral and assessment of adults for heart transplantation. Heart 2011;97:1520–7.
92. Weiss ES, Nwakanma LU, Patel ND, Yuh DD. Outcomes in patients older than 60 years of age undergoing orthotopic heart transplantation: an analysis of the UNOS database. J Heart Lung Transplant 2008;27:184–91.
93. Almuti K, Haythe J, Tsao L, et al. Does renal function deteriorate more rapidly in diabetic cardiac transplant recipients? Transplantation 2007;83:550–3.
94. Hamour IM, Omar F, Lyster HS, et al. Chronic kidney disease after heart transplantation. Nephrol Dial Transplant 2009;24:1655–62.
95. Bizouarn P, Ausseur A, Desseigne P, et al. Early and late outcome after elective cardiac surgery in patients with cirrhosis. Ann Thorac Surg 1999;67:1334–8.
96. Filsoufi F, Salzberg SP, Rahmanian PB, et al. Early and late outcome of cardiac surgery in patients with liver cirrhosis. Liver Transpl 2007;13:990–5.
97. Ailawadi G, Lapar DJ, Swenson BR, et al. Model for end-stage liver disease predicts mortality for tricuspid valve surgery. Ann Thorac Surg 2009;87:1460–7.
98. Chokshi A, Cheema FH, Schaefle KJ, et al. Hepatic dysfunction and survival after orthotopic heart transplantation: application of the MELD scoring system for outcome prediction. J Heart Lung Transplant 2012;31:591–600.
99. Erdoes LS, Hunter GC, Venerus BJ, et al. Prospective evaluation of peripheral vascular disease in heart transplant recipients. J Vasc Surg 1995;22:434–40.
100. Takayama H, Salerno CT, Aldea GS, Verrier ED. Characteristics of extracoronary vascular disease in heart transplant recipient. J Card Surg 2008;23:459–63.
101. Rogers CA, Ganesh JS, Banner NR, Bonser RS; Steering Group. Cumulative risk adjusted monitoring of 30-day mortality after cardiothoracic transplantation: UK experience. Eur J Cardiothorac Surg 2005;27:1022–9.
102. Russo MJ, Rana A, Chen JM, Hong KN, et al. Pretransplantation patient characteristics and survival following combined heart and kidney transplantation: an analysis of the United Network for Organ Sharing Database. Arch Surg 2009;144:241–6.
103. Takayama H, Nathens AB, Merry H, et al. Is pre-transplant vascular disease a risk factor for mortality and morbidity after heart transplantation? Eur J Cardiothorac Surg 2007;31:457–61.
104. Patlolla V, Mogulla V, DeNofrio D, et al. Outcomes in patients with symptomatic cerebrovascular disease undergoing heart transplantation. J Am Coll Cardiol 2011;58:1036–41.
105. Russo MJ, Chen JM, Hong KN, et al.; Columbia University Heart Transplant Outcomes Research Group. Survival after heart transplantation is not diminished among recipients with uncomplicated diabetes mellitus: an analysis of the United Network of Organ Sharing database. Circulation 2006 21;114:2280–7.
106. Almuti K, Haythe J, Tsao L, et al. Does renal function deteriorate more rapidly in diabetic cardiac transplant recipients? Transplantation 2007;83:550–3.
107. Birkmeyer NJ, Charlesworth DC, Hernandez F, et al. Obesity and risk of adverse outcomes associated with coronary artery bypass surgery. Northern New England Cardiovascular Disease Study Group. Circulation 1998;97:1689–94.
108. Fasol R, Schindler M, Schumacher B, et al. The influence of obesity on perioperative morbidity: retrospective study of 502 aortocoronary bypass operations. Thorac Cardiovasc Surg 1992;40:126–9.
109. Weiss ES, Allen JG, Russell SD, et al. Impact of recipient body mass index on organ allocation and mortality in orthotopic heart transplantation. J Heart Lung Transplant 2009;28:1150–7.
110. Lietz K, John R, Burke EA, et al. Pretransplant cachexia and morbid obesity are predictors of increased mortality after heart transplantation. Transplantation 2001;72:277–83.
111. Clark AL, Knosalla C, Birks E, et al. Heart transplantation in heart failure: the prognostic importance of body massindex at time of surgery and subsequent weight changes. Eur J Heart Fail 2007;9:839–44.
112. Gellad ZF, Alexander BD, Liu JK et al. Severity of Clostridium difficile-associated diarrhea in solid organ transplant patients. Transpl Infect Dis 2007;9:276–80.
113. Uriel N, Jorde UP, Cotarlan V, et al. Heart transplantation in human immunodeficiency virus-positive patients. J Heart Lung Transplant 2009;28:667–9.
114. Carbone M, Mutimer D, Neuberger J. Hepatitis C virus and nonliver solid organ transplantation. Transplantation 2013;95:779–86.
115. Shafii AE, Su JW, Smedira NG, et al. The effect of recipient hepatitis C virus infection on outcomes following heart transplantation. Transplant Proc 2010;42:1784–7.
116. Chen YC, Chuang MK, Chou NK, et al. Twenty-four year single-center experience of hepatitis B virus infection in heart transplantation. Transplant Proc 2012;44:910–12.
117. Wu RS, Gupta S, Brown RN, et al. Clinical outcomes after cardiac transplantation in muscular dystrophy patients. J Heart Lung Transplant 2010;29:432–8.
118. Engels EA, Pfeiffer RM, Fraumeni JF Jr, et al. Spectrum of cancer risk among US solid organ transplant recipients. JAMA 2011;306:1891–901.
119. Martinez OM, de Gruijl FR. Molecular and immunologic mechanisms of cancer pathogenesis in solid organ transplant recipients. Am J Transplant 2008;8:2205–11.
120. Oliveira GH, Hardaway BW, Kucheryavaya AY, et al. Characteristics and survival of patients with chemotherapy-induced cardiomyopathy

undergoing heart transplantation. 1. J Heart Lung Transplant 2012;31:805–10.
121. Akashi H, Kato TS, Takayama H, et al. Outcome of patients with cardiac sarcoidosis undergoing cardiac transplantation—single-center retrospective analysis. J Cardiol 2012;60:407–10;11.
122. Zaidi AR, Zaidi A, Vaitkus PT. Outcome of heart transplantation in patients with sarcoid cardiomyopathy. J Heart Lung Transplant 2007;26:714–17.
123. Ruberg FL, Berk, JL. Transthyretin (TTR) Amyloidosis. Circulation 2012;126:1286–300.
124. Dubrey SW, Comenzo RL. Amyloid diseases of the heart: current and future therapies. Q J Med 2012;105:617–31.
125. Dey BR, Chung SS, Spitzer TR, et al. Cardiac transplantation followed by dose-intensive melphalan and autologous stem-cell transplantation for light chain amyloidosis and heart failure. Transplantation 2010;90:905–11.
126. Maurer MS, Raina A, Hesdorffer C, et al. Cardiac transplantation using extended-donor criteria organs for systemic amyloidosis complicated by heart failure. Transplantation 2007;83:539–45.
127. DePasquale EC, Nasir K, Jacoby DL. Outcomes of adults with restrictive cardiomyopathy after heart transplantation. J Heart Lung Transplant 2012;31:1269–75.
128. Radovancevic B, Poindexter S, Birovljev S, et al. Risk factors for development of accelerated coronary artery disease in cardiac transplant recipients. Eur J Cardiothorac Surg 1990;4:309–12.
129. Potaris K, Radovancevic B, Thomas CD, et al. Lung cancer after heart transplantation: a 17-year experience. Ann Thorac Surg 2005;79:980–3.
130. Botha P, Peaston R, White K, et al. Smoking after cardiac transplantation. Am J Transplant 2008;8:866–71.
131. Corbett C, Armstrong MJ, Neuberger J. Tobacco smoking and solid organ transplantation. Transplantation 2012;94(10):979–87.
132. Steinman TI, Becker BN, Frost AE, et al.; Clinical Practice Committee, American Society of Transplantation. Guidelines for the referral and management of patients eligible for solid organ transplantation. Transplantation 2001;71:1189–204.
133. Presberg BA, Levenson JL, Olbrisch ME, Best AM. Rating scales for the psychosocial evaluation of organ transplant candidates. Comparison of the PACT and TERS with bone marrow transplant patients. Psychosomatics 1995;36:458–61.
134. Maldonado JR, Dubois HC, David EE, et al. The Stanford Integrated Psychosocial Assessment for Transplantation (SIPAT): anew tool for the psychosocial evaluation of pre-transplant candidates. Psychosomatics 2012;53:123–32.
135. Mehra MR. The cardiac allograft is going up in smoke: a call to action. Am J Transplant 2008;8:737–8.
136. Dew MA, DiMartini AF, De Vito Dabbs A, et al. Rates and risk factors for nonadherence to the medical regimen after adult solid organ transplantation. Transplantation 2007;83:858–73.
137. Dobbels F, De Geest S, van Cleemput J, et al. Effect of late medication non-compliance on outcome after heart transplantation: a 5-year follow-up. J Heart Lung Transplant 2004;23:1245–51.
138. Butler JA, Peveler RC, Roderick P, et al. Modifiable risk factors for non-adherence to immunosuppressants in renal transplant recipients: a cross-sectional study. Nephrol Dial Transplant 2004 19:3144–9.
139. Dew MA, DiMartini AF, Steel J, et al. Meta-analysis of risk for relapse to substance use after transplantation of the liver or other solid organs. Liver Transplant 2008;14:159–72.
140. Dobbels F, Vanhaecke J, Dupont L, et al. Retransplant predictors of posttransplant adherence and clinical outcome: evidence base for pretransplant psychosocial screening. Transplantation 2009;87:1497–504.
141. George TJ, Beaty CA, Ewald GA, et al. Reoperative sternotomy is associated with increased mortality after heart transplantation. Ann Thorac Surg 2012;94:2025–32.
142. Hull MC, Morris CG, Pepine CJ, Mendenhall NP. Valvular dysfunction and carotid, subclavian, and coronary artery disease in survivors of Hodgkin lymphoma treated with radiation therapy. JAMA 2003;290:2831–7.
143. Chang AS, Smedira NG, Chang CL, et al. Cardiac surgery after mediastinal radiation: extent of exposure influences outcome. J Thorac Cardiovasc Surg 2007;133:404–13.
144. Uriel N, Vainrib A, Jorde UP, et al. Mediastinal radiation and adverse outcomes after heart transplantation. J Heart Lung Transplant 2010;29:378–81.
145. Wanaka K, Matsuo T, Matsuo M, et al. Re-exposure to heparin in uremic patients requiring hemodialysis with heparin-induced thrombocytopenia. J Thromb Haemost 2010;8:616.
146. Pötzsch B, Klövekorn WP, Madlener K. Use of heparin during cardiopulmonary bypass in patients with a history of heparin-induced thrombocytopenia.N Engl J Med 2000;343:515.
147. Selleng S, Haneya A, Hirt S, et al. Management of anticoagulation in patients with subacute heparin-induced thrombocytopenia scheduled for heart transplantation. Blood 2008;112:4024–7.
148. Welsby IJ, Um J, Milano CA, et al. Plasmapheresis and heparin reexposure as a management strategy for cardiac surgical patients with heparin-induced thrombocytopenia. Anesth Analg 2010;110:30–5.
149. Zucker MJ, Sabnani I, Baran DA, et al. Cardiac transplantation and/or mechanical circulatory support device placement using heparin anti-coagulation in the presence of acute heparin-induced thrombocytopenia. J Heart Lung Transplant 2010;29:53–60.
150. Patel ND, Weiss ES, Nwakanma LU, et al. Impact of donor-to-recipient weight ratio on survival after heart transplantation: analysis of the United Network for Organ Sharing Database. Circulation 2008;118(14 Suppl):S83–8.
151. Weiss ES, Allen JG, Patel ND, et al. The impact of donor-recipient sex matching on survival after orthotopic heart transplantation: analysis of 18 000 transplants in the modern era. Circ Heart Fail 2009;2:401–8.
152. Kittleson MM, Shemin R, Patel JK, et al. Donor-recipient sex mismatch portends poor 10-year outcomes in a single-center experience. J Heart Lung Transplant 2011;30:1018–22.
153. Khush KK, Kubo JT, Desai M. Influence of donor and recipient sex mismatch on heart transplant outcomes: analysis of the International Society for Heart and Lung Transplantation Registry. J Heart Lung Transplant 2012;31:459–66.
154. Patel ND, Weiss ES, Allen JG, et al. Heart transplantation for adults with congenital heart disease: analysis of the United network for organ sharing database. Ann Thorac Surg 2009;88(3):814–21; discussion 821–2.
155. Tambur AR, Pamboukian SV, Costanzo MR, et al. The presence of HLA-directed antibodies after heart transplantation is associated with poor allograft outcome. Transplantation 2005;80:1019–25.
156. Topilsky Y, Gandhi MJ, Hasin T, et al. Donor-specific antibodies to class II antigens are associated with accelerated cardiac allograft vasculopathy: a three-dimensional volumetric intravascular ultrasound study. Transplantation 2013;95:389–96.
157. Taylor DO, Yowell RL, Kfoury AG, et al. Allograft coronary artery disease: clinical correlations with circulating anti-HLA antibodies and the immunohistopathologic pattern of vascular rejection. J Heart Lung Transplant 2000;19:518–21.
158. Smith JD, Brunner VM, Jigjidsuren S, et al. Lack of effect of MICA antibodies on graft survival following heart transplantation. Am J Transplant 2009;9:1912–19.
159. Smith JD, Brunner VM, Jigjidsuren S, et al. Clinical relevance of complement-fixing antibodies in cardiac transplantation. Hum Immunol 2009;70:605–9.
160. Daniels G, Poole J, de Silva M, et al. The clinical significance of blood group antibodies. Transfus Med 2002;12:287–95.
161. Reid MR, Lomas-Francis C. The Blood Group Antigen Facts Book. New York: Harcourt Brace; 1997.
162. Cooper DK. A clinical survey of cardiac transplantation between ABO blood group-incompatible recipients and donors. Transplant Proc 1990;22:1457.

163. West LJ, Pollock-Barziv SM, Dipchand AI, et al. ABO-incompatible heart transplantation in infants. N Engl J Med 2001;344:793–800.
164. Fong SW, Qaqundah BY, Taylor WF. Developmental patterns of ABO isoagglutinins in normal children correlated with the effects of age, sex and maternal isoagglutinins. Transfusion 1974;14:551–9.
165. Springer GF, Horton RE. Blood group isoantibody stimulation in man by feeding blood group-active bacteria. J Clin Invest 1969;48:1280–91.
166. Irving C, Gennery A, Kirk R. Pushing the boundaries: the current status of ABO-incompatible cardiac transplantation. J Heart Lung Transplant 2012;31:791–6.
167. Padmanabhan A, Ratner LE, Jhang JS, et al. Comparative outcome analysis of ABO-incompatible and positive crossmatch renal transplantation: a single-center experience. Transplantation 2009;87:1889–96.
168. Tydén G, Hagerman I, Grinnemo KH, et al. Intentional ABO-incompatible heart transplantation: a case report of 2 adult patients. J Heart Lung Transplant 2012;31:1307–10.
169. Klein J, Sato A. The HLA system. First of two parts and second of two parts. N Engl J Med 2000;343:702–9 and 782–6.
170. Eng HS, Leffell MS. Histocompatibility testing after fifty years of transplantation. J Immunol Methods 2011;369:1–21.
171. Halloran PF, Wadgymar A, Autenried P. The regulation of expression of major histocompatibility complex products. Transplantation 1986;41:413–20.
172. Terasaki PI.Humoral theory of transplantation. Am J Transplant 2003;3:665–73.
173. Ho EK, Vlad G, Vasilescu ER, et al. Pre- and posttransplantation allosensitization in heart allograft recipients:major impact of de novo alloantibody production on allograft survival. Hum Immunol 2011;72:5–10.
174. Smith JD, Banner NR, Hamour IM, et al. De novo donor HLA-specific antibodies after heart transplantation are an independent predictor of poor patient survival. Am J Transplant 2011;11:312–19.
175. Tait BD, Süsal C, Gebel HM, et al. Consensus guidelines on the testing and clinical management issues associated with HLA and non-HLA antibodies in transplantation. Transplantation 2013;95:19–47.
176. Zeevi A, Girnita A, Duquesnoy R. HLA antibody analysis: sensitivity, specificity, and clinical significance in solid organ transplantation. Immunol Res 2006;36:255–64.
177. Tinckam K. Histocompatibility methods. Transplant Rev (Orlando) 2009;23:80–93.
178. Gebel HM, Bray RA.The evolution and clinical impact of human leukocyte antigen technology. Curr Opin Nephrol Hypertens 2010;19:598–602.
179. Roelen DL, Doxiadis II, Claas FH. Detection and clinical relevance of donor specific HLA antibodies: a matter ofdebate. Transpl Int 2012;25:604–10.
180. Chin C, Chen G, Sequeria F, et al. Clinical usefulness of a novel C1q assay to detect immunoglobulin G antibodies capable of fixing complement in sensitized pediatric heart transplant patients. J Heart Lung Transplant 2011;30:158–63.
181. Cecka JM. Calculated PRA (CPRA): the new measure of sensitization for transplant candidates. Am J Transplant 2010;10:26–9.
182. <http://optn.transplant.hrsa.gov/resources/professionalResources.asp>.
183. Zeevi A, Lunz J, Feingold B, et al. Persistent strong anti-HLA antibody at high titer is complement binding and associated with increased risk of antibody-mediated rejection in heart transplant recipients. J Heart Lung Transplant 2013;32:98–105.
184. Hawkins JA, Hillman ND, Lambert LM, et al. Immunogenicity of decellularized cryopreserved allografts in pediatric cardiac surgery: comparison with standard cryopreserved allografts. J Thorac Cardiovasc Surg 2003;126:247–52.
185. Kneib C, von Glehn CQ, Costa FD, et al. Evaluation of humoral immune response to donor HLA after implantation of cellularized versus decellularized human heart valve allografts. Tissue Antigens 2012;80:165–74.
186. Locke JE, Zachary AA, Warren DS, et al. Proinflammatory events are associated with significant increases in breadth and strength of HLA-specific antibody. Am J Transplant 2009;9:2136–9.
187. Brown G, Biberfeld P, Christensson B, Mason DY. The distribution of HLA on human lymphoid, bone marrow and peripheral blood cells. Eur J Immunol 1979;9:272–5.
188. Triulzi DJ, Kleinman S, Kakaiya RM, et al. The effect of previous pregnancy and transfusion on HLA alloimmunization in blood donors: implications for a transfusion-related acute lung injury risk reduction strategy. Transfusion 2009;49:1825–35.
189. Scornik JC, Meier-Kriesche HU. Blood transfusions in organ transplant patients: mechanisms of sensitization and implications for prevention. Am J Transplant 2011;11:1785–91.
190. Rebibou JM, Chabod J, Alcalay D, et al. Flow cytometric evaluation of pregnancy-induced anti-HLA immunization and blood transfusion-induced reactivation. Transplantation 2002;74:537–40.
191. Regan L, Braude PR, Hill DP. A prospective study of the incidence, time of appearance and significance of anti-paternal lymphocytotoxic antibodies in human pregnancy. Hum Reprod 1991;6:294–8.
192. Konoeda Y, Terasaki PI, Wakisaka A, et al. Public determinants of HLA indicated by pregnancy antibodies. Transplantation 1986;41:253–9.
193. Urban M, Gazdic T, Slimackova E, et al. Alloimmunosensitization in left ventricular assist device recipients and impact on posttransplantation outcome. ASAIO J 2012;58:554–61.
194. Drakos SG, Stringham JC, Long JW, et al. Prevalence and risks of allosensitization in HeartMate left ventricular assist device recipients: the impact of leukofiltered cellular blood product transfusions. J Thorac Cardiovasc Surg 2007;133:1612–19.
195. John R, Lietz K, Schuster M, Naka Y, et al. Immunologic sensitization in recipients of left ventricular assist devices. J Thorac Cardiovasc Surg 2003;125:578–91.
196. Drakos SG, Kfoury AG, Kotter JR, et al. Prior human leukocyte antigen-allosensitization and left ventricular assist device type affect degree of post-implantation human leukocyte antigen-allosensitization. J Heart Lung Transplant 2009;28:838–42.
197. Nikaein A, El-Awar N, Hunt J, et al. Clinically irrelevant circulating human leukocyte antigen antibodies in the presence of ventricular assist devices. J Heart Lung Transplant 2012;31:443–7.
198. Kaufman RM, Schlumpf KS, Wright DJ, Triulzi DJ; NHLBI Retrovirus Epidemiology Donor Study-II (REDS-II). Does Rh immune globulin suppress HLA sensitization in pregnancy? Transfusion 2013;53(9):2069–77.
199. Stehlik J, Islam N, Hurst D, et al. Utility of virtual crossmatch in sensitized patients awaiting heart transplantation. J Heart Lung Transplant 2009;28:1129–34.
200. Itescu S, Burke E, Lietz K, et al. Intravenous pulse administration of cyclophosphamide is an effective and safe treatment for sensitized cardiac allograft recipients. Circulation 2002;105:1214–19.
201. Jordan SC, Toyoda M, Vo AA. Regulation of immunity and inflammation by intravenous immunoglobulin: relevance to solid organ transplantation. Expert Rev Clin Immunol 2011;7:341–8.
202. Jordan SC, Peng A, Vo AA. Therapeutic strategies in management of the highly HLA-sensitized and ABO-incompatible transplant recipients. Contrib Nephrol 2009;162:13–26.
203. Vo AA, Lukovsky M, Toyoda M, et al. Rituximab and intravenous immune globulin for desensitization during renal transplantation. N Engl J Med 2008;359:242–51.
204. Montgomery RA, Zachary AA, Racusen LC, et al. Plasmapheresis and intravenous immune globulin provides effective rescue therapy for refractory humoral rejection and allows kidneys to be successfully transplanted into cross-match-positive recipients. Transplantation 2000;70:887–95.
205. Patel J, Everly M, Chang D, et al. Reduction of alloantibodies via proteasome inhibition in cardiac transplantation. J Heart Lung Transplant 2011;30:1320–6.

206. Kobashigawa J, Mehra M, West L, et al. Consensus Conference Participants. Report from a consensus conference on the sensitized patient awaiting heart transplantation. J Heart Lung Transplant 2009;28:213–25.
207. Loh E, Bergin JD, Couper GS, Mudge GH Jr. Role of panel-reactive antibody cross-reactivity in predicting survival after orthotopic heart transplantation. J Heart Lung Transplant 1994;13:194–201.
208. Kobashigawa JA, Sabad A, Drinkwater D, et al. Pretransplant panel reactive-antibody screens. Are they truly a marker for poor outcome after cardiac transplantation? Circulation 1996;94(9 Suppl):II294–7.
209. R, Rajasinghe H, Chen JM, Weinberg AD, et al. Impact of current management practices on early and late death in more than 500 consecutive cardiac transplant recipients. Ann Surg 2000;232:302–11.
210. Schaffer JM, Singh SK, Reitz BA, et al. Heart transplant graft survival is improved after a reduction in panel reactive antibody activity. J Thorac Cardiovasc Surg 2013;145:555–64;.
211. Kobashigawa JA, Patel JK, Kittleson MM, et al. The long-term outcome of treated sensitized patients who undergo heart transplantation. Clin Transplant 2011;25:E61–7.
212. Arnaoutakis GJ, George TJ, Kilic A, et al. Effect of sensitization in US heart transplant recipients bridged with a ventricular assist device: update in a modern cohort. J Thorac Cardiovasc Surg 2011;142:1236–45.
213. George JF, Taylor DO, Blume ED, et al. Minimizing infection and rejection death: clues acquired from 19 years of multi-institutional cardiac transplantation data. J Heart Lung Transplant 2011;30:151–7.
214. Taylor DO, Bristow MR, O'Connell JB, et al. Improved long-term survival after heart transplantation predicted by successful early withdrawal from maintenance corticosteroid therapy. J Heart Lung Transplant 1996;15:1039–46.
215. Mehra MR, Uber PA, Park MH, et al. Corticosteroid weaning in the tacrolimus and mycophenolate era in heart transplantation: clinical and neurohormonal benefits. Transplant Proc 2004;36:3152–5.
216. Deng MC, Eisen HJ, Mehra MR, et al. CARGO Investigators. Noninvasive discrimination of rejection in cardiac allograft recipients using gene expression profiling. Am J Transplant 2006;6:150–60.
217. Pham MX, Teuteberg JJ, Kfoury AG, et al. IMAGE Study Group. Gene-expression profiling for rejection surveillance after cardiac transplantation. N Engl J Med 2010;362:1890–900.
218. Stehlik J, Starling RC, Movsesian MA, et al. Cardiac Transplant Research Database Group. Utility of long-term surveillance endomyocardial biopsy: a multi-institutional analysis. J Heart Lung Transplant 2006;25:1402–9.
219. Mancini D, Pinney S, Burkhoff D, et al. Use of rapamycin slows progression of cardiac transplantation vasculopathy. Circulation 2003;108:48–53.
220. Keogh A, Richardson M, Ruygrok P, et al. Sirolimus in de novo heart transplant recipients reduces acute rejection and prevents coronary artery disease at 2 years: a randomized clinical trial. Circulation 2004;110:2694–700.
221. Page RL 2nd, Miller GG, Lindenfeld J. Drug therapy in the heart transplant recipient: part IV: drug-drug interactions. Circulation 2005;111:230–9.

CHAPTER 17

Immunosuppression strategies

Jon A. Kobashigawa MD

Introduction

Initial efforts in human cardiac transplantation were thwarted by poor outcomes that resulted from suboptimum immunosuppressive regimens, yielding either overwhelming infection or allograft rejection. Survival at 1 year in the 1970s was only around 50%.[1] In the past two decades, refinement of donor and recipient selection methods, better donor heart management, and the introduction of cyclosporine, followed by even more successful immunosuppressive regimens, has significantly improved survival. With a 1-year survival approaching 90%, a 5-year survival rate of approximately 70%, and a median survival in excess of 10 years, heart transplantation is now a valuable option for selected patients with end-stage heart failure.[2]

Minimizing immunosuppression and immunosuppression-associated complications without sacrificing efficacy are the goals of post-transplantation management. The true art of immunosuppression strategy lies in the employment of a combination of immunosuppressive agents since each affects a different pathway of T-cell activation (Figure 17.1). Currently, there is still no standard immunosuppressive protocol in heart transplantation (Figure 17.2) despite several multicenter randomized clinical trials seeking to optimize immunosuppression regimens.

Conventional immunosuppression agents

Immunosuppressive drugs result in three possible outcomes: the desired immunosuppressive effects, adverse effects of immunodeficiency such as infection and malignancy, and nonimmune toxicities such as diabetes, hypertension, and renal insufficiency. Infectious complications, frequent after cardiac transplantation, are a common cause of death in the first year after transplantation and continue to be a significant problem even after the first year.[3] Malignancy is another significant problem after cardiac transplantation. An important risk factor for post-transplant malignancy is impaired immunoregulation, which is synergistic with carcinogens such as nicotine or ultraviolet light exposure, and oncogenic viruses such as the Epstein–Barr virus (EBV) and the papilloma virus (HPV).[3] Lymphoproliferative diseases, skin cancers, and Kaposi sarcoma have a particularly high incidence relative to the general population. A relatively common cause of death after the first year following transplantation, malignancies account for 24% of deaths after 5 years.[4] All immunosuppressive drugs contribute to the risk of malignancy, with the possible exception of steroids. The cumulative amount of immunosuppression, especially OKT3 and polyclonal anti-lymphocyte preparations, is positively correlated with the risk of malignancy.[6] However, data in animals suggest that the antigrowth properties of a newer immunosuppressive drug, sirolimus, may result in fewer malignancies.[5]

Immunosuppressive agents commonly used in heart transplant patients and their mechanisms of action and common side effects are listed in Table 17.1 which gives trade names, pharmacology, necessary adjustments for renal or hepatic dysfunction, and dosing and general monitoring guidelines for each of the drugs. Table 17.2 lists the major adverse effects of immunosuppressive drugs.

Corticosteroids (steroids)

Steroids, among the first immunosuppressive agents used in clinical transplantation, have remained a central component in the management of transplantation. They are essential in the induction phase following transplantation and are the first line of therapy during acute rejection episodes. Glucocorticoids exert potent immunosuppressive and anti-inflammatory effects by altering transcriptional regulation of a number of genes that affect leukocytes (T and B lymphocytes, granulocytes, macrophages, and monocytes) as well as endothelial cell[7] function. The major effect on lymphocytes is mediated by inhibition of the transcription factor activator protein 1 and nuclear factor kappa B (NF-κB), which affect expression of several genes, including those controlling growth factors, cytokines, and adhesion molecules. In nonlymphoid cells, steroids cause a decrease in the production of vasoactive and chemoattractant factors and lipolytic and proteolytic enzymes. This results in inhibition of neutrophil adhesion to endothelial cells, prevention of macrophage differentiation, and downregulation of endothelial function, including decreases in myosin heavy chain expression. Some of the anti-inflammatory effects of steroids are regulated through the release of lipocortin, which acts by inhibiting phospholipase A2, thus inhibiting the production of leukotrienes and prostaglandins.[8,9]

Steroid therapy is a standard component of induction, maintenance, and antirejection therapy in heart transplant recipients. High-dose steroids are generally administered intraoperatively and postoperatively with gradual tapering of doses over months. Pulse steroids, either oral or intravenous, are generally the first treatment for moderate rejection (grade 3A or 3B) without hemodynamic compromise. Approximately 80–85% of these rejection episodes respond to the initial corticosteroid regimen.[10,11] Treatment with an oral prednisone bolus and taper appears to be as effective as intravenous methylprednisolone in asymptomatic patients with rejection.[12]

Steroids are associated with the largest number of long-term adverse effects. Hypertension, emotional lability, cataracts, gastric

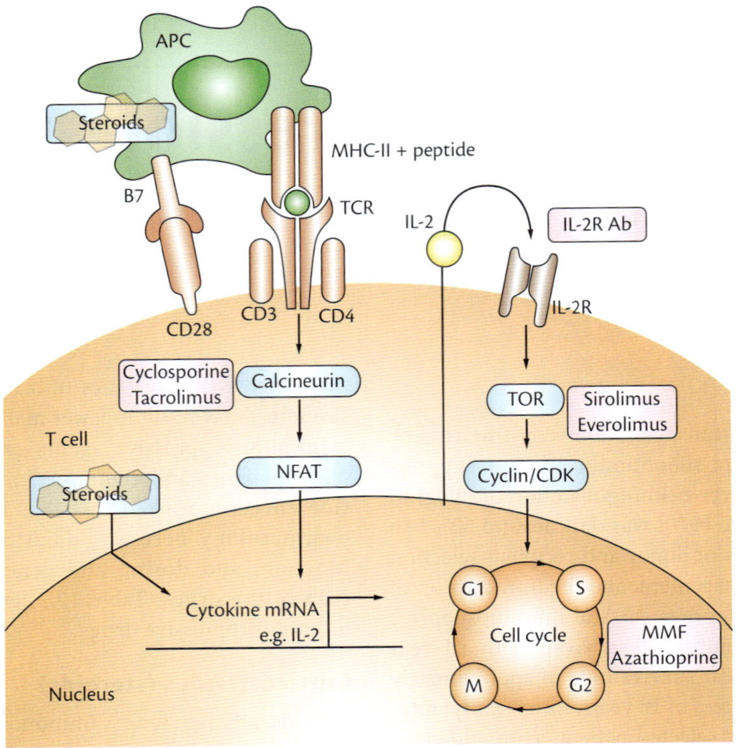

Fig. 17.1 Schematic of mechanisms of action of immunosuppressive drugs. T-cell proliferation results from activation after presentation of donor antigen (peptide) by antigen-presenting cells in conjunction with the MHC class II and B7 complex. This mechanism results in activation of calcineurin, which leads to production of IL-2. Autocrine stimulation by IL-2 results in cell proliferation by a pathway involving target of rapamycin (TOR) and cyclin/cyclin-dependent kinase. Immunosuppressive agents (shown in pink boxes) exert their effects at a number of different targets to prevent T-cell proliferation. G1 (first growth phase), S (synthesis of DNA), G2 (second growth phase), and M (cell division) represent the phases of the cell cycle. APC, antigen-presenting cell; CDK, cyclin-dependent kinase; IL-2, interleukin-2; IL-2R, interleukin-2 receptor; IL-2R Ab, interleukin-2-receptor antibody; MHC, major histocompatibility complex; MMF, mycophenolate mofetil; mRNA, messenger RNA; NF-AT, nuclear factor of activated T cells; TCR, T-cell receptor; TOR, target of rapamycin protein.[218]

Halloran PF, Gourishankar S. Principles and overview of immunosuppression. In: Norman DJ, Turka LA, eds. Primer on Transplantation, edn 2. Mount Laurel: American Society of Transplantation; 2001: 87–98.

ulcer, poor wound healing, and proximal myopathy are all associated with steroid therapy. Cosmetic effects including hirsutism, acne, easy bruising, skin fragility, moon face, buffalo hump, weight gain, and truncal obesity are particularly troubling to many patients. Important metabolic effects are hyperlipidemia, salt and water retention, diabetes mellitus, osteopenia, and growth retardation in children.[9,13] Long-term administration of steroids may result in chronic adrenal suppression, and adrenal insufficiency can follow a steroid taper or "stress" (illness, surgical procedures, infections).

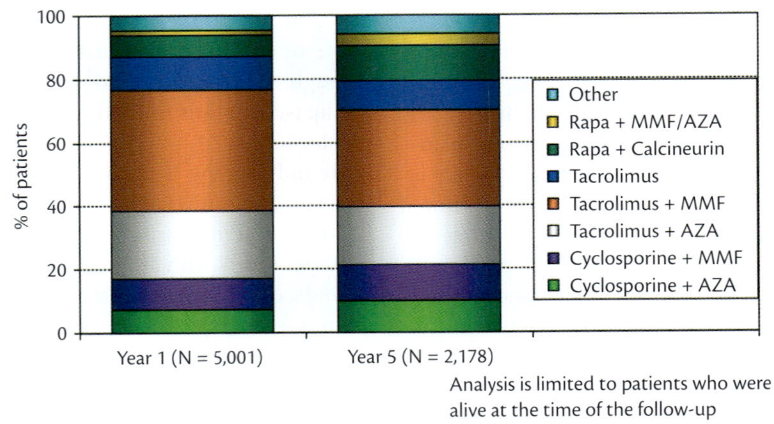

Fig. 17.2 Various maintenance immunosuppression regimens after heart transplantation at 1- and 5-year follow-up.[219]

Reprinted from Journal of Heart and Lung Transplantation, 27(9), Taylor DO, Edwards LB, Aurora P, Christie JD, Dobbels F, Kirk R, et al. Registry of the International Society for Heart and Lung Transplantation: twenty-fifth official adult heart transplant report—2008, 943–56, copyright (2008) with permission from Elsevier.

ATG, anti-thymocyte globulin; CNI, calcineurin inhibitor; ECMO, extracorporeal membrane oxygenation; EF, ejection fraction; IABP, intra-aortic balloon pump; IVIG, IV immune globulin.

Reprinted from The Surgeon, 9(3), Patel JK, Kittleson M, Kobashigawa JA. Cardiac allograft rejection, 160–7, copyright (2011) with permission from Elsevier.

Table 17.1 Commonly used oral (and intravenous) immunosuppressive drugs

Drugs	Trade name	Pharmacology	Adjustment for renal/ hepatic dysfunction	Dosing			Monitoring
				Oral	Intravenous	Comments	
Prednisone	Deltasone Generic	Processed in the liver and metabolites excreted in the urine	Consider prednisolone if hepatic dysfunction	×		Intra and post: Solumedrol 5–10 mg/kg pre- or intraoperatively and 5–7 mg/kg in 3 divided doses over next 24 h; then rapidly tapered from 1 to 0.3 mg/kg/day at 3–6 mo to 0.1 mg/kg/day at 6 mo For rejection: prednisone 1–3 mg/kg/day PO for 3–7 day or solumedrol 3–10 mg/kg/day IV; Lower doses have been used successfully	No currently available monitoring tool except clinical response
Prednisolone	Generic	Prednisone is converted to Prednisolone in liver	No	×			
Methylprednisolone	Medrol	Prednisone and Prednisolone have 4–5 times potency of hydrocortisone	No	×			
	Solumedrol			×			
Azathioprine	Imuran	Converted in liver to 6-mercaptopurine, which is inactivated by xanthine oxidase or TMPT predominantly in the liver	Decrease doses for renal dysfunction and lower dose range for hepatic dysfunction	×	×	1–2 mg/kg per day PO or IV Rarely used >3 mg/kg IV and oral the same dose	Monitoring of levels not clinically available Dose is decreased if white blood cells <3000–4000 Major drug interaction with allopurinol Polymorphisms in *TMPT* may increase effect
MMF	◆ Cellcept ◆ Generic	Rapidly hydrolyzed to mycophenolic acid (MPA) and MPA to its gluronide, which is excreted in urine and bile	≤1000 mg BID	×	×	500–1500 mg BID Higher doses have been used when monitoring trough MPA levels IV and oral the same dose	◆ Monitoring of MPA levels is controversial, but trough levels of 2.5–5.0 μg/mL have been suggested CSA inhibits enterohepatic circulation of MPA, decreasing exposure and levels
CNIs:							
CSA:							
Oil-based	◆ Sandimmune ◆ Generic	Oil-based formulation has unpredictable absorption secondary to need for emulsification by bile salts	Hepatic dysfunction: Decrease dose by half and follow levers	4–8 mg/kg per day in 2 divided doses	1–2 mg/kg per day in 2 divided doses or as continuous infusion	Dosing is high early after transplantation and gradually decreases over time Drugs that inhibit CYP-3A4 and p-GP may result in significantly higher levels IV dose is 1/3–1/4 of oral dose IV may be best administered in 2–6 h infusions	Abbott TDX assay most commonly used CSA trough levels have been routinely used with levels of 300–350 ng/ml early postoperatively decreasing to ~200 at 2 years Levels at 2 h postdose appear to more accurately estimate area under the curve and may result in lower doses
Modified (oil-based formulation is not bioequivalent to modified preparation)	◆ Neoral ◆ Gengraf ◆ Other-generics	Modified for more predictable absorption Both forms extensively metabolized by CYP-3A4 and are substrates and inhibitors of p-GP					

(continued)

Table 17.1 Continued

Tacrolimus	◆ Prograf ◆ Generic	Metabolized by CYP-3A4 and are substrates and inhibitors of p-GP	Follow levels for hepatic dysfunction	0.05–0.1 mg/kg per day in 2 divided doses	0.01–0.02 mg/kg per day in 2 divided doses or as continuous infusion	Doses are high early after transplantation and decrease over time Drugs that inhibit CYP3A4 or p-GP may result in higher levels	Whole-blood levels of 10–15 ng/ml early after transplantation and 5–10 ng/ml at 2 years are targets
TOR inhibitors:							
Sirolimus	Rapamune	CYP-3A4 and p-GP substrate	≤33% ↓ if hepatic dysfunction	×		2 mg/day in 1 dose (may be preceded by a single 6-mg loading dose)	Whole-blood trough levels of 5–15 ng/ml Coadministration with CSA may increase CSA levels as much as 100% Dose 4 hour apart with CSA or tacrolimus
Everolimus	Zotress (US) Certican (EU)	CYP-3A4 and p-GP substrate	≤33% ↓ if hepatic dysfunction	×		0.75 mg BID	Therapeutic drug monitor is 3–8 ng/ml Early renal insufficiency seen when used with sd-CSA. rd-CSA recommended

CNI, calcineurin inhibitor; CSA, cyclosporine; CYP, cytochrome P450; MMF, mycophenolate mofetil; p-GP, p-glycoprotein; rd-CSA, reduced-dose cyclosporine; sd-CSA, standardized-dose cyclosporine; TOR, target of rapamycin; TMPT, thiopurine methyltransferase.

Lindenfeld J, Miller GG, Shakar SF, Zolty R, Lowes BD, Wolfel EE, et al. Drug Therapy in the Heart Transplant Recipient: Part II: Immunosuppressive Drugs. Circulation 2004;110(25);3858–65.

Table 17.2 Major adverse effects of immunosuppressive drugs[214]

	Steroid	AZA	MMF	CSA	TAC	SIR	EVR	OKT3	Atgam	Thymo
Potential for drug–drug interactions	1	1	1	4	4	4	4			
Hypertension	2			4	3	2		3	3	3
Diabetes	3			1–2	2–3					
Obesity	2									
Hyperlipidemia[a]	2			3	3	3–4	3–4			
Renal insufficiency				3	3		4[b]			
Osteoporosis	3			1–2	1–2		1–2			
Avascular necrosis	1									
Poor wound healing	2					2[c]	1–2			
Neurological minor tremors, paresthesias				3	3					
Neurological major seizures, cerebritis				1	1			1	1	1
Hirsutism	2			3						
Alopecia		1			2					
Gingival hyperplasia				3						
GI[d]		2	3	2	3	3	3	3	2	3
Hepatic toxicity		2		1	2	1	1		1	
Hypomagnesmia				3	3					
Hyperkalemia				2	2	2				
Hyperuricemia				3	3	3				
Anemia		2	3			3	3			
Thrombocytopenia		1	2		3	3	3		3	3
Neutropenia		3	3			3	3	1	1	1
Cushingoid features	3									
Cytokine release syndrome—mild								4	3–4	3–4
Cytokine release syndrome—severe								1–2	0–1	0–1
Serum sickness									1	0–1

AZA, azithoprine; BAS, basiliximab; CSA, cyclosporine; EVR, everolimus; GI, gastrointestinal; MMF, mycophenolate mofetil; OKT3, muromonab-CD3; SIR, sirolimus; TAC, tacrolimus; Thymo, thymoglobulin.

1, rare (<5%); 2, common (5%-15%); 3, very common; 4, most patients.

[a] Hyperlipidemia (↑ total cholesterol, ↑↑LDL cholesterol, ↑ tr glycerides) (16%–50%).

[b] When used concomitantly with cyclosporine.

[c] Wound healing (especially early after operation), >50%.

[d] GI problems: diarrhea, nausea, vomiting.

Lindenfeld J, Miller GG, Shakar SF, Zolty R, Lowes BD, Wolfel EE, et al. Drug Therapy in the Heart Transplant Recipient: Part II: Immunosuppressive Drugs. Circulation 2004;110(25);3858–65.

Calcineurin inhibitors

Currently available calcineurin inhibitors (CNIs) include cyclosporine and tacrolimus. CNIs have become the cornerstone of maintenance therapy. Cyclosporine is a lipophilic undecapeptide. Both cyclosporine and tacrolimus act by blocking calcium-activated calcineurin (see Figure 17.1).[14,15] Cyclosporine and tacrolimus enter the cell primarily through diffusion and bind to different immunophilins: cyclosporine to cyclophilin and tacrolimus to FK binding protein-12 (FKBP-12). The complex of drug and immunophilin binds to calcineurin, a phosphatase that dephosphorylates multiple molecules, including nuclear factor of activated T cells (NF-AT). Dephosphorylated NF-AT translocates to the nucleus, where it binds to specific DNA sites in the promoter regions of several cytokine genes, including interleukin (IL)-2. Thus, both cyclosporine and tacrolimus inhibit transcription of IL-2 and other cytokines.[16] Cyclosporine also stimulates transforming growth factor-β (TGFβ) production, which contributes to its immunosuppressive activity.[17]

The advent of cyclosporine resulted in a a major improvement in transplant outcomes. In 1982, this agent was found to suppress delayed-type hypersensitivity skin reactions to tuberculin in guinea-pig but seemed to have no effect on antibody synthesis, which suggested a mechanism of immunosuppression that was specific to T cells. By 1998, more than 2800 heart transplant procedures were performed annually, with actuarial survival rates at 1 year and 5 years of 85% and 75%, respectively.[18] However, cyclosporine treatment also suppressed the clinical signs and symptoms of acute allograft rejection, making endomyocardial biopsy essential for rejection surveillance. A modified microemulsion formulation of cyclosporine demonstrated greater bioavailability and more predictable pharmacokinetics than oil-based preparations.[19] Randomized studies demonstrated equivalent graft and patient survival at 24 months,[20] but lower rates of rejection requiring treatment when the microemulsion formulation was used.[21,22,23] This microemulsion preparation was also better tolerated: so that there were fewer discontinuations of the study drug, and lower average doses of corticosteroids were required than with oil-based cyclosporine. Therapeutic monitoring of cyclosporine levels 2 hours after dosing was reported to be a better indicator of immunosuppressive efficacy than trough levels.[24,25]

Cyclosporine causes dose-related nephrotoxicity that can be acute, or chronic resulting in arteriolar sclerosis and tubulo-interstitial fibrosis (see Table 17.2). Rarely, cyclosporine nephrotoxicity may be manifested as a hemolytic uremic syndrome. Hypertension and hyperlipidemia occur in most patients.[26] De novo diabetes mellitus at 1 year develops in as many as 10% of patients. Neurological toxicity includes tremor, paresthesias, headache, seizures, mental status changes, visual symptoms, and insomnia. cyclosporine can cause nausea, vomiting, cholestasis, and cholelithiasis and contributes to the development of osteoporosis. Hypertrichosis, which occurs in at least 50% of patients, and gingival hyperplasia are side effects seen with cyclosporine that do not occur with tacrolimus.

Tacrolimus (previously known as FK506) is a macrolide and is produced by the fungus *Streptomyces tsukubaensis*. It has a similar mode of action to cyclosporine and is used as an alternative to it. Initial uncontrolled studies in cardiac transplantation suggested that tacrolimus results in a lower incidences of rejection and fewer adverse effects compared with cyclosporine.[27,28] A number of randomized controlled trials have also been performed that have compared tacrolimus and oil-based[29,30] or microemulsion[31,32] cyclosporine. Although compared with oil-based cyclosporine, patient and allograft survival were not significantly different in the tacrolimus group,[29,30] the incidence of moderate to severe cellular rejection at 6 months was significantly lower for tacrolimus compared with microemulsion cyclosporine.[31] However, the incidence of new-onset diabetes mellitus was significantly higher compared with microemulsion cyclosporine, while the incidences of post-transplant arterial hypertension and dyslipidemia were all lower with tacrolimus compared with cyclosporine. Infection and renal function were comparable at all study endpoints. Recent long-term follow-up studies[32,33] have confirmed the side effect profile of tacrolimus. Tacrolimus might be effective as monotherapy following cardiac transplantation.[34,35] This drug was also effective for rescue from steroid-resistant rejection.[36,37] Currently, tacrolimus is widely used as primary therapy or to treat recurrent acute rejection or as a subsitute for cyclosporine when cyclosporine-related toxic effects occur.[38]

The side effects of tacrolimus are similar to those of cyclosporine although the incidence of hypertension and hyperlipidemia are somewhat lower (see Table 17.2).[29] Hyperglycemia and neurological toxicity are more common with tacrolimus than with cyclosporine. Hyperglycemia is especially problematic at high doses and in some subgroups such as women and patients of African origin.[38] Diabetes may be more common when tacrolimus is given with azathioprine than with mycophenolate mofetil (MMF).[39] Hirsutism and gingival hypertrophy do not occur with tacrolimus; indeed, alopecia may be a side effect of tacrolimus.

Antiproliferative immunosuppressants

In addition to a CNI, an antiproliferative agent is usually used in current immunosuppressive regiments. Azathioprine and mycophenolate mofetil (MMF) are the commonly used antiproliferative agents.

Azathioprine

Azathioprine is a prodrug that is converted rapidly by plasma esterases or nonenzymatically by glutathione to 6-mercaptopurine, which is further converted to thioinosine monophosphate, its active metabolite (see Figure 17.1). Thioinosine monophosphate is converted to a purine analog and incorporated into DNA, inhibiting its synthesis and the proliferation of both T and B lymphocytes.

Azathioprine is generally used as maintenance therapy in combination with steroids and a CNI; it has US Food and Drug Administration (FDA) approval as an adjunct for the prevention of rejection in renal transplantation. Early initial immunosuppressive protocols during the 1970s in human heart transplantation used azathioprine combined with prednisone, resulting in a 1-year survival of 60–65% and 5-year actuarial survival of 35–40%.[40,41] The development of cyclosporine resulted in substantial increases in survival.[42] Cyclosporine in combination with either prednisone or azathioprine is less effective than therapy with all three agents.[41] Compared with dual therapy, triple therapy has been shown to have a decreased incidence of renal failure, infections, use of cytolytic drugs, and lymphoproliferative diseases.[43]

The major side effect of azathioprine is myelosuppression, including leukopenia, anemia, and thrombocytopenia (see Table 17.2). These side effects are generally dose dependent and resolve in 7–10 days with dose reduction. Pancreatitis, hepatitis, and hepatic veno-occlusive disease can occur but are rare. Skin cancers, once thought to be related primarily to azathioprine, are now thought to be related to the overall level of immunosuppression.[44]

Mycophenolate mofetil

MMF is a noncompetitive inhibitor of inosine monophosphate dehydrogenase, a key enzyme in the de novo synthesis of guanine nucleotides. Proliferating lymphocytes are dependent on this pathway because it is their only pathway for the purine synthesis and DNA replication. Other cells use both de novo and salvage pathways for purine synthesis. Therefore, MMF is a selective inhibitor of lymphocyte proliferation. In vivo and in vitro mycophenolic acid inhibits lymphocyte proliferation in response to allogeneic stimulation without inhibiting the growth of other cell lines.[45]

Initial human clinical trials in heart transplant recipients suggested that MMF was well tolerated and as efficacious as azathioprine with less myelosuppression.[45]A subsequent large prospective multicenter randomized trial compared azathioprine and MMF in combination with cyclosporine and steroids. In this study 11% of the patients withdrew before receiving drug because an intravenous form was not available.[46] In an intention-to-treat analysis, there was no difference in survival or rejection, but in an analysis of treated patients, there was a reduction in mortality at 1 year (6.2% vs. 11.4%; $p = 0.031$) and a reduction in rejection requiring treatment (65.7% vs. 73.7%; $p = 0.026$) in the MMF patients. The Joint UNOS/International Society for Heart and Lung Transplantation (ISHLT) Thoracic Registry has been analyzed for differences in the effects of MMF and azathioprine in patients on a cyclosporine-based regimen.[47] Patients treated with MMF had an actuarial survival benefit (1 year, 96% vs. 93%; 3 year, 91% versus 86%; $p = 0.0012$). These results are similar to those in renal transplant recipients. MMF is effective in reversing recurrent rejection when used in place of azathioprine.[48,49] In patients with chronic renal dysfunction, switching from azathioprine to MMF in combination with cyclosporine reduction or withdrawal to improve renal function has also been used as an effective strategy.[50]

MMF is usually well tolerated (see Table 17.2). Major side effects include nausea, vomiting, and diarrhea, which usually are responsive to a decrease in dosage.[51] The toxicity of MMF may be more closely related to the mycophenolic acid levels than the dose. The risk of opportunistic infections appears to be higher in patients treated with MMF when compared with azathioprine (53.3% vs. 43.6% $p = 0.025$ at 1 year).[46]

Proliferation signal inhibitors

Proliferation signal inhibitors include sirolimus and everolimus (everolimus).

Sirolimus

Sirolimus, first isolated in soil samples from Rapa-Nui (Easter Island), is a natural product of the actinomycete *Streptomyces hygroscopicus*.[52,53] A macrolide antibiotic, sirolimus has a structure similar to that of tacrolimus. Sirolimus binds to the same family of immunophilins as tacrolimus, the FKBPs, but rather than blocking calcineurin dependent T-cell activation, FKBP-sirolimus inhibits a kinase, the target of rapamycin (TOR) (see Figure 17.1). The action of these inhibitors is, therefore, complementary to the CNIs. TOR phosphorylates proteins that are important in the regulation of the cell cycle, thus playing a critical role in connecting signals from the growth factor receptors to the cell nucleus for stimulation of growth and proliferation of T and B lymphocytes.[54,55] Activation of TOR also signals proliferation of smooth muscle cells and endothelial cells in response to growth factors.[53] This latter mechanism may explain why sirolimus inhibits arterial smooth muscle cell and endothelial cell proliferation and has been shown to prevent graft atherosclerosis in rat cardiac allografts, to prevent intimal hyperplasia after coronary stenting in native coronary artery disease, and to inhibit tumor growth in animal models.[55,56,57]

Sirolimus has been shown to effectively prevent acute graft rejection and inhibit treatment-refractory acute graft rejection in heart transplant recipients.[58] In an Australian randomized open-label trial of sirolimus compared with azathioprine, sirolimus was associated with a reduced rejection rate.[59] No significant difference in 1-year mortality was noted, but sirolimus significantly worsened renal function and was associated with a raised frequency of hypertension. Importantly, sirolimus, which is also known to have antiproliferative effects on smooth muscle cells, was shown to decrease the development of cardiac allograft vasculopathy (CAV), as assessed by intravascular ultrasound (IVUS) at 6 months; the benefit was maintained at 2 years.[59] In another angiographic study of cardiac transplant patients with established CAV, sirolimus was also shown to slow disease progression.[60] The immunosuppressed state following organ transplantation is associated with an increased risk of malignancy, which is a major cause of death after cardiac transplantation in the long term. The anti-tumor effects of the proliferation signal inhibitors, in particular sirolimus, might offer prophylactic benefit. In a study in renal transplant patients who developed Kaposi's sarcoma, switching medication from cyclosporine to sirolimus was shown to significantly reduce tumor burden.[61]

The early use of proliferation signal inhibitors following transplantation, however, will probably be limited because of concerns related to delayed wound healing, resulting from the potent antiproliferative effects of this class of agents. Use of sirolimus in patients who have recently had lung transplantation has been associated with airway anastomosis dehiscence,[62] and a prospective analysis in renal transplant patients showed a significant increase in wound-healing complications following early use of this drug.[63] Other major adverse effects of sirolimus include hyperlipidemia with hypertriglyceridemia and increased LDL cholesterol, thrombocytopenia, neutropenia, and anemia (see Table 17.2).[64,65,66,67,68,68] Hypercholesterolemia and hypertriglyceridemia are at least partially responsive to dose reduction.[64] Sirolimus-induced hyperlipidemia also responds to conventional treatment with HMG-CoA reductase inhibitors (statins) and fibric acid derivatives (fibrates).[69] However, there may be significant interactions with sirolimus and these drugs as a result of competitive metabolism via CYP3A.[70] Therefore, heightened awareness is necessary for potential hepatic and muscular toxicity with statins or fibrates in conjunction with sirolimus. Overall, the tendency of sirolimus to promote hyperlipidemia must be balanced against the putative anti-artherogenic effects of the mTOR inhibitors. Thrombocytopenia seems to be dose related and is reversible. Severe thrombocytopenia is rare. Neutropenia may also occur, but in the phase 3 multicenter studies, no patient developed absolute neutropenia. Sirolimus exacerbates the adverse renal and other effects of cyclosporine but does not appear to result in renal dysfunction or diabetes when given without a CNI. Sirolimus has been used in place of a CNI with improved renal function.[71] A noninfectious pneumonitis has been reported with sirolimus.[64]

Everolimus

Everolimus is an analog of sirolimus that has recently been approved for kidney transplant. The preliminary reports from a number of studies in heart transplant recipients demonstrated positive results. In a previous randomized double-blind prospective trial, 634 cardiac transplant recipients were assigned to receive azathioprine or 2 doses of everolimus (1.5 mg or 3 mg daily, in 2 divided doses).[72] At 6 months, the proportion of patients who had reached the primary efficacy endpoint (a composite of death, graft loss or retransplantation, loss to follow-up, biopsy-proven severe acute rejection, or rejection with hemodynamic compromise) was significantly smaller in both the low-dose and high-dose everolimus groups (36.4% and 27.0%) than in the group receiving azathioprine (46.7%). The study result was robust in demonstrating that all IVUS parameters were reduced in those patients treated with everolimus versus azathioprine at 12 months. The rates of cytomegalovirus (CMV) infection were significantly lower in everolimus groups (7.7%, 7.6%, and 21.5%, respectively). Serum creatinine levels were also significantly higher in the two everolimus groups (both $p = 0.001$ at month 3) than in the azathioprine group, particularly when used in combination with cyclosporine: at 1 year serum creatinine was

168 μmol/L (1.9 mg/dl) in the low-dose everolimus-treated group, 172 μmol/L (2 mg/dl) in the high-dose everolimus-treated group, and 141 μmol/L (1.6 mg/dl) in the azathioprine-treated group). These study results were also confirmed by the most recent phase 3 clinical trial in heart transplantation,[73] which suggested the favorable effect of everolimus in reducing CAV.

Overall, everolimus seemed to effectively reduce rejection and CAV, but the findings suggested that serum creatinine levels should be carefully monitored in patients receiving concomitant cyclosporine. In a recent clinical trial of 176 heart transplant patients, the use of everolimus with low-dose cyclosporine (to prevent the observed renal insufficiency) compared to MMF with standard-dose cyclosporine was shown not to worsen renal function.[74] Similar results were observed in a larger clinical trial of 721 patients randomized to everolimus with low-dose cyclosporine or to MMF with standard-dose cyclosporine.[75] Renal function was comparable between groups in centers that achieved the lower cyclosporine target levels.

Statins

A number of studies have now confirmed the benefit of 3-hydroxy-3-methylglutaryl coenzyme A inhibitors (statins) in cardiac transplantation.[76,77] These studies showed not only a decrease in the development of CAV and improved survival, but also a surprising reduction in the number of rejection episodes. One randomized trial involved 97 cardiac transplant patients who were treated with or without pravastatin. Significant first-year benefits in terms of cholesterol levels, survival, rejection with hemodynamic compromise, the development of CAV, and decreased natural-killer (NK) cell cytotoxic effects were seen in the statin-treated patients.[76] This study suggested an immunomodulatory effect of statins in cyclosporine-treated cardiac transplant patients. Subsequently the pravastatin-treated group had greater 10-year survival than the control group (68% vs. 48%; $p = 0.026$) and greater 10-year freedom from the combined endpoint of angiographic graft vasculopathy, death, or both (43% vs. 20%; $p = 0.009$).[78] Similar results were observed in 72 heart transplant patients randomized to simvastatin or no statin.[77]

Previous studies suggested that statins had an immunosuppressive effect.[77,78,79,80] Statins reduce cholesterol production and isoprenylation of certain proteins, such as Ras and Ras-related proteins, which seem to be important in T-cell activation and effector function and are pivotal in the development of allograft rejection during organ transplantation.[81,82,83] Pravastatin was also been reported to decrease coronary artery intimal lesions while depressing IgG alloantibody levels, suggesting a role for the humoral immune response in the development of CAV.[84–86] Kwak and colleagues[79] reported that statins effectively repress the induction of major histocompatibility complex class II (MHC-II) expression by interferon-γ in a dose-dependent manner. The authors used messenger RNA experiments to establish that the specific mechanism by which MHC-II induction is inhibited by statins is a selective, repressive effect on the induction of expression of the promoter IV region of the MHC-II transactivator (*CIITA*) gene. They concluded that inhibition of inducible expression of MHC-II molecules in the considerable variety of cells that normally become MHC-II-positive by the effect of interferon-γ has multiple functional consequences. Such conditions include repression of the activation of endogenous CD4+ T lymphocytes and recognition of MHC-II molecules by CD4+ T lymphocytes in an allogeneic context after organ transplantation. Given these beneficial effects, early statin therapy (regardless of cholesterol level) is now an integral part of the immunosuppressive regimen in cardiac transplantation.

Immunosuppresion strategies and regimen

Induction therapy versus noninduction therapy

Immunosuppression regimens are generally defined as induction, maintenance, or rejection regimens. Induction therapy consists of intense perioperative immunosuppression and is currently used in approximately 40% of cardiac transplant patients.[87] The main benefit of this therapy is a marked reduction in rejection in the early postoperative period (the first 4–6 weeks after transplantation), when graft dysfunction and renal dysfunction are problematic. Induction therapy also allows later introduction of CNIs, thus avoiding exacerbation of renal dysfunction.[88,89] In general, induction therapy can be divided into two categories: depleting antibodies and nondepleting antibodies or fusion proteins with natural binding properties currently being studied.[90] Depleting antibodies markedly reduces alloreactive T cells at the time of transplantation making the host unresponsive to the allograft. Depleting antibodies include both monoclonal (anti-CD3 antibodies [OKT3] and alemtuzumab) and polyclonal (anti-thymocyte globulin, ATG) antibodies. Nondepleting antibodies inhibit critical T-cell activities (i.e., IL-2-driven cell proliferation) without causing their depletion. Anti-IL-2 receptor (CD-25) antibodies (daclizumab and basiliximab) and fusion proteins with natural binding properties are currently being studied, e.g., CTLA4-Ig (belatacept). Table 17.3 summarizes trade names, pharmacology, necessary adjustments for renal or hepatic dysfunction, and dosing and general monitoring guidelines for commonly used intravenous immunosuppressive drugs. Common adverse events of drugs for both induction therapy and maintenance therapy are included in Table 17.2.

Polyclonal antibodies

Polyclonal anti-lymphocyte antibodies are available in two ATG formulations: Atgam (equine ATG) and Thymoglobulin (rabbit ATG) polyclonal antibodies that result in substantial lymphocyte depletion.[91] These preparations contain antibodies to many surface T- and B-cell molecules, including HLA.[92] Antibodies to CD45, a protein that plays a role in T-cell activation, may be particularly important in reversing rejection and inducing tolerance.[9] Treatment results in complement-dependent opsonization and eventual cell lysis and may contribute to apoptosis of these cells. There may be binding to granulocytes and platelets and a reduction of these cells in peripheral blood. The xenogeneic origin of these polyclonal antibodies can induce a host antibody response that results in acute hypersensitivity response or serum sickness on subsequent exposure. Because batches of polyclonal antibodies vary in potency, monitoring of T cells with flow cytometry is helpful in assessing effectiveness and adjusting dosing.

Lympholytic agents (Atgam, Thymoglobulin), generally given for 7–14 days postoperatively, have been standard induction drugs. Polyclonal antibodies are also used for the treatment of steroid-resistant rejection in heart transplant recipients. Both Atgam and Thymoglobulin have FDA approval for the management of acute rejection in renal transplant recipients. The few comparisons between Atgam and Thymoglobulin appear predominantly

Table 17.3 Commonly used intravenous-only immunosuppressive drugs[215]

Drugs	Trade name	Pharmacology	Adjustment for renal/hepatic dysfunction	Dosing	Monitoring
Polyclonal anti-lymphocyte preparations		Elimination by protein degradation and antibody formation to equine (ATGAM) or rabbit (Thymoglobulin) protein	No		ATGAM requires skin test before first dose. Premedication[†] is required. Monitoring is done by following CD3 counts. Various targets include CD3 at 5%-10% baseline, <50 CD3+ cells/ml, 50–100 CD3+ cells/ml Repeating daily dose when CD3+ cells increase may decrease number of daily doses, especially with Thymoglobulin
Anti-thymocyte globulin	ATGAM			10–15 mg/kg/day IV over 6–8 hours for 3–14 days	
	Thymoglobulin			1.5 mg/kg/day IV over 6–8 hours for 3–14 days	
Monoclonal[b]					
Muromonab CD3	Orthoclone, OKT3	Elimination by protein degradation and binding to target cells with opsonization and phagocytosis	No	5 mg/day for 7–14 days	Premedication[a] is required Monitoring CD3+ cells as above Lower doses may be used if monitoring CD3+ cells HAMA may result in an increase of CD3+ cells HAMA should be checked. before a repeated course is given
Alemtuzumab	Campath	CD52 antibody, depleting T cells, as well as B cells and other lymphoid subsets	No	30 mg IV over 2 hours once intraoperatively	Premedication[a] is required. Monitoring total lymphocyte counts
Anti-cytokine receptor antibodies		Elimination vias protein degradation similar to IgG	No		CD3 counts do not change. IL-2R+ lymphocytes may be measured but are not generally followed clinically Rare cases of hypersensitivity to basilixmab have been reported
Daclizumab	Zenapzx			1 mg/kg per day within 24 hour of transplantation and q14days for 4 additional doses. Other dose schedules have been reported.	
Basiliximab	Simulect			20 mg within 2 hours of surgery and 4 day postoperatively	

HAMA, anti-human mouse antibodies.

[a] Premedication for cytokine release syndrome includes antipyretics, intravenous steroids, antihistamines, and H_2 blockers.

[b] Generally administered through central line, although Thymoglobulin has been administered through a peripheral line.

Lindenfeld J, Miller GG, Shakar SF, Zolty R, Lowes BD, Wolfel EE, et al. Drug Therapy in the Heart Transplant Recipient: Part I: Immunosuppressive Drugs. Circulation 2004;110(25);3734–40.

in the renal transplantation literature. From the limited data available, Thymoglobulin appears to be moderately more efficacious than Atgam when used for induction therapy or for treating steroid-resistant rejection.[93,94] Thymoglobulin was associated with greater long-term event-free survival.[95,96] Lympholytic agents are also used in the early perioperative management of patients with worsening renal insufficiency when treatment with CNIs is delayed to prevent the development of acute renal failure. With the introduction of more potent drugs for maintenance immunosuppression, induction therapy, especially with lympholytic agents, is often reserved for patients at highest risk of rejection or renal failure.

Although induction therapy was originally designed to induce tolerance to the graft, this goal has not been realized. Because ATGs are foreign proteins, there is a risk of allergic reactions. Urticaria is more common with Atgam, and fever, chills, and rash may occur with both compounds, especially after the first dose. The cytokine release syndrome, more common with OKT3, can occur with the polyclonal antibodies. Hypertension, diarrhea, and headache are common. Serum sickness can occur, especially with the equine-derived Atgam. Leukopenia and thrombocytopenia may require either a reduction in dose or termination of therapy. There is an increased incidence of either primary or reactivation CMV infections with the use of both monoclonal and polyclonal antibodies, and prophylactic doses of ganciclovir are given during and for up to 3 months after the course of intravenous anti-lymphocyte therapy.[9] Lymphocyte-depleting antibodies have been clearly shown, as a group, to increase the risk of malignancy, mainly of virally induced cancers. The cumulative load of immunosuppression appears to be a primary determinant of the incidence of non-Hodgkin's lymphoma early after transplantation.[97] Induction therapy in general is also associated with high cost.

Monoclonal antibodies

Monoclonal anti-lymphocyte antibodies currently include muromonab-CD3 (OKT3) and alemtuzumab.

OKT3 is a murine antibody that recognizes the ε chain of the CD3 molecule on T cells. CD3 is required for the TCR to generate the intracellular signals that activate T cells.[98] The binding of OKT3 to CD3 renders the T cell unable to respond to an antigen challenge or to bind to target cells. T cells bound to OKT3 are opsonized and removed from the circulation by macrophages in the spleen and liver. Initial binding of OKT3 to the TCR-CD3 complex results in activation of the T cells with release of multiple cytokines. This cytokine release syndrome represents an important aspect in the adverse effect profile of this antibody.

OKT3 has FDA approval for the treatment of acute allograft rejection in renal transplant patients and for the treatment of steroid-resistant acute allograft rejection in cardiac and hepatic transplant patients. In heart transplant recipients, OKT3 has been used primarily for treatment of steroid-refractory rejection, especially when it is associated with hemodynamic compromise, and for induction therapy in recipients at greater risk of rejection.[99] OKT3 has a 90% rate of complete or partial reversal of biopsy-proven steroid-resistant rejection in heart transplant recipients.[100] The experience with induction therapy with OKT3 has not been as promising as the original studies indicated. Although the incidence of early cellular rejection is lower than with conventional triple drug therapy, there is an increased incidence of late rejection, a higher rate of humoral (vascular) rejection, and no overall benefit at 1 year after cardiac transplantation.[101] OKT3 is no longer available in the United States due to dwindling use.

Alemtuzumab is a lymphocyte-depleting monoclonal antibody specific for the lymphocyte surface antigen CD52 on human lymphocytes, which depletes T cells (most potently), as well as B cells and other lymphoid subsets, thus may decrease the dosage or need for concurrent maintenance immunosuppressive agents. Alemtuzumab is not yet approved by FDA for use in solid organ transplantation. Although routine use of alemtuzumab in cardiac transplant recipients reportedly facilitates a steroid-free regimen, significant adverse effects, especially decline in renal function and increase in antibody-mediated rejection (AMR) also may occur.[102] In some patients, CD4+ and CD8+ counts did not return to baseline levels within 1 year after discontinuation.

Anti-cytokine receptor antibodies used in transplantation are basiliximab and daclizumab. Basiliximab is a chimeric (mouse/human) anti-IL-2R monoclonal antibody with mouse variable regions fused to the constant regions of a human IgG. Daclizumab is a humanized anti-IL-2R (CD25) monoclonal antibody that has the murine antigen-binding sequences molecularly engrafted onto a human antibody.

Both basiliximab and daclizumab bind the α subunit of IL-2R expressed on antigen-activated T cells. This prevents binding of IL-2 to the IL-2R, inhibiting proliferation of T cells.[103,104] However, this action alone is not sufficient to prevent rejection, and there appear to be other important, although incompletely understood, actions of these antibodies.[9,105]

Basiliximab is FDA approved for the prophylaxis of acute organ rejection in patients receiving renal transplants in a regimen that includes cyclosporine and corticosteroids. Some centers reserve this therapy only for high-risk recipients. In a double-blind randomized controlled trial comparing daclizumab with placebo in 434 heart transplant recipients, there was a significant increase in mortality caused by infection due to a flaw in study design where some patients received double induction with a cytolytic agent plus daclizumab.[106] To date, the daclizumab trial was the only multicenter randomized induction versus noninduction clinical trial in cardiac transplantation. Unfortunately, daclizumab is no longer available.

Other side effects of anti-cytokine receptor antibodies include hypersensitivity. Cytokine release syndrome does not occur after administration of this type of drug, and there has been no reported increased risk of malignancy.[103,104,106,107] Hypersensitivity has been reported with initial exposure and re-exposure to both basiliximab and daclizumab. The second dose should be withheld if complications such as hypersensitivity occur.[108]

Clinical utility of induction therapy

Although the use of induction therapy has been commonplace for more than 20 years, there is not yet a large and well-designed definitive clinical trial examining the clinical utility of induction therapy. From the latest ISHLT registry data,[2] 52% of heart transplant recipients received immunosuppressive induction. IL-2R antagonists were used in 30% of patients, polyclonal anti-lymphocytic antibodies were used in 20%, and induction with alemtuzumab was used in 3% of patients. Use of OKT3 has become negligible. Interestingly, there are marked geographic variations in the use of immunosuppressive induction therapy. In Europe, induction therapy is used in 76% of patients, whereas in North America, induction therapy is used in 51% of patients. However, patients receiving immunosuppressive induction therapy had a higher risk of rejection between discharge and 1 year after transplant compared with patients not receiving induction therapy—31% in polyclonal antibody induction, 35% in IL-2R antagonist induction, and 28% in no induction ($p < 0.05$).[2] This difference may have resulted from selective use of immunosuppressive agents in patients with a known elevated risk of rejection. Reviewing major clinical trials of immunosuppressants that allowed induction therapy in the protocol,[46,72] none of them indicated significant difference in the incidence of rejection between induction group and the overall study population. Thus the disadvantages and benefits of induction therapy following heart transplantation need to be carefully weighed.

Major clinical trials of immunosuppression regimen

Relatively few heart transplant procedures, about 4500 worldwide, are performed each year, limiting the number of randomized clinical trials available to guide treatment decisions. As a result, most guideline recommendations are class IIa or IIb and based on level B or C evidence.

The major study endpoints of the immunosuppression randomized clinical trials in heart transplantation have included the following either alone or in combination: survival, rejection, CAV, and adverse events. Although survival is the most important endpoint, heart transplant studies are relatively small and have not been powered to demonstrate a mortality benefit. The clinical endpoints mentioned above directly or indirectly affect mortality as well as morbidity and quality of life. Therefore, these appear to be clinically reasonable endpoints to compare the immunosuppressive regimens used in these heart transplant trials.

The major randomized clinical trials of immunosuppressive therapy in heart transplantation are listed in Table 17.4. In these trials, there has been no demonstrated difference in survival among the various immunosuppressive regimens, with is one exception. In the intent-to-treat analysis of the multicenter MMF trial in 1998,[46] there was no 1-year survival benefit in patients on MMF therapy compared to azathioprine therapy. However, in this study, patients were randomized to treatment prior to transplant and perioperative morbidity/mortality led to 11% of patients never receiving the study drug with more deaths occurring by chance in the MMF group. This appears to have negated a survival benefit in the MMF group in the intent-to-treat analysis. For patients who received at least one dose of MMF (treated-patient analysis), there was a significant 1-year survival benefit.

Several immunosuppressive agents have been shown to decrease the incidence of rejection (Table 17.4). However, many of these trials including the MMF,[46] everolimus[72] and sirolimus[59] trials used azathioprine as the comparator. In the European tacrolimus/cyclosporine[30] and the US tacrolimus/cyclosporine[29] trials both in combination with azathioprine, there was no difference in rejection between tacrolimus and cyclosporine-treated patients. However, a tacrolimus/cyclosporine trial reported by Grimm et al.[31] revealed a significantly lower rejection rate at 6 months for tacrolimus compared to cyclosporine (both in combination with azathioprine). More recently, a three-arm trial compared regimens of tacrolimus/MMF, tacrolimus/sirolimus, and cyclosporine/MMF[109] and found that both regimens involving tacrolimus had significantly less treated rejection at 6 months than the regimen with cyclosporine/MMF. Furthermore, tacrolimus/MMF when compared only to cyclosporine/MMF had significantly less cellular rejection (ISHLT grade>2R/3A) as well as any-treated rejections. Of interest, Tacrolimus In Combination, Tacrolimus Alone Compared (the TICTAC trial)[35,110] demonstrated that tacrolimus monotherapy had comparable rejection compared to tacrolimus/MMF-treated patients. These findings also suggested that early corticosteroid weaning, tacrolimus monotherapy, or dual therapy are potential viable options for selected heart transplant patients. Recently, it was reported that everolimus with reduced-dose cyclosporine compared to MMF with standard-dose cyclosporine had comparable 1-year rejection incidence.[75]

Several of the recent randomized immunosuppressive trials including the MMF,[46] everolimus,[72,73] and sirolimus[59] trials demonstrated benefit in the first-year IVUS results which were performed to assess CAV. The progressive development of intimal thickening by IVUS in the first year after heart transplant is predictive of development of angiographically apparent CAV. Rapidly progressive CAV, defined as an increase of 0.5 mm or more in maximal intimal thickness within the first year after heart transplant, is associated with a significantly increased risk of 5-year all-cause death, myocardial infarction, and the subsequent development of angiographically severe CAV. The performance of IVUS at 1 and 12 months after heart transplant is therefore increasingly used to identify patients at high risk for future cardiovascular events, and may aid in allowing therapeutic adjustment of immunosuppression.[111] The everolimus study was the most robust in demonstrating first-year IVUS benefit of everolimus in several IVUS parameters (intimal area, intimal volume, intimal index along with maximum intimal thickness >0.5 mm).[73] The MMF study showed benefit for MMF therapy using maximum intimal thickness greater than 0.3 mm, whereas at 0.5 mm significant benefit was no longer seen. The sirolimus study showed IVUS data benefit for sirolimus therapy; however, patients were studied at baseline and at 6 months (not at 1 year) after heart transplantation. In a single-center angiographic (no IVUS) randomized study of cardiac transplant patients with established CAV, sirolimus was shown to slow disease progression.[60]

While survival, rejection, and development of CAV appear fairly comparable among most of the newer immunosuppressive agents, adverse events are what distinguish the various drug regimens. The mTOR inhibitors, everolimus[72] and sirolimus[59] as a group have worse renal function in the combination with standard-dose cyclosporine therapy, along with higher lipid levels and poorer wound healing compared to the azathioprine-treated group. Also sirolimus-treated patients had more anemia, thrombocytopenia, diarrhea, and mouth ulcers than azathioprine-treated patients. In contrast, it was demonstrated that everolimus with reduced-dose cyclosporine compared to MMF with standard-dose cyclosporine had comparable renal function at 1 year,[74] although a more recent clinical trial using this regimen continued to show inferior renal function.[75] There is also evidence from nonrandomized studies showing that conversion from CNI-based immunosuppression to sirolimus-based immunosuppression results in improved renal function.[112,113] A recent multicenter randomized trial has demonstrated that conversion to CNI-free immunosuppression (MMF, sirolimus) is superior to CNI-reduced immunosuppression in improving renal failure in late heart transplant recipients with renal insufficiency.[114] Patients treated with everolimus and sirolimus also demonstrated fewer CMV infections than the azathioprine-treated patients.

Table 17.4 Major multicenter randomized immunosuppressive clinical trials in heart transplantation and significant differences in primary endpoints and adverse effects between study groups[216]

Study	*n*	Follow-up	Survival	Rejection	CAV by IVUS	Renal function	Infections	Cholesterol and triglycerides	Hypertension	Hematologic	GI disorders	Other
Kobashigawa[46] 1998 MMF vs. AZA	650	3 years	*MMF = higher survival	MMF = less rejection	NS; **MMF = less CAV at 1 year		MMF = more any opportunistic infection			AZA = more leukopenia	MMF = more diarrhea and esophagitis	NS for hyperglycemia treatment
Reichart[30] 1998 TAC vs. CSA	82	1 year	NS	NS		NS	NS		CSA = more hypertension			NS for glucose intolerance
Taylor[29] 1999 TAC vs. CSA	85	1 year	NS	NS		NS	NS	CSA = higher chol & tri	CSA = more hypertension	NS		
Eisen[72] 2003 EVR vs. AZA	634	1 year	NS	EVR groups = less rejection	EVR groups = less CAV	EVR groups = worse renal function	EVR groups = lower viral/ CMV but more bacterial infections	EVR groups = higher chol & tri	NS	NS	NS	NS for wound infection
Keogh[59] 2004 SIR vs. AZA	136	2 years	NS	SIR groups = less rejection at 6 months	SIR groups = less CAV	SIR groups = worse renal function	SIR groups = lower CMV but more pneumonia	NS for chol; SIR groups = higher trig	NS	SIR groups= more anemia & thrombocytopenia	AZA = more nausea; SIR groups = more diarrhea	AZA = more arrhythmia and atrial fibrillation; SIR groups = more mouth ulcers & abnormal healing
Grimm[31] 2006 TAC vs. CSA	314	1.5 year	NS	TAC = less rejection at 6 months		NS	NS	CSA = higher chol & tri	CSA = more hypertension	TAC = more anemia	CYA = more cholelithiasis	TAC = more diabetes mellitus & tremor; CSA = more gum hyperplasia & hirsutism
Kobashigawa[109] 2006 TAC/MMF vs. TAC/ SIR vs. CSA/MMF	343	1 year	NS	NS; TAC groups = lower any treated rejection		TAC/MMF = best renal function	TAC/SIR = lower viral but more fungal infections	NS for chol; TAC/MMF = lower trig	NS	NS		TAC/SIR = more insulin therapy & impaired wound healing; NS for diabetes mellitus

Baran[110] 2007 TAC/MMF vs. TAC	58	1 year	NS	NS	NS	NS	TAC/ MMF = more hospitalized infections			NS		NS for malignancy
Lehmkuhl[74] 2008 EVR/rd-CSA vs. MMFsd-CSA	176	1 year	NS	NS		NS	EVR = Less CMV infections			MMF = more leukopenia		
Baran[35] 2011 TAC/MMF vs. TAC alone	150	5 years	NS	NS	NS	NS; TAC alone group = numerically better renal function	TAC/ MMF = more hospitalized infections			TAC alone = higher mean white blood cell count, but not clinically meaningful		
Eisen[75] 2012 EVR-CSA vs. MMF-CSA (unpublished)	721	1 years	NS	EVR groups = numerically more rejection	EVR groups = less CAV	EVR groups = worse renal function	EVR = Less CMV infections	EVR groups = higher chol & tri	NS	NS	NS	EVR groups = higher overall rate of discontinuation due to severe adverse events

*Treated-patient population (see text).

**Reanalysis of MMF IVUS data

AZA, azathioprine, CSA, cyclosporine, EVR, everolimus, MMF, mycophenolate mofetil, rd-CSA, reduced-dose cyclosporine, sd-CSA, standard-dose cyclosporine, SIR, sirolimus; TAC, tacrolimus.

MMF-treated patients from the MMF trial[46] had more opportunistic infections, diarrhea, and esophagitis than azathioprine-treated patients. From the tacrolimus versus cyclosporine trials,[29,30,31] patients on cyclosporine had higher cholesterol and triglyceride levels, and more hypertension, cholelithiasis, gum hyperplasia, and hirsutism than tacrolimus-treated patients. However, tacrolimus-treated patients had more diabetes mellitus, tremor, and anemia than cyclosporine-treated patients. From the three-arm trial,[109] the regimen of tacrolimus/MMF compared to tacrolimus/sirolimus and cyclosporine/MMF had the best renal function and lowest triglyceride levels. The tacrolimus/sirolimus group had a higher incidence of poor wound healing and the most patients on insulin therapy.

Selection of immunosuppression after heart transplantation by each program appears to be based on experience and their interpretation of the randomized clinical trials. In addition, individualization of immunosuppression is practiced throughout the heart transplant community according to patient characteristics and perceived risks for complications. Specific immunosuppressive drug regimens may be appropriate for one patient and not another due to particular patient characteristics. The multicenter randomized clinical trials of immunosuppression offer information that the practicing clinician can apply to their patients to select the best immunosuppressive regimen for optimal outcome.

One must use caution in the interpretation of the various randomized immunosuppressive clinical trials as there are other factors that can affect outcome. For example, the most appropriate dose of each of the medications is not known, so that clinical trials outcomes may be different with different dose combinations of the same drugs. Foremost, it is the immunosuppressive drug regimen (each regimen usually has 2–3 drugs) and not necessarily the individual drug that leads to the clinical outcome. Adverse effects may be caused by drug–drug interaction. For example, everolimus and sirolimus are not nephrotoxic alone but they appear to augment the nephrotoxicity effects of the CNIs. There are also concerns regarding study design. Several studies[29,30] did not standardize postoperative care outcome and are difficult to assess. Another concern is that several of the studies' comparator drugs included azathioprine, which is rarely used in the current era. The meaning of these results is unclear in the presence of newer immunosuppressive medications with improved efficacy. Finally, the randomized clinical trials included a lower risk population with several studies having many exclusion criteria (to exclude high risk patients) including renal dysfunction, older age and the presence of elevated circulating antibodies. However, taking these concerns into account, there are important findings that can be taken from the results of the randomized clinical trials.

Survival appears to be comparable in all the randomized clinical trials in heart transplantation. However, none of the studies were powered to demonstrate a true survival difference between study groups. The other study endpoints of rejection, CAV, and adverse events have demonstrated differences between immunosuppressive regimens in several trials.

The rejection data from the clinical trials suggest that tacrolimus-based regimens may have benefit over cyclosporine-based regimens (class IIb/level B).[31,109] When one compares contemporary immunosuppressive regimens of tacrolimus/MMF and cyclosporine/MMF from the three-arm trial,[109] the rejection data suggest that tacrolimus/MMF may have benefit over cyclosporine/MMF (class IIb/level B). However, diabetes appears more prevalent with tacrolimus-based therapy. The third arm of this three-arm trial[109] demonstrated that tacrolimus/sirolimus-treated patients had lower rejection but adverse events of nephrotoxicity and poor wound healing, perhaps making this regimen less desirable compared with tacrolimus/MMF. everolimus with reduced-dose cyclosporine which was shown to have comparable rejection to the regimen of MMF with standard-dose cyclosporine while maintaining renal function,[112] although a recent randomized trial does not confirm this.[72] Everolimus with reduced-dose cyclosporine has not been compared to tacrolimus/MMF in a randomized trial.

The CAV benefit of MMF, everolimus, and sirolimus-based immunosuppressive regimens by IVUS appears important and suggests these drugs should be considered for inclusion (class IIb, level B).[30,72,115] However, the renal dysfunction reported in the everolimus and sirolimus trials with standard-dose cyclosporine dampens the enthusiasm for the use of this drug regimen. Of note, there are differences in IVUS study design and IVUS results. The multicenter IVUS validation study (using first-year IVUS MIT >0.5 mm) can only validate the IVUS results of the everolimus trial (similar IVUS protocol) in terms of suggesting longer-term outcomes benefit which includes improved 5-year survival, freedom from nonfatal-MACE and CAV. This does not diminish the CAV benefits from the IVUS data in the MMF and sirolimus trials.

The various adverse events experienced in the randomized clinical trials further underscore the need for individualization of immunosuppression. For example, patients with high risk for CMV infection might benefit from everolimus- or sirolimus-based immunosuppression; patients with gingival hyperplasia may benefit from tacrolimus-based regimen; or patients with excess tremors/peripheral neuropathy may benefit from a cyclosporine-based regimen. The adverse events listed in Table 17.4 (along with the results of the clinical trials) can be used to determine what immunosuppressive drugs would best serve patients with specific characteristics in the selection of a particular immunosuppression regimen.

In summary, the choice of immunosuppression remains individualized depending on the characteristics and risks of the heart transplant recipient and on the interpretation of the results from the randomized clinical trials. As immunosuppressive regimens continue to evolve, the choice of immunosuppression in heart transplantation will change, depending on the results of future immunosuppressive randomized clinical trials.

Minimization of immunosuppression

Steroid weaning

Steroid therapy is associated with glucose intolerance, dyslipidemia, hypertension, osteoporosis, and infection. Steroid-free immunosuppression regimens have previously been associated with adverse long-term outcomes. Five-year survival was reported to be similar according to Keogh et al., being 82% with prednisone and 85% without prednisone.[116] However, rejection rates were significantly higher in the steroid-free group and almost half the patients were converted to maintenance steroids. In a recent study, however, 32 low-risk cardiac transplant patients were randomized to receive either an ATG-based corticosteroid-avoidance regimen or a long-term corticosteroid-based regimen with no antibody induction as a control group.[117] Pulse steroid therapy was used for the treatment of acute cellular rejection (ACR) in both groups. At 1 year, there was no significant difference in the mean incidence of ACR (ISHLT ≥2R/3A) episodes between two groups. Importantly, the steroid-avoidance patients had significant improvement in muscle strength and less bone loss compared with the control patients during the first 6 months after transplantation. The authors reported that the steroid-avoidance regimen with ATG induction appeared to be safe and effective in cardiac transplantation. However, further studies are required to demonstrate the long-term safety and benefits of such a regimen.

Yacoub initially described the utility of a low-dose steroid regimen and complete withdrawal of corticosteroids in patients treated with ATG.[118] Patients at low risk of rejection, including those without circulating antibodies, women without a history of multiple pregnancies, those without a history of rejection, and older transplant recipients may be considered for steroid withdrawal. Generally, two strategies have been utilized. Early withdrawal of prednisone has been achieved during the first month of transplantation in conjunction with cytolytic induction. Long-term outcomes have been variable, with success in 49% to 70% of patients.[119,120,121] However, given that the majority of acute rejection episodes occur during the first 6 months after transplantation, steroid withdrawal after this period has generally been more successful with steroid withdrawal being achieved in up to 80%, even without the use of induction therapy.[122,123]

To determine the safety of gradual weaning from prednisone maintenance, 68 patients (>6 months from transplantation) were weaned from 5 mg/day by decreasing the daily dose by 1 mg each month, with monthly biopsies, in a study by Kobashigawa.[122] Asymptomatic moderate rejection occurred in 13 compliant patients. Rejection with hemodynamic compromise occurred in two patients with documented medication noncompliance, who were excluded from further analysis. Successful weaning without rejection was possible in 53 of 66 (80%) compliant patients. All moderate rejection episodes responded to oral steroid pulse therapy. The two serious rejections after noncompliance responded to OKT3. There were no symptoms from steroid withdrawal that required taper alteration.

A randomized trial comparing tacrolimus monotherapy to tacrolimus with MMF saw both groups wean from corticosteroids between 8 and 12 weeks after transplant.[35] All patients were successfully weaned and no patient required later reinstitution of corticosteroids. Steroid weaning after cardiac transplantation is now commonplace, with the most recent registry data showing that over 40% of heart transplant recipients are successfully maintained off steroids at 5 years.[2]

Calcineurin inhibitor minimization (renal-sparing protocol)

The cumulative incidence of chronic renal failure in heart transplant recipients has been reported at 10.9% over 5 years[124] and has been chiefly attributed to the use of CNI. From experience of renal transplantation, cyclosporine and tacrolimus contribute to chronic allograft nephropathy to a similar degree.[125] A number of trials have addressed the feasibility of CNI reduction or elimination in cardiac transplantation (Table 17.5).[50,113,127,128,129,130,131,132,136,137,138,139]

Lower rejection rates and improved outcomes with MMF over azathioprine have permitted successful lowering of CNI exposure. In a recent sequential study,[126] 240 cardiac transplant patients were treated with either MMF (n = 119) or azathioprine (n = 121) both in combination with cyclosporine and corticosteroids after rabbit ATG induction. By protocol, lower cyclosporine levels were targeted in the MMF group during the first year (e.g., 203 ± 52 ng/ml MMF vs. 236 ± 59 ng/ml azathioprine, p = 0.0006 at 6 months). Patient survival at 1 year and at 3 years was similar in both groups. The cumulative probability of receiving antirejection treatment within 1 year was lower in the MMF group, as was biopsy-proven acute rejection with ISHLT grade ≥3A (24% vs. 35%, p = 0.03). The MMF group also had fewer episodes requiring cytolytic therapy (6% vs. 13%, p = 0.04) and more patients had steroids withdrawn by 1 year (66% vs. 32%, p < 0.001). Renal function was significantly better in the MMF group with lower creatinine levels and creatinine clearance (CrCl) at 1 year, presumably reflecting the lower levels of CNI used. These results suggest that immunosuppression with MMF rather than azathioprine following induction therapy allows lower cyclosporinee level, better renal function, and increased steroid weaning at 1 year while also achieving better control of acute rejection.

In another prospective multicenter study,[127] MMF was substituted for azathioprine prior to cyclosporine reduction in 109 patients and compared to a control group of 52 patients whose treatment remained unchanged. At 8 months there was a significant decrease (p <0.0001) in serum creatinine (SCr) in the intervention arm (23.3 ± 50.7 μmol/L) compared to a modest increase in the control group (7.3 ± 46.9 μmol/L). In the intervention arm, the cyclosporine level was 57 ± 24 vs. 116 ± 36 ng/ml in controls. The presence of diabetes did not affect the change in renal function in the intervention arm. Cyclosporine reduction was associated with a significant decrease in blood pressure (about 5 mmHg lower both systolic and diastolic average during day and night-time) in the intervention group compared with the control group.

A number of smaller single-center studies have also suggested a component of reversible renal function with cyclosporine dose reduction in conjunction with a change from azathioprine to MMF.[128,129,130] Late cyclosporine reduction in heart transplant recipients without adjunctive therapy appears not to improve renal function, however; in a study of pediatric recipients with a creatinine clearance (CrCl) of around 70 ml/min, this was essentially unchanged at more than 5-year follow-up.[131] The substitution of sirolimus for azathioprine also seems to be of limited benefit in the setting of CNI minimization, given that agents of this class (proliferation signal inhibitors) tend to exacerbate CNI nephrotoxicity. The use of proliferation signal inhibitors with CNIs generally requires CNI dose reduction to prevent nephrotoxicity. In one study, CrCl improved in the first 3 months in the minimization group but was similar to baseline values by 6 months.[132] In another nonrandomized study of 38 patients[133] who were a median of 82 months from transplant, the only predictors of benefit at 6 months in CrCl from the introduction of sirolimus with concomitant CNI dose reduction were better renal function 3 months before conversion and a shorter time from transplant to conversion. A recent pilot study with everolimus and reduced-dose cyclosporine in recipients more than 1 year from transplantation[134] was associated with no significant decline in renal function, and no indication of increased rejection at 3 months post conversion.

Monitoring of cyclosporine levels at 2 hours after dosing (C2) may be a better indicator of immunosuppression efficacy than trough levels and may be associated with lower CNI exposure. In a longitudinal study of 114 stable cardiac allograft recipients

Table 17.5 Summary of renal function outcomes in studies reporting calcineurin inhibitor (CNI)-sparing strategies in heart transplantation[217]

Author	Population	CNI strategy	Time post-transplant	Treatment arm	Control	Follow-up	Renal function		
							Treatment	Control	p value vs. control
Angermann[127]	Adult, CRD, ITT	Minimization	≥6 months	Azathioprine to mycophenolate mofetil switch (n = 109)	CNI maintained (n = 52)	8 months	CrCl ↑7.6 ml/min from baseline (p <0.001)	CrCl ↑ 0.9 mL/min from baseline (p = NS)	p < 0.001
Baryalei[129]	Adult, SCr above 1.7 mg/dl	Minimization	≥3 months	Azathioprine to mycophenolate mofetil switch (n = 14)	CNI maintained (n = 10)	Mean 177–242 days	SCr ↓29.6% from baseline (p = 0.001)	SCr ↓4.2% from baseline (p = NS)	p = 0.02
Tedoriya[130]	Adult, CRD	Minimization	90 months	Azathioprine to mycophenolate mofetil switch (n = 30)	Baseline	12 months	SCr ↓17.9%	NA	p < 0.01
Arizon del Prado[128]	Adult, CRD	Minimization	Mean 5 yearsr	Azathioprine to mycophenolate mofetil switch (n = 31)	Pre-decrease of cyclosporine	NA	SCr of 1.83 ± 0.24 mg/dL	SCr 2.05 ± 0.55 mg/dl	p < 0.01
Aleksic[50]	Adult, de novo	Minimization	111–1813 days	Azathioprine to mycophenolate mofetil switch (n = 12)	Pre-MMF therapy	81–315 days after MMF therapy	SCr of 1.9 ± 0.6 mg/dl; CrCl of 61 ± 41	SCr of 2.5 ± 0.8 mg/dl; CrCl of 43 ± 18	p = 0.02, p = 0.015
Rice[131]	Pediatric, CrCl ~70 ml/min	Minimization	12 months	CNI reduction only (n = 25)	12 months	>72 months	GFR ↑2.7%	NA	p = NS
Trösch[132]	Adult, SCr above 2.5 mg/dl	Minimization	≥4 years	Azathioprine to sirolimus switch (n = 12)	Baseline Baseline	3 months 6 months	CrCl ↑34.2% CrCl similar	NA NA	p = 0.003 p = NS
Meiser[137]	Adult, de novo	Avoidance	De novo	Sirolimus, mycophenolate mofetil, corticosteroids (n = 8)	Baseline	3 months	SCr ↓26.7%	NA	Not reported
Zakliczynski[138]	Adult, CRD	Withdrawal	Mean 5 years	Sirolimus (n = 5)	Baseline	2 months	SCr ↑50.3%, all required dialysis	NA	Not reported
Hunt[140]	Adult, SCr ~2 mg/dl	Withdrawal	Mean 4.78 years	Sirolimus, mycophenolate mofetil (n = 30)	Baseline	Mean 304 days	SCr ↓19.6%	NA	p < 0.001
Groetzner[139]	Adult,SCr above 1.9 mg/dl	Withdrawal	≥2 months	Sirolimus, mycophenolate mofetil (n = 30)	CNI maintained (n = 33)	12 months	SCr ↓30.1% from baseline(p = 0.001)	SCr ↑ 35.1% from baseline (p = 0.02)	Not reported
Kushwaha[141]	Adult, C_i 25–50 ml/min	Withdrawal	1–14 years	Sirolimus, azathioprine or mycophenolate mofetil (n = 34)	CNI maintained (n = 24)	1 year	C_i ↑ from 36.08± ± 2.4 to 48.67 ± 4.1 ml/min	Ci ↓ from 40.04 ± 1.86 to 34.63 ± 1.6 ml/min	Not reported

C_i, iothalamate clearance; CNI, calcineurin inhibitor; CrCl, creatinine clearance; CRD, chronic renal dysfunction; GFR, glomerular filtration rate; ITT, intent to treat; NA, not applicable; NS, not significant; SCr, serum creatinine.

Flechner SM, Kobashigawa J, Klintmalm G. Calcineurin inhibitor-sparing regimens in solid organ transplantation: focus on improving renal function and nephrotoxicity. Clin Transplant. 2008;22(1):1–15, Wiley.

more than a year out from transplantation, patients were initially followed for about a year with C2 monitoring (target range 300–600 μg/L).[24] The patients were then switched to trough level (C0) monitoring (target range 100–200 μg/L). During C2 monitoring, cyclosporine dosage, C0 levels, C2 and creatinine decreased by 26%, 56%, 45% and 2.3% respectively compared to baseline. When changed to C0 monitoring, these variables increased by 24%, 56%, 38% and 10% respectively (p <0.0001). In a more recent randomized controlled trial of 125 patients, C2 monitoring compared to C0 monitoring allowed a significant cyclosporine dose reduction without compromising patient outcome in stable heart transplant patients.[25] Catarovich recently reported that C2 monitoring could be safely used in de-novo heart transplant recipients and a low C2 range in combination with basiliximab induction resulted in preserved renal function without increased risk of acute rejection.[135] These studies suggest that C2 monitoring allows a safe reduction in cyclosporine exposure without the risk of acute rejection. However, whether this translates into long-term benefit remains to be determined. In renal transplant recipients with CNI minimization, persistent damage is observed on biopsies for the duration that the CNIs are continued.[136]

CNI avoidance

Despite the pivotal role of CNIs in the success of cardiac transplantation, efforts have been made to avoid this class of agents all together. Initial small studies suggested that CNI avoidance may be possible. A pilot study evaluated the efficacy of sirolimus, MMF, and corticosteroids in 11 de-novo patients. With a follow-up of 3–12 months, patient survival (n = 8) was 100% and freedom from rejection 75%. Mean creatinine levels initially decreased and remained stable thereafter. Adverse events included moderate myelosuppression, elevated cholesterol and triglyceride levels, pericardial effusion, and peripheral edema.[137] Larger randomized studies have yet to be performed, however,and the true safety of avoiding CNI use in cardiac transplantation remains to be established.

CNI withdrawal

Withdrawal of CNI using SIR[138] or sirolimus with MMF[139,140,141] has been evaluated in a number of studies. Groetzner[139] studied cardiac transplant patients with late post-transplantation renal impairment with conversion from CNI to MMF and sirolimus. In this study 31 patients with CNI-based immunosuppression and serum creatinine (SCr) greater than 1.9 mg/dL were started with sirolimus and the dose was adjusted to achieve target trough levels between 8 and 14 ng/mL. MMF was continued with trough level adjusted between 1.5 and 4 μg/mL. Subsequently, the CNIs were tapered down and stopped. Survival was 90% after a mean follow-up of 13 ± 95 months. No acute rejection episode was detected during the study period. Renal function improved significantly after conversion: creatinine preconversion versus postconversion was 3.14 ± 0.76 mg/dl vs. 2.14 ± 0.83 mg/dl, p = 0.001. In three patients, hemodialysis therapy was stopped completely after conversion.

Similarly, in 2005, 80 heart transplant patients (range 1–14 years post-transplantation) with renal dysfunction had their CNIs abruptly discontinued and were switched to sirolimus at 5 mg twice daily for 2 days and then 2 mg daily in a study by Kushwaha.[141] The treatment goal was a trough level of 6–12 ng/ml, and all patients were also managed with MMF at 1000 mg twice daily. At a mean of 304 days after conversion, the mean SCr decreased from 2.04 ± 0.57 mg/dl before conversion to 1.64 ± 0.48 mg/dl (p <0.001). In patients whose SCr was less than 2.5 mg/dL before conversion, the mean SCr level decreased from 1.81 ± 0.39 to 1.62 ± 0.5 mg/dl after conversion (p = 0.01), with no patient developing end-stage renal disease. In patients with SCr 2.5 mg/dl or higher before conversion, the SCr decreased from 2.85 ± 0.29 to 1.73 ± 0.43 mg/dL (p = 0.001) at a mean of 304 days after conversion. However four patients developed end-stage renal disease requiring dialysis despite conversion.

The substitution of CNIs with sirolimus also appears to have no adverse effect on cardiac function and rejection in cardiac transplant recipients with renal dysfunction.[140] Thirty-four stable cardiac transplant recipients with CNI-induced nephrotoxicity (CrCl 25–50 ml/min) or CAV were enrolled. Twelve patients were prospectively enrolled for renal dysfunction, and the remaining patients were converted to sirolimus on clinical grounds because of poor renal function or the presence of CAV. A further 24 patients were retrospective controls, stable (range 2–10 years post-transplantation), and maintained on a standard CNI-based immunosuppressant regimen. CNI was withdrawn gradually over 12 weeks, adjunct immunosuppression was left unchanged, and sirolimus was started at 1 mg/day, with titration over 2 weeks to achieve levels of 10–15 ng/ml. CrCl improved significantly in both sirolimus-treated groups without exacerbating rejection or compromising cardiac function. In the control group, however, the baseline renal clearance declined significantly over the course of 1 year.

In a non-randomized study[142] in heart transplant recipients with renal dysfunction (GFR ≤50 ml/min) and/or CAV detected by annual angiography, 78 patients were changed to a sirolimus-based immunosuppression with complete CNI withdrawal a mean of 3.8 years after transplantation. The study demonstrated an improvement in CAV progression by intravascular ultrasound with sirolimus treatment without an increase in rejection at 12 months. Although there was a significant decrease in creatinine at 12 months, calculated GFR remained unchanged in the sirolimus group. Additionally there was a significant increase in proteinuria in the sirolimus arm at 12 months. In the CNI group, proteinuria did not change at 12 months. The difference in proteinuria between the sirolimus and CNI groups was significant. Blood albumin level did not change in patients treated with sirolimus, and no patients developed edema or hematuria.

In contrast to the above studies, in five patients with chronic renal disease, replacement of cyclosporine with sirolimus resulted in a 50% increase in SCr and universal dialysis requirement.[138] However, from all studies mentioned, it appears that CNI withdrawal is successful, particularly when withdrawal is initiated at a time when SCr is not excessively elevated and withdrawal is not initiated too early after transplantation.

Data of greatest concern relating to sirolimus as a primary immunosuppressant, however, comes from the Heart Save the Nephron (STN) clinical trial that prompted premature termination of the study.[143] This study aimed to assess the potential renal-sparing impact of sirolimus in heart transplantation as early as 12 weeks after transplantation. Patients were initially treated with CNIs but then at 12 weeks were randomized to either CNIs or sirolimus; MMF and prednisone were adjunctive immunosuppressants. The study was terminated prematurely because four of seven patients randomized to sirolimus experienced a ISHLT grade 2R/3A rejection episode. Three of four episodes occurred at one transplant center, and one patient experienced hemodynamic compromise. Low blood levels of sirolimus were recorded in two patients. It appears therefore that the introduction of sirolimus may not be safe in the absence of CNI use in the acute phases of heart transplantation, at a time when the risk of rejection is highest and therapeutic immunosuppression is of greatest importance, an area where CNIs have been of proven efficacy.

CNI immunotherapy

Although minimization of CNI and corticosteroid use has been the focus of a number of clinical trials, very few studies have investigated the safety and efficacy of CNI monotherapy in cardiac transplant recipients. An initial retrospective study[144] reported in 2001 revealed that of 43 patients initiated with tacrolimus and prednisone alone, 32 patients were subsequently weaned off steroids at a mean of 246 days after transplantation (range 106–730 days). The freedom from treated rejection (ISHLT 3A/3B and grade 2 rejection in the first 90 days) was 69% at 90 days and 52% at 1 year. In a subsequent follow-up report[34] 90 of 124 patients initially treated with tacrolimus and corticosteroids were weaned to tacrolimus monotherapy without the use of an anti-proliferative agent, resulting in an overall success rate of 75% at an average of 271 ± 8 days after transplantation. The remaining 69 recipients were treated with other tacrolimus- or cyclosporine-based regimens. Survival was significantly greater in the tacrolimus monotherapy group. The prevalence of high-grade rejection within the first year and incidence of CAV were similar between groups. Ten patients (11%) in the monotherapy group required recommencement of combination immunosuppression at an average of 768 ± 772 days. The investigators concluded that CNI monotherapy is acceotable in the majority of cardiac transplant recipients. Patients who tolerated reduced immunosuppression enjoyed greater survival than those treated with other regimens, without additional high-grade rejection or vasculopathy.

These promising results prompted a randomized study, the TICTAC trial.[35] In 2011, the median 3-year follow-up of the TICTAC trial (n = 150, 79 in the monotherapy group, 71 in the combination group) was reported.[34] All patients received oral tacrolimus, MMF, and corticosteroids. Induction therapy was not routinely used. Patients were then randomized to a group where MMF was maintained or to a group where it was discontinued 14 days after transplantation. Tacrolimus levels were maintained between 9 and 11 ng/dl. Corticosteroids were rapidly withdrawn in both groups between 8 and 12 weeks. The primary endpoint, mean 6-month ISHLT biopsy score, was 0.70 ± 0.44 in the monotherapy group and 0.65 ± 0.40 in the combination therapy group (p = NS). The freedom from rejection (grade ≥2R) at 6 months was 85.9% in the monotherapy group and and 94.4% in the combination therapy group. At 12 months, the freedom from rejection was 85.9% in the monotherapy group and 93.1% in the combination therapy group (p = NS). AMR occurred in two patients (one in each group), both within the first 90 days after transplant. Nine patients who were changed from the monotherapy to combination therapy group because of rejection and 26 patients were withdrawn from MMF therapy (usually because of neutropenia unresponsive to MMF dose reduction). There are no significant difference between groups in 3-year survival (92.4% in the monotherapy group and 97% in the combination therapy group, p = NS) and the development of CAV by coronary angiography and IVUS (42 patients in the trial had an early baseline IVUS and a matching follow-up study). Renal function and rates of infection at 12 months are comparable between the two groups.

In the TICTAC report, the authors speculate on the advantage of early lower immunosuppression and good outcome by mentioning an interesting protocol for administering immunosuppression. The 100% success of corticosteroid weaning without any patient requiring reinstitution of corticosteroids in this study is especially laudable. Certainly, this form of therapy cannot be broadly extended to all heart transplant patients. Nonetheless, it is encouraging to know that tacrolimus monotherapy or dual therapy early after transplant can be considered an option if this is needed for special cases such as intolerance to antiproliferative medications, severe infections, and severe existing side effects to corticosteroid therapy. There is growing conviction that today's "standard" immunosuppression will someday be replaced by immunosuppression individualized for each patient on the basis of genomic profile, baseline risks for rejection and infection, and perhaps serial assessments of immune response after transplantation.

Monitoring

Minimization of immunosuppression requires close vigilance to avoid the risk of rejection. Therapeutic drug monitoring becomes increasingly important as the number of maintenance drugs decreases, especially when weaning occurs relatively early post-transplantation. In the TICTAC trial, tacrolimus levels were carefully maintained at between 9 and 11 ng/ml.[35,110] Clinical status, endomyocardial biopsy, and echocardiography remain the principal tools for rejection monitoring during drug weaning. With prednisone tapering at our institution, patients are weaned 1 mg/month with monthly endomyocardial biopsies and echocardiograms.[145] Although gene expression profiling from peripheral blood (AlloMap; CareDx, Inc, Brisbane, CA, USA) has recently become available as an alternative to endomyocardial biopsy for the detection of ACR,[146] its utility and safety has yet to be demonstrated for the purpose of immunosuppression weaning.

Another peripheral whole-blood assay which assesses the net state of immunosuppression in transplant recipients is also clinically available. In a meta-analysis of 504 solid organ transplant recipients (heart, kidney, kidney–pancreas, liver, and small bowel) from 10 US centers, the Cylex ImmuKnow assay (Viracor-IBT Laboratories, Inc., Lee's Summit, MO, USA) was performed at various times after transplantation and compared with clinical course (stable, rejection, infection).[147] In this analysis, 39 biopsy-proven cellular rejections and 66 diagnosed infections occurred. Odds ratios of infection or rejection were calculated based on measured immune response values. A recipient with an immune response value of 25 ng/ml ATP was 12 times (95% confidence of 4–36) more likely to develop an infection than a recipient with a stronger immune response. Similarly, a recipient with an immune response of 700 ng/ml ATP was 30 times (95% confidence of 8–112) more likely to develop a cellular rejection than a recipient with a lower immune response value. The intersection of odds ratio curves for infection and rejection in the moderate immune response zone was 280 ng/ml ATP. This intersection of risk curves provides an immunological target of immune function for solid organ recipients. These data suggest that the Cylex ImmuKnow assay has a high negative predictive value and provides a target immunological response zone for minimizing risk and managing patients to stability.

In a large study of almost 300 heart transplant recipients who had 864 Cylex ImmuKnow assays performed, a low score was predictive of infection risk, although in this study, due to the low number of rejection episodes, the association between a high score and rejection risk was inconclusive.[148] Lower white blood cell count and African American ethnicity have been correlated with a lower Cylex ImmuKnow response. The assay shows some promise in monitoring the immune status in cardiac transplant recipients with post-transplantation lymphoproliferative disorder (PTLD) in whom minimization of immunosuppression is the predominant treatment strategy.[149] Cylex ImmuKnow has not been used in patients being routinely weaned off immunosuppressive agents and its clinical utility in this regard remains unclear.

The level of immunosuppression used after transplantation is generally determined by the pre- and post-transplant risk for rejection. A higher number of HLA mismatches have been shown to be a marker for adverse outcomes with steroid weaning in cardiac transplantation.[145] Pretransplantation panel reactive antibodies are also correlated with post-transplantation adverse outcomes in heart transplant recipients.[150,151] Detection of anti-HLA antibodies by flow cytometry both before and after transplantation has been shown to be more predictive of rejection compared with complement-dependent cytotoxicity assay.[150] Interestingly, in this study, the majority of pretransplantation HLA antibodies were not directed against donor antigens. These non-donor-directed antibodies are likely surrogate markers that correspond to previous T cell activation and thus the rejection episodes that occur in these patients may be in response to donor-derived MHC peptides that share cryptic determinants with the HLA antigens that initially sensitized the patient. Routine periodic monitoring of flow-panel reactive antibodies (flow-PRAs) may therefore provide a useful marker in a strategy to minimize immunosuppression. Quantitation of flow-PRAs is also now possible with measurement of mean fluorescence intensities which may further help stratify risk in patients with circulating antibodies. The presence of post-transplantation antibodies is also a marker for the subsequent development of CAV.[152] Detection of post-transplantation alloantibodies may therefore determine the type and strength of ongoing immunosuppression utilized.

Special considerations in immunosuppression

Management of cardiac allograft vasculopathy

CAV, characterized by a proliferation of the allograft vascular intima, remains one of the leading causes of death in cardiac transplant recipients at 5 years post-transplantation, accounting for up to 30% of deaths.[4] The pathophysiology of CAV is closely linked to immunologic mechanisms, such as the activation of alloreactive T cells and antibodies, and nonimmunologic factors, including history of pretransplantation coronary artery disease and CMV infection of the donor, older age of the donor and recipient, hyperlipidemia, ischemia, or reperfusion injury.[153,154] Since clinically apparent CAV is associated with a poor prognosis, prevention is important. Preventive strategies include treatment of nonimmunologic factors associated with CAV progression and optimization of immunosuppressive therapy.

Immunosuppressive agents may affect the development of CAV in a number of ways. The indirect effects of long-term steroid therapy on lipid metabolism have already been described. This effect is enhanced with the use of cyclosporine, although there is some evidence that substitution of cyclosporine with tacrolimus may counter the rise in serum lipids.[28] The number and severity of episodes of acute rejection likely contributes to the subsequent development of CAV.[155,156] More effective immunosuppressive regimens may therefore have a beneficial impact on the development of CAV.

Tacrolimus has been studied extensively in liver transplantation and shown to be superior to cyclosporine in preventing chronic rejection.[157] In cardiac transplantation, while it has been demonstrated to cause less hypertension and hyperlipidemia than cyclosporine,[29] data on preventing CAV has been less conclusive. In one study treatment with tacrolimus has been associated with the lower incidence of anti-endothelial antibodies.[158] In another study, there was a trend toward more CAV by IVUS in patients treated with tacrolimus compared to cyclosporine.[159] In a long-term follow-up of patients randomized to tacrolimus or cyclosporine under a standardized noninduction protocol, there was no difference in the development of angiographic CAV between these two agents.[32]

MMF has been shown to be effective at reducing cardiac allograft rejection and post-transplantation mortality.[46] More recent studies suggest that it may also be effective at reducing CAV.[115,160,161] This effect may be related at least in part to the ability of MMF to reduce B-cell responses as patients treated with this agent developed lower anti-vimentin titers and this was correlated with the lower incidence of CAV by IVUS. MMF may also inhibit the production of reactive oxidant species which contributes to endothelial cell dysfunction.[162]

Another class of agents, the proliferation signal inhibitors, or mammalian target of rapamycin (mTOR) inhibitors, which inhibit T-cell and B-cell proliferation driven primarily by interleukins,[163] have significantly expanded therapeutic options. Sirolimus has been shown to slow the progression of CAV in nonrandomized[60] and randomized[59] clinical trials. Mancini et al.[60] studied 46 patients with newly diagnosed CAV who were randomly assigned to treatment with sirolimus ($n = 22$) versus continued current immunosuppression (azathioprine or MMF; $n = 24$). Primary endpoints of that study were death, need for angioplasty or bypass surgery, myocardial infarction, and greater than 25% worsening of the catheterization score (graded with the use of a semiquantitative scale and repeated annually). Three patients in the sirolimus group reached primary endpoints compared with 14 in the control group ($p < 0.001$). A study by Keogh et al.[59] showed that intimal progression by IVUS was absent for up to 2 years in de-novo heart transplant patients who received sirolimus. Importantly, the studies on sirolimus were done in comparison to azathioprine, which is no longer used in many programs compared with MMF.

The use of everolimus in de-novo heart transplant patients has been shown to slow intimal thickness by IVUS at 1 year.[72] The latter study was the most robust in demonstrating that all first-year IVUS parameters were reduced in those patients treated with everolimus versus azathioprine. The incidence of vasculopathy (first-year maximal intimal thickness >0.5 mm) was significantly lower in the 1.5 mg group (35.7%, $p = 0.045$) and the 3.0 mg group (30.4%, $p = 0.01$) than in the azathioprine group (52.8%).[72,164] These initial findings were confirmed by a 2-year and 4-year follow-up IVUS substudy,[155,156] as well as the most recent phase 3 everolimus clinical trial in comparison with MMF.[72] Interestingly, administration of everolimus was associated with a lower incidence of acute rejection and fewer episodes of CMV infection, two well-known risk factors for CAV.[72,75,156]

Once CAV is established, pharmacological treatment options are limited. The only pharmacological approach that has shown promise is with sirolimus.[59] Optimization of drug combinations for the treatment of CAV must take into account multiple factors. An ideal regimen will be one that is hypolipidemic, reduces blood pressure, has a positive effect on hemodynamics, and does not compromise CMV status or renal function.[16]

Management of malignancy

According to the ISHLT registry,[2] the cumulative prevalence of malignancy (all types combined) in recipients of heart transplants is higher than in the general population. By 15 years after transplantation, close to 50% of heart transplant recipients are diagnosed with some form of malignancy. The commonly observed malignancies after heart transplantation are the tumors of skin, involving up to 29% of patients, and solid organ carcinomas (e.g., lung, gut, and prostate), involving up to 18% of patients by 15 years after transplantation. PTLD is much more common in transplant patients than in the general population, typically involves younger patients, is often related to viral oncogene (EBV), and may affect 6% of patients during the first 15 years after transplantation.

Important in addressing post-transplantation malignancy is the reducing the burden of net immunosuppression, incorporating decisions on minimization or withdrawal of CNI.

For patients at high risk of acute rejection, defined as having experienced two or more episodes of grade 2R, or hemodynamic compromise with or without positive biopsy, introduction of a proliferation signal inhibitor (sirolimus or everolimus), with gradual reduction but not complete withdrawal of CNI therapy should be considered. In patients who are at low risk of acute rejection (i.e., who have never experienced ≥2R rejections), proliferation signal inhibitors may be safely considered in combination with a gradual reduction and ultimate withdrawal of CNIs, replacing them with mycophenolate acid agents. Although CNI withdrawal may not be considered a standard in heart transplantation, reasonable safety has been reported in CNI-free protocols with sirolimus.[112] However, it is recommended to strictly follow these patients with invasive (patients who had multiple rejections in their post-transplant history) or noninvasive (patients with low or intermediate risk of acute rejection) tools to monitor the risk of graft rejection, after CNI withdrawal.[113,146,147]

In all instances of post-transplantation malignancy, consideration should be given to withdrawal of azathioprine.[166] There are important practicalities which should be considered to ensure the safe introduction of the proliferation signal inhibitors and avoid adverse drug–drug interactions. The recommended therapeutic targeted trough blood level for proliferation signal inhibitors coadministered with cyclosporine is 3–8 ng/ml for everolimus[165] and 5–15 ng/mL for sirolimus.[167] It is essential for all the physicians involved in the care of these patients to be aware of potential interactions between proliferation signal inhibitors and other drugs, particularly chemotherapy agents.

Specifically for PTLD, given the pathologic and clinical heterogeneity of the disorder, treatment is often individualized. Reduction in immune suppression has been a mainstay in the treatment of PTLD for over 40 years.[168,169] Outside of early lesions and/or low tumor burden, however, reduction of immune suppression alone is associated with cure in a minority of subjects. Additional therapeutic options for PTLD include rituximab (chimeric anti-CD20 monoclonal antibody), chemotherapy, antiviral therapy, cytokine therapy, adoptive immunotherapy, surgery, and radiation either as single agents or as combined modality.

Treatment of patients with high circulating antibodies/sensitization

The management of allosensitized cardiac transplant candidates presents steep challenges for transplantation cardiologists and surgeons. The differences in specificity of different antibody detection techniques, the uncertainty about which antibody specificities are relevant, and the incomplete understanding of B-cell immunity in allotransplantation make solid progress in this area difficult. It is clear that allosensitized patients experience delays to transplantation because of the relatively limited acceptable donor pool imposed by their anti-HLA antibody specificities.[170,171] Not all patients with an elevated PRA level will need desensitization, but those with high PRA and true specificities are typically considered for therapy.

Conventional approaches of desensitization include polyclonal cytolytics,[172] intravenous immunoglobulin (IVIg),[173] plasmapheresis,[174] MMF,[175,176,177,178,179,180] and cyclophosphamide.[181,182,183] The use of induction in heart transplantation remains controversial, and many of the trials excluded patients with elevated PRA. Desensitization strategies have evolved significantly over the last decade. Current protocols typically involve a two-pronged approach in which anti-HLA antibodies are removed from circulation and drugs are administered to halt their production. Both rabbit and equine polyclonal cytolytic preparations of IgG target a broad range of T-cell surface epitopes and induce profound depletion of those particular subsets within 24 hours of administration of the first dose.[172]

IVIg is a product of pooled IgG antibodies (immunoglobulin) extracted from the plasma of multiple blood donors. Following reports of use in antibody-mediated diseases, IVIg was used to desensitize patients awaiting renal transplants and ultimately found to be effective in a multicenter double blinded placebo-controlled randomized trial.[173]

Plasma exchange, or plasmapheresis, involves the removal of circulating antibodies by exchanging the patient's plasma for either donor plasma or albumin. As antibody removal without addressing underlying antibody production is felt to be an inadequate strategy, plasmapheresis is typically combined with the use of another immunomodulatory agent.[174]

Both clinical and experimental data support the effect of MMF on B-cell proliferation and immunoglobulin production.[175,176,177] However, there is only one study of the effects of MMF as desensitization therapy in sensitized adults awaiting heart transplantation,[178] though several studies have reported a successful decrease in anti-HLA antibodies in the post-transplantation period using MMF.[160,179,180]

Immunomodulation of an alloimmunized heart transplant candidate with cyclosporine and IVIg was reported by De Marco et al.[181] The rationale for adding cyclosporine is to minimize rebound in B-cell proliferation following IVIg. Cyclosporine has also been used with plasmapheresis for the treatment of humoral heart transplant rejection with hemodynamic compromise,[182] although 4/6 patients had an additional rejection episode, suggesting insufficient maintenance protection against B-cell proliferation and antibody production. More recent data in a series of 26 alloimmunized patients who received intravenous pulse administration of cyclosporine suggested that it was effective in reducing IgG anti-HLA alloreactivity, shortened waiting time to transplantation, and was superior to MMF in reducing rejection with a comparable safety profile.[183]

Recently, novel immunosuppressants such as rituximab and bortezomib have focused on as new desensitization agents. Rituximab, a chimeric anti-CD20 (anti-B-cell) monoclonal antibody, has been proven to be effective as a desensitization regimen in combination with IVIg for kidney transplant patients awaiting a transplant from either a living donor or a deceased donor.[184] Rituximab has been shown to expand the transitional B-cell compartment upon reconstitution.[185] A clinical trial applying rituximab in heart transplant patient is currently under way.[186] Bortezomib is a 26S proteosome inhibitor that has proapoptotic effects on plasma cells and has been shown to decrease antibody production. Some early experience in renal transplantation has shown variable efficacy of bortezomib in the treatment of AMR and desensitization.[187] In a pilot study, use of plasmapheresis and bortezomib appeared to decrease circulating antibodies in sensitized patients awaiting heart transplantation.[188] Bortezomib may be a promising addition to the therapies currently available to treat this increasingly prevalent high-risk group. The use of this strategy, however, is associated with an increased risk of adverse events, especially infection.

Published data to guide the management of immunosuppression following transplant in a sensitized recipient are limited and typically based on single-center experience. Ideally, an organ without unacceptable HLA antigens can be identified. However, there is a tendency to use a more aggressive regimen in the early postoperative period, as the increased risk of adverse outcome in allosensitized patients is well established. Many centers will administer polyclonal cytolytics, and close monitoring of donor-specific antibodies, graft function, and examination for histologic evidence of AMR with C3d and C4d staining is typical. The development of donor-specific antibodies after transplant has also been noted to predict increased risk of biopsy-proven rejection and vasculopathy at 5 and 10 years.[189] Identification of de-novo donor-specific antibodies thus may be an opportunity to modify immunosuppression and mitigate long-term consequences.

Treatment of cardiac allograft rejection

A number of therapeutic options are available once a diagnosis of allograft rejection has been made. The choice of treatment is generally guided by the severity of rejection noted clinically and the type and grade of rejection noted histologically from the endomyocardial biopsy (Figure 17.3). The treatment of asymptomatic AMR is not established although long-term follow-up of these patients suggests that they are prone to increased mortality or the development of CAV.[191,192] These patients are generally followed more closely with higher targeted calcineurin levels and maintenance steroid therapy continued indefinitely. For patients with evidence of cardiac dysfunction, intravenous pulse dose steroids are usually indicated to minimize the extent of myocardial injury. Patients on cyclosporine should be switched to tacrolimus.[36,190] Patients with AMR who have evidence of cardiac dysfunction need a more aggressive approach with pulse dose steroids and may be considered for treatment with IVIg. The use of targeted B-cell therapy with rituximab or plasma cells with the proteosome inhibitor bortezomib is currently the focus of investigation. Patients may present with symptomatic cardiac dysfunction from either ACR or AMR. As the severity of rejection progresses there is usually histological evidence for both ACR and AMR. Patients may present with a spectrum of symptoms from heart failure to overt cardiogenic shock. A comprehensive approach utilizing all or some modalities including high-dose intravenous steroids, cytolytic therapy with polyclonal ATG, plasmapheresis, and IVIg may be needed. In patients with hemodynamic compromise, support with inotropic therapy, intra-aortic balloon pump or even extracorporeal membrane oxygenation may help facilitate the augmented immunosuppressive therapies, although mortality remains high in these patients.

	Asymptomatic	Reduced ejection fraction	Heart failure/shock
Cellular	Target higher CNI levels Oral steroid bolus + taper	Oral steroid bolus/taper or IV pulse steroids	IV pulse steroids Cytolytic therapy (ATG) Plasmapheresis IVIg Inotropic therapy IABP or ECMO support
Humoral	No treatment?	Oral steroid bolus/taper or IV pulse steroids ± IVIg	

Fig. 17.3 Treatment options for acute cellular rejection and antibody-mediated rejection according to severity.[220]

ATG, anti-thymocyte globulin; CNI, calcineurin inhibitor; ECMO, extracorporeal membrane oxygenation; EF, ejection fraction; IABP, intra-aortic balloon pump; IVIG, IV immune globulin. Reprinted from The Surgeon, 9(3), Patel JK, Kittleson M, Kobashigawa JA. Cardiac allograft rejection, 160–7, copyright (2011) with permission from Elsevier.

For patients with recurrent acute rejection, defined as three or more consecutive episodes of moderate/severe acute rejection, the usual therapeutic strategies involve high doses of steroids or globulin, which often lead to a number of side effects, especially in patients with infections or referred to surgery. The use of photopheresis, also called photochemotherapy, allows significant reduction of rejection episodes and of conventional immunosuppressive regimens.[193] Photopheresis was originally largely used in the treatment for cutaneous T-cell lymphoma and autoimmune diseases.[194] It involves ex-vivo separation of leukocytes from erythrocytes and exposure of the leukocytes to 8-methoxypsoralen and ultraviolet light. The leukocytes that are rapidly proliferating (such as T cells responding to alloantigens) are preferentially damaged. The damaged cells are returned to the patient and presumably induce counterimmune responses such as T-cell vaccination. Photopheresis is usually performed twice a week for 4 weeks. When given to reverse cardiac transplant rejection, photopheresis appears to be as effective as high-dose methylprednisolone without the side effects of corticosteroids.[195] Photopheresis has also been successful in several reports in reversing refractory rejection and in reducing the frequency of recurrence of rejection in patients who are frequent rejectors.[196,197,198] Alternative immunosuppressive agents have shown some benefit in the reversal of recurrent or recalcitrant cardiac allograft rejection.

Adjustment of immunosuppression with infectious comorbidity

Infectious disease after transplantation remains a field in evolution. Antimicrobial therapies are often more complex in these patients than in others because of the urgency to initiate empiric therapy and the frequency of drug toxicity and drug interactions (see Table 17.2). In the circumstances of significant clinical infection, the dose of immunosuppressants are usually globally decreased, in order to increase the net state of immunosuppression. At our center, we consider Cylex ImmuKnow immune monitoring score lower than 200 ng ATP/ml as a predictor of excessiveimmunosuppression, given recent results from the Cylex clinical study.[199] Based on our experience, when confronting a clinically significant infection we would decrease 25–50% of the dose of agents with antiproliferative effects, typically MMF, sirolimus and everolimus, of patients with normal cardiac function and no recent history of rejection within the past 3 months.

The initiation or cessation of antimicrobial therapies may alter the levels of CNI, antifungal agents, and other drugs. Drug interactions and drug toxicity are common. Cyclosporine, tacrolimus, and sirolimus are extensively metabolized by cytochrome P450 3A4 enzymes in the gut wall and liver. Drugs that inhibit cytochrome P450 3A4 (e.g., erythromycin) may decrease the metabolism of these agents and cause increased plasma concentrations. The azole antifungals also inhibit p-glycoprotein (voriconazole > ketoconazole > itraconazole > fluconazole). Individual members of each class of antimicrobial agents alter drug levels to different degrees; the effects in individual patients vary. Thus, it is critical to consider downward adjustments of cyclosporine and tacrolimus dosing at the initiation of azole therapy. Conversely, the metabolism of cyclosporine and tacrolimus is upregulated by drugs such as rifampin, isoniazid, and nafcillin. This results in lower blood levels with a given dose of the immunosuppressive agent and an increased risk of rejection.

Novel immunosuppressive agents

Inhibition of CD28/B7 T-cell costimulatory receptors could be a highly specific way of immunosuppression, which obviates the undesirable side effects of most immunosuppressants. CD28 is an important costimulatory molecule involved in T-cell proliferation at the time of antigen recognition by T cells.[200] Inhibition of CD28 results in reduced T-cell proliferation and prolonged allograft survival in animal models of transplantation. Cytotoxic T lymphocyte antigen-4 (CTLA-4) or CD152, a homolog of CD28, is transiently expressed after T-cell activation. A combination of CTLA-4 and immunoglobulins results in a fusion protein, CTLA-4 immunoglobulin, or abatacept, which has been shown to block T-cell proliferation in response to antigen stimulation and to prolong allograft survival in animal models of transplantation by competing with the B7 ligands for their receptors. An alternative compound, LEA29Y or belatacept, was developed by site-targeted mutagenesis to bind rapidly but have a slower dissociation rate than CTLA-4 immunoglobulin and, thus, be potentially more potent.[201] Belatacept was approved by the FDA in 2011 for use in renal transplantation.[202] The goal of such an approach would be to maintain patients on very low-dose, long-term immunosuppression without CNI, after administration of costimulatory pathway inhibitor therapy. Clinical trials of LEA29Y combination therapy in renal transplantation versus standard cyclosporine combination therapy have shown significantly improved renal function and more ideal blood pressure management in the LEA29Y group.[203] However, belatacept patients are at increased risk for developing PTLD, predominantly involving the central nervous system.[204] Recipients without immunity to EBV (i.e., seronegative) are at particularly increased risk. Tuberculosis was also more frequently observed in patients receiving belatacept.[167,205]

Eculizumab is a humanized monoclonal antibody directed against the terminal complement protein C5. It blocks the cleavage of C5 and halts the formation of the membrane attack complex. It is currently for use in patients with paroxysmal nocturnal hemoglobinuria.[206] In sensitized renal transplant recipients with high levels of donor-specific alloantibody, post-transplantation eculizumab treatment is associated with significant decreased incidence of early AMR.[207] There have also been case reports suggesting that eculizumab can be safely and effectively be used as rescue therapy in AMR[208] and in post-transplant hemolytic uremic syndrome.[209,210]

Other new drugs under evaluation include drugs for maintenance therapy (anti-protein kinase C,[211] anti- Janus kinase-3,[212] B-lymphocyte stimulator,[213] and novel CNIs).

Conclusion

The success of cardiac transplantation is largely attributable to the development of effective immunosuppressive regimens. The use of CNIs was responsible for a significant reduction in the frequency of acute rejection resulting in improved early survival. CAV, however, remains a significant late problem following transplantation. The newer agents, including MMF and the proliferation signal inhibitors, show promise in having a significant beneficial impact not only on this late complication, but also further reducing episodes of acute rejection. The role of cytolytic induction therapy remains unclear and awaits further clinical randomized trials, although its use would seem to be most appropriate in patients at high risk of renal failure to enable delayed initiation of CNI. Of the current commonly used immunosuppressive regimens, tacrolimus in combination with MMF seems most beneficial. A number of immunosuppressive agents being developed and tested show great promise, but clinical studies in cardiac transplantation have yet to be performed.

References

1. Caves PK, Stinson EB, Griepp RB, et al. Results of 54 cardiac transplants. Surgery 1973;74(2): 307–14.
2. Stehlik J, Edwards LB, Kucheryavaya AY, et al. The registry of the International Society for Heart and Lung Transplantation: Twenty-eighth adult heart transplant report—2011. J Heart Lung Transplant 2011;30(10):1078–94.
3. Penn I. Post-transplant malignancy: the role of immunosuppression. Drug Saf 2000;23(2):101–13.
4. Taylor DO, Edwards LB, Mohacsi PJ, et al. The registry of the International Society for Heart and Lung Transplantation: twentieth official adult heart transplant report—2003. J Heart Lung Transplant 2003;22(6):616–24.
5. Guba M, von Breitenbuch P, Steinbauer M, et al. Rapamycin inhibits primary and metastatic tumor growth by antiangiogenesis: involvement of vascular endothelial growth factor. Nat Med 2002;8(2):128–35.
6. Swinnen LJ, Costanzo-Nordin MR, Fisher SG, et al. Increased incidence of lymphoproliferative disorder after immunosuppression with the monoclonal antibody OKT3 in cardiac-transplant recipients. N Engl J Med 1990;323(25):1723–8.
7. Cohen DJ. Action, efficacy and toxicities: corticosteroids. In: Norman DJ, Turka LA, ed. Primer on Transplantation. Mount Laurel, NJ: American Society of Transplantation; 2001, pp. 146–51.
8. Hollaran PF, Gourishankar S. Principals and overview of immunosuppression. In: Norman DJ, Turka LA, ed. Primer on Transplantation. Mount Laurel, NJ: American Society of Transplantation; 2001:87–98.

9. George J. Immunosuppressive modalities. In: Kirklin JK, Young JB, McGiffen DC, ed. Heart Transplantation. New York, NY: Churchill Livingstone; 2002, pp. 390–463.
10. Park MH, Starling RC, Ratliff NB, et al. Oral steroid pulse without taper for the treatment of asymptomatic moderate cardiac allograft rejection. J Heart Lung Transplant 1999;18(12):1224–7.
11. Hosenpud JD, Norman DJ, Pantely GA. Low-dose oral prednisone in the treatment of acute cardiac allograft rejection not associated with hemodynamic compromise. J Heart Transplant.1990;9(3 Pt 2):292–6.
12. Kobashigawa JA, Stevenson LW, Moriguchi JD, et al. Is intravenous glucocorticoid therapy better than an oral regimen for asymptomatic cardiac rejection? A randomized trial. J Am Coll Cardiol 1993;21(5):1142–4.
13. Schimmer BP, Parker KL. Adrenocortical steroids and their synthetic analogs. In: Hardman JG, Limbard LE, Molinoff PB, Ruddar RW, Goodman AG, ed. Goodman & Gilman: The Pharmacological Basis of Therapeutics. 9th ed. New York, NY: McGraw-Hill; 1996, p. 1459.
14. Kahan BD. Cyclosporine. N Engl J Med 1989;321(25):1725–38.
15. Clipstone NA, Crabtree GR. Identification of calcineurin as a key signaling enzyme in T-lymphocyte activation. Nature 1992;357(6380):695–7.
16. Reem GH. Molecular mode of action of cyclosporine and FK506 in human thymocytes. J Autoimmun 1992;5(suppl A):159–65.
17. Shin GT, Khanna A, Ding R, et al. In vivo expression of transforming growth factor-beta1 in humans: stimulation by cyclosporine. Transplantation 1998;65(3):313–18.
18. Cheung A, Menkis AH. Cyclosporine heart transplantation. Transplant Proc 1998;30(5):1881–4.
19. Cooney GF, Jeevanandam V, Choudhury S, et al. Comparative bioavailability of Neoral and Sandimmune in cardiac transplant recipients over 1 year. Transplant Proc 1998;30(5):1892–4.
20. Eisen HJ, Hobbs RE, Davis SF, et al. Safety, tolerability, and efficacy of cyclosporine microemulsion in heart transplant recipients: a randomized, multicenter, double-blind comparison with the oil-based formulation of cyclosporine: results at 24 months after transplantation. Transplantation 2001;71(1):70–8.
21. Carrier M, White M, Pellerin M, et al. Comparison of Neoral and Sandimmune cyclosporine for induction of immunosuppression after heart transplantation. Can J Cardiol 1997;13(5):469–73.
22. Maccherini M, Bernazzali S, Diciolla F, et al. Neoral versus Sandimmun: clinical impact and modification of immunosuppressive therapy in cardiac transplantation. Transplant Proc 1998;30(5):1904–5.
23. Yonan NA, Aziz T, el-Gamel A, et al. Long-term safety and efficacy of Neoral in heart transplantation. Transplant Proc 1998;30(5):1906–9.
24. Cantarovich M, Elstein E, de Varennes B, Barkun JS. Clinical benefit of neoral dose monitoring with cyclosporine 2-hr post-dose levels compared with trough levels in stable heart transplant patients. Transplantation 1999;68(12):1839–42.
25. Mathias HC, Ozalp F, Will MB, et al. A randomized, controlled trial of C0- Vs C2-guided therapeutic drug monitoring of cyclosporine in stable heart transplant patients. J Heart Lung Transplant 2005;24(12):2137–43.
26. Valantine H. Neoral use in the cardiac transplant recipient. Transplant Proc 2000;32(3A Suppl):27S–44S.
27. Pham SM, Kormos RL, Hattler BG, et al. A prospective trial of tacrolimus (FK 506) in clinical heart transplantation: intermediate-term results. J Thorac Cardiovasc Surg 1996;111(4):764–72.
28. Armitage JM, Kormos RL, Morita S, et al. Clinical trial of FK 506 immunosuppression in adult cardiac transplantation. Ann Thorac Surg 1992;54(2): 205–10.
29. Taylor DO, Barr ML, Radovancevic B, et al. A randomized, multicenter comparison of tacrolimus and cyclosporine immunosuppressive regimens in cardiac transplantation: decreased hyperlipidemia and hypertension with tacrolimus. J Heart Lung Transplant 1999;18(4):336–45.
30. Reichart B, Meiser B, Viganò M, et al. European multicenter tacrolimus heart pilot study: three year follow-up. J Heart Lung Transplant 2001;20(2):249–50.
31. Grimm M, Rinaldi M, Yonan NA, et al. Superior prevention of acute rejection by tacrolimus vs. cyclosporine in heart transplant recipients—a large European trial. Am J Transplant 2006;6(6):1387–97.
32. Kobashigawa JA, Patel J, Furukawa H, et al. Five-year results of a randomized, single-center study of tacrolimus vs microemulsion cyclosporine in heart transplant patients. J Heart Lung Transplant 2006;25(4):434–9.
33. Garlicki M, Czub P, Labuś K, et al. Conversion from cyclosporine to tacrolimus improves renal function and lipid profile after cardiac transplantation. Ann Transplant 2006;11(1):24–7.
34. Lubitz SA, Baran DA, Alwarshetty MM, et al. Long-term results of tacrolimus monotherapy in cardiac transplant recipients. J Heart Lung Transplant 2006;25(6):699–706.
35. Baran DA, Zucker MJ, Arroyo LH, et al. A prospective, randomized trial of single-drug versus dual-drug immunosuppression in heart transplantation: the tacrolimus in combination, tacrolimus alone compared (TICTAC) trial. Circ Heart Fail 2011;4(2):129–37.
36. Mentzer RM Jr, Jahania MS, Lasley RD. Tacrolimus as a rescue immunosuppressant after heart and lung transplantation. The U.S. Multicenter FK506 Study Group. Transplantation 1998;65(1):109–13.
37. Meiser BM, Uberfuhr P, Fuchs A, et al. Tacrolimus: a superior agent to OKT3 for treating cases of persistent rejection after intrathoracic transplantation. J Heart Lung Transplant 1997;16(8):795–800.
38. Taylor DO, Barr ML, Meiser BM, et al. Suggested guidelines for the use of tacrolimus in cardiac transplant recipients. J Heart Lung Transplant 2001;20(7):734–8.
39. Montori VM, Basu A, Erwin PJ, et al. Posttransplantation diabetes: a systematic review of the literature. Diabetes Care 2002;25(3):583–92.
40. Lu CY, Sicher SC, Vazquez MA. Prevention and treatment of renal allograft rejection: new therapeutic approaches and new insights into established therapies. J Am Soc Nephrol 1993;4(6):1239–56.
41. Copeland JG, Mammana RB, Fuller JK, et al. Heart transplantation: four years' experience with conventional immunosuppression. JAMA 1984;251(12):1563–6.
42. Hosenpud JD, Novick RJ, Breen TJ, et al. The Registry of the International Society for Heart and Lung Transplantation: twelfth official report: 1995. J Heart Lung Transplant 1995;14(5):805–15.
43. Olivari MT, Kubo SH, Braunlin EA, et al. Five-year experience with triple-drug immunosuppressive therapy in cardiac transplantation. Circulation 1990;82(5 Suppl):IV276–80.
44. Euvrard S, Kanitakis J, Claudy A. Skin cancers after organ transplantation. N Engl J Med 2003;348(17):1681–91.
45. Ensley RD, Bristow MR, Olsen SL, et al. The use of mycophenolate mofetil (RS-61443) in human heart transplant recipients. Transplantation 1993;56(1):75–82.
46. Kobashigawa J, Miller L, Renlund D, et al. A randomized active-controlled trial of mycophenolate mofetil in heart transplant recipients: Mycophenolate Mofetil Investigators. Transplantation 1998;66(4):507–15.
47. Hosenpud JD, Bennett LE. Mycophenolate mofetil versus azathioprine in patients surviving the initial cardiac transplant hospitalization: an analysis of the Joint UNOS/ISHLT Thoracic Registry. Transplantation 2001;72(10):1662–5.
48. Kirklin JK, Bourge RC, Naftel DC, et al. Treatment of recurrent heart rejection with mycophenolate mofetil (RS-61443): initial clinical experience. J Heart Lung Transplant 1994;13(3):444–50.
49. Taylor DO, Ensley RD, Olsen SL, et al. Mycophenolate mofetil (RS-61443): preclinical, clinical, and three-year experience in heart transplantation. J Heart Lung Transplant 1994;13(4):571–82.
50. Aleksic I, Baryalei M, Busch T, et al. Improvement of impaired renal function in heart transplant recipients treated with mycophenolate mofetil and low-dose cyclosporine. Transplantation 2000;69(8):1586–90.
51. Renlund DG, Gopinathan SK, Kfoury AG, Taylor DO. Mycophenolate mofetil (MMF) in heart transplantation: rejection prevention and treatment. Clin Transplant 1996;10(1 Pt 2):136–9.
52. Vezina C, Kudelski A, Sehgal SN. Rapamycin (AY-22,989), a new antifungal antibiotic, I: taxonomy of the producing streptomycete and isolation of the active principle. J Antibiot (Tokyo) 1975;28(10):721–26.

53. Sehgal SN, Baker H, Vezina C. Rapamycin (AY-22,989), a new antifungal antibiotic, II: fermentation, isolation and characterization. J Antibiot (Tokyo) 1975;28(10):727–32.
54. Heitman J, Movva NR, Hall MN. Targets for cell cycle arrest by the immunosuppressant rapamycin in yeast. Science 1991;253(5022):905–9.
55. Guba M, von Breitenbuch P, Steinbauer M, et al. Rapamycin inhibits primary and metastatic tumor growth by antiangiogenesis: involvement of vascular endothelial growth factor. Nat Med 2002;8(2):128–35.
56. Poston RS, Billingham M, Hoyt EG, et al. Rapamycin reverses chronic graft vascular disease in a novel cardiac allograft model. Circulation 1999;100(1):67–74.
57. Degertekin M, Serruys PW, Foley DP, et al. Persistent inhibition of neointimal hyperplasia after sirolimus-eluting stent implantation: long-term (up to 2 years) clinical, angiographic, and intravascular ultrasound follow-up. Circulation 2002;106(13):1610–13.
58. Radovancevic B, Vrtovec B. Sirolimus therapy in cardiac transplantation. Transplant Proc 2003;35(3 Suppl): 171S–6S.
59. Keogh A, Richardson M, Ruygrok P, et al. Sirolimus in de novo heart transplant recipients reduces acute rejection and prevents coronary artery disease at 2 years: a randomized clinical trial. Circulation 2004;110(17):2694–700.
60. Mancini D, Pinney S, Burkhoff D, et al. Use of rapamycin slows progression of cardiac transplantation vasculopathy. Circulation 2003;108(1):48–53.
61. Stallone G, Schena A, Infante B, et al. Sirolimus for Kaposi's sarcoma in renal-transplant recipients. N Engl J Med 2005;352:1317–23.
62. King-Biggs MB, Dunitz JM, Park SJ, et al. Airway anastomotic dehiscence associated with use of sirolimus immediately after lung transplantation. Transplantation 2003;75:1437–43.
63. Dean PG, Lund WJ, Larson TS, et al. Wound-healing complications after kidney transplantation: a prospective, randomized comparison of sirolimus and tacrolimus. Transplantation 2004;77:1555–61.
64. Kahan BD, Camardo JS. Rapamycin: clinical results and future opportunities. Transplantation 2001;72(7):1181–93.
65. Ponticelli C, MacDonald AS, Rajagopalan P, et al. Phase III trial of Rapamune versus placebo in primary renal allograft recipients. Transplant Proc 2001;33(3):2271–2.
66. Kahan BD. Efficacy of sirolimus compared with azathioprine for reduction of acute renal allograft rejection: a randomised multicentre study: the Rapamune US Study Group. Lancet 2000;356(9225):194–202.
67. Groth CG, Backman L, Morales JM, et al. Sirolimus (rapamycin)-based therapy in human renal transplantation: similar efficacy and different toxicity compared with cyclosporine: Sirolimus European Renal Transplant Study Group. Transplantation 1999;67(7):1036–42.
68. Kreis H, Cisterne JM, Land W, et al. Sirolimus in association with mycophenolate mofetil induction for the prevention of acute graft rejection in renal allograft recipients. Transplantation 2000;69(7): 1252–60.
69. Blum CB. Effects of sirolimus on lipids in renal allograft recipients: an analysis using the Framingham risk model. Am J Transplant 2002;2(6): 551–9.
70. Barshes NR, Goodpastor SE, Goss JA. Sirolimus-atorvastatin drug interaction in the pancreatic islet transplant recipient. Transplantation 2003;76 (11): 1649–50.
71. Snell GI, Levvey BJ, Chin W, et al. Sirolimus allows renal recovery in lung and heart transplant recipients with chronic renal impairment. J Heart Lung Transplant 2002;21(5):540–6.
72. Eisen HJ, Tuzcu EM, Dorent R, et al. Everolimus for the prevention of allograft rejection and vasculopathy in cardiac-transplant recipients. N Engl J Med 2003;349(9):847–58.
73. Kobashigawa J, Pauly D, Ross H, et al. Reduction of cardiac allograft vasculopathy with everolimus over mycophenolate mofetil: intravascular ultrasound results of a randomized multicenter trial. J Heart Lung Transplant 2011;30(4, Supplement): S24.
74. Lehmkuhl HB, Arizon J, Viganò M, et al. Results of a 12-month, multicenter, randomized trial of everolimus with reduced-exposure cyclosporine versus MMF and standard-exposure cyclosporine in de novo cardiac transplant recipients. Transplantation 2009;88(1):115–22.
75. Eisen H, Pauly D, Starling R, et al. Everolimus with reduced CsA vs MMF with standard CsA exposure in de novo heart transplant recipients: 12 month efficacy and safety analysis. J Heart Lung Transplant 2011;30(4, Supplement): S25.
76. Kobashigawa JA, Katznelson S, Laks H, et al. Effect of pravastatin on outcomes after cardiac transplantation. N Engl J Med 1995;333:621–7.
77. Wenke K, Meiser B, Thiery J, et al. Simvastatin initiated early after heart transplantation: 8-year prospective experience. Circulation 997;107(1): 93–7.
78. Kobashigawa JA, Moriguchi JD, Laks H, et al. Ten-year follow-up of a randomized trial of pravastatin in heart transplant patients. J Heart Lung Transplant 2005;24(11):1736–40.
79. Kwak B, Mulhaupt F, Myit S, Mach F. Statins as a newly recognized type of immunomodulator. Nat Med 2000;6(12): 1399–402.
80. Kobashigawa JA. Statins in solid organ transplantation: is there an immunosuppressive effect? Am J Transplant 2004;4(7): 1013–18.
81. Downward J, Graves JD, Warne PH, et al. Stimulation of p21ras upon T-cell activation. Nature 1990;346(6286):719–23.
82. Wei X, Si MS, Imagawa DK, Ji P, et al. Perillyl alcohol inhibits TCRmediated [Ca2+]i signaling, alters cell shape and motility, and induces apoptosis in T lymphocytes. Cell Immunol 2000;201(1):6–13.
83. Maggard MA, Johnson C, Wang T, et al. Inhibition of transplant vasculopathy by pravastatin is associated with attenuated host allo-antibody response. Transplant Proc 1999;31(1–2):728–9.
84. Rose EA, Smith CR, Petrossian GA, et al. Humoral immune responses after cardiac transplantation correlation with fatal rejection and graft atherosclerosis. Surgery 1989;106(2):203–7; discussion 207–8.
85. Park MH, Young JB, Tuzcu EM, et al. Anti-donor HLA antibodies associated with allograft arteriopathy detected using intravascular ultrasound. Transplantation 1998;65(12):S26.
86. Maggard MA, Ke B, Wang T, et al. Effects of pravastatin on chronic rejection of rat cardiac allografts. Transplantation 1998;65(2):149–55.
87. Baran DA, Galin ID, Gass AL. Current practices: immunosuppression induction, maintenance, and rejection regimens in contemporary post-heart transplant patient treatment. Curr Opin Cardiol 2002;17(2):165–70.
88. Delgado DH, Miriuka SG, Cusimano RJ, et al. Use of basiliximab and cyclosporine in heart transplant patients with pre-operative renal dysfunction. J Heart Lung Transplant 2005;24(2):166–9.
89. Cantarovich M, Metrakos P, Giannetti N, et al. Anti-CD25 monoclonal antibody coverage allows for calcineurin inhibitor "holiday" in solid organ transplant patients with acute renal dysfunction. Transplantation 2002;73(7):1169–72.
90. Baran DA. Induction therapy in cardiac transplantation: when and why? Heart Fail Clin 2007;3(1):31–41.
91. Bonnefoy-Berard N, Revillard JP. Mechanisms of immunosuppression induced by antithymocyte globulins and OKT3. J Heart Lung Transplant 1996;15(5):435–42.
92. Bourdage JS, Hamlin DM. Comparative polyclonal antithymocyte globulin and antilymphocyte/antilymphoblast globulin anti-CD antigen analysis by flow cytometry. Transplantation 1995;59(8):1194–200.
93. Gaber AO, First MR, Tesi RJ, et al. Results of the double-blind, randomized, multicenter, phase III clinical trial of Thymoglobulin versus ATGAM in the treatment of acute graft rejection episodes after renal transplantation. Transplantation 1998;66(1):29–37.
94. Brennan DC, Flavin K, Lowell JA, et al. A randomized, double-blinded comparison of Thymoglobulin versus ATGAM for induction immunosuppressive therapy in adult renal transplant recipients. Transplantation 1999;67(7):1011–18.
95. Hardinger KL, Schnitzler MA, Miller B, et al. Five-year follow-up of thymoglobulin versus ATGAM induction in adult renal transplantation. Transplantation 2004;78(1):136–41.

96. Hardinger KL, Rhee S, Buchanan P, et al. A prospective, randomized, double-blinded comparison of thymoglobulin versus Atgam for induction immunosuppressive therapy: 10-year results. Transplantation 2008;86(7):947–52.
97. Opelz G, Döhler B. Lymphomas after solid organ transplantation: a collaborative transplant study report. Am J Transplant 2004;4(2):222–30.
98. Caillat-Zucman S, Blumenfeld N, Legendre C, et al. The OKT3 immunosuppressive effect: in situ antigenic modulation of human graft-infiltrating T cells. Transplantation 1990;49(1):156–60.
99. Hooks MA, Wade CS, Millikan WJ Jr. Muromonab CD-3: a review of its pharmacology, pharmacokinetics, and clinical use in transplantation. Pharmacotherapy 1991;11(1):26–37.
100. Haverty TP, Sanders M, Sheahan M. OKT3 treatment of cardiac allograft rejection. J Heart Lung Transplant 1993;12(4):591–8.
101. Adamson R, Obispo E, Dychter S, et al. Long-term outcome with the use of OKT3 induction therapy in heart transplant patients: a single-center experience. Transplant Proc 1998;30(4):1107–9.
102. Teuteberg JJ, Shullo MA, Zomak R, et al. Alemtuzumab induction prior to cardiac transplantation with lower intensity maintenance immunosuppression: one-year outcomes. Am J Transplant 2010;10(2):382–8.
103. Beniaminovitz A, Itescu S, Lietz K, et al. Prevention of rejection in cardiac transplantation by blockade of the interleukin-2 receptor with a monoclonal antibody. N Engl J Med 2000;342(9):613–19.
104. Kahan BD, Rajagopalan PR, Hall M. Reduction of the occurrence of acute cellular rejection among renal allograft recipients treated with basiliximab, a chimeric anti-interleukin-2-receptor monoclonal antibody: United States Simulect Renal Study Group. Transplantation 1999;67(2):276–84.
105. ter Meulen CG, Baan CC, Hene RJ, et al. Two doses of daclizumab are sufficient for prolonged interleukin-2R alpha chain blockade. Transplantation 2001;72(10):1709–10.
106. Hershberger RE, Starling RC, Eisen HJ, et al. Daclizumab to prevent rejection after cardiac transplantation. N Engl J Med 2005;352(26):2705–13.
107. Nashan B, Moore R, Amlot P, et al. Randomised trial of basiliximab versus placebo for control of acute cellular rejection in renal allograft recipients: CHIB 201 International Study Group. Lancet 1997;350:1193–8.
108. Leonard PA, Woodside KJ, Gugliuzza KK, et al. Safe administration of a humanized murine antibody after anaphylaxis to a chimeric murine antibody. Transplantation 2002;74(12):1697–700.
109. Kobashigawa JA, Miller LW, Russell SD, et al. Tacrolimus with mycophenolate mofetil (MMF) or sirolimus vs. cyclosporine with MMF in cardiac transplant patients: 1-year report. Am J Transplant 2006;6(6):1377–86.
110. Baran DA, Zucker MJ, Arroyo LH, et al. Randomized trial of tacrolimus monotherapy: tacrolimus in combination, tacrolimus alone compared (the TICTAC trial). J Heart Lung Transplant 2007;26(10):992–7.
111. Kobashigawa JA, Tobis JM, Starling RC, et al. Multicenter intravascular ultrasound validation study among heart transplant recipients: outcomes after five years. J Am Coll Cardiol 2005;45(9):1532–7.
112. Raichlin E, Khalpev Z, Kremers W, et al. Replacement of calcineurin-inhibitors with sirolimus as primary immunosuppression in stable cardiac transplant recipients. Transplantation 2007;84(4):467–74.
113. Groetzner J, Meiser B, Landwehr P, et al. Mycophenolate mofetil and sirolimus as calcineurin inhibitor-free immunosuppression for late cardiac-transplant recipients with chronic renal failure. Transplantation 2004;77(4):568–74.
114. Groetzner J, Kaczmarek I, Shulz U, et al. Mycophenolate and sirolimus as calcineurin inhibitor-free immunosuppression improves renal function better than calcineurin inhibitor-reduction in late cardiac transplant recipients with chronic renal failure. Transplantation 2009;87(5):726–33.
115. Kobashigawa JA, Tobis JM, Mentzer RM, et al. Mycophenolate mofetil reduces intimal thickness by intravascular ultrasound after heart transplant: reanalysis of the multicenter trial. Am J Transplant 2006;6(5 Pt 1):993–7.
116. Keogh A, Macdonald P, Harvison A, et al. Initial steroid-free versus steroid-based maintenance therapy and steroid withdrawal after heart transplantation: two views of the steroid question. J Heart Lung Transplant 1992;11(2 Pt 2):421–7.
117. Yamani MH, Taylor DO, Czerr J, et al. Thymoglobulin induction and steroid avoidance in cardiac transplantation: results of a prospective, randomized, controlled study. Clin Transplant 2008;22(1):76–81.
118. Yacoub M, Alivizatos P, Khaghani A, Mitchell A. The use of cyclosporine, azathioprine and anti-thymocyte globulinwith or without lowdose steroids for immunosuppression of cardiac transplant patients. Transplant Proc 1985;17:221–2.
119. Esmore DS, Spratt PM, Keogh AM, Chang VP. Cyclosporine and azathioprine immunosuppression without maintenance steroids: a prospective randomized trial. J Heart Transplant 1989;8(3):194–9.
120. Lee KF, Pierce JD, Hess ML, et al. Cardiac transplantation with corticosteroid-free immunosuppression: long-term results. Ann Thorac Surg 1991;52(2):211–17; discussion 18.
121. Renlund DG, O'Connell JB, Gilbert EM, et al. Feasibility of discontinuation of corticosteroid maintenance therapy in heart transplantation. J Heart Transplant 1987;6(2):71–8.
122. Kobashigawa JA, Stevenson LW, Brownfield ED, et al. Initial success of steroid weaning late after heart transplantation. J Heart Lung Transplant 1992;11(2 Pt 2):428–30.
123. Miller LW, Wolford T, McBride LR, et al. Successful withdrawal of corticosteroids in heart transplantation. J Heart Lung Transplant 1992;11(2 Pt 2):431–4.
124. Ojo AO,Held PJ, Port FK, et al. Chronic renal failure after transplantation of a nonrenal organ. N Engl J Med 2003;349(10):931–40.
125. Flechner SM, Kobashigawa J, Klintmalm G. Calcineurin inhibitor-sparing regimens in solid organ transplantation: focus on improving renal function and nephrotoxicity. Clin Transplant 2008;22(1):1–15.
126. Hamour IM, Lyster HS, Burke MM, et al. Mycophenolate mofetil may allow cyclosporine and steroid sparing in de novo heart transplant patients. Transplantation 2007;83(5):570–6.
127. Angermann CE, Stork S, Costard-Jackle A, et al. Reduction of cyclosporine after introduction of mycophenolate mofetil improves chronic renal dysfunction in heart transplant recipients—the IMPROVED multicentre study. Eur Heart J 2004;25(18):1626–34.
128. Arizon del Prado JM, Aumente MD, Lopez Granados A, et al. Use of mycophenolate mofetil in patients with transplanted heart and renal insufficiency: the relevance of the pharmacokinetic study. Transplant Proc 2002;34(1):144–5.
129. Baryalei M, Zenker D, Pieske B, et al. Renal function and safety of heart transplant recipients switched to mycophenolate mofetil and lowdose cyclosporine. Transplant Proc 2003;35(4):1539–42.
130. Tedoriya T, Keogh AM, Kusano K, et al. Reversal of chronic cyclosporine nephrotoxicity after heart transplantation-potential role of mycophenolate mofetil. J Heart Lung Transplant 2002;21(9):976–82.
131. Rice JE, Shipp AT, Carlin JB, et al. Late reduction in cyclosporine dosage does not improve renal function in pediatric heart transplant recipients. J Heart Lung Transplant 2002;21(10):1109–12.
132. Trösch F, Rothenburger M, Schneider M, et al. First experience with rapamycin-based immunosuppression to improve kidney function after heart transplantation. Thorac Cardiovasc Surg 2004;52(3):163–8.
133. Gustafsson F, Ross HJ, Delgado MS, et al. Sirolimus-based immunosuppression after cardiac transplantation: predictors of recovery from calcineurin inhibitor-induced renal dysfunction. J Heart Lung Transplant 2007;26(10):998–1003.
134. Ross H, Pflugfelder P, Haddad H, et al. Cyclosporine reduction in the presence of everolimus: 3-month data from a Canadian pilot study of maintenance cardiac allograft recipients. J Heart Lung Transplant 2008;27(2):197–202.

135. Cantarovich M, Ross H, Arizon JM, et al. Benefit of Neoral C2 monitoring in de novo cardiac transplant recipients receiving basiliximab induction. Transplantation 2008;85(7):992–9.
136. Serón D, Moreso F, Fulladosa X, et al. Reliability of chronic allograft nephropathy diagnosis in sequential protocol biopsies. Kidney Int 2002;61(2):727–33.
137. Meiser B, Reichart B, Adamidis I, et al. First experience with de novo calcineurin-inhibitor-free immunosuppression following cardiac transplantation. Am J Transplant 2005;5(4 Pt 1):827–31.
138. Zakliczynski M, Nozynski J, Zakliczynska H, et al. Deterioration of renal function after replacement of cyclosporine with sirolimus in five patients with severe renal impairment late after heart transplantation. Transplant Proc 2003;35(6):2331–2.
139. Groetzner J, Kaczmarek I, Landwehr P, et al. Renal recovery after conversion to a calcineurin inhibitor-free immunosuppression in late cardiac transplant recipients. Eur J Cardiothorac Surg 2004;25(3):333–41.
140. Hunt J, Lerman M, Magee MJ, et al. Improvement of renal dysfunction by conversion from calcineurin inhibitors to sirolimus after heart transplantation. J Heart Lung Transplant 2005;24(11):1863–7.
141. Kushwaha SS, Khalpey Z, Frantz RP, et al. Sirolimus in cardiac transplantation: use as a primary immunosuppressant in calcineurin inhibitor-induced nephrotoxicity. J Heart Lung Transplant 2005;24(12):2129–36.
142. Raichlin E, Bae JH, Khalpey Z, et al. Conversion to sirolimus as primary immunosuppression attenuates the progression of allograft vasculopathy after cardiac transplantation. Circulation 2007;116(23):2726–33.
143. Hunt J, Bedanova H, Starling R, et al. Premature termination of a prospective, open label, randomized, multicenter study of sirolimus to replace calcineurin inhibitors (CNI) in a standard care regimen of CNI, MMF and corticosteroids early after heart transplantation. J Heart Lung Transplant 2007;26(suppl 2):398.
144. Baran DA, Segura L, Kushwaha S, et al. Tacrolimus monotherapy in adult cardiac transplant recipients: intermediate-termresults. J Heart Lung Transplant 2001;20(1):59–70.
145. Kobashigawa JA, Stevenson LW, Brownfield ED, et al. Corticosteroid weaning late after heart transplantation: relation to HLADR mismatching and long-term metabolic benefits. J Heart Lung Transplant 1995;14(5):963–7.
146. Deng MC, Eisen HJ, Mehra MR, et al. Noninvasive discrimination of rejection in cardiac allograft recipients using gene expression profiling. Am J Transplant 2006;6(1):150–60.
147. Kowalski RJ, Post DR, Mannon RB, et al. Assessing relative risks of infection and rejection: a meta-analysis using an immune function assay. Transplantation 2006;82(5):663–8.
148. Kobashigawa JA, Kiyosaki KK, Patel JK, et al. Benefit of immune monitoring in heart transplant patients using ATP production in activated lymphocytes. J Heart Lung Transplant 2010;29(5):504–508.
149. Gautam A, Morrissey PE, Brem AS, et al. Use of an immune function assay to monitor immunosuppression for treatment of posttransplant lymphoproliferative disorder. Pediatr Transplant 2006;10(5):613–16.
150. Nwakanma LU, Williams JA, Weiss ES, et al. Influence of pretransplant panel-reactive antibody on outcomes in 8,160 heart transplant recipients in recent era. Ann Thorac Surg 2007;84(5):1556–62, discussion 62–3.
151. Tambur AR, Bray RA, Takemoto SK, et al. Flow cytometric detection of HLA-specific antibodies as a predictor of heart allograft rejection. Transplantation 2000;70(7):1055–9.
152. Tambur AR, Pamboukian SV, Costanzo MR, et al. The presence of HLA-directed antibodies after heart transplantation is associated with poor allograft outcome. Transplantation 2005;80(8):1019–25.
153. Grattan MT, Moreno-Cabral CE, Starnes VA, et al. Cytomegalovirus infection is associated with cardiac allograft rejection and atherosclerosis. JAMA 1989;261:3561–6.
154. Kirklin JK, Young JB, McGiffin DC, et al. Cardiac allograft vasculopathy (chronic rejection). In: Kirklin JK, Young JB, McGiddin DC, ed. Heart Transplantation. New York: Churchill Livingstone; 2002, pp. 615–65.
155. Oni AA, Ray J, Hosenpud JD. Coronary venous intimal thickening in explanted cardiac allografts. Evidence demonstrating that transplant coronary artery disease is a manifestation of a diffuse allograft vasculopathy. Transplantation 1992;53(6):1247–51.
156. Hornick P, Smith J, Pomerance A, et al. Influence of acute rejection episodes, HLA matching, and donor/recipient phenotype on the development of "early" transplant-associated coronary artery disease. Circulation 1997;96(9 Suppl):II-148–53.
157. Williams R, Neuhaus P, Bismuth H, et al. Two-year data from the European multicentre tacrolimus (FK506) liver study. Transpl Int 1996;9 Suppl 1:S144–50.
158. Jurcevic S, Dunn MJ, Crisp S, et al. A new enzyme-linked immunosorbent assay to measure anti-endothelial antibodies after cardiac transplantation demonstrates greater inhibition of antibody formation by tacrolimus compared with cyclosporine. Transplantation 1998;65(9):1197–202.
159. Klauss V, König A, Spes C, et al. Cyclosporine versus tacrolimus (FK 506) for prevention of cardiac allograft vasculopathy. Am J Cardiol 2000;85(2):266–9.
160. Kaczmarek I, Ertl B, Schmauss D, et al. Preventing cardiac allograft vasculopathy: long term beneficial effects of mycophenolate mofetil. J Heart Lung Transplant 2006;25(5): 550–5.
161. Rose ML, Danskine A, Smith JD, et al. Mycophenolate mofetil (MMF) depresses antibody production after cardiac transplantation. Circulation 2000;102(18S):II.490.
162. Krotz F, Keller M, Derflinger S, et al. Mycophenolate acid inhibits endothelial NAD(P)H oxidase activity and superoxide formation by a Rac1-dependent mechanism. Hypertension 2007;49(1):201–8.
163. Segovia J, Gomez-Bueno M, Alonso-Pulpon L. Treatment of allograft vasculopathy in heart transplantation. Expert Opin Pharmacother 2006;7:2369–83.
164. Eisen H. Long-term cardiovascular risk in transplantation: insights from the use of everolimus in heart transplantation. Nephrol Dial Transplant 2006;21(suppl 3):iii-9–iii-13.
165. Mehra MR, Uber PA. TOR inhibitors and cardiac allograft vasculopathy: Is inhibition of intimal thickening an adequate surrogate of benefit? J Heart Lung Transplant 2003;22:501–4.
166. Starling RC, Hare JM, Hauptman P et al. Therapeutic drug monitoring for everolimus in heart transplant recipients based on exposure-effect modeling. Am J Transplant 2004;4(12):2126–31.
167. Mahalati K, Kahan BD. Clinical pharmacokinetics of sirolimus. Clin Pharmacokinet 2001;40(8):573–85.
168. Starzl TE, Porter KA, Iwatsuki JT, et al. Reversibility of lymphomas and lymphoproliferative lesions developing under cyclosporine-steroid therapy. Lancet 1984;17:583–7.
169. Reshef R, Vardhanabhuti S, Luskin MR, et al. Reduction of immunosuppression as initial therapy for posttransplantation lymphoproliferative disorder. Am J Transplant 2011;11:336–47.
170. Itescu S, Schuster M, Burke E, et al. Immunobiologic consequences of assist devices. Cardiol Clin 2003;21(1):119–33, ix–x.
171. Drakos SG, Stringham JC, Long JW, et al. Prevalence and risks of allosensitization in HeartMate left ventricular assist device recipients: the impact of leukofiltered cellular blood product transfusions. J Thorac Cardiovasc Surg 2007;133:1612–19.
172. Guttmann RD, Caudrelier P, Alberici G, Touraine JL. Pharmacokinetics, foreign protein immune response, cytokine release, and lymphocyte subsets in patients receiving thymoglobuline and immunosuppression. Transplant Proc 1997:29:24S.
173. Jordan SC, Tyan D, Stablein D, et al. Evaluation of intravenous immunoglobulin as an agent to lower allosensitization and improve transplantation in highly sensitized adult patients with end-stage renal disease: report of the NIH IG02 trial. J Am Soc Nephrol 2004;15:3256–62.
174. Pisani BA, Mullen GM, Malinowska K, et al. Plasmapheresis with intravenous immunoglobulin G is effective in patients with elevated

panel reactive antibody prior to cardiac transplantation. J Heart Lung Transplant 1999;18:701–6.
175. Allison AC, Eugui EM. Mycophenolate mofetil and its mechanisms of action. Immunopharmacology 2000;47(2–3):85–118.
176. Grailer A, Nichols J, Hullett D, et al. Inhibition of human B cell responses in vitro by RS-61443, cyclosporine A and DAB486 IL-2. Transplant Proc 1991;23(1 Pt 1):314–15.
177. Theruvath TP, Saidman SL, Mauiyyedi S, et al. Control of antidonor antibody production with tacrolimus and mycophenolate mofetil in renal allograft recipients with chronic rejection. Transplantation 2001;72(1):77–83.
178. Schmid C, Garritsen HS, Kelsch R, et al. Suppression of panel-reactive antibodies by treatment with mycophenolate mofetil. Thorac Cardiovasc Surg 1998;46(3):161–2.
179. Weigel G, Griesmacher A, Karimi A, et al. Effect of mycophenolate mofetil therapy on lymphocyte activation in heart transplant recipients. J Heart Lung Transplant 2002;21(10):1074–9.
180. Lietz K, John R, Schuster M, et al. Mycophenolate mofetil reduces anti-HLA antibody production and cellular rejection in heart transplant recipients. Transplant Proc 2002;34(5):1828–9.
181. De Marco T, Damon LE, Colombe B, et al. Successful immunomodulation with intravenous gamma globulin and cyclophosphamide in an alloimmunized heart transplant recipient. J Heart Lung Transplant 1997;16(3):360–5.
182. Grauhan O, Knosalla C, Ewert R, et al. Plasmapheresis and cyclophosphamide in the treatment of humoral rejection after heart transplantation. J Heart Lung Transplant 2001 20(3):316–21.
183. Itescu S, Burke E, Lietz K, et al. Intravenous pulse administration of cyclophosphamide is an effective and safe treatment for sensitized cardiac allograft recipients. Circulation 2002;105(10):1214–19.
184. Vo AA, Lukovsky M, Toyoda M, et al. Rituximab and intravenous immune globulin for desensitization during renal transplantation. N Engl J Med 2008;359:242–51.
185. Kopchaliiska D, Zachary AA, Montgomery RA, Leffell MS. Reconstitution of peripheral allospecific CD19+ B-cell subsets after B-lymphocyte depletion therapy in renal transplant patients. Transplantation 2009, 87:1394–401.
186. National Institute of Allergy and Infectious Diseases. Prevention of cardiac allograft vasculopathy using rituximab (Rituxan) therapy in cardiac transplantation. <http://clinicaltrials.gov/ct2/show/NCT01278745(2011)>.
187. Walsh RC, Everly JJ, Brailey P, et al. Proteasome inhibitor-based primary therapy for antibody-mediated renal allograft rejection. Transplantation 2010;89:277–84.
188. Patel J, Everly M, Chang D, et al. Reduction of alloantibodies via proteosome inhibition in cardiac transplantation. J Heart Lung Transplant 2011;30:1320–6.
189. Kaczmarek I, Deutsch MA, Kauke T, et al. Donor-specific HLA alloantibodies: long-term impact on cardiac allograft vasculopathy and mortality after heart transplant. Exp Clin Transplant 2008;6:229–35.
190. Onsager DR, Canver CC, Jahania MS, et al. Efficacy of tacrolimus in the treatment of refractory rejection in heart and lung transplant recipients. J Heart Lung Transplant 1999;18:448–55.
191. Wu GW, Kobashigawa JA, Fishbein MC, et al. Asymptomatic antibody-mediated rejection after heart transplantation predicts poor outcomes. J Heart Lung Transplant 2009;28:417–22.
192. Kfoury AG, Hammond ME, Snow GL, et al. Cardiovascular mortality among heart transplant recipients with asymptomatic antibody-mediated or stable mixed cellular and antibody-mediated rejection. J Heart Lung Transplant 2009;28:781–4.
193. Giunti G, Schürfeld K, Maccherini M, et al. Photopheresis for recurrent acute rejection in cardiac transplantation. Transplant Proc 1999;31(1–2):128–9.
194. Holloway KB, Flowers FP, Ramos-Caro FA. Therapeutic alternatives in cutaneous T-cell lymphoma. J Am Acad Dermatol 1992;27(3):367–78.
195. Costanzo-Nordin MR, McManus BM, Wilson JE, et al. Efficacy of photopheresis in the rescue therapy of acute cellular rejection in human heart allografts: a preliminary clinical and immunopathologic report. Transplant Proc 1993;25(1 Pt 2):881–3.
196. Lehrer MS, Rook AH, Tomaszewski JE, DeNofrio D. Successful reversal of severe refractory cardiac allograft rejection by photopheresis. J Heart Lung Transplant 2001;20(11):1233–6.
197. Dall'Amico R, Livi U, Milano A, et al. Extracorporeal photochemotherapy as adjuvant treatment of heart transplant recipients with recurrent rejection. Transplantation 1995;60(1):45–9.
198. Barr ML, Meiser BM, Eisen HJ, et al. Photopheresis for the prevention of rejection in cardiac transplantation. Photopheresis Transplantation Study Group. N Engl J Med 1998;339(24):1744–51.
199. Kobashigawa JA, Kiyosaki KK, Patel JK, et al. Benefit of immune monitoring in heart transplant patients using ATP production in activated lymphocytes. J Heart Lung Transplant 2010;29:504–8.
200. Kokko KE, Newell KA, Pearson TC, et al. Enhanced immunosuppression induced by targeted mutation of cytotoxic T lymphocyte antigen-4 immunoglobulin. Curr Opin Organ Transplant 2005;10(4):265–9.
201. Larsen CP, Pearson TC, Adams AB, et al. Rational development of LEA29Y (belatacept), a high-affinity variant of CTLA4-lg with potent immunosuppressive properties. Am J Transplant 2005;5:443–53.
202. Bristol-Myers Squibb. Indication and important safety information, Nulojix (belatacept). <http://www.nulojix.com/hcp/index.aspx>.
203. Larsen CP, Knechtle SJ, Adams A, et al. A new look at T cell costimulation: a therapeutic strategy for long-term maintenance immunosuppression. Am J Transplant 2006;6:876–83.
204. Vincenti F, Larsen C, Durrbach A, et al. Co-stimulation blockade with belatacept in renal transplantation. N Engl J Med 2005;353(8):770–81.
205. Grinyó J, Charpentier B, Pestana JM, et al. An integrated safety profile analysis of belatacept in kidney transplant recipients. Transplantation 2010;90(12):1521–7.
206. Hillmen P, Young NS, Schubert J, et al. The complement inhibitor eculizumab in paroxysmal nocturnal hemoglobinuria. N Engl J Med 2006;355(12):1233–43.
207. Stegall MD, Diwan T, Raghavaiah S, et al. Terminal Complement Inhibition Decreases Antibody-Mediated Rejection in Sensitized Renal Transplant Recipients. Am J Transplant 2011;11(11):2405–13.
208. Locke JE, Magro CM, Singer AL, et al. The use of antibody to complement protein C5 for salvage treatment of severe antibody-mediated rejection. Am J Transplant 2009;9(1):231–5.
209. Chatelet V, Fremeaux-Bacchi V, Lobbedez T, et al. Safety and long-term efficacy of eculizumab in a renal transplant patient with recurrent atypical hemolytic-uremic syndrome. Am J Transplant 2009;9(11): 2644–5.
210. Larrea CF, Cofan F, Oppenheimer F, et al. Efficacy of eculizumab in the treatment of recurrent atypical hemolytic-uremic syndrome after renal transplantation. Transplantation 2010;89(7): 903–4.
211. Matz M, Weber U, Mashreghi MF, et al. Effects of the new immunosuppressive agent AEB071 on human immune cells. Nephrol Dial Transplant 2010;25(7):2159–67.
212. Djamali A, Pietrangeli CE, Gordon RD, Legendre C. Potential of emerging immunosuppressive strategies to improve the posttransplant cardiovascular risk profile. Kidney Int Suppl 2010;(118):S15–21.
213. Oropallo MA, Kiefer K, Marshak-Rothstein A, Cancro MP. Beyond transitional selection: New roles for BLyS in peripheral tolerance. Drug Dev Res 2011;72(8):779–87.
214. Lindenfeld J, Miller GG, Shakar SF, et al. Drug therapy in the heart transplant recipient: Part II: immunosuppressive drugs. Circulation 2004;110(25);3858–65.
215. Lindenfeld J, Miller GG, Shakar SF, et al. Drug therapy in the heart transplant recipient: Part I: immunosuppressive drugs. Circulation 2004;110(25);3734–40.
216. Costanzo MR, Dipchand A, Starling R, et al. The International Society of Heart and Lung Transplantation Guidelines for the care of heart transplant recipients. J Heart Lung Transplant 2010;29(8):914–56.

217. Flechner SM, Kobashigawa J, Klintmalm G. Calcineurin inhibitor-sparing regimens in solid organ transplantation: focus on improving renal function and nephrotoxicity. Clin Transplant 2008;22(1):1–15.
218. Halloran PF, Gourishankar S. Principles and overview of immunosuppression. In: Norman DJ, Turka LA, ed. Primer on Transplantation, 2nd edn. Mount Laurel: American Society of Transplantation; 2001, pp. 87–98.
219. Taylor DO, Edwards LB, Aurora P, et al. Registry of the International Society for Heart and Lung Transplantation: twenty-fifth official adult heart transplant report—2008. J Heart Lung Transplant 2008;27(9):943–56.
220. Patel JK, Kittleson M, Kobashigawa JA. Cardiac allograft rejection. Surgeon 2011;9(3):160–7.

CHAPTER 18

Rejection surveillance: Types and treatment

Natasha Lipson Altman MD and Sean P. Pinney MD

Introduction

Long-term survival following heart transplantation has been achieved through refinements in patient and donor selection and in postoperative management. Without doubt, the single greatest advance has been the development of effective immune suppression, which has extended median survival to more than 10 years and transformed heart transplantation from a curiosity to its present position as the therapy of choice for advanced heart failure. The introduction of cyclosporine in the early 1980s was a breakthrough which directly led to this improvement in patient survival and ushered in the widespread implementation of heart transplantation throughout North America and Europe. The calcineurin inhibitor (CNI) tacrolimus has largely replaced cyclosporine in present-day immunosuppressive regimens because of advantages that it offers in individualizing therapy and minimizing drug-specific side effects. Therefore, a primary role of the transplant physician is immune surveillance, specifically balancing the risk of allograft rejection against treatment-related adverse events, specifically infection, renal dysfunction, and other side effects.

Frequency of allograft rejection

Cardiac allograft rejection is a common occurrence. More than one-quarter of all recipients will experience rejection within the first year with a little more than half of the episodes requiring specific drug treatment or hospitalization.[1] A sequential review of the International Society for Heart and Lung Transplantation (ISHLT) registry over time clearly shows a continuing decline in the frequency of treated rejection. For example, for those patients transplanted between 1994 and 2000, 41% needed hospitalization for rejection treatment within the first year. By comparison, only 26% of those transplanted between 2001 and 2009 required hospitalization and treatment.[2] Some general observations can be made about the frequency of allograft rejection as it relates to age, gender, and choice of immune suppression. First, rejection occurs more commonly in younger as compared to older recipients. Second, women, particularly black women, have higher rates of rejection than men. Finally, cyclosporine-treated patients experience greater rates of rejection and treated rejection than tacrolimus-treated patients, but the rates of graft loss are similar.[1,3] The frequency of allograft rejection can be viewed as a time-dependent variable with the highest incidence occurring within the first 6 months following transplantation and quickly tapering down to fewer than 0.02 rejection episodes per month by 1 year.[4] While allograft rejection episodes decrease with the passage of time, late episodes occur, resulting in a cumulative frequency distribution that approaches an asymptote after the first year.[4]

There is now general acceptance about the presence and severity of antibody-mediated rejection (AMR) (Table 18.1), but a lack of consensus surrounding its definition and diagnostic criteria have limited attempts to quantify its occurrence in the general heart transplant population.[5,6] Often, patients will experience AMR during the first few weeks following transplantation accompanied by a rise in donor-specific antibodies. Compared to acute cellular rejection (ACR), AMR tends to develop in a more dramatic fashion, frequently presenting with acute allograft dysfunction, hemodynamic instability, ST-segment elevation on surface electrocardiogram, or with ventricular tachyarrhythmias. Allosensitized patients with detectable levels of circulating anti-HLA antibodies

Table 18.1 The 2013 ISHLT working formulation for pathologic diagnosis of cardiac antibody-mediated rejection

Grade	Definition	Substrates
pAMR 0	Negative for pathologic AMR	Histologic and immunopathologic studies are both negative
pAMR 1 (H+)	Histopathologic AMR alone	Histologic findings are present and immunopathologic findings are negative
pAMR 1 (I+)	Immunopathologic AMR alone	Histologic findings are negative and immunopathologic findings are positive (CD68+ and/or C4d+)
pAMR 2	Pathologic AMR	Histologic and immunopathologic findings are both present
pAMR 3	Severe pathologic AMR	Interstitial hemorrhage, capillary fragmentation, mixed inflammatory infiltrates, endothelial cell pyknosis, and/or karyorrhexis, and marked edema and immunopathologic findings are present. These cases may be associated with profound hemodynamic dysfunction and poor clinical outcomes

AMR, antibody-mediated rejection.

Reproduced from Berry *et al.* The 2013 International Society for Heart and Lung Transplantation Working Formulation for the standardization of nomenclature in the pathologic diagnosis of antibody-mediated rejection in heart transplantation. *J Heart Lung Transplant* 2013: 32(12) with permission from Elsevier.

before transplantation may experience AMR as early as 2–7 days after transplantation. Two-thirds of these patients will subsequently develop graft dysfunction and face an increased risk of developing cardiac allograft vasculopathy (CAV).[7,8,9] Patients experiencing late-onset AMR experience a more benign course with only 13% of such patients developing graft dysfunction.[7]

Association of rejection with outcomes

Acute rejection is a major cause of death early after transplantation. Approximately 10% of the deaths at 1 and 3 years are directly attributable to acute rejection, but over time the cumulative incidence of death due to acute rejection is no more than 2%.[1] Death due to acute rejection is age-dependent, accounting for one-fifth of 1-year mortalities in those aged 18–39 years, but only for 5% of those patients 60 years of age or older.[1] Those patients having experienced an episode of treated rejection within the first year are at higher risk of dying in the following years. As a group, those treated for rejection experienced a 5-year survival of 80% compared to 87% for those not experiencing rejection.[1] Longer-term consequences of rejection include higher rates of CAV, the need for greater immune suppression, and the associated adverse sequelae.[10]

Endomyocardial biopsy

Endomyocardial biopsy (EMB) is the gold standard for diagnosing allograft rejection. Initially introduced by Caves in 1973, EMB quickly replaced other diagnostic modalities, such as the measurement of electrocardiographic voltage, and has remained the diagnostic tool of choice for detecting rejection.[11] Timely performance of EMB allows direct microscopical evaluation of the myocardium, providing a snapshot of the state of immune activation. The presence of an inflammatory infiltrate within the myocardium reflects the final pathway of allograft rejection which is itself a complex series of immune reactions. Although the essential reactions of alloantigen recognition and immune activation cannot be classified through a biopsy, an EMB can serve to confirm or exclude the presence of an inflammatory infiltrate; specify whether ACR, AMR, or both are present; and quantify the severity of the infiltrate. For this reason, EMB remains the technique of choice, particularly in the early months after transplantation, to tailor immunosuppressive therapy and guide decisions regarding the treatment of allograft rejection.

In spite of these strengths, EMB remains an imperfect tool. The technique is labor intensive, requiring either fluoroscopic or echocardiographic guidance to properly site the bioptome, and it is invasive, which produces some degree of risk as well as patient anxiety and discomfort. Even though EMB has a low complication rate, usually less than 1%, serious adverse events do occur.[12] These include the inadvertent tearing of chordae producing tricuspid valve insufficiency, right ventricular free wall perforation, vascular trauma to the femoral or carotid artery, and errant biopsies, especially of the liver.

The histopathological grading system first introduced by Dr. Margaret Billingham and later revised and standardized by the ISHLT (Table 18.2) has some noticeable shortcomings.[13,14] Although considered the gold standard, this system has itself never been independently validated against another system for biopsy assessment.[14] The grading system consists essentially of a series of descriptions of histological patterns which lend themselves to some inherent inconsistencies. For example, a biopsy which shows an extensive lymphocytic infiltrate throughout the myocardium and interstitium, but possesses only a single focus of myocyte necrosis, would be scored a 1R, and treated as inconsequential, whereas a sample containing a sparse infiltrate but two areas of myocyte necrosis would be scored a 2R, encouraging a more aggressive therapeutic response. Another of the system's limitations is the occasional disconnect between allograft dysfunction and the histopathologic pattern seen on biopsy, referred to in common parlance as "biopsy-negative rejection." This is because the causes, mediators, and cellular changes associated with cardiac allograft dysfunction are incompletely described.[15]

Inflammation, with T-lymphocyte and macrophage infiltration, is likely to be an important, cause of graft dysfunction, but certainly not the only one: ischemic injury, CAV, and other undiscovered mechanisms contribute as well. Recent investigations exploring the association between allograft gene expression, histopathology, and clinical findings have highlighted these inconsistencies.[14,16] Certain lesions classified as diagnostic for ACR show little correlation with the clinical and molecular phenotype defined by specific pathogenesis-based gene transcripts.[14] Furthermore, transcriptional profiling of endomyocardial samples has shown heterogeneity within the 1R classification with a small number of overlapping pathways being shared in common with the more advanced moderate and severe grades of rejection, suggesting common physiological underpinnings.[16] Finally, in spite of the presence of a uniform and standardized grading system, discordance of biopsy interpretation between pathologists continues to exist.[17] Proper interpretation of biopsy samples is

Table 18.2 Histopathology grading systems for endomyocardial biopsies

Description 2004		Description 1990	
Grade 0R	**No rejection**	**Grade 0**	**No rejection**
1R, mild	Interstitial and/or perivascular infiltrate with up to 1 focus of myocyte damage	1, mild 1A, focal	Focal perivascular and/or interstitial infiltrate without myocyte damage
		1B, diffuse	Diffuse infiltrate without myocyte damage
		2, moderate (focal)	One focus of infiltrate with associated myocyte damage
2R, moderate	Two or more foci of infiltrate with associated myocyte damage	3, moderate 3A, focal	Multifocal infiltrate with myocyte damage
3R, severe	Diffuse infiltrate with multifocal myocyte damage ± edema, ± hemorrhage ± vasculitis	3B, diffuse	Diffuse infiltrate with myocyte damage
		4, severe	Diffuse, polymorphous infiltrate with extensive myocyte damage ± edema, ± hemorrhage ± vasculitis

"R" denotes revised grade to avoid confusion with the 1990 scheme.

Table 18.3 Example of a typical endomyocardial biopsy schedule

Time post transplant	Frequency of endomyocardial biopsy
1 month	Weekly
2 months	Biweekly
3–6 months	Monthly
7–12 months	Every 2 months
12–18 months[a]	Every 3 months
2–5 years[b]	Yearly

[a] May consider stopping after 1 year in appropriately selected low-risk patients.

[b] The utility of endomyocardial biopsy after 5 years is less certain.

enhanced by review by specialized cardiac pathologists, particularly those affiliated with high-volume transplant centers.

The timing and frequency of EMB is predicated on understanding the frequency and likelihood of detecting allograft rejection. Since allograft rejection may often be present in the absence of symptoms, protocolized biopsies are performed at set intervals designed to match the risk of rejection (Table 18.3). Such biopsies are particularly useful within the first year to guide immune suppressive medication dosing and the tapering of corticosteroids. The utility of extending protocolized biopsies beyond the first year in the majority of transplant recipients has been questioned.[18] In the present era of effective immune suppression, the incidence of rejection outside the first transplant year is so low that finding it in the absence of symptoms is unusual. Furthermore, it is not entirely clear that discovering an inflammatory infiltrate in an asymptomatic recipient necessarily correlates with adverse outcomes. For example, some have suggested that late-occurring moderate-to-severe rejection is a unique entity which may undergo spontaneous resolution in the absence of treatment.[19] Nonetheless, late rejection occurs with sufficient frequency to define a subgroup of individuals at higher risk of such occurrences. These include patients with multiple prior episodes of rejection, those with a shorter time interval from a previous rejection episode, young recipients, and African American recipients.[20]

Generally speaking, the likelihood of detecting allograft rejection (ACR, AMR, or both) in biopsy is greater when rejection is clinically suspected.[14,21] The clinical manifestations of rejection are protean and the presentation can be subtle. Constitutional symptoms including malaise, lethargy, and fever represent systemic responses to the local immune activation. Cell death and inflammation, which result from acute rejection, produce myocardial edema which leads to increased ventricular wall stiffness and diastolic dysfunction. Over time, progressive cell death and cytokine activation may result in systolic dysfunction. With increased left ventricular filling pressures, typical symptoms of pulmonary and venous congestion occur, including exertional dyspnea, orthopnea, paroxysmal nocturnal dyspnea, and lower extremity swelling. When rejection is associated with a compromise in allograft function, an S3 or S4 gallop may be auscultated and the neck veins may be distended. Echocardiography can document diminished ventricular function. The new onset of atrial arrhythmias, particularly atrial fibrillation or flutter, often correlates with rejection episodes, whereas ventricular arrhythmias do not unless accompanied by severe hemodynamic compromise or AMR.[22] Bradyarrhythmias and atrioventricular conduction block may also occur due to myocardial edema, as can a pericardial friction rub and pericardial effusion. Other clues to the presence of rejection include a reduction in QRS voltage on the ECG, usually the result of myocardial edema, and the new ability to control hypertension which was previously refractory to medical therapy.

Gene expression profiling

The recognition that host responses of immune activation and leukocyte trafficking could be detected as changes in peripheral blood mononuclear cell (PBMC) gene expression led to the development, approval and clinical adoption of the first, and only, noninvasive test for rejection surveillance. The AlloMap (CareDx, Inc., Brisbane, CA, USA) gene expression profiling (GEP) test was developed to discriminate between ISHLT rejection grade 0 (quiescence) and grade 3A (2R) or greater (nonquiescence).[23] Starting with a customized microarray consisting of 7370 genes and coupled with the addition of genes known to be involved or associated with immune activation and transplant rejection, a total of 252 candidate genes were identified. Next, in the diagnostic development phase, real-time polymerase chain reaction (PCR) assays were set up for each of the 252 candidate genes and performed on 145 samples obtained from 36 rejection and 109 quiescent samples. Analysis of these PCR data yielded 68 genes which discriminated well between rejection and quiescence samples. Six genes were eliminated due to significant variability based upon sample processing time. From the remaining 62 genes, 20 metagenes were constructed by combining genes whose expression acted in a concordant manner. Finally, a linear discriminant equation was derived by sequentially fitting the gene expression data to maximize agreement with the biopsy sample results. This final equation yields a score between 0 and 40 based upon the expression of 11 genes (3 metagenes and 4 single genes) which best distinguished between rejection and quiescence.

Prospective validation of this linear discriminant equation was carried out on two separate cohorts. Using a discriminant score of 20, where lower scores reflect quiescence, the receiver operating characteristic (ROC) area under the curve (AUC) for the primary validation cohort of 63 unique patient samples was 0.72 ± 0.06. Analysis of this group revealed that time after transplant was the single greatest factor affecting the score. A second validation set in patients 6 months or more and 1 year or more after transplantation was performed with improved ROC characteristics. Using a threshold value of 28 for patients 6 months or more following transplantation yielded an improved ROC AUC of 0.80 ± 0.114. For samples obtained from patients 1 year or more following transplantation, a threshold value of 30 could discriminate quiescence from nonquiescence with a positive predictive value of 6.8% and negative predictive value of 99.6%. The area under the ROC curve was 0.86 ± 0.09. The strength of this test therefore lies in its high negative predictive value (NPV) where scores below threshold have a very high probability of confirming quiescence, thereby excluding rejection. For this particular validation sample, 68% of the test scores were less than 30.

In spite of these strengths, there are some notable technical and clinical limitations which have emerged from the CARGO trial. First, the utility of the test is predicated on the assumption that signals from heart allograft rejection will be reflected in PBMC gene expression, but this limits candidate genes to only those expressed in leukocytes and potentially excludes other more important genome-wide interactions. Preliminary studies surveying whole-blood genomic markers have highlighted this limitation by identifying other classifier genes whose transcripts appear to differentiate quiescence from nonquiescence with better performance metrics than those from PBMCs alone.[24] Second, real differences were observed between the microarray and PCR methods for gene significance. Perhaps this was due to the elimination of certain genes which displayed minor changes in gene expression not detectable by microarray, but which would have been discovered with the amplification which comes from PCR. Finally, the derivation of the discriminant equation was highly dependent upon the proper grading of EMBs by the core pathologists, but, as discussed above, interobserver variability exists between independent observers with much of the uncertainty around specific biopsies being generated by the presence of Quilty lesions.[17,25]

In spite of the search for a noninvasive strategy of rejection surveillance to replace EMB, only one alternative has emerged with the necessary high NPV to confidently exclude allograft rejection. The IMAGE investigators randomized 602 patients between 6 months and 5 years after transplantation without antecedent moderate–severe ACR or AMR to a strategy incorporating GEP along with clinical and echocardiographic monitoring to the standard one using protocolized EMBs.[26] Over a median follow-up of 19 months in this event-driven trial, the GEP strategy was noninferior to that of EMB with respect to the primary composite endpoint of rejection with hemodynamic compromise, graft dysfunction due to other causes, death, or retransplantation. There was a significant reduction in the number of biopsies performed with those in the GEP pathway who underwent 0.5 biopsies per patient-year of follow-up compared to 3.0 biopsies per patient-year in the EMB arm. Not surprisingly, patient satisfaction was significantly greater in the GEP group. There were greater numbers of treated asymptomatic rejection episodes in the EMB arm, and one might assume that the GEP strategy may have failed to detect all the cases of asymptomatic rejection, but there was no noticeable difference in the 2-year outcome of graft dysfunction, death, or retransplantation. One implication from this observation is the possibility that not all cases of asymptomatic rejection require therapy. However, the long-term sequelae from untreated rejection, potentially including graft fibrosis or CAV, are unknown.

There are several important limitations to the IMAGE trial which may prevent the widespread adoption of GEP as an alternative rejection surveillance strategy. First, the subjects were a low-risk group. The eligible population for this trial was enrolled at least 6 months following transplantation, a time when rejection risk is receding. Two-thirds of patients were enrolled between 1 and 3 years after transplantation and roughly 15% were enrolled between 3 and 5 years after transplantation when rejection risk is low. Only 20% of eligible patients were enrolled, suggesting that physicians eschewed high-risk candidates, allowing only low-risk patients to participate. Also, few black patients, a population known to be at higher risk of experiencing rejection, were enrolled. As a group, black patients comprised 12% of the study population, but were disproportionately randomized to the EMB strategy, making it difficult to draw conclusions about the GEP strategy in this vulnerable population. A second limitation is the relatively low statistical power of this trial. The investigators chose wide confidence margins to demonstrate noninferiority between the GEP and EMB pathways, which does not exclude the possibility of as much as a 68% increase in experiencing the primary endpoint in the GEP arm. Additionally, by including graft dysfunction, death, and retransplantation in the primary endpoint, conditions which may be the result of factors other than rejection, the investigators may have further diluted the study's predictive power. Finally, it is interesting to note that only 6 of the 34 treated rejection episodes in the GEP arm were detected by the GEP test. It appears that most were detected on clinical grounds alone. Besides raising questions about the utility of the GEP test, these observations may lead one to consider a strategy of rejection surveillance based solely on clinical and echocardiographic means of detection, at least in a low-risk population. Taken together, these limitations to the IMAGE investigation preclude the adoption of GEP as the sole means of rejection surveillance.

In order for a GEP strategy to replace EMB, not only will there need to be a larger trial than IMAGE with narrower confidence intervals and longer follow-up, but there will also need to be proof that PBMC sampling can discriminate quiescence from nonquiescence in the early period following transplant when rejection risk is highest. This early period is characterized by the administration of relatively high doses of corticosteroids. This has a direct effect upon the AlloMap score since the expression of at least three genes (*IL1R2, FLT3, ITGAM*) surveilled by the test are sensitive to corticosteroid dosing.[27] Using a lower discriminant score in this early period may allow the use of AlloMap in this period without lessening the test's NPV. In a small single-center trial, 60 patients less than 1 year after transplantation were randomized to a standard surveillance strategy using EMB versus a GEP strategy, similar to IMAGE, but using a time-dependent threshold test value.[28] For patients who were between 2 and 6 months after transplantation, a threshold score greater than 30 would prompt an EMB while a score greater than 34 would be required to biopsy those who had received transplant more than 6 months before. In this pilot trial, there was no difference in the primary composite endpoint of hemodynamically significant rejection, allograft dysfunction, death, or retransplantation. The results of intravascular ultrasound for CAV detection at 1 year have not been released. This pilot study provides some encouragement that GEP starting at 2 months appears to be comparable to EMB without compromising cardiac function at 1 year, and offers the advantage of increased patient satisfaction by minimizing the number of biopsies performed.

Noninvasive assessment

Driven by a desire to avoid the invasive EMB with its attendant risks and associated patient discomfort, clinicians have long searched for a reliable noninvasive alternative which could reduce, if not entirely eliminate, the need for biopsy. Such a test should allow early detection of rejection before any significant myocardial necrosis has occurred, be widely available, minimize resource use, and possess sufficient sensitivity and specificity to be clinically relevant.[29] Many noninvasive tests have shown promise, but most lack effective discriminating characteristics to be reproducible. Only PBMC, GEP, and ventricular evoked response (VER) monitoring have been endorsed by the ISHLT as an alternative to EMB in appropriately selected candidates.[30] Others, described below, are often clinically useful, but do not serve as a replacement for EMB.

Echocardiography

Echocardiography facilitates heart transplant care by gauging ventricular function, detecting valvular insufficiency, guiding bioptome placement during EMB and, when combined with pharmacologic or exercise stress testing, screening for CAV. However, no single echocardiographic variable has proven effective in diagnosing or excluding rejection.[31] Several investigators have pointed to the impaired diastolic function which accompanies allograft rejection as being a potential surrogate marker detectable by the use of standard Doppler and tissue Doppler echocardiography.[31,32,33,34,35] Early diastolic peak velocity of the basal left ventricular wall was shown in one study[35] to have a high sensitivity (90%) for detecting clinical rejection, but, as has often been the case with echocardiography, this finding was not confirmed in other studies.[31] A recent review of the published literature concluded that a lack of evidence exists to support using diastolic indices as a screening test for allograft rejection.[36] In another study, five echocardiographic parameters (presence of a pericardial effusion, E/A ratio of mitral inflow velocity, diameter of inferior vena cava, duration of pulmonary atrial reversal, and isovolumic relaxation time) were shown to be univariate predictors of rejection. When present, the likelihood of rejection increased from 40% to 52% and 71%, for one, two, and three variables, respectively. The likelihood of rejection being present was considered high enough in those patients with two or more predictors more than 6 months from transplantation to consider avoiding biopsy altogether. Although the potential of this approach to decrease the number of surveillance biopsies is attractive, the lack of prospective validation studies obviates its adoption.

Cardiac MRI

The appeal of cardiac MRI (CMR) is the ability of a single study to quantify allograft function and characterize tissue composition.[37,38,39,40] Myocardial edema, which is known to be associated with acute myocardial infarction and myocarditis, may be produced by the inflammatory response generated by allograft rejection and is detectable using T2-weighted imaging. Since the 1980s there have been several small trials testing the ability of CMR to detect allograft rejection using T-2 weighted imaging.[37,38,39] These studies have been variably successful as they were limited by older imaging techniques, low magnet strength, and poor resolution. More recently, quantitative T-2 mapping using a stronger (1.5 T) magnet has shown greater promise of being able to detect allograft rejection.[40] In a study of 53 patients, all within the first year of transplantation, the measurement of a prolonged T-2 relaxation time was directly correlated with the presence of allograft rejection. Using a conservative cutoff value of 56 ms, the investigators were able to demonstrate a test sensitivity of 86.5%, specificity of 94.6%, and ROC AUC of 0.89. These findings are furthered strengthened by the fact that the presence of myocardial edema was not influenced by the type of rejection as CMR was able to detect both ACR and AMR as well as two cases of hemodynamically significant rejection which were not further characterized by EMB. CMR thus holds promise for being an alternative to EMB if these initial results can be confirmed in larger, prospective trials.

Ventricular evoked response

Long-term monitoring of VER signals to programmed electrical stimulation has been used in a small number of centers for rejection surveillance.[41,42] Recorded signals from telemetric pacemakers implanted during the transplant surgery can be analyzed for changes in the evoked T-wave amplitude following a period of programmed stimulation. Intramyocardial edema, cellular infiltrates, and cell necrosis are believed to alter ion channels which can delay cellular repolarization. This may be reflected as a reduction in the maximum negative slope in the descending part of the repolarization phase of the intramyocardial electrogram. In certain centers with proven expertise, the use of VER monitoring has performed very well in rejection screening with both a high sensitivity and NPV. Its use has been endorsed by the ISHLT for use in low-risk patients.

Risk profiling and immune monitoring

One of the challenges for transplant physicians is to properly balance the risk of infection against the need to prevent rejection. As one considers tailoring immune suppression to individual patients it is helpful to consider the influences of age, gender, and time from transplantation on the risk of rejection.[43] For example, patients transplanted between 10 and 30 years of age are more likely than elderly patients to experience rejection. Conversely, patients older than 60 years seem more susceptible to death from infection than rejection. While it would seem prudent to target higher immunosuppressive drug levels for young patients, particularly women and African Americans, it may be more important to minimize exposure in elderly patients. Clinical risk scores which incorporate these and other variables such as HLA matching provide a more granular accounting of risk, but offer little more clinical utility than that provided by good practical sense.[44]

Few tools are available for clinicians to quantitatively assess the degree of immune suppression. Therapeutic drug level monitoring is helpful in preventing drug toxicities, but fails to adequately gauge global immune response. One promising new tool is an immune monitoring assay (ImmuKnow; Cylex, Columbia, MD, USA) which is approved by the US Food and Drug Administration (FDA) for the detection of cell-mediated immunity in immunosuppressed patients. This assay measures the ATP release from activated lymphocytes and correlates with the degree of immune responsiveness. In a single-center retrospective evaluation, those patients experiencing an infection episode had an average score below that of patients measured during steady state.[45] Higher scores, reflective of a more robust immune system, did not correlate with rejection episodes, but these were too few in number to provide adequate statistical power. Other biomarkers such as soluble CD30 and interleukin-5 may have more utility.[46] While immune monitoring may ultimately assist physicians in personalizing immunosuppressive medication dosing to minimize the risks of infection and rejection, its utility first needs to be proven in prospective trials before its broader acceptance into clinical practice can be endorsed.

Treatment

Acute cellular rejection

Strategies for the treatment of rejection differ significantly from one center to another (Table 18.4). Factors influencing the decision to treat include the grade of rejection, the state of cardiac function (as determined by echocardiogram and/or right heart catheterization), and time from transplantation. In general, ISHLT grade 0R and 1R biopsies do not require treatment in the absence of symptoms or abnormal hemodynamics. Care should be taken to ensure that doses and levels of immunosuppressive medications are at their therapeutic targets. Patients with symptomatic rejection should receive corticosteroids. Patients with significant histologic signs of rejection (≥grade 2R) require specialized care. Patients with grade 2R rejection who are less than 6 months after transplantation or who have hemodynamic dysfunction should be admitted for intravenous corticosteroids (e.g., methylprednisolone 1 g daily for 3 days). An echocardiogram, to evaluate ventricular function and to exclude pericardial effusion, should be performed at initiation of therapy and repeated 1 week later. EMB should be repeated within 7–14 days. Patients with grade 2R rejection and

Table 18.4 Example of a rejection treatment protocol

Grade	Treatment options for allograft rejection
0R	No alteration in immunosuppression required Patients receiving corticosteroids may have dose reduced
1R	
Asymptomatic, normal LVEF	Optimize immunosuppressive dosing Repeat biopsy per protocol Wean corticosteroids, if applicable
Symptomatic, reduced LVEF	Oral steroid bolus/taper or IV pulse steroids
2R	
< 6 months following transplant, reduced LVEF or hemodynamic compromise	IV pulse steroids (methylprednisolone 1 gram daily x 3 days) Oral steroid taper Target higher CNI level
> 6 months following transplant with normal hemodynamics and LVEF	Oral steroid bolus (Prednisone 50 mg bid × 3 days) Consider steroid taper Optimize immunosuppressive dosing (CNI, anti-metabolite)
3R	
All patients	IV pulse corticosteroids
Reduced LVEF	Cytolytic therapy (thymoglobulin)
Heart failure/shock	Inotropic therapy IABP, percutaneous LVAD or ECMO
Co-existent AMR	Plasmapheresis IV immune globulin
AMR1	Oral or IV corticosteroids IV immune globulin Plasmapheresis Consider rituximab or bortezomib

AMR, antibody-mediated rejection; bid, twice daily; CNI, calcineurin inhibitor; ECMO, extracorporeal membrane oxygenation; IABP, intra-aortic balloon pump; IV, intravenous; LVAD, left ventricular assist device; LVEF, left ventricular ejection fraction.

normal hemodynamics who are longer than 6 months from transplantation should be given oral corticosteroids (e.g., prednisone 50 mg twice daily for 3 days), which may be followed by a tapering dose. An echocardiogram should be performed within 7 days and EMB repeated in 7–14 days. ISHLT 3R or hemodynamically severe rejection occurs in less than 5% of patients, but requires in-patient admission and treatment with high-dose corticosteroids and thymoglobulin. In-patient admission and hemodynamic monitoring are essential as such patients are at risk of rapidly progressing cardiac failure and circulatory collapse.

Antibody-mediated rejection

Treatment of AMR is targeted at three distinct processes: clearance or neutralization of circulating antibodies, eradication of plasma cells, and prevention of sensitized B cells from transforming into plasma cells. Plasmapheresis with plasma exchange can quickly remove circulating alloantibodies, and allow graft function to recover.[47] Up to 40% of circulating IgG may not be cleared by plasmapheresis, but may be neutralized or cleared by administering intravenous immunoglobulin (IVIg). A non-sucrose-containing preparation may be selected in order to avoid nephrotoxicity. Although not formally endorsed by the ISHLT guidelines, the anti-CD20 monoclonal antibody rituximab (Genentech, San Francisco, CA, USA), a chimeric humanized antibody directed against the pan-B-cell surface molecule CD20, has been used frequently as a component of therapy. It targets sensitized B cells and interferes with their ability to transform into antibody-producing plasma cells. Ultimately, rituximab may provide long-term benefit by eliminating "memory" B cells and preventing the adverse late sequelae of humoral rejection. Clinical investigations with the proteasome inhibitors bortezomib and carfilzomib for AMR treatment are under way. Heparin may be infused to reduce thrombus formation in the cardiac microvasculature.

References

1. Lund LH, Edwards LB, Kucheryavaya AY, et al. The registry of the International Society for Heart and Lung Transplantation: thirtieth official adult heart transplant report—2013; focus theme: age. J Heart Lung Transplant 2013;32:951–64.
2. Mehra MR. Balancing the tightrope of cardiac allograft rejection: equations or experience? Circulation 2012;125:2971–4.
3. Kobashigawa JA, Miller LW, Russell SD, et al. Tacrolimus with mycophenolate mofetil (MMF) or sirolimus vs. cyclosporine with MMF in cardiac transplant patients: 1-year report. Am J Transplant 2006;6:1377–86.
4. Kubo SH, Naftel DC, Mills RM, et al. Risk factors for late recurrent rejection after heart transplantation: a multi-institutional, multivariable analysis. J Heart Lung Transplant 1995;14:409–18.
5. Kobashigawa J, Crespo-Leiro MG, Ensminger SM, et al. Report from a consensus conference on antibody-mediated rejection in heart transplantation. J Heart Lung Transplant 2011;30:252–69.
6. Berry GJ, Burke MM, Andersen C, et al. The 2013 International Society for Heart and Lung Transplantation Working Formulation for the standardization of nomenclature in the pathologic diagnosis of antibody-mediated rejection in heart transplantation. J Heart Lung Transplant 2013;32:1147–62.
7. Reed EF, Demetris AJ, Hammond E, et al. Acute antibody-mediated rejection of cardiac transplants. J Heart Lung Transplant 2006;25:153–9.
8. Barr ML, Cohen DJ, Benvenisty LA, et al. Effect of anti-HLA antibodies on the long-term survival of heart and kidney allografts. Transplant Proc 1993;25:262–4.
9. Reed EF, Hong B, Ho E, et al. Monitoring of soluble HLA alloantigens and anti-HLA antibodies identifies heart allograft recipients at risk of transplant-associated coronary artery disease. Transplantation 1996;61:566–72.
10. Raichlin E, Edwards BS, Kremers WK, et al. Acute cellular rejection and the subsequent development of allograft vasculopathy after cardiac transplantation. J Heart Lung Transplant 2009;28:320–7.
11. Caves PK, Stinson EB, Graham AF, et al. Percutaneous transvenous endomyocardial biopsy. JAMA 1973;225:288–91.
12. Holzmann M, Nicko A, Kühl U, et al. Complication rate of right ventricular endomyocardial biopsy via the femoral approach: a retrospective and prospective study analyzing 3048 diagnostic procedures over an 11-year period. Circulation 2008;118:1722:8.
13. Stewart S, Winters GL, Fishbein MC, et al. Revision of the 1990 working formulation for the standardization of nomenclature in the diagnosis of heart rejection. J Heart Lung Transplant 2005;24:1710–20.
14. Mengel M, Sis B, Kim D, et al. The molecular phenotype of heart transplant biopsies: relationship to histopathological and clinical variables. Am J Transplant 2010;10:2105–15.

15. Marboe CC. The molecular phenotype of heart transplant biopsies. Am J Transplant 2010;10:1957–58.
16. Holweg CT, Potena L, Luikart H, et al. Identification and classification of acute cardiac rejection by intragraft transcriptional profiling. Circulation 2011;123:2236–43.
17. Crespo-Leiro MG, Zuckermann A, Bara C, et al. Concordance among pathologists in the second Cardiac Allograft Rejection Gene Expr Observational Study (CARGO II). Transplantation 2012;94:1172–7.
18. Patel JK, Kobashigawa JA. Should we be doing routine biopsy after heart transplantation in a new era of anti-rejection? Curr Opin Cardiol 2006;21:127–31.
19. Klingenberg R, Koch A, Schnabel PA, et al. Allograft rejection of ISHLT >/= 3A occurring late after heart transplantation: a distinct entity? J Heart Lung Transplant 2003;22:1005–13.
20. Stehlik J, Starling RC, Movsesian MA, et al. Utility of long-term surveillance endomyocardial biopsy: a multi-institutional analysis. J Heart Lung Transplant 2006;25:1402–9.
21. Levi DS, DeConde AS, Fishbein MC, et al. The yield of surveillance endomyocardial biopsies as a screen for cellular rejection in pediatric heart transplant patients. Pediatr Transplant 2004;8:22–8.
22. Cui G, Tung T, Kobashigawa J, et al. Increased incidence of atrial flutter associated with the rejection of heart transplantation. Am J Cardiol 2001;88:280–84.
23. Deng MC, Eisen HJ, Mehra MR, et al. Noninvasive discrimination of rejection in cardiac allograft recipients using gene expression profiling. Am J Transplant 2006;6:150–60.
24. Lin D, Hollander Z, Ng RT, et al. Whole blood genomic biomarkers of acute cardiac allograft rejection. J Heart Lung Transplant 2009;28:927–35.
25. Marboe CC, Billingham M, Eisen H, et al. Nodular endocardial infiltrates (Quilty lesions) cause significant variability in the diagnosis of ISHLT rejection grades 2 and 3A in endomyocardial biopsies from cardiac allograft recipients. J Heart Lung Transplant 2005;24:S219–26.
26. Pham MX, Teuteberg JJ, Kfoury AG, et al. Gene-expression profiling for rejection surveillance after cardiac transplantation. N Engl J Med 2010; 362(20):1890–900.
27. Mehra MR, Kobashigawa JA, Deng MC, et al. Transcriptional signals of T-cell and corticosteroid-sensitive genes are associated with future acute cellular rejection in cardiac allografts. J Heart Lung Transplant 2007;26:1255–63.
28. Kobashigawa J, Patel J, Kittleson M, et al. Results of a randomized trial of Allomap vs. heart biopsy in the 1st year after heart transplantation: Early Invasive Monitoring Attenuation through Gene Expr Trial. J Heart Lung Transplant 2013;32(Supplement):S203.
29. Patel JK, Kittleson M, Kobshigawa JA. Cardiac allograft rejection. Surgeon 2011;9;160–7.
30. Costanzo MR et al. The International Society of Heart and Lung Transplantation Guidelines for the care of heart transplant recipients. J Heart Lung Transplant 2010;29:914–56.
31. Sun JP, Abdalla IA, Asher CR, et al. Non-invasive evaluation of orthotopic heart transplant rejection by echocardiography. J Heart Lung Transplant 2005;24:160–5.
32. Desruennes M, Solis E, Cabrol A, et al. Doppler echocardiography: an excellent noninvasive method for the detection of acute cardiac allograft rejection. Transplant Proc 1989;21:3634–8.
33. Morocutti G, DiChiara A, Proclemer A, et al. Signal-averaged electrocardiography and Doppler echocardiographic study in predicting acute rejection in heart transplantation. J Heart Lung Transplant 1995;14:1065–72.
34. Valantine H, Fowler M, Hatle L, et al. Doppler echocardiographic indices of diastolic function as markers of acute cardiac rejection. Transplant Proc 1987;19:2556–59.
35. Dandel M, Hummel M, Muller J, et al. Reliability of tissue Doppler wall motion monitoring after heart transplantation for replacement of invasive routine screenings by optimally timed cardiac biopsies and catheterizations. Circulation 2001;104:I184–91.
36. Mena C, Wencker D, Krumholz HM, et al. Detection of heart transplant rejection in adults by echocardiographic diastolic indices: a systematic review of the literature. J Am Soc Echocardiagr 2006;19:1295–300.
37. Smart FW, Young JB, Weilbaecher D, et al. Magnetic resonance imaging for assessment of tissue rejection after heterotopic heart transplantation. J Heart Lung Transplant 1993;12:403–10.
38. Marie PY, Angioi M, Carteaux JP, et al. Detection and prediction of acute heart transplant rejection with myocardial T2 determination provided by black-blood magnetic resonance imaging sequence. J Am Coll Cardiol 2001;37:825–31.
39. Butler CR, Thompson R, Haykowsky M, et al. Cardiovascular magnetic resonance in the diagnosis of acute heart transplant rejection: a review. J Cardiovasc Magn Reson 2009;11:7.
40. Usman AA, Taimen K, Wasielewski M, et al. Cardiac magnetic resonance T2 mapping in the monitoring and follow-up of acute cardiac transplant rejection: a pilot study. Circ Cardiovasc Imaging 2012;5:782–90.
41. Mahaux V, Demoulin JC, Biessaux Y, et al. Heart graft monitoring by the ventricular evoked response. PACE 2000;23[Pt.II]:2003–5.
42. Schweiger M, Wasler A, Prenner G, et al. The prognostic validity of the ventricular evoked response (VER) signals in cardiac transplantation. J Heart Lung Transplant 2005;24:1730–5.
43. George JF, Taylor DO, Blume ED, et al. Minimizing infection and rejection death: clues acquired from 19 years of multi-institutional cardiac transplantation data. J Heart Lung Transplant 2011;30:151–7.
44. Kilic A, Weiss ES, Allen JG, et al. Simple score to assess the risk of rejection after orthotopic heart transplantation. Circulation 2012;125:3013–21.
45. Kobashigawa JA, Kiyosaki KK, Patel JK, et al. Benefit of immune monitoring in heart transplant patients using ATP production in activated lymphocytes. J Heart Lung Transplant 2010;29:504–8.
46. Heikal NM, Bader FM, Martins TB, et al. Immune function surveillance: association with rejection, infection and cardiac allograft vasculopathy. Transplant Proc 2013;45:376–82.
47. Olivari MT, May CB, Johnson NA, et al. Treatment of acute vascular rejection with immunoadsorption. Circulation 1994;90:II70–3.

CHAPTER 19

Complications after cardiac transplantation

Howard J. Eisen MD

Introduction

Cardiac transplantation provides definitive therapy for advanced heart failure refractory to other therapies and was first introduced in 1967. It took an additional 15–16 years for adequate immunosuppressive therapy to be developed to enable prolonged survival while reducing the morbidity and mortality of the early post-transplantation complications, acute cellular rejection (ACR) and infection (these only became available once there was a more complete understanding of the alloimmune responses to the allograft). Over the subsequent 30 years, improvements in the management of infectious diseases, intensive care unit management, and immunosuppressive and adjunctive post-transplantation therapy, as well as an understanding of how to use these therapies more effectively, resulted in improved outcomes especially in the first 6 months after transplantation (Figure 19.1).[1] Despite this, long-term outcomes are not comparable to those of demographically comparable nontransplant patients. As early post-transplantation outcomes have improved, major efforts are now directed at diagnosing, treating, and perhaps preventing the later post-transplantation complications such as cardiac allograft vasculopathy (CAV) and malignancy, which represent the major obstacles to long-term survival in cardiac transplant recipients.

Acute cellular rejection

One of the majors causes of morbidity and mortality in the early post-transplantation period is ACR. This is the result of the alloimmune response of the recipient immune system to donor heart antigens on the surface of endothelial and other cells of the allograft. Recipient CD4+ and CD8+ cells recognize donor major histocompatibility complex (MHC) antigens through the direct pathway by directly binding to allo-MHC antigens on the surface of allogeneic antigen presenting cells (APCs).[2,3] CD4+ cells can also recognize peptides derived from the donor MHC presented bound to recipient MHC antigens by recipient APCs (Figure 19.2).[4,5] This interaction is referred to as Signal 1. When there are concurrent interactions between CD40 on the surface of the APC and CD40 ligand on the T-cell surface, referred to as Signal 2, this results in changes in gene expression culminating in production of cytokines such as interleukin-2 (IL-2) with subsequent proliferation and activation of T cells and enhancement of the alloimmune response (Figure 19.3). If left unimpeded or not completely inhibited, rejection can result in severe damage to the cardiac allograft, resulting in heart failure or death.

Since the mid 1970s, the diagnosis of ACR has been made by endomyocardial biopsy (EMB) where a cardiac bioptome is directed through the right internal jugular or less commonly, right femoral vein, toward the right ventricle where four to eight pieces of cardiac tissue are obtained. After staining, the samples are examined under the microscope and the severity of rejection is defined by extent of lymphocyte and inflammatory infiltration into the myocardium and extent of myocyte necrosis; an example of International Society for Heart and Lung Transplantation (ISHLT) grade 2R is shown in Figure 19.4. Rejection is graded by the ISHLT nomenclature which was revised from a prior nomenclature (Table 19.1).[6] Severity of rejection is based on the extent and type of leukocyte infiltrate in the myocardium and the extent of myocyte necrosis. Treatment for ACR usually begins with ISHLT grade 2R. Though invasive, this procedure is very safe and only rarely associated with complications such as cardiac perforation and arrhythmias.[7] ACR is most common in the first 3 months after transplantation followed by the next 3 months after transplantation and becomes less frequent afterward. The frequency of EMB reflects the frequency of ACR. A typical EMB schedule is weekly for 4 weeks beginning 1 week after transplantation, then every 2 weeks for the next 2 months, monthly for the next 3 months and then every other month for the last 6 months of the first year after transplantation. Beyond the first year, the frequency of obtaining surveillance biopsies varies by program from every 3 months for years to every 6 months for 3–5 years to none at all. Of course, patients presenting with clinical evidence of rejection such as heart failure symptoms, atrial or ventricular arrhythmias, or a decrease in left ventricular function will undergo EMB. Estimates from the ISHLT registry are that up to 50% of patients have had a biopsy-proven rejection although this percentage has been declining.[1] Recent immunosuppression clinical trials also demonstrate a decline in the frequency of biopsy-proven rejection.[8] Having a rejection episode impacts survival, and this is especially true of rejection with hemodynamic compromise.[9]

Maintenance immunosuppression for prevention of acute cellular rejection

Immunosuppression is directed toward inhibition of the alloimmune response to the cardiac allograft. The mainstay of modern immunosuppression is triple therapy of which calcineurin inhibitors, specifically cyclosporine and tacrolimus, are the most potent components. These agents inhibit calcineurin; cyclosporine does this by binding to cyclophilin while tacrolimus binds to the FK binding complex.[2,5] Through dephosphorylated NF-AT, transcription of

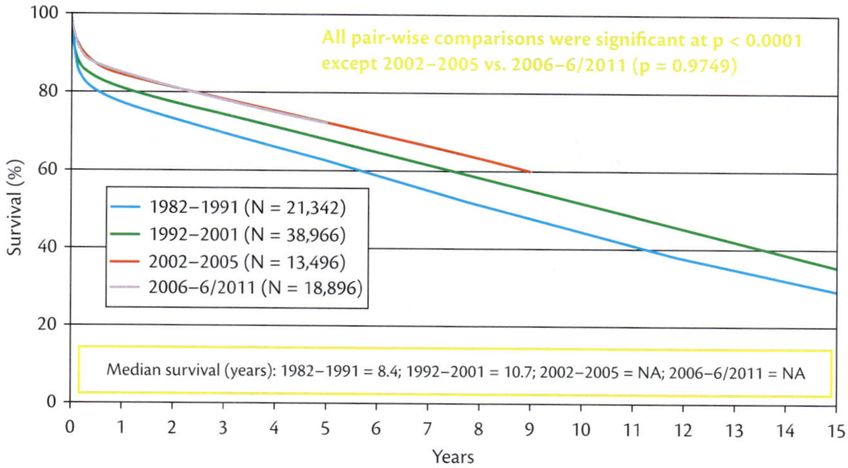

Fig. 19.1 Survival of adult heart transplant recipients by era, showing improvement over the past 30 years.

Reprinted from Journal of Heart and Lung Transplantation, 32, Lund LH, Edwards LB, Kucheryavaya AY, et al; The Registry of the International Society for Heart and Lung Transplantation: thirtieth official adult heart transplant report—2013; focus theme: age. International Society for Heart and Lung Transplantation, 951–64, copyright (2013) with permission from Elsevier.

the IL-2 genes is inhibited, resulting in blunting of T-cell activation and proliferation.[2,5]

The second arm of triple therapy is the antiproliferative agents, of which azathioprine (AZA) and mycophenolate mofetil (MMF) have historically been most commonly used. Azathioprine, which was originally developed to treat leukemia, is a prodrug for 6-mercaptopurine, a purine analog that is incorporated into DNA, inhibiting DNA synthesis and lymphocyte proliferation.[10] MMF inhibits inosine monophosphate dehydrogenase, which is involved in de-novo purine synthesis in T and B cells and therefore inhibits their proliferation in response to allogeneic stimulation from MHC antigens on the surface of cells in the cardiac allograft.[10] MMF has largely replaced azathioprine as the antiproliferative agent of choice in maintenance immunosuppressive therapy after cardiac transplantation as it has been shown in a large randomized double-blind comparison to azathioprine to reduce rejection frequency, including the frequency of rejection with hemodynamic compromise, as well as improving survival.[11,12]

The third component of triple maintenance immunosuppressive therapy after heart transplantation is corticosteroids. They have

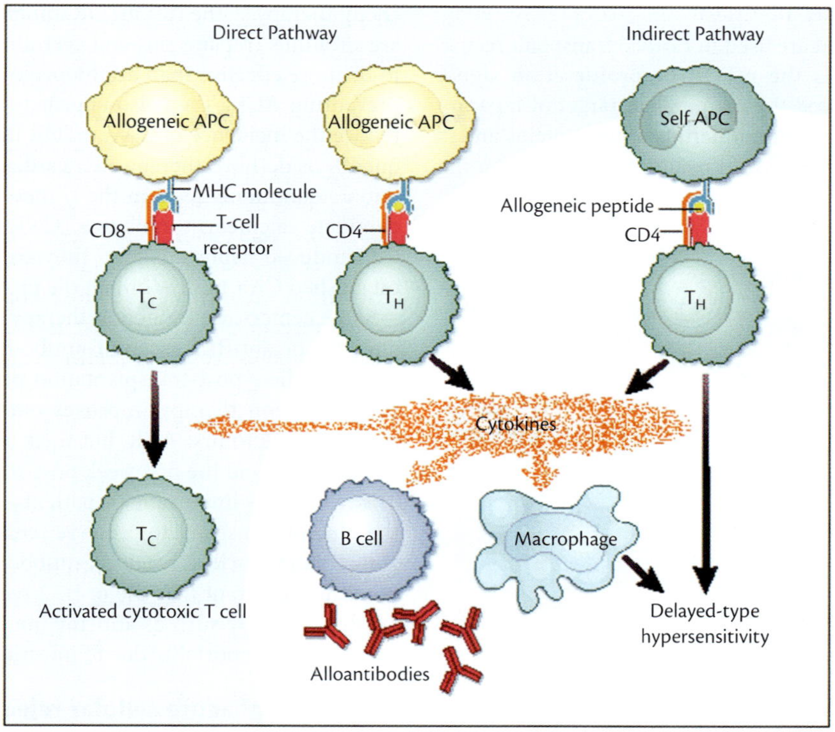

Fig. 19.2 Direct and indirect pathways of recognition of allogeneic MHC antigens on allograft cell surfaces by recipient's T cells.

From New England Journal of Medicine, Sayegh M and Turka L, Mechanisms of Disease: The Role of T-Cell Costimulatory Activation Pathways in Transplant Rejection, 338:1813–21, Copyright © (1998) Massachusetts Medical Society. Reprinted with permission from Massachusetts Medical Society.

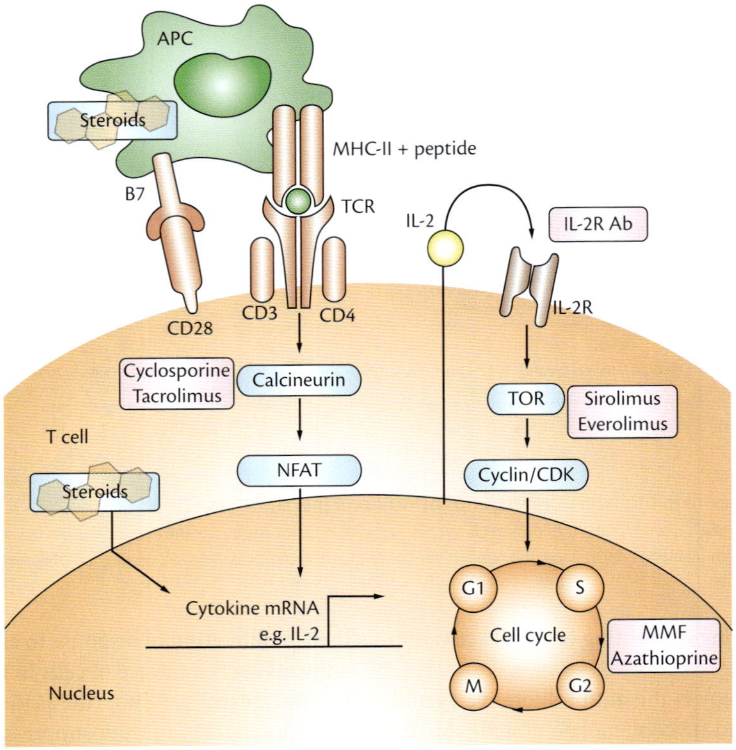

Fig. 19.3 Recognition of allogeneic MHC antigens, Signal 2 interactions, and subsequent IL-2 elaboration and T-cell activation.
Halloran PF, Gourishankar S. Principles and overview of immunosuppression. In: Norman DJ, Turka LA, eds. Primer on Transplantation, edn 2. Mount Laurel: American Society of Transplantation; 2001: 87–98.

pleiotropic effects on the alloimmune response and because they freely diffuse across the cell membrane, they can have intracellular effects including modulation of cytokine genes. They may also have a lympholytic effect.[2,5,10]

Another class of drugs that are used in cardiac transplant recipients to prevent rejection is the mTOR or proliferation signal inhibitors (PSIs). These inhibit the mammalian target of rapamycin (mTOR), which interacts with numerous other proteins and is involved in cell proliferation.[2,5,10] As a result of their effect on the mechanisms of proliferation, mTOR inhibitors are used to prevent transplant rejection, restenosis after angioplasty and stent deployment (delivered locally via drug-eluting stents) and as cancer chemotherapy.[13] The two mTOR inhibitors used in transplantation are sirolimus (rapamycin) and everolimus. They have been shown to be more effective than azathioprine and as effective as MMF in preventing ACR. They also appear to attenuate the severity and reduce the incidence of CAV. mTOR inhibitors are used more frequently as de-novo therapy after cardiac transplantation in Europe but are commonly used in the United States to help minimize or eliminate calcineurin inhibitors (CNI) in transplant patients with CNI-induced nephrotoxicity. They are also used in patients with established CAV to slow or halt the progression of this disease.

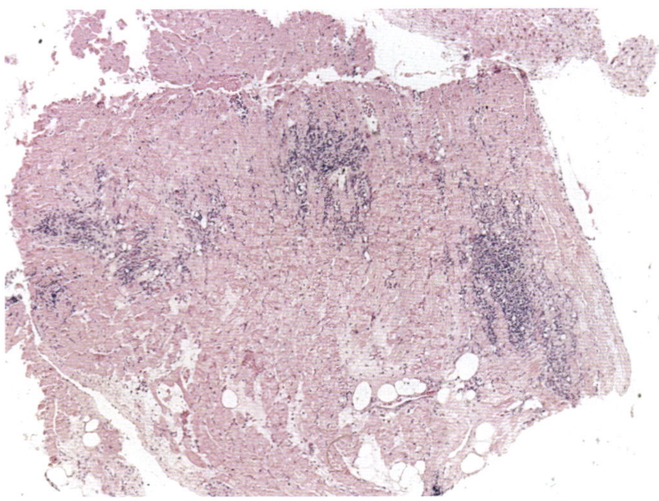

Fig. 19.4 Photomicrograph of ISHLT grade 2R biopsy specimen from endomyocardial biopsy showing myocyte necrosis and diffuse lymphocyte infiltration.

Some centers use induction therapy with either anti-thymocyte globulin or anti-IL2 receptor antibodies, usually basiliximab, in the immediate post-transplantation period. There is no evidence that induction therapy improves outcomes other than perhaps delaying time to first ACR, but their use allows delay of CNI initiation to beyond the first week post-transplantation (Figure 19.5). This would be important in patients with renal insufficiency at the time of transplant to preserve renal function. From the daclizumab (another IL-2 receptor antibody) cardiac transplant study, it became apparent that use of IL-2 receptor antibodies and other cytolytic therapy such as anti-thymocyte globulin was associated with increased mortality due to infection.[14]

Treatment of acute cellular rejection

ACR without hemodynamic compromise is treated with a short (3-day) course of oral corticosteroids. There is no advantage to using intravenous steroids in these patients. CNI doses are

Table 19.1 International Society for Heart and Lung Transplantation standardized cardiac biopsy grading for acute cellular rejection[a]

2004 grading		1990 grading	
Grade 0R[b]	No rejection	Grade 0	No rejection
Grade 1R, mild	Interstitial and/or perivascular infiltrate with up to 1 focus of myocyte damage	Grade 1, mild	
		A—Focal	Focal perivascular and/or interstitial infiltrate without myocyte damage
		B—Diffuse	Diffuse infiltrate without myocyte damage
		Grade 2 moderate (focal)	One focus of infiltrate with associated myocyte damage
Grade 2R, moderate	Two or more foci of infiltrate with associated myocyte damage	Grade 3, moderate	
		A—Focal	Multifocal infiltrate with myocyte damage
Grade 3R, severe	Diffuse infiltrate with multifocal myocyte damage ± edema, ± hemorrhage ± vasculitis	B—Diffuse	Diffuse infiltrate with myocyte damage
		Grade 4, severe	Diffuse, polymorphous infiltrate with extensive myocyte damage ± edema, ± hemorrhage + vasculitis

[a] The presence or absence of acute antibody-mediated rejection (AMR) may be recorded as AMR 0 or AMR 1, as required.

[b] "R" denotes revised grade to avoid confusion with 1990 scheme.

Reprinted from Journal of Heart and Lung Transplantation, 24, Stewart S et al., Revision of the 1990 working formulation for the standardization of nomenclature in the diagnosis of heart rejection, 1710–20, copyright (2005) with permission from Elsevier.

optimized based on therapeutic drug monitoring of drug levels. Patients receiving cyclosporine may be switched to tacrolimus. ACR associated with hemodynamic compromise is treated more aggressively with cytolytic therapy with anti-thymocyte globulin and intravenous corticosteroids.[15] Hemodynamic compromise is defined as a fall in left ventricular ejection fraction of more than 25%, a cardiac index less than 2.0 L min^{-1} m^{-2}, or the need for inotropic support. Hemodynamic support with inotropic therapy and circulatory support with intra-aortic balloon counterpulsation or temporary mechanical support may be required as well, especially if the patient is hypotensive and has a diminished cardiac index.

Antibody-mediated rejection

T-cell-mediated damage to the cardiac allograft is not the only mechanism of immune assault. B-cell-initiated damage to the transplant resulting in antibody-mediated rejection (AMR) has often been difficult to diagnose in the past but the diagnosis has been systematized as a result of the ISHLT AMR nomenclature (Box 19.1).[16] The histopathologic characteristics of AMR include intravascular infiltration of macrophages (defined by CD68 staining), capillary endothelial swelling, and nuclear enlargement.[16] AMR is also often characterized by capillary endothelial and myocardial deposition of the complement fragment C4d and less commonly C3d. The ISHLT nomenclature defines severity of AMR based on the presence or absence of histopathology and immunopathology findings and AMR3 is defined by these features and interstitial hemorrhage, capillary fragmentation, mixed inflammatory infiltrates, endothelial pyknosis, and severe edema.[16] AMR3 is often associated with hemodynamic compromise as defined above. Therapy is generally reserved for AMR2 or greater and consists of corticosteroids and intravenous immunoglobulin (IVIg). AMR associated with a

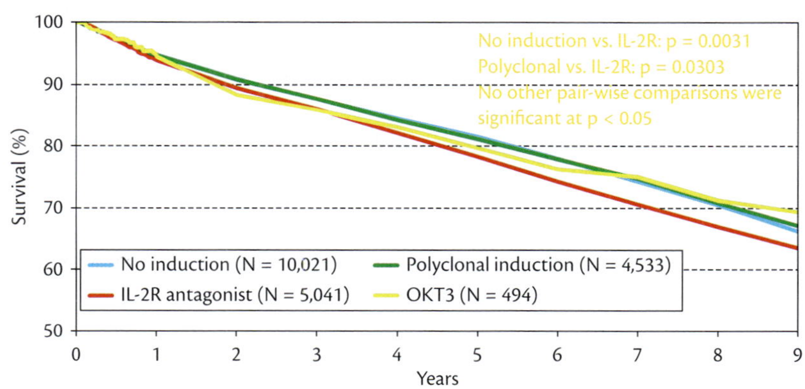

Fig. 19.5 Kaplan–Meier survival of heart transplant recipients by induction type or the absence of induction.

Reprinted from Journal of Heart and Lung Transplantation, 32, Lund LH, Edwards LB. Kucheryavaya AY, et al; The Registry of the International Society for Heart and Lung Transplantation: thirtieth official adult heart transplant report—2013; focus theme: age. International Society for Heart and Lung Transplantation, 951–64, copyright (2013) with permission from Elsevier.

Box 19.1 ISHLT working formulation for pathologic diagnosis of antibody-mediated rejection in heart transplantation

- pAMR 0 Negative for pathologic AMR; histologic and immunopathologic studies both negative
- pAMR 1 Suspicious for pathologic AMR; histologic findings positive, immunopathologic findings negative (pAMR 1-h), or immunopathologic findings positive, histologic findings negative (pAMR 1-i)
- pAMR 2 Positive pathologic AMR; histologic *and* immunopathologic findings both present
- pAMR 3 Severe pathologic AMR; interstitial hemorrhage, capillary fragmentation, mixed inflammatory infiltrates, endothelial cell pyknosis, and/or karyorrhexis and marked edema

Reprinted from Journal of Heart and Lung Transplantation, 30, Berry GJ et al., The ISHLT working formulation for pathologic diagnosis of antibody-mediated rejection in heart transplantation: evolution and current status (2005–2011), 601, copyright (2011) with permission from Elsevier.

decline in ventricular function and with anti-donor antigen specific antibodies is treated with intravenous corticosteroids, cytolytic therapy, IVIg, plasmapheresis, and rituximab.[17] This therapy would also be used in cardiac transplant patients presenting with cardiogenic shock where the actual results of the EMB might provide information regarding etiology but would not alter therapy.

Therapy for both ACR and AMR is empiric and may vary from center to center, as there have been no randomized clinical trials of any of these approaches.

Toxicity from immunosuppressive therapy

When discussing the option of cardiac transplantation with a patient, the term "trading one disease (advanced heart failure) for another (the post-transplantation state)" is often used and this reflects the two-edged sword of immunosuppressive therapy. While modern immunosuppressive therapy has reduced the mortality from rejection and made cardiac transplantation a viable and highly successful option for patients with advanced heart failure who have exhausted other options, it comes with a price, which are its numerous toxicities. Chief among these toxicities are the adverse renal effects of the CNIs, cyclosporine and tacrolimus. The CNIs have both acute and chronic effects. When these drugs are administered in the immediate post-transplantation period many if not most patients will experience a rise in their creatinine and in some cases, oliguria; these may happen even in patients with normal baseline renal function before transplantation. This effect is thought to be due to renal arterial vasoconstriction[18,19,20,21] and usually resolves within a few weeks after transplantation. The chronic effects are more insidious and develop over time. These chronic effects result from scarring and fibrosis in the kidney but may also be due to chronic vasoconstriction, which may explain why the chronic renal insufficiency observed in cardiac transplant recipients often improves with reduction or elimination of CNIs. It is clear that nephrotoxicity from CNIs has adverse prognostic implications and patients with elevated serum creatinine above 2.5 mg/dl beyond the first year after transplantation may have worse survival than those with lower creatinine (Figure 19.6).[18]

CNIs also cause hypertension as a result of their renovascular effects and activation of the renin–angiotensin–aldosterone system. It is estimated that over 90% of patients receiving cyclosporine and over 50% of those receiving tacrolimus are hypertensive, in spite of these patients being relatively hypotensive before transplantion. The post-transplantation hypertension may be resistant to therapy, often requiring multiple drugs to control it.

Other toxicities from CNIs include seizures, peripheral neuropathies, and posterior reversible encephalopathy syndrome (PRES).[22,23] Seizures and PRES are often exacerbated by elevated levels of CNI and may improve with reduction in CNI doses. PRES is caused in part by the hypertension that results from CNIs; mitochondrial dysfunction may also play a role.[24] In contrast, peripheral neuropathies develop after chronic use of CNIs and over a prolonged period of time. The peripheral neuropathy is seldom reversible but its progression may be slowed by reduction in CNI doses.

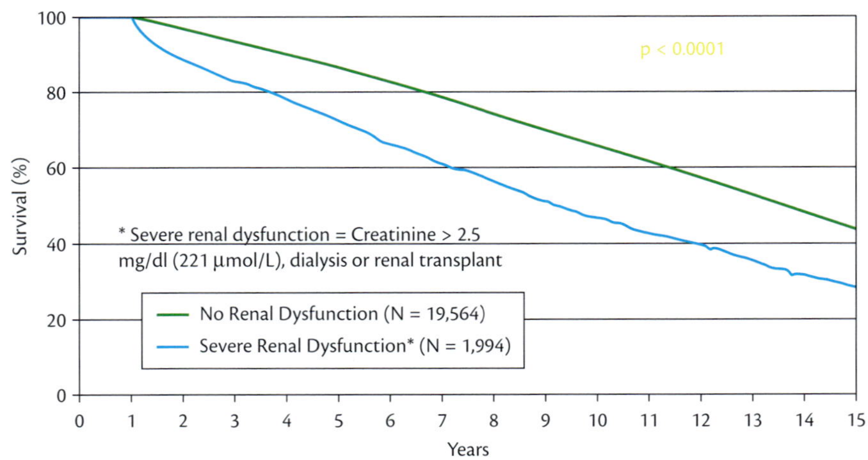

Fig. 19.6 Kaplan–Meier survival of heart transplant recipients by the presence or absence of severe renal dysfunction defined as a creatinine level greater than 2.5 mg/dl conditional on survival to 1 year.

Reprinted from Journal of Heart and Lung Transplantation, 32, Lund LH, Edwards LB, Kucheryavaya AY, et al; The Registry of the International Society for Heart and Lung Transplantation: thirtieth official adult heart transplant report—2013; focus theme: age. International Society for Heart and Lung Transplantation, 951–64, copyright (2013) with permission from Elsevier.

While not life threatening, gout is a frequent, painful, and debilitating sequel of organ transplantation.[25] Gout in these patients may occur more frequently than in nontransplant patients, may be more severe in its symptoms, and is more likely to develop in joints other than the podagra (great toes of the feet) including knees and joints of the upper extremities. Treatment is similar to the approaches used in nontransplant patients and includes intra-articular injection of corticosteroids and colchicine. Concomitant use of allopurinol and azathioprine should be avoided because of synergistic inhibitory effects on lymphocyte DNA synthesis, resulting in profound leukopenia.

Cyclosporine can cause hirsutism and gingival hyperplasia, both reversible when the cyclosporine doses are decreased. Tacrolimus in contrast causes alopecia and does not cause hirsutism. Switching from cyclosporine to tacrolimus can ameliorate the gingival hyperplasia.[5,10]

MMF can cause reversible leukopenia, which is usually mild. More frequent and more likely to result in cessation of MMF are the gastrointestinal side effects which can include diarrhea, abdominal pain, constipation, nausea, anorexia, and reflux-type symptoms. These side effects may occur in over 50% of patients receiving MMF.[11,12] The mechanism of the gastrointestinal side effects appears to be apoptosis of colonic crypt and duodenal, gastric, and esophageal cells.[26,27] These side effects are also reversible with dose reduction or cessation of MMF. Enteric-coated mycophenolic acid was introduced in the hope that it would result in fewer gastrointestinal side effects and this preparation may relieve gastrointestinal symptoms in some patients.[28]

MMF has been associated with increased first-trimester pregnancy loss and increased risk of congenital abnormalities of the external ear, facial, limb, kidney, heart, and esophagus and has been assigned to pregnancy category D by the US Food and Drug Administration (FDA).[29] Cleft palate, in particular, has been noted. A Risk Evaluation and Mitigation Strategy for MMF has been mandated by the FDA to inform healthcare providers about the risks of using MMF during pregnancy and its continued use during pregnancy should only occur if there are no alternatives.[29] Transplant patients interested in becoming pregnant should be switched from MMF to another agent.

Azathioprine has largely, though not completely, been supplanted by MMF because of the latter's demonstrated superiority in preventing rejection and improving survival.[11,12] Azathioprine may produce the same gastrointestinal side effects and leukopenia as MMF. Of particular significance is the potentiation of the risk of developing cancer in patients receiving azathioprine. It is thought that 6-thioguanine, a metabolite of azathioprine, may accumulate in skin cells and, in conjunction with ultraviolet light exposure or prior injury for ultraviolet light, result in the development of basal and squamous cell carcinomas.[30,31] Squamous cell carcinomas are 65–250 times more likely to develop in patients receiving azathioprine.[30,31]

The mTOR inhibitors (or PSIs) have a variety of side effects that can complicate post-transplantation patient care. When either sirolimus or everolimus is used with full-dose cyclosporine, renal insufficiency with elevated serum creatinine and reduced glomerular filtration rate (GFR) can occur.[32] Consequently, efforts should be made to reduce CNI doses beyond the first month after transplantation in patients also receiving mTOR inhibitors. In most cases, the renal insufficiency will abate with reduction in CNI dose. mTOR inhibitors may also affect wound healing. Early use of sirolimus postoperatively in de-novo heart transplant recipients resulted in an increased likelihood of surgical wound healing complications.[33] Three everolimus clinical trials did not show an increased risk of wound healing problems but the largest of these studies showed that de-novo transplant recipients receiving everolimus in the early post-transplantation period were more likely to develop significant pericardial effusions including those requiring drainage.[32,34,35] mTOR inhibitors can also cause leukopenia and rarely pancytopenia. These are reversible when mTOR inhibitor doses are decreased. Rashes and edema can also occur, especially with sirolimus. Perhaps the most dangerous side effect is pulmonary fibrosis and inflammation, which can occur abruptly and be highly debilitating as well as life threatening. Although rare, pulmonary toxicity from everolimus and sirolimus can require mechanical ventilation. It also is usually reversible after cessation of mTORs; they should not be reinitiated in patients who have had pulmonary toxicity.

Infection

Infections remain a threat throughout the lifetime of transplant recipients, as a consequence of the immunosuppression required to prevent rejection. This is particularly true in the first year after transplantation when infection is one of the three major causes of death (along with rejection and primary graft dysfunction).[1] The types of infection seen in cardiac transplant recipients vary depending on the time after transplantation (Figure 19.7).[36] Nosocomial infections most commonly occur in the first month after transplantation and are due to mechanical ventilation, intravascular lines, Foley catheters, and wound infections, paralleling the common postsurgical infections. These infections may be particularly lethal given the emergence of bacteria highly resistant to a variety of antibiotics. For example, certain strains of klebsiella are now sensitive only to colistin. Care needs to be taken to minimize exposure to infectious diseases by removing catheters and unnecessary intravenous lines and extubating patients as quickly as possible. An increasingly common sequela of antibiotic treatment of infections is *Clostridium difficile* colitis. A high index of suspicion should be maintained for the diagnosis of this sometimes fatal infection in patients who develop diarrhea during or after a course of antibiotics.

Infections in cardiac transplant recipients can be from fungi, viruses, and protozoans as well as bacteria and of these, fungal infections carry the highest mortality. During the period of most intense immunosuppression, which is during the first year and particularly during the first 6 months after transplantation, efforts are made to prevent these infections. Trimethoprim sulfamethoxazole is used to prevent pneumocystis pneumonia and also can prevent listeria and toxoplasmosis infections.[15] Patients allergic to sulfa drugs should receive either atovaquone or dapsone. Clotrimoxazole should be used for 3 months to prevent oral candidiasis. Cytomegalovirus (CMV) is a significant cause of post-transplantation morbidity and mortality. These infections develop after the first month post-transplantation. Valganciclovir is used for prophylaxis and the duration of therapy depends on the CMV serologic status of the donor and recipient.[15,36] CMV-positive patients who receive either CMV seropositive or seronegative donor hearts should receive valganciclovir for 6 months. The highest-risk patients, CMV-negative patients who receive hearts from CMV-positive donors should receive valgancyclovir for 1 year, given the high risk of transmission

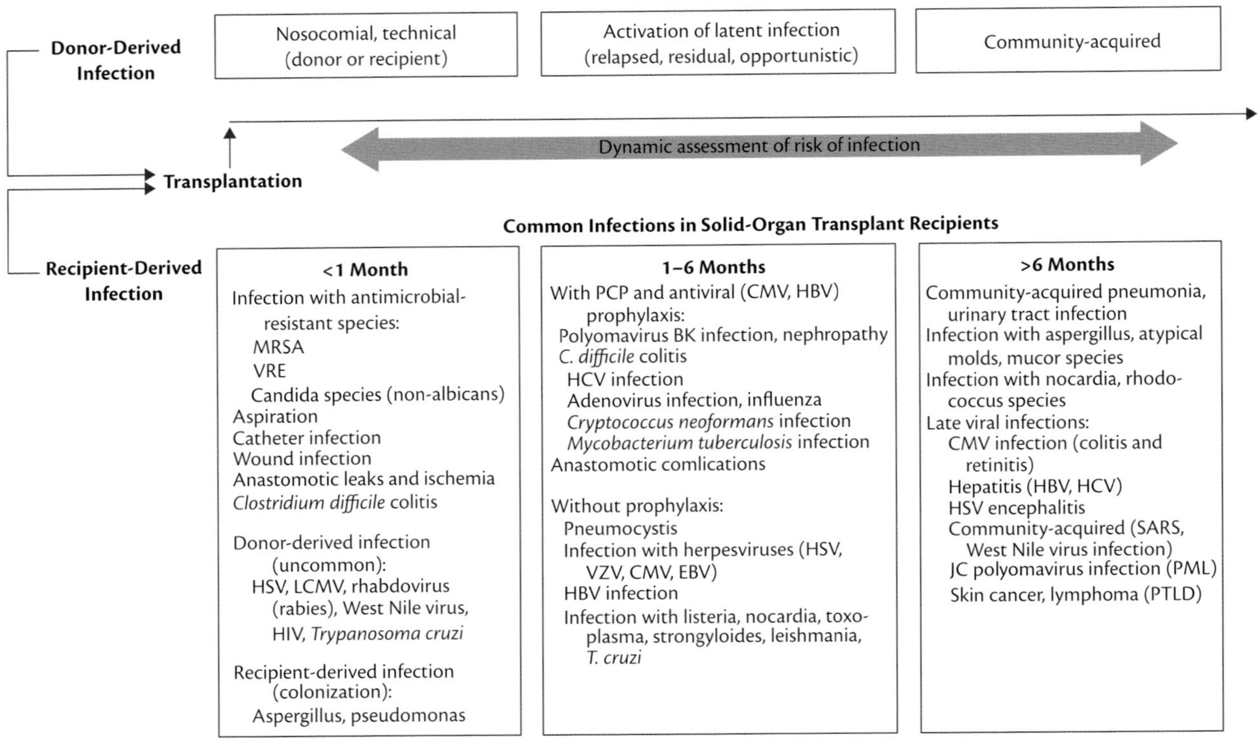

Fig. 19.7 Types of infection in solid organ transplant recipients based on time after transplantation.
From New England Journal of Medicine, Fishman J, Medical Progress: Infection in Solid-Organ Transplant Recipients, 357:2601–14, Copyright © Massachusetts Medical Society. Reprinted with permission from Massachusetts Medical Society.

and the likely development of primary CMV infections. If not prevented, these are often associated with significant morbidity and mortality, including CMV febrile illness and tissue invasion of the lungs, colon and gastrointestinal tract, liver, heart, and brain. In contrast, the lowest-risk patients for CMV, serologically negative recipients of serologically negative donor hearts, can potentially forgo valgancyclovir altogether and receive aciclovir for 3 months instead (which should also prevent herpes simplex infections). CMV infections can still occur after CMV prophylaxis has been completed. In patients presenting with a febrile illness or clinical syndromes that suggest CMV tissue invasion, documentation of the infection can be made by polymerase chain reaction (PCR) quantification of CMV viral copies and, for tissue infection, by biopsy of the organ in question (e.g., bronchoscopy for suspected pneumonitis). Treatment should be either valganciclovir or intravenous ganciclovir and response to therapy should be monitored by clinical improvement and reduction in CMV viral copies by PCR.

Epstein–Barr virus (EBV) infections, either as primary infections or reactivation, can cause mononucleosis type syndromes with fever, malaise, fatigue, and pancytopenia. They can also cause post-transplantation lymphoproliferative syndrome (PTLD) that is discussed further in the malignancy section.[37,38] Rituximab, an anti-CD20 antibody, is used to treat the severe febrile illness as well as PTLD.[39] EBV PCR can be used to to manage PTLD by monitoring the response to reductions in immunosuppression and to rituximab.[40] There are no specific antiviral agents for EBV.

Fungal infections are associated with a higher mortality than other infections. Candidiasis most commonly involves the esophagus but can also cause pneumonitis and can infect other organs. It can be treated with fluconazole. Aspergillus infections most commonly cause pneumonia, though other organs may be involved. This is usually treated with voriconoazole. Aspergillus infection prophylaxis is employed by some transplant programs, but not all, because of the rarity of these infections and the potential toxicities of antifungal agents.

Reduction of immunosuppression is critical to reducing the risk of infection in cardiac transplant recipients but this has to be balanced against the risk of developing ACR, AMR, or CAV. One approach has been to use a commercially available assay of ATP release from activated lymphocytes in peripheral blood. Lower assay scores are associated with the development of infections within 1 month of the assay measurement and thus may suggest over-immunosuppression.[41,42] Some groups have used these assays to reduce immunosuppression by decreasing MMF or CNI doses when lower scores are obtained.

Chronic renal failure

CNIs have dramatically improved clinical outcomes and have become the cornerstone of modern immunosuppression. They have, however, appropriately been referred to as a two-edged sword because of their toxicities. Significant nephrotoxicity is one of the most frequent. CNI toxicity can be acute, occurring within the first few days after transplantation when the recipient first receives CNIs. While acute nephrotoxicity usually improves, a more chronic form of CNI nephrotoxicity (defined as a GFR <29 ml min^{-1} 1.73 m^{-2} body surface area) was observed in 16.5% of 69 321 nonrenal transplant patients identified from the Scientific Registry of Transplant Recipients (SRTR); 28.9% of patients with nephrotoxicity needed chronic dialysis or renal transplantation.[18] For cardiac transplant recipients, the risk was 10.9% at 5 years. Risk factors for the development of renal failure after transplantation included increasing age, female sex, hypertension, diabetes, and postoperative acute renal failure. Chronic renal failure was associated with increased mortality in these patients. For cardiac transplant recipients, there was no difference in the risk of renal failure based on the type of CNI used. Beyond the mechanisms associated with CNI-induced nephrotoxicity such as renal arteriolar vasoconstriction from enhanced endothelin, and reduced nitric oxide production, other mechanisms for chronic nephrotoxicity include interstitial fibrosis, tubular atrophy, and hyalinosis of renal arterioles.[43,44] Hemodynamic compromise with diminished renal perfusion before transplantation can also set the stage for post-transplantation nephrotoxicity. Greater awareness of the adverse consequences of post-transplantation chronic renal failure has resulted in efforts to reduce CNI doses more aggressively and to develop reduced CNI or even CNI-sparing immunosuppressive protocols.[45,46] The timing of when to initiate changes in immunosuppression to improve renal function is not clear and an increased risk of ACR has been observed during the conversion to CNI-sparing or CNI-free protocols.[45,46]

Diabetes mellitus

The use of corticosteroids, specifically high-dose corticosteroids, in the first few weeks after transplantation can exacerbate, or result in the development, of diabetes mellitus, making efforts to reduce and wean patients off corticosteroids within the first 6 months to 1 year after transplantation a priority. Pretransplantation risk factors for new onset of diabetes mellitus (NODM) include increased age, obesity, family history of diabetes mellitus, abnormal glucose tolerance, and the metabolic syndrome, as well as Hispanic or African American ethnicity.[47,48] CNIs, particularly tacrolimus, which may decrease β-cell secretion of insulin, have increasingly been recognized as contributory.[49] The weight gain seen after transplantation as a result of corticosteroid use can also increase insulin resistance. Strategies for mitigating NODM include aggressive steroid weaning, efforts to promote weight loss after transplantation including exercise programs, and switching from tacrolimus to cyclosporine. Specific treatment regimens for NODM have not been defined and consultation with an endocrinologist is important.

Hyperlipidemia

Ischemic cardiomyopathy is a common cause of the heart failure that results in patients requiring cardiac transplantation. Consequently, many patients have hyperlipidemia before cardiac transplantation. This may only become worse after transplantation and many patients without prior hyperlipidemia become hyperlipidemic afterward. This can be accounted for by the immunosuppression used. Corticosteroids increase the synthesis of free fatty acids as well as insulin receptors.[49] CNIs bind to LDL receptors and thus increase serum LDL.[49] mTOR inhibitors cause hypercholesterolemia and hyperlipidemia, for reasons that are not entirely clear. Triglycerides also increase as a result of increased insulin resistance. The relationship of hyperlipidemia to the development of CAV is tenuous and certainly weaker than for nontransplant coronary artery atherosclerosis, but hyperlipidemia can predispose to atherosclerosis in other vascular beds such as the cerebrovascular and peripheral circulation, putting patients at risk for strokes and peripheral vascular disease. HMG-CoA reductase inhibitors are routinely used in all cardiac transplant recipients and this is a class I indication in the ISHLT heart transplant guidelines.[15] Their benefits extend beyond a reduction in LDL cholesterol, and pravastatin and simvastatin have been shown to improve survival, reduce the incidence of CAV and ACR, and reduce the severity of CAV.[50,51] These beneficial effects appear to be due to the anti-inflammatory effects of statins.[52] The actual LDL targets for treatment have not been defined in cardiac transplant recipients and so targets from nontransplant patients are often extrapolated to transplant patients. Simvastatin, but not pravastatin, is metabolized by CYP 3A4, as are the CNIs, and concomitant use can result in an increased risk of rhabdomyolysis. Therefore, lower doses of statins, such as simvastatin, should be used and an effort should be made to prescribe doses used in clinical trials.

Hypertension

Hypertension is frequent in cardiac transplant recipients and is due primarily to CNIs which increase endothelin levels and also cause renal insufficiency. Post-transplantation hypertension lacks the diurnal variation seen in nontransplant patients with hypertension. Tacrolimus-treated patients are less likely to develop hypertension.[53] Post-transplantation hypertension is often difficult to treat and may require multiple antihypertensive medications. As CNI doses are decreased over time, fewer medications may be required to treat the hypertension.

Osteoporosis

Many patients with advanced heart failure are osteopenic before heart transplantation as a result of relative malnutrition and vitamin D deficiency.[54] This is exacerbated after transplantation as a result of corticosteroids and osteoporosis often progresses, especially in the first 12 months post-transplantation. Weaning of corticosteroids mitigates this bone loss. Cardiac transplant recipients are often treated with vitamin D and calcium supplements. Biphosphonates are also often used to treat osteoporosis.[55]

Malignancy

One of the two major causes of death after the first year post-transplantation is malignancy (Figure 19.8).[1] By 8 years after transplantation, 26% of patients have developed malignancies.[56] The risk of malignancy in cardiac transplant recipients is substantially higher than in the nontransplant population. The malignancies occurring in cardiac transplant recipients are a heterogeneous group but the most frequent are squamous cell carcinomas which occur in 18% of cardiac transplant recipients.[56] Transplant patients are also susceptible to a unique type of malignancy, post-transplant lymphoproliferative disorder (PTLD), which is usually caused by EBV.[57] Kaposi sarcoma is caused by human herpesvirus 8 and occurs more frequently in transplant recipients than in the nontransplant population.[58] Other carcinogenic factors whose effects may be enhanced after transplant include ultraviolet light (for skin cancers) and smoking (for lung cancer). Among the malignancies PTLD and lung cancer are major causes of death, but any malignancy occurring in transplant recipients may have a more aggressive course. Certain malignancies such as breast, prostate,

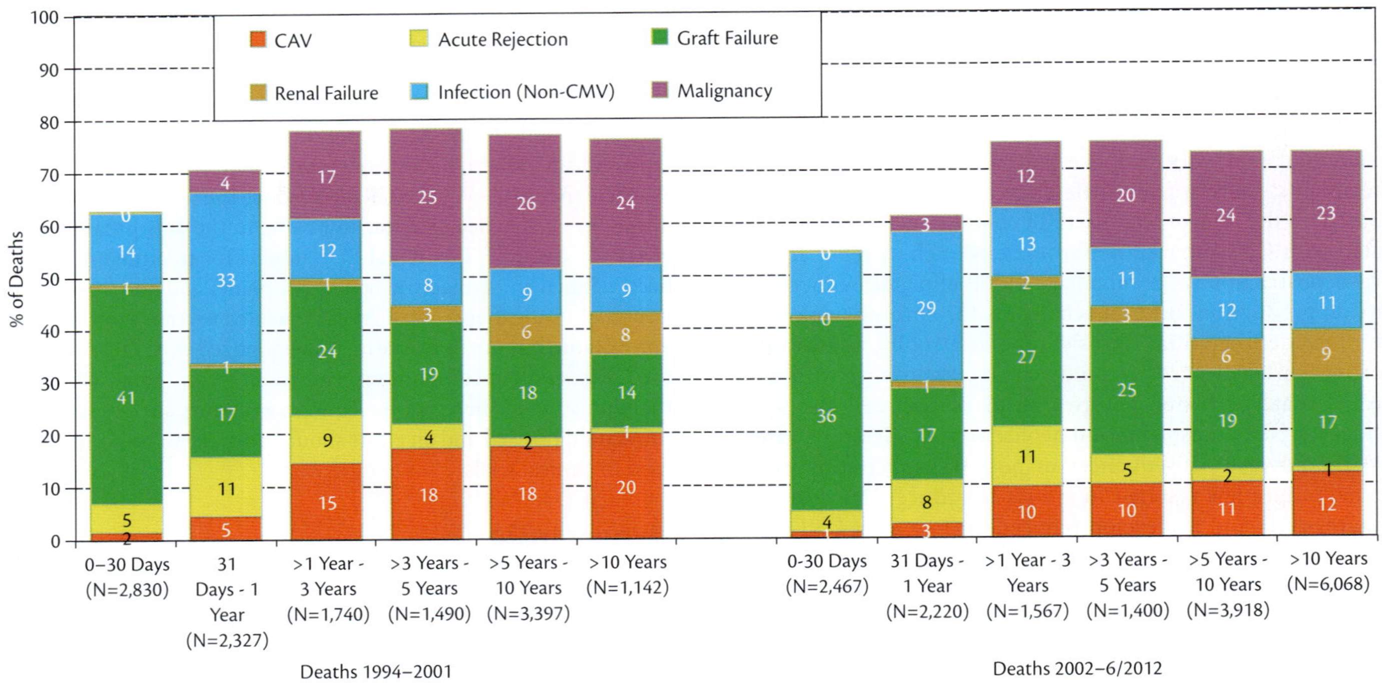

Fig. 19.8 Leading causes of death based on time after transplantation. Most late graft failures are due to cardiac allograft vasculopathy.
Reprinted from Journal of Heart and Lung Transplantation, 32, Lund LH, Edwards LB, Kucheryavaya AY, et al; The Registry of the International Society for Heart and Lung Transplantation: thirtieth official adult heart transplant report—2013; focus theme: age International Society for Heart and Lung Transplantation, 951–64, copyright (2013) with permission from Elsevier.

and colon cancer do not have an increased incidence in transplant recipients.[59]

The increased risk of malignancy is related to immunosuppression and inhibition of both immune surveillance and anti-tumor responses, usually mediated by T cells. The risk of malignancy is further increased by the totality of the immunosuppression used. Long courses of induction with OKT-3, for example, have been associated with a high risk of PTLD.[60,61] Certain immunosuppressive agents are more likely to increase the risk of developing malignancies. Azathioprine is associated with a markedly increased risk of squamous cell carcinoma and this may be related to direct DNA damage in these cells.[61,62] CNIs may also increase the risk of developing malignancies.[63,64] In contrast, the use of mTOR inhibitors may be associated with a reduced risk of malignancy.[65,66,67,68] mTOR is involved in proliferation of cells, including malignant cells, so its inhibition would be expected to reduce proliferation of malignant cells. A retrospective analysis of SRTR data showed that renal transplant recipients receiving either CNI and mTOR inhibitors or mTOR inhibitors without CNI were significantly less likely to develop malignancies than those receiving CNIs without mTOR inhibitors.[69] Conversion of renal transplant recipients with Kaposi sarcoma from CNI-based immunosuppression to mTOR-based immunosuppression resulted in regression of the sarcoma.[70] mTOR inhibitors (in higher doses) are also used and FDA approved as adjunctive therapy for patients with renal cell carcinoma and breast cancer.[13]

Screening for malignancy in cardiac transplant recipients generally follows the recommendations of the American Cancer Society although it is not clear if modifications should be made in this algorithm. For example, chest CT scans may be a reasonable addition for cardiac transplant recipients who were smokers. Patients with a history of skin cancers should undergo more frequent evaluations by dermatologists: at the author's institution, a transplant dermatology clinic has been established to aggressively screen patients for recurrent or de-novo skin cancers in patients with fair skin and significant prior sun exposure. Patients are also advised to use the highest-strength sun block.

Once a malignancy has been diagnosed, in addition to the appropriate medical and surgical therapy for that malignancy, immunosuppression should be reduced and mTOR inhibitors are often added for their antiproliferative and presumptive antimalignancy effects. There have been no clinical trials to verify the utility of this approach.

Cardiac allograft vasculopathy

CAV represents the other major cause of death beyond the first year after transplantation and, along with malignancy, represents one of the significant factors limiting long-term survival in many cardiac transplant recipients.[1] CAV is a disease that is specific to cardiac transplant recipients. Histologically, it resembles restenosis after angioplasty with smooth muscle cell proliferation, but is far more extensive than restenosis (Figure 19.9).[71] This would indicate that, as with restenosis, CAV is a response to injury although the exact type of injury is not clear. Potential causes of vascular injury include the alloimmune responses to the donor heart vasculature, specifically ACR and AMR. The number and severity of acute rejection episodes and the presence of anti-endothelial antibodies increase the risk of developing CAV.[72,73,74,75,76,77] Hyperlipidemia and CMV infections are associated with the development of CAV but the mechanism by which they contribute to pathogenesis is unclear.[78,79,80,81,82] Nonimmunologic events and factors associated

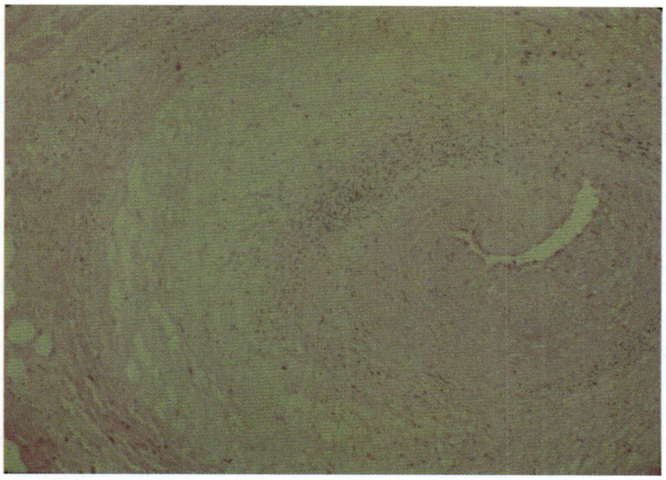

Fig. 19.9 Photomicrograph of cross-section of left anterior descending coronary artery from patient who died of cardiac allograft vasculopathy, showing intimal hyperplasia.

with the development of CAV include ischemia–reperfusion injury at the time of organ procurement and transplant as well as the physiology attending donor brain death.[83] These result in the elaboration of cytokines, growth factors, and other inflammatory factors. It is likely the sum total of injuries to the allograft determine the risk of developing CAV.

Histologically, CAV is very different from the atherosclerosis seen in nontransplant patients. It is panvscular as opposed to restricted largely to the epicardial vessels. Progression is rapid and obliteration of the arterial lumen can occur in just a few years as opposed to the decades that it takes for "garden variety" atherosclerosis to develop. CAV lesions are concentric and lipid poor while nontransplant atherosclerosis lesions are eccentric and lipid-rich. Calcification occurs early in nontransplant atherosclerosis but if it occurs at all in CAV, it is late. Finally, arterial dilatation, a form of compensatory remodeling that is observed in nontransplant atherosclerosis, is not seen in CAV.

The extent of CAV in post-transplantation patients has been determined from a number of sources. Using coronary angiography, the most widely available vascular imaging technique, the Cardiac Transplant Research Database (CTRD) reviewed 4736 angiograms in 2609 patients from 39 institutions and found that 42% of patients had angiographic evidence of CAV at 5 years but only 7% had severe disease, defined as more than 70% stenosis in the left main artery, two or more primary epicardial arteries, or three branch arteries in all three coronary arteries.[84] Overall 7% of patients died or needed retransplantation but in the severe CAV groups two-thirds reached either of these endpoints. The United Network for Organ Sharing (UNOS) registry reported a prevalence of 23% at 5 years.[85] The ISHLT registry noted a prevalence of 8%, 30%, and 51% respectively of CAV for patients 1, 5 and 10 years after transplant and noted a decline in CAV incidence in the 2001–07 time period compared to the 1994–2001 time period.[56]

The transplanted heart is denervated, so ischemic events are usually silent. Some patients reinnervate their transplanted hearts several years after transplantation and may therefore develop chest pain although their symptoms may be atypical.[86,87] Electrocardiography may also demonstrate atypical patterns of ischemia. Consequently, patients undergo routine coronary angiography for at least the first 5 years after transplantation to detect the presence of CAV.[15] Angiography should also be performed in patients with dyspnea and with arrhythmias suggestive of left ventricular dysfunction not attributable to either type of rejection. The presence or any angiographic disease indicates a 3.4-fold increased risk of major adverse cardiac events and a 4.6-fold increased likelihood of death at 3.5 years follow-up.[88]

A variety of diagnostic modalities that have been employed to detect CAV, but the most widely available is coronary angiography. The ISHLT therefore developed a nomenclature to define the presence and severity of CAV.[89] Severity is defined by the extent of disease, severity of stenosis, and the presence of restrictive heart disease (Box 19.2).The severity of CAV as defined by the ISHLT nomenclature correlates with prognosis.

Intravascular ultrasound (IVUS) provides useful morphologic and prognostic information regarding CAV. IVUS can provide volumetric measures such as luminal area as well as cross-sectional

Box 19.2 ISHLT cardiac allograft vasculopathy nomenclature

ISHLT CAV0	Not significant	No detectable angiographic lesion
ISHLT CAV1	Mild	Angiographic left main (LM) <50%,[a] or primary vessel[b] with maximum lesion of <70%, or any branch stenosis <70% (including diffuse narrowing) without allograft dysfunction
ISHLT CAV2	Moderate	Angiographic LM ≥50%; a single primary vessel ≥70%, or isolated branch stenosis ≥70% in branches of two systems, without allograft dysfunction
ISHLT CAV3	Severe	Angiographic LM ≥50%, or two or more primary vessels ≥70% stenosis, or isolated branch stenosis ≥70% in all three systems; or ISHLT CAV1 or CAV2 with allograft dysfunction (defined as LVEF ≤45%) or evidence of significant restrictive physiology[c]

[a] Normal graft function.

[b] A primary vessel denotes the proximal and middle 33% of the left anterior descending artery, the left circumflex, the ramus, and the dominant or codominant right coronary artery with the posterior descending and posterolateral branches. A secondary branch vessel includes the distal 33% of the primary vessels or any segment within a large septal perforator, diagonals and obtuse marginal branches, or any portion of a nondominant right coronary artery.

[c] Restrictive cardiac allograft physiology is defined as symptomatic heart failure with echocardiographic E/A velocity ratio >2 (>1.5 in children), shortened isovolumetric relaxation time (<60 ms), shortened deceleration time (<150 ms), or restrictive hemodynamic values (right atrial pressure >12 mmHg, pulmonary capillary wedge pressure >25 mmHg, cardiac index <2 L $min^{-1}m^{-2}$).

measures such as intimal area. Changes over time can be carefully assessed from serial IVUS studies. One parameter, change in maximal intimal thickness from baseline to 1 year on IVUS studies, has been shown to have robust prognostic implications. A change in maximal intimal thickness of 0.5 mm or more from the baseline to the 1-year study has been shown to predict major adverse cardiac events and reduced survival at 5 years after transplantation.[90,91,92] IVUS is often used in clinical trials of immunosuppression as a surrogate marker of CAV. However, the procedure is invasive, requires the use of contrast material and is usually not reimbursed by insurance, so its use is primarily for research.

Noninvasive approaches have also been utilized to diagnose CAV but lack the prognostic and morphometric effectiveness of the invasive procedures. Of the noninvasive tests, dobutamine stress-echocardiography (DSE) is the most commonly used and validated approach with a sensitivity of 85% for the presence of CAV; patients with negative DSEs have a good prognosis.[93,94,95] One role for DSE is as a screen to decide whether patients should proceed to angiography but this should not be used as an alternative in the first 5 years after transplantation.

As opposed to ACR, CAV has proved to be impervious to traditional immunosuppressive agents. Two randomized clinical trials of statins (pravastatin or simvastatin) demonstrated that these agents reduce the incidence and severity of CAV.[50,51] This represented the first evidence that medical therapy could affect the development of CAV. The multicenter randomized trial of MMF versus azathioprine showed minimally significant changes in maximal intimal thickness and no significant changes in other IVUS measures or in angiographic severity of disease.[11,12] Beyond the use of statins, no significant change in immunosuppression to treat or reverse CAV occurred until the mTOR inhibitors were introduced in clinical trials.

A randomized clinical trial of pravastatin started within 4 days after transplantation compared to placebo (both in conjunction with standard immunosuppression) showed a significant reduction in the severity of CAV defined by IVUS and by angiography as well as an improvement in 1-year survival.[50] Similar results were published 8 years later in a randomized trial of simvastatin compared to placebo.[51]

An earlier randomized clinical trial of diltiazem compared to placebo showed benefits in the effect on CAV severity but this was determined using quantitative angiography and not IVUS.[96] A retrospective analysis showed that statins but not diltiazem reduced the progression of CAV.[97]

The randomized double-blind clinical trial of MMF compared to azathioprine showed a trend toward a significant reduction in change in maximal intimal thickness determined by IVUS, but no trends or statistically significant differences in other IVUS parameters or the results of quantitative angiography were shown between the two groups.[11,12] A post-hoc analysis of the IVUS data from the MMF–azathioprine study using more contemporary methods of analysis showed a reduction in change of maximal intimal thickness from baseline to 1-year of 0.3 mm but no difference for the more robust and validated change of 0.5 mm between baseline and 1-year IVUS.[98]

Vitamin C and E when added to standard immunosuppressive therapy reduced the progression of CAV, as shown by IVUS in a small group of patients.[99]

mTOR or PSIs have been compared to other antiproliferative agents in a number of clinical trials. Two different doses of sirolimus were compared to azathioprine in an open-label study in Australia and New Zealand.[100] Progression of CAV defined by the change in a number of IVUS parameters, including maximal from baseline to 6 months after transplantation, was significantly reduced in sirolimus-treated but not azathioprine-treated patients. Despite similar cyclosporine trough levels, serum creatinines were significantly elevated in the sirolimus-treated patients. Biopsy-proven ISHLT grade 2R rejection was also significantly reduced in the sirolimus-treated patients.

A larger randomized double-blind trial compared the mTOR inhibitor everolimus (either 1.5 mg or 3.0 mg daily) to azathioprine in 634 patients from Europe and North and South America.[32] Biopsy-proven ISHLT grade 2R rejection and viral infections, including CMV, were significantly reduced in the everolimus-treated patients compared to the azathioprine-treated patients. Bacterial infections and hypertriglyceridemia were more frequent in the everolimus-treated patients. Everolimus significantly attenuated the increases in maximum intimal thickness from baseline to 1-year after transplantation as measured by IVUS and favorably affected other IVUS parameters. The incidence of CAV defined by IVUS was also significantly reduced in the two everolimus groups compared to the azathioprine group. As in the previously mentioned sirolimus study, serum creatinines were increased and GFRs were decreased in the everolimus groups despite similar cyclosporine trough levels, suggesting potentiation of the nephrotoxic effects of cyclosporine by the mTOR inhibitors. The everolimus trial was amended to allow for reduced target trough levels of cyclosporine to improve renal function. Rejection frequency in the everolimus-treated patients after the first 2 weeks after transplantation was not affected by cyclosporine trough levels between 50 and 400 ng/ml provided the everolimus level was in the 3–8 ng/ml range.[101]

A criticism of both of these studies was that they used azathioprine as a comparator when MMF was more potent and ultimately displaced azathioprine as the antiproliferative of choice. At the time that these trials commenced, MMF was not universally available. A 176-patient randomized open-label trial compared everolimus (3–8 ng/ml) with reduced dose and target trough levels of cyclosporine to MMF and standard cyclosporine dose and trough levels.[34] No difference was seen in the frequency of ISHLT grade 2R rejection but CMV infections were less frequent. The GFR was only 3.1 ml/min less in the everolimus group at month 12. IVUS was not performed in this study.

A 24-month open-label comparison of everolimus (1.5 mg or 3.0 mg daily) with reduced dose and target trough levels of cyclosporine to MMF and standard cyclosporine dose and trough levels was performed in 721 patients from Europe, Asia, Australia, and North and South America.[8] There was no difference in the incidence of biopsy-proven ISHLT grade 2R rejection between the groups. The 3.0 mg everolimus group was stopped early due to numerically increased mortality. Mortality was also higher up to month 3 in the 1.5 mg everolimus-treated patients receiving anti-thymocyte globulin; no difference was seen in everolimus-treated patients who did not receive induction therapy. By month 24, mortality was similar between the 1.5 mg everolimus-treated and MMF groups. As was observed before, CMV infections were less common but bacterial infections, though not sepsis, were more common in the 1.5 mg everolimus patients. Pericardial effusions, including those requiring drainage, were more common in the everolimus group. Renal function was inferior in the entire 1.5 mg everolimus group compared to the MMF group and this was accounted for by centers that failed to achieve the predefined reduction in trough cyclosporine levels; patients who did achieve these predefined reductions had comparable GFRs to the MMF patients. Most notable in this study was the IVUS-documented attenuation of CAV with a reduction in the change in maximum intimal thickness from baseline to 1 year in the everolimus-treated 1.5 mg patients compared to the MMF patients. The incidence of CAV was also significantly reduced in patients receiving everolimus. These findings were observed regardless of sex, age, diabetic status, donor disease, and the presence of hyperlipidemia.[102]

While everolimus is approved by the FDA for renal and liver transplantation, it has not been approved for heart transplantation (it is approved in Europe and elsewhere). Sirolimus has been available for over a decade in the US but when used in the early post-transplantation period, it has been associated with more post-surgical wound healing complications and pleural and pericardial effusions.[33] Kushwaha and colleagues used three-dimensional IVUS to evaluate progression of CAV in heart transplant patients and found that the switch to sirolimus (mean 3.8 ± 3.5 years post-transplant) both with CNI and in CNI-free regimens was associated with attenuation of this progression.[103] A subsequent study by this group retrospectively analyzed patients switched to sirolimus (mean 1.2 years) with complete CNI withdrawal and found that CAV progression assessed by IVUS was attenuated and 5-year survival and freedom from major adverse cardiac events was improved in these patients compared to controls.[104] These studies suggest that benefits can still be derived from mTOR inhibitors even when they are started more than a year after transplantation although a more recent study suggested that there was no benefit past 2 years post-transplantation.

The options for patients with established CAV are somewhat limited, with less clinical data upon which to make decisions than in patients with nontransplant atherosclerosis. Because of their antiproliferative effects, mTOR inhibitors have been studied in small series of cardiac transplant patients with established CAV. Mancini and colleagues showed that adding sirolimus to the immunosuppressive regimen of these patients resulted in attenuation of CAV progression defined by IVUS, angiography, and clinical events.[105] Segovia used IVUS to assess CAV progression over 1 year in cardiac transplant patients identified angiographically with either a 50% or more lesion in a major coronary artery or 70% or more lesions in two branch arteries. They found reduced progression or even regression after initiation of everolimus compared to controls taking standard therapy with mTOR inhibitors.[106,107] No difference in major adverse cardiac events was noted in this small study. Ultimately, the efficacy of mTOR inhibitors in the treatment of established CAV in heart transplant recipients will need to be established in larger randomized clinical trials.

Percutaneous and surgical revascularization therapies have been used in cardiac transplant patients with established CAV. Early success rates are excellent for single-vessel percutaneous coronary interventions (PCI) but restenosis rates at least equal if not exceed those observed in nontransplant atherosclerosis.[108,109,110] Retrospective analyses of bare metal versus drug-eluting stents suggests that the latter were associated with less restenosis and lumen loss than the former in cardiac transplant patients.[111,112]

Coronary artery bypass graft surgery has been used in only a small number of cardiac transplant recipients because of the diffuse nature of CAV, which makes many arteries poor targets for this procedure, and because of inferior outcomes compared to non-transplant recipients.[113]

The only definitive treatment for CAV is retransplantation, which can provide excellent outcomes in carefully selected patients with CAV.[114] Retransplantation should be avoided as a treatment for ACR or AMR with hemodynamic compromise as the outcomes in these patients are poor. Whether it is ethical to retransplant a patient whose allograft is failing is controversial given the scarcity of donor organs.

Summary

The management of cardiac transplant recipients has improved dramatically over the past several decades. Factors that contribute to this improvement include better postoperative intensive care management, more effective prevention of ACR and opportunistic infections after transplantation, more effective treatment of nosocomial infections, and more accurate assessments of antibody cross-reactivity between donor and recipient resulting in less early AMR. Outcomes have improved significantly but these have mainly occurred in the first 6 months after transplantation. Long-term complications, including toxicity from immunosuppressive agents, malignancy, and CAV, remain a challenge. New immunosuppressive agents and more effective ways of utilizing immunosuppressive agents as well as novel strategies for assessing immune system response to the transplant and modulating immunosuppression accordingly may improve long-term outcomes and reduce adverse events.

References

1. Lund LH, Edwards LB, Kucheryavaya AY, et al. The Registry of the International Society for Heart and Lung Transplantation: thirtieth official adult heart transplant report—2013; focus theme: age International Society for Heart and Lung Transplantation. J Heart Lung Transplant 2013;32:951–64.
2. Halloran PD. Immunosuppressive drugs for kidney transplantation. N Engl J Med 2004;351:2715–29.
3. Liu Z, Colovai AI, Tugulea S, et al. Indirect recognition of donor HLA-DR peptides in organ allograft rejection. J Clin Invest 1996;98:1150.
4. Vella JP, Magee C, Vos L, et al. Cellular and humoral mechanisms of vascularized allograft rejection induced by indirect recognition of donor MHC allopeptides. Transplantation 1999;67:1523.
5. Lindenfeld J, Miller GG, Shakar, et al. Drug therapy in the heart transplant recipient: part I: cardiac rejection and immunosuppressive drugs. Circulation 2004;110:3734–40.
6. Stewart S, Winters GL, Fishbein MC, et al. Revision of the 1990 working formulation for the standardization of nomenclature in the diagnosis of heart rejection. J Heart Lung Transplant 2005;24:1710–20.
7. Saraiva F, Matos V, Goncalves L, et al. Complications of endomyocardial biopsy in heart transplant patients: a retrospective study of 2117 consecutive procedures. Transplant Proc 2011;43:1908–12.
8. Eisen HJ, Kobashigawa J, Starling RC, et al. Everolimus versus mycophenolate mofetil in heart transplantation: a randomized, multicenter trial. Am J Transplant 2013;13:1203–16.
9. Mills Jr. RM, Naftel D, Kirklin J, et al. Cardiac transplant rejection with hemodynamic compromise: a multi-institutional study of risk factors and endomyocardial cellular infiltrate. J Heart Lung Transplant 16:813 1997.

10. Lindenfeld J, Miller GG, Shakar SF, et al. Drug therapy in the heart transplant recipient: part II: immunosuppressive drugs. Circulation 2004;110:3858–65.
11. Kobashigawa J, Miller L, Renlund D, et al. A randomized active-controlled trial of Mycophenolate mofetil in heart transplant recipients. Transplantation 1998;66:507–15.
12. Eisen HJ, Kobashigawa J, Keogh A, et al. Three-year results of a randomized, double-blind, controlled trial of mycophenolate mofetil versus azathioprine in cardiac transplant recipients. J Heart Lung Transplant 2005;24:517–25.
13. Baselga J, Campone M, Piccart M. Everolimus in postmenopausal hormone-receptor–positive advanced breast cancer. N Engl J Med 2012;366:520–9.
14. Hershberger RE, Starling RC, Eisen HJ, et al. Daclizumab to prevent rejection after cardiac transplantation. N Engl J Med 2005;352:2705–13.
15. Costanzo MR, Dipchand A, Starling R, et al. The International Society of Heart and Lung Transplantation Guidelines for the care of heart transplant recipients. International Society of Heart and Lung Transplantation Guidelines. J Heart Lung Transplant 2010;29:914–56.
16. Berry GJ, Angelini A, Burke MM, et al. The ISHLT working formulation for pathologic diagnosis of antibody-mediated rejection in heart transplantation: evolution and current status (2005–2011). J Heart Lung Transplant 2011;30:601–11.
17. Kobashigawa J, Crespo-Leiro MG, Ensminger SM, et al. Report from a consensus conference on antibody-mediated rejection in heart transplantation. J Heart Lung Transplant 2011;30:252–69.
18. Ojo AO, Held PJ, Port FK, et al. Chronic renal failure after transplantation of a nonrenal organ. N Engl J Med 2003;349:931–40.
19. Greenberg A, Thompson ME, Griffith BJ, et al. Cyclosporine nephrotoxicity in cardiac allograft patients—a seven-year follow-up. Transplantation 1990;50:589–93.
20. Sehgal V, Radhakrishnan J, Appel GB, et al. Progressive renal insufficiency following cardiac transplantation: cyclosporine, lipids, and hypertension. Am J Kidney Dis 1995;26:193–201.
21. Bennett WM. Insights into chronic cyclosporine nephrotoxicity. Int J Clin Pharmacol Ther 1996;34:515–19.
22. Serkova NJ, Christians U, Benet LZ. Biochemical mechanisms of cyclosporine neurotoxicity. Mol Interv 2004;4:97.
23. Kou R, Greif D, Michel T. Dephosphorylation of endothelial nitric-oxide synthase by vascular endothelial growth factor. Implications for the vascular responses to cyclosporin A. J Biol Chem 2002;277:29669.
24. Beal MF. Mitochondrial dysfunction in neurodegenerative diseases. Biochim Biophys Acta 1998;1366:211.
25. Stamp LK, Chapman PT. Gout and organ transplantation. Curr Rheumatol Rep 2012;14:165–72.
26. Papadimitriou JC, Drachenberg CB, Wiland A, et al. Histolological morphology of colitis associated with mycophenolate mofetil (MMF) in renal allograft recipients: Acute graft versus host disease (GVH)-like features (abstract). Transplantation 1999;67(Suppl):256.
27. Ducloux D, Ottignon Y, Semhoun-Ducloux S, et al. Mycophenolate mofetil-induced villous atrophy. Transplantation 1998;66:1115–16.
28. Lehmkuhl H, Hummel M, Kobashigawa J, et al. Enteric-coated mycophenolate-sodium in heart transplantation: efficacy, safety, and pharmacokinetic compared with mycophenolate mofetil. Transplant Proc 2008;40:953–5.
29. Kim M, Rostas S, Gabardi S. Mycophenolate fetal toxicity and risk evaluation and mitigation strategies. Am J Transplant 2013 13:1383–9.
30. Greenberg JN, Zwald FO. Management of skin cancer in solid-organ transplant recipients: a multidisciplinary approach. Dermatol Clin 2011;29:231–41.
31. Moloney FJ, Comber H, O'Lorcain P, et al. A population-based study of skin cancer incidence and prevalence in renal transplant recipients. Br J Dermatol 2006;154:498–504.
32. Eisen, HJ, Tuzcu, EM, Dorent, R, et al. Everolimus for the prevention of allograft rejection and vasculopathy in cardiac-transplant recipients. N Engl J Med 2003;349:847–58.
33. Kuppahally S, Al-Khaldi A, Weisshaar D, et al. Wound healing complications with de novo sirolimus versus mycophenolate mofetil-based regimen in cardiac transplant recipients. Am J Transplant 2006;6(5 Pt 1):986–92.
34. Lehmkuhl HB, Arizon J, Viganò M, et al. Everolimus with reduced cyclosporine versus MMF with standard cyclosporine in de novo heart transplant recipients; 2411 Study Investigators. Transplantation 2009;88:115–22.
35. Eisen HJ, Kobashigawa J, Starling RC, et al. Everolimus versus mycophenolate mofetil in heart transplantation: a randomized, multicenter trial. Am J Transplant 2013;13:1203–16.
36. Fishman JA. Infection in solid-organ transplant recipients. N Engl J Med 2007;357(25):2601–14.
37. Fishman JA. Infection in solid-organ transplant recipients. N Engl J Med 2007;357(25):2601–14.
38. Liebowitz D. Epstein-Barr virus and a cellular signaling pathway in lymphomas from immunosuppressed patients. N Engl J Med 1998;338:1413.
39. Worth A, Conyers R, Cohen J, et al. Pre-emptive rituximab based on viraemia and T cell reconstitution: a highly effective strategy for the prevention of Epstein-Barr virus-associated lymphoproliferative disease following stem cell transplantation. Br J Haematol 2011;155:377.
40. Worth A, Conyers R, Cohen J, et al. Pre-emptive rituximab based on viraemia and T cell reconstitution: a highly effective strategy for the prevention of Epstein-Barr virus-associated lymphoproliferative disease following stem cell transplantation. Br J Haematol 2011;155:377.
41. Kowalski RJ, Post DR, Mannon RB, et al. Assessing relative risks of infection and rejection: a meta-analysis using an immune function assay. Transplantation 2006;82:663–8.
42. Kobashigawa JA, Kiyosaki KK, Patel JK, et al. Benefit of immune monitoring in heart transplant patients using ATP production in activated lymphocytes. J Heart Lung Transplant 2011;29:504–8.
43. Myers BD. Cyclosporine nephrotoxicity. Kidney Int 1986;30:964–74.
44. Puschett JB, Greenberg A, Holley J, McCauley J. The spectrum of ciclosporin nephrotoxicity. Am J Nephrol 1990;10:296–309.
45. Flechner SM, Kobashigawa J, Klintmalm G. Calcineurin inhibitor-sparing regimens in solid organ transplantation: focus on improving renal function and nephrotoxicity. Clin Transplant 2008;22(1):1–15.
46. Gustafsson F, Ross HJ. Renal-sparing strategies in cardiac transplantation. Curr Opin Organ Transplant 2009;14:566–70.
47. Russo MJ, Chen JM, Hong KN, et al. Survival after heart transplantation is not diminished among recipients with uncomplicated diabetes mellitus: an analysis of the United Network of Organ Sharing database. Columbia University Heart Transplant Outcomes Research Group. Circulation 2006;114:2280–7.
48. Wilkinson A, Davidson J, Dotta F, et al. Guidelines for the treatment and management of new-onset diabetes after transplantation. Clin Transplant 2005;19:291–8.
49. Lindenfeld J, Page RL 2nd, Zolty R, et al. Drug therapy in the heart transplant recipient: Part III: common medical problems. Circulation 2005;111:113–17.
50. Kobashigawa, JA, Katznelson, S, Laks, H, et al. Effect of pravastatin on outcomes after cardiac transplantation. N Engl J Med 1995;333:621.
51. Wenke, K, Meiser, B, Thiery, J, et al. Simvastatin initiated early after heart transplantation: 8-year prospective experience. Circulation 2003;107:93.
52. Katznelson S Immunosuppressive and antiproliferative effects of HMG-CoA reductase inhibitors. Transplant Proc 1999;31(3B Suppl):22S–24S.
53. Ye F, Ying-Bin X, Yu-Guo W, Hetzer R. Tacrolimus versus cyclosporine microemulsion for heart transplant recipients: a meta-analysis. J Heart Lung Transplant 2009;28:58–66.
54. Ebeling PR. Approach to the patient with transplantation-related bone loss. J Clin Endocrinol Metab 2009;94:1483–90.
55. Shane E, Addesso V, Namerow PB, et al. Alendronate versus calcitriol for the prevention of bone loss after cardiac transplantation. N Engl J Med 2004;350:767–76.

56. Stehlik J, Edwards LB, Kucheryavaya AY, et al. The Registry of the International Society for Heart and Lung Transplantation: twenty-seventh official adult heart transplant report—2010. J Heart Lung Transplant 2010;29:1089–103.
57. Hanto DW. Classification of Epstein-Barr virus-associated posttransplant lymphoproliferative diseases: implications for understanding their pathogenesis and developing rational treatment strategies. Annu Rev Med 1995;46:381.
58. Emond JP, Marcelin AG, Dorent R, et al. Kaposi's sarcoma associated with previous human herpesvirus 8 infection in heart transplant recipients. J Clin Microbiol 2002;40:2217.
59. Engels EA, Pfeiffer RM, Fraumeni JF Jr, et al. Spectrum of cancer risk among US solid organ transplant recipients. JAMA 2011;306:1891.
60. Swinnen LJ, Costanzo-Nordin MR, Fisher SG, et al. Increased incidence of lymphoproliferative disorder after immunosuppression with the monoclonal antibody OKT3 in cardiac-transplant recipients. N Engl J Med 1990;323:1723.
61. Buell JF, Gross TG, Woodle ES. Malignancy after transplantation. Transplantation 2005;80:S254.
62. Swann PF, Waters TR, Moulton DC, et al. Role of postreplicative DNA mismatch repair in the cytotoxic action of thioguanine. Science 1996;273:1109.
63. Hojo M, Morimoto T, Maluccio M, et al. Cyclosporine induces cancer progression by a cell-autonomous mechanism. Nature 1999;397:530.
64. Imao T, Ichimaru N, Takahara S, et al. Risk factors for malignancy in Japanese renal transplant recipients. Cancer 2007;109:2109.
65. Campistol JM, Eris J, Oberbauer R, et al. Sirolimus therapy after early cyclosporine withdrawal reduces the risk for cancer in adult renal transplantation. J Am Soc Nephrol 2006;17:581.
66. Mathew T, Kreis H, Friend P. Two-year incidence of malignancy in sirolimus-treated renal transplant recipients: results from five multicenter studies. Clin Transplant 2004;18:446.
67. Salgo R, Gossmann J, Schöfer H, et al. Switch to a sirolimus-based immunosuppression in long-term renal transplant recipients: reduced rate of (pre-)malignancies and nonmelanoma skin cancer in a prospective, randomized, assessor-blinded, controlled clinical trial. Am J Transplant 2010;10:1385.
68. Euvrard S, Morelon E, Rostaing L, et al. Sirolimus and secondary skin-cancer prevention in kidney transplantation. N Engl J Med 2012;367:329.
69. Kauffman HM, Cherikh WS, Cheng Y, et al. Maintenance immunosuppression with target-of-rapamycin inhibitors is associated with a reduced incidence of de novo malignancies. Transplantation 2005;80:883.
70. Stallone G, Schena A, Infante B, et al. Sirolimus for Kaposi's sarcoma in renal-transplant recipients. N Engl J Med 2005;352:1317.
71. Tanaka, H, Swanson, SJ, Sukhova, G, et al. Early proliferation of medial smooth muscle cells in coronary arteries of rabbit cardiac allografts during immunosuppression with cyclosporine A. Transplant Proc 1995;27:2062.
72. Stoica, SC, Cafferty, F, Pauriah, M, et al. The cumulative effect of acute rejection on development of cardiac allograft vasculopathy. J Heart Lung Transplant 2006;25:420.
73. Raichlin, E, Edwards, BS, Kremers, WK, et al. Acute cellular rejection and the subsequent development of allograft vasculopathy after cardiac transplantation. J Heart Lung Transplant 2009;28:320.
74. Reed, EF, Demetris, AJ, Hammond, E, et al. Acute antibody-mediated rejection of cardiac transplants. J Heart Lung Transplant 2006;25:153.
75. Fredrich, R, Toyoda, M, Czer, LS, et al. The clinical significance of antibodies to human vascular endothelial cells after cardiac transplantation. Transplantation 1999;67:385.
76. Gullestad, L, Simonsen, S, Ueland, T, et al. Possible role of proinflammatory cytokines in heart allograft coronary artery disease. Am J Cardiol 1999;84:999.
77. Miller, GG, Davis, SF, Atkinson, JB, et al. Longitudinal analysis of fibroblast growth factor expression after transplantation and association with severity of cardiac allograft vasculopathy. Circulation 1999;100:2396.
78. Chang, G, DeNofrio, D, Desai, S, et al. Lipoprotein(a) levels and heart transplantation atherosclerosis. Am Heart J 1998;136:329.
79. Kapadia, SR, Nissen, SE, Ziada, KM, et al. Impact of lipid abnormalities in development and progression of transplant coronary disease: a serial intravascular ultrasound study. J Am Coll Cardiol 2001;38:206.
80. Shi, C, Lee, WS, Russell, ME, et al. Hypercholesterolemia exacerbates transplant arteriosclerosis via increased neointimal smooth muscle cell accumulation: studies in apolipoprotein E knockout mice. Circulation 1997;96:2722.
81. Fateh-Moghadam, S, Bocksch, W, Wessely, R, et al. Cytomegalovirus infection status predicts progression of heart-transplant vasculopathy. Transplantation 2003;76:1470.
82. Potena, L, Grigioni, F, Ortolani, P, et al. Relevance of cytomegalovirus infection and coronary-artery remodeling in the first year after heart transplantation: a prospective three-dimensional intravascular ultrasound study. Transplantation 2003;75:839.
83. Mehra, MR, Uber, PA, Ventura, HO, et al. The impact of mode of donor brain death on cardiac allograft vasculopathy: an intravascular ultrasound study. J Am Coll Cardiol 2004;43:806.
84. Costanzo, MR, Naftel, DC, Pritzker, MR, et al. Heart transplant coronary artery disease detected by coronary angiography: a multiinstitutional study of preoperative donor and recipient risk factors. Cardiac Transplant Research Database. J Heart Lung Transplant 1998;17:744.
85. Nagji, AS, Hranjec, T, Swenson, BR, et al. Donor age is associated with chronic allograft vasculopathy after adult heart transplantation: implications for donor allocation. Ann Thorac Surg 2010;90:168.
86. Wilson, RF, McGinn, AL, Johnson, TH, et al. Sympathetic reinnervation after heart transplantation in human beings. J Heart Lung Transplant 1992;11:S88.
87. Stark, RP, McGinn, AL, Wilson, RF. Chest pain in cardiac-transplant recipients. Evidence of sensory reinnervation after cardiac transplantation. N Engl J Med 1991;324:1791.
88. Uretsky BF, Kormos RL, Zerbe TR, Lee A, Tokarczyk TR, Murali S, et al. Cardiac events after heart transplantation: incidence and predictive value of coronary arteriography. J Heart Lung Transplant 1992;11(3 Pt 2):S45–51.
89. Mehra, MR, Crespo-Leiro, MG, Dipchand, A, et al. International Society for Heart and Lung Transplantation working formulation of a standardized nomenclature for cardiac allograft vasculopathy-2010. J Heart Lung Transplant 2010;29:717.
90. Tuzcu, EM, Kapadia, SR, Sachar, R, et al. Intravascular ultrasound evidence of angiographically silent progression in coronary atherosclerosis predicts long-term morbidity and mortality after cardiac transplantation. J Am Coll Cardiol 2005;45:1538.
91. Mehra, MR, Ventura, HO, Stapleton, DD, et al. Presence of severe intimal thickening by intravascular ultrasonography predicts cardiac events in cardiac allograft vasculopathy. J Heart Lung Transplant 1995;14:632.
92. Kobashigawa, JA, Tobis, JM, Starling, RC, et al. Multicenter intravascular ultrasound validation study among heart transplant recipients: outcomes after five years. J Am Coll Cardiol 2005;45:1532.
93. Akosah, KO, McDaniel, S, Hanrahan, JS, Mohanty, PK. Dobutamine stress echocardiography early after heart transplantation predicts development of allograft coronary artery disease and outcome. J Am Coll Cardiol 1998;31:1607.
94. Akosah, KO, Mohanty, PK, Funai, JT, et al. Noninvasive detection of transplant coronary artery disease by dobutamine stress echocardiography. J Heart Lung Transplant 1994;13:1024.
95. Spes, CH, Klauss, V, Mudra, H, et al. Diagnostic and prognostic value of serial dobutamine stress echocardiography for noninvasive assessment of cardiac allograft vasculopathy: a comparison with coronary angiography and intravascular ultrasound. Circulation 1999;100:509.
96. Schroeder, JS, Gao, SZ, Alderman, EL, et al. A preliminary study of diltiazem in the prevention of coronary artery disease in heart-transplant recipients. N Engl J Med 1993;328:164.
97. Carrier, M, Rivard, M, Kostuk, W, et al. The Canadian Study of Cardiac Transplantation. Atherosclerosis. Investigators of the CASCADE Study. Can J Cardiol 1999;15:1337.

98. Li H, Tanaka K, Chhabra A, et al. Vascular remodeling 1 year after cardiac transplantation.J Heart Lung Transplant 2007;26:56–62.
99. Fang, JC, Kinlay, S, Beltrame, J, et al. Effect of vitamins C and E on progression of transplant-associated arteriosclerosis: a randomised trial. Lancet 2002;359:1108.
100. Keogh, A, Richardson, M, Ruygrok, P, et al. Sirolimus in de novo heart transplant recipients reduces acute rejection and prevents coronary artery disease at 2 years: a randomized clinical trial. Circulation 2004;110:2694.
101. Starling RC, Hare JM, Hauptman P, et al. Therapeutic drug monitoring for everolimus in heart transplant recipients based on exposure-effect modeling. Am J Transplant 2004;4:2126–31.
102. Kobashigawa JA, Pauly DF, Starling RC, et al. Cardiac allograft vasculopathy by intravascular ultrasound in heart transplant patients: substudy from the everolimus versus mycophenolate mofetil randomized, multicenter trial. JACC Heart Fail 2013;1:389–99.
103. Raichlin E, Bae JH, Khalpey Z, Edwards BS, et al. Conversion to sirolimus as primary immunosuppression attenuates the progression of allograft vasculopathy after cardiac transplantation.Circulation 2007;116:2726–33.
104. Topilsky Y, Hasin T, Raichlin E, et al. Sirolimus as primary immunosuppression attenuates allograft vasculopathy with improved late survival and decreased cardiac events after cardiac transplantation. Circulation 2012;125:708–20.
105. Mancini D, Pinney S, Burkhoff D, et al. Use of rapamycin slows progression of cardiac transplantation vasculopathy. Circulation 2003;108:48.
106. Segovia J, Fernandez-Yanez J, Gonzalez-Vichez, et al. Clinical effects of introducing everolimus in the immunosuppressive regimen of patients with established cardiac allograft vasculopathy (CAV): efficacy analysis of a randomized, multicenter study (abstract). J Heart Lung Transplant 2012;31:S121.
107. Segovia J, Gomez-Bueno M, Goicolea J, et al. Effect of everolimus in patients with established cardiac allograft vasculopathy: results of a randomized, multicenter intravascular ultrasound study (abstract). J Heart Lung Transplant 2012;31:S77.
108. Benza, RL, Zoghbi, GJ, Tallaj, J, et al. Palliation of allograft vasculopathy with transluminal angioplasty: a decade of experience. J Am Coll Cardiol 2004;43:1973.
109. Wong PM, Piamsomboon C, Mathur A, et al. Efficacy of coronary stenting in the management of cardiac allograft vasculopathy. Am J Cardiol 1998;82:239.
110. Jain SP, Ramee SR, White CJ, et al. Coronary stenting in cardiac allograft vasculopathy. J Am Coll Cardiol 1998;32:1636.
111. Lee MS, Kobashigawa J, Tobis J. Comparison of percutaneous coronary intervention with bare-metal and drug-eluting stents for cardiac allograft vasculopathy. JACC Cardiovasc Interv 2008;1:710–15.
112. Azarbal B, Arbit B, Ramaraj R, et al. Clinical and angiographic outcomes with everolimus eluting stents for the treatment of cardiac allograft vasculopathy. J Interv Cardiol 2014;27(1):73–9.
113. Bhama, JK, Nguyen, DQ, Scolieri, S, et al. Surgical revascularization for cardiac allograft vasculopathy: Is it still an option? J Thorac Cardiovasc Surg 2009;137:1488.
114. Johnson, MR, Aaronson, KD, Canter, CE, et al. Heart retransplantation. Am J Transplant 2007;7:2075.

CHAPTER 20

Right heart failure: Anatomy, physiology, and pathobiology

Thomas G. Di Salvo MD MPH MBA
and Simon Maltais MD PhD

Right ventricular structure and function

Embryology

The human heart develops from two sources of cells.[1] The primary or first heart field cells (FHF) give rise to the entire left ventricle (LV), parts of the right ventricle (RV), and parts of the inflow regions of the heart.[2] The second heart field (SHF) cells give rise to all the outflow tracts, parts of the RV, and parts of the inflow regions.[1] Thus, the LV derives exclusively from the FHF, the outflow tracts entirely from the SHF, and the RV from both the FHF and SHF.[2]

Distinct from FHF cells, SHF cells are marked by expression of Isl1+ (insulin gene enhancer protein, a LIM homeodomain transcription factor). SHF cells also express the transcription factors Isl1 and Tbx1 and the growth factors Fgf8 and Fgf10.[2] Thus, a substantial part of the RV and all of the RV outflow tract (RVOT) develop from SHF (RV sinus from the primitive heart tube, infundibulum from the conus cordis) from Isl1+ progenitors regulated in part via Wnt/β-catenin signaling.[3] Foxh1, Mef2c, HAND1, HAND2, and BOP transcription factors also play critical roles in RV development.[1]

Fetal and early postnatal life

In utero, the RV has same mass as the LV and is capable of equivalent free-wall thickening and force development due to the elevated pulmonary vascular resistance (PVR) during fetal life.[4,5] Pulmonary blood flow in utero is diverted from the lungs by the patent ductus arteriosus (PDA), which in utero is a channel as large as the aorta. With birth, inflation of lungs sharply reduces PVR. PDA constriction and PDA closure by day 2–3 of life result in the complete separation of the pulmonary and systemic circulations.[4] RV mass thenceforth regresses in parallel to the reduction in PVR, which falls to adult levels within 2 weeks. RV "in utero hypertrophy" thus regresses after birth and the RV remodels itself to the normal adult crescent-shaped RV (except in selected congenital lesions such as pulmonary stenosis (PS) and congenitally corrected transposition of the great arteries (cCTGA) where "protective" fetal molecular, metabolic, and structural RV phenotype is preserved).[5]

Adult right ventricular anatomy

Shape

The three-dimensional shape of the RV is complex compared to the conical LV, as illustrated in Figure 20.1.[6] When viewed from the front, the RV appears triangular and when viewed in cross-section it appears crescentic.[7] Goor and Lilehi described three RV segments: the sinus inflow, trabecular portion, and infundibulum.[8] The RV also has three bands (partietal, septomarginal, and moderator) and a ventriculoinfundibular fold which separates the pulmonary

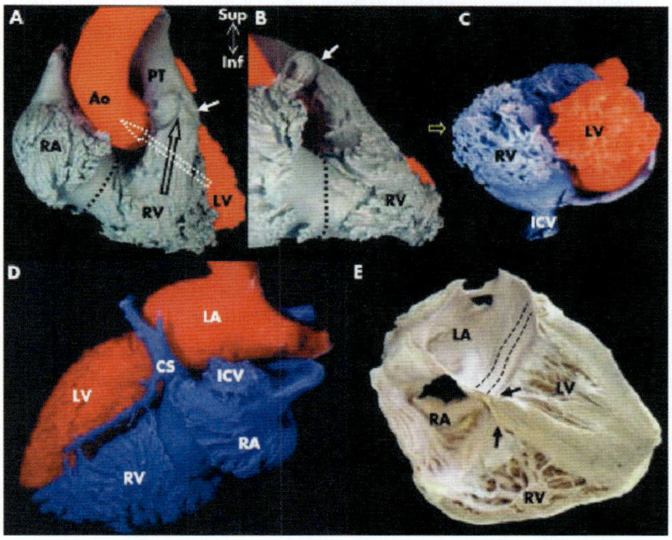

Fig. 20.1 Anatomy of the right ventricle. An endocast of a normal heart with right heart chambers colored blue and left heart chambers colored red is viewed from different perspectives to display the spatial relationships between cardiac chambers. (A) Viewed from the anterior aspect, the crossover arrangement between left and right ventricular outflow tracts (dotted arrow and open arrow respectively) is apparent. The pulmonary valve (solid arrow) is situated most superiorly. (B) This view from right and anterior shows the triangular shape of the right ventricle delimited by the tricuspid (dotted line) and pulmonary (arrow) valves. (C) Viewed from the apex, the right ventricle is crescentic, wrapping round the LV. The open arrow marks the acute margin. The coronary sinus is related to the inferior wall of the left atrium. (D) This view from the diaphragmatic aspect shows the course of the coronary sinus and the cardiac crux. (E) This four-chamber section through a heart shows the offset arrangement of the hingelines of the tricuspid and mitral valves (arrows) with the tricuspid valve attached closer to the cardiac apex than the mitral valve. The broken lines trace the course of the coronary sinus passing along the inferior aspect of the left atrium. Ao, aorta; CS, coronary sinus; ICV, inferior caval vein; LA, left atrium; LV, left ventricle; PT, pulmonary trunk; RA, right atrium; RV, right ventricle.

Table 20.1 MRI differences: structure and function of the right and left ventricles

Parameter	Right ventricle	Left ventricle
End-diastolic volume (ml)	138 ± 40	121 ± 34
End-systolic volume (ml)	54 ± 21	40 ± 14
Stroke volume (ml)	84 ± 24	82 ± 23
Ejection fraction (%)	61 ± 7	67 ± 5
Free wall mass (g)	46 ± 11	104 ± 27
Interventricular mass (g)	—	54 ± 13
Total ventricular mass (g)	46 ± 11	158 ± 39
Total ventricular mass/end-diastolic volume (g/ml)	0.35 ± 0.06	1.33 ± 0.18

Reprinted with permission of Macmillan Publishers Ltd: Nature Reviews Cardiology, Mertens LL, Friedberg MK. 7:551–63, copyright (2010).

and tricuspid valves.[7] The normal thickness of the RV free wall is 3–5 mm exclusive of RV trabeculations and bands (Table 20.1).[6] In healthy adults, the RV volume exceeds LV volume, and the total RV free wall mass is approximately one-fourth of the total LV mass including the interventricular septum (Table 20.2).[9] Owing to its tissue composition and geometry, the RV has greater chamber distensibility than the LV.[10]

Fiber orientation

Grossly, the RV exhibits superficial subepicardial transverse fibers extending roughly parallel to the atrioventricular (AV) groove, with the remaining deeper fibers extending in a mostly longitudinal orientation relative to the RV long axis.[6] In reality, the myocytes in both ventricles are aggregated as a much more complex three-dimensional meshwork embedded in a supporting matrix of connective tissue rather than as discrete "fibers" or anatomic "layers."[11,12] It has been difficult by dissection to identify the relative orientation of human myocytes due to dissection-induced disruption of the meshwork.[11] In the LV, current consensus supports three predominant meshwork populations.[12] The first population exhibits spiraling alignment of myocyte long axis tangential to the epicardial and endocardial borders with rather marked variation in the angulation relative to the ventricular equator. These myocytes produce the major unloading of blood during systole. The second population exhibits myocyte alignment at angles of up to 40° from the epicardium toward the endocardium. These myocytes produce auxotonic forces during the cardiac cycle. The third population exhibits centrally located myocytes with roughly circumferential alignment.

Table 20.2 Summary of structural and hemodynamic differences between the right and left ventricles

Characteristic	Right ventricle	Left ventricle
End-diastolic volume (ml/m^2)	75 ± 13	66 ± 12
Mass (g/m^2)	26 ± 5	87 ± 12
Thickness (mm)	2–5	7–11
Pressures (mmHg)	25/4	130/8
Ejection fraction (%)	61 ± 7	67 ± 5
Emax (mmHg/mL)	1.30 ± 0.84	5.48 ± 1.23
PVR vs. SVR (dyne s^{-1} cm^{-5})	70 (20–130)	1100 (700–1600)
SWI (g m^{-2} beat^{-1})	8 ± 2	50 ± 20
Adaptation to disease state	Volume	Pressure

PVR, pulmonary vascular resistance; SVR, systemic vascular resistance; SWI, stroke work index.

Unlike the adult LV, the normal adult RV is largely composed of transverse and longitudinal meshwork myocytes and lacks these central circumferentially oriented myocytes, although there are some RV myocytes with circumferential orientation in the subepicardium and in the infundibulum.[12,13] The presence of a thick middle layer of circular myocytes in the hypertrophied hearts of patients with tetralogy of Fallot supports the notion that the congenitally overloaded human RV may either (1) remodel in part by adopting LV structural characteristics or (2) not undergo the normal perinatal involution of central circumferential RV myocytes as PVR drops after birth and the RV normally remodels.[14] In animal models of acquired pulmonary hypertension, the RV does not appear to develop de-novo central circumferentially oriented myocytes like the LV.[13] In the normal RV, there are common RV–LV fibers at RV attachment sites, including the inferior and posterior interventricular septum. This is in keeping with the broader concept that the heart is in fact arrayed more like a modified blood vessel with each myocyte linked to neighboring myocytes in a supporting connective tissue matrix with continuity of helical fibers from apex to base, rather than like a skeletal muscle with discrete fibers and points of origin and insertion.[11]

The RV and LV are bound together by interlacing helical muscle bundles to form an integrated and interdependent contractile organ conjoined by a common interventricular septum (Figure 20.2).[15] Septal segments and architecture mirror the LV free wall, namely obliquely oriented fibers from the descending and ascending segments of the apical loop. The septum comprises approximately 40% of LV myocardial mass and functions as a single LV free-wall-like unit. The septum is surrounded by the wrapping of the right segment of the basal loop which contains the predominantly transversely oriented fibers comprising the RV free wall along with the more longitudinal fibers.

Right ventricular cardiomyocytes

Relatively few or significant intrinsic structural differences between normal RV and LV isolated cardiomyocytes have been reported in most animal studies.[16] In healthy adult pigs, for example, mitochondial:myofibril volume ratios were increased in LV and interventricular septum cardiomyoctes compared to RV cardiomyocytes although the differences were quite modest (e.g., in LV 65.9% myofibrils vs. 67.9% mitochondria and in RV 22.2% myofibrils vs. 22.1% mitochondria).[17] In pigs, the interventricular septum exhibits a mitochondrial density and mitochondria:myofibril ratio similar to that of the LV. The relative proportions of cardiomyocyte volume (66.3% myofibril, 21.9% mitochondrial, 1.6% T-system, sarcoplasmic reticulum (SR) 2.3%, and 3.2% clear intracellular space 3.2%) were also not substantially different between LV and RV cardiomyocytes. The investigators concluded from this morphologic study that the relative homogeneity of the cytoplasmic volumes of myofibrils, mitochondria, T-system, SR, and clear

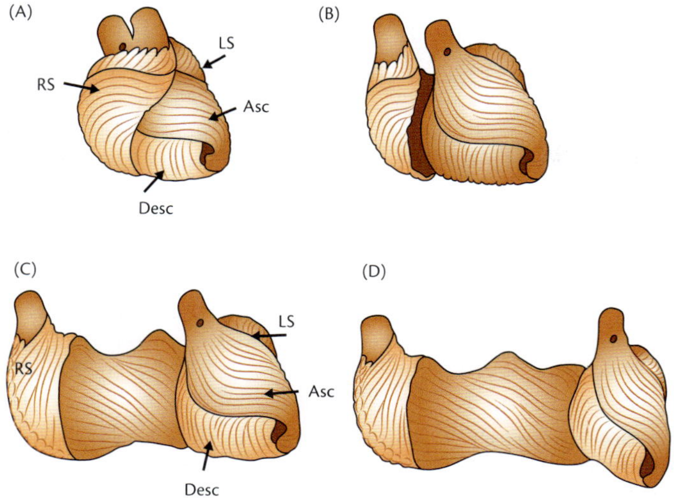

Fig. 20.2 Unfolding of the heart model to show (A) the intact ventricle with transverse RV fibers and oblique ascending and descending LV fibers; (B) detachment of the PA to begin unfolding the basal segment (note underlying obliquely oriented descending and ascending segment of septum); (C) complete unfolding of basal loop of the right ventricle with the genu, posteriorly, separated from the left ventricular segment of the basal loop (note transverse fiber orientation of the free wall); and (D) the entire basal loop with the entire genu in the midst of the transverse basal loop segment (left side RV, right side LV). Note the basal loop that surrounds the obliquely oriented fibers within the descending and ascending segments of the apical loop that is responsible for septal motion.
Saleh S, Liakopoulos OJ, Buckberg GD. The septal motor of biventricular function. European Journal of Cardiothoracic Surgery, (2006) 29 Suppl 1:S126-38 by permission of Oxford University Press.

intracellular space with slightly higher values for the LV cardiomyocytes indicated the greater workload and higher rate of oxidation in the LV compared to the RV.

In the mouse, the RV and LV proteomes are very similar qualitatively as well as quantitatively with less than 1% of proteome proteins exhibiting twofold or greater differences in expression.[18] The investigators concluded that the mouse LV and RV proteomes exhibited "negligible differences" but could not exclude differences in lower abundant proteins and/or protein post-translational modifications. In healthy rabbits and pigs, the RV and LV proteomes exhibited only minor differences without evidence for greater than 20% differences in expression for the vast majority of proteins or significant post-translational modifications.[19] After removal of RV connective tissue and fat (up to one-third the gross RV wet weight), the LV versus RV mg protein/g wet weight values were quite similar, 150 ± versus 153 ± 8 (pigs) and 156 ± 1 versus 178 ± 5 (rabbit). No differences in LV vs. RV cytochrome protein levels, mitochondrial content, oxidative phosphorylation enzymatic activities, or metabolic rate were found when LV and RV were normalized to mg protein/g tissue after removal of RV connective tissue and fat. The investigators concluded that the metabolic and mechanical potential of RV and LV cardiomyocyte cytosol is nearly identical and that differences in net workload and metabolic needs between the ventricles appear to be matched by the amount of cytosol and cardiac muscle. The authors postulated that both RV and LV cardiomyocytes exhibit a fixed, optimized ratio of contractile proteins and energetic machinery such that cellular aerobic capacity is matched between ventricles, and that the maximum capacity for metabolic flux is the same per gram of either RV or LV cardiac tissue. The difference between the RV and LV, the investigators concluded, resided not in the cardiomyocyte, but in (1) the lesser RV mass, (2) different RV chamber geometry conferring RV adaptation to low-impedance volume work, and (3) RV fiber orientation also conferring RV adaptation for the same reason.

Despite the absence of striking morphologic or proteomic changes in the normal resting RV versus LV, in animals isolated RV cardiomyocytes exhibit generally lesser maximal sarcomere shortening and smaller peak calcium transients despite little change in the expression levels of major calcium handling proteins.[16] At the molecular level, the RV exhibits greater expression of α-myosin heavy chain isozyme, greater cholinergic density, generally lesser responsiveness to α-agonists, and greater responsiveness in the RVOT to β-agonist stimulation compared to the LV.[16] Finally, the rapidly expanding body of experimental evidence in animal models and humans supports that RV adaptive and maladaptive remodeling and the transition to RV failure has several pathobiological features distinct from those described to date in the LV, as discussed in detail later.[7,10,20,21]

Right ventricular cardiodynamics

Right ventricular cardiac contraction cycle

RV contraction is sequential and "peristaltic," sweeping from inlet to RV free wall and apical trabecular myocardium to the infundibulum.[10,22] The infundibulum contracts 30–50 ms after the RV free wall and the duration of infundibular contraction exceeds that of the other RV segments.[7,22] Normal contractile RV function is illustrated in Figures 20.3 and 20.4. As RV "fails", this normal "peristaltic" RV contraction pattern is lost and the RV contraction pattern evolves into a more "LV-like" contractile sequence and hemodynamic pressure–flow pattern as illustrated in Figure 20.5.[23]

Four separate mechanisms contribute to overall RV contraction and ejection:

1. RV free wall inward movement toward the septum due to shortening of RV transverse fibers (a "bellows-like" effect)
2. shortening along the RV long axis from base toward the apex due to shortening of the RV longitudinal fibers accompanied by later systolic twisting of the RV basal segment
3. shortening and twisting of the obliquely arrayed interventricular septum fibers which provides both RV free wall septal traction via RV free wall septal attachments and likely translation of an "impelling" force to the RV blood pool due to septal twisting
4. "peristaltic-like" sequential contraction of the RV inflow, apical, and outflow regions which assists in impelling blood from the RV into the pulmonary artery (PA).[10,22]

Owing to the largely transverse and longitudinal rather than oblique array of RV fibers, systolic and diastolic radial and torsional motion is less prominent in the RV than in the LV except at the base of the heart.[24,25,26] Since RV free wall shortening ends before both the (1) cessation of forward pulmonary blood flow and (2) minimization of the RV free wall to interventricular septum distance, there is an important and substantial "late" systolic contribution of the interventricular septum to RV ejection.[10,27] RV shortening is greater longitudinally than radially such that the radius of RV curvature and the RV surface area do not change appreciably during contraction.[28] Since radial and torsional movements do not contribute as significantly to RV ejection,[7] the lack of RV systolic

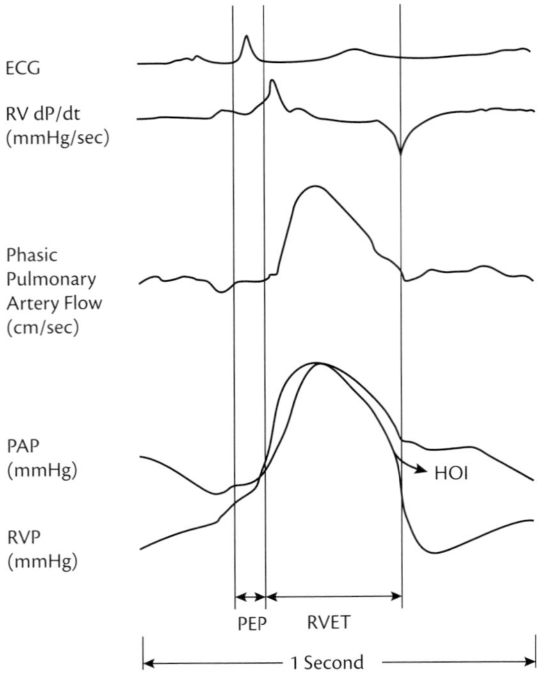

Fig. 20.3 Normal right ventricle (RV) hemodynamics. Simultaneously recorded electrocardiogram (ECG), RV analog signal of pressure development (dP/dt), phasic pulmonary artery flow, pulmonary artery pressure (PAP) and RV pressures (RVP) in a human subject. Vertical lines show the pre-ejection period (PEP) and RV ejection time (RVET). The hangout interval (HOI) represents the time interval between the pulmonary incisura and the RV pressure wave form, caused by ejection in to the compliant pulmonary vasculature.

Reprinted from Cardiology Clinics, 30, Dell'Italia L, Anatomy and physiology of the right ventricle, 167–87, copyright (2012) with permission from Elsevier.

and diastolic radial and torsional contraction in addition to lesser RV myocardial mass and RV chamber configuration are likely all key mechanisms which render the RV vulnerable to significant increases in afterload, unlike the LV.

Compared to the LV, the RV exhibits (1) an earlier peaking and more rapidly declining systolic pressure, (2) a much shorter isovolumic contraction and isovolumic relaxation time, and (3) a longer ejection phase.[7,10,22] PA blood flow may continue despite pulmonary valve closure and a negative RV–PA pressure gradient (the so called "hangout interval") due to RVOT bolus momentum.[29] The hangout interval correlates inversely with peak PA pressure and RV end-systolic pressure, and does not correlate with RV ejection time.[29]

The RV end-systolic pressure–volume relation (RV ESPVR) follows a linear time-varying elastance model and is responsive to inotropic agents as illustrated in Figure 20.6.[30] Normal RV maximal elastance is 1.30 ± 0.84 mmHg/ml.[23] RV maximal elastance rather than the traditional "Emax" as defined by the onset of isovolumic contraction at end-systole is a more sensitive measure of RV contractility, since RV ejection continues well beyond end-systole.[31] The traditionally derived RV ESPVR, given by the ratio of PA–dicrotic notch pressure or RV peak pressure to end-ejection volume, thus underestimates end-systolic pressure and volume in the RV as determined from maximal elastance.[23,30] The degree to which RV ESPVR and RV maximal elastance, like LV ESPVR and Emax, are affected by RV afterload, RV size, RV shape, and ventricular interaction is not well understood.[32] Compared to the LV, RV

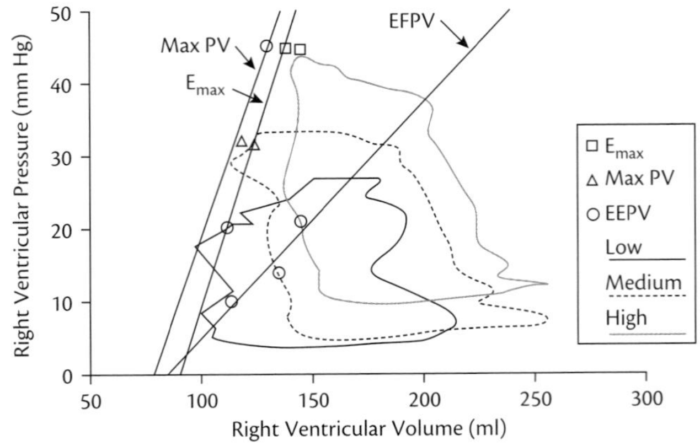

Fig. 20.4 Right ventricle (RV) cardiodynamics and pressure–volume relationships. The slopes of maximum time-varying elastance (Emax), maximum pressure/volume ratio (maxPV), and end-ejection pressure/volume (EEPV) are displayed for the RV by lines of best fit by passing through three points of each pressure–volume loop.

Reprinted from Cardiology Clinics, 30, Dell'Italia L, Anatomy and physiology of the right ventricle, 167–87, copyright (2012) with permission from Elsevier.

time-varying elastance exhibits a lower slope and higher V_0, likely due to lower RV pressure, larger RV volumes and lower RV mass.[10]

RV systolic function reflects mostly contractility, afterload, and preload, but also heart rhythm, ventricular contractile synchrony, RV force–interval relationship, ventricular interdependence, valvular regurgitation, and shunt flow.[7] Normal mean right ventricular

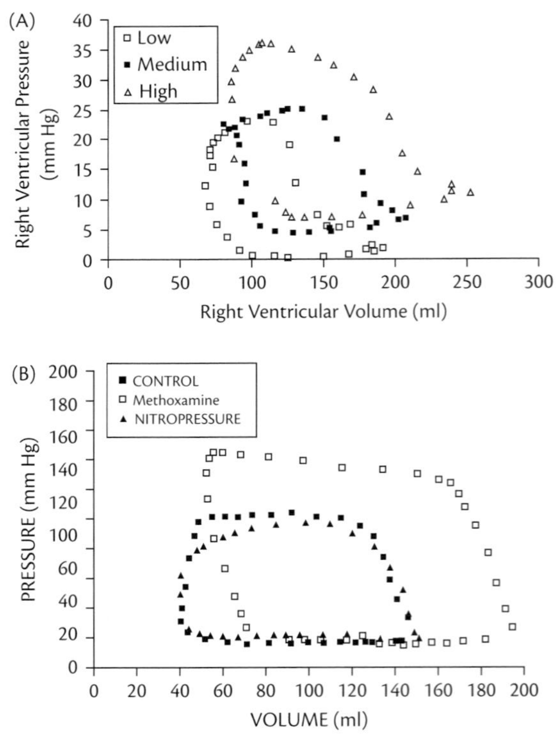

Fig. 20.5 Right and left ventricle (RV and LV) pressure–volume loops under varying conditions. RV (A) pressure–volume loops and LV (B) pressure–volume loops under high (open triangles), medium (black circles), and low (open squares) loading conditions, showing that the differences in RV and LV ejection dynamics at low loads and the similarity of RV and LV ejection dynamics at high loads.

Reprinted from Cardiology Clinics, 30, Dell'Italia L, Anatomy and physiology of the right ventricle, 167–87, copyright (2012) with permission from Elsevier.

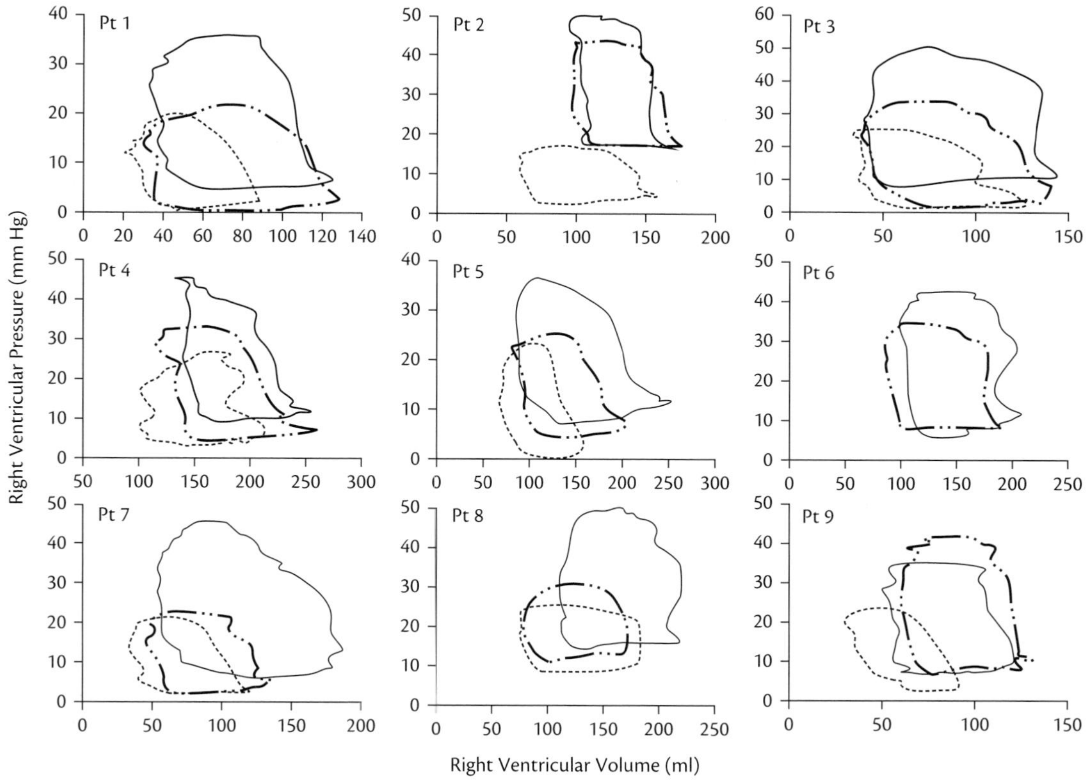

Fig. 20.6 Right ventricle (RV) response to nitroprusside and phenylephrine. RV pressure–volume loops for nine study patients having simultaneous high-fidelity RV pressure and RV biplane cineangiography, showing a parallel upward shift of the RV diastolic pressure–volume relation with changes in RV loading achieved with nitroprusside (dotted line), baseline (dashed dotted line), and phenylephrine (solid line).

ejection fraction (RVEF) is 61% by MRI, slightly lower than the normal mean left ventricular ejection fraction (LVEF) of 67% in healthy volunteers (Table 20.3).[9] RV stroke work is less than LV stroke work since the PVR is normally less than systemic vascular resistance in a ratio of 1:10. RV and LV stroke volume is the same in absence of semilunar regurgitation.[9] In acute RV infarction, RV dysfunction is exacerbated by loss of atrial systole and the resultant decreased preload reserve.[33]

Regulation of right ventricular function

Heart rate, Frank–Starling mechanism, and autonomic nervous system acutely regulate RV function. The mechanism of postextrasystolic potentiation in the RV results from a preload-dependent mechanism rather than enhanced contractility.[34] In a study of 11 subjects, postextrasystolic beats resulted in an increase in RVEF (61 ± 10% to 68 ± 4%, p <0.001), RV stroke volume (99 ± 18 ml to 128 ± 20 ml, p <0.001) without change in RV end-systolic volume, RV end-systolic pressure, or RV + dP/dt_{max} (318 ± 102 mmHg/s vs. 294 ± 82 mmHg/s, p = NS).[34] However, central venous pressure (CVP) in excess of 15 mmHg does not recruit additional RV contractile reserve.[7,10,35,36]

The autonomic nervous system has differential effects on inflow and outflow regions: vagal stimulation prolongs the sequence of activation and sympathetic stimulation may abolish the usual delay or even reverse it. The inotropic response of the infundibulum is greater than that of inflow tract. The normal RV exhibits a negative inotropic response to α-agonists, but the failing RV exhibits a positive inotropic response.[10]

Importance of pulmonary vascular impedance in determining right ventricular ejection

To eject, the RV must overcome pulmonary vascular impedance (PVI), the sum of all of the resistive, capacitative, inertial, pulse wave reflection, anatomic, hydraulic, and hemodynamic features and forces which oppose RV ejection.[10,37] In clinical practice, PVI is typically equated to the PVR,[37] but in reality PVR typically underestimates PVI, often markedly so, as in instances of advanced pulmonary artery remodeling[37] or in instances of postcapillary pulmonary hypertension.[38] In the intact circulation, PVI is determined by heart rate, pulmonary vessel configuration and viscoelastic stiffness, pulmonary wave reflections, RV geometry, RV function, RV interventricular pressures, ventricular interaction, and LV pressures.[10,37] Models of the intact pulmonary vasculature integrating all these passive and dynamic impedance components have yet to be developed for wide clinical use. As discussed in detail later in this chapter, postcapillary pulmonary hypertension due to LV dysfunction increases RV afterload and PVI and is a critical therapeutic target in clinical RV dysfunction of any cause.[38]

Increased afterload and limits of acute compensation

Normally, the RV is coupled to a low-impedance pulmonary vascular system. The normal low pulmonary impedance results from the absence of pulmonary vascular remodeling, normal LV function, low resultant PVR and a higher PA distensibility and pulmonary peripheral pulse wave reflection coefficient approximately one-half that of the systemic arterial circulation.[10,37,39,40,41] There is an approximate linear relationship between PA pressure and RV peak

Table 20.3 Assessment of right ventricular systolic function

Parameter	Normal value	Load dependence	Clinical utility
RVEF (%) (by MRI)	61 ± 7% (47–76%)	+ + +	Clinical validation, wide acceptance
RVFAC (%)	>35%	+ + +	Good correlation with RVEF
TAPSE (mm)	>16	+ + +	Prognostic value in MI, CABG, PAH
Doppler TV Sm annular (cm/s)	>10	+ + +	Good sensitivity and specificity for RVEF <50%
Strain	Basal 19 ± 6 Mid: 27 ± 6 Apical: 32 ± 6	+ + +	Correlates with stroke volume
RIMP (IVCt + IVRt/EJt)	>0.40 (pulsed Doppler)	+ +	Less reliable with arrhythmia, MI
dP/dt (mmHg/s)	100–250	+ +	Not reliable index of contractility
IVA (m/s²) (Vmax/time to PV)	1.4±0.5	+	Promising new index of contractility
Max elastance (mmHg/ml)	1.30±0.84	+	Most reliable index of contractility

CABG, coronary artery bypass graft; EJt, ejection time; IVA, isovolumic acceleration; IVCt, isovolumic contraction time; IVRt, isovolumic relaxation time; MI, myocardial infarction; PAH, pulmonary hypertension; RIMP, right ventricular index of myocardial performance; RVEF, right ventricular ejection fraction; RVFAC, right ventricular fractional area change; TAPSE, tricuspid valve systolic annular plane excursion; TV Sm annular, tricuspid *annular* systolic myocardial velocity.

Adapted from Haddad et al. 2008 and Rudski et al. 2010.

$+dP/dt_{max}$ in both normal subjects and subjects with pulmonary hypertension.[42] In response to intravenous phenylephrine, the RV exhibits an increase in peak RV $+dP/dt_{max}$, PA pressure, duration of isovolumic contraction, and increase in RVEDP.[23] Figure 20.7 illustrates the inverse relationship between RVEF and RV wall stress.

The RV, however, demonstrates a much greater sensitivity to afterload change than does the LV, as illustrated in Figure 20.8. The RV adapts much better to (1) chronic rather than acute and (2) volume rather than pressure overload. Compared to the LV, the RV "vulnerability" to pressure overload is due to multiple factors: lesser RV mass, lower time-varying elastance, predominant longitudinal shortening with lack of twist/torsion, lesser resistance to acute chamber dilatation and resultant "functional" tricuspid regurgitation and enhanced septal ventricular interaction in acute RV overload states. Given these structural and functional limitations, the previously "normal" RV is incapable of acutely generating a mean pulmonary artery pressure (PAP) greater than 40 mmHg. In classic animal models of acute pulmonary hypertension, sufficiently rapid and severe elevation of mean PAP precipitates circulatory collapse, due to failure of the RV to maintain adequate stroke work.

Right ventriculardiastolic filling and function

The driving force for RV diastolic filling is the diastolic pressure gradient along the entire RV inlet, from the high right atrium

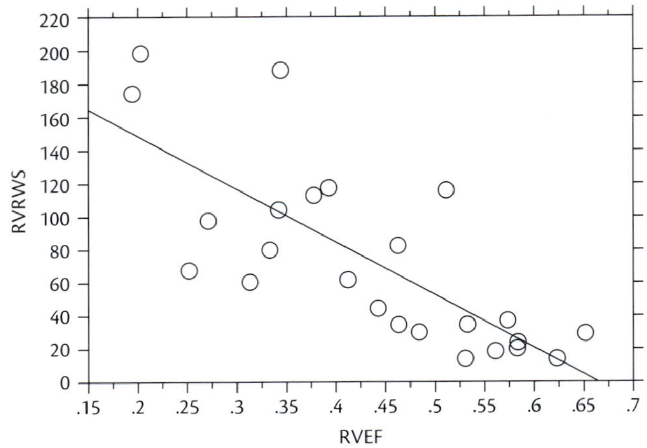

Fig. 20.7 Inverse relationship between a calculated measure of end-systolic circumferential right ventricular wall stress (RVWS) and right ventricular systolic function as measured by ejection fraction.

Voelkel N, Quaife R, Leinwand L, et al. Right ventricular function and failure: Report of a National Heart, Lung, Blood Institute Working Group on cellular and molecular mechanisms of right heart failure. Circulation 2006;114:1883–91.

(RA) to the RV apex (the RV filling pressure difference, RVFPD).[43] In the presence of a normal tricuspid valve, the mean RVFPD is close to 0 mmHg when measured between the high RA and the RV apex, with a peak RVFPD of 1.4 mmHg (95% CI 2.0–2.6) in normal health controls and a peak RVFPD of 1.0 mmHg (95% CI 0.8–1.2) in patients with dilated cardiomyopathy.[43] The LV peak filling pressure difference (LVFDP) is 3.5–4 mmHg, and slower relaxation of the RV compared to the LV may account for the lower peak RVFDP.[43] Early peak RVFPD correlated directly with mean RA pressure and inversely with the time constant *t* of RV relaxation. The RVFPD results almost completely from inertial forces across a normal tricuspid valve. Convective forces are minimal due to the low velocities present during RV filling and to the "hourglass" shape of RA–RV inflow.[43]

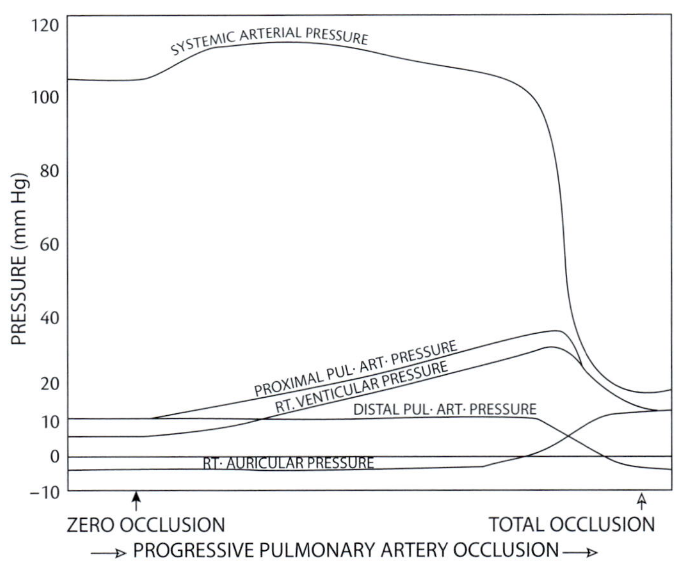

Fig. 20.8 Right ventricle vulnerability to pressure overload.

Greyson, CR. Pathophysiology of right ventricular failure. Crit Care Med 2008;36(Suppl 1):S57–S65.

The rate and degree of RV relaxation are major determinants of RV filling. There is likely early diastolic "suction" during early RV diastole, during which time RV intracavitary pressure falls below RA pressure.[44] RVFPD is 30–40% lower in dilated cardiomyopathy compared to controls.[43]

RV filling starts before and finishes after LV filling, RV isovolumic relaxation time is shorter, and both RV and filling velocities (E and A) and the RV E/A ratio are lower in the RV than in the LV.[10,22] As stated, the RV follows a force–interval relationship (stroke volume increases with longer diastolic filling periods). Within physiological limits, increased RV preload (CVP up to 15 mmHg) improves RV contractility. Beyond these physiological limits, excessive RV preload may compress LV and diminish cardiac output (via ventricular interdependence during diastole).

Diastolic RV dysfunction is common in patients with RV failure (Table 20.4). Compared to normal subjects, patients with heart failure (HF) exhibit a high prevalence of lower E/A ratios, lower peak E-wave velocity, and prolonged RV isovolumic times.[32] Tricuspid E-wave deceleration time was shorter only in patients with LV restrictive filling pattern.[32] The RA volume index (RAVI) is associated with worse RV systolic dysfunction, LVEF, and LV diastolic dysfunction, with a more modest correlation with tricuspid early/late velocities ratio and hepatic vein systolic/diastolic ratio, and no correlation with tricuspid early/tricuspid annular early velocities.[45] RV diastolic function is also abnormal in patients with pulmonary hypertension (PAH) in proportion to RV mass and mean pulmonary pressures, with increased isovolumic relaxation time, decreased E-wave and E/A wave velocities, and increased A wave velocities by echocardiography.[46,47]

Table 20.4 Assessment of right ventricular diastolic function

Index	Normal values	Clinical utility—comment
Pressures (mmHg)	RA mean: 3 (1–5) RVEDP: 4 (1–7)	High values suggest diastolic dysfunction
Inferior vena cava	Diameter ≤1.7 cm, collapse index (CI) ≥50%	Estimates of RA pressure (mmHg): IVC ≤1.7 cm, CI ≥50%: 0–5 IVC >1.7 cm, CI ≥50%: 6–10 IVC >1.7 cm, CI <50%: 10–15 IVC >1.7, fixed: ≥15
Diastolic E/A velocity	1.50 ± 0.3	E/A >2 suggests restriction
E deceleration time (ms)	198 ± 23	DT <160 ms suggests restriction
Hepatic vein S/D velocity ratio	>1 in sinus rhythm, <1 in AF	Reversal of flow seen in severe diastolic dysfunction or severe TR
Diastolic pulmonary flow	Absent	Presence suggests "restriction" in TOF
End-diastolic compliance	Not well defined	Limited data available in humans

AF, atrial fibrillation; CI, cardiac index; DT, deceleration time; IVC, inferior vena cava; RA, right atrium; RVEDP, right ventricular end-diastolic pressure; S/D, systolic to diastolic; TOF, tetralogy of Fallot; TR, tricuspid regurgitation.

Haddad F, Hung S, Rosenthal D, Murphy D. Right ventricular function in cardiovascular disease, Part I: Anatomy, physiology, aging, and functional assessment of the right ventricle. Circulation 2008;117:1436–48.

Ventricular interdependence

Ventricular interdependence (VI) results from the structural contiguity and functional continuity of the human RV and LV: i.e., both ventricles share common encircling muscle fibers, an interventricular septum, and a pericardial space while maintaining a similar cardiac output (Figure 20.9).[48] The RV free wall attaches to the anterior and posterior septum.[49] VI occurs during both diastole and systole and affects both ventricles. Independent loading of either ventricle during diastole shifts the contralateral ventricle diastolic pressure–volume relationship upward and leftward, even in the absence of pericardium.[50] Diastolic VI occurs on a beat-to-beat basis, and is most marked with abrupt changes in ventricular volume.

Systolic VI also occurs on an immediate beat-to-beat basis. Increasing the systolic pressure or volume in one ventricle results in an increase in both diastolic and systolic pressure in the contralateral ventricle and a decrease in pressure or volume in one ventricle results in an immediate decrease in pressure or volume in the contralateral ventricle.[48] In an experimental model of VI, LV systolic pressure was predominantly due to LV contraction (93%), but RV systolic pressure (and pulmonary blood flow) was predominantly due to LV contraction (64%).[51] Based on an overview of available experimental models, approximately 20–40% of RV systolic pressure and RV outflow likely results from LV contraction, and approximately 4–10% of LV systolic pressure and outflow likely results from RV contraction.[48] The contribution of LV contraction to RV contraction is typically "masked" by the normal near synchrony of LV and RV contraction, and likely is due to both (1) transmission of tension via shared fibers to the RV free wall and (2) an increased left-to-right trans-septal pressure gradient that buttresses the septum thereby augmenting RV free wall contraction.[52]

The septum thus plays a critical role in VI,[48] and in determining RV function in particular. The septum and RV free wall contribute approximately equally to overall RV function.[49] Alterations in systolic and diastolic loading can deform septal shape and position. RV systolic hypertension results in progressive leftward systolic shift of the septum during systole, and RV diastolic overload results in leftward shift of the septum during diastole. During diastole, this leftward septal shift results in relative LV compression, upward shift of LV diastolic P–V relationship (decreased LV distensibility), diminished LV preload, increased LV end-diastolic pressure, and subsequent decline in cardiac output. Chronic RV pressure overload reduces both septal and LV lateral wall longitudinal and circumferential strain rates and impairs LV torsion.[53]

The importance of the septum is underscored in experimental models of acute RV infarction and clinical studies in humans.[54] The normally contracting septum can maintain circulatory stability in the presence of acute RV free wall infarction if the RV is not dilated.[33,55] The loss of atrial systole and resultant decreased RV preload results in hemodynamic compromise in acute RV infarction.[33]

RV compliance is greater than LV compliance and thus the pericardium imposes greater constraint on the RV than the LV.[48] The pericardium likely affects diastolic VI to a greater extent than systolic VI.[56,57]

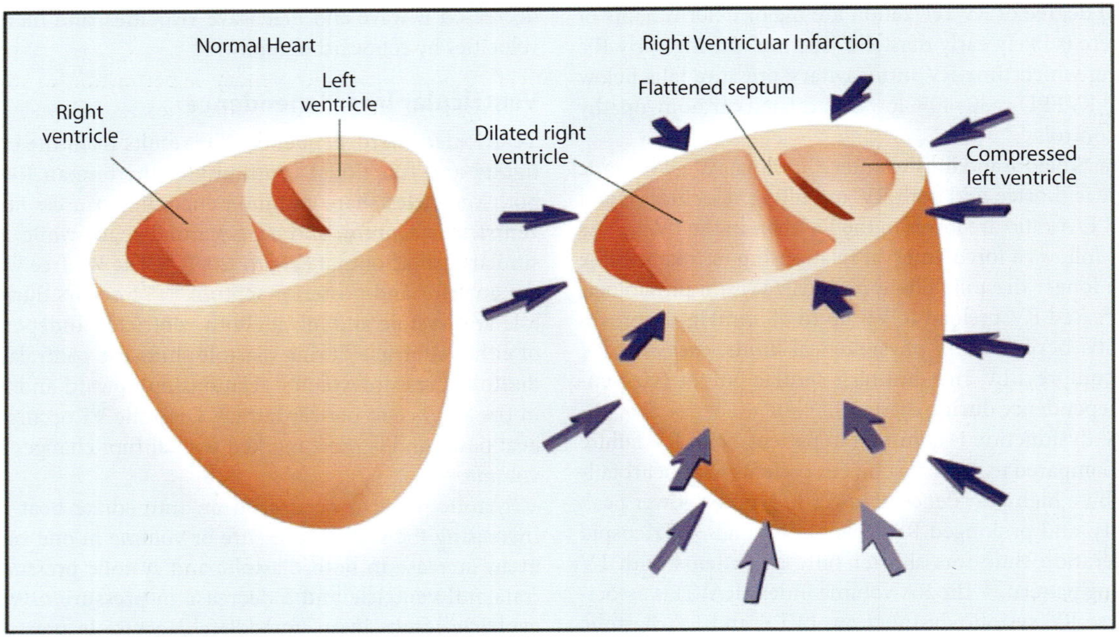

Fig. 20.9 Ventricular interdependence. The combination of pericardial constraint, right ventricular dilation, and leftward septal flattening and/or displacement results in left ventricular compression.

Right ventricular coronary demand and supply

The stroke work of the normal RV is approximately one-fourth that of the normal LV given the normally lower pulmonary versus system vascular resistance.[7] Accordingly, in dogs, right coronary artery flow rates to the normal RV (46 ± 6 ml min^{-1} 100 g^{-1}) and hypertrophied RV (53 ± 11 ml min^{-1} 100 g^{-1}) are both less the left anterior descending flow rate (88 ± 10 ml min^{-1} 100 g^{-1}) to the normal LV [58,59]. The myocardial oxygen consumption of the normal resting RV (4.0 ± 0.5 ml min^{-1} 100 g^{-1}) and hypertrophied RV (4.3 ± 0.7 ml min^{-1} 100 g^{-1}) are both approximately half that of the normal resting LV (7.8 ± 1.3 ml min^{-1} 100 g^{-1}).[58,59] An increase in RV oxygen requirement results in an increase in both RV coronary flow and RV oxygen extraction, in contrast to the LV, when an increase in LV oxygen requirement results in an increase in coronary blood flow without significant increase in the near-maximal resting oxygen extraction.[58,59] Compared to the LV, the RV exhibits lower oxygen requirements at rest and exercise, lower resting coronary blood flow and conductance, "equal" systolic and diastolic coronary flow, less effective pressure–flow autoregulation, greater effect of flow and pressure on oxygen demand, greater oxygen extraction reserve, higher dependency on NO to regulate resting right coronary artery (RCA) flow, and similar reductions in subepicardial and subendocardial flows during hypoperfusion.[7,10,35,54] The relative resistance of the RV to irreversible ischemic injury results from lower oxygen consumption, more extensive collateral circulation (moderator band artery, a branch of first septal perforator) and the ability to increase oxygen extraction due to RV "oxygen extraction reserve" under ischemic conditions.[10] This has led some experienced investigators to conclude that "RV myocardial infarction is a misnomer".[54]

Major anatomic and functional differences between the left and right ventricles

The RV differs in a variety of ways from the LV, as summarized in Box 2.1. The RV has a different embryological origin as the RVOT, and part of RV myocardium are both derived from the anterior heart field. Unlike the LV, the RV undergoes a process of dynamic remodeling following birth, including rapid regression of total mass and increase in compliance. Compared to that of the LV, adult RV adult structure is marked by functionally and anatomically separate inflow and outflow regions, a higher surface area to volume ratio, larger volume (~10 mL/m^2), one-quarter the total mass, thinner walls, triangular/crescentic configuration, presence of a prominent moderator band and less predictable papillary muscle relations.

Compared to integrated LV cardiodynamics, integrated RV cardiodynamics is marked by adaptation for volume rather than pressure work, less pressure development during systole, less discrete isovolumic contraction and relaxation periods, lower ventricular stroke work index, lower time-varying elastance, and lower net vascular impedance. More than the LV, the RV relies upon the interventricular septum for efficient ejection and exhibits overall greater sensitivity than the LV to ventricular interaction. RVOT peristaltic contraction helps propel the RV ejection bolus into the PA. Compared to the LV, the RV has lower resting coronary perfusion, lower oxygen extraction, greater extraction reserve, and lower susceptibility to ischemic injury.

Adaptive and maladaptive ventricular remodeling

RV adverse remodeling and RV transition to failure play key roles in diverse human cardiovascular disease states and conditions, including all types of LV failure (where RV function independently predicts survival), all types of pulmonary hypertension (primary and secondary—where RV function is a much more important determinant of clinical outcome and survival than the degree of pulmonary hypertension or altered PVR), tricuspid and pulmonary valve disease, childhood and adult congenital heart disease, and common acquired lung diseases (e.g., emphysema, pulmonary embolism).[7,35]

Box 20.1 Summary of differences between the right and left ventricle

- Embryology
  - RV embryological origin (RVOT, part of RV myocardium from anterior heart field)
- Remodeling
  - Physiologic "involution" following birth: increase in compliance, regression of mass
- Structure
  - Higher surface area to volume ratio than LV
  - Larger volume than LV (~ 10 mL/m^2)
  - 1/4 LV mass
  - Thinner walls
  - Triangular configuration
  - Moderator band
  - Less predictable papillary muscle relations
- Cardiodynamics
  - Evolved for pressure, not volume work
  - Less pressure generation during cardiac cycle
  - Lower stroke work index
  - Lower time-varying elastance
  - Lower vascular impedance
  - Importance of septum for ejection
  - Importance of free wall for ejection
  - Vigorous outflow tract contraction to "impel" ejection bolus
- Perfusion
  - Lower resting coronary perfusion
  - Lesser resting oxygen extraction ("extraction reserve")
  - Lesser susceptibility to ischemic injury
- Molecular cardiology: RV isolated myocytes
  - Maximal sarcomere shortening less than LV myocytes
  - Smaller peak calcium transients than LV myocytes
- Molecular cardiology: RV
  - Greater expression of a-myosin heavy chain isozyme
  - Greater cholinergic adrenergic receptor density than in LV
  - Possible negative inotropic effect of α-adrenergic stimulation
  - Inotropic response of RVOT exceeds response of RV inflow tract
- Molecular cardiology: RV remodeling
  - Different gene expression signatures (animal pressure/volume overload models)

Despite the lack of correlative mechanistic data, there are some intriguing observations regarding human RV remodeling derived from patients with pulmonary hypertension of diverse cause.[20] First, genetic heterogeneity underlies RV adaptation to pressure overload. Not all patients with similar degrees of pulmonary hypertension develop the same degree of right ventricular hypertrophy (RVH). Second, as described below, the human RV remodeled by pressure overload possesses considerable plasticity, as evidenced by the resolution of RV dysfunction due to chronic pressure overload following lung transplantation for parenchymal lung disease and surgery for chronic thromboembolic pulmonary hypertension. Third, the human RV appears more "resistant" to the effects of acute or chronic ischemia than the LV.[54]

Despite an increasing number of studies of explanted human myocardium in children and adults with congenital heart disease, no study to date has focused exclusively on the RV mRNA or miRNA transcriptome or proteome in human adult heart failure. The fundamental features of RV maladaptive remodeling and RV transition to failure pathobiology are thus unknown in human adult heart failure, including the degree of similarity (or not) to LV pathobiology.[20] Since many of the mechanisms of RV remodeling likely share similarities and/or are identical to mechanisms implicated in LV remodeling, a brief overview of LV remodeling is in order, followed by review of the available evidence to date of RV adaptive and maladaptive remodeling and the transition to RV failure.

Left ventricular remodeling

When presented with acute or chronic pressure and/or volume overload or injury of diverse cause, the human LV undergoes complex adaptations termed remodeling.[60] During remodeling, molecular, cellular, and extracellular matrix changes lead to changes in the size, shape, and function of the heart.[61] LV remodeling involves a complex series of interrelated events, including:

1. cardiomyocyte hypertrophy and sarcomere reorganization with accompanying changes in cardiomyocyte electrical properties and excitation–contraction coupling, calcium cycling, myofilament function, bioenergetics and metabolism, contractile function, cell survival signaling, and viability
2. increased rates of extracellular matrix protein synthesis and degradation (particularly collagenolysis via metalloproteinases) ultimately resulting in fibrosis and ventricular dilatation and shape change
3. changes in myocardial perfusion and energetics, typically an insufficient increase in capillary density for the degree of hypertrophy, changeover from fatty acid to glucose as the preferential metabolic substrate, mitochondrial remodeling, and a general increase in metabolically derived reactive oxygen species.[62,63]

During remodeling, the LV passes through an initially adaptive phase marked by cardiomyocyte and ventricular hypertrophy.[63] In experimental models of LV remodeling, LV pressure versus volume overload adaptive remodeling results in distinct remodeling phenotypes characterized by differential gene expression signatures, type and degree of extracellular matrix fibrosis, and ventricular size and shape adaptations.[64] Adaptive ventricular remodeling aims to restore circulatory homostasis following myocardial injury or constitutive overload. These changes in response to pathologic conditions are different from the ventricular physiologic remodeling responses to physical exercise.[63] With a sufficient degree of initial injury, subsequent injury and/or persistently severe pressure and/or volume overload, the initially adaptive ventricular remodeling phase transitions to a maladaptive phase, typically marked by progressive cardiomyocyte loss, increasing extracellular matrix fibrosis, progressive ventricular dilatation and shape distortion, and systolic and diastolic dysfunction.[63] The clinical syndrome of heart failure then supervenes. Over time, maladaptive ventricular remodeling may transition to inexorable ventricular failure despite current therapies.[62]

In most, but not all, studies of explanted human myocardium the ischemic and nonischemic LV have not exhibited distinctive mRNA transcriptomic signatures.[65,66,67,68,69,70,71,72,73] Considerable transcriptome heterogeneity and overlap exists between patients due to multiple factors, including disease duration, disease severity, comorbid conditions, pharmacologic and/or device therapies, and environmental factors. A generally reciprocal relationship between myocardial signaling pathways (especially through the "hub" protein STAT3) and myocardial oxidative phosphorylation metabolic pathways was recently reported in a meta-analysis of all available human LV myocardial transcriptome datasets.[65] The LV transcriptome differences reported in this meta-analysis were hypothesized to result mostly from HF disease duration and severity, with more long-standing and severely affected hearts exhibiting more consistently similar transcriptomes.

The transcriptomic signatures of LV myocardial pressure and volume overload differ in animal models[64] and humans,[61] and vary according to overload duration and severity. Recent work focused on miRNA modulation of mRNA translation.[74,75,76,77,78] miRNAs have been previously reported by other investigators to play an important role in LV hypertrophy, LV adaptive and maladaptive remodeling, and LV failure in humans.[76,79] The miRNA signatures of ischemic versus nonischemic human HF differ[80] and specific circulating miRNAs may hold promise as biomarkers of the clinical syndrome of HF.[81]

Animal models of right ventricular remodeling

Animal models of pulmonary hypertension have provided insights into RV eccentric and concentric remodeling. In response to volume overload, the RV remodels by eccentric hypertrophy. Following 7 weeks of exercise in rats, there was a 25% increase in RV area, 22% increase in RV weight, 26% lengthening of RV myocytes, no change in sarcomere length, mitochondria:mitofibril volume ratio or RV midwall thickness, a 16% increase in RV capillary density, a 41% increase in total capillary length, and a 10% reduction in maximum diffusion distance from capillary wall to mitochondria due to capillary proliferation.[82] This pattern of proportional eccentric hypertrophy coupled with structural adaptations of the capillary bed improves the diffusion and transport of oxygen within the tissue. In a chronic AV shunt dog model at 3 months, there were significant increases in RV systolic pressures, end-diastolic pressures, and end-diastolic volume without changes in baseline contractility.[83] However, stepwise increases in RV afterload from 35 to 50 mmHg in this model led to greater stepwise increases in contractility in control (2.73 ± 0.30 mmHg/ml and 4.15 ± 0.30 mmHg/ml) than in volume-overloaded hearts (2.11 ± 0.38 mmHg/ml and 2.99 ± 0.29 mmHg/ml, p <0.05 vs. controls) consistent with impaired inotropic adaptation to increased afterload in the volume-overloaded hearts.[83] In a transannular patch RV volume overload sheep model at 3 months, dobutamine increased contractility (1.2 ± 0.5 mmHg/ml vs. 2.8 ± 1.7 mmHg/ml, p = 0.03) but to a lesser extent than in pulmonary-banded RV pressure-overload sheep (1.44 ± 0.7 mmHg/ml vs. 4.0 ± 2.0 mmHg/ml, p = 0.022 compared to change in volume-overloaded sheep).[84]

In response to pressure overload, the RV remodels by concentric hypertrophy. In a monocroataline-induced pulmonary hypertension rat model at 4 weeks, the RV to LV weight ratio increased from 0.29 ± 0.05 to 0.49 ± 0.10 g (p <0.001), RV wall thickness increased from 0.98 ± 0.25 to 1.43 ± 0.41 mm (p <0.01) and RVEF declined from 49 ± 6% to 26 ± 6% (p <0.05).[85] RV systolic and diastolic volumes, filling pressures, and wall stress approximately doubled and cardiac output significantly decreased.[85] In a PA banding model in goats at 4 days, there was a 66% increase in RV free wall thickness, 27% increase in RV myocyte perimeter, and 69% increase in RV myocyte area in banded animals.[86] In a cat model with PA banding, RV pressure overload, and atrial septal defect RV volume overload, cardiomyocyte cross-sectional area increased in both types of overload compared to controls but the increase was greatest in pressure overload pressure and attributable to a more "rounded" cardiomyocyte profile rather than cardiomyocyte lengthening.[87] There were no differences in the proportion of organelles or volume densities of either mitochondria or myofibrils. Both pressure and volume overload exhibited a comparable degree of increase in RV weight but the volume density of cardiomyocytes in pressure-overload papillary muscles was significantly decreased with a significantly increased proportion of connective tissue and collagen.[87] The investigators concluded that in RV pressure overload (1) while overall RV mass increases, RV cardiomyocyte mass does not increase proportionally to overall RV mass; (2) this lack of proportional increase in RV cardiomyocyte mass contributes to RV systolic dysfunction; and (3) increased RV diastolic stiffness in RV pressure overload is attributable at least in part to increased RV connective tissue and collagen deposition.[87] In a progressive PA banding model in dogs at 3 months, RV elastance and stiffness both increased (p <0.05), consistent with preserved systolic function but impaired diastolic function.[88] In this model RA elastance increased as did RA reservoir function and distensibility, likely to maintain filling of the stiffened RV.[88] Interestingly, in a PA banding pig model, diffusion tensor MRI imaging showed (1) RV hypertrophy but no difference in RV endocardial and epicardial helical angles or RV myocardial fiber pathways in RV hypertrophy hearts compared to RV control hearts, and (2) lack of extensive zone of circular myocytes in both control hearts and RV hypertrophy hearts compared to the normal LV.[13] The investigators concluded that the hypertrophied but "preserved" normal RV three-dimensional architecture found in RV hypertrophy rendered the hypertrophied RV vulnerable to a sustained or progressive increase in afterload, unlike the LV.[13]

Remodeling in human disease and the transition to right ventricular failure

The normal human RV accommodates a large increase in venous return during exercise mostly by increasing RV stroke volume as the RV end-diastolic volume does not typically change.[89] The normal human RV is well-adapted to large-volume stroke work, due to (1) RV recruitable work reserve, (2) RV diastolic distensibility, (3) exercise-induced augmentation in septal contraction with application of greater RV free wall traction, and (4) the normal drop in PVR with exercise.[10] In human disease, chronic RV volume overload (e.g., right-to-left shunt lesion, tricuspid regurgitation, or pulmonary regurgitation) results in eccentric hypertrophy and adaptive RV remodeling that may sustain the circulation for decades. As in animal models, RV cardiomyocytes lengthen by increasing sarcomeres in series with appropriate proportional increases in myofibrils, mitochondrial mass, and capillary supply. Unrelenting volume overload, however, results in an eventual adverse chain of events: (1) progressive RV dilatation increases RV wall stress with adverse effects on cardiomyocyte and extracellular structure, function, and coupling; (2) increase in oxygen consumption may not be met by an insufficiently developed capillary bed with ever greater RV hypertrophy; (3) tricuspid annular dilation with secondary tricuspid regurgitation begets greater RV volume overload and RV wall stress: and (4) severe RV dilation may result in leftward septal movement, impaired LV filling due to adverse VI, elevation of LV filling pressure with commensurate elevation of RV afterload, and reduction in cardiac output due to LV underfilling.

In patients with pulmonary hypertension, concentric RV hypertrophy and RV remodeling is typically proportional to the degree of elevation of PAP and most advanced in patients with overt RV failure.[89] Cardiomyocyte remodeling occurs largely via increased sarcomeres added in series, in an attempt to normalize the increased systolic wall stress borne by cardiomyocytes. Regional heterogeneity of remodeling is frequently observed, with greater hypertrophy often of the RVOT.[90] Concentric hypertrophy results in an increase in RV mass and oxygen consumption. RV ischemia may play a greater role in maladaptive concentric remodeling, as the higher RV systolic pressures reduce the aortic root–RV systolic pressure systolic coronary perfusion gradient.[89] As noted above, in animal models of RV pressure overload, extracellular remodeling is prominent. In infant human hearts with congenital RV pressure overload, increased subendocardial collagen deposition is apparent by several months of life compared to normal infant hearts or the hearts of infants born with congenital volume overload.[91] In adults dying of massive pulmonary emboli with acute severe RV pressure overload, RV fibrosis is also apparent in addition to patchy myocyte necrosis with an accompanying unique macrophage, T-cell, and neurophilic inflammatory infiltrate distinct from epicardial coronary artery myocardial infarction or myocarditis, perhaps due to progressively severe RV wall stress and global myocardial hypoxia.[92]

Cardiodynamic and geometric aspects of remodeling

Further insight into fundamental cardiodynamic and geometric aspects of human adaptive and maladaptive RV remodeling has been provided by evolving hemodynamics, echocardiography, and cardiac MRI (CMR) applications and the major clinical factors determining RV remodeling listed in Box 20.2.[26] RV dilation (RVEDVI >110 ml/m^2 in males, >100 ml/m^2 in females) is often the first sign of RV volume and/or pressure overload.[26] RVEF (normal >44%, 95% CI 38–50% by 2D or 3D echocardiography and >61 ± 7% by CMR, although in wide clinical practice 40–45% is used) and percent fractional RV area change (normal >40%) are both typically reduced.[93] Progressive RV systolic dysfunction results in greater prolongation of RV isovolumic contraction and RV diastolic dysfunction results in greater prolongation of RV isovolumic relaxation.[10] The ratio of the RV isovolumic relaxation plus the RV isovolumic contraction divided by the RV total ejection time—the myocardial performance index (MPI) or Tei ratio—increases with RV pressure and volume overload as RV isovolumic periods, which are normally very short, progressively prolong.[26] MPI predicts disease progression in primary pulmonary hypertension and congenital heart disease.[26] RV fibrosis is commonly detected by delayed contrast-enhancement CMR in patients with zzzzzzzz (ARVD) and congenital heart disease, with the extent of fibrosis correlating with regional and global RV dysfunction.[26] In

Box 20.2 Major clinical factors involved in the transition to right ventricular failure

- Unrelieved acute or chronic RV injury/stress
- Progressive intrinsic RV myocardial contractile dysfunction
  - Cardiomyopathy (e.g., ARVD, cardiomyopathy, congenital heart disease)
  - RV infarction
- Unrelieved RV pressure overload and RV–PA uncoupling
  - Intrinsic pulmonary vascular disease
  - Pulmonary vascular remodeling
  - LV dysfunction
- Unrelieved RV volume overload
  - Primary TR
  - Secondary TR from progressive tricuspid annular dilatation
  - Left-to-right shunt
  - PR
- RV ischemia
  - RV hypertrophy with insufficient capillary hypertrophy
  - RV marginal stenosis/occlusion
  - Low aortic root pressure
  - Low cardiac output
- Interventricular septum dysfunction or displacement
- Dysrhythmia
  - Lack of coordinated atrial transport (e.g., atrial fibrillation)
  - RV dyssynchrony (e.g., bundle branch block, regional contractile heterogeneity)
- Degree and severity of pre-existing RV dysfunction
- Degree and severity of pre-existing pulmonary vascular disease
- Degree and severity of pre-existing intrinsic pulmonary parenchymal disease
- Hypoxemia
  - Intrinsic lung disease
  - Obstructive sleep apnea/obesity–hypoventilation syndrome
- Medical comorbidities
  - Diabetes mellitus
  - Chronic kidney disease
  - Chronic liver disease
- Genomic heterogeneity

predominant pressure overload, the RV free wall may exhibit concentric hypertrophy (RV wall thickness >5 mm).[94]

With progressive RV dysfunction, tricuspid valve systolic annular plane excursion (TAPSE) and tissue Doppler velocity (S) both decrease, indicative of lesser RV longitudinal shortening in the absence of changes in RV afterload.[26] RV strain (degree of deformation) and strain rate (rate of deformation over time) measured by either tissue velocity or ultrasound speckle tracking, while load dependent, are reduced progressively with progressive RV dysfunction and failure.[95] RV strain and strain rate mapping often exhibits regional heterogeneity, particularly in pulmonary hypertension, with particular reduction in apical RV region.[26] A less load-dependent measure of RV systolic function, the slope of myocardial acceleration during isovolumic contraction (IVA) by tissue Doppler, correlates with RV end-systolic elastance and is depressed in progressive RV failure.[95]

RV mechanical dyssynchrony implies the loss of the normal sequential peristaltic RV contraction pattern from inflow, apical to outflow regions.[26] Although right bundle branch block does not appear to result in substantial RV dyssynchrony (as assessed by time to peak strain of the RV lateral wall and interventricular septum), RV dyssynchrony alone and RV and interventricular RV–LV dyssynchrony (as assessed by time to peak strain in RV vs. LV free wall) are frequently observed in patients with pulmonary hypertension and associated with poorer functional capacity and greater disease severity.[26]

RA dilatation occurs with chronic elevation of RV pressures in the absence of tricuspid regurgitation, and Doppler indices of RV diastolic function (from tricuspid inflow velocities, early diastolic strain rate) are frequently abnormal in patients with RV failure from diverse causes, as discussed above.[26,93,95]

Possible molecular mechanisms of the transition to right ventricular failure

The molecular mechanisms occasioning the transition of the remodeled RV to failure are unknown. To date, the molecular aspects of RV remodeling have mostly been studied in animal models of pressure overload and in studies of explanted human myocardium in children with congenital heart disease.[96] In mice, the normal RV evidences differential mRNA expression as compared to the normal LV,[97] and differential functional and molecular responses as compared to the LV to pressure versus volume overload.[98] In mouse models of RV pressure overload, the RV evidences a gene expression pattern (1) distinct from the normal RV[97,99] and (2) mostly concordant to the pattern observed in the pressure-overloaded LV[100] except for significant differences in expression of members of the Wnt signaling pathway, annexin A7, clusterin/apolipoprotein J, Nbl1, Fnbp4, and LOX.[99] In a mouse Sugen5416/hypoxia model, the failing RV exhibits a gene expression "signature" distinct from the pressure-overloaded RV marked by (1) decreased expression of angiogenic factors (VEGF, IGF-1, apelin, angiopoeitin-1) and miRNA 113a and (2) increased expression of glycolytic enzymes and regulators (including HK1, ADH7, and Ucp2) and genes encoding fibrosis-controlling proteins (including TGF-β1, TGF-β2, Smad4, MAPK3, forkhead box A2).[97] miRNAs play an key role in RV remodeling in animal models of both pulmonary hypertension[97] and congenital heart disease[101] and in human infants with congenital heart disease.[102,103] From the available evidence in animal models and in human congenital heart disease, then, RV remodeling pathobiology appears (1) distinct from LV pathobiology; (2) dependent upon type, duration and severity of RV injury and/or overload; (3) distinguishable by mRNA transcriptome signatures (cell growth, angiogenesis, fibrosis, and energy metabolism); and (4) subject to miRNA regulation of mRNA translation.

Neurohormonal signaling

In a dog model of stressed RV[104] and in human RV failure, β-adrenergic receptor density is decreased and there is decreased activity of the catalytic subunit of adenylate cyclase.[105] Analogous to the β-receptor downregulation and receptor upcoupling characteristic of chronic LV failure, this may be an adaptive response.[106] In failing adult rat RV myocardium, α_1 agonists result in a positive inotropic response, in contrast to the negative inotropic response in nonfailing adult RV myocardium.[107] In human PAH with isolated RV failure, elevated catecholamine levels are significantly correlated with higher PAP ($r = 0.66$), higher PVR ($r = 0.69$) and lower cardiac index ($r = -0.56$).[108] There is loss of RV responsiveness to the inotropic effects of antiotensin II (ATII) and uncoupling of angiotensin I (ATI) receptors to downstream signaling pathways, both of which are attenuated by angiotensin converting enzyme (ACE) inhibitors and/or angiotensin receptor antagonists.[109] PAH patients with non-DD genotype have reported to have worse survival.[110] Changes also occur in endothelin signaling systems. Increase in vascular and RV expression of ET-1 and ET receptors are found in both rat PAH models[111] and in humans with PAH and decreased RV function in association with higher circulating ET-1 levels.[108,112]

Cytokine signaling

Cytokine-mediated inflammation plays an important role in ischemic and inflammatory heart failure[113] and pulmonary hypertension.[114] Proinflammatory cytokines, such as TNFα, IL-1β, IL-6, cardiotrophin, and IL-8 can modulate (1) contractile performance directly via effects on electromechanical coupling, NOS3, activity and β-adrendergic sensitivity; (2) matrix metalloproteinase activity and ventricular remodeling; and (3) cardiomyocyte survival.[115] Less is known about the cardiac roles of anti-inflammatory cytokines such as IL-10 and thrombospondin-1.[116] Although proinflammatory cytokine circulating levels are biomarkers of HF severity and clinical outcome, clinical trials of anti-TNFα therapies failed to provide benefit to patients with chronic HF, likely due to the complexity of innate immune signaling in the heart and paracrine cross-talk between myocardial cell types.[62,117] Recent attention in LV heart failure has turned away from inhibiting proinflammatory cytokines to (1) augmenting growth and trophic cytokines such as granulocyte colony-stimulating factor (G-CSF) and erythropoietin [118] and (2) modulating Toll-like receptors which mediate the innate myocardial immune signaling response.[119] Although cytokines are generally felt to play an important role in RV remodeling, experimental evidence specifying both the exact role and relative importance of cytokines in RV remodeling and both acute and chronic RV failure is lacking.[7,16,20,35,96,120]

Nitric oxide signaling

In animal models of LV pressure overload, blocking cGMP catabolism by chronic treatment with the phosphodiesterase-5a (PDE5) inhibitor sildenafil suppresses LV hypertrophy by deactivating multiple hypertrophy signaling pathways including calcineurin/NFAT,

PI3K/AKT, and ERK 1/2.[121] In small trials in patients with systolic and diastolic heart failure and pulmonary hypertension, sildenafil improves exercise hemodynamics and performance[122,123,124,125,126] and LV systolic and diastolic function and attenuates indices of adverse LV and RV remodeling.[127,128] Large, multicenter efficacy trials of PDE5-I in patients with chronic LV failure and secondary pulmonary hypertension are under way, but the outcomes are unpredictable.[129,130]

PDE5 inhibitors such as sildenafil are currently approved for use in primary pulmonary hypertension as a pulmonary arterial vasodilator.[131] In clinical trials of patients with PAH, sildenafil in dose-related fashion increased cardiac output.[132] PDE5 expression is minimal in the normal RV[133] but undergoes marked upregulation in the hypertrophied and failing RV.[134] The effects of chronic PDE5 inhibition on RV remodeling in particular may provide a new therapeutic strategy to attenuate RV maladaptive remodeling and the transition to RV failure.[130,131,135]

Bioenergetics and mitochondrial remodeling

Substantial changes occur in RV bioenergetics and metabolism in both pulmonary hypertension (PH) and RV failure.[136] RV hypertrophy and RV failure are both marked by a reduction in normal 60–90% predominance of mitochondrial fatty acid oxidation and an increase in cytosolic glycolysis for ATP synthesis.[89] Since glucose metabolism requires less oxygen consumption for an equivalent amount of ATP synthesis, stressed myocardium typically evidences a shift toward preferential glucose uptake and metabolism rather than fatty acid metabolism to minimize oxygen requirement.[136] RV glucose uptake is increased in patients with PH,[137] indicative of the relative switch to RV cytosolic glycolysis rather than mitochondrial oxidative phosphorylation.[96] Nonmetabolized fatty acids and/or incompletely metabolized toxic fatty acid intermediates accumulate in failing RV myocardium and may further impair function.[136]

In animal models, gene expression profiles are compatible with multilevel impairment of fatty acid metabolism (decreased expression of PPAR-1α, PPAR-α, and ERR-α) and significant mitochondrial dysfunction.[138] Mitochondial membrane potential is increased in RV tissue obtained from patients with PH,[139] leading to mitochondrial hyperpolarization.[140] Mitochondrial hyperpolarization is felt to confer protection against mitochondrial-dependent apoptosis[89] by moving the mitochondrial transition pore away from the apoptotic threshold.[140] However, mitochondrial hyperpolarization "stalls" oxidative phosphorylation and shifts energy production further toward cytosolic glycolysis.[140] This metabolic and mitochondrial remodeling in RV hypertrophy and RV failure may result in relative protection from ischemia and mitochondrial-dependent apoptosis, but may be at the expense of reduced contractility, since mitochondrial oxidative phosphorylation of fatty acids yields more ATP than cytosolic glycolysis.[89] Evolving evidence supports a potential therapeutic role for pharmacologic metabolic modulators to reverse the glycolytic phenotype, such as dichloroacetate (DCA), a phosphodiesterase kinase inhibitor.[96] In animal models of PAH, DCA promotes reverse remodeling of the pressure-overloaded RV and improves RV contractility.[139]

Excitation–contraction coupling

Sarcolemmal depolarization upon arrival of an action potential opens the voltage-sensitive sarcolemma L-type calcium channel and results in an influx of a small amount of calcium through the channel into a local junctional cleft functional microdomain composed of T-tubules and ryanodine sarcoplasmic reticulum receptors (RyRs).[141] Calcium influx into the junctional cleft occasions the opening of RyRs in turn which release a larger amount of calcium sequestered by calsequestrin in the SR into the cytosol.[142] Via this process of calcium-induced calcium release (CICR) trhough the SR RyRs, cytosolic calcium typically rises from 0.1–0.2 mM to 2–10 mM.[143] Phosphorylation of RyRs by phosphokinase A (PKA) and/or CaMKII increases SR calcium release.[142] Calcium released into the cytosol then acts in multiple ways as a critical second messenger:

1. Calcium initiates actin–myosin cross-bridge cycling directly (calcium binds to TnC and "pulls" TnI off the troponin complex actin binding site; in so doing, the troponin–tropomyosin complex is also reconfigured permitting myosin-head binding to actin; myosin-head binding to actin in the presence of ATP then initiates actin–myosin cross-bridge cycling).
2. Calcium uptake into mitochondria provides an important energy supply and demand feedback signal.
3. Calcium binding to calmodulin (Ca-CaM) provides transcriptional regulation of cardiomyocyte hypertrophy via the Ca-CaM-CaMKII-HDAC (histone deacetylase) and Ca-CaM-calcineurin-NFAT (nuclear factor of activated T cells) pathways. [141]

In these ways, calcium is linked to critical aspects of cardiomyocyte contractile function, metabolism, and gene transcription. Following release from the SR, calcium is then actively transported back into the SR by sarcoplasmic reticulum ATPase (SERCA2) and is also extruded from the cardiomyocyte via a sarcolemmal sodium–calcium exchanger (NCX).[142] SERCA2 activity in turn is inhibited by unphosphorylated phospholamban (PLN). Phosphorylation of PLN by PKA and/or CaMKII increases SERCA2 activity. In this manner, excitation–contraction coupling (EC coupling) occurs within cardiomyocytes.

A welter of EC coupling and calcium handling abnormalities have been well described in the failing heart: alteration in all components essential for CICR, blunted CICR with loss of EC coupling "gain" (since conductance of L-type calcium channels and RyRs is unchanged in heart failure, loss of EC coupling "gain" is thought to result from either dysregulation of CICR component kinetics/stoichiometry and/or anatomic microenvironment ultrastructural defects), decreased SR calcium content, PKA-induced RyR hyperphosphorylation, reduced RyR SR calcium release with an increase in RyR "leaks" and calcium "sparks," reduced amplitude of intracellular calcium transients with resultant blunted force generation, blunted decay of the global intracelluar calcium transient, elevation of end-diastolic calcium concentration, SERCA2 loss of function and reduced rate of SERCA2 calcium reuptake, PLN gain of function with associated increase in PLN:SERCA2 ratio and PLN hypophosphorylation due at least in part to increased activity of PP1, NCX gain of function and increased mitochondrial calcium uptake.[141,142,143,144,145] The SERCA/PLN ensemble in particular has provided an attractive target for new therapies, including gene transfer of SERCA2 to "rescue" the HF phenotype.[145]

EC coupling and alterations of calcium cycling and their effects on RV function have been relatively little studied to date.[16,146] In mice, RVH induced by PA constriction results in deceased myocyte tension development and reduced calcium responsiveness.[147] The force generation of RV papillary muscle per unit mass is less than that of LV papillary muscle.[16] The contraction velocities of RV intact ventricular muscle strips and RV isolated single cells are both more rapid than in the corresponding LV tissues.[148]

Contractile proteins

In LV heart failure, there is a reduction in volume of myofibrils per cell.[106] Although changes in contractile protein expression may occur, most of the functional alterations of contractile proteins in the failing heart are thought to more likely result from isoform shifts; post-translational modification, particularly altered phosphorylation states; and perhaps enhanced rates of proteolysis.[149] Changes in contractile protein isoform expression have been reported for myosin heavy chain (MHC, α to β isoform), myosin light chain (ventricular to atrial isoform), troponin T (adult to fetal isoform), and titin (stiff N2B to compliant N2BA isoform).[151,152,153,154,155]

As in the LV, the alterations in the complex signaling pathways that alter human RV contractile protein phosphorylation will exhibit undoubted diversity based upon disease etiology, duration, severity, neurohormonal "cross-talk", coexistent and/or comorbid medical conditions, pharmacologic and device interventions, and genotype.

Cytoskeletal proteins and the extracellular matrix

Cytoskeletal disorganization is present in animal models of RV failure. In neonatal calves with severe PH and RV failure, there was histologic loss and disorganization of costameres and intercalated disks and in myocytes, vinculin and desmin were redistributed diffusely in the cytosol and metavinculin was present in disorganized clumps.[156] Increased reactive oxidative species may activate matrix metalloproteinases and induce mitophagy due to mitochondrial damage from reactive oxidative species.[157]

Cell survival: necrosis, apoptosis, and autophagy

Since cardiomyocytes are both terminally differentiated and replication-deficient, the heart likely does not exhibit programmed cardiac myocyte loss, unlike other organs as part of normal homeostatic renewal. Apoptosis is observed in the pressure-overloaded RV, as is cyclic expression of genes and proteins in both apoptosis (e.g, Fas/CD95, Bcl-2, Bax, caspase-3) and cell proliferation (e.g., cyclin A and E) pathways.[99] Although frequently cited as a possible mechanism of maladaptive RV remodeling and transition to RV failure, the specific role and importance of RV cardiomyocyte apoptosis has yet to be established in animal models or human disease.[20,96]

Right ventricular features unique to human disease

In human disease, the RV exhibits unique aspects of adaptive and maladaptive ventricular remodeling and the transition to failure. First, unlike the LV, the RV can adaptively remodel for prolonged periods under certain chronic overload conditions, particularly in selected congenital cardiac lesions. Congenital PS (severe RV pressure overload) and cCTGA (where RV functions as the systemic ventricle) may be well tolerated for many decades, perhaps due to preservation of RV "fetal phenotype" and/or "RV training" due to chronic RV overload. Patients with the Eisenmenger syndrome may tolerate suprasystemic pulmonary arterial pressures for decades. The RV that does not undergo the usual postnatal "involution" thus has the capability of performing sustained levels of pressure–volume work. Distinctive factors of the RV that likely contribute to these intriguing observations are (1) embryology, (2) structure (shape, fiber layers), (3) physiology, (4) genetic remodeling repertoire. The adult RV, having passed through the normal postnatal RV involution, is much less adaptable to similar degrees of acquired overload.

Second, in acquired diseases, the RV can exhibit a greater degree of plasticity than the LV. Dramatic RV reverse modeling with resolution of RV dysfunction may follow lung transplantation for diverse causes of end-stage parenchymal lung disease, and successful PA thromboendarterectomy for PH induced by chronic thromboembolic pulmonary embolic disease. The adult RV is also much more resistant to irreversible ischemic injury due to coronary artery occlusion and/or acute or chronic ischemia than the LV. This relative resistance to the effects of ischemia is due to multiple factors, including lower RV mass, greater oxygen extraction reverse, more collaterals, and less obligate pressure–volume work.

Third, survival is possible without an RV or an RV-like right-sided contractile chamber. The Fontan repair for obliterative RV structural congenital heart lesions permits pulmonary blood flow and left heart filling as long as pulmonary impedance remains low. In some instances of refractory RV failure, RV disarticulation can be performed successful with normal PVR.

References

1. Buckingham M, Meilhad S, Zaffran S. Building the mammalian heart from two sources of myocardial cells. Nat Rev Genet 2005;6:826–35.
2. Rochais F, Mesbah K, Kelly R. Signaling pathways controlling second heart field development. Circ Res 2009;104:933–42.
3. Klaus A, Saga U, Taketo M, Tzahor E, Birchmeier W. Distinct roles of Wnt/β-catenin and Bmp signaling during early cardiogenesis. Proc Natl Acad Sci U S A 2007;104:18351–6.
4. Rudolph A. The changes in the circulation after birth: Their importance in congenital heart disease. Circulation 1970;41:343–59.
5. Smolich JJ, Walker AM, Campbell GR, Adamson TM. Left and right ventricular myocardial morphometry in fetal, neonatal, and adult sheep. Am J Physiol 1989;257:H1–9.
6. Ho S, Nihoyannopoulos P. Anatomy. echocardiography, and normal right ventricular dimensions. Heart 2006;92:i2–i13.
7. Haddad F, Hung S, Rosenthal D, Murphy D. Right ventricular function in cardiovascular disease, Part I: Anatomy, physiology, aging, and functional assessment of the right ventricle. Circulation 2008;117:1436–48.
8. Goor D, Lillehei C. Congenital Malformations of the Heart. New York: Grune and Stratton; 1975, pp. 1–37.
9. Lorenz C, Walker E, Morgan V, et al. Normal human right and left ventricular mass, systolic function, and gender differences by cine magnetic resonance imaging. J Cardiovasc Magn Reson 1999;1:7–21.
10. Dell'Italia L. Anatomy and physiology of the right ventricle. Cardiol Clin 2012;30:167–87.
11. Anderson RH, Sanchez-Quintana D, Redmann K, Lunkenheimer PP. How are the myocytes aggregated so as to make up the ventricular mass? Seminars in thoracic and cardiovascular surgery. Pediatr Card Surg Annu 2007:76–86.
12. Anderson R, Smerup M, Sanchez-Quintana D, et al. The three-dimensional arrangement of the myocytes in the ventricular walls. Clin Anat 2009;22:64–76.
13. Nielsen E, Smerup M, Agger P, et al. Normal right ventricular three-dimensional architecture, as assessed with diffusion tensor magnetic resonance imaging, is preserved during experimentally induced right ventricular hypertrophy. Anat Rec (Hoboken) 2009;292:640–51.
14. Sanchez-Quintana D, Anderson R, Ho S. Ventricular myocarchitecture in tetralogy of Fallot. Heart 1996;76:280–6.
15. Saleh S, Liakopoulos OJ, Buckberg GD. The septal motor of biventricular function. Eur J Cardiothorac Surg 2006;29(Suppl 1):S126–38.
16. Walker L, Buttrick P. The right ventricle: Biologic insights and response to disease. Curr Cardiol Rep 2009;5:22–8.

17. Singh S, White F, Bloor C. Myocardial morphometric characteristics in swine. Circ Res 1981;1981:434–41.
18. Scholten A, Mohammed S, Low TY, et al. In-depth quantitative cardiac proteomics combining electron transfer dissociation and the metalloendopeptidase Lys-N with the SILAC mouse. Mol Cell Proteomics 2011;10:O111 008474.
19. Phillips D, Aponte AM, Covian R, et al. Homogenous protein programming in the mammalian left and right ventricle free walls. Physiol Genomics 2011;43:1198–206.
20. Bogaard H, Abe K, Noordegraaf A, Voelkel N. The right ventricle under pressure: Cellular and molecular mechanisms of right-heart failure in pulmonary hypertension. Chest 2009;135:794–804.
21. Warnes CA. Adult congenital heart disease importance of the right ventricle. J Am Coll Cardiol 2009;54:1903–10.
22. Dell'Italia L. The right ventricle: anatomy, physiology and clinical importance. Curr Probl Cardiol 1991;16:653–720.
23. Dell'Italia L, Walsh R. Application of a time varying elastance model to right ventricular performance in man. Cardiovasc Res 1988;1988:864–74.
24. Haber I, Metaxas DN, Geva T, Axel L. Three-dimensional systolic kinematics of the right ventricle. Am J Physiol Heart Circ Physiol 2005;289:H1826–33.
25. Carlsson M, Ugander M, Heiberg E, Arheden H. The quantitative relationship between longitudinal and radial function in left, right, and total heart pumping in humans. Am J Physiol Heart Circ Physiol 2007;293:H636–44.
26. Mertens LL, Friedberg MK. Imaging of the right ventricle—current state of the art. Nat Rev Cardiol 2010;7:551–63.
27. Pouler H, Lefevre J, Mechelen H, et al. Free-wall shortening and relaxation during ejection in the canine right ventricle. Am J Physiol 1980;329:H601–13.
28. Petitjean C, Rougon N, Cluzel P. Assessment of myocardial function: a review of quantification methods and results using tagged MRI. J Cardioavsc Magn Reson 2005;7:501–16.
29. Dell'Italia L, Walsh R. Acute determinants of the hangout interval in the pulmonary circulation. Am Heart J 1988;116:1289–97.
30. Brown K, Ditchey R. Human right ventricular end-systolic pressure-volume relation defined by maximal elastance. Circulation 1988;78:81–91.
31. Maughan W, Shoukas A, Sagawa K, Weisfeldt W. Intravenous pressure-volume relationship of the canine right ventricle. Circ Res 1979;44:309–15.
32. Kass D, Maughan W. From "Emax" to pressure-volume relations: a broader view. Circulation 1988;77:1203–12.
33. Goldstein J, Barzilai B, Rosamond T, et al. Determinants of hemodynamic compromise with severe right ventricular infarction. Circulation 1990;82:359–68.
34. Dell'Italia L. Mechanism of postextrasystolic potentiation in the right ventricle. Am J Cardiol 1990;65:736–41.
35. Haddad F, Doyle R, Murphy D, Hunt S. Right ventricular function in cardiovascular disease part II: Pathophysiology, clinical importance and management of right ventricular failure. Circulation 2008;117:1717–31.
36. Vlahakes GJ. Right ventricular failure after cardiac surgery. Cardiol Clin 2012;30:283–9.
37. Champion H, Michelakis E, Hassoun P. Comprehensive invasive and non-invasive approach to the right ventricle-pulmonary circulation unit: State of the art and clinical and research implications. Circulation 2009;120:992–1007.
38. Tedford RJ, Hassoun PM, Mathai SC, et al. Pulmonary capillary wedge pressure augments right ventricular pulsatile loading. Circulation 2012;125:289–97.
39. Murgo J, Westerhof N. Imput impedance of the pulmonary arterial system in normal man. Effects of respiration and comparison to systemic impedance. Circ Res 1984;54:666–73.
40. Caro C, Harrison G, Mognoni P. Pressure wave transmission in the human pulmonary circulation. Cardiovasc Res 1967;1:91–100.
41. Reuben S. Wave transmission in the pulmonary arterial system in disease in man. Circ Res 1970;27:523–9.
42. Gleason W, Braunwald E. Studies on the first derivative of the ventricular pressure pulse in man. J Clin Invest 1962;41:80–91.
43. Cortina C, Bermejo J, Yotti R, et al. Noninvasive assessment of the right ventricular filling pressure gradient. Circulation 2007;116:1015–23.
44. Sun Y, Belenkie I, Wang J, Tyberg J. Assessment of right ventricular diastolic suction in dogs using wave-intensity analysis. Am J Physiol Heart Circ Physiol 2006;291:H3114–21.
45. Sallach J, Tang W, Borowski A, et al. Right atrial volume index in chronic systolic heart failure and prognosis. JACC Cardiovasc Imaging 2009;2:527–34.
46. Mauritz G, Marcus J, Westerhof N, et al. Prolonged right ventricular post-systolic isovolumic period in pulmoanry arterial hypertension is not a reflection of diastolic dysfunction. Heart 2011;97:473–8.
47. Gan C, Holverda S, Marcus J, et al. Right ventricular diastolic dysfunction and the acute effects of sildenafil in pulmonary hypertension patients. Chest 2007;132:11–17.
48. Santamore W, Dell'Italia L. Ventricular interdependence: Significant left ventricular contributions to right ventricular systolic function. Prog Cardiovasc Dis 1998;40:289–308.
49. Voelkel N, Quaife R, Leinwand L, et al. Right ventricular function and failure: Report of a National Heart, Lung, Blood Institute Working Group on cellular and molecular mechanisms of right heart failure. Circulation 2006;114:1883–91.
50. Weber K, Janicki J, Shroff S, Fishman A. Contractile mechanisms and interaction of the right and left ventricles. Am J Cardiol 1981;47:686–95.
51. Damiano J, La Follette P, Cox J, et al. Significant left ventricular contribution to right ventricular systolic function. Am J Physiol 1991;261:1514–24.
52. Feneley M, Gavaghan T, Baron D, et al. Contribution of left ventricular contraction to the generation of right ventricular systolic pressure in the human heart. Circulation 1985;71:473–80.
53. Puwanant S, Park M, Popovic ZB, et al. Ventricular geometry, strain, and rotational mechanics in pulmonary hypertension. Circulation 2010;121:259–66.
54. Goldstein J. Acute right ventricular infarction. Cardiol Clin 2012;30:219–32.
55. Goldstein J, Tweddell J, Barzilai B, et al. Importance of left ventricular function and systolic interaction to right ventricular performance during acute right heart ischemia. J Am Coll Cardiol 1992;19:704–11.
56. Schertz C, Pinsky M. Effect of the pericardium on systolic ventricular interdepence in the dog. J Crit Care 1993;8:17–23.
57. Farrar D, Chow E, Brown C. Isolated systolic and diastolic ventricular interactions in pacing-induced dilated cardiomyopathy and effects of volume loading and pericardium. Circulation 1995;88:720–5.
58. Kusachi S, Nighiyama O, Yasuhara K, et al. Right and left ventricular oxygen metabolism in open-chest dogs. Am J Physiol 1982;243:H716–66.
59. Saito D, Tani H, Kusachi S, et al. Oxygen metabolism of the hypertrophic right ventricle in open chest dogs. Cardiovasc Res 1991;25:731–9.
60. Hill J, Olson E. Cardiac plasticity. New Engl J Med 2008;358:1370–80.
61. Kehat I, Molkentin J. Molecular pathways underlying cardiac remodeling during pathophysiological stimulation. Circulation 2010;122:2727–35.
62. Shah A, Mann D. In seach of new therapeutic targets and strategies for heart failure: recent advances in basic science. Lancet 2011;378:704–12.
63. Koitabashi N, Kass D. Reverse remodeling in heart failure—mechanisms and therapeutic oppotunities. Nat Rev Cardiol 2011;10:1–11.
64. Toischer K, Rokita A, Unsold B, et al. Differential cardiac remodeling in preload versus afterload. Circulation 2010;122:993–1003.
65. Barth A, Kumordzie A, Frangakis C, et al. Reciprocal transcriptional regulation of metabolic and signaling pathways correlates with disease severity in heart failure. Circ Cardiovasc Genet 2011;4:475–83.

66. Barth A, Kuner R, Buness A, et al. Identification of a common gene expression signature in dilated cardiomyopathy across independent microarray studies. J Am Coll Cardiol 2006;48:1610–17.
67. Cooper LJ, Onuma O, Sagar S, et al. Genomic and proteomic analysis of myocarditis and dilated cardiomyopathy. Heart Fail Clin 2010;6:75–85.
68. Kittleson M, Ye S, Irizarry R, et al. Identification of a gene expression profile that differentiates between ischemic and nonischemic cardiomyopathy. Circulation 2004;110:3444–51.
69. Kuner R, Barth A, Ruschhaput M, et al. Genomic analysis reveals poor separation of human cardiomyopathies of ischemic and nonischemic etiologies. Physiol Genomics 2008;34:88–94.
70. Nenni L, Romauldi C, Maseri A, Lanfranchi G. Differential gene expression profiling in genetic and multifactorial cardiovascular diseases. J Mol Cell Cardiol 2006;41:934–48.
71. Sanoudou D, Vafiadaki E, Arvanitis D, et al. Array lessons from the heart: focus on the genome and transcriptome of cardiomyopathies. Physiol Genomics 2005;21:131–43.
72. Sarwar R, Cook S. Genomic analysis of left ventricular remodeling. Circulation 2009;120:437–44.
73. Tan F, Moravec C, Li J, et al. The gene expression fingerprint of human heart failure. Proc Natl Acad Sci U S A 2002;99:11387–92.
74. Ebert M, Sharp P. Roles for micro-RNAs in conferring robustness to biological processes. Cell 2012;149:515–24.
75. Pritchard C, Cheng H, Twari M. MicroRNA profiling: approaches and considerations. Nat Rev Genet 2012;13:358–69.
76. Small E, Frost R, Olson E. MicroRNAs add a new dimension to cardiovascular disease. Circulation 2010;121:1022–32.
77. Small E, Olson E. Pervasive roles of microRNAs in cardiovascular biology. Nature 2011;469:336–42.
78. van Rooij E. The art of microRNA research. Circ Res 2011;108:219–34.
79. Dorn G. Decoding the cardiac message. Circ Res 2012;110:755–63.
80. Topkara V, Mann D. Role of microRNAs in cardiac remodeling and heart failure. Cardiovasc Drugs Ther 2011;25:171–82.
81. Tijsen A, Creemers E, Moerland P, et al. MiR423-5p as a circulating biomarker for heart failure. Circ Res 2010;10:1035–9.
82. Anversa P, Levicky V, Beghi C, et al. Morphometry of exercise-induced right ventricular hypertrophy in the rat. Circ Res 1983;52:57–64.
83. Szabo G, Soos P, Bahrle S, et al. Adaptation of the right ventricle to an increased afterload in the chronically volume overloaded heart. Ann Thorac Surg 2006;82:989–95.
84. Yerebakan C, Klopsch C, Niefeldt S, et al. Acute and chronic response of the right ventricle to surgically induced pressure and volume overload—an analysis of pressure-volume relations. Interact Cardiovasc Thorac Surg 2010;10:519–25.
85. Hessel MH, Steendijk P, den Adel B, et al. Characterization of right ventricular function after monocrotaline-induced pulmonary hypertension in the intact rat. Am J Physiol Heart Circ Physiol 2006;291:H2424–30.
86. Dias CA, Assad RS, Caneo LF, et al. Reversible pulmonary trunk banding. II. An experimental model for rapid pulmonary ventricular hypertrophy. J Thorac Cardiovasc Surg 2002;124:999–1006.
87. Marino TA, Kent RL, Uboh CE, et al. Structural analysis of pressure versus volume overload hypertrophy of cat right ventricle. Am J Physiol 1985;249:H371–9.
88. Gaynor SL, Maniar HS, Bloch JB, et al. Right atrial and ventricular adaptation to chronic right ventricular pressure overload. Circulation 2005;112:I212–18.
89. Rich S. Right ventricular adaptation and maladaption in chronic pulmonary arterial hypertension. Cardiol Clin 2012;30:257–69.
90. Simon M, Pinsky M. Right ventricular dysfunction and failure in chronic pressure overload. Cardiol Res Prac 2011;.
91. Schwartz SM, Gordon D, Mosca RS, et al. Collagen content in normal, pressure, and pressure-volume overloaded developing human hearts. Am J Cardiol 1996;77:734–8.
92. Orde MM, Puranik R, Morrow PL, Duflou J. Myocardial pathology in pulmonary thromboembolism. Heart 2011;97:1695–9.
93. Brittain E, Hemnes A, Keebler M, et al. Right venticular plasticity and functional imaging. Pulmonary circulation 2012;2:309–26.
94. Rudski LG, Lai WW, Afilalo J, et al. Guidelines for the echocardiographic assessment of the right heart in adults: a report from the American Society of Echocardiography endorsed by the European Association of Echocardiography, a registered branch of the European Society of Cardiology, and the Canadian Society of Echocardiography. J Am Soc Echocardiogr 2010;23:685–713; quiz 86–8.
95. Karas MG, Kizer JR. Echocardiographic assessment of the right ventricle and associated hemodynamics. Prog Cardiovasc Dis 2012;55:144–60.
96. Haddad F, Ahsley E, Michelakis E. New insights for the diagnosis and management of right ventricular failure, from molecular imaging to targeted right ventricular therapy. Curr Opin Cardiol 2010;25:131–40.
97. Drake J, Bogarrd H, Mizuno S, et al. Molecular signature of a right heart failure program in chronic severe pulmonary hypertension. Am J Respir Cell Mol Biol 2011;45:1239–47.
98. Bartelds B, Borgdorff M, Smit-van Oosten A, et al. Differential responses of the right ventricle to abnormal loading conditions in mice: pressure vs. volume load. Eur J Heart Failure 2011;13:1275–82.
99. Urashima T, Zhao M, Wagner R, et al. Molecular and physiological characterization of RV remodeling in a murine model of pulmonary stenosis. Am J Physiol Heart Circ Physiol 2008;295:H1351–H68.
100. Kreymborg K, Uchida S, Gellert P, et al. Identification of right heart-enriched genes in a murine model of chronic outflow tract obstruction. J Mol Cell Cardiol 2010;49:598–605.
101. Reddy S, Zhao M, Hu D, et al. Dynamic microRNA expression during the transition from right ventricular hypertrophy to failure. Physiol Genomics 2012;44:562–75.
102. Bittel C, Butler M, Kibiryeva N, et al. Gene expression in cardiac tissues from infants with idiopathic conotruncal defects. BMC Med Genomics 2011;4:1–10.
103. O'Brien J, Kibiryeva N, Zhou X, et al. Noncoding RNA expression in myocardium from infants with Tetralogy of Fallot. Circ Cardiovasc Genet 2012;5:279–86.
104. Fan TH, Liang CS, Kawashima S, Banerjee SP. Alterations in cardiac beta-adrenoceptor responsiveness and adenylate cyclase system by congestive heart failure in dogs. Eur J Pharmacol 1987;140:123–32.
105. Bristow MR, Minobe W, Rasmussen R, et al. Beta-adrenergic neuroeffector abnormalities in the failing human heart are produced by local rather than systemic mechanisms. J Clin Invest 1992;89:803–15.
106. Mann D. Pathophysiology of heart failure. In: Libby P, Bonow RO, Mann DL, Zipes DP, ed., Braunwald's Heart Disease: A Textbook of Cardiovascular Medicine, 8th edn, Chapter 22. Philadelphia, PA: Saunders Elsevier; 2008, pp. 541–60.
107. Wang GY, Yeh CC, Jensen BC, et al. Heart failure switches the RV alpha1-adrenergic inotropic response from negative to positive. Am J Physiol Heart Circ Physiol 2010;298:H913–20.
108. Nootens M, Kaufmann E, Rector T, et al. Neurohormonal activation in patients with right ventricular failure from pulmonary hypertension: relation to hemodynamic variables and endothelin levels. J Am Coll Cardiol 1995;26:1581–5.
109. Rouleau JL, Kapuku G, Pelletier S, et al. Cardioprotective effects of ramipril and losartan in right ventricular pressure overload in the rabbit: importance of kinins and influence on angiotensin II type 1 receptor signaling pathway. Circulation 2001;104:939–44.
110. Abraham WT, Raynolds MV, Gottschall B, et al. Importance of angiotensin-converting enzyme in pulmonary hypertension. Cardiology 1995;86(Suppl 1):9–15.
111. Ueno M, Miyauchi T, Sakai S, et al. Effects of physiological or pathological pressure load in vivo on myocardial expression of ET-1 and receptors. Am J Physiol 1999;277:R1321–30.
112. Bolger AP, Sharma R, Li W, et al. Neurohormonal activation and the chronic heart failure syndrome in adults with congenital heart disease. Circulation 2002;106:92–9.
113. Coggins M, Rosenzweig A. The fire within: Cardiac inflammatory signaling in health and disease. Circ Res 2012;110:116–25.

114. Schermuly R, Ghofrani H, Wilkins M, Grimminger F. Mechanisms of disease: Pulmonary arterial hypertension. Nat Rev Cardiol 2011;8:443–55.
115. Probhu S. Cytokine-induced modulation of cardiac function. Circ Res 2004;95:1140–53.
116. Lecour S, James R. When are pro-inflammatory cytokines safe in heart failure? Eur Heart Journal 2011;32:680–5.
117. Anker S, Coats S. How to RECOVER from RENAISSANCE? The sigificance of RECOVER, RENAISSANCE, RENEWAL and ATTACH. Int J Cardiol 2002;86:123–30.
118. Nagai T, Komuro I. Gene and cytokine therapy for heart failure: Molecular mechanisms in the improvement of cardiac function. Am J Physiol Heart Circ Physiol 2012;303:H501–12.
119. Mann D. THe emerging role of innate immunity in the heart and vascular system: For whom the cell tolls. Circ Res 2011;108:1133–45.
120. Banerjee D, Haddad F, Zamanian R, Nagendran J. Right ventricular failure: A novel era of targeted therapy. Curr Heart Fail Rep 2010;7:202–11.
121. Takimoto E, Champion H, Li M, et al. Chronic inhibition of cyclic GMP phosphodiesterase 5A prevents and reverses cardiac hypertrophy. Nat Med 2005;11:214–22.
122. Behling A, Rohde L, Colombo F, et al. Effects of 5′-phosphodiesterase four-week long inhibition with sildenafil in patients with chronic heart failure: a double-blin, placebo-controlled clinical trial. J Card Fail 2008;14:189–97.
123. Guazzi M, Samaja M, Arena R, et al. Long-term use of sildenafil in the therapeutic management of heart failure. J Am Coll Cardiol 2007;50:2136–44.
124. Guazzi M, Tumminello G, Di Marco F, et al. The effects of phospodiesterase-5 inhibition with sildenafil on pulmonary hemodynamics and diffusion capacity, exercise ventilory efficiency, and oxygen uptake kinetics in chronic heart failure. J Am Coll Cardiol 2004;44:2339–48.
125. Lewis G, Shah R, Shahzad K, et al. Sildenafil improves exercise capacity and quality of life in patients with systolic heart failure and secondary pulmonary hypertension. Circulation 2007;116:1555–62.
126. Lewis G, Lachmann J, Camuso J, et al. Sildenafil improves exercise hemodynamics and oxygen uptake in patients with systolic heart failure. Circulation 2007;115:59–66.
127. Guazzi M, Vicenzi M, Arena R, Guazzi M. PDE5 inhibition with sildenafil improves left ventricular diastolic function, cardiac geometry, and clinical status in paitents with stable heart failure: Results of a 1-year, prospective, randomized, placebo-controlled trial. Circ Heart Fail 2011;4:8–17.
128. Guazzi M, Vicenzi M, Arena R, Guazzi M. Pulmonary hypertension in heart failure with preserved ejection fraction: A target of phosphodiesterase-5 inhibition in a 1-year study. Circulation 2011;124:164–74.
129. Hoeper M, Barbera A, Channick R, et al. Diagnosis, assessment and treatment of non-pulmonary arterial hypertension pulmonary hypertension. J Am Coll Cardiol 2009;54:S85–96.
130. Kass D. Cardiac role of cyclic-GMP hydrolyzing phosphodiesterase type 5: From experimental models to clinical trials. Curr Heart Fail Rep 2012;9:192–9.
131. Archer S, Michelakis E. Phosphodiesterase type 5 inhibitors for pulmonary arterial hypertension. N Engl J Med 2009;361:1864–71.
132. Galie N, Ghofrani H, Torbicki A, et al. Sildenafil citrate therapy for pulmonary arterial hypertension. New Engl J Med 2005;353:2148–57.
133. Guazzi M. Clinical use of phosphodiesterase-5 inhibitors in chronic heart failure. Circ Heart Fail 2008;1:272–80.
134. Shan X, Qualie M, Monk J, et al. Differential expression of PDE5 in failing and nonfailing human myocardium. Cir Heart Fail 2012;5:79–86.
135. Kass D. Res-erection of Viagra as a heart drug. Circ Heart Fail 2011;4:2–4.
136. Altin SE, Schulze PC. Metabolism of the right ventricle and the response to hypertrophy and failure. Prog Cardiovasc Dis 2012;55:229–33.
137. Oikawa M, Kagaya Y, Otani H, et al. Increased [^{18}F]fluorodeoxyglucose accumulation in right ventricular free wall in patients with pulmonary hypertension and the effect of epoprostenol. J Am Coll Cardiol 2005;45:1849–55.
138. Gomez-Arroyo J, Mizuno S, Szczepanek K, et al. Metabolic gene remodeling and mitochondrial dysfunction in failing right ventricular hypertrophy due to pulmonary arterial hypertension. Circ Heart Fail 2013;6:136–44.
139. Nagendran J, Gurtu V, Fu DZ, et al. A dynamic and chamber-specific mitochondrial remodeling in right ventricular hypertrophy can be therapeutically targeted. J Thorac Cardiovasc Surg 2008;136:168–78, 78 e1–3.
140. Michelakis E. Mitochondrial medicine: A new era in medicine opens new windows and brings new challenges. Circulation 2008;117:2431–4.
141. Bers D. Calcium cycling and signaling in cardiac myocytes. Annu Rev Physiol 2008;70:23–49.
142. Lehnart S, Maier L, Hasenfuss G. Abnormalities of calcium metabolism and myocardial contractility in the failing heart. Heart Fail Rev 2009;14:213–24.
143. Del Monte F, Hajjar R. Intraceullar devastation in heart failure. Heart Fail Rev 2008;13:151–62.
144. Lou Q, Janardhan A, Efimov I. Remodeling of calcium handling in human heart failure. Adv Exp Med Biol 2012;740:1145–74.
145. Kranias E, Hajjar R. Modulation of cardiac contractility by the phospholamban/SERCA2 regulatome. Circ Res 2012;110:1646–60.
146. Walker LA, Walker JS, Glazier A, et al. Biochemical and myofilament responses of the right ventricle to severe pulmonary hypertension. Am J Physiol Heart Circ Physiol 2011;301:H832–40.
147. Fan D, Wannenburg T, de Tombe P. Decreased myocyte tension development and calcium responsiveness in rat right ventricular pressure overload. Circulation 1997;95:2312–17.
148. Harding S, O'Gara P, Jones S, et al. Species dependence of contraction velocity in signel isolated cardiac myocytes. Cardioscience 1990;1:49–53.
149. Katz A. Cell biochemistry: Abnormal excitation-contraction coupling, contraction, and relaxation; arrhythmias; energy starvation. In: Heart Failure: Pathophysiology, Molecular Biology, and Clinical Management. Chapter 3. Phildelphia, PA: Lippincott, Williams and Wilkins; 2000, pp. 71–108.
150. Lowes B, Minobe W, Abraham W, et al. Changes in gene expression in the intact human heart: Downregulation of α-myosin heavy chain in hypertrophic, failing ventricular myocardium. J Clin Invest 1997;100:2315–24.
151. Hamdani N, Kooij V, van Dijk S, et al. Sarcomeric dysfunction in heart failure. Cardiovasc Res 2008;77:649–58.
152. Nassar R, Malouf N, Mao L, et al. cTnT1, a cardiac troponin T isoform, decreases myofilament tension and affects the left ventricular pressure waveform. Am J Physiol Heart Circ Physiol 2005;288:H1147–56.
153. Nagueh S, Shah G, Wu Y, et al. Altered titin expression, myocardial stiffnessn and left ventricular function in patients with dilated cardiomyopathy. Circulation 2004;2004:155–62.
154. LeWinter M. Functional consequences of sarcomeric protein abnormalities in failing myocardium. Heart Fail Rev 2005;10:249–57.
155. Neagoe C, Kulke M, del Monte F, et al. Titin isoform switch in ischemic human heart disease. Circulation 2002;106:1333–41.
156. Lemler M, Bies R, Frid M, et al. Myocyte cytoskeletal disorganization and right heart failure in hypoxia-induced neonatal pulmonary hypertension. Am J Physiol Heart Circ Physiol 2000;279:H1365–76.
157. Qipshidze N, Tyagi N, Metreveli N, et al. Autophagy mechanism of right ventricular remodeling in murine model of pulmonary artery constriction. Am J Physiol Heart Circ Physiol 2012;302:H688–96.

CHAPTER 21

Right ventricular failure: Clinical features and management

Thomas G. Di Salvo MD MPH MBA
and Simon Maltais MD PhD

Clinical definition of right ventricular failure

Right ventricular (RV) failure may be defined as the presence of an otherwise unexplained elevated mean right atrial pressure (RAP) of 8 mmHg or more or a RAP/pulmonary capillary wedge pressure (PCW) of 0.8 mmHg or more, typically accompanied by a low cardiac index ($\leq$2.2 L min^{-1} m^{-2}). RV failure typically does not occur in the absence of acute or chronic RV pressure overload, RV volume overload, or significant interventricular septum displacement and/or contractile dysfunction. Reduction in RV contractility may not by itself result in RV failure because even severe isolated RV ischemia, or replacement of the RV by a patch, may be tolerated.

Etiologies and differential diagnosis of right ventricular failure

Box 21.1 summarizes the more common etiologies and differential diagnosis of both acute and chronic RV failure. The single most common cause of RV failure is chronic RV afterload elevation due to left ventricular (LV) systolic or diastolic dysfunction or failure. Other causes of RV pressure-overload induced RV failure include acute and chronic pulmonary thromboembolism, right ventricular outflow tract (RVOT) obstruction in congenital heart disease (e.g., tetraology of Fallot), pulmonary stenosis, primary pulmonary vascular disease (precapillary pulmonary artery hypertension [PAH]) and/or secondary pulmonary vascular remodeling (chronic, severe postcapillary PAH), branch pulmonary stenosis in congenital heart disease, peripheral pulmonic stenosis (PS), and secondary pulmonary vascular disease due to congenital heart disease (e.g., Eisenmenger syndrome).

Tricuspid regurgitation is the most common cause of RV failure due to volume overload. Additional etiologies of RV volume overload resulting in RV failure include chronic left-to-right shunts (atrial septal defect, ventricular septal defect, anomalous pulmonary venous drainage, sinus of Valsalva aneurysm rupture into the RV, coronary artery fistula), carcinoid, and rheumatic valvular disease. Occlusion of the right coronary artery proximal to the origin of the RV marginal branches, which supply the RV free wall, may result in acute ischemic injury and RV failure. In addition, severe acute RV pressure overload (e.g., acute massive pulmonary embolism) may be accompanied by substantial ischemic RV dysfunction due to reduction in RV perfusion and severe pressure-overload induced necrosis, as discussed in following sections of this chapter.

RV failure may result from selective or predominant involvement of the RV in an idiopathic cardiomyopathy that does not fulfill criteria for the diagnosis of arrhythmogenic RV cardiomyopathy (ARVC). In such patients, significant arterial pulmonary hypertension should be excluded. ARVC may first present with RV failure, as discussed in a subsequent section of this chapter.

Transient RV failure, like LV failure, may result from overwhelming sepsis, likely due to the effects of circulating cytokines which suppress ventricular systolic function without prominent necrosis. Transient RV failure may also result from profound transient hypoxemia or hypotension. Given reduced resting oxygen extraction and coronary perfusion, the RV is more resistant to hypoxia and to global coronary hypoperfusion than is the LV.

RV inflow obstruction from tricuspid or superior vena cava (SVC) stenosis or occlusion may mimic many of the symptoms and signs of RV failure. Pericardial disease (tamponade, constrictive pericarditis) may also mimic the symptoms and signs of RV failure without alteration in intrinsic RV myocardial function.

Complex congenital heart disease (e.g., Ebstein anomaly, tetralogy of Fallot, d- and l-transposition of the great arteries, hypoplastic left heart syndrome) may result in RV failure due to RV or RVOT structural alterations or positioning of the anatomic RV as the systemic subaortic ventricle. In the latter instance, RV dysfunction typically evolves after a variable period of RV adaptation.

Symptoms of right ventricular failure

The symptoms and signs of RV failure are nonspecific (Table 21.1). The sensitivity and specificity of any of these individual symptoms in the diagnosis of RV failure has not been established.

Patients with predominant RV volume overload lesions, tricuspid regurgitation, and significant RV eccentric remodeling tend to present initially with symptoms attributable to systemic venous congestion, followed by later curtailment of functional capacity. Patients with predominant RV pressure overload lesions tend to present with earlier symptoms of reduced functional capacity and exertional intolerance followed later by symptoms of systemic venous congestion. Frequently in minimally symptomatic patients with advanced RV remodeling, a new-onset arrhythmia such as atrial fibrillation prompts medical attention. Patients with acute severe RV pressure overload (e.g., massive pulmonary embolism)

Box 21.1 Common etiologies of acute right ventricular failure

Acute severe right ventricular pressure overload

- LV ventricular dysfunction (ventricular interaction, postcapillary PAH, arrhythmia)
- Acute exacerbation of severe PAH of any cause
- Acute massive PE
- ARDS
- Mechanical ventilation
- Severe hypoxic-induced pulmonary vasoconstriction
- Acute RVOT obstruction

Acute severe right ventricular volume overload

- Acute tricuspid regurgitation
  - Trauma
  - Infective endocarditis
  - MI
- Acute intracardiac left-to-right shunting (e.g., postinfarction VSD)

Acute intrinsic right ventricular myocardial dysfunction

- Ischemic injury
  - RV myocardial infarction
- Sepsis (cytokine-induced)
- Postpericardiotomy injury
- Post-LVAD implantation

Impeded right ventricular filling

- Cardiac tamponade
- Mechanical obstruction to RV filling (SVC syndrome, TS)

Arrhythmias

- Any arrhythmia associated with loss of coordinated atrial transport or ventricular synchrony

ARDS, acute respiratory distress syndrome; LV, left ventricle; LVAD, left ventricular assist device; MI, myocardial infarction; PAH, pulmonary arterial hypertension; PE, pulmonary embolism; RVOT, right ventricular outflow tract; SVC, superior vena cava; TS, tricuspid stenosis; VSD, ventricular septal defect.

Adapted from Lahm et al. 2010, Sayer et al. 2012 and Haddad et al. 2008.

or chronic thromboembolic pulmonary hypertension and RV dysfunction may present with prominent dyspnea, tachycardia, exertional chest discomfort, and near-syncope or syncope. Patients with ARVC may present with palpitations, near-syncope, syncope, or sustained ventricular arrhythmias in the absence of symptoms or signs of RV failure. Patients presenting with disproportionate or marked volume overload (anasarca, ascites) should be evaluated for possible concurrent or predominant kidney disease (e.g., nephrotic syndrome, renal failure), hepatic disease (e.g., advanced cirrhosis), and other cardiac conditions (e.g., constrictive pericarditis, restrictive cardiomyopathy).

Table 21.1 Right ventricular failure: general symptoms and signs

	Symptoms	Signs
Acute RV failure	Dyspnea Light-headedness Chest pain	Hypotension Tachycardia Cyanosis Elevated jugular venous pressure Right parasternal heave RV third heart sound increase with inspiration, best heard left lower sternal border TR murmur Accentuated second heart sound
Chronic RV failure	Exertional intolerance and dyspnea Fatigue Right upper quadrant abdominal discomfort or bloating Lower extremity edema	Acute signs as above may be present Hepatic enlargement, pulsatile liver (severe TR) or ascites Lower extremity edema

TR, tricuspid regurgitation.

Adapted from Piazza et al 2005.

Physical examination signs of right ventricular failure

The physical examination signs of RV failure are etiology-dependent (see Box 21.2). The sensitivity and specificity of any of these individual signs in the diagnosis of RV failure has not been established. The most important aspects of the physical examination are to ascertain rest and exertional vital signs (blood pressure, heart rate, respiratory rate, oxygen saturation), weight, the adequacy of systemic perfusion, jugular venous pressure and waveform, signs of pulmonary hypertension, signs of tricuspid regurgitation and the degree of systemic venous volume overload. Serial ambulatory measures of functional capacity (e.g., 6 minute walk test with exertional oximetry) can be helpful ancillary assessments of interval changes in overall circulatory function and response to specific therapies. Since patients with significant RV failure will typically require diuretic therapy, a goal weight range representing optimal RV preload should be maintained and serially assessed in all patients with established RV failure. Reduction in weight without change in systemic venous volume should prompt consideration of cardiac cachexia and, ominously progressive heart failure.

Laboratory assessment of right ventricular failure

Laboratory evaluation of patients with RV failure includes measurement of serum electrolytes, renal function, hepatic function, complete blood count and selected biomarkers including brain naturietic peptide (BNP) and cardiac enzymes (troponin I). Deterioration in renal function and elevation of hepatic function tests due to progressive hepatic congestion may result from tricuspid regurgitation or worsening RV function.[1,2] BNP is elevated

Box 21.2 Physical signs suggestive of specific etiologies of right ventricular failure

Blood pressure

- *Pulsus paradoxus*: defined as inspiratory fall in systolic blood pressure >10 mmHg:
  - Cardiac tamponade (virtually 100%)
  - Any cause of marked increased in inspiratory negative intrathoracic pressure (e.g., severe bronchoconstriction or obstructive lung disease)
  - Severe RV failure, RV infarction or potentially any condition marked by advanced ventricular interdependence

Jugular venous pressure

- *Kussmaul's sign:* defined as an inspiratory distention of neck veins
  - TS, restrictive cardiomyopathy, constrictive pericarditis, SVC syndrome, RV infarction
- *Prominent jugular a wave*: TS, RH hypertrophy, RV diastolic dysfunction, RV failure of diverse cause
- *Blunted jugular x descent*: TR
- *Prominent jugular c-v wave*: TR (most prominently), ASD, RV failure of any cause
- *Prominent x and y descents*: restrictive cardiomyopathy, "pseudo-restriction"
- *Blunted y descent*: cardiac tamponade

Palpation

- *RV heave:* Diverse causes of RV pressure and volume overload, most prominent in RV pressure overload states

Auscultation

- *Loud P2:* defined as P2 audible in LLSB or at apex
  - PH of diverse cause
- *Soft P2*
  - PR
- *Wide or "fixed" splitting of second heart sound:* defined as S2 split changes <0.02 s with quiet respiration
  - Delayed RV electrical activation: RBBB, LV pacing
  - Prolonged RV ejection time: acute PE, PH, PS
  - Increased RV volume: ASD
  - Early aortic closure: MR, VSD
- *RV S3 gallop:* defined as S3 heard best at LLSB with intensity augmentation with inspiration
  - Any condition associated with rapid RV filling (bolus deceleration) and/or decreased RV distensibility
- *RV S4 gallops*: defined as S4 heard best at LLSB with intensity augmentation with inspiration
  - Diverse causes of RV hypertrophy or diastolic dysfunction
- *Holosystolic murmur 4th–5th L ICS*: with augmentation with either inspiration (Carvallo's sign) or hepatic compression (Vitums's sign)
  - Primary or secondary tricuspid regurgitation
- *Diastolic rumble 4th–5th ICS*: with augmentation with inspiration
  - TS (opening snap of TS is typically inaudible)
- *Diastolic murmur*: heard in 2nd ICS
  - Primary PR (e.g., repaired TOF)
  - Secondary PR due to PH and/or main PA dilation of diverse cause (Graham Steell murmur)
- *Pulmonary ejection murmur*: with augmentation during inspiration
  - Primary PS
  - RVOT obstruction of diverse cause
- *Pulmonary valve ejection click*: with decrease in intensity with inspiration
  - Primary (congenital) PS

Abdomen

- *Hepatomegaly*:
  - When hepatomegaly is pulsatile, sensitivity is 20% for TR
- *Hepatojugular reflux*:
  - Sensitivity is 66% for TR; may also belie elevated LV pressures
- *Ascites*:
  - Diverse causes of RV failure

Extremities

- *Edema*:
  - Diverse causes of RV failure
- *Cyanosis*:
  - Low cardiac output
  - Right-to-left shunt

ASD, atrial septal defect; ICS, intercostal space; LLSB, lower left sternal border; LV, left ventricle; MR, mitral regurgitation; PA, pulmonary artery; PE, pulmonary embolism; PH, pulmonary hypertension; PR, pulmonary regurgitation; PS, pulmonary stenosis; RBBB, right bundle branch block; RV, right ventricle; RVOT, RV outflow tract; SVC, superior vena cava; TOF, tetralogy of Fallot; TR, tricuspid regurgitation; TS, tricuspid stenosis; VSD, ventricular septal defect.

in both RV volume and overload states, but has not been as thoroughly studied as in LV volume and pressure overload states.[3,4,5] Nevertheless, significant changes in BNP likely reflect changes in RV function and load.[3,4] Elevations of both BNP and troponin I (TnI) are prognostically important in patients with group 1 PAH.[6] The role of genetic testing in familial or idiopathic cardiomyopathies and ARVC is evolving.[7] Laboratory evaluation in different etiologies of RV failure is discussed in more detail in subsequent sections of this chapter.

Electrocardiography in right ventricular failure

Commonly encountered electrocardiographic findings in RV failure appear in Boxes 21.3 and 21.4. The sensitivity and specificity of any of these ECG features is not well established in RV failure, however. Figure 21.1 illustrates relatively specific ECG features in RV hypertrophy, acute RV infarction, acute pulmonary embolism, and ARVC.

Chest radiography in right ventricular failure

Commonly encountered radiographic features of RV failure are listed in Table 21.2. Figure 21.2 provides examples from patients with different etiologies of RV enlargement. Typical signs of RV enlargement include a boot-shaped heart and filling in of the retrosternal airspace by the dilated RV. On a lateral chest radiograph, if more than one-third the distance from the suprasternal notch to the tip of the xiphoid is occupied by soft tissue density, RV enlargement is likely present in the absence of retrosternal adenopathy, mediastinal mass, scarring from prior stenotomy, or marked dilation of either the main pulmonary artery or the aortic root.[8]

Box 21.4 Common ECG criteria for diagnosis of right ventricular hypertrophy

- R in V_1 0.7 mV
- QR in V_1
- R/S in $V_1 > 1$ with R > 0.5 mV
- R/S in V_5 or $V_6 < 1$
- S in V_5 or $V_6 > 0.7$ mV
- R in V_5 or $V_6 \geq 0.4$ mV with S in $V_1 \leq 0.2$ mV
- Right axis deviation (> 90°)
- S_1Q_3 pattern
- $S_1S_2S_3$ pattern
- P pulmonale pattern

The sensitivities, specificities and diagnostic accuracy of these criteria are not well established as they were proposed from small, selective populations.

Adapted from the American Journal of Cardiology, Vol 53, Issue 8, Murphy, Marvin L et al., Reevaluation of electrocardiographic criteria for left, right and combined cardiac ventricular hypertrophy, 1140–1147, copyright (1984) with permission from Elsevier.

Box 21.3 ECG changes in right ventricular failure

Rhythm

- Sinus tachycardia
- Atrial fibrillation

Axis

- Right axis deviation (QRS axis >90°) or indeterminate axis

Right ventricular hypertrophy

Other

- T-wave inversion in leads III, aVF, V_{1-4}
- Incomplete or complete right bundle branch block
- $S_1Q_{III}T_{III}$: Concurrent deep S wave in lead 1, Q-wave and T-wave inversion in lead III (pulmonary embolism)
- Qr pattern in V_1
- S waves >1.5 mm in leads I and aVL
- Q waves in leads III and aVF but not in lead II
- Transition zone shift to late precordial leads (e.g., V_5)
- Low limb lead voltage

Adapted from Piazza et al. 2005.

Cardiac catheterization in right ventricular failure

Current American Heart Association (AHA)/American College of Cardiology (ACC) treatment guidelines altered prior recommendations for pulmonary artery catheterization (PAC) in the management of heart failure to class IIB, recommending that PAC might be reasonable to guide therapy in selected patients with refractory endstage heart failure (level of evidence C).[9] While routine PAC does not change outcomes in patients with acutely decompensated LV systolic dysfunction, the role of PAC in the diagnosis and management of RV failure has not been studied.[9] Definitive diagnosis of precapillary versus postcapillary PAH requires PAC and PAC is therefore recommended by consensus guidelines in the evaluation and management of patients with PAH,[6] and is helpful in many patients with RV failure. Figure 21.3 presents a useful algorithm for the hemodynamic evaluation of RV failure.

Normal right ventricular stroke work index (RVSWI) is greater than 600 mmHg ml^{-1} m^{-2} RVSWI predicts duration of inotropic support following pulsatile LVAD implantation and RVSWI less than 300 ml^{-1} m^{-2} independently predicts risk of RV failure following LVAD implantation.[10]

Common and challenging hemodynamic scenarios in right ventricular failure

Commonly encountered evolving differential diagnosis scenarios based upon hemodynamic findings are listed in Box 21.5. Several relatively common challenging scenarios also bear additional brief content.

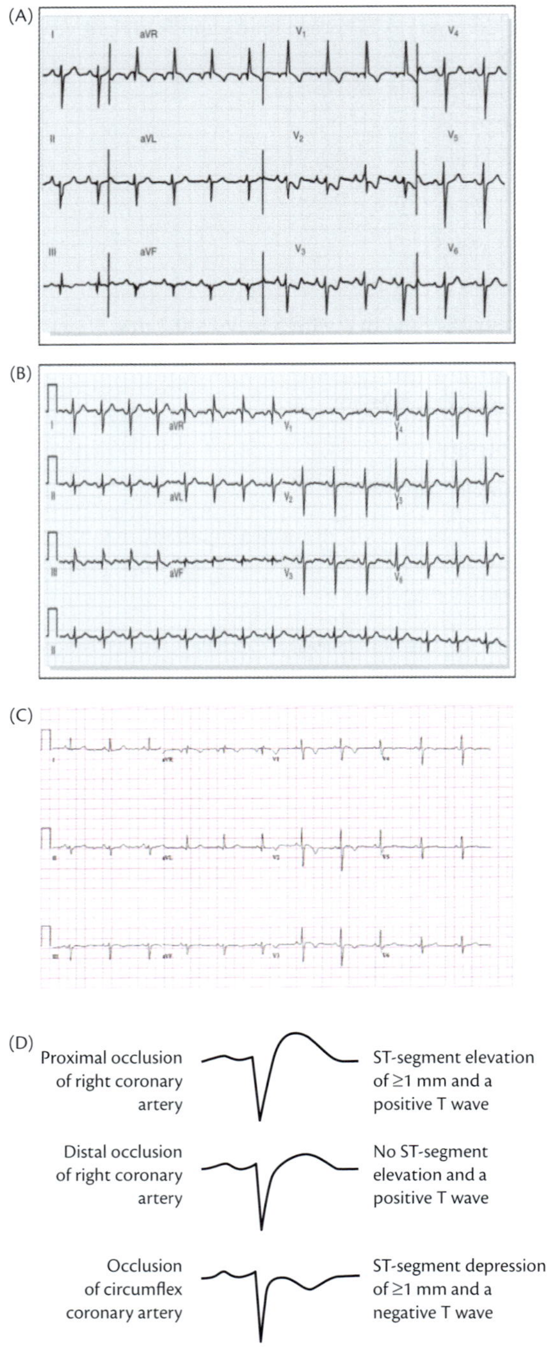

Fig. 21.1 Illustrative examples of electrocardiography in right ventricular (RV) failure. (A) RV hypertrophy. This pattern is most consistent with RV pressure overload: tall R in V_1, right axis deviation, T-wave inversions V_{1-4}, delayed precordial transition zone (rS in v6), right atrial enlargement and S_1Q_3 pattern. (B) Acute RV myocardial infarction. Three different ST-segment and T-wave configurations that can be identified by lead V_4R in patients with acute inferoposterior myocardial infarction. (C) Arrhythmogenic RV cardiomyopathy. Note the prominent inverted precordial T waves in V_{1-4}, now a major criterion for the diagnosis of arrhythmogenic RV cardiomyopathy. (D) Acute pulmonary embolism. Note the $S_1Q_3T_3$ pattern, incomplete right bundle block, inverted and/or flattened precordial T waves V_{1-4}.

(A) Reprinted with permission from Bonow: Braunwald's Heart Disease—A Textbook of Cardiovascular Medicine, 9th ed. Saunders, 2011. (B) Reprinted with permission from Wellens HJJ 1999. (C) Reprinted with permission from Ellinor et al 2010. (D) Reprinted with permission from Bonow: Braunwald's Heart Disease—A Textbook of Cardiovascular Medicine, 9th ed. Saunders, 2011.

Table 21.2 Chest radiographic findings in RV failure

RA and/or RV enlargement	Pulmonary arteries	Other
Cardiomegaly in anterior projection (RA and/or RV enlargement)	Dilation of proximal pulmonary arteries	Inferior vena cava and/or azygous vein dilatation
Increased curvature of right heart border due to right atrial dilatation in anterior projection	Abrupt tapering of distal pulmonary artery branches	Pleural and/or pericardial effusions
Filling of retrosternal space in lateral projection due to RV enlargement		

Adapted from Piazza et al 2005.

Scenario 1: Equalization of left and right heart pressures: right ventricular failure related "pseudo-restriction"

Equalization of right and left heart pressures with early rapid ventricular filling and a "dip and plateau" waveform pattern occurs in a variety of conditions marked by severe or acute volume overload and pericardial constraint, including severe tricuspid regurgitation (TR), severe decompensated LV failure, acute RV dilation from infarction or injury, acute mitral regurgitation due to chordae rupture, restrictive cardiomyopathy, constrictive pericarditis, and cardiac tamponade.[11] In clinical practice, patients with biventricular heart failure, marked systemic venous congestion, and acute or incrementally worse RV volume overload frequently present with near-equalization or equalization of right and left heart filling pressures when measurement of pressures is performed prior to aggressive medical management and/or when severe tricuspid regurgitation, advanced pulmonary vascular remodeling, or advanced ventricular interdependence persist despite aggressive medical therapy. This scenario can pose particularly difficult diagnostic challenges in patients with (1) known or suspected primary restrictive cardiomyopathies, (2) moderate to severe TR, (3) multiple cardiac surgeries with pericardial and mediastinal adhesions and fibrosis, (4) advanced pulmonary vascular remodeling, and (5) advanced ventricular interdependence. Narrowing the differential diagnosis of equalization of right and left heart filling pressures requires careful clinical contextualization, cardiac imaging, and serial assessment of hemodynamics following aggressive medical therapy.

Scenario 2: Constrictive pericarditis versus restrictive cardiomyopathy versus right ventricular failure

While it is beyond the scope of this chapter to discuss distinguishing restrictive cardiomyopathy from constrictive pericarditis in detail, the differential diagnosis not infrequently arises in clinical practice as both conditions present with elevation of right heart pressures and/or equalization of right and left heart pressures.[11] Distinguishing the two conditions can be challenging, and involves both traditional and dynamic respiratory criteria. Historical traditional criteria with relatively poor specificity pointing to restrictive cardiomyopathy include (1) LVEDP greater than RVEDP by 5 mmHg or more, (2) PASP greater than 50 mmHg, and (3) RVEDP less than 0.3 RV systolic pressure. More accurate distinction relies on measures of dynamic ventricular interdependence during respiration. Patients with constrictive pericarditis exhibit dissociation of intrathoracic and intracardiac

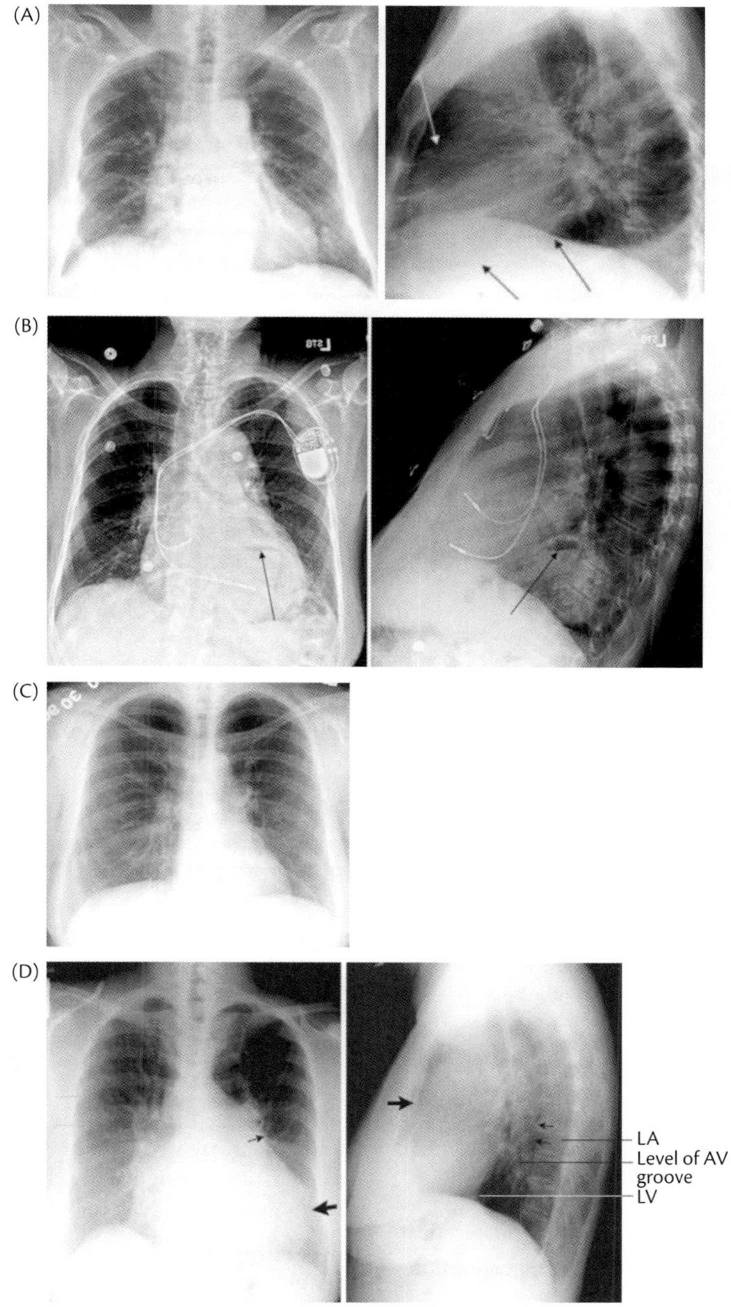

Fig. 21.2 Chest radiographs illustrative of right ventricular (RV) failure. (A) Biventricular hypertrophy (note boot-shaped heart on PA view, arrows on lateral view), marked pulmonary vascular redistribution (note haziness and loss of definition of margins of pulmonary vessels throughout), and right pleural effusion. (B) Heart failure, biventricular dilation, large hiatus hernia (arrows; note air–fluid level), and pacemaker leads in the right atrium and RV. (C) Small and asymptomatic atrial septal defect. The PA view shows a normal cardiac contour, with mild pulmonary vascular plethora at the periphery of the lung fields. Mitral stenosis. **A,** PA view shows enlarged cardiac silhouette, prominent convexity of the left atrial (LA) appendage (small arrow), slightly elevated cardiac apex (large arrow) suggestive of RV (rather than LV) enlargement. **B,** The lateral view confirms marked RV (arrow) and left atrial (small arrows) enlargement. Note filling in of the retrosternal airspace. LA, left atrium; LV, left ventricle.

chamber pressures because the pericardial "scar" does not permit complete transmission of intrathoracic pressures to the intracardiac chambers.[11] In constrictive pericarditis, the septum bulges leftward during inspiration and rightward during expiration, resulting in inspiratory decreases in PCW and LV pressures and increases in right atrial (RA) and RV pressures and the reciprocal pressure changes during expiration. The hemodynamic hallmarks of pericardial constriction are interdependent reciprocal changes in RV versus LV peak systolic pressure, stroke volume, and pulse pressures due to pericardial constraint of total ventricular volume by the noncompliant pericardium and incomplete transmission of intrathoracic pressures to the intracardiac chambers. Ventricular interdependence in constrictive pericarditis can be quantified by the systolic area index (SAI) which yields the ratio of areas

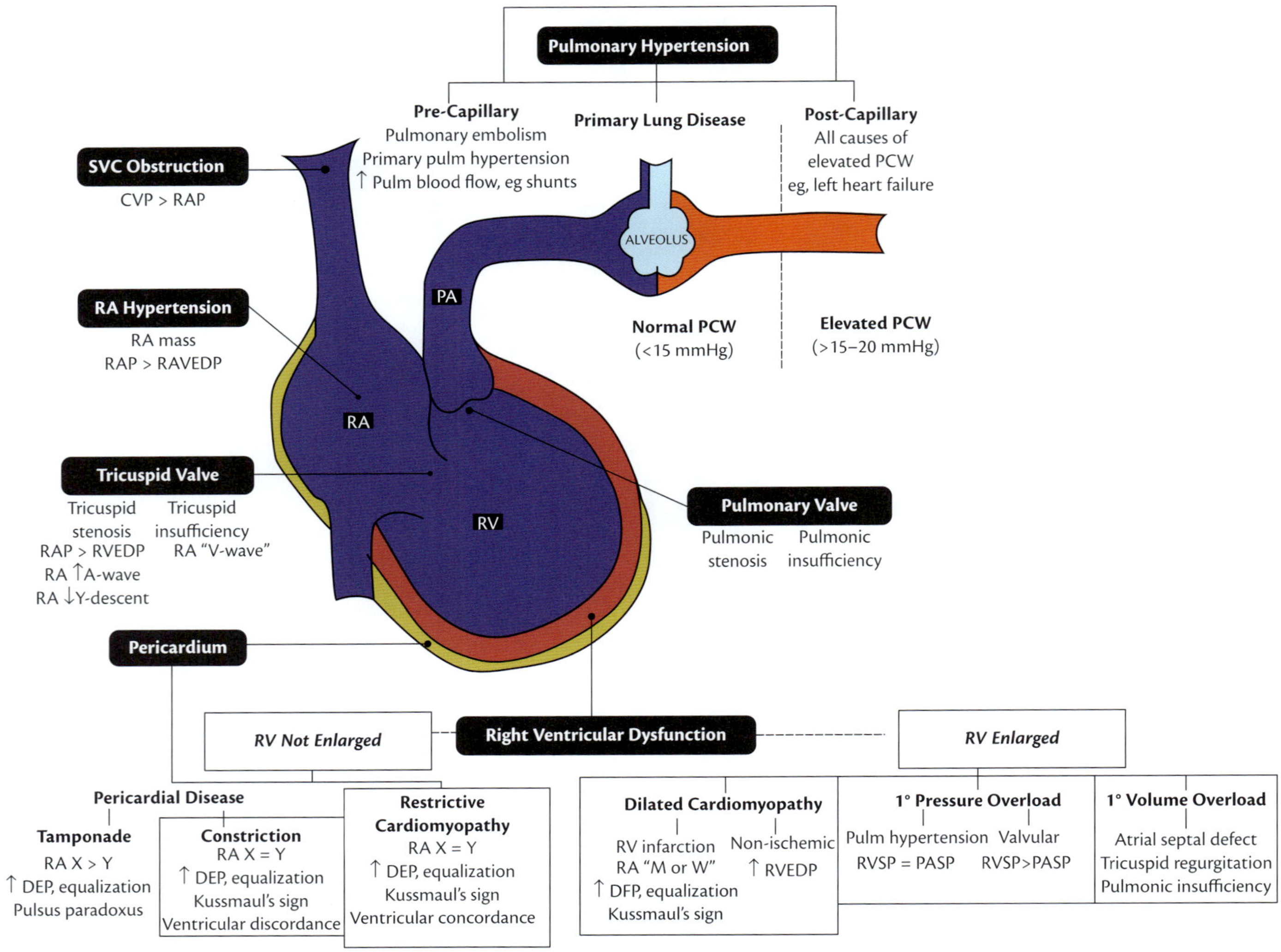

Fig. 21.3 Hemodynamic evaluation of right ventricular failure.
Reprinted with permission from Goldstein et al 2011.

(mmHg × s) under the RV and LV systolic pressure waveforms during inspiration vs. expiration:

$$\text{SAI} = \frac{\text{RV area during inspiration / LV area during inspiration}}{\text{RV area during expiration / LV area during expiration}}$$

An SAI ratio greater than 1.1 has 97% sensitivity and 100% predictive accuracy for identifying surgically proven constrictive pericarditis.[12]

Scenario 3: Dynamic tricuspid regurgitation

Patients with RV failure often present with significant systemic venous volume overload and elevated RV filling pressures resulting in acute or incrementally worse RV volume overload. RV volume overload may result in greater RV morphologic deformation and worse secondary TR. Aggressive reduction of systemic venous volume overload commonly reduces secondary TR by one or two echocardiographic grades and permits more precise assessment of RV mechanics. At catheterization, analysis of RV waveform inspiratory changes can help differentiate severe TR from constrictive pericarditis.[13,14] In severe TR, the pericardium is not as rigid, and enhanced RV diastolic filling during inspiration is marked by a rapid increase in RV diastolic filling pressures, rapid flow waves, accentuation of height and slope of RV early rapid filling wave, and widening of LV and RV diastolic pressures.[13,14]

Integrating hemodynamic and imaging information in right ventricular failure

Box 21.5 lists the more commonly encountered clinical scenarios based upon an integration of hemodynamics and RV imaging. Table 21.3 tabulates typical hemodynamic profiles of commonly encountered RV failure conditions.

Right ventricular imaging

RV imaging has been reviewed in both RV failure and pulmonary hypertension.[15,16,17,18,19,20,21] Different RV imaging modalities including transthoracic two-dimensional Doppler echocardiography (TTE), cardiac MRI (CMR), and CT may provide complementary diagnostic and prognostic information in selected instances of RV dysfunction or failure.[17,20]

Right ventricular morphology and systolic function

Echocardiography

RV morphology and function can generally be described qualitatively by TTE in most patients except when transthoracic imaging

Box 21.5 Evolving clinical differential diagnosis: three scenarios

Scenario #1: JVP >8 mmHg, no RV enlargement, mPAP <25 mmHg

- SVC occlusion
- RA "obstruction" (e.g., mass, vegetation, thrombus)
- TV obstruction (TS from rheumatic or carcinoid heart disease)
- Pericardial disease
- Primary RV diastolic dysfunction (RVH, ischemia, restrictive cardiomyopathy)

Scenario #2: JVP > 8 mmHg, RV enlargement, mPAP < 25 mmHg

- Primary RV volume overload:
  - Primary or secondary TR
  - Primary or secondary PR
  - Left-to-right shunt (e.g., ASD)
- Primary myocardial injury:
  - RV ischemia or infarction
  - RV "stunning" (e.g., hypoxemia, sepsis)

Scenario #3: JVP > 8 mmHg, RV enlargement, mPAP > 25 mmHg

- Postcapillary PAH (group 2 PAH):
  - LVrEF, LVpEF
  - Mitral valve disease (MR, MS)
- Precapillary PH (group 1, 3, 4, 5 PAH):
  - Pulmonary vascular remodeling of diverse etiology

ASD, atrial septal defect; JVP, jugular venous pressure; LVpEF, left ventricular preserved ejection fraction; LVrEF, left ventricular reduced ejection fraction; mPAP, mean pulmonary artery pressure; MR, mitral regurgitation; MS, mitral stenosis; PAH, pulmonary arterial hypertension; PH, pulmonary hypertension; PR, pulmonary regurgitation; RA, right atrium; RV, right ventricle; RVH, right ventricular hypertrophy; SVC, superior vena cava; TR, tricuspid regurgitation; TS, tricuspid stenosis; TV, tricuspid valve.

windows are suboptimal, and presently TTE is the mainstay of initial and subsequent evaluation of RV function and morphology. RV imaging by TEE, CMR, or CT is typically reserved for patients who require more precise evaluation of RV function, morphology or tissue composition to render a specific diagnosis (e.g., ARVC, congenital heart disease, acute pulmonary embolism).[21] Echocardiographic findings in PAH[15,18] and RV failure[16] have been reviewed extensively. Table 21.4 summarizes the American Society of Echocardiograph guideline reference limits for recommended measures of RV structure and function. Figure 21.4 provides examples of representative echocardiographic findings in RV failure.

Table 21.3 Hemodynamic profiles of acute and chronic right ventricular failure

Cause	RAP	PAP	PCWP	TPG	PVR	Examples
Isolated RV failure	↑	↓	↓	↓	↓	ARVC
Precapillary PAH	↑	↑	↓	↓	↓	Idiopathic PAH, chronic thromboembolic pulmonary hypertension, congenital heart disease
Postcapillary PAH	↑	↑	↑	↓	↓	Left heart failure
Mixed PH (pre- and postcapillary)	↑	↑	↑	↑	↑	Left heart failure

ARVC, arrhythmogenic right ventricular cardiomyopathy; PAH, pulmonary artery hypertension; PAP, pulmonary artery pressure; PCWP, pulmonary capillary wedge pressure; PH, pulmonary hypertension; PVR, pulmonary vascular resistance; RAP, right atrial pressure; RV, right ventricle; TPG, transpulmonary pressure gradient.

Reprinted from Cardiology Clinics, 30, Sayer GT, Semigran MJ, Right ventricular performance in chronic congestive heart failure, 271–82, copyright (2012) with permission from Elsevier.

Cardiac MRI

CMR is currently the second-line modality after TTE for comprehensive RV assessment, and is indicated when TTE imaging windows are suboptimal. In addition, CMR is the current reference standard for assessment of RV volume, ejection fraction, wall thickness, noninvasive tissue characterization, and complex congenital heart disease.[17,20] Table 21.5 tabulates CMR RV morphologic and functional parameters and Figure 21.5 illustrates representative CMR findings in RV failure.

CT

Due to nephrotoxic contrast agent risks and radiation exposure, CT is infrequently used for RV assessment except in instances where both echocardiographic and CMR are suboptimal or contraindicated (e.g., poor echocardiographic windows in patients with permanent pacemakers or ICDs).[19] CT can provide assessment of RV size, volume, free wall thickening/hypertrophy, septal movement, and pulmonary vasculature.[21] CT has lower temporal resolution than CMR, and tends to overestimate RV end-systolic and end-diastolic volumes.[21] Contrast-enhanced CT evidence of significant RV dilatation (RV/LV maximum diameter ratio >0.9) provides prognostic information in patients with acute pulmonary embolism.[19]

Nuclear techniques

Nuclear imaging modalities are not widely used for RV imaging, although first-pass radionuclide ventriculography can assess RVEF during rest and exercise conditions. Positron emission tomography (PET) or SPECT scanning is normally limited by the relatively lower RV than LV counts, but may be of value in assessment of RV metabolism and perfusion in PAH-associated RV hypertrophy.[21]

Table 21.4 Summary of American Society of Echocardiography reference limits for recommended echocardiographic measures of right heart structure and function

Measure	Abnormal
Chamber dimensions	
RV basal diameter	>4.2 cm
RV mid-cavity diameter	>3.5 cm
RV longitudinal diameter	>8.6 cm
RV end-diastolic area	>25 cm^2
RV end-systolic area	>14 cm^2
RV end-diastolic volume index	>80 ml/m^2
RV end-systolic volume index	>46 ml/m^2
RV subcostal wall thickness	>0.5 cm
RVOT PSAX distal diameter	>2.7 cm
RVOT PLAX proximal diameter	>3.3 cm
RA major dimension	>5.3 cm
RA minor dimension	>4.4 cm
RA end-systolic area	>18 cm^2
Systolic function	
TAPSE	<1.6 cm
Pulsed Doppler peak velocity at the annulus	<10 cm/s
Pulse Doppler MPI	>0.40
Tissue Doppler MPI	>0.55
FAC (%)	<35
Diastolic function	
E/A ratio	<0.8 or >2.1
E/E′ ratio	>6
Deceleration time	<120 ms
IVC diameter	<2.1 cm
IVC collapse with sniff (%)	>50%

FAC, fractional area change; MPI, myocardial performance index; PLAX, parasternal long-axis; PSAX, parasternal short axis; RA, right atrium; RV, right ventricle; RVD, right ventricular diameter; RVOT, right ventricular outflow tract; TAPSE, tricuspid annular plane systolic excursion.

Reprinted from the Journal of the American Society of Echocardiography, 23, Rudski LG, Lai WW, Afilalo J, et al. Guidelines for the echocardiographic assessment of the right heart in adults, 685–713, copyright (2010) with permission from Elsevier.

Right ventricular diastolic function

In clinical practice RV diastolic function is assessed by integrating TTE size, volume, and Doppler associations.

Integrated right ventricular imaging approach

Table 21.6 summarizes the RV parameters that can be assessed by specific imaging modalities across different diseases and conditions. Table 21.7 summarizes representative studies of various RV imaging modalities with a focus on the prognostic value of selected RV structural and/or functional parameters in diverse conditions. Box 21.6 provides an algorithmic approach to imaging the RV in suspected or known instances of RV dysfunction or failure.

Acute right ventricular failure

This section focuses on the presentation, evaluation, and general management principles of acute severe RV failure.[22,23,24,25,26,27,28,29,30,31,32] Etiologies of acute severe RV failure with specific therapies (acute RV infarction, acute massive pulmonary embolism, acute lung injury/adult respiratory distress syndrome, post cardiac surgery) are discussed in greater detail in subsequent sections of this chapter.

Clinical presentation

Acute RV failure typically occurs in five settings: (1) abrupt, severe increases in RV afterload, (2) abrupt, severe increases in RV volume, (3) diffuse RV injury, (4) abrupt onset of impeded RV filling, and (5) acute arrhythmias. Figures 21.6 and 21.7 illustrate the pathophysiology of acute RV failure. The most common etiologies of acute, severe RV failure in the intensive care unit (ICU) setting include LV failure, acute RV infarction, acute massive pulmonary embolism, sepsis, acute lung injury/adult respiratory distress syndrome, cardiac tamponade, and post cardiac surgery (LVAD implantation, cardiac transplantation).

Clinical evaluation

The most important principles of clinical evaluation of acute severe RV failure include assessment of (1) RV and LV structure and function (see Box 8.7), (2) pulmonary artery pressure and pulmonary vascular resistance, (3) ventricular interaction, (4) specific underlying cause(s), and (5) common exacerbating factors (e.g., intravascular volume, mechanical ventilation). The sensitivity and specificity of the signs, symptoms, and ECG and imaging features in acute severe RV failure have not been well established except in particular conditions (e.g., echocardiographic Westermark's sign in acute pulmonary embolism, ECG aVR3–4 ST-segment elevation in acute RV infarction). See Table 21.8 and Box 21.7.

In the ICU setting, the most relevant clinical information is obtained from RV imaging (TTE, TEE, or CMR) and pulmonary artery catheterization (PAC) (see Box 21.8).[27] Although PAC does not improve outcomes in acute lung injury[33] or decompensated LV failure,[34] PAC provides essential hemodynamic characterization of RV function (cardiac output, RV stroke work index), RV load (CVP, PVR), pulmonary vasculature (PVR, capacitance), LV load (PCWP, SVR), LV function (cardiac output, LVSWI) and ventricular interaction in the following settings: (1) severely or critically ill patients who fail to respond to initial therapeutic measures, (2) patients with complex or mixed pre- and postcapillary pulmonary hypertension and (3) patients with suspected or known significant ventricular interaction. See Box 21.8.

General management principles of acute right ventricular failure

The management of RV failure is largely empiric, as few trials have focused exclusively on pharmacologic or device therapy of RV failure alone.[31] Stepwise principles for managing acute and/or chronic severe RV failure are summarized in Box 21.9. The unique anatomic and physiologic features of the RV and the critical roles played by RV–PA coupling RV–LV ventricular interdependence determine the outcome of severe, acute RV failure. Successful management of acute, severe RV failure thus necessitates three major tasks: (1) meticulous evaluation of the relative roles of RV structure and function, RV–PA coupling, and RV–LV ventricular interdependence, (2) treatment of underlying precipitants and exacerbating conditions, and (3) optimization of RV preload, afterload, and contractility.[28,31] If RV failure persists (by clinical course or persistent elevation of CVP >12–15 mmHg), then aggressive afterload reduction and inotropes are often required.[28] Figure 21.8presents an acute RV management algorithm.

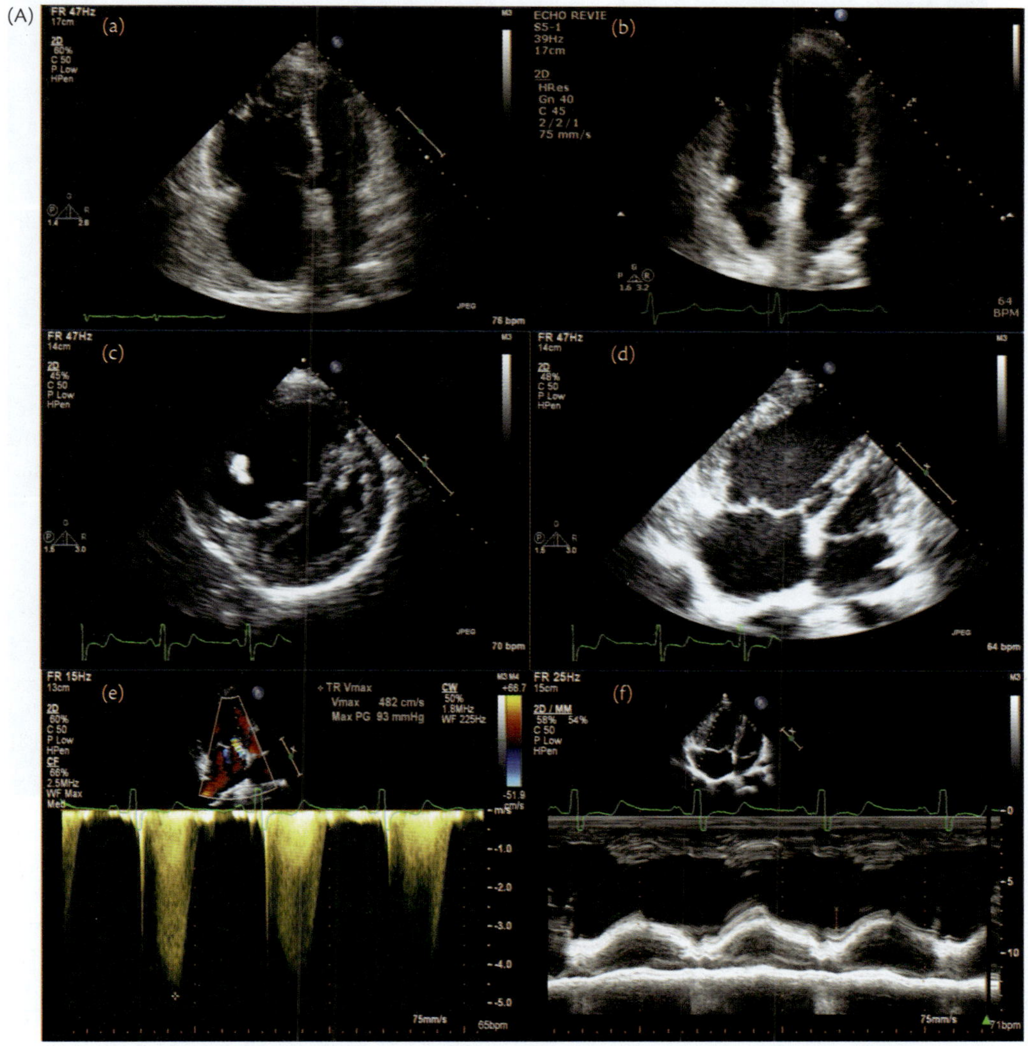

Fig. 21.4 (A) Representative echocardiographic findings in right ventricular (RV) dysfunction. (a) RV enlargement and hypertrophy in patient with CTEPH. (b) Normal RV size 6 months after pulmonary thromboendarterectomy in same patient as in (a). (c) Parasternal short-axis view demonstrating RV dilation and hypertrophy and displacement of septum toward the left ventricle (LV). (d) Apical four-chamber view demonstrating RV enlargement and hypertrophy and RA dilation. (e) Tricuspid regurgitation jet demonstrating severe PH in patient with PAH. (f) Peak systolic velocity of tricuspid annulus borderline depressed at 10 cm/s. TAPSE in patient with PAH. (B) Assessment of RV function by echocardiography. (a) %FAC, calculated from measures from the apical four-chamber view. The importance of longitudinal shortening can be appreciated in this image. (b) MPI, calculated by measuring the ejection time (ET) on the pulmonary artery tracing and the time between closure and opening of the tricuspid valve on the tricuspid inflow tracing. MPI = (TCOT − ET)/ET. In this patient, the MPI was normal after tetralogy of Fallot repair. (c) TAPSE. An M-mode echocardiogram through the tricuspid annulus is obtained and the excursion of the tricuspid annulus is measured as illustrated. This index enables assessment of longitudinal RV function. (d) Tissue Doppler velocities of the tricuspid annulus. Pulsed tissue Doppler measurements can be used to calculate tissue velocities. Systolic velocities can be used as a parameter for systolic longitudinal RV function. (e) Longitudinal strain measurements of the RV, made using speckle tracking technology. By convention, systolic longitudinal shortening is represented as a negative value and can be measured in six different segments. The mean values of these segments are used to trace a mean longitudinal strain curve (white dotted line). The value at end-systole is then measured. (f) Color tissue Doppler echocardiogram at the lateral tricuspid valve annulus and measurement of IVA. Aortic valve opening and closure are depicted by green lines for event timing. The timing of these events may be taken as that of pulmonary valve opening and closure. The slope of IVA is shown. Note that IVA occurs within the QRS complex and peaks before pulmonary valve opening in the isovolumic period. A′, late-diastolic tissue velocity; AVC, aortic valve closure; AVO, aortic valve opening; E′, early-diastolic tissue velocity; ET, ejection time; %FAC, percentage fractional area change; IVA, isovolumic acceleration; MPI, myocardial performance index; S′, systolic tissue velocity; TAPSE, tricuspid annular systolic plane excursion; TCOT, tricuspid valve closure–opening time.

(A) Reprinted with permission from Brittain et al 2012. (B) Reprinted with permission from Mertens et al 2010.

(B)

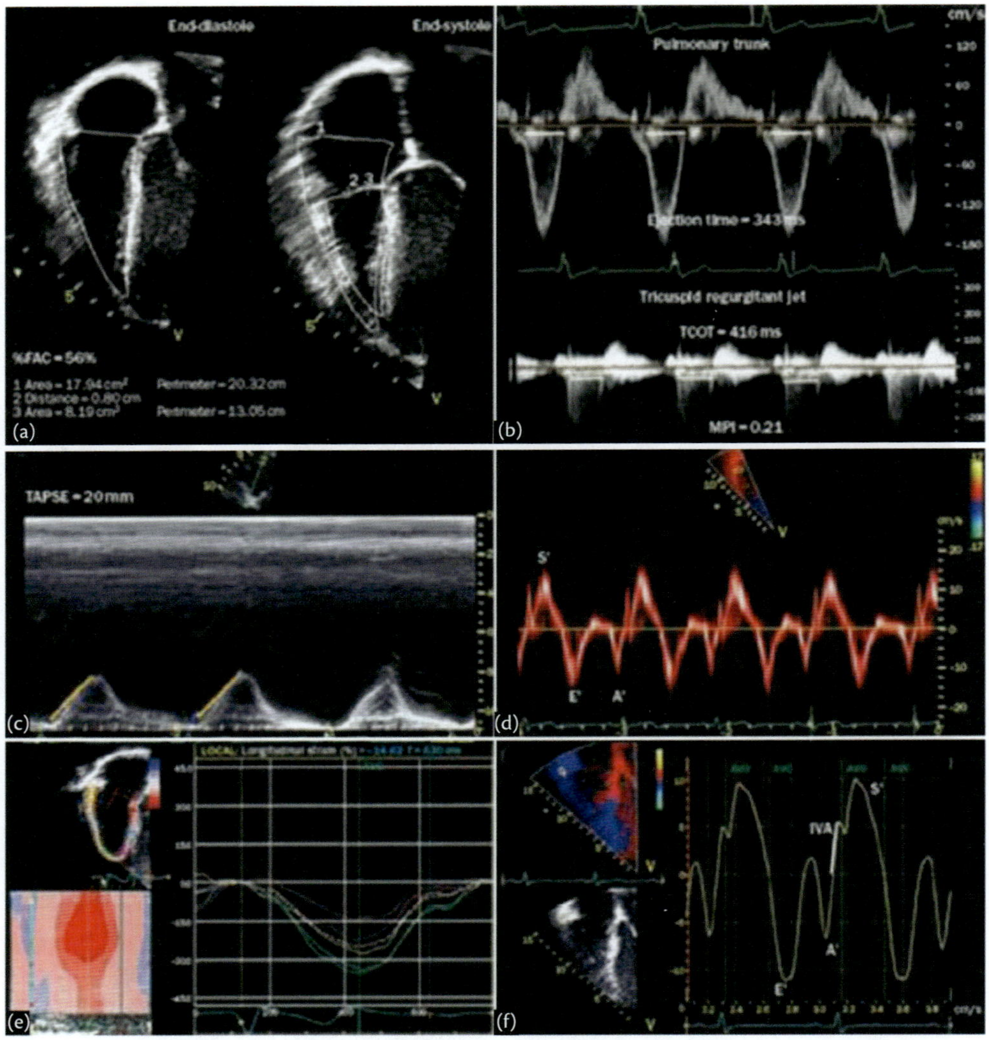

Fig. 21.4 Continued

Table 21.5 Right ventricular morphology and functional MRI parameters

Parameter	Acquisition sequence	Normal value	Clinical comment
RVEF (%)	Conventional breath-hold cine MRI	61 ± 7	>40–45 used in clinical practice
RV mass (g/m²)	Conventional breath-hold cine MRI	26 ± 5	
RVEDV (ml/m²)	Conventional breath-hold cine MRI	75 ± 13	
TR/PR volume/ severity	Velocity-encoded cine MRI	None or physiological	Mild: < 20 ml Moderate: 20–50 ml Severe: > 50 ml
Shunt fraction	Velocity-encoded cine MRI	Absent	Q_p/Q_s <1.5 hemodynamically insignificant
Myocardial delayed enhancement	Contrast-enhanced inversion recovery gradient echo	Absent	Predicts arrhythmia and exercise tolerance in TOF patients Correlates with RV WMA in patients with RVMI
Pulmonary transit time (s)	Dynamic first-pass contrast-enhanced saturation-recovery gradient echo	6 ± 1.4 7.2 ± 1.2	Limited normative data Prolongation correlates with degree of LVEF, PH

CHD, congenital heart disease; LVEF, left ventricular ejection fraction; PH, pulmonary hypertension; Q_p/Q_s, pulmonary flow/systemic flow; TOF, tetralogy of Fallot; RV, right ventricle; RVMI, right ventricular myocardial infarction; WMA, wall motion abnormality.

Brittain E, Hemnes A, Keebler M, Lawson J, Byrd B, Di Salvo TG. Right venticular plasticity and functional imaging. Pulmonary circulation 2012;2:309-26.

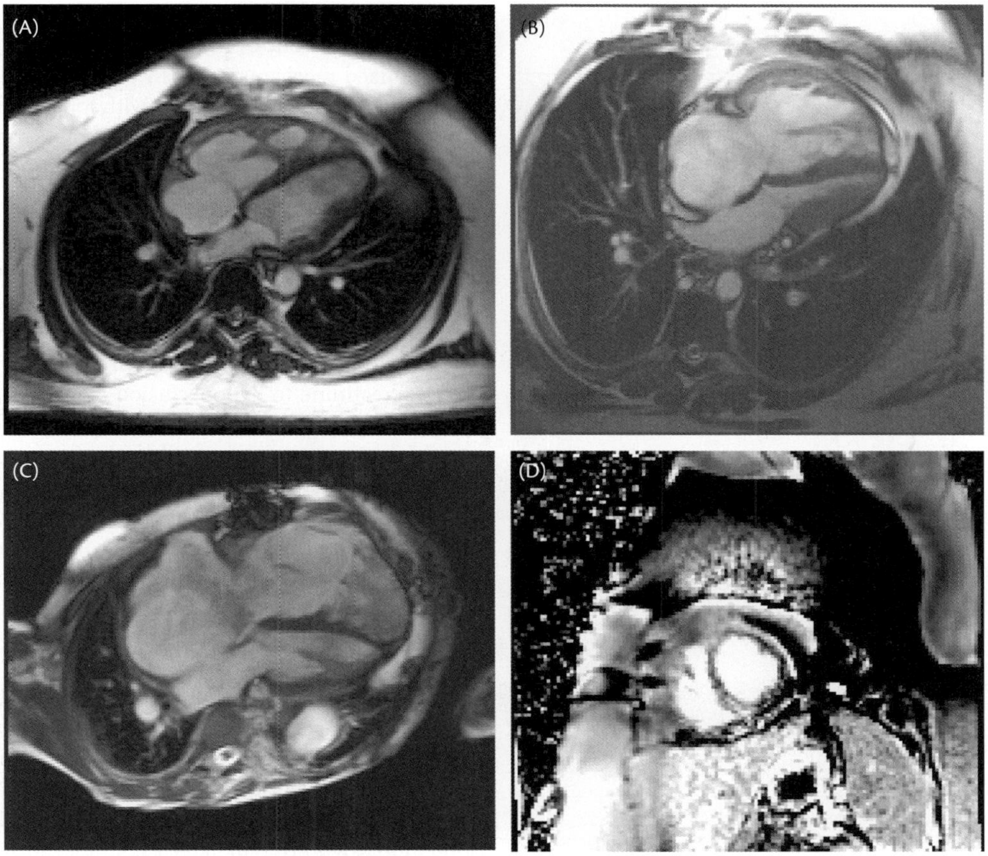

Fig. 21.5 Representative CMR findings in right ventricular (RV) dysfunction. (A) Mild RV and RA dilation with RV hypertrophy and prominent hypertrophy of moderator band. (B) Severe RV and RA dilation with RVH and compression of left-sided chambers by interventricular septal deviation. (C) End-stage RV failure with marked RV and RA dilation and thinned-out RV free wall. (D) Late gadolinium enhanced short-axis image demonstrating fibrosis at the RV septal insertion point.
Reprinted with permission from Brittain et al 2012.

Oxygen delivery

Hypoxia induces both (1) pulmonary artery vasoconstriction with further elevation of RV afterload and (2) RV ischemia due to arterial oxygen desaturation.[30,32] Arterial oxygen saturation should therefore be maintained at or above 90% in all patients with acute, severe RV failure.[30,32] Maintaining hemoglobin level above 10 g/dl is also recommended in instances of acute severe RV failure to ensure adequate tissue oxygen delivery, but this is controversial.[30,32]

Right ventricular perfusion

In acute RV pressure overload, a greater proportion of RV perfusion occurs during diastole. Therefore, a suitable aortic root pressure (mean arterial systolic pressure >60 mmHg) should be maintained to prevent progressive RV ischemia. Since RV free wall blood flow is largely provided by RV marginal branches, sufficient patency of both the right coronary artery (RCA) and RV marginal branches is required to provide adequate RV free wall perfusion.

Maintenance of sinus rhythm and atrioventricular synchrony

In RV failure, loss of coordinated atrial systole may result in a 30% decline in RV filling and reduction in RV output. Although RV dyssynchrony has not been studied as widely as LV dyssynchrony, RV dyssynchrony in animal models reduces RV mechanical systolic efficiency.[22] In more chronic RV failure, resynchronization reduces pulmonary artery pressures[35,36] and induces reverse RV remodeling.[37,38,39]

Mechanical ventilation

Intubation and mechanical ventilation should be avoided whenever possible in patients with acute, severe RV failure due to the deleterious effects of mechanical ventilation on RV function.[26] Since the pulmonary capillaries are intra-alveolar vessels, they are stressed by alveolar positive mechanical ventilation pressures.[40] Cyclic (tidal ventilation) or continuous (PEEP application) positive airway pressure increases the alveolar transpulmonary pressure and increases PVR, resulting in greater RV afterload.[41,42] In addition, cyclic or continuous positive airway pressure (CPAP) increases pleural pressure and thus increases RV effective elastance leading to decreased RV diastolic filling in the absence of a proportional rise in central venous pressure.[41] In instances of acute severe RV failure, peak plateau airway pressures less than 30 cmH_2O, tidal volume 6–8 ml kg^{-1} min^{-1}, minimal PEEP to ensure adequate oxygenation, and avoidance of hypercarbia, acidosis and auto-PEEP minimize the adverse effects of mechanical ventilation on RV contractile function and load.

Minimization of "mechanical" intrapulmonary influences

Coupling of the RV to the pulmonary circulation may be adversely affected by structural or mechanical factors that influence pulmonary pressures, resistance, or ventilation. Large pleural effusions should be evacuated. It is important to recognize and reduce V/Q mismatch, intrapulmonary shunting, hypotentilation-induced hypoxia/hypercarbia, and auto-PEEP in patients with advanced obstructive lung disease.[27]

Table 21.6 Summary of right ventricle parameters assessed by specific imaging modalities in various diseases

Parameter	Modality	Disease
RV anatomy	TTE CMR (SSFP) CT	All CHD
RV dimensions	TTE CMR (SSFP, volumetry) CT	All CHD ARVC (RVOT)
Pulmonary valve	TTE CMR (phase contrast imaging)	CHD
Pulmonary arteries	CMR (angiography, 3D SSPFT) CT TTE/TEE (proximal segments)	CHD PAH Acute/chronic PE
Tricuspid valve	TTE 3D echocardiography	All
RV volumes	CMR (SSFP)	All
RV ejection fraction	CMR Gated blood-pool SPECT CT (TTE not recommended for quantitative assessment)	All
Regional RV function and RV dyssynchrony[a]	Tissue Doppler strain and strain rate imaging[a]	All
Myocardial velocities[a]	TTE speckle tracking[a]	
Strain/strain rate[a]	TTE Tissue Doppler strain/strain rate[a], speckle tracking[a]	
RV ischemia	CMR (late enhancement, edema) TTE (wall motion) SPECT (perfusion)	RV infarction RV failure
RV scar/ fibrosis	CMR (late enhancement) SPECT	
Coronary arteries	Angiography MDCT PET/CT	RV infarction Coronary disease

ARVC, arrhythmogenic right ventricular cardiomyopathy; CHD, congenital heart disease; CMR, cardiac magnetic resonance imaging; MDCT, multidetector computed tomography; RVOT, right ventricular outflow tract; PAH, pulmonary arterial hypertension; PET, positron emission tomography; SPECT, single-photon electron CT; SSFP, steady-state free precession sequence; TEE, transesophageal echocardiography; TTE, transthoracic echocardiography.

[a] Evolving and/or investigational at present.

Valsangiacomo Buechel ER, Mertens LL. Imaging the right heart: the use of integrated multimodality imaging. European Heart Journal (2012);33:949–60 by permission of Oxford University Press.

Determination of PAH elevation mechanism and PAH reversibility

Patients with acute RV failure typically have significant PAH. It is critical to determine the predominant mechanism of PAH, usually by TTE and right heart catheterization.[27,28,31] PAH may arise from (1) intrinsic pulmonary vascular disease (precapillary PAH), (2) left heart systolic or diastolic dysfunction (postcapillary PAH), or (3) mixed mechanisms (both precapillary and postcapillary).[31] In instances of acute RV failure with long-standing PAH, it is also important to determine if PAH is reversible or fixed.[6,31]

Target and management strategy for right ventricular preload and the cardiorenal syndrome

Elevation of CVP beyond 15 mmHg incurs the risk of RV overdistension and adverse RV–LV ventricular interaction.

Patients with RV failure and venous congestion may develop the cardiorenal syndrome.[2,43,44,45] It is a common error in the management of acute, severe RV failure to attribute an elevation in serum creatinine to hypoperfusion alone in patients with significant venous congestion.[23,45] Relief of venous congestion improves renal function independent of blood pressure, pulmonary capillary wedge pressure (PCWP), cardiac index, and glomerular filtration rate (GFR).[46,47] In patients with acute on chronic RV failure, the typical gradual rise in RV pressures during the month preceding the acute presentation[46,47] may have already elevated systemic venous pressures substantially and occasioned greater renal dysfunction, which is frequently reversible with reduction in systemic venous congestion.[44]

Management of the cardiorenal syndrome is evolving.[1,2,48,49] The mainstay of currently recommended therapy is aggressive diuretic therapy using a stepped pharmacologic algorithm. The stepped pharmacologic algorithm employed in the CARRESS trial is shown in Box 21.10[50] and a summary of the pharmacokinetic properties of loop diuretics is given in Table 21.9. Most hospitalized patients initially require intravenous loop diuretics at typically twice the usual outpatient dosage, due to delayed or insufficient oral absorption and/or splanchnic hypoperfusion.[48,49] The DOSE trial did not show a difference in bolus versus continuous intravenous administration of furosemide.[51] Inotropes (e.g., dobutamine) and/or inodilators (e.g., milrinone) have not been consistently shown to improve renal function in the cardiorenal syndrome compared to diuretic therapy alone.[1,2,48,49,52,53,54] Use of inotropes and inodilators should be restricted to settings in which cardiorenal syndrome is most clearly related to renal hypoperfusion, and such agents should be used for the shortest practical duration given adverse effects.[49] Low-dose dopamine (<2 mg kg^{-1} min^{-1}) acts relatively selectively on DA1 receptors without substantial β_1 receptor agonism, and may effect augmentation of renal blood flow via renal vasodilation in patients with acute heart failure.[55,56] Nesiritide is not recommended as standard therapy in acute heart failure (HF), including acute HF complicated by the cardiorenal syndrome, given the lack of efficacy with nesiritide in the randomized controlled ASCEND trial.[57] Oral tolvaptan, a vasopressin V2 receptor antagonist, reduces symptoms and edema compared to conventional therapy in patients hospitalized with HF, but is not associated with long-term improved outcomes.[58] The adenosine A1 receptor antagonist rolofylline did not demonstrate beneficial effects on outcomes or renal function in patients hospitalized with acute HF and volume overload.[59] The role of (1) novel agents such as intravenous vasopressin antagonists and serelaxin (relaxin) and (2) adjunctive intravenous agents such as low-dose dopamine and nesiritide in combination with loop diuretics in the management of acute HF and the cardiorenal syndrome is rapidly evolving and a major focus of the NHLBI Heart Failure Network Clinical Research program.

Table 21.7 Illustrative examples of right ventricle imaging in diverse conditions

Disease	Study	Parameter assessed	Population	Outcome
MI	Engstrom et al. 2010	TAPSE, S′	STEMI patients with cardiogenic shock	TAPSE ≤ 14 had HR of 2.1 for death S′ = 7.8 vs. 10 in IMI with and without RV involved
	Antoni et al. 2010	TAPSE, RVFAC, RV strain	Inferior MI	TAPSE ≤ 1.5, RVFAC <32%, and RV Strain <−22.1% predicted death/MI/HF readmission
	Ozdemir et al. 2003	RIMP	Acute MI	RIMP > 0.70 has sensitivity and specificity of 94% and 80% for RVMI
	Kumar et al. 2006	RV LGE on CMR	STEMI	RV LGE outperformed exam, ECG, and echocardiogram for detection of RVMI
PAH	Forfia et al. 2006	TAPSE	All forms of PH	One year survival with TAPSE > 1.8 cm of 94% vs. 60% for TAPSE <1.8 cm
	Yeo et al. 1998	RIMP	IPAH	5-year survival free of cardiac death or lung transplant with RIMP < .83 vs. ≥ 0.83, 74% vs. 4%
	Sachdev et al. 2011	RV strain	WHO Group 1 PAH	RV free wall strain worse than −12.5% predicted 1–4-year mortality
	McGann et al. 200 and Shehata et al. 2011	RV LGE on MRI	All forms of PH	Extent of RV LGE correlated directly with RV mass index and inversely with RVEF
	van Wolferen et al. 2007, 2011	RVEDVI, SVI on CMR	IPAH	RVEDVI ≥ 84 ml/m^2 and SVI ≤ 25 ml/m^2 predict mortality SV increase of 10 ml after treatment considered clinically relevant
	van Wolferen et al. 2007, 2011 and Wilkins et al. 2005	RV mass after therapy	WHO Group 1 PAH	Significant decrease in RV mass, increase in CI on sildenafil/bosentan combination but not bosentan alone
CTEPH and post-lung transplant	Menzel et al. 2002	RV volume and EF by 3DE	CTEPH	RVEDV decreased from 121 ml to 80 and RVEF increased from 25% to 36% post-PTE
	Menzel et al. 2002	RIMP	CTEPH	RIMP decreased from 0.55 to 0.37 post-PTE
	Reesink et al. 2007	RV volume and mass by CMR	CTEPH	RV volume normalized and RV mass decreased significantly post-PTE
	Katz et al. 1996	RV volume and FAC	Post-lung transplant	RV volume decreased significantly but FAC did not improve immediately post-transplant
	Kramer et al. 1994	RVEF by radionuclide angiography	Post-lung transplant	RVEF increased from 23% to 48% at 3–6 months
	Frist et al. 1995	RVEF and RV mass by CMR	Post-lung transplant	RVEF near-normal at 3 months, RV mass normalized by 1 year
LVAD	Topilsky et al. 2011	FAC	Pre-LVAD implant	FAC <20% predicts postoperative RV failure
	Puwanant et al. 2008	TAPSE	Pre-LVAD implant	TAPSE <7.5 mm predicts RV failure (sensitivity 91%, specificity 46%)
	Topilsky et al. 2011	Corrected TR duration (TRDc)	Pre-LVAD implant	TRDc ≤ 461 ms is associated with decreased 1- and 2-year survival
	Kukucka et al. 2011	RV-to-LV end-diastolic diameter ratio	Pre-LVAD or BiVAD implant	R/L > 0.72 predicted RV failure (OR 11.4)
	Topilsky et al. 2011	S′ and septal deviation	30 days post-LVAD implant	Decreased S′ (OR 0.70) and septal deviation to left (OR 3.0) associated with 90 day mortality, HF readmission, or NYHA ≥ 3

3DE, tridimensional echocardiography; BiVAD, biventricular assist device; CI, cardiac index; CMR, cardiac magnetic resonance imaging; CTEPH, chronic thromboembolic pulmonary hypertension; ECG, electrocardiogram; HF, heart failure; HR, hazard ratio; IDC, idiopathic dilated cardiomyopathy; IPAH, idiopathic pulmonary arterial hypertension; IVA, isovolumic acceleration; LGE, late gadolinium enhancement; LVAD, left ventricular assist device; MI, myocardial infarction; NYHA, New York Heart Association; OR, odds ratio; PASP, pulmonary artery systolic pressure; PH, pulmonary hypertension; PTE, pulmonary thromboendarterectomy; RIMP, right ventricular index of myocardial performance; RV, right ventricle; RVAD, right ventricular assist device; RVEDVI, right ventricular end-diastolic volume index; RVEF, right ventricular ejection fraction; RVFAC, right ventricular fractional area change; S′, myocardial velocity at the lateral tricuspid annulus; STEMI, ST-segment myocardial infarction; SVI, stroke volume index; TAPSE, tricuspid annular plane systolic excursion; TDI, tissue Doppler imaging; TR, tricuspid regurgitation; TRDc, tricuspid regurgitation duration (corrected for heart rate); WHO, World Health Organization.

Brittain E, Hemnes A, Keebler M, Lawson J, Byrd B, Di Salvo TG. Right ventricular plasticity and functional imaging. Pulmonary Circulation 2012;2:309–26.

Box 21.6 Proposed algorithm for the assessment of right ventricular function

Echocardiography

- Recommended for screening test for known/suspected RV dysfunction or failure
- Useful for serial assessment of RV function, response to therapy
- Parameters assessed:
  - Dimensions

    RV size

    RA size
  - ASE recommended for assessment of RV function (at least one):

    Fractional area change

    TAPSE

    S′ (PW TDI)

    RV index of myocardial performance
  - Consider in patients with RV dysfunction:

    dP/dT

    Isovolumic acceleration

    Diastolic function (E/A, E/E′)
  - RV/pulmonary hemodynamics:

    PASP

    RA pressure estimate (from IVC dimensions)
  - Consider:

    PADP

    PVR
  - Additional parameters:

    RV free wall and septal strain

    Pulmonary acceleration time

Cardiac MRI

- Consider if:
  - Echo is technically difficult and/or discrepancy exists among echo parameters
  - Discrepancy between echo results and clinical impression
  - MRI is indicated for assessment of biventricular failure, RV-specific etiology (ARVC), pericardial disease, unexplained syncope
- Parameters assessed:
  - Dimensions:

    RV size and volume

    RV mass

    RA size
  - RV ejection fraction
  - Volume and severity of TR, PR
  - LGE
  - Pulmonary vascular assessment

    Pulmonary transit time

    Pulmonary blood volume

    Capacitance
  - Additional parameters

    Myocardial strain

Radionuclide ventriculography

- Consider if echo inconclusive and MRI contraindicated
- Parameters assessed:
  - RV ejection fraction
  - Pulmonary transit time
  - Diastolic function

Multidetector CT

- Consider if echo inconclusive and MRI contraindicated
- Modality of choice in suspected PE
- Parameters assessed:
  - Possible pulmonary emboli
  - RV size and volume
  - Coronary artery calcification

ARVC, arrhythmogenic right ventricular cardiomyopathy; ASE, American Society of Echocardiography; IVC, inferior vena cava; LGE, late gadolinium enhancement; PADP, pulmonary artery diastolic pressure; PASP, pulmonary artery systolic pressure; PE, pulmonary embolism; PR, pulmonary regurgitation; PVR, pulmonary vascular resistance; PW TDI, pulse wave tissue Doppler imaging; RA, right atrium; RV, right ventricle; TAPSE, tricuspid annular plane systolic excursion; TR, tricuspid regurgitation.

Brittain E, Hemnes A, Keebler M, Lawson J, Byrd B, Di Salvo TG. Right ventricular plasticity and functional imaging. Pulmonary circulation 2012;2:309–26.

Despite favorable outcomes in small earlier studies,[60,61,62] the randomized CARRESS-HF study found (1) no change in body weight, (2) worse serum creatinine, and (3) increased adverse events in patients hospitalized with acute heart failure treated with ultrafiltration rather than with a stepped-therapy pharmacologic algorithm (Box 21.10).[50]

Target and management strategy for right ventricular afterload

In acute RV failure in general, the therapeutic target should be normalization of PVR or at least reduction of PVR to less than 3 Wood units. In clinical practice, achieving this PVR target requires adequate oxygenation, optimization of pulmonary mechanics and ventilator strategy, and aggressive pulmonary vasodilator therapy.[22,26]

Inhalational administration of pulmonary vasodilators minimizes the V/Q mismatch that may result from systemic administration

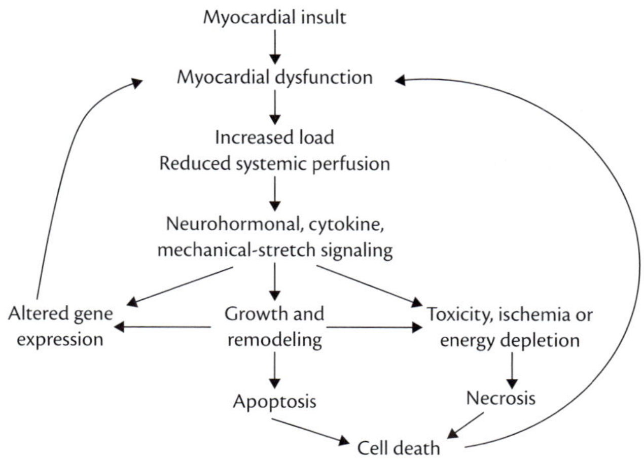

Fig. 21.6 Pathophysiology of chronic right ventricular failure.
Reprinted with permission from Haddad et al 2008.

of nonselective pulmonary vasodilators.[22] In acute RV failure due to chronic LV failure, post-LVAD or following cardiac transplantation, cardiotomy, or acute RV infarction, inhaled nitric oxide (iNO) 5–80 ppm reduces PVR and RV filling pressures, increases cardiac output and potentiates inodilator efficacy when used adjunctively.[24] In patients with decompensated LV failure and elevated PCWP pressures (typically >20–25 mmHg), however, iNO administration may result in acute pulmonary edema due to augmented LV filling.[25] Use of iNO is also limited by risk of methemoglobinemia, reactive oxygen species, rebound pulmonary hypertension upon discontinuation, and cost.

In acute RV failure following cardiac surgery or cardiac transplantation, inhaled prostacyclins (epoprostenol, iloprost, treprostinil) reduce PVR and RV filling pressures and improve RV function.[27,30,61] Inhaled prostacyclins are relatively easy to administer, less expensive than iNO, and may provide synergistically greater reductions in PVR and PAP and increases in cardiac output when used with sildenafil.[27] Inhaled milrinone potentiates the pulmonary vasodilatory effects of inhaled prostacyclin following cardiac surgery.[62]

Intravenous epoprostenol is indicated in patients with primary pulmonary vascular disease and normal LV function.[6] Intravenous epoprostenol is contraindicated in patients with LV dysfunction, as a randomized trial of intravenous epoprostenol therapy in patients with LV dysfunction resulted in higher morbidity and mortality.[63]

Oral endothelin antagonists and PDE5 inhibitors have not been studied in patients with acute severe RV failure cared for in critical care settings.[22,27] Chronic oral endothelin antagonist therapy resulted in increased morbidity and mortality in chronic LV systolic dysfunction.[64,65,66,67]

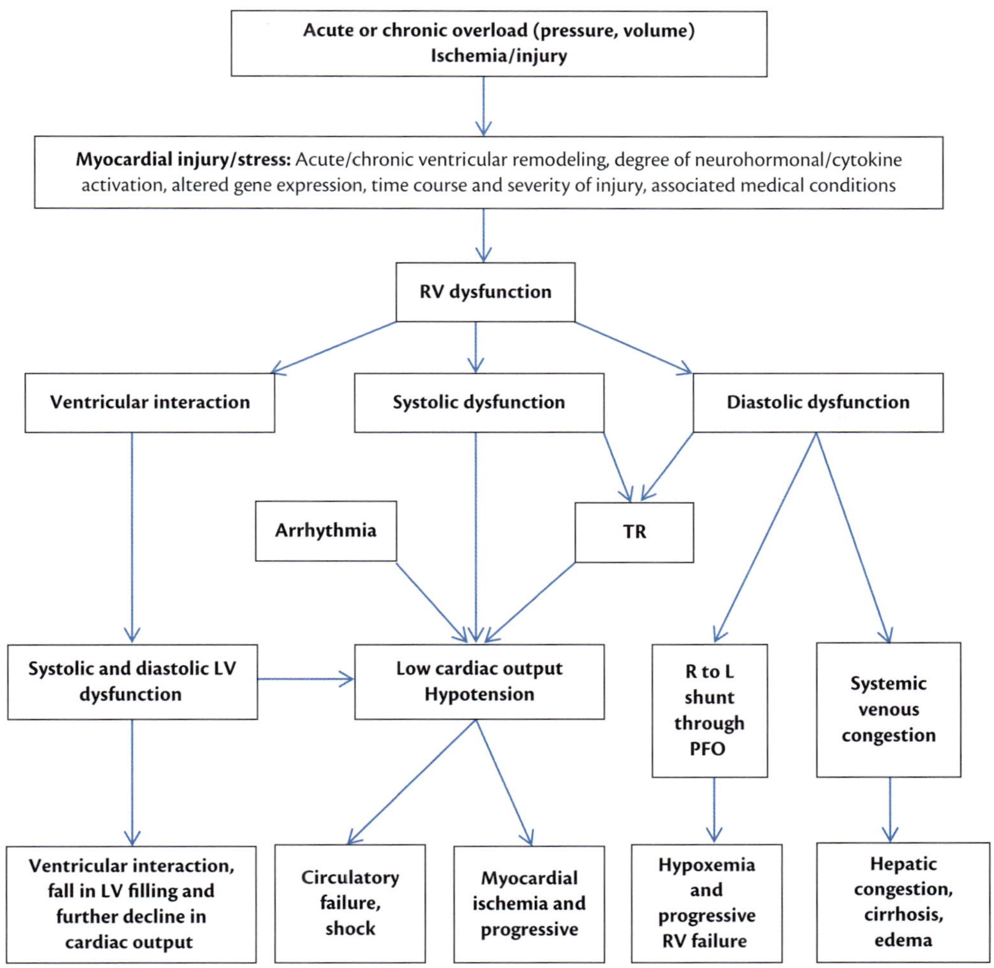

Fig. 21.7 Pathophysiology of acute right ventricular failure.
Figure adapted from Haddad et al 2008.

Table 21.8 Echocardiographic features in acute right ventricular failure

Chamber size/ hypertrophy	Function	Pulmonary artery	Other
RV dilatation More concentric rather than normal crescentic RV morphology RV free wall hypertrophy Leftward septal shift with left ventricular deformation Reduction in left ventricular volume Right atrial enlargement RV dysfunction	RV hypokinesis (reduction in RV percent area change, tricuspid annular plane systolic excursion, tricuspid annular plane systolic velocity, myocardial performance index, longitudinal strain) Paradoxical septal motion Tricuspid regurgitation	Pulmonary artery dilation Elevated pulmonary artery pressure	Dilated inferior vena cava with lack of normal inspiratory collapse Pleural and/or pericardial effusion

Adapted from Piazza et al. 2005.

Target and management strategy for right ventricular contractile performance

In acute RV failure, the cardiac index therapeutic target should generally be 2.2 L $min^{-1}m^{-2}$ or greater. In instances of acute severe RV failure associated with (1) significant PAH where optimization of RV preload and afterload does not improve cardiac index or (2) primary RV myocardial dysfunction with or without PAH, inotropic therapy is often indicated to achieve this target cardiac index. Table 21.10 lists the effects of various inotropes used in RV failure.

In normotensive patients with RV failure and acute or chronic elevation of PAP and/or PVR, the PDE3 inhibitor and inodilator milrinone is generally the preferred agent, due to greater reductions in PAP and PVR achieved than with adrenergic agonist agents.[22,27,68] In patients with severe LV dysfunction, bolus milrinone reduces mean PAP by 12%, PVR by 31%, PCW by 16% and increases cardiac output by 42%.[69] In patients with severe LV dysfunction, bolus milrinone thus provides an assessment of the reversibility of pulmonary hypertension.[69] Compared to nitroprusside, milrinone increases cardiac output to a greater degree given a similar reduction in systemic vascular resistance.[70] Compared to dobutamine, milrinone reduces SVR to a greater degree for a given effect on dP/dt.[71] Milrinone can therefore result in substantial systemic vasodilation and hypotension which, when marked, may worsen RV perfusion.[68]

In hypotensive patients with acute or chronic elevation of PAP and/or PVR or in patients with primary RV dysfunction (e.g., acute RV myocardial infarction), the β-agonist dobutamine is generally preferred.[22,27] Dobutamine augments contractility with

Box 21.7 MRI findings in acute right ventricular failure

Chambers

- Increase in RV volume
- Decrease in RV ejection fraction
- More concentric rather than normal crescentic RV morphology
- RV free wall hypertrophy
- Paradoxical septal motion
- Leftward septal shift with left ventricular deformation
- Reduction in left ventricular volume

Tricuspid regurgitation

Vessels

- Pulmonary artery dilation
- Dilated inferior vena cava

Other

- Right atrial enlargement
- Pleural and/or pericardial effusion

Adapted from Piazza et al. 2005.

Box 21.8 Cardiac catheterization findings in acute right ventricular failure

Acute right ventricular myocardial infarction

- Elevation of RA pressure with increased a wave, sharp x descent, blunted y descent
- Elevation of RV diastolic pressure
- Equalization of RV and LV diastolic pressures with "dip and plateau" configuration
- Depressed RV systolic pressure
- Reduction in cardiac index

Predominant right ventricular pressure overload

- RV systolic and diastolic pressures increased
- Elevated pulmonary artery pressures
- Elevated pulmonary vascular resistance
- With advanced RV failure, equalization of diastolic pressures with steep a wave, rapid y descent, steep x descent and resulting "W" configuration
- Reduction in cardiac index

Predominant right ventricular volume overload

- RV diastolic pressures increased
- Elevated pulmonary artery pressures
- Variable degree of elevation of pulmonary vascular resistance depending on LV function
- Large systolic v wave due to tricuspid regurgitation
- Reduction in cardiac index

Box 21.9 Stepwise principles of managing acute and/or chronic severe right ventricular failure

1. Set hemodynamic targets:

   CVP <15 mmHg: little further RVSW recruitment, minimize VI
   PVR <3 Woods units: reduce RV afterload
   CI >2.2 L min^{-1} m^{-2}: ensure adequate organ perfusion
   MAP >60 and normal SVR: ensure adequate RV perfusion

2. Ensure adequate oxygenation and oxygen delivery:

   Arterial oxygen saturation >90%: blunt hypoxic pulmonary vasoconstriction, organ hypoxia
   Hemoglobin >10 g/dl: ensure adequate oxygen delivery

3. Minimize adverse RV preload and afterload hemodynamic effects of mechanical ventilation:

   Peak plateau airway pressures <30 cmH_2O
   Tidal volume 6–8 ml kg^{-1} min^{-1}
   Minimal PEEP to ensure adequate oxygenation
   Minimize effects of permissive hypercarbia/acidosis on RV contractile function and PVR
   Avoid auto-PEEP

4. Maintain normal sinus rhythm to ensure adequate RV loading (particularly when RV pressures elevated)
5. Minimize effects of RV apical pacing on RV function
6. Ensure adequate RV perfusion

   RCA anatomy, adequate aortic root pressure and SVR

7. Minimize "mechanical" intrapulmonary influences on RV function and/or RV–PA coupling:

   Treat large pleural effusions
   Manage V/Q mismatch, intrapulmonary shunting, hypotentilation-induced hypoxia/hypercarbia
   Manage auto-PEEP in patients with advanced obstructive lung disease

8. Determine primary mechanism(s) responsible for elevation of PAH and degree of PAH reversibility:

   PAH due pulmonary vascular disease (precapillary PAH)
   PAH due to left heart disease (postcapillary PAH)
   Mixed PAH (both precapillary and postcapillary mechanisms)
   Reversible vs. fixed PAH

9. Evolve strategies for simultaneous management:

   RV preload
   RV afterload
   RV contractility

10. Recognize and minimize adverse ventricular interaction:

   RV volume overload with equalization of RV and LV pressures ("pseudo-restriction")
   RV pressure overload with leftward septa shifting and LV underfilling
   LV systolic or diastolic failure with elevation
   Dyssynchrony

11. Make serial assessment of hemodynamic goals and degree of ventricular interdependence

CI, cardiac index; CVP, central venous pressure; LV, left ventricle; MAP, mean arterial pressure; PA, pulmonary artery; PAH, pulmonary arterial hypertension; PEEP, positive end-expiratory pressure; PVR, pulmonary vascular resistance; RCA, right coronary artery; RV, right ventricle; RVSW, right ventricular stroke work; SVR, systemic vascular resistance; V/Q, ventilation/perfusion ratio.

lesser effects on both systemic and pulmonary resistance than milrinone.[22,27,68] In acute PAH, doses of dobutamine > 5 μg/kg/min fail to effect greater reductions in PAP.[32,72,73] The β-agonist inotropes norepinephrine and epinephrine increase cardiac output and systemic and pulmonary vascular resistance.[22] Given their effects on pulmonary vascular resistance, norepinephrine and epinephrine are typically reserved as second-line and/or "rescue" inotropes in patients who fail to respond to either milrinone or dobutamine. High-dose dopamine and neosynephrine are relatively contraindicated in patients with acute severe RV failure complicated by acute or chronic elevation of PAP and/or PVR due to the prominent pulmonary vasoconstriction accompanying their administration.[27] In animal studies of RV failure, levosimendan, a calcium-sensitizing inotropic agent, was superior to dobutamine in reducing PVR and increasing RV contractility.[74,75] When inotropic support fails, then RV mechanical support is indicated. Indications and options for RV mechanical support are discussed in detail in this chapter in the section on RV failure following cardiac surgery.

Serial assessment of the degree and influence of ventricular interaction

Interaction between the RV and LV plays an important role in determining the outcome of acute, severe RV failure and may evidence varying mechanisms and influence (1) at presentation, (2) following specific therapies or interventions, and (3) during evolution of a multisystem illness. Serial assessment of the mechanisms and influence of ventricular interaction is therefore an integral part of the overall management of acute, severe RV failure.

Treatment of underlying specific responsible etiologies

Treatment of the underlying specific etiologies responsible for acute, severe RV failure is discussed in detail in subsequent chapters that discuss treatment of pulmonary hypertension. However, specific management issues in ischemic syndromes as well with LVADs are detailed below.

Left ventricular assist device implantation

LVAD implantation should be considered to promote reduction of PVR in potential cardiac transplant recipients whose persistent elevated PVR despite pharmacologic interventions and CRT otherwise precludes transplantation.[24] In the observational studies to date, implantation of both pulsatile or nonpulsatile LVADs in potential transplant candidates can reduce mean PAP, transpulmonary gradient, and PVR by up to 50% within several months.[76,77,78]

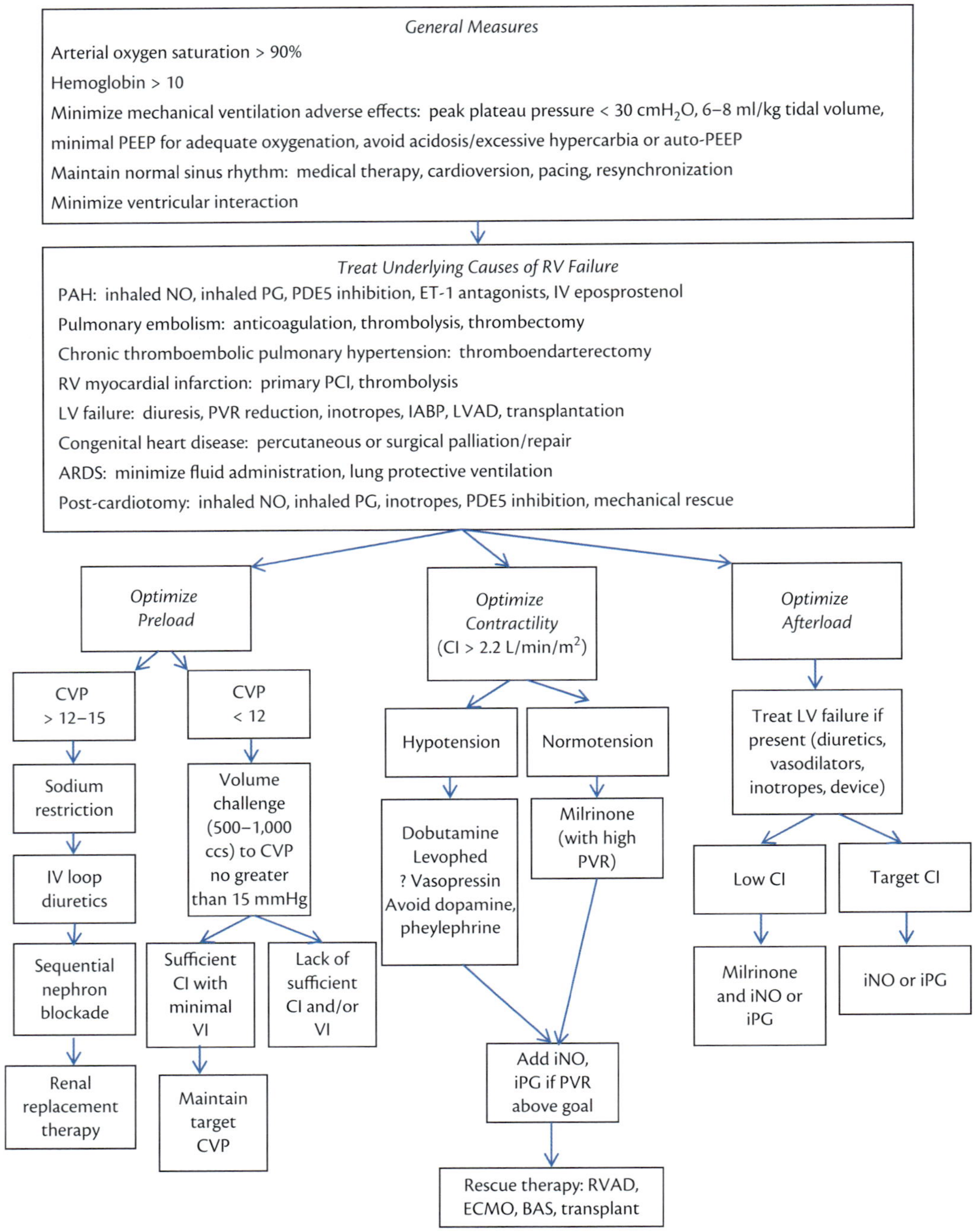

Fig. 21.8 Acute severe right ventricular failure: management algorithm.

In patients whose PVR does not decrease following LVAD implantation, adjunctive therapy with PDE5 inhibitor post-LVAD may reduce mPAP and PVR by up to 50%.[79]

Right ventricular failure in right ventricular myocardial infarction

Definition and incidence

RV free wall (RVFW) ischemia occurs in 40–50% of acute ST-segment elevation inferoposterior LV infarcts.[80,81] RV myocardial infarction (RVMI) is typically associated with transmural inferoposterior infarction resulting from proximal occlusion of a dominant RCA and resultant hypoperfusion of at least one large RV marginal branch.[82,83,84] RVMI is an independent predictor of worse outcome following an LV inferoposterior MI,[85,86] and RVMI resulting in cardiogenic shock has mortality similar to shock from LVMI.[81,87,88]

Effect of ischemia on right ventricular function

The degree of acute RVFW ischemia and the integrity of the RV free wall–interventricular septum interaction both determine the severity of hemodynamic sequelae of RVMI.[80] Significant hypoperfusion of a large portion of the RV free wall results in RV free wall dyskinesis, acute RV dilatation, reduced RV systolic performance, and attendant reductions in LV preload, cardiac output, and

Box 21.10 CARRESS trial: stepped pharmacologic therapy in acute decompensated heart failure

UO >5 L/day—reduce current diuretic regimen if desired
UO 3–5 L/day—continue current diuretic regimen
UO <3 L/day—see table

	Current dose		Suggested dose	
	Loop	**Thiazide**	**Loop (/day)**	**Thiazide**
A	≤80	+ or −	40 mg IV bolus + 5 mg/h	0
B	81–160	+ or −	80 mg IV bolus + 10 mg/h	5 mg metolazone QD
C	161–240	+ or −	80 mg IV bolus + 20 mg/h	5 mg metolazone BID
D	>240	+ or −	80 mg IV bolus + 30 mg/h	5 mg metolazone BID

At 24 h—Stepped pharmacologic care arm

- Persistent volume overload present:

  UO >5 L/day—reduce current diuretic regimen *if desired*
  UO 3–5 L/ day—continue current diuretic regimen
  UO <3 L/day—advance to next step on table

At 48 hrs—Stepped pharmacologic care arm

- Persistent volume overload present:

  UO >5 L/day—reduce current diuretic regimen *if desired*
  UO 3–5 L/day—continue current diuretic regimen
  UO <3 L/day—advance to next step on table

- Dopamine or dobutamine at 2 mg kg^{-1} h^{-1} if SBP <110 mmHg and EF <40% or RV systolic dysfunction. Nitroglycerin or nesiritide if SBP >120 (any EF) and severe symptoms.

At 72 h—Stepped pharmacologic care arm

- Persistent volume overload present:

  UO > 5 L/day—reduce current diuretic regimen *if desired*
  UO 3–5 L/day—continue current diuretic regimen
  UO <3 L/day—advance to next step on table

- Dopamine or dobutamine at 2 mg kg^{-1} h^{-1} if SBP <110 mmHg and EF <40% or RV systolic dysfunction. Nitroglycerin or nesiritide if SBP >120 (any EF) and severe symptoms
- Advanced cardiorenal therapy: hemodynamic guided IV therapy, LVAD, dialysis or UF cross-over

At 96 h—Stepped pharmacologic care arm

- Persistent volume overload present:

  UO >5 L/day—reduce current diuretic regimen *if desired*
  UO 3–5 L/day—continue current diuretic regimen
  UO < 3 L/day—advance to next step on table

- Dopamine or dobutamine at 2 mg kg^{-1} h^{-1} if SBP <110 mmHg and EF < 40% or RV systolic dysfunction. Nitroglycerin or nesiritide if SBP > 120 (any EF) and severe symptoms
- Advanced cardiorenal therapy: hemodynamic guided IV therapy, LVAD, dialysis or UF cross-over

EF, ejection fraction; LVAD, left ventricular assist device; RV, right ventricle; SBP, systolic blood pressure; UF, ultrafiltration; UO, urine output.

systemic blood pressure[89] in addition to reversed septal curvature and equalization of RV and LV filling pressures.[90] Diastolic RV filling pressures rise abruptly and steeply due to the decreased distensibility of the acutely ischemic RV.[91] Acute RV dilatation and rising RV diastolic pressure with a noncompliant pericardium may incur

Table 21.9 Pharmacokinetics of the loop diuretics used in acute right ventricular failure

Property	Furosemide	Bumetanide	Torsemide
Relative IV potency (mg)	40	1	20
Bioavailability (%)	10–100 (average, 50)	80–100	80–100
Oral to intravenous conversion	2:1	1:1	1:1
Initial outpatient total daily oral dose (mg)	20–40	0.5–1	5–10
Maintenance outpatient total daily oral dose (mg)	40–240	1–5	10–200
Maximum daily intravenous dose (mg)	400–600	10	200
Onset (min)			
Oral	30–60	30–60	30–60
Intravenous	5	2–3	10
Peak serum concentration after oral administration (h)	1	1–2	1
Affected by food	Yes	Yes	No
Metabolism	50% renal conjugation	50% hepatic	80% hepatic
Half-life (h)			
Normal	1.5–2	1	3–4
Renal dysfunction	2.8	1.6	4–5
Hepatic dysfunction	2.5	2.3	8
Heart failure	2.7	1.3	6
Average duration of effect (h)	6–8	4–6	6–8
Approximate cost for oral 30 day supply (community pharmacy), $	4	4	19–23

Table 21.10 Inotrope agents in acute right ventricular failure

Inotrope	CI	PVR	SVR	PVR/SVR	Comments
Milrinone	↑↑	↓↓	↓↓	↓	Preferred agent in (1) normotension, (2) acute or chronic elevation of PAP and/or PVR
Dobutamine	↑↑	↓	↓	↑/↓	Preferred agent in (1) hypotension or (2) primary RV dysfunction
Vasopressin	↑/↓	↓	↑↑	↓	Attractive hemodynamic profile, sparse data on efficacy and outcomes
Norepinephrine	↑	↑	↑↑	↑/↓	Second-line or rescue agent
Epinephrine	↑↑↑	↑	↑↑	↑/↓	Second-line or rescue agent
Dopamine	↑	↑	↑	↑/↓	Relatively contraindicated
Phenyleprine	↑	↑↑	↑	↑	Relatively contraindicated
Isoproterenol	↑↑	↑	↑	↑/↓	Second-line or rescue agent (rarely used)
Levosimendan	↑↑	↓	↑/↓	↓	Not as well studied as milrinone or beta-agonists

Green EM, Givertz MM. Management of acute right ventricular failure in the intensive care unit. Curr Heart Fail Rep 2012;9:228–35.

leftward diastolic shift of the interventricular septum, further compromising LV loading and compliance.[92] The aggregation of these effects results in the equalized RV and LV diastolic pressures and the characteristic "dip and plateau" pressure waveform obtained at cardiac catheterization in an acute RVMI.[91]

Despite the high mortality associated with RVMI complicated by shock, given (1) the relative resistance of the RV myocardium to infarction in both animal models and patients, likely due to the preservation of relatively viable RV myocardium, and (2) the spontaneous improvement in RV function over time with or without infarct-related artery patency,[83,93,94] RV infarction has been termed a relative misnomer by experienced investigators.[80] Factors conferring the relative resistance of RV compared to LV myocardium to infarction include lower oxygen demand (lower mass, preload, impedance, stroke work than LV), dual coronary supply including left system branches (particularly the anterior RVFW), a more abundant system of Thebesian veins, lower coronary resistance, and lower oxygen extraction at rest.[95,96] The management principles therefore revolve around rapid reperfusion, maintenance of AV interaction, and interventricular associations.

Arrhythmogenic right ventricular cardiomyopathy

Right ventricular arrthythmogenic cardiomyopathy (ARVC) is a clinically and genetically heterogeneous disorder of cardiac muscle with a prevalence of 1 in 2000 to 1 in 5000.[98,99,100,101,102,103] ARVC was formerly termed arrhythmogenic right ventricular dysplasia due to the prominent and frequent nature of RV involvement. More recent reports substantiating biventricular and/or predominant LV involvement in have occasioned introduction of the broader diagnostic term "arrhythmogenic cardiomyopathy" (AC).[98]

Etiology and pathogenesis

AC is primarily a disorder of cardiac desmosomes, symmetrical protein complexes which (1) anchor intermediate cytoskeleton filaments to the cell surface and (2) form gap junctions between adjacent cells via a middle section which spans adjacent cell membranes.[100] In addition to their structural functions, desmosomes play important roles in diverse biological processes, including development, cell polarity, intracellular signal transduction via nuclear cross-talk, and intracellular calcium handling.[98,99,100,101,103] AC results most commonly from autosomal dominant inheritance of a mutation in one of five key desmosome protein genes: palkoglobin (JUP), desmoplakin (DSP), plakophilin-2 (PKP2), demoglein-2 (DSG2), or desmocollin-2 (DSC2).[98] AC-like cardiomyopathies may also result from abnormalities in nondesmosomal genes, including ryanodine receptor 2 (RYR2), desmin (DES), titin (TTN), TGFβ3, and TMEM43, an adipogenic pathway gene.[100]

The main pathologic feature of AC is loss of RV or LV myocardium with replacement by fibrofatty tissue.[99] Fibrofatty replacement is progressive and may results in ventricular wall thinning and/or aneurysm formation. The "defective desmosome" hypothesis of AC posits that genetically determined disruption and/or dysfunction of the desmosome promotes myocyte detachment at the intercalated disc under mechanical stress.[99] Periodic bursts ("hot phases") of myocyte detachment and degeneration with associated myocarditis-like inflammation and eventual fibrofatty replacement are felt to underlie disease progression.[98,99] Progressive (1) gap junction remodeling and (2) electromechanical myocyte uncoupling sets the stage for conduction delay, reentry, and progressive electrical instability.[99]

Clinical presentation and features

Patients with AC typically present between the second and fourth decades of life with asymptomatic or symptomatic RV-origin (LBBB pattern) ventricular arrhythmias.[103] Patients with ARVC most often present with palpitations or presyncope.[101] Arrhythmias are typically worse during or just after exercise, and AC accounts for 10% of all sudden deaths in individuals under the age of 35 years.[103] Patients may present with ECG ε waves, RBBB, late potentials, and reentrant ventricular tachycardia (VT);[102] however, AC may also present with incidental RV dilation or dysfunction, predominant RV failure, predominant LV failure, or biventricular HF indistinguishable from other etiologies, and clinical features vary with age, disease stage, and disease severity.[7] LV involvement is present in at least 50% of cases.[102] In early stages, structural changes may be absent or subtle and confined to localized regions of the RV, typically the inflow tract, outflow tract or RV apex, the "triangle of dysplasia".[7] Later progression is the rule, with more diffuse RV and LV involvement, particularly of the LV posterior lateral wall.[7] In late stages, biventricular cardiomyopathy and HF may evolve.[7]

Complications of AC include cardiac arrest from VT/VF and progressive RV, LV, or biventricular HF.[98,99,100] AC accounts for 10–15% of all sudden deaths under age 35.[103] Young age, prior cardiac arrest, rapid VT, different morphologies, syncope, severe RV failure, and biventricular involvement all portend higher risk of sudden death and worse outcome.[99]

Clinical diagnosis

Given the nonspecific clinical features of AC, an international task force proposed initial diagnostic guidelines in 1994 and subsequently revised them in 2010.[7] The 2010 guideline revision aimed to improve diagnostic sensitivity for the detection of early and familial disease. The diagnostic guidelines, which include structural, histological, ECG, arrhythmic, and familial features divided into major and minor criteria, are shown in Box 21.11. In the 2010 revised guidelines, a diagnosis of definite AC requires either (1) two major or (2) one major and two minor criteria or (3) four minor criteria from different categories. A diagnosis of borderline AC requires either (1) one major and one minor or (2) three minor criteria from different categories. A diagnosis of possible AC requires (1) one major or (2) two minor criteria from different categories.

Management

ICD implantation

The management of AC focuses mostly on the prevention of sudden cardiac death.[98,99,101,102,103] ICD implantation confers the greatest reduction in risk of sudden death in patients with AC. The current 2008 ACC/AHA/HRS guidelines recommend ICD implantation for secondary prevention of sudden cardiac arrest in AC.[104] The guidelines highlight the lack of consensus regarding the role of ICD implantation in the primary prevention of sudden cardiac death in AC, pointing out (1) lack of established predictive markers, risk-stratification algorithms and clinical trial data, (2) conflicting reports of the prognostic valve of inducible VT at programmed stimulation, and (3) limited prognostic role of genotype.[104] The guidelines state that

> . . . Some authorities have proposed that an ICD should be implanted in patients with ARVD/C and an increased risk for SCD based on the presence of a previous cardiac arrest, syncope due to VT, evidence of extensive RV disease, LV involvement, or presentation with polymorphic CT and RCA aneurysm . . . individualized decisions for primary prevention of SCD must be based on experience, judgment, and the available data. In considering this decision, the clinician should be mindful that in patient with ARVD/C/the ICD has proved safe and reliable in sensing and terminating sustained ventricular arrhythmias. Sudden death is rare in the available clinical series, whereas appropriate ICD shocks are common.[104]

Based upon prior observational studies and the expanding role of prophylactic ICD implantation, in many centers patients who fulfill Task Force criteria for a definite diagnosis of AC typically undergo ICD implantation for primary prevention.[101,105,106,107,108,109] Some experts, however, do not recommend prophylactic ICD implantation in asymptomatic patients with no or minimal manifestations of the disease or in healthy gene carriers.[102,109] Many patients with syncope/presyncope and left bundle branch block (LBBB) NSVT or VT present with Task Force borderline or possible AC.[101] In such

Box 21.11 2010 Task Force criteria for diagnosis of arrhythmogenic right ventricular cardiomyopathy

Global or regional dysfunction and structural alterations

Major criteria

- By 2D echo: Regional RV akinesis, dyskinesis, aneurysm and one of the following (end-diastole):
  1. PLAX RVOT ≥32 mm
  2. PSAX ≥36 mm
  3. fractional area change ≤33%
- By MRI: Regional RV akinesis, dyskinesis, or dyssynchronous RV contraction and one of the following:
  1. ratio of RV end-diastolic volume to BSA ≥110 ml/m^2 (male) or ≥ 100 ml/m^2 (female)
  2. RV ejection fraction ≤40%
- By RV angiography: Regional RV akinesis, dyskinesis, aneurysm

Minor criteria

- By 2D echo: Regional RV akinesis or dyskinesis, aneurysm, and one of the following (end-diastole):
  1. PLAX RVOT ≥29 and <32 mm
  2. PSAX ≥32 to <36 mm
  3. fractional are change >33% to <40%
- By MRI: Regional RV akinesis, dyskinesis or dyssynchronous RV contraction and 1 of the following:
  1. ratio of RV end-diastolic volume to BSA ≥100 to <110 ml/m^2 (male) or ≥90 to <100 ml/m^2 (female)
  2. RV ejection fraction 40% to ≤45%

Tissue characterization of wall

Major criterion

- Residual myocytes <60% by morphometric analysis (or <50% if estimated), with fibrous replacement of the RV free wall myocardium in ≥1 sample, with or without fatty replacement of tissue on endomyocardial biopsy

Minor criterion

- Residual myocytes 60–75% by morphometric analysis (or 50–65% if estimated), with fibrous replacement of the RV free wall myocardium in ≥1 sample, with or without fatty replacement of tissue on endomyocardial biopsy

Repolarization abnormalities

Major criterion

- Inverted T waves in right precordial leads (V1, V2, V3) or beyond in individuals >14 years of age (in the absence of complete RBBB QRS ≥ 120 ms)

Minor criteria

- Inverted R waves in leads V1 and V2 in individuals >14 years of age (in the absence of complete RBBB) or in V4, V5, or V6

- Inverted T waves in leads V1, V2, V3, and V4 in individuals > 14 years of age in the presence of complete RBBB

Depolarization/conduction abnormalities

Major criterion

- Epsilon wave (reproducible low-amplitude signals between end of QRS complex to onset of the T-wave) in the right precordial leads (V1 to V3)

Minor criteria

- Late potentials by SAECG in ≥ 1 of 3 parameters in the absence of a QRS duration of ≥ 110 ms on the standard ECG
- Filtered QRS duration (fQRS) ≥ 144 ms
- Duration of terminal QRS < 40 μV (low-amplitude signal duration) ≥ 38 ms
- Root-mean-square voltage of terminal 40 ms ≤ 20 μV
- Terminal activation duration of QRS ≥ 55 ms measured from the nadir of the S wave to the end of the QRS, including R', in V1, V2 or V3, in the absence of complete RBBB

Arrhythmias

Major criterion

- Nonsustained or sustained ventricular tachycardia of LBBB morphology with superior axis (negative or indeterminate QRS axis in leads II, III, and aVF and positive in lead aVL)

Minor criteria

- Nonsustained or sustained ventricular tachycardia of RV outflow configuration, LBBB morphology with inferior axis (positive QRS in leads II, III, and aVF and negative in lead aVL) or of unknown axis
- >500 ventricular extrasystoles per 24 hours (Holter)

Family history

Major criteria

- ARVC/D confirmed in a first-degree relative who meets current Task Force criteria
- ARVC/D confirmed pathologically at autopsy or surgery in a first-degree relative
- Identification of a pathogenic mutation categorized as associated or probably associated with ARVC/D in the patient under evaluation

Minor criteria

- History of ARVC/D in a first-degree relative in whom it is not possible or practical to determine whether the family member meets current Task Force criteria
- Premature sudden death (<35 years of age) due to suspected ARVC/D in a first-degree relative
- ARVC/D confirmed pathologically or by current Task Force criteria in second-degree relative

ARVC/D, arrhythmogenic right ventricular cardiomyopathy/dysplasia; BSA, body surface area; LBBB, left bundle branch block; PLAX, parasternal long-axis view; PSAX, parasternal short-axis view; RBBB, right bundle branch block; RV, right ventricle; RVOT, right ventricular outflow tract; SAECG, signal-averaged electrocardiography.

Marcus FI, McKenna WJ, Sherrill D, et al. Diagnosis of arrhythmogenic right ventricular cardiomyopathy/dysplasia: proposed modification of the task force criteria. Circulation 2010;121:1533–41.

patients the practice of ICD implantation is evolving in the context of Task Force criteria, results of endomyocardial biopsy, and detailed electrophysiological evaluation to exclude other cardiomyopathies and/or RVOT tachycardias.[101]

Medical management

Affected individuals should be counseled to avoid strenuous physical exercise and competitive athletics, although most sudden deaths occur during normal activities.[98,101] Symptomatic arrhythmias in patients with ICDs may be treated with adjunctive sotalol (first line) or amiodarone (second line).[98,101] The role of β-adrenergic antagonists and angiotensin converting enzyme (ACE) inhibitors in reducing ventricular arrhythmias and/or attenuating adverse ventricular remodeling is not established in AC, but it is reasonable to treat with such agents in patients with advanced remodeling and/or clinical HF.[101] Catheter ablation of fibrofatty scar is evolving in the earlier management of VT.[98] Heart transplantation is reserved for patients with either refractory ventricular arrhythmias or patients with endstage RV, LV, or biventricular HF.[98]

Right ventricular failure in adult congenital heart disease

RV failure occurs frequently in adult congenital heart disease (ACHD) and poses particular challenges in diagnosis and management.[110,111,112,113,114,115,116] The complexities of ACHD anatomic features, prior surgical and catheter-based interventions, ventricular function assessment, functional capacity and exercise performance assessment, and arrhythmia diagnosis and management are all best addressed in specialized ACHD referral centers.[115,116,117,118,119,120,121] However, HF/transplant cardiologists and surgeons will increasingly comanage such patients with ACHD specialists, given the palliative nature of many ACHD surgical and catheter-based interventions.

This brief discussion focuses on the most common RV management issues in ACHD.[110,111] Detailed guidelines for ACHD management have been published by the ACC/AHA, European Society of Cardiology, and Canadian Cardiovascular Society.[115,116,117,118,119,120]

Pressure-overloaded adult right ventricle

Pulmonary stenosis

Pulmonary stenosis (PS) accounts for 80–90% of all RVOT obstructive lesions in ACHD. PS most commonly results from a classically "domed" stenotic pulmonary valve (80–90%), a more dysplastic valve (10–20%), or much less commonly from subvalvular or supravalvular stenoses.[110] A dynamic "secondary" stenosis due to RVOT hypertrophy may evolve in PS.[110] In the absence of additional volume overload and preservation of sinus rhythm, the pressure-overloaded RV may be compensated until the fourth or fifth decade of life, and hence the diagnosis of PS is not uncommonly made in adult life. Progressive RV dilation in patients with uncorrected PS suggests an associated lesion, such as an atrial septal defect (ASD) or pulmonary regurgitation (PR).[120] When RV pressure exceeds 50% systemic pressure, symptoms of dyspnea, fatigue chest pain, and exertional dizziness typically supervene. The treatment of choice for PS is percutaneous balloon valvotomy, indicated when peak instantaneous PV gradient is greater than 60 mmHg or mean gradient greater than 40 mmHg even in the absence of symptoms.[120]

An important long-term management issue is the evolution of significant PR following surgical or percutaneous valvotomy or due to bioprosthetic pulmonary valve degeneration.[120] PR may precipitate RV dilatation, dysfunction, and failure decades after the initial surgery. The ACC/AHA guidelines recommend PV replacement prior to the evolution of severe RV enlargement, any more than mild RV dysfunction, deterioration in exercise capacity, or the onset of atrial or ventricular arrhythmias.[120]

Double-chambered right ventricle

In the double-chambered RV, anomalous muscle bundles partition the RV into a higher-pressure proximal chamber and lower-pressure distal chamber.[111] The morphologic features are quite diverse, and degree of RVOT obstruction progresses over time.[120] It may be associated with valvular PS, tetralogy of Fallot, ventricular septal defect, or double-outlet RV. Reparative surgery is recommended for patients with peak midventricular gradient greater than 60 mmHg or mean gradient greater than 40 mmHg, regardless of symptoms.[120]

Volume-overloaded adult right ventricle

Atrial septal defect

An ASD may occur in the fossa ovalis (secundum ASD, 75%), near the crux of the heart (primum ASD, 15–20% and seen primarily in trisomy 21), sinus venosus (sinus venosus ASD, 5–10%), or coronary sinus septum (1%).[120,122] Additional malformations occur in 30% of patients. ASDs are common and may present at any age.[122] Chronic left-to-right shunting through a sizeable ASD (as a rule, an ASD ≥10 mm in diameter) results in RV volume overload, increased pulmonary blood flow, RV failure arrhythmias, and increased mortality.[122,123,124] The size of the shunt depends on RV/LV compliance, ASD size, and left atrial (LA)/RA pressure.[115,122] Adult patients may occasionally present with RV failure, typically with significant tricuspid valve (TV) annular dilatation and TR and PAH of varying severity due to long-standing pulmonary overcirculation from left-to-right shunting.[122] Small defects (<10 mm) may remain asymptomatic until the fourth or fifth decade of life until the decrease in LV compliance due to age, hypertension, coronary or valvular disease increases left-to-right shunting.[120] Small shunts without RV dilatation or PAH are typically asymptomatic and require no medical therapy.[120]

The ACC/AHA guidelines recommend that ASDs large enough to cause PAH should be closed given (1) pulmonary vascular reactivity and (2) net left-to-right shunting.[120] The ACC/AHA guidelines also recommend ASD closure for RA and RV enlargement with or without symptoms. Small ASDs (<5 mm) without evidence of RV volume overload do not require closure in the absence of paradoxical embolism. The European guidelines recommend consideration of ASD closure in in patients with PVR at least 5 Wood units but less than two-thirds SVR, or PAP less than two-thirds systemic pressure and evidence of net left-to-right shunting with Qp:Qs greater than 1.5.[115] In an older series, surgical repair was associated with 74% 30-year survival.[125] In the current era, device percutaneous closure has become the treatment of choice for secundum ASDs except in patients with stretched ASDs larger than 36 mm, inadequate atrial rims, or ASD proximity to AV valves.[122] Following ASD closure, reduction in RA and RV volume is observed within 24 hours and RV reverse remodeling continues for up to a year.[122,126,127,128] ASD closure is associated with a reduced prevalence of atrial arrhythmias.[129]

Ventricular septal defect

Ventricular septal defect (VSD) is the commonest congenital heart lesion at birth (30–40%).[130] VSDs are typically categorized by location: (1) perimembranous (80%), (2) muscular/trabecular (15–20%), (3) outlet/supracristal (5%) and (4) inlet/AV canal (Down syndrome).[120] Multiple defects may occur and spontaneous closure is most common with muscular/trabecular and perimembranous VSDs.[130] The magnitude and direction of shunting is a function of PVR, VSD size, LV/RV systolic and diastolic function, and presence of RVOT obstruction. Small defects associated with small shunts (typically <25% of the aortic annulus) result in neither LV volume overload or PAH; moderate defects (25–75% of the aortic annulus) typically result in mild of moderate LV overload and mild to moderate PAH; and large defects (>75% of the aortic annulus) are most likely associated with LV volume overload and PAH. Unrepaired VSDs may result in several problems in adult life, including LV volume overload and LV failure, double-chambered RV, PAH with resultant RV dilation and RV failure. In the ACC/AHA and European guidelines, VSD closure is indicated with (1) Qp:Qs 2.0 or more, with clinical evidence of LV volume overload; (2) net left-to-right shunting (Qp:Qs >1.5) and PAP or PVR and less than two-thirds systemic values; and (3) net left-to-right shunting at Qp:Qs >1.5 with LV systolic of diastolic failure. Unrepaired nonrestrictive VSDs may result in Eisenmenger syndrome and RV failure, as discussed below.

Tetralogy of Fallot

The tetralogy of Fallot (TOF) consists of (1) subpulmonary infundibular stenosis and RVOT obstruction, (2) VSD, (3) an aorta which overrides the VSD, and (4) RV hypertrophy.[120,131,132,133] TOF exhibits considerable morphologic and functional heterogeneity and associated anomalies include PA hypoplasia and/or stenosis of both the PA trunk and branches, ASD, AVSD, right aortic arch, and LAD arising from right coronary cusp.

Unrepaired TOF has a poor prognosis, with more than 95% mortality before age 40. Adult patients may be treated with a palliative shunting procedure in childhood to augment pulmonary blood flow (Blalock–Taussig, Waterston, Potts shunts) prior to primary repair and occasional adults with TOF continue to present after palliative shunting alone. Primary TOF repair between 6 and 18 months of age is routine at present with a 35-year survival of 85%. Primary repair consists of (1) VSD closure and (2) relief of RVOT obstruction by infundibular resection and, when indicated, RVOT augmentation by a transannular patch or extracardiac conduit. PV valvotomy or replacement may be required if the PV is abnormal, and repair with a RVOT transannular patch results in PR of varying severity.

Key postoperative management issues in the adult with repaired TOF include (1) RV volume overload resulting in RV dilatation and dysfunction from residual (and frequently progressive) PR with or without TR from PR-induced RV dilation, (2) RV pressure overload from residual RVOT obstruction with or without branch pulmonary artery stenosis, (3) arrhythmias (both supraventricular and ventricular), and (4) risk stratification for sudden cardiac death. LV dysfunction may result from prolonged cyanosis before repair, prolonged cardiopulmonary bypass, and/or poor myocardial preservation, LAD trauma at the time of surgery (since it crosses to RVOT when arising anomalously from the right coronary cusp) or secondary to severe RV dysfunction and is an independent risk factor for increased mortality.[134]

Given the incidence of PR-induced RV dysfunction in particular following TOF repair, current guidelines recommend that patients are followed annually at centers with expertise in ACHD. CMR has evolved as the imaging modality of choice in patients with repaired TOF for serial assessment of RV function and PR.[135,136] Essential components of CMR in repaired TOF include assessments of (1) quantitative RV and LV volume, mass, stroke volume, and ejection fraction, (2) regional wall motion abnormalities, (3) RVOT and PA, and (4) quantification of PR and TR.[136]

The most common management issues in repaired adult TOF patients are (1) the appropriateness and timing of PV replacement in patients with severe PR and RV dysfunction and (2) risk stratification and prevention of sudden cardiac death.[120] According to the ACC/AHA guidelines, PV replacement is indicated for severe PR and symptoms or decreased exercise tolerance. PV replacement is deemed reasonable in adults with severe PR and any one of the following: (1) moderate to severe RV dysfunction, (2) moderate to severe RV enlargement, (3) symptomatic or sustained atrial or ventricular arrhythmias, or (4) moderate to severe TR. The ACC/AHA guidelines do not provide a specific quantitative threshold for RV dysfunction and/or RV enlargement for PV replacement. The European Society of Cardiology guidelines recommend PV replacement when the RV end-diastolic index exceeds 160 ml/m^2 and the Canadian Cardiovascular Society recommends PV replacement when the RV end-diastolic index exceeds 170 mL/m^2. Single-center studies have reported that even markedly dilated RVs favorably remodel following PVR, but that normalization of RV end-diastolic volume is most likely when preoperative end-diastolic volume is less than 150 ml/m^2.[137,138,139] In a single-center matched cohort study, late PV replacement for symptomatic PVR or RV dilatation did not reduce the incidence of VT or death.[140]

The risk of sudden cardiac death (SCD) following TOF repair is reported as 1–6% in series with variable durations of follow-up with an incidence of 2.5% per decade of follow-up. Sudden death accounts for about a third of all late deaths. To date, no single generally accepted risk-stratification scheme has emerged, although clear clinical risk factors for increased risk of SCD have been rather consistently demonstrated across multiple centers, including long-standing palliative shunts, older age at primary repair, abnormal RV hemodynamics (due to PR or residual obstruction), LV dysfunction, extensive ventricular fibrosis on CMR, high-grade ectopy on Holter monitoring, inducible VT at electrophysiologic study, and QRS duration greater than 180 ms.[141,142] For patients followed in experienced ACHD centers, the presence of such clinical risk factors prompts consideration of implantation of a primary prevention ICD, although management is not yet standardized. Patients with unexplained syncope should undergo hemodynamic and electrophysiologic evaluation and an ICD should be considered in the absence of a defined or reversible cause. ICDs should be implanted in patients for secondary prevention following documented sustained VT or cardiac arrest.

Ebstein anomaly

Ebstein anomaly, a complex and heterogenous malformation with variable severity which may first present in adult life with RV dysfunction and/or failure, is rare and accounts for less than 1% of all congenital heart disease.[143,144] Ebstein anomaly results from failure of delamination of tricuspid valve tissue and is characterized by (1) adherence of the septal and posterior TV leaflets directly to RV myocardium; (2) over 8 mm/m^2 body surface area apical displacement of the TV septal leaflet relative to the mitral annular plane; (3) dilation of an "atrialized" portion of the RV; (4) redundancy, fenestration and tethering of the anterior RV leaflet; and (5) dilatation of the right AV junction ("true" TV annulus).[143] Two-thirds of hearts show RV dilatation, which may involve both the atrialized RV and the RV apex and RV outflow tract. A greater echocardiographic ratio of combined RA plus atrialized RV area to functional RV and LV area is incorporated into a severity grading score which predicts prognosis.[143,145] Associated anomalies are common, and include an ASD (80–94%), bicuspid or atretic aortic valve, pulmonary artery atresia or hypoplasia, RVOT obstruction, subaortic stenosis, coarctation, pulmonary stenosis, VSD, LV dilatation, and LV noncompaction. An accessory conduction pathway is present in 6–36% of cases.

Hemodynamic severity is dependent on the extent of TV leaflet distortion and severity of TR, RV size and function, extent of intra-atrial shunting (when present), PA or PV anomalies, and LV structure and function. Typical symptoms at adult presentation may include exertional intolerance, progressive exertional cyanosis, fatigue, right-sided HF, arrhythimas (atrial and ventricular), and sudden death or paradoxical embolism.[143]

Progressive RV enlargement, RV dysfunction, progressive TR, and progressive cyanosis should prompt consideration of surgical repair. The repair is often complex, but typically consists of TV repair or replacement, ASD closure, plication of the atrialized RV, and directed antiarrhytmia procedures.[143] ACC/AHA guidelines currently recommend tricuspid repair or replacement with concomitant ASD closure for Ebstein anomaly complicated by (1) symptoms, (2) deteriorating exercise capacity, (3) cyanosis (oxygen saturation <90%), (4) paradoxical embolism, (5) progressive cardiomegaly on chest radiograph, (6) progressive RV dilatation or reduction in RV systolic function, and (7) in patients with severe TR after repair with progressive RV dilatation, RV systolic dysfunction, and appearance/progression of atrial and/or ventricular arrhythmias. Early surgical mortality is 5–10% and 10–15-year survival is 80–92% for both (1) primary repair/replacement and (2) following reoperation for recurrent TR or TV bioprosthetic deterioration. In patients in whom repair is not feasible, either cavopulmonary modified Fontan connection or transplantation may be warranted.

Systemic right ventricular anomalies

d-Transposition of the great arteries (dTGA)

dTGA consists of AV concordance with ventriculoarterial discordance, hence the pulmonary artery arises from the LV which serves as the subpulmonary ventricle and the aorta arises from the RV which serves as the systemic ventricle.[146] Since the systemic and pulmonary circulations in dTGA run in parallel, a communication at the atrial (AS), ventricular (VSD), or great vessel (PDA) level must be present for dTGA to be compatible with life. In dTGA, the morphologic TV functions as the systemic AV valve and frequently becomes regurgitant over time.

Virtually all adults with dTGA will have undergone one or more surgical procedures in childhood. Since the mid-1980s, the surgical therapy of choice has been the arterial switch operation (ASO or Jatene operation), typically performed in the first month of life.[147] ASO involves (1) transection of the aorta and main PA with anastomosis of the aorta to the LV and the main PA to the RV and (2) reimplantation of the coronary arteries. Survival following ASO is 90% at 10 years and children undergoing ASO experience improved exercise capacity compared to children undergoing other dTGA surgical approaches. Adult ASO survivors may experience coronary insufficiency and myocardial ischemia, great vessel anastomosis stenosis (aortic or pulmonary stenosis), aortic or PR, and ventricular dysfunction. ACC/AHA guidelines recommend surgery for ASO patients with (1) RVOT obstruction greater than 50 mmHg peak to peak or RV:LV pressure ratio greater than 0.7, (2) coronary arterial abnormalities, (3) severe neoaortic valve regurgitation, and (4) neoaortic root dilatation greater than 55 mm.

Prior to the mid-1980s, adult dTGA patients during childhood typically underwent either (1) the atrial switch (Senning or Mustard) procedures or (2) the Rastelli procedure. In the atrial switch procedure, an atrial baffle of either autologous tissue (Senning) or synthetic material (Mustard) is created to baffle venous return to the contralateral AV valve and ventricle (i.e., deoxygenated caval return is baffled through the MV into the subpulmonary LV, oxygenated pulmonary venous return is baffled through the TV into the systemic RV). Late survival is 65% at 25 years. Atrial switch procedures are, however, associated with characteristic late problems, including (1) baffle leaks (25%) and/or obstruction, which depending on size and location may result in SVC or IVC obstruction or paradoxical embolism and require revision or closure, (2) subpulmonary stenosis due to LV compression by the enlarged systemic RV, (3) arrhythmias (supraventricular and ventricular) which prove particularly challenging in management, (4) systemic RV dilation, dysfunction and failure, and (5) progressive TR resulting from systemic RV dilation. Assessment and management of progressive systemic RV dilation dysfunction and failure in particular necessitate lifelong follow-up in experienced ACHD centers. ACC/AHA guidelines recommend surgery for atrial switch procedure patients with (1) moderate to severe systemic (morphologic tricuspid) AV valve regurgitation without significant ventricular dysfunction; (2) baffle leak with left-to-right shunt greater than 1.5:1, right-to-left shunt with arterial desaturation at rest or with exercise, symptoms, and progressive ventricular dilatation that is not amenable to device intervention; (3) SVC or IVC obstruction not amenable to device intervention; (4) pulmonary venous pathway obstruction not amenable to device intervention; and (5) symptomatic severe subpulmonary stenosis.

dTGA patients with a large subaortic VSD and PS may have undergone the Rastelli procedure in which (1) a surgically placed patch directs blood from the LV through the VSD to the aorta, (2) the pulmonary valve is oversewn and (3) a valved conduit establishes continuity between the RV and main PA.[146] With the Rastelli repair, the LV serves as the systemic ventricle. However, conduit degeneration and dysfunction is inevitable with the need for reoperation. Complications of the Rastelli repair include (1) frequent atrial and ventricular arrhythmias including sudden death, (2) RVOT and/or conduit obstruction with acute or chronic RV failure, and (3) RV or LV failure. ACC/AHA guidelines recommend surgery following Rastelli repair for (1) RVOT obstruction with peak to peak gradient greater than 50 mmHg or RV/LV pressure ratio greater than 0.7; (2) severe conduit regurgitation with symptoms or declining exercise tolerance, severe RV dysfunction, severe RV dilation, development/progressive of atrial or ventricular arrhythmias, and more than moderate TR; (3) residual VSD closure with Qp:Qs greater than 1.5, systolic PA pressure greater than 50 mmHg, increasing LV size from volume overload, decreasing RV function from pressure overload, RVOT obstruction or net left-to-right shunt greater than 1.5:1.

l-Transposition of the great arteries (lTGA)

lTGA or congenitally corrected transposition consists of AV discordance and ventriculoarterial discordance, hence the RV enters to morphologic LV which gives rise to the PA and the LA enters the morphologic RV which gives rise to the aorta.[147] In lTGA, venous return flows through the "right" atria and "right" great vessel but through the "wrong" ventricle, as the LV is the subpulmonary ventricle and the RV the systemic ventricle. Associated anomalies include VSD (70%, usually perimembranous), PS (40%, usually subvalvular), progressive systemic AV (morphologic tricuspid) valve dysfunction (90%, including commonly Ebstein-like displacement toward apex) and conduction system dysfunction (spontaneous complete heart block incidence 2%/year). Given the anatomic and hemodynamic heterogeneity, clinical presentation of lTGA is quite varied and depends on function of the systemic (morphologic RV) ventricle, systemic (morphologic tricuspid) valve function, and associated abnormalities. Patients with less complex forms of lTGA may present in adulthood, particularly due to systemic (morphologic tricuspid) valve regurgitation with advanced systemic (morphologic RV) ventricular dysfunction and/or clinical HF.

The major problem in adults with lTGA is progressive systemic (morphologic RV) failure.[148,149,150] Adults who may have undergone earlier "conventional" operations for repair of associated anomalies (e.g., VSD closure, PS repair) in complex lTGA still remain at high risk of systemic (morphologic RV) failure.[149] In a multicenter observational series of lTGA patients, one-third of adults without associated anomalies developed HF by age 45 and two-thirds of adults with associated defects and/or prior surgery developed HF by age 45.[149] Systemic (morphologic RV) failure is likely multifactorial in lTGA.[151] Risk factors for RV dysfunction and failure include increasing age, associated anomalies, arrhythmias, pacemaker implantation, and prior surgery including tricuspid repair or replacement. Degeneration and regurgitation of the systemic (morphologic tricuspid) valve, a nearly universal feature of lTGA, most likely contributes foremost to systemic (morphologic RV) dilatation, dysfunction, and failure.[152] Systemic ventricular dilatation or dysfunction in lTGA should always prompt consideration of progressive AV (morphologic TV) regurgitation. Coronary anatomy in lTGA is concordant and the systemic (morphologic RV) ventricle is typically supplied by only a single coronary artery (morphologic RCA).[153] Patients with lTGA may demonstrate myocardial perfusion defects and/or diminished coronary flow reserve and RV ischemia, infarction, or inadequate coronary flow reserve may each play pathophysiologic roles.[154,155,156] Finally, although survival into the seventh or eighth decade of life is possible with lTGA, in most patients the morphologic RV is likely inherently incapable of serving as the lifelong systemic ventricle.

Management of adult lTGA is focused on (1) systemic (morphologic RV) dysfunction and in particular the appropriateness and timing of systemic AV valve replacement, (2) coexisting anomalies, and (3) arrhythmia management. Medical therapy with ACE inhibitors and β-adrenergic antagonists has not been shown to prevent progressive systemic (morphologic RV) dysfunction and failure in lTGA. As noted, decline in (systemic morphologic RV) function should always prompt consideration of progressive systemic (morphologic tricuspid) valve regurgitation. Since lTGA adults have a high incidence of complete heart block necessitating permanent pacing, pacing from the subpulmonary LV apex may induce systemic RV dyssynchrony and progressive systemic RV dysfunction. In such instances, biventricular pacing (which may be technically challenging, given variation in coronary sinus anatomy in lTGA patients) should be considered.

Indications for surgical intervention of adult lTGA without associated unrepaired anomalies include onset of symptoms attributable to (1) severe systemic valve regurgitation or (2) systemic ventricular dysfunction. Systemic valve replacement should be performed before systemic ventricular ejection fraction declines to less than 45%.[157] Recommended surgical options in adult lTGA patients with associated unrepaired anomalies in which the subpulmonary LV is functioning at systemic pressure depends on the type and severity of unrepaired anomalies: (1) "complete" anatomic repair with a "double switch" operation (simultaneous atrial and arterial switch) or (2) Rastelli-like repair with an appropriately located nonrestrictive VSD. Indications for surgery in patients who have undergone prior operations include (1) repair of replacement of systemic AV valve when nonanatomic repair has been previously done and (2) conduit replacement and/or LVOT obstruction resection in patients with prior Rastelli-like repair.

Eisenmenger syndrome

The Eisenmenger syndrome results from chronic elevation of pulmonary pressure and flow from an unrestrictive left-to-right shunt, functional and structural alterations in the pulmonary vasculature with advanced pulmonary vascular remodeling, elevation of pulmonary vascular resistance, and reversal of shunt flow to right-to-left with resultant arterial hypoxemia and cyanosis.[158,159] Eisenmenger syndrome is most common with unrepaired post-tricuspid unrestrictive left-to-right shunts (truncus arteriosus, AV canal, transposition, large VSD, large PDA) and less frequently from pretricuspid nonrestrictive left-to-right shunt (large ASD).[160] The pulmonary vasculature evolves progressive endothelial dysfunction and histological changes similar to advanced idiopathic pulmonary hypertension, including plexiform lesions. RV volume overload from left-to-right shunt flow and RV pressure overload from severe elevation of PVR results in RV hypertrophy, dilatation, dysfunction, and inexorable failure.[161]

Frequent complications include supraventricular and ventricular arrhythmias, endocarditis, cerebral abscess, iron deficiency, and hyperviscosity from volume depletion in the setting of secondary erythocytosis.[158,159,160,161,162] Low functional class, history of arrhythmia, RV dysfunction, RVH on ECG, and elevated serum creatinine all are associated with increased mortality. Sudden death and HF are the most common causes of death. In a recent echocardiographic study, tricuspid annular plane systolic excursion (TAPSE) less than 15 mm, RV systolic:diastolic effective duration ratio 1.5 or greater, RA area 25 cm^2 or greater, and RA:LA area ratio 1.5 or greater were highly predictive of mortality in an echocardiographic predictive score.[161]

Clinical evaluation should include defect type, defect dimension, net shunt directionality, associated cardiac and extracardiac anomalies, and prior surgical or catheter-based interventions. Detailed review to identify all possible PAH triggers is required. Patients with Eisenmenger syndrome have the lowest exercise capacity among patients with ACHD, due to progressive right-to-left shunting, not necessarily limitation of total cardiac output. Precise documentation of the extent, severity, and potential reactivity of pulmonary hypertension and PVR is required. Patients with Eisenmenger's may demonstrate acute pulmonary vascular reactivity with provocative testing with inhaled nitric oxide or epoprostenol and such patients may have a more favorable prognosis.

Recent studies have established a role for pulmonary artery remodeling therapies in patients with Eisenmenger syndrome. The absence of pulmonary vascular reactivity should not, however, preclude therapy with such agents, due to their antiproliferative effects. Bosentan reduced PVR and improved 6 minute walk test performance in a small randomized trial.[163] In an open-label study, sildenafil reduced mean PAP and PVR, and improved 6 minute walk test performance.[164] Case reports and small uncontrolled studies of prostacyclin and prostacyclin analogs have reported similar benefits. Such therapies should be initiated only in centers with expertise in ACHD. Heart–lung transplantation is associated with better outcomes than lung transplantation with cardiac corrective surgery,[165] but transplantation for Eisenmenger syndrome overall is associated with higher perioperative mortality than transplantation for other heart diseases.

Fontan circulation

Increasing numbers of ACHD patients born with tricuspid atresia/single-ventricle congenital anomalies have had Fontan repairs when biventricular repair was not possible. In post-Fontan patients, there is not a subpulmonary ventricle.[166] In the Norwood procedure for hypoplastic left heart syndrome, the morphologic RV is used to support the systemic circulation with a Fontan-like diversion of systemic venous return directly into the pulmonary arterial circuit.[167] In such patients, the RV serving as the systemic ventricle may fail similar to the systemic (morphologic RV) in lTGA. In anomalies with an absent or severely hypoplastic RV or nonrepairable RVOT anatomy, the LV serves as the systemic ventricle with a similar diversion of systemic venous return directly into the pulmonary arterial circuit.

Fontan patients pose unique and complex management challenges due to the palliative nature of the Fontan circulation and the absence of right-sided hydraulic pump to augment pulmonary arterial flow and systemic ventricle loading. Fontan patients live with chronic, nonpulsatile systemic venous congestion to a variable degree due to reduced venous compliance, increased microvascular filtration pressures, increase venous tone, and altered splanchnic hemodynamics. Exercise capacity is reduced.[168] Although the patients lack a subpulmonary ventricle, they evolve complications analogous to chronic RV failure. A high percentage of Fontan patients evolve hepatic cirrhosis, which may preclude cardiac transplantation.[169,170] Patients may evolve protein-losing enteropathy, which has a high associated mortality. The lack of pulsatile flow raises PVR, maldistributes pulmonary blood flow, may induce subclinical thromboembolism, and contributes to systemic ventricular failure and systemic AV valvular regurgitation. Systemic ventricular function is largely determined by the preload limitation imposed by the Fontan circulation and/or failure of the systemic ventricle (morphologic RV). The "failed Fontan" evidences complex venous anatomy (Fontan repair itself, aortopulmonary and systemic venous collaterals), malnutrition due to protein-losing enteropathy, and systemic ventricular (morphologic RV) failure. Lifelong post-surgical vigilance is required to refer patients for transplantation before the evolution of cirrhosis.[171,172]

Right ventricular failure from tricuspid regurgitation

The appropriateness, type, and timing of surgery for TR in particular remain a complex management challenge—and frequent dilemma—for reflective clinical cardiologists and cardiac surgeons alike. This section reviews the epidemiology, anatomy, pathophysiology and management of primary and secondary TR. Various controversies are discussed.

Controversial topics

Tricuspid valve repair versus replacement

The ACC/AHA guidelines for surgical management of TR as listed in Box 21.12. Surgical management of TV disease must be individualized, based upon clinical status, etiology, and TV apparatus.[173,174] Depending on such factors, either TV replacement or repair is recommended for primary severe TR. TV repair is recommended for secondary severe TR with concurrent MV disease requiring MV surgery, with TV replacement reserved for secondary severe TR when the TV apparatus is not amenable to repair. In general, TV repair rather than replacement is preferred, with TV replacement clearly indicated when TV leaflets are diseased, abnormal, or destroyed in either primary or secondary TR.[174,175] Although overall survival with bioprosthetic and mechanical valves is similar, the ACC/AHA guidelines recommend bioprosthetic valves in general to reduce rate of thromboembolic complications.

Box 21.12 2008 ACC/AHA guidelines for surgical management of tricuspid regurgitation

Class I

1. Tricuspid valve repair is beneficial for severe TR in patients with MV disease requiring MV surgery
   (Level of evidence: B)

Class IIa

1. Tricuspid valve replacement or annuloplasty is reasonable for severe primary TR when symptomatic
   (Level of evidence: C)
2. Tricuspid valve replacement is reasonable for severe TR secondary to diseased/abnormal tricuspid valve leaflets not amenable to annuloplasty or repair
   (Level of evidence: C)

Class IIb

1. Tricuspid annuloplasty may be considered for less than severe TR in patients undergoing MV surgery when there is pulmonary hypertension or tricuspid annular dilatation

   (Level of evidence: C)

Class III

1. TV replacement or annuloplasty is not indicated in asymptomatic patients with TR whose pulmonary artery systolic pressure is less than 60 mmHg in the presence of a normal MV

   (Level of evidence: C)
2. TV replacement or annuloplasty is not indicated in patients with mild primary TR

   (Level of evidence: C)

MV, mitral valve; TR, tricuspid regurgitation; TV, tricuspid valve.

Adapted from Bonow RO, Carabello BA, Kanu C, et al. ACC/AHA 2006 guidelines for the management of patients with valvular heart disease. Circulation 2006;114:e84–231; Bonow RO, Carabello BA, Chatterjee K, et al. 2008 Focused update incorporated into the ACC/AHA 2006 guidelines for the management of patients with valvular heart disease, Circulation 2008;118:e523–661.

Tricuspid regurgitation associated with transtricuspid pacemaker or ICD leads

Patients with transtricuspid pacemaker and/or defibrillator leads may evolve significant lead-related TR and pose management challenges. Echocardiographic TR worsens by 1 or more grades in 24% of patients following implantation of transtricuspid leads and evolves to moderate to severe in 18%. Following successful TV repair, the presence of a transtricuspid lead doubles (to 42%) the incidence of severe TR at 5 years. Placement of an epicardial rather than transtricuspid leads at the time of TV surgery may reduce incidence of late repair failure.[175] Up to 10–15% of patients undergoing either TV repair or replacement may require postoperative permanent pacemakers due to heart block.

Tricuspid regurgitation associated with left ventricular assist devices

TR can worsen after LVAD implantation due to (1) increased venous return and preload to the RV resulting in RV volume overload,[176,177] and (2) distortion of RV geometry.[178] Severe TR should be addressed at the time of LVAD implant to improve RV function and remodeling. Compared to patients with grade 2$^+$ TR or more, patients with severe TR and gross preoperative RV dysfunction have consistently been identified to be at increased risks for prolonged inotropic support, need for RVADs, and mortality.[179] TR repair at the time of LVAD implantation has reduced the incidence of RV failure after implantation of the HeartMate II LVAD.[180,181,182,183,184] Table 21.11 lists the studies supporting concomitant surgical treatment of secondary TR at the time of LVAD implantation.

Percutaneous approaches in tricuspid regurgitation

Percutaneous treatment for TV disease is evolving. Over the past few years there has been considerable progress with the percutaneous approach to the aortic and mitral valves, but there is little data to support the same approach for the TV.[185]

Table 21.11 Additional contemporary peer-reviewed studies supporting the concomitant treatment of functional tricuspid regurgitation at the time of a left-sided surgery

	Year	Type of study	Patients (*n*)	Reported outcomes /main conclusions	Median follow-up (years)	Level of evidence
Benedetto et al. 2012	2012	Randomized controlled trial	44	≤2+ TR correction in pts with TV annular dilatation ≥40 mm reduces TR progression, increased RV function and functional outcome (IIb)	1	B
Van de Veire et al. 2011	2011	Retrospective	182	Echocardiographic outcomes warrants that concomitant TV annuloplasty during MVP should be considered in pts with TV annular dilatation and ≤ 2+ TR (IIb)	24	C
Navia et al. 2010	2010	Retrospective	2277	Patients with ≥ 2+ TR and rigid annuloplasty alone (standard or 3D) had the least increase of 3+/4+ TR following left-sided procedures	5	C
Bernal et al. 2010	2010	Retrospective	153	In patients with severe rheumatic mitral and tricuspid valve disease, the incidence of reoperation was increased in the absence of a TV prosthetic ring annuloplasty (IIB)	15.8	C
Chan et al. 2009	2009	Retrospective	624	TV repair is indicated to improve symptoms in pts with ≥ 2+ TR undergoing MVP (I) Increased TV annular dimensions alone in the absence of significant TR (≤ 1+ TR) should not dictate TV repair (IIb)	6.8	B C
Di Mauro et al. 2009	2009	Retrospective	165	Patients with untreated ≥ 2+ TR at the time of MVP had a lower survival compared to patients with ≤ 2+ TR (IIb)	7.2	C
Calafiore et al. 2009	2009	Retrospective	110	Triscuspid annuloplasty is mandatory in pts with≥ 2+ TR undergoing MVP (I)	5.7	C
Kwak et al. 2008	2008	Retrospective	615	The incidence of late TR was 26.9% in patients without TR undergoing MVP The presence of AF was the only independent predictor of development of late TR	11.6	C

AF, atrial fibrillation; BSA, body surface area; MVP, mitral valve procedure; PPM: permanent pacemaker; RV, right ventricle; TAD, tricuspid annulus diameter; TR, tricuspid regurgitation; TV, tricuspid valve.

Right ventricular failure and left ventricular assist devices

RV failure is a significant cause of increased morbidity and mortality following implantation of a LVAD. In the largest study to date, early RV failure after LVAD implantation was associated with a 20% reduction in 1-year survival, longer length of hospital stay, and decreased chance of cardiac transplantation.[179] Clinical trials and observational series to date have most often used two different definitions of early RV failure: (1) presence of any one of the following: postoperative inotropic support for more than 14 days, inhaled nitric oxide for more than 48 hours, need for RV mechanical support, and/or hospital discharge on an inotropic agent; and (2) presence of two or more of the following in the first 48 hours post-LVAD implantation: mean arterial pressure less than 55 mmHg, central venous pressure greater than 16 mmHg, mixed venous oxygen saturation less than 55%, cardiac index less than 2.0 L $min^{-1}m^{-2}$, inotropic support in excess of 20 units by the inotropic score.[186]

The reported incidence of RV failure following LVAD implantation has varied in clinical trials and observational series, with a reasonable summary estimate of 15–25% for a diverse array of devices.[186,187,188,189] In the HeartMate I XVE bridge to transplant (BTT) trial, 11% of patients required RVAD support.[190,191] In the HeartMate II BTT trial, 6% of patients required RVAD support and the overall incidence of RV failure was 20% (defined as RVAD support or inotropic support starting after 14 days).[192] In the HeartMate II destination (DT) trial, 4% of patients required RVAD support.[193] Thus, the incidence of acute RV failure requiring RV mechanical support following LVAD has fallen, due to improvement in patient selection and pre-, intra-, and postoperative management with a focus on optimization of RV function prior to LVAD.[194,195,196] In recent studies of continuous-flow LVADs, the incidence of acute RV failure overall has been 5–6%. Since RV function typically stabilizes or improves following LVAD placement, late RV failure accounts for a small proportion of late morbidity and mortality. The risk of long-term RV failure post-VAD appears to be 4–15%.[197–199] and 8% of DT patients die of RV failure.[200]

Right ventricular physiology following LVAD implantation

RV failure post-LVAD is dependent on the chronicity and severity of preoperative RV remodeling and dysfunction, perioperative complications (e.g., myocardial preservation), adequacy of early postoperative medical therapy targeting the RV (e.g., volume, reduction of pulmonary impedance, inotropic support), and course and success of RV accommodation to the acute and chronic alterations in RV load and contractile state that a LVAD necessarily imposes. Implantation of an LVAD results in three prominent and immediate effects on RV function: (1) decrease in RV impedance due to LV unloading, (2) increase in RV preload due to increased cardiac output, and (3) alteration of RVFW contraction due to bowing of the interventricular septum away from the RVFW into the decompressed LV with repositioning of the interventricular septum "hinge" required for normal RVFW contraction. Of these, the RVFW–interventricular septum interaction is the most subtle to diagnose and the most challenging to manage.

LVADs exert a beneficial acute and chronic effect on RV function by reducing LA pressure, LV diastolic pressure, PVR, and RV impedance. These RV unloading effects are potent, as even patients with apparent "fixed" secondary pulmonary hypertension typically have significant reduction in pulmonary hypertension post-LVAD.[201] This beneficial acute effect on RV impedance is partially offset by acute RV volume loading due to a post-LVAD increase in cardiac output compounded by perioperative intravenous fluids and blood transfusions. In the chronic phase, changes in RV volume load due to inadequate medical therapy and/or suboptimal LVAD settings may also increase RV preload, leading to TR annular dilation and worsening TR and RV adverse RV remodeling. Additionally, the acute rise in cardiac output and preload may unmask RV dysfunction masked by the pre-LVAD state of low cardiac output.

More important than these acute changes in preload and impedance likely is the RVFW–interventricular septal hinge necessary for normal RV contraction, since up to half of overall RV systolic function is derived from the interventricular septum. As the LV is unloaded immediately by the continuous-flow LVAD, the interventricular septum is "sucked" leftward, resulting in RV dilatation and less efficient traction applied to the RVFW by the septum. Initiation of LVAD support, therefore, should be done with low flows to avoid abrupt leftward septum shift. Adjustment of pump speed to achieve flows appropriate for the RV is more challenging with continuous-flow devices than with pulsatile devices. Ineffective LV unloading (high RV impedance), excessive LV unloading (leftward septal bowing and loss of RVFW–interventricular hinge) and/or persistent RV dysfunction all portend worse outcome post-LVAD.[202,203] By echocardiography, inefficient unloading of the LV marked by increased estimated LA pressure, persistent RV dysfunction, short mitral deceleration index, and leftward deviation of the septum are all associated with worse outcomes post-LVAD.

Clinical predictors of right ventricular failure

A variety of patient risk scores have been developed for VAD implantation,[204,205,206,207] including the INTERMACS profile,[208] Heart Failure Survival Score,[209] Seattle Heart Failure Model,[210] Lietz–Miller Destination Therapy Risk Score, and Columbia risk scores.[211] Given the high morbidity and mortality associated with acute and chronic RV, a variety of RV risk models have also been developed, mostly from single centers. Box 21.13 summarizes the most consistently identified risk factors from available studies.

Early experience with early pulsatile BTT LVADs reported that patients who required biventricular assist devices (BiVADs) developed RV failure post-VAD or were less likely to survive to discharge had (1) lower cardiac indices, worse renal function, urgent implants, and higher utilization of mechanical ventilation;[212] (2) preoperative circulatory support, female gender, nonischemic etiology;[213] and (3) preoperative RV failure.[214] Subsequent studies have confirmed these early findings. Fukamachi reported that post-LVAD RVAD was more common in younger patients, female patients, smaller patients, myocarditis patients with lower preoperative PAP and lower RVSWI.[215] Dang reported that following HeartMate XVE, RV failure was more common in females but that elevated intraoperative CVP was the only independent predictor of RV failure.[216] Santambrogio reported preoperative mechanical ventilation, worse renal and hepatic function, and lower mean PAP as risk factors.[217] Preoperative echocardiographic predictors of RV failure include an RV failure risk score derived from preoperative LV echocardiographic measures (smaller LV size, higher LVEF, higher of LA:LV diameter ratio),[218] higher short:long RV axis ratio, and grade III–IV TR,[219] larger TV annulus with or without TR, smaller LV or early systolic equalization of RV and RA pressure,[220] lower tricuspid annular systolic excursion,[221] and more severe RV dysfunction.[222]

More recent studies have derived RV failure or RV implantation risk scores from preoperative characteristics. Investigators at the University of Pennsylvania showed multivariate predictors of RVAD implantation included CI 2.2 L $min^{-1}m^{-2}$ or less, RVSWI 0.25 mmHg L^{-1}/m^{-2} or less, severe preoperative RV dysfunction, preoperative Cr 1.9 mg/dl or more, previous cardiac surgery, and systolic blood pressure 96 mmHg or less.[223] Investigators from the University of Michigan derived a RV failure risk point score containing vasopressor requirement (4 points), aspartate aminotransferase 80 IU or more (2 points), bilirubin 2.0 mg/dl or more (2.5 points), creatinine 2.3 mg/dl or more (3 points), with the highest risk of RV failure associated with score 5.5 or more with proportionally reduced survival.[224] In the 484 patients enrolled in the HeartMate II BTT trial, CVP:PCWP ratio greater than 0.63, preoperative ventilator support, and blood urea nitrogen greater than 39 mg/dl were independent predictors of RV failure post-VAD. In a smaller multi-institutional study of 175 consecutive LVAD recipients (42% of patients for destination therapy), preoperative need for intra-aortic balloon pump (IABP) support, increased PVR, and VAD implantation as destination therapy were independent factors included in a point risk score.[225]

Management of right ventricular failure post-VAD

Preoperative management and planning

Planning for the management of RV dysfunction and failure at the time of LVAD implantation should focus on prevention, including timing of implantation ideally prior to the evolution of RV risk factors.[226] Following detailed study of RV function and the risk of acute and long-term RV failure, two surgical considerations in particular are of vital importance: (1) indication for biventricular versus LV support alone and (2) approach to tricuspid regurgitation. Early planned institution of biventricular mechanical support results in improved hospital and 1-year survival compared to delayed (until it is an emergency) conversion of LVAD to a biventricular device (29% vs. 51%, $p < 0.05$).[227] The surgical approach should therefore be proactive and planned, rather than reactive. Since tricuspid annular dilation independent of TR grade and grade III–IV TR[228] both increase the risk of acute and long-term RV failure post-LVAD, a concomitant TV procedure to promote RV reverse remodeling should be considered and performed in appropriate candidates. Selected patients with severe proximal RCA disease should be considered for revascularization. Given the importance of the interventricular septum, thought should also be given to the adequacy of interventricular septal perfusion.

Currently, most patients undergo hemodynamic optimization prior to LVAD implantation. A pulmonary artery catheter is

Box 21.13 Major risk factors for right ventricular failure identified in studies to date

Patient characteristics

- Smaller body size
- Female gender
- Nonischemic etiology
- Prior cardiac surgery

Clinical course

- Severe clinical RV preoperative dysfunction
- Preoperative ventilator support
- Preoperative inotropic or vasopressor use
- Preoperative intra-aortic balloon use ("bridge to a bridge")

Hepatic and renal function

- Bilirubin ≥2.0 mg/dl
- AAT >80 IU/L
- BUN >39 mg/dl
- Creatinine ≥2.3 mg/dl

Hemodynamics

- RA or CVP >15 mmHg
- CVP/PCWP ratio >0.63
- Low PAP
- Low RVSWI (<300 mmHg × ml/m^2)
- PVR >4 Wood units
- Cardiac index ≤2.2 L/min/m^2
- Systolic blood pressure ≤96 mmHg

RV dimensions

- RVEDV >200 ml
- RVESV >177 ml

Echocardiography

- Severe RV dysfunction
- Moderate to severe TR
- RV short/long-axis ratio >0.6
- TAPSE <7.5 mm

AAT, aspartate aminotransferase; BUN, blood urea nitrogen; CVP, central venous pressure; PAP, pulmonary artery pressure; PCW, pulmonary capillary wedge pressure; PVR, pulmonary vascular resistance; RA, right atrium; RV, right ventricle; RVEDV, right ventricular end-diastolic volume; RVESV, right ventricular end-systolic volume; RVSWI, right ventricular stroke work index; TAPSE, tricuspid annular plane systolic excursion; TR, tricuspid regurgitation.

Data from Lund et al. 2010, Rich J 2012, Slaughter et al. 2010, Kaczorowski et al. 2011.

typically inserted 24–48 hours or so before the planned surgical date, to optimize cardiac output, reduce RA pressure to less than 15 mmHg, and address elevation of PVR if present, thereby reducing RV preload and impedance and minimizing hepatic congestion before surgery. In patients with moderate or greater risk of acute RV failure, an IABP may be implanted for several days before the surgical date, to determine RV contractile reserve and optimize cardiac output. Lack of increase in TAPSE and PA systolic pressure during dobutamine infusion predicts patients at higher risk of RV failure.[229] In patients in cardiogenic shock (INTERMACS I or II), temporary univentricular or biventricular support may be required.

Intraoperative phase

As discussed, before LVAD implantation, plans for the management of TR, RV ischemia due to RCA disease, and the need for temporary or long-term biventricular support should have been addressed and finalized. During the operation, echocardiography is standard for assessing the RV, LV, and the device itself. The CVP should be maintained below 16–18 mmHg to avoid RV volume overload but above 10 mmHg to avoid RV underfilling. Ventilation and oxygenation strategies should aim to avoid pulmonary vasoconstriction due to acidosis or hypoxia. Inotropic support with milrinone, epinephrine, isoproterenol, or vasopressin is indicated in cases associated with mild to moderate RV dysfunction. Inhaled nitric oxide and inhaled prostacyclin are both beneficial to reduce PVR with residual elevated PVR. Pacing should aim to maintain atrial transport at an appropriate rate, typically 90–100 beats per minute. Coagulation is typically reversed completely following bypass for 48 hours, to minimize acute bleeding risks.

Once the device is implanted, it is crucial to start the continuous-flow pump speed slowly to avoid septal suction, acute RV dilatation and dysfunction, and LV collapse. A ramped speed study by echocardiography is valuable to determine optimal pump speed based upon the cardiac index, RV and LV size, and septal position. Typically, speed is adjusted when possible to maintain a normal LV end-diastolic dimension and midline septal position, mean arterial blood pressure 70–80 mmHg, pulse pressure 10–20 mmHg, and echocardiographic opening of the aortic valve every third heart beat or so. Real-time echocardiography is routinely performed (in our center via an indwelling transesophageal probe while the patient is intubated) to assess RV and LV function and dimensions, septal position, and the pericardium in the early postoperative phase. A comprehensive echocardiographic RV examination should be possible in 80% of VAD echo studies.[230]

If significant suspected or observed RV failure is a complication, some instances of RV dysfunction may be improved by short-term intraoperative reinstitution of RV bypass with progressive attempts at weaning on more aggressive medical therapy. Leaving the sternum open for 24–36 hours may reduce CVP when elevated. In more refractory instances, temporary RVAD support should be considered before leaving the operating room if these interventions do not result in CI greater than 2.0 L min^{-1} m^{-2} and CVP less than 20 mmHg. Currently, the CentriMag or Thoratec LVAD (Thoratec Corp., Pleasanton, CA, USA) are devices commonly employed for RV support.

Postoperative: hospital phase

In clinical practice, achieving equilibrium between LV unloading and RV contraction is an iterative and empiric art, dependent on VAD settings, intravascular volume, RV size and function, degree of TR, pulmonary mechanics, pulmonary and systemic vascular impedance, LV size and function, and LV performance. Inotropic support is typically maintained post-LVAD for a variable period of 5–7 days, as volume re-equilibration occurs. Inotropic support is gradually weaned, pending clinical course. The persistence of grade III–IV TR and RV dysfunction is associated with a higher risk of RV failure post-LVAD and worsening of RV function is an indication for upgrading BTT patient status on the Eurotransplant waiting list.[228] Signs of RV failure post-LVAD include typical physical examination findings, echocardiographic progressive RV dilatation or TR, suction events (displayed continuous-flow pump speed falls significantly below fixed speed setting), and decreased pump flow.[183] Postoperative RV failure by echocardiography is marked by RV enlargement, significant TR, elevated RA pressure (interatrial septal bowing to left, tricuspid diastolic inflow, inferior vena cava dilatation, reversal of hepatic vein flow), a typically small LV chamber, or collapse of the LV with suction events.[231]

To prevent or treat mild to moderate post-LVAD RV failure, management strategies for (1) optimizing RV preload, (2) minimizing RV impedance, and (3) optimizing RV contractile state should be separately developed. CVP should be maintained below 15 mmHg, to minimize TV annulus and RV dilatation. Minimizing RV impedance in the more chronic phase with PDE5 inhibition is an attractive option in patients with an elevated PVR. Although even severe elevation in PVR declines in time in most instances post-VAD, sildenafil potentiates LVAD-associated reductions in PVR at 12–15 weeks. Optimization of RV contractility requires a multifaceted strategy, including (1) the duration and weaning course of RV inotropic support and (2) echocardiographically guided optimization of VAD speed and effects on LV size, interventricular septum position, and resultant effects on RV load, dimension, and function. Evidence-based medical therapies for LV systolic failure are routinely reintroduced as tolerated over time post-LVAD (angiotensin II inhibitors, β-receptor antagonists, aldosterone inhibitors), although the benefit of combined neurohormonal antagonism in treating "isolated" RV failure post-VAD is not well established.

Postoperative: intermediate and late phases

In the majority of patients with pulsatile LVADs, RV systolic function measured by RV fractional area change improves over time.[231,232] At 4–6 months following placement of continuous-flow LVADs, reported reductions in RA pressure, RVSWI, tricuspid annular motion, mean PAP and PVR, and TR all likely result from RV unloading and/or improvement in RV function. Since LVADs reduce mean systolic and diastolic PAP and PVR, RV impedance is significantly reduced.[233] Improvement in RV function post-LVAD is associated with improved renal function and reduced mortality.[234] Post-LVAD intermediate-term survival is adversely affected by preoperative TV annular dilatation and a higher RV failure risk score computed from echocardiographic LV measurements (smaller LV dimension, higher LVEF, higher LA:LV end-diastolic diameter ratio). Persistent postoperative RV dysfunction predicts lower exercise capacity measured by peak oxygen uptake[235] and increased mortality.

Right ventricular failure in chronic pulmonary thromboembolism

Epidemiology

Chronic thromboembolic pulmonary hypertension (CTPH) is one of the leading causes of severe pulmonary hypertension and typically presents with symptoms and signs of RV failure. CTPH has a reported incidence of 1–3.8% at 2–3 years following pulmonary embolism (PE).[236,237,238] CTPH is more frequent in young patients, patients with prior PE, patents with idiopathic PE and PE associated with larger perfusion defects. Evidence of prior PE is lacking in 42–63% of patients with CTPH, so CTPH is necessary to include in the differential diagnosis of "unexplained" PH and/or RV failure. Such patients may have inherited thrombotic disorders (anti-phospholipid antibody syndrome, lupus anticoagulant, factor V Leiden, increased factor VII levels), prior splenectomy, ventriculoatrial shunts, or chronic inflammatory disorders (inflammatory bowel disease, osteomylelitis, infected cardiac devices).

Pathophysiology

CPTH results from the chronic obstruction of pulmonary arterial branches following PE with incomplete resolution of thrombus and the evolution of pulmonary vascular remodeling including vessel fibrosis. The severity of CTPH is not explained by the degree of pulmonary vascular occlusion due to thromboembolism alone.[239] Distal and/or microvascular changes may result from (1) subsegmental elastic artery occlusion, (2) "classic" plexiform arteriopathy of patent small muscular arteries similar to other types of pulmonary hypertension, or (3) arteriopathy of arterioles distal to total or partially occluded vessels and (4) in-situ thrombosis which may occur in CTPH as it occurs in other forms of severe pulmonary hypertension. Both the proximal occlusions and secondary small-vessel ateriopathy contribute to elevation in PVR. Hemodynamic benefit from surgical thomboendarterectomy is greater with less distal arteriopathy. As in other cases of PH, differential genetic susceptibility to the more distal pulmonary vascular remodeling exists.

Mortality and prognosis

Reported 5-year mortality in CTPH is as high as 70% overall and reported 3-year mortality is as high as 90% in patients with mean PAP greater than 50 mmHg. Prognosis is dependent primarily on the degrees of RV dysfunction and the elevation of PVR rather than the degree of elevation of PAP. RV failure evolves during CTPH due to chronic RV pressure overload, and the diagnosis is often first suggested following echocardiography.[240,241] Pulmonary resistance greater than 1000 dynes cm^{-5} predicts worse survival and higher perioperative risk. Right heart catheterization is therefore essential in the evaluation of such patients, to determine RV filling pressures, cardiac output, and PVR in preparation of surgical correction.

Clinical presentation

CTPH presents nonspecifically with moderate to severe symptoms attributable to pulmonary hypertension and/or right HF, including exertional dyspnea, fatigue, chest pain, or syncope.[242] Given the nonspecific presentation, in a large registry the median time from symptom onset to CTPH diagnosis was 14.1 months and the median time from last acute PE to CTPH diagnosis was 12.5 months. As noted, up to 63% of patients have no clear prior history of PE. Physical signs depend on the severity of PH and RV failure and may include elevated JVP, right parasternal RV heave, accentuated P2, murmur of TR, hepatomegaly, ascites, peripheral edema, and cyanosis. Signs of RV failure signify a late state of the disease associated with high mortality. A rare pathognomic sign found in only 10% of cases is bruits due to turbulent flow through partially occluded vessels over the peripheral lower lung fields.

CTPH should be a consideration in the differential diagnosis of all patients who present with unexplained PH and/or RV dysfunction, especially in patients with a history of PE. Following PE, since up to 50–60% of patients may exhibit significant residual perfusion defect on ventilation/perfusion (V/Q) scanning and/or CT angiography and 2–44% of patients have persistent pulmonary hypertension and/or RV hypokinesis following PE, the diagnosis of CTPH also necessitates the demonstration of precapillary pulmonary hypertension. In the European Respiratory Society pulmonary hypertension guidelines, follow-up echocardiography is recommended in 3–6 months following hospital discharge for PE to determine whether or not pulmonary hypertension has resolved and/or CTPH is evolving.

Diagnosis

The chest radiograph may be normal, or demonstrate pulmonary artery enlargement, attenuation of segmental pulmonary arterial branches, and cardiomegaly. Echocardiography permits assessment of PAP and evidence of RV remodeling including RV and RA dilatation, RV pressure overload, and TR. Prospective studies have not yet validated the most appropriate diagnostic approach to cases of suspected CTPH, but most suggest V/Q scanning followed by CT angiography whenever V/Q scanning shows abnormal perfusion. A V/Q scan is recommended in all suspected instances of CTPH as a diagnostic screening test. A normal V/Q scan essentially excludes the diagnosis as 98.7% of patients with CTPH have abnormal perfusion and 19.0% abnormal ventilation by V/Q scanning.[242]

Patients with suspected CTPH who have abnormal perfusion scans should undergo pulmonary angiography.[179] CT angiography has replaced conventional pulmonary angiography given safety concerns, although conventional pulmonary angiography remains the gold standard for diagnosis. CT angiography shows proximal lesions in 60.4%, dilation of bronchial arteries in 68.4%, and mosaic perfusion pattern in 76.6% of cases and conventional pulmonary angiography shows proximal lesions in 63%. CT angiography may also demonstrate organized thrombi, abrupt tapering or occlusion of branch vessels, intraluminal vascular webs, and bronchial artery collaterals. Lack of central pulmonary artery visible lesions does not rule out CTPH.

Right heart catheterization is indicated in patients with positive pulmonary angiography to assess RV function and PVR. In the CTPH registry, the mean PAP was 47 mmHg, PVR 709 dyne cm^{-5} and cardiac index 2.2 L $min^{-1}m^{-2}$ at RHC. The final diagnosis of CTPH is based upon demonstrating (1) precapillary pulmonary hypertension (mean PA >25 mmHg, mean PCW <15 mmHg, PVR > 2–3 Wood units) at RHC and (2) multiple chronic/organized/occlusive thrombi and/or emboli in the elastic pulmonary arteries (main, lobar, segmental, subsegmental) despite at least 3 months of effective, uninterrupted anticoagulation. PVR elevated "out of proportion" to angiographic disease is typically indicative of distal disease less predictably responsive to good surgical outcome.

Management: pulmonary thromboendarteretomy

Surgical pulmonary thromboendartectomy is the treatment of choice for CTPH and should not be delayed for trials of medical therapy in operative candidates. Patients who present with CTPH without or without history of PE have progressive disease despite appropriate anticoagulation and have a high risk of dying from RV failure. Up to 40% of patients with CPTH may, however, not be candidates for surgical thromboendartecomy, due to predominant distal or inaccessible disease or extensive comorbidities.

Surgical evaluation should be conducted by an experienced multidisciplinary team made up of pulmonologists, radiologists, cardiologists, anesthesiologists, and surgeons. Best surgical outcomes are associated with (1) greater surgeon and center experience, (2) concordance between PVR and anatomic disease, (3) preoperative PVR less than 1000–1200 dyn s cm^{-5} (100–120 MPa s m^{-3}) and (4) absence of selected comorbidities (e.g., splenectomy, ventriculoatrial shunt). There is an approximate linear relationship between preoperative PVR and perioperative mortality. Operative mortality has been reported as 4–15% and is dependent on preoperative PVR, with mortality of 10.1% in patients with preoperative PVR greater than 1000 dyne s cm^{-5} and mortality 1.3% in patients with PVR less than 1000 dyn s cm^{-5} In the current era in the most experienced centers, operative mortality is as low as 4% and neither severe preoperative RV dysfunction nor severe elevation of PVR should preclude surgical candidacy.

Successful surgery typically results in rapid and often dramatic improvement in PA pressure, PVR, RV function, and symptoms. In approximately 10–15% of patients, PH does not regress substantially and prognosis is worse with postoperative PVR greater than 500 dyn s cm^{-5}. Successful surgery typically yields substantial if not "complete" reverse RV remodeling as assessed by echocardiography or MRI and normalization of RV systolic wall stress. The 5-year survival exceeds 75%.

Management: medical therapy

Lifelong anticoagulation to a target INR of 2–3 is indicated in patients with CTPH to prevent both in-situ thrombosis and recurrent PE. Anticoagulation will not, however, affect significant regression of PH. Medical therapy for CTPH is reserved for nonsurgical candidates and is used in approximately 40% of CTPH patients overall. Diuretics and oxygen provide symptomatic relief. To date, randomized trials of medical therapy in CTPH have been small and typically uncontrolled, and the benefits of traditional therapies for primary pulmonary hypertension (WHO group 1) are not well established. In a randomized trial, bosentan reduced PVR by 24% and increased cardiac index by 0.3 L min^{-1} m^{-2} without improvement in 6 minute walk test performance. Medical therapy may be beneficial in four instances: (1) surgery not possible due to distal disease; (2) therapeutic bridge to surgery in high-risk patients (intravenous epoprostenol in patients NYHA symptoms, mPAP >50 mmHg, PVR >1000 dyn s cm^{-5}); (3) persistent PH and/or distal disease following surgery (10–15% of patients); and (4) nonsurgical candidates due to comorbidities. In the CTPH registry, PDEV inhibitors were used in 17.5%, endothelin antagonists in 21.7%, prostacyclin analogs in 2.7%, and combination therapies in 4% overall.

References

1. Ronco C. Cardio-renal syndromes: from foggy bottoms to sunny hills. Heart Fail Rev 2011;16:509–17.
2. Ronco C, Haapio M, House AA, et al. Cardiorenal syndrome. J Am Coll Cardiol 2008;52:1527–39.

3. Motiwala SR, Januzzi JL, Jr. The role of natriuretic peptides as biomarkers for guiding the management of chronic heart failure. Clin Pharmacol Therapeut 2013;93(1):57–67.
4. O'Donoghue M, Braunwald E. Natriuretic peptides in heart failure: should therapy be guided by BNP levels? Nat Rev Cardiol 2010;7:13–20.
5. Porapakkham P, Zimmet H, Billah B, Krum H. B-type natriuretic peptide-guided heart failure therapy: A meta-analysis. Arch Int Med 2010;170:507–14.
6. McLaughlin VV, Archer SL, Badesch DB, et al. ACCF/AHA 2009 expert consensus document on pulmonary hypertension: a report of the American College of Cardiology Foundation Task Force on Expert Consensus Documents and the American Heart Association: developed in collaboration with the American College of Chest Physicians, American Thoracic Society, Inc., and the Pulmonary Hypertension Association. Circulation 2009;119:2250–94.
7. Marcus FI, McKenna WJ, Sherrill D, et al. Diagnosis of arrhythmogenic right ventricular cardiomyopathy/dysplasia: proposed modification of the task force criteria. Circulation 2010;121:1533–41.
8. Bettmann M. The chest radiograph in cardiovascular disease. In: Bonow RO, Mann DL, Zipes DP, Libby P, ed., Braunwald's Heart Disease: A Textbook of Cardiovascular Medicine, 9th ed, Chapter 16. Philadelphia, PA: Elsevier Saunders; 2011.
9. Kahwash R, Leier CV, Miller L. Role of the pulmonary artery catheter in diagnosis and management of heart failure. Cardiol Clin 2011;29:281–8.
10. Slaughter MS, Pagani FD, Rogers JG, et al. Clinical management of continuous-flow left ventricular assist devices in advanced heart failure. J Heart Lung Transplant 2010;29:S1–39.
11. Sorajja P. Invasive hemodynamics of constrictive pericarditis, restrictive cardiomyopathy, and cardiac tamponade. Cardiol Clin 2011;29:191–9.
12. Talreja DR, Nishimura RA, Oh JK, Holmes DR. Constrictive pericarditis in the modern era: novel criteria for diagnosis in the cardiac catheterization laboratory. J Am Coll Cardiol 2008;51:315–19.
13. Jaber WA, Sorajja P, Borlaug BA, Nishimura RA. Differentiation of tricuspid regurgitation from constrictive pericarditis: novel criteria for diagnosis in the cardiac catheterisation laboratory. Heart 2009;95:1449–54.
14. Studley J, Tighe DA, Joelson JM, Flack JE, 3rd. The hemodynamic signs of constrictive pericarditis can be mimicked by tricuspid regurgitation. Cardiology in review 2003;11:320–6.
15. Badano LP, Ginghina C, Easaw J, et al. Right ventricle in pulmonary arterial hypertension: haemodynamics, structural changes, imaging, and proposal of a study protocol aimed to assess remodelling and treatment effects. Eur J Echocardiogr 2010;11:27–37.
16. Jurcut R, Giusca S, La Gerche A, et al. The echocardiographic assessment of the right ventricle: what to do in 2010? Eur J Echocardiogr 2010;11:81–96.
17. Mitoff PR, Beauchesne L, Dick AJ, et al. Imaging the failing right ventricle. Curr Opin Cardiol 2012;27:148–53.
18. Roberts J, Forfia P. Diagnosis and assessment of pulmonary vascular disease by Doppler echocardiography. Pulmonary Circ 2012;2:160–81.
19. Sanz J, Conroy J, Narula J. Imaging of the right ventricle. Cardiol Clin 2012;30:189–203.
20. Stevens GR, Fida N, Sanz J. Computed tomography and cardiac magnetic resonance imaging in pulmonary hypertension. Prog Cardiovasc Dis 2012;55:161–71.
21. Valsangiacomo Buechel ER, Mertens LL. Imaging the right heart: the use of integrated multimodality imaging. Eur Heart J 2012;33:949–60.
22. Green EM, Givertz MM. Management of acute right ventricular failure in the intensive care unit. Curr Heart Fail Rep 2012;9:228–35.
23. Greyson CR. Right heart failure in the intensive care unit. Curr Opin Crit Care 2012;18:424–31.
24. Guazzi M, Arena R. Pulmonary hypertension with left-sided heart disease. Nat Rev Cardiol 2010;7:648–59.
25. Guazzi M, Castelvecchio S, Bandera F, Menicanti L. Right ventricular pulmonary hypertension. Curr Heart Fail Rep 2012;9:303–8.
26. Hoeper MM, Granton J. Intensive care unit management of patients with severe pulmonary hypertension and right heart failure. American J Respir Crit Care Med 2011;184:1114–24.
27. Lahm T, McCaslin C, Wozniak T, et al. Medical and surgical treatment of acute right ventricular failure. J Am Coll Cardiol 2010;56:1435–46.
28. McDonald MA, Ross HJ. Trying to succeed when the right ventricle fails. Curr Opin Cardiol 2009;24:239–45.
29. Piazza G, Goldhaber SZ. The acutely decompensated right ventricle: pathways for diagnosis and management. Chest 2005;128:1836–52.
30. Poor HD, Ventetuolo CE. Pulmonary hypertension in the intensive care unit. Prog Cardiovasc Dis 2012;55:187–98.
31. Sayer GT, Semigran MJ. Right ventricular performance in chronic congestive heart failure. Cardiol Clin 2012;30:271–82.
32. Zamanian RT HF, Doyle RL, et al. Management strategies for patients with pulmonary hypertension in the intensive care unit. Crit Care Med 2007;35:2037–50.
33. Wheeler AP, Bernard GR, Thompson BT, et al. Pulmonary-artery versus central venous catheter to guide treatment of acute lung injury. N Engl J Med 2006;354:2213–24.
34. Binanay C, Califf RM, Hasselblad V, et al. Evaluation study of congestive heart failure and pulmonary artery catheterization effectiveness: the ESCAPE trial. JAMA 2005;294:1625–33.
35. Healey J, Davies R, Tang A. Improvement of apparently fixed pulmonary hypertension with cardiac resynchronization therapy. J Heart Lung Transplant 2004;23:650–2.
36. Shalaby A, Voigt A, El-Saed A, Saba S. Usefulness of pulmonary artery pressure by echocardiography to predict outcome in patients receiving cardiac resynchronization therapy Am J Cardiol 2008;101:238–41.
37. Bleeker G, Schalij M, Nihoyannopoulos P, et al. Left ventricular dyssnchrony predicts right ventricular remodeling after cardiac resychronization therapy. J Am Coll Cardiol 2005;46:2264–9.
38. Rajagopalan N, Suffoletto M, Tanabe M, et al. Right ventricular function following cardiac resynchronization therapy. Am J Cardiol 2007;100:1434–6.
39. Verhaert D, Grimm R, Puntawangkoon C, et al. Long-term reverse remodeling with cardiac resynchronization therapy. J Am Coll Cardiol 2010;55:1788–95.
40. Jardin F, Vieillard-Baron A. Is there a safe plateau pressure in ARDS? The right heart only knows. Intensive Care Med 2007;33:444–7.
41. Jardin F, Vieillard-Baron A. Right ventricular function and positive pressure ventilation in clinical practice: from hemodynamic subsets to respirator settings. Intensive Care Med 2003;29:1426–34.
42. Fougeres E, Teboul JL, Richard C, et al. Hemodynamic impact of a positive end-expiratory pressure setting in acute respiratory distress syndrome: importance of the volume status. Crit Care Med 2010;38:802–7.
43. Bock JS, Gottlieb SS. Cardiorenal syndrome: new perspectives. Circulation 2010;121:2592–600.
44. Tang WH, Mullens W. Cardiorenal syndrome in decompensated heart failure. Heart 2010;96:255–60.
45. Ross EA. Congestive renal failure: the pathophysiology and treatment of renal venous hypertension. J Card Fail 2012;18:930–8.
46. Mullens W, Abrahams Z, Francis GS, et al. Importance of venous congestion for worsening of renal function in advanced decompensated heart failure. J Am Coll Cardiol 2009;53:589–96.
47. Testani JM, Khera AV, St John Sutton MG, et al. Effect of right ventricular function and venous congestion on cardiorenal interactions during the treatment of decompensated heart failure. Am J Cardiol 2010;105:511–16.
48. Felker GM, Mentz RJ. Diuretics and ultrafiltration in acute decompensated heart failure. J Am Coll Cardiol 2012;59:2145–53.
49. Lazzarini V, Felker GM. Management of the cardiorenal syndrome in acute heart failure. Curr Treat Options Cardiovasc Med 2012;14:342–55.
50. Bart BA, Goldsmith SR, Lee KL, et al. Ultrafiltration in decompensated heart failure with cardiorenal syndrome. N Engl J Med 2012 ;367:2296–304.

51. Felker GM, Lee KL, Bull DA, et al. Diuretic strategies in patients with acute decompensated heart failure. N Engl J Med 2011;364:797–805.
52. Cuffe MS, Califf RM, Adams KF, Jr., et al. Short-term intravenous milrinone for acute exacerbation of chronic heart failure: a randomized controlled trial. JAMA 2002;287:1541–7.
53. Felker GM, Benza RL, Chandler AB, et al. Heart failure etiology and response to milrinone in decompensated heart failure: results from the OPTIME-CHF study. J Am Coll Cardiol 2003;41:997–1003.
54. Kurien S, Warfield KT, Wood CM, Miller WL. Effects of standard heart failure therapy and concomitant treatment with intravenous furosemide or inotropes (dobutamine, dopamine, and/or milrinone) on renal function and mortality in patients treated with nesiritide. Am J Cardiol 2006;98:1627–30.
55. Elkayam U, Ng TM, Hatamizadeh P, et al. Renal vasodilatory action of dopamine in patients with heart failure: magnitude of effect and site of action. Circulation 2008;117:200–5.
56. Giamouzis G, Butler J, Starling RC, et al. Impact of dopamine infusion on renal function in hospitalized heart failure patients: results of the Dopamine in Acute Decompensated Heart Failure (DAD-HF) Trial. J Card Fail 2010;16:922–30.
57. O'Connor CM, Starling RC, Hernandez AF, et al. Effect of nesiritide in patients with acute decompensated heart failure. N Engl J Med 2011;365:32–43.
58. Konstam MA, Gheorghiade M, Burnett JC, Jr., et al. Effects of oral tolvaptan in patients hospitalized for worsening heart failure: the EVEREST Outcome Trial. JAMA 2007;297:1319–31.
59. Massie BM, O'Connor CM, Metra M, et al. Rolofylline, an adenosine A1-receptor antagonist, in acute heart failure. N Engl J Med 2010;363:1419–28.
60. Bart BA, Boyle A, Bank AJ, et al. Ultrafiltration versus usual care for hospitalized patients with heart failure: the Relief for Acutely Fluid-Overloaded Patients With Decompensated Congestive Heart Failure (RAPID-CHF) trial. J Am Coll Cardiol 2005;46:2043–6.
61. De Wet CJ, Affleck DG, Jacobsohn E, et al. Inhaled prostacyclin is safe, effective, and affordable in patients with pulmonary hypertension, right heart dysfunction, and refractory hypoxemia after cardiothoracic surgery. J Thorac Cardiovasc Surg 2004;127:1058–67.
62. Haraldsson A, Kieler-Jensn N, Ricksten S. The additive pulmonary vasodilatory effects of inhaled prostacyclin and inhaled milrinone in postcardiac surgical patients with pulmonary hypertension. Anesth Analg 2001;93:1439–45.
63. Califf R, Adams K, McKenna W, et al. A randomized controlled trial of epoprostenol thearpy for severe congestive heart failure: the Flolan International Randomized Survival Trial (FIRST). Am Heart J 1997;134:44–54.
64. Anand I, McMurray J, Cohn JN, et al. Long-term effects of darusentan on left-ventricular remodelling and clinical outcomes in the EndothelinA Receptor Antagonist Trial in Heart Failure (EARTH): randomised, double-blind, placebo-controlled trial. Lancet 2004;364:347–54.
65. Kalra PR, Moon JC, Coats AJ. Do results of the ENABLE (Endothelin Antagonist Bosentan for Lowering Cardiac Events in Heart Failure) study spell the end for non-selective endothelin antagonism in heart failure? Int J Cardiol 2002;85:195–7.
66. Luscher TF, Enseleit F, Pacher R, et al. Hemodynamic and neurohumoral effects of selective endothelin A (ET(A)) receptor blockade in chronic heart failure: the Heart Failure ET(A) Receptor Blockade Trial (HEAT). Circulation 2002;106:2666–72.
67. Packer M, McMurray J, Massie BM, et al. Clinical effects of endothelin receptor antagonism with bosentan in patients with severe chronic heart failure: results of a pilot study. J Card Fail 2005;11:12–20.
68. Metra M, Bettari L, Carubelli V, Cas LD. Old and new intravenous inotropic agents in the treatment of advanced heart failure. Prog Cardiovasc Dis 2011;54:97–106.
69. Givertz M, Hare J, Loh E, et al. Effect of bolus milrinone on hemodynamic variables and pulmonary vascular resistance in paitents with severe left ventricular dysfunction: a rapid test for resersibility of pulmonary hypertension. J Am Coll Cardiol 1996;28:1775–80.
70. Jaski BE, Fifer MA, Wright RF, et al. Positive inotropic and vasodilator actions of milrinone in patients with severe congestive heart failure. Dose-response relationships and comparison to nitroprusside. J Clin Invest 1985;75:643–9.
71. Colucci WS, Wright RF, Jaski BE, et al. Milrinone and dobutamine in severe heart failure: differing hemodynamic effects and individual patient responsiveness. Circulation 1986;73:III175–83.
72. Kerbaul F, Rondelet B, Motte S, et al. Effects of norepinephrine and dobutamine on pressure load-induced right ventricular failure. Crit Care Med 2004;32:1035–40.
73. Vizza CD, Rocca GD, Roma AD, et al. Acute hemodynamic effects of inhaled nitric oxide, dobutamine and a combination of the two in patients with mild to moderate secondary pulmonary hypertension. Crit Care 2001;5:355–61.
74. Kerbaul F, Rondelet B, Demester JP, et al. Effects of levosimendan versus dobutamine on pressure load-induced right ventricular failure. Crit Care Med 2006;34:2814–19.
75. Missant C, Rex S, Segers P, Wouters PF. Levosimendan improves right ventriculovascular coupling in a porcine model of right ventricular dysfunction. Crit Care Med 2007;35:707–15.
76. Guglin M, Khan H. Pulmonary hypertension in heart failure. J Cardiac Fail 2010;16:461–74.
77. Etz CD, Welp HA, Tjan TD, et al. Medically refractory pulmonary hypertension: treatment with nonpulsatile left ventricular assist devices. Ann Thorac Surg 2007;83:1697–705.
78. Zimpfer D, Zrunek P, Roethy W, et al. Left ventricular assist devices decrease fixed pulmonary hypertension in cardiac transplant candidates. J Thorac Cardiovasc Surg 2007;133:689–95.
79. Tedford RJ, Hemnes AR, Russell SD, et al. PDE5A inhibitor treatment of persistent pulmonary hypertension after mechanical circulatory support. Circ Heart Fail 2008;1:213–19.
80. Goldstein JA. Pathophysiology and management of right heart ischemia. J Am Coll Cardiol 2002;40:841–53.
81. Goldstein JA. Right versus left ventricular shock. J Am Coll Cardiol 2003;41:1280–2.
82. Andersen HR, Falk E, Nielsen D. Right ventricular infarction: frequency, size and topography in coronary heart disease: a prospective study comprising 107 consecutive autopsies from a coronary care unit. J Am Coll Cardiol 1987;10:1223–32.
83. Bowers TR, O'Neill WW, Pica M, Goldstein JA. Patterns of coronary compromise resulting in acute right ventricular ischemic dysfunction. Circulation 2002;106:1104–9.
84. Isner JM, Roberts WC. Right ventricular infarction complicating left ventricular infarction secondary to coronary heart disease. Frequency, location, associated findings and significance from analysis of 236 necropsy patients with acute or healed myocardial infarction. Am J Cardiol 1978;42:885–94.
85. Zehender M, Kasper W, Kauder E, et al. Right ventricular infarction as an independent predictor of prognosis after acute inferior myocardial infarction. N Engl J Med 1993;328:981–8.
86. Hamon M, Agostini D, Le Page O, Riddell JW. Prognostic impact of right ventricular involvement in patients with acute myocardial infarction: meta-analysis. Crit Care Med 2008;36:2023–33.
87. Pfisterer M. Right ventricular involvement in myocardial infarction and cardiogenic shock. Lancet 2003;362:392–4.
88. Jacobs AK, Leopold JA, Bates E, et al. Cardiogenic shock caused by right ventricular infarction: a report from the SHOCK registry. J Am Coll Cardiol 2003;41:1273–9.
89. Tani M. Roles of the right ventricular free wall and ventricular septum in right ventricular performance and influence of the parietal pericardium during right ventricular failure in dogs. Am J Cardiol 1983;52:196–202.
90. Laster SB, Shelton TJ, Barzilai B, Goldstein JA. Determinants of the recovery of right ventricular performance following experimental chronic right coronary artery occlusion. Circulation 1993;88:696–708.
91. Goldstein JA, Barzilai B, Rosamond TL, et al. Determinants of hemodynamic compromise with severe right ventricular infarction. Circulation 1990;82:359–68.

92. Goldstein JA, Vlahakes GJ, Verrier ED, et al. The role of right ventricular systolic dysfunction and elevated intrapericardial pressure in the genesis of low output in experimental right ventricular infarction. Circulation 1982;65:513–22.
93. Dell'Italia LJ, Lembo NJ, Starling MR, et al. Hemodynamically important right ventricular infarction: follow-up evaluation of right ventricular systolic function at rest and during exercise with radionuclide ventriculography and respiratory gas exchange. Circulation 1987;75:996–1003.
94. Lim ST, Marcovitz P, Pica M, et al. Right ventricular performance at rest and during stress with chronic proximal occlusion of the right coronary artery. Am J Cardiol 2003;92:1203–6.
95. Farrer-Brown G. Vascular pattern of myocardium of right ventricle of human heart. Br Heart J 1968;30:679–86.
96. Ohzono K, Koyanagi S, Urabe Y, et al. Transmural distribution of myocardial infarction: difference between the right and left ventricles in a canine model. Circ Res 1986;59:63–73.
97. Goldstein JA, Harada A, Yagi Y, et al. Hemodynamic importance of systolic ventricular interaction, augmented right atrial contractility and atrioventricular synchrony in acute right ventricular dysfunction. J Am Coll Cardiol 1990;16:181–9.
98. Basso C, Bauce B, Corrado D, Thiene G. Pathophysiology of arrhythmogenic cardiomyopathy. Nat Rev Cardiol 2012;9:223–33.
99. Corrado D, Basso C, Pilichou K, Thiene G. Molecular biology and clinical management of arrhythmogenic right ventricular cardiomyopathy/dysplasia. Heart 2011;97:530–9.
100. Delmar M, McKenna WJ. The cardiac desmosome and arrhythmogenic cardiomyopathies: from gene to disease. Circ Res 2010;107:700–14.
101. Ellinor PT, MacRae CA, Thierfelder L. Arrhythmogenic right ventricular cardiomyopathy. Heart Fail Clin 2010;6:161–77.
102. Basso C, Corrado D, Marcus FI, et al. Arrhythmogenic right ventricular cardiomyopathy. Lancet 2009;373:1289–300.
103. Muthappan P, Calkins H. Arrhythmogenic right ventricular dysplasia. Prog Cardiovasc Dis 2008;51:31–43.
104. Epstein AE, DiMarco JP, Ellenbogen KA, et al. ACC/AHA/HRS 2008 Guidelines for Device-Based Therapy of Cardiac Rhythm Abnormalities: a report of the American College of Cardiology/American Heart Association Task Force on Practice Guidelines (Writing Committee to Revise the ACC/AHA/NASPE 2002 Guideline Update for Implantation of Cardiac Pacemakers and Antiarrhythmia Devices): developed in collaboration with the American Association for Thoracic Surgery and Society of Thoracic Surgeons. Circulation 2008;117:e350–408.
105. Hulot JS, Jouven X, Empana JP, et al. Natural history and risk stratification of arrhythmogenic right ventricular dysplasia/cardiomyopathy. Circulation 2004;110:1879–84.
106. Lemola K, Brunckhorst C, Helfenstein U, et al. Predictors of adverse outcome in patients with arrhythmogenic right ventricular dysplasia/cardiomyopathy: long term experience of a tertiary care centre. Heart 2005;91:1167–72.
107. Wichter T, Paul M, Wollmann C, et al. Implantable cardioverter/defibrillator therapy in arrhythmogenic right ventricular cardiomyopathy: single-center experience of long-term follow-up and complications in 60 patients. Circulation 2004;109:1503–8.
108. Bhonsale A, James CA, Tichnell C, et al. Incidence and predictors of implantable cardioverter-defibrillator therapy in patients with arrhythmogenic right ventricular dysplasia/cardiomyopathy undergoing implantable cardioverter-defibrillator implantation for primary prevention. J Am Coll Cardiol 2011;58:1485–96.
109. Corrado D, Calkins H, Link MS, et al. Prophylactic implantable defibrillator in patients with arrhythmogenic right ventricular cardiomyopathy/dysplasia and no prior ventricular fibrillation or sustained ventricular tachycardia. Circulation 2010;122:1144–52.
110. Alonso-Gonzalez R, Dimopoulos K, Ho S, et al. The right heart and pulmonary circulation (IX). The right heart in adults with congenital heart disease. Rev Esp Cardiol 2010;63:1070–86.
111. Davlouros PA, Niwa K, Webb G, Gatzoulis MA. The right ventricle in congenital heart disease. Heart 2006;92 Suppl 1:i27–38.
112. Rhodes JF, Hijazi ZM, Sommer RJ. Pathophysiology of congenital heart disease in the adult, part II. Simple obstructive lesions. Circulation 2008;117:1228–37.
113. Sommer RJ, Hijazi ZM, Rhodes JF. Pathophysiology of congenital heart disease in the adult: part III: Complex congenital heart disease. Circulation 2008;117:1340–50.
114. Sommer RJ, Hijazi ZM, Rhodes JF, Jr. Pathophysiology of congenital heart disease in the adult: part I: Shunt lesions. Circulation 2008;117:1090–9.
115. Baumgartner H, Bonhoeffer P, De Groot NM, et al. ESC Guidelines for the management of grown-up congenital heart disease (new version 2010). Eur Heart J 2010;31:2915–57.
116. Silversides CK, Dore A, Poirier N, et al. Canadian Cardiovascular Society 2009 Consensus Conference on the management of adults with congenital heart disease: shunt lesions. Can J Cardiol 2010;26:e70–9.
117. Silversides CK, Kiess M, Beauchesne L, et al. Canadian Cardiovascular Society 2009 Consensus Conference on the management of adults with congenital heart disease: outflow tract obstruction, coarctation of the aorta, tetralogy of Fallot, Ebstein anomaly and Marfan's syndrome. Can J Cardiol 2010;26:e80–97.
118. Silversides CK, Marelli A, Beauchesne L, et al. Canadian Cardiovascular Society 2009 Consensus Conference on the management of adults with congenital heart disease: executive summary. Can J Cardiol 2010;26:143–50.
119. Silversides CK, Salehian O, Oechslin E, et al. Canadian Cardiovascular Society 2009 Consensus Conference on the management of adults with congenital heart disease: complex congenital cardiac lesions. Can J Cardiol 2010;26:e98–117.
120. Warnes CA, Williams RG, Bashore TM, et al. ACC/AHA 2008 Guidelines for the Management of Adults with Congenital Heart Disease: a report of the American College of Cardiology/American Heart Association Task Force on Practice Guidelines (Writing Committee to Develop Guidelines on the Management of Adults with Congenital Heart Disease). Circulation 2008;118:e714–833.
121. Kilner PJ. The role of cardiovascular magnetic resonance in adults with congenital heart disease. Progr Cardiovasc Dis 2011;54:295–304.
122. Webb G, Gatzoulis MA. Atrial septal defects in the adult: recent progress and overview. Circulation 2006;114:1645–53.
123. Campbell M. Natural history of atrial septal defect. Br Heart J 1970;32:820–6.
124. Craig RJ, Selzer A. Natural history and prognosis of atrial septal defect. Circulation 1968;37:805–15.
125. Murphy JG, Gersh BJ, McGoon MD, et al. Long-term outcome after surgical repair of isolated atrial septal defect. Follow-up at 27 to 32 years. N Engl J Med 1990;323:1645–50.
126. Salehian O, Horlick E, Schwerzmann M, et al. Improvements in cardiac form and function after transcatheter closure of secundum atrial septal defects. J Am Coll Cardiol 2005;45:499–504.
127. Schussler JM, Anwar A, Phillips SD, et al. Effect on right ventricular volume of percutaneous Amplatzer closure of atrial septal defect in adults. Am J Cardiol 2005;95:993–5.
128. Veldtman GR, Razack V, Siu S, et al. Right ventricular form and function after percutaneous atrial septal defect device closure. J Am Coll Cardiol 2001;37:2108–13.
129. Vecht JA, Saso S, Rao C, et al. Atrial septal defect closure is associated with a reduced prevalence of atrial tachyarrhythmia in the short to medium term: a systematic review and meta-analysis. Heart 2010;96:1789–97.
130. Penny DJ, Vick GW, 3rd. Ventricular septal defect. Lancet 2011;377:1103–12.
131. Apitz C, Webb GD, Redington AN. Tetralogy of Fallot. Lancet 2009;374:1462–71.
132. Huehnergarth KV, Gurvitz M, Stout KK, Otto CM. Repaired tetralogy of Fallot in the adult: monitoring and management. Heart 2008;94:1663–9.
133. Shinebourne EA, Babu-Narayan SV, Carvalho JS. Tetralogy of Fallot: from fetus to adult. Heart 2006;92:1353–9.

134. Diller GP, Kempny A, Liodakis E, et al. Left ventricular longitudinal function predicts life-threatening ventricular arrhythmia and death in adults with repaired tetralogy of fallot. Circulation 2012;125:2440–6.
135. O'Meagher S, Munoz PA, Alison JA, et al. Exercise capacity and stroke volume are preserved late after tetralogy repair, despite severe right ventricular dilatation. Heart 2012; 98:1595–9.
136. Geva T. Repaired tetralogy of Fallot: the roles of cardiovascular magnetic resonance in evaluating pathophysiology and for pulmonary valve replacement decision support. J Cardiovasc Magn Reson 2011;13:9.
137. Dave HH, Buechel ER, Dodge-Khatami A, et al. Early insertion of a pulmonary valve for chronic regurgitation helps restoration of ventricular dimensions. Ann Thorac Surg 2005;80:1615–20; discussion 20–1.
138. Oosterhof T, van Straten A, Vliegen HW, et al. Preoperative thresholds for pulmonary valve replacement in patients with corrected tetralogy of Fallot using cardiovascular magnetic resonance. Circulation 2007;116:545–51.
139. Therrien J, Provost Y, Merchant N, et al. Optimal timing for pulmonary valve replacement in adults after tetralogy of Fallot repair. Am J Cardiol 2005;95:779–82.
140. Harrild DM, Berul CI, Cecchin F, et al. Pulmonary valve replacement in tetralogy of Fallot: impact on survival and ventricular tachycardia. Circulation 2009;119:445–51.
141. Gatzoulis MA, Balaji S, Webber SA, et al. Risk factors for arrhythmia and sudden cardiac death late after repair of tetralogy of Fallot: a multicentre study. Lancet 2000;356:975–81.
142. Gatzoulis MA, Till JA, Somerville J, Redington AN. Mechanoelectrical interaction in tetralogy of Fallot. QRS prolongation relates to right ventricular size and predicts malignant ventricular arrhythmias and sudden death. Circulation 1995;92:231–7.
143. Attenhofer Jost CH, Connolly HM, Dearani JA, et al. Ebstein's anomaly. Circulation 2007;115:277–85.
144. Paranon S, Acar P. Ebstein's anomaly of the tricuspid valve: from fetus to adult: congenital heart disease. Heart 2008;94:237–43.
145. Celermajer DS, Bull C, Till JA, et al. Ebstein's anomaly: presentation and outcome from fetus to adult. J Am Coll Cardiol 1994;23:170–6.
146. Warnes CA. Transposition of the great arteries. Circulation 2006;114:2699–709.
147. Hornung TS, Calder L. Congenitally corrected transposition of the great arteries. Heart 2010;96:1154–61.
148. Connelly MS, Liu PP, Williams WG, et al. Congenitally corrected transposition of the great arteries in the adult: functional status and complications. J Am Coll Cardiol 1996;27:1238–43.
149. Graham TP, Jr., Bernard YD, Mellen BG, et al. Long-term outcome in congenitally corrected transposition of the great arteries: a multi-institutional study. J Am Coll Cardiol 2000;36:255–61.
150. Dimas AP, Moodie DS, Sterba R, Gill CC. Long-term function of the morphologic right ventricle in adult patients with corrected transposition of the great arteries. Am Heart J 1989;118:526–30.
151. Graham TP, Jr., Markham L, Parra DA, Bichell D. Congenitally corrected transposition of the great arteries: an update. Current Treat Options Cardiovasc Med 2007;9:407–13.
152. Prieto LR, Hordof AJ, Secic M, et al. Progressive tricuspid valve disease in patients with congenitally corrected transposition of the great arteries. Circulation 1998;98:997–1005.
153. Ismat FA, Baldwin HS, Karl TR, Weinberg PM. Coronary anatomy in congenitally corrected transposition of the great arteries. Int J Cardiol 2002;86:207–16.
154. Hornung TS, Bernard EJ, Celermajer DS, et al. Right ventricular dysfunction in congenitally corrected transposition of the great arteries. Am J Cardiol 1999;84:1116–9, A10.
155. Hornung TS, Bernard EJ, Jaeggi ET, et al. Myocardial perfusion defects and associated systemic ventricular dysfunction in congenitally corrected transposition of the great arteries. Heart 1998;80:322–6.
156. Hauser M, Bengel FM, Hager A, et al. Impaired myocardial blood flow and coronary flow reserve of the anatomical right systemic ventricle in patients with congenitally corrected transposition of the great arteries. Heart 2003;89:1231–5.
157. van Son JA, Danielson GK, Huhta JC, et al. Late results of systemic atrioventricular valve replacement in corrected transposition. J Thorac Cardiovasc Surg 1995;109:642–52; discussion 52–3.
158. Beghetti M, Galie N. Eisenmenger syndrome a clinical perspective in a new therapeutic era of pulmonary arterial hypertension. J Am Coll Cardiol 2009;53:733–40.
159. Diller GP, Gatzoulis MA. Pulmonary vascular disease in adults with congenital heart disease. Circulation 2007;115:1039–50.
160. Rosenzweig EB, Barst RJ. Congenital heart disease and pulmonary hypertension: pharmacology and feasibility of late surgery. Progr Cardiovasc Dis 2012;55:128–33.
161. Moceri P, Dimopoulos K, Liodakis E, et al. Echocardiographic predictors of outcome in Eisenmenger syndrome. Circulation 2012;126:1461–8.
162. Kumar RK, Sandoval J. Advanced pulmonary vascular disease: the Eisenmenger syndrome. Cardiology Young 2009;19:622–6.
163. Galie N, Beghetti M, Gatzoulis MA, et al. Bosentan therapy in patients with Eisenmenger syndrome: a multicenter, double-blind, randomized, placebo-controlled study. Circulation 2006;114:48–54.
164. Zhang ZN, Jiang X, Zhang R, et al. Oral sildenafil treatment for Eisenmenger syndrome: a prospective, open-label, multicentre study. Heart 2011;97:1876–81.
165. Waddell TK, Bennett L, Kennedy R, et al. Heart-lung or lung transplantation for Eisenmenger syndrome. J Heart Lung Transplant 2002;21:731–7.
166. Deal BJ, Jacobs ML. Management of the failing Fontan circulation. Heart 2012;98:1098–104.
167. d'Udekem Y, Iyengar AJ, Cochrane AD, et al. The Fontan procedure: contemporary techniques have improved long-term outcomes. Circulation 2007;116:I157–64.
168. Kempny A, Dimopoulos K, Uebing A, et al. Reference values for exercise limitations among adults with congenital heart disease. Relation to activities of daily life—single centre experience and review of published data. Eur Heart J 2012;33:1386–96.
169. Baek JS, Bae EJ, Ko JS, et al. Late hepatic complications after Fontan operation; non-invasive markers of hepatic fibrosis and risk factors. Heart 2010;96:1750–5.
170. Kiesewetter CH, Sheron N, Vettukattill JJ, et al. Hepatic changes in the failing Fontan circulation. Heart 2007;93:579–84.
171. Bernstein D, Naftel D, Chin C, et al. Outcome of listing for cardiac transplantation for failed Fontan: a multi-institutional study. Circulation 2006;114:273–80.
172. Griffiths ER, Kaza AK, Wyler von Ballmoos MC, et al. Evaluating failing Fontans for heart transplantation: predictors of death. Ann Thorac Surg 2009;88:558–63; discussion 63–4.
173. Bonow RO, Carabello BA, Chatterjee K, et al. 2008 Focused update incorporated into the ACC/AHA 2006 guidelines for the management of patients with valvular heart disease: a report of the American College of Cardiology/American Heart Association Task Force on Practice Guidelines (Writing Committee to Revise the 1998 Guidelines for the Management of Patients With Valvular Heart Disease): endorsed by the Society of Cardiovascular Anesthesiologists, Society for Cardiovascular Angiography and Interventions, and Society of Thoracic Surgeons. Circulation 2008;118:e523–661.
174. Bonow RO, Carabello BA, Kanu C, et al. ACC/AHA 2006 guidelines for the management of patients with valvular heart disease: a report of the American College of Cardiology/American Heart Association Task Force on Practice Guidelines (writing committee to revise the 1998 Guidelines for the Management of Patients With Valvular Heart Disease): developed in collaboration with the Society of Cardiovascular Anesthesiologists: endorsed by the Society for Cardiovascular Angiography and Interventions and the Society of Thoracic Surgeons. Circulation 2006;114:e84–231.

175. Tang GH, David TE, Singh SK, et al. Tricuspid valve repair with an annuloplasty ring results in improved long-term outcomes. Circulation 2006;114:I577–81.
176. Firstenberg MS, Sai-Sudhakar CB, Anyanwu A. Valvular disease in patients requiring long-term left ventricular assist devices: pathophysiology and therapeutic options. Expert Rev Cardiovasc Ther 2012;10:205–13.
177. Stainback RF, Croitoru M, Hernandez A, et al. Echocardiographic evaluation of the Jarvik 2000 axial-flow LVAD. Texas Heart Inst J 2005;32:263–70.
178. Kukucka M, Stepanenko A, Potapov E, et al. Impact of tricuspid valve annulus dilation on mid-term survival after implantation of a left ventricular assist device. J Heart Lung Transplant 2012;31:967–71.
179. Kormos RL, Teuteberg JJ, Pagani FD, et al. Right ventricular failure in patients with the HeartMate II continuous-flow left ventricular assist device: incidence, risk factors, and effect on outcomes. J Thorac Cardiovasc Surg 2010;139:1316–24.
180. Krishan K, Nair A, Pinney S, et al. Liberal use of tricuspid-valve annuloplasty during left-ventricular assist device implantation. Eur J Cardiothoracic Surg 2012;41:213–17.
181. Piacentino V, 3rd, Troupes CD, Ganapathi AM, et al. Clinical impact of concomitant tricuspid valve procedures during left ventricular assist device implantation. Ann Thorac Surg 2011;92:1414–18; discussion 18–19.
182. Piacentino V, 3rd, Williams ML, Depp T, et al. Impact of tricuspid valve regurgitation in patients treated with implantable left ventricular assist devices. Ann Thorac Surg 2011;91:1342–6; discussion 1346–7.
183. Pinney SP. The role of tricuspid valve repair and replacement in right heart failure. Curr Opin Cardiol 2012;27:288–95.
184. Saeed D, Kidambi T, Shalli S, et al. Tricuspid valve repair with left ventricular assist device implantation: is it warranted? J Heart Lung Transplant 2011;30:530–5.
185. Roberts PA, Boudjemline Y, Cheatham JP, et al. Percutaneous tricuspid valve replacement in congenital and acquired heart disease. J Am Coll Cardiol 2011;58:117–22.
186. Rich JD. Right ventricular failure in patients with left ventricular assist devices. Cardiol Clin 2012;30:291–302.
187. Craig ML. Management of right ventricular failure in the era of ventricular assist device therapy. Curr Heart Fail Rep 2011;8:65–71.
188. Kaczorowski DJ, Woo YJ. Who needs an RVAD in addition to an LVAD? Cardiol Clin 2011;29:599–605.
189. Mangi AA. Right ventricular dysfunction in patients undergoing left ventricular assist device implantation: predictors, management, and device utilization. Cardiol Clin 2011;29:629–37.
190. Frazier OH, Rose EA, Oz MC, et al. Multicenter clinical evaluation of the heartmate; vented electric left ventricular assist system in patients awaiting heart transplantation. J Heart Lung Transplant 2001;20:201–2.
191. Rose EA, Gelijns AC, Moskowitz AJ, et al. Long-term use of a left ventricular assist device for end-stage heart failure. N Engl J Med 2001;345:1435–43.
192. Miller LW, Pagani FD, Russell SD, et al. Use of a continuous-flow device in patients awaiting heart transplantation. N Engl J Med 2007;357:885–96.
193. Slaughter MS, Rogers JG, Milano CA, et al. Advanced heart failure treated with continuous-flow left ventricular assist device. N Engl J Med 2009;361:2241–51.
194. Genovese EA, Dew MA, Teuteberg JJ, et al. Incidence and patterns of adverse event onset during the first 60 days after ventricular assist device implantation. Ann Thorac Surg 2009;88:1162–70.
195. John R, Naka Y, Smedira NG, et al. Continuous flow left ventricular assist device outcomes in commercial use compared with the prior clinical trial. Ann Thorac Surg 2011;92:1406–13; discussion 1413.
196. Slaughter MS, Meyer AL, Birks EJ. Destination therapy with left ventricular assist devices: patient selection and outcomes. Curr Opin Cardiol 2011;26:232–6.
197. Lee S, Kamdar F, Madlon-Kay R, et al. Effects of the HeartMate II continuous-flow left ventricular assist device on right ventricular function. J Heart Lung Transplant 2010;29:209–15.
198. Park SJ, Milano CA, Tatooles AJ, et al. Outcomes in advanced heart failure patients with left ventricular assist devices for destination therapy. Circ Heart Fail 2012;5:241–8.
199. Starling RC, Naka Y, Boyle AJ, et al. Results of the post-U.S. Food and Drug Administration-approval study with a continuous flow left ventricular assist device as a bridge to heart transplantation: a prospective study using the INTERMACS (Interagency Registry for Mechanically Assisted Circulatory Support). J Am Coll Cardiol 2011;57:1890–8.
200. Lietz K, Long JW, Kfoury AG, et al. Outcomes of left ventricular assist device implantation as destination therapy in the post-REMATCH era: implications for patient selection. Circulation 2007;116:497–505.
201. Mikus E, Stepanenko A, Krabatsch T, et al. Reversibility of fixed pulmonary hypertension in left ventricular assist device support recipients. Eur J Cardiothorac Surg 2011;40:971–7.
202. Topilsky Y, Hasin T, Oh JK, et al. Echocardiographic variables after left ventricular assist device implantation associated with adverse outcome. Circ Cardiovasc Imaging 2011;4:648–61.
203. Topilsky Y, Oh JK, Shah DK, et al. Echocardiographic predictors of adverse outcomes after continuous left ventricular assist device implantation. JACC Cardiovasc Imaging 2011;4:211–22.
204. Gilotra NA, Russell SD. Patient selection for mechanical circulatory support. Heart Fail Rev 2013;18:27–34.
205. Lund LH, Matthews J, Aaronson K. Patient selection for left ventricular assist devices. Eur J Heart Fail 2010;12:434–43.
206. Miller LW, Lietz K. Candidate selection for long-term left ventricular assist device therapy for refractory heart failure. J Heart Lung Transplant 2006;25:756–64.
207. Schaffer JM, Allen JG, Weiss ES, et al. Evaluation of risk indices in continuous-flow left ventricular assist device patients. Ann Thorac Surg 2009;88:1889–96.
208. Kirklin JK, Naftel DC, Kormos RL, et al. Third INTERMACS Annual Report: the evolution of destination therapy in the United States. J Heart Lung Transplant 2011;30:115–23.
209. Aaronson KD, Schwartz JS, Chen TM, et al. Development and prospective validation of a clinical index to predict survival in ambulatory patients referred for cardiac transplant evaluation. Circulation 1997;95:2660–7.
210. Levy W, Mozaffaraian D, Linker D, et al.; REMATCH Investigators. Can the Seattle Heart Failure Score be used to risk-stratify heart failure patients for potential left ventricular assist device therapy? J Heart Lung Transplant 2009;28:231–6.
211. Rao V, Oz MC, Flannery MA, et al. Revised screening scale to predict survival after insertion of a left ventricular assist device. J Thorac Cardiovasc Surg 2003;125:855–62.
212. Farrar DJ, Hill JD, Pennington DG, et al. Preoperative and postoperative comparison of patients with univentricular and biventricular support with the thoratec ventricular assist device as a bridge to cardiac transplantation. J Thorac Cardiovasc Surg 1997;113:202–9.
213. Ochiai Y, McCarthy PM, Smedira NG, et al. Predictors of severe right ventricular failure after implantable left ventricular assist device insertion: analysis of 245 patients. Circulation 2002;106:I198–202.
214. Deng MC, Loebe M, El-Banayosy A, et al. Mechanical circulatory support for advanced heart failure: effect of patient selection on outcome. Circulation 2001;103:231–7.
215. Fukamachi K, McCarthy PM, Smedira NG, Vargo RL, Starling RC, Young JB. Preoperative risk factors for right ventricular failure after implantable left ventricular assist device insertion. Ann Thorac Surg 1999;68:2181–4.
216. Dang NC, Topkara VK, Mercando M, et al. Right heart failure after left ventricular assist device implantation in patients with chronic congestive heart failure. J Heart Lung Transplant 2006;25:1–6.

217. Santambrogio L, Bianchi T, Fuardo M, et al. Right ventricular failure after left ventricular assist device insertion: preoperative risk factors. Interact Cardiovasc Thorac Surg 2006;5:379–82.
218. Kato TS, Farr M, Schulze PC, et al. Usefulness of two-dimensional echocardiographic parameters of the left side of the heart to predict right ventricular failure after left ventricular assist device implantation. Am J Cardiol 2012;109:246–51.
219. Potapov EV, Stepanenko A, Dandel M, et al. Tricuspid incompetence and geometry of the right ventricle as predictors of right ventricular function after implantation of a left ventricular assist device. J Heart Lung Transplant 2008;27:1275–81.
220. Topilsky Y, Maltais S, Oh JK, et al. Focused review on transthoracic echocardiographic assessment of patients with continuous axial left ventricular assist devices. Cardiology Res Pract 2011;2011:187434.
221. Puwanant S, Hamilton KK, Klodell CT, et al. Tricuspid annular motion as a predictor of severe right ventricular failure after left ventricular assist device implantation. J Heart Lung Transplant 2008;27:1102–7.
222. Neragi-Miandoab S, Goldstein D, Bello R, et al. Right ventricular dysfunction following continuous flow left ventricular assist device placement in 51 patients: predicators and outcomes. J Cardiothorac Surg 2012;7:60.
223. Fitzpatrick JR, 3rd, Frederick JR, Hsu VM, et al. Risk score derived from pre-operative data analysis predicts the need for biventricular mechanical circulatory support. J Heart Lung Transplant 2008;27:1286–92.
224. Matthews JC, Koelling TM, Pagani FD, Aaronson KD. The right ventricular failure risk score a pre-operative tool for assessing the risk of right ventricular failure in left ventricular assist device candidates. J Am Coll Cardiol 2008;51:2163–72.
225. Drakos SG, Janicki L, Horne BD, et al. Risk factors predictive of right ventricular failure after left ventricular assist device implantation. Am J Cardiol 2010;105:1030–5.
226. Patel CB, Rogers JG. Durable mechanical circulatory support devices. Prog Cardiovasc Dis 2011;54:132–43.
227. Fitzpatrick JR, 3rd, Frederick JR, Hiesinger W, et al. Early planned institution of biventricular mechanical circulatory support results in improved outcomes compared with delayed conversion of a left ventricular assist device to a biventricular assist device. J Thorac Cardiovasc Surg 2009;137:971–7.
228. Potapov EV, Stepanenko A, Krabatsch T, Hetzer R. Managing long-term complications of left ventricular assist device therapy. Curr Opin Cardiol 2011;26:237–44.
229. Deswarte G, Kirsch M, Lesault PF, et al. Right ventricular reserve and outcome after continuous-flow left ventricular assist device implantation. J Heart Lung Transplant 2010;29:1196–8.
230. Lam KM, Ennis S, O'Driscoll G, et al. Observations from non-invasive measures of right heart hemodynamics in left ventricular assist device patients. J Am Soc Echocardiogr 2009;22:1055–62.
231. Estep JD, Stainback RF, Little SH, et al. The role of echocardiography and other imaging modalities in patients with left ventricular assist devices. JACC Cardiovasc Imaging 2010;3:1049–64.
232. Maybaum S, Mancini D, Xydas S, et al. Cardiac improvement during mechanical circulatory support: a prospective multicenter study of the LVAD Working Group. Circulation 2007;115:2497–505.
233. John R, Liao K, Kamdar F, et al. Effects on pre- and posttransplant pulmonary hemodynamics in patients with continuous-flow left ventricular assist devices. J Thorac Cardiovasc Surg 2010;140:447–52.
234. Maeder MT, Leet A, Ross A, et al. Changes in right ventricular function during continuous-flow left ventricular assist device support [corrected]. J Heart Lung Transplant 2009;28:360–6.
235. Simon MA, Kormos RL, Gorcsan J, 3rd, et al. Differential exercise performance on ventricular assist device support. J Heart Lung Transplant 2005;24:1506–12.
236. Pengo V, Lensing AW, Prins MH, et al. Incidence of chronic thromboembolic pulmonary hypertension after pulmonary embolism. N Engl J Med 2004;350:2257–64.
237. Becattini C, Agnelli G, Pesavento R, et al. Incidence of chronic thromboembolic pulmonary hypertension after a first episode of pulmonary embolism. Chest 2006;130:172–5.
238. Auger WR, Kim NH, Trow TK. Chronic thromboembolic pulmonary hypertension. Clin Chest Med 2010;31:741–58.
239. Hoeper MM, Mayer E, Simonneau G, Rubin LJ. Chronic thromboembolic pulmonary hypertension. Circulation 2006;113:2011–20.
240. Kline JA, Steuerwald MT, Marchick MR, et al. Prospective evaluation of right ventricular function and functional status 6 months after acute submassive pulmonary embolism: frequency of persistent or subsequent elevation in estimated pulmonary artery pressure. Chest 2009;136:1202–10.
241. Ribeiro A, Lindmarker P, Johnsson H, et al. Pulmonary embolism: one-year follow-up with echocardiography Doppler and five-year survival analysis. Circulation 1999;99:1325–30.
242. Pepke-Zaba J, Delcroix M, Lang I, et al. Chronic thromboembolic pulmonary hypertension (CTEPH): results from an international prospective registry. Circulation 2011;124:1973–81.

CHAPTER 22

Pulmonary arterial hypertension

Myung H. Park, MD

Introduction

The past decade has witnessed unprecedented advances in the field of pulmonary arterial hypertension (PAH). Once considered a uniformly fatal disease with no effective treatment, there are currently fourteen therapies approved by the United States Food and Drug Administration (FDA), with more agents under investigation. This has been the result of unparalleled increase in understanding of the mechanisms and pathology of the disease, coupled with increase in the awareness of PAH and concerted efforts to diagnose the disease through a systematic approach. All this progress has resulted in improvements in quality of life and survival; however, PAH remains a devastatingly progressive disease with high morbidity and mortality. Indeed, though much has been accomplished in management of this rare condition, many more challenges lie ahead to improve outcome and attain a cure.

Historical view

The historical journey of PAH is a fascinating tale of misconceptions woven in with brilliant studies and observations spanning over five centuries in the areas of the right ventricle (RV) and pulmonary vascular hemodynamics. The initial insight into RV function and pulmonary circulation dates to the work of William Harvey (*Exercitatio anatomica de motu cordis et sanguinis in animabilus*, 1628).[1] Harvey deduced from his observations of blood flow and dissections that the blood circulates from the heart via the arteries and back from the tissues through the veins and through the lungs. He also commented on the function and limitations of the RV, stating that: "Thus, the right ventricle may be said to be made for the sake of transmitting blood through the lungs, not for nourishing them." This initial work was followed by occasional descriptions of the involvement of the RV in pulmonary disease processes by various researchers including Laennec in 1826, describing RV hypertrophy in the setting of emphysema,[2] and Virchow reporting dilated RV after pulmonary embolism in 1846.[1,3]

Physicians continued to describe sporadic cases involving pulmonary circulation and the heart. Ernst von Romberg was the first to describe a patient with pulmonary vascular lesions in 1891 as "sclerosis of the pulmonary arteries" from autopsy findings.[4] Osler soon followed with a list of causes of RV hypertrophy from his series of patients, including mitral valve disease, emphysema, and "obliteration of pulmonary arteries" in 1893, though no further discussion was given.[5] These insightful descriptions were followed by three decades of speculations and misconceptions regarding the etiology of "pulmonary vascular lesions". A similar clinical syndrome consisting of cyanosis, dyspnea, and polycythemia was described by Ayerza (working in Argentina), and the disease was referred to as Ayerza's disease by one of his students, Arrillaga.[6,7] Ayerza attributed the condition to syphilitic pulmonary endarteritis which spurred further controversy involving the spirochete as the etiology of the disease. It was Oscar Brenner, a British physician, who accurately concluded that the clinical manifestations of Ayerza's disease were those of heart failure secondary to pulmonary disease, based on past published reports and his own observations.[8] However, he was not able to make the connection between the pulmonary vascular disease and the RV hypertrophy, describing each unit as a separate entity due to "an unknown cause."[7,8,9]

It would take another half-century of innovation and research for the pathology and hemodynamics of the disease to be better understood and the relationship between the pulmonary vascular lesions and RV physiology to be elucidated. The seminal innovation was obtaining measurements of the inaccessible pulmonary circulation. Werner Forssman, a German physician who catheterized himself in 1929 via the antecubital vein and published a picture of the catheter in his heart, is credited with disproving the belief that placing a catheter in the body would cause fatal complications.[10] Richards and Cournand, from Columbia University College, New York, took this many steps further by placing catheters in animals and then in humans in 1940, demonstrating that the procedure was safe.[11] This led to an explosion of information about flow and pressure relationships in health and variety of disease states.

Forssman, Cournand, and Richards were awarded the Nobel Prize in 1956 for their innovative discoveries. Their contributions revolutionized the practice of cardiopulmonary medicine until the present day.

Physicians were eager to use catheterization techniques to study the physiology of patients presenting with "pulmonary vascular lesions." Using this method, Dresdale and colleagues in 1951 used the term primary pulmonary hypertension (PPH) to describe a patient with hypertensive vasculopathy of pulmonary vessels of unknown cause.[12] Paul Wood contributed to the understanding of the possible etiology of this disease by observing that a reduction in pulmonary artery pressure (PAP) was seen in response to intravenous (IV) administration of acetylcholine in patients with pulmonary hypertension secondary to mitral stenosis, eliciting a proposal that a "vasoconstrictive factor" may be a cause.[13] However, it was an alarming increased incidence of pulmonary hypertension in Europe in the late 1960s which galvanized the medical community to learn more about this fatal condition. Since then, the rapid evolution and progress in the field of PAH have been unprecedented, marked by five world symposiums, nine FDA-approved treatments, national and international registries, and ongoing research and clinical trials exploring new treatment pathways.

Classification and epidemiology

The clinical classification of pulmonary hypertension (PH) has undergone significant modifications since the initial meeting 1973 in Geneva, Switzerland, in response to a sudden increase in incidence of PH in Europe related to use of the diet drug aminorex. The World Health Organization (WHO) assembled a group of experts to determine the current state of knowledge, which resulted in a classification scheme for PH consisting of two categories, primary (PPH) and secondary PH.[14] In order to gather data on this rare disease, the National Heart, Lung and Blood Institute (NHLBI) created a National Registry of Patients with PPH from 1981 to 1987, enrolling 187 patients from 32 clinical centers in the US. This registry has had a monumental impact in providing epidemiological and clinical information which has paved the way for subsequent studies. The results showed that PPH is a rare condition, with an incidence of 2–5 per million per year when strictly defined in the absence of any possible contributing substrates. It occurs more frequently in women than men (1.7:1) with a mean age of diagnosis of 36 years; when left untreated, it was shown to be a progressive disease with high mortality, with a median survival of 2.8 years.[15,16] Based on estimates obtained from the proportional-hazards models, an equation was devised to predict a patient's likelihood of survival according to baseline hemodynamic measurements, which has been utilized widely as a comparator in survival analysis.[16] In addition, this study brought to attention a significant delay in making the diagnosis from onset of symptoms (2.5 years), a factor which has prompted efforts in increasing awareness of PH.

The 2nd World Symposium on PH was held in Evian, France in 1998 to commemorate the 25th anniversary of the first meeting. The development of the "Evian Classification" brought significant revisions, dividing PH into five categories based on pathobiologic and clinical features. Further modifications were made in Venice, Italy at the 3rd World Symposium in 2003. This meeting was held in the midst of tremendous advances in the field of molecular and genetic sciences in pulmonary vascular diseases, as well as development of effective PAH-targeted therapies, which changed the understanding and practice of PAH.[17] The Venice Classification of Pulmonary Hypertension replaced the term PPH with idiopathic pulmonary arterial hypertension (IPAH) and moved pulmonary veno-occulsive disease and pulmonary capillary hemangiomatosis into a single subcategory of PAH based on similar pathological and clinical course.

The "Dana Point Classification", which was derived from the 4th World Symposium in 2008, maintained the general architecture with minor changes to group 1 PAH.[17] However, it should be noted that group 1 PAH, although classified under one category, covers a diverse spectrum of diseases that share underlying pulmonary vasculopathy as a common feature but the clinical course is greatly influenced and governed by the associated systemic conditions.[19] Recent registry reports and studies highlight that diseases grouped together, such as congenital heart disease and connective tissue disease within group 1 PAH, have vastly different epidemiological and clinical features and outcomes.

The most recent 5th World Symposium on Pulmonary Hypertension held in 2013 held in Nice, France, resulted in several modifications (Box 22.1).[20] To reflect the recent discoveries in the field of genetics in PAH, the "Nice Classification" included a list of new gene mutations discovered to be associated with PAH

Box 22.1 Updated classification of pulmonary hypertension (Nice 2013)

1. Pulmonary arterial hypertension
   - 1.1 Idiopathic PAH
   - 1.2 Heritable PAH
     - 1.2.1 BMPR2
     - 1.2.2 ALK1, ENG, **SMAD9, CAV1, KCNK3**
     - 1.2.3 Unknown
   - 1.3 Drug- and toxin-induced
   - 1.4 Associated with
     - 1.4.1 Connective tissue diseases
     - 1.4.2 HIV infection
     - 1.4.3 Portal hypertension
     - 1.4.4 Congenital heart diseases
     - 1.4.5 Schistosomiasis

1′ Pulmonary veno-occlusive disease and/or pulmonary capillary hemangiomatosis

1″ Persistent pulmonary hypertension of the newborn (PPHN)

2. Pulmonary hypertension due to left heart disease
   - 2.1 Left ventricular systolic dysfunction
   - 2.2 Left ventricular diastolic dysfunction
   - 2.3 Valvular disease
   - 2.4 Congenital/acquired left heart inflow/outflow tract obstruction and congenital cardiomyopathies
3. Pulmonary hypertension due to lung diseases and/or hypoxia
   - 3.1 Chronic obstructive pulmonary disease
   - 3.2 Interstitial lung disease
   - 3.3 Other pulmonary diseases with mixed restrictive and obstructive pattern
   - 3.4 Sleep-disordered breathing
   - 3.5 Alveolar hypoventilation disorders
   - 3.6 Chronic exposure to high altitude
   - 3.7 Developmental lung disease
4. Chronic thromboembolic pulmonary hypertension (CTEPH)
5. Pulmonary hypertension with unclear and/or multifactorial mechanisms
   - 5.1 Hematologic disorders: **chronic hemolytic anemia**, myeloproliferative disorders, splenectomy
   - 5.2 Systemic disorders: sarcoidosis, pulmonary histiocytosis, lymphangioleiomyomatosis
   - 5.3 Metabolic disorders: glycogen storage disease, Gaucher disease, thyroid disorders

5.4 Others: tumoral obstruction, fibrosing mediastinitis, chronic renal failure **segmental PH**

BMPR = bone morphogenic protein receptor type II; CAV1 = caveolin-1; ENG = endoglin; HIV – human acquired immunodeficiency virus; PAH = pulmonary arterial hypertension
Simonneau G, Gatzoulis MA, Adatia I, et al. Updated clinical classification of pulmonary hypertension. Journal of the American College of Cardiology, 2013; 62 :D34–41.

for the heritable PAH group, of which caveolin-1 (CAV1) and KCNK3 represent mutations not related to TGF-β family providing new insights into the pathogenesis of PAH. Several drugs were added to the list of toxin-induced PAH: benfluorex (a derivative of fenfluramine) and SSRIs for definite association; interferon alpha and beta and amphetamine-like drugs for possible; and dasatinib, a tyrosine-kinase inhibitor used in treatment of chronic myeloproliferative (CML) disorders with likely association. The congenital heart disease (CHD) category was updated to encompass the four different phenotypes of the disease to offer a clinically useful way to approach CHD. Sickle cell disease (SCD) was moved to group 5 (unclear multifactorial mechanisms) as a result of recent findings that SCD has markedly different characteristics than other forms of PAH in pathologic findings from autopsies, hemodynamic profiles, and response to PAH-specific treatments. The other main change was designating persistent pulmonary hypertension of the newborn (PPHN) as number 1 to designate that it carries more differences than similarities with other types of PAH.[20]

Idiopathic pulmonary arterial hypertension

PAH can be idiopathic, hereditary, the result of drug or toxin exposure, or associated with conditions such as connective tissue disease (CTD) (see Box 22.1). Idiopathic PAH is PAH of unknown cause, a diagnosis of exclusion determined after a thorough evaluation. The estimate of PAH prevalence in the current era is 15 per million persons, with IPAH accounting for approximately 39–46% of cases.[21,22,23,24] Recently national and international registries have done much to advance our understanding of the current epidemiology and demographics of PH. The French registry gathered data from 17 French university hospitals from 2002 to 2003, enrolling 674 patients.[21,22] The mean age was 50 ± 15 years, with a 1.9:1 female/male ratio. Body mass index (BMI) was normal (24.4 ± 5.5) with BMI above 30 seen in 14.8% of the cases, a proportion reported to be similar to that of the adult French population. The time of onset of symptoms to diagnosis was 27 months, and a majority of patients had severe symptoms at presentation (75% in New York Heart Association [NYHA] functional class III or IV) with 1-year survival of the cohort reported as 82.9% (Figure 22.1). The Registry to Evaluate Early and Long-term Pulmonary Arterial Hypertension Disease and Management (REVEAL) comes from 54 US centers, collecting data between 2006 and 2007 and is the largest registry of WHO group I PAH patients reported to date.[23,24] The baseline characteristics were analyzed from 2525 patients, showing mean age to be 53 ± 14 years and 78% female (F:M ratio 4.1:1 for IPAH and 3.8:1 for associated PAH [APAH]). The mean duration between symptom onset and diagnostic catheterization was 2.8 years (median 13.6 months) and 73.6% of patients were in NYHA functional class III or IV.

Some interesting differences emerged among the PAH populations reported. The REVEAL patients were older at

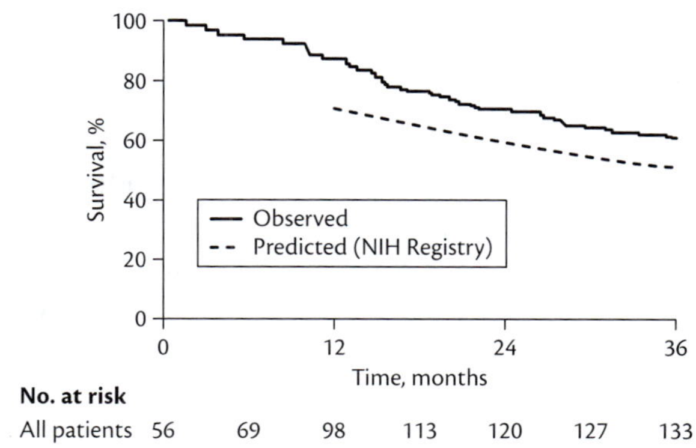

Fig. 22.1 Kaplan–Meier survival estimates in the combined estimates in the combined population of patients with pulmonary arterial hypertension. When the predictive modeling approach of the NIH registry was used, the estimated survival (gray line) was around 10% lower than what was actually observed.
Humbert M, Sitbon O, Chaouat A, et al. Survival in patients with idiopathic, familial, and anorexigen-associated pulmonary arterial hypertension in the modern management era. Circulation 2010;122:156–163.

diagnosis compared with the National Institutes of Health (NIH) registry (44.9 ± 0.6 vs. 36.4 ± 1.1 years) and more likely to be women (78.7 ± 1.2% vs 63.1 ± 3.5%). Indeed, recent studies corroborate these findings by demonstrating that the age range of affected individuals is increasing, as cases of IPAH have been reported in many patients over 70 years of age.[25] Comparison of the two modern registries show that the REVEAL patient population were similar in age and severity of disease to the ones reported in the French registry, but REVEAL patients were more likely to be women (79.8 ± 0.8% vs. 65.3 ± 1.8%) and obese (BMI ≥30 kg/m^2, 32.5 ± 1.0% vs. 14.8 ± 1.4%). Other contemporary US-based registries have reported a similar degree of female preponderance.[24] The cause of the different gender ratio between Europe and the US or between the US in the 1980s (as reported in the NIH study),[16] and now, has yet to be determined.

Associated pulmonary arterial hypertension

The term familial PAH has been replaced by heritable PAH (HPAH) since specific gene mutations have been identified in sporadic cases with no family history.[18] Heritable forms of PAH include clinically sporadic IPAH with germline mutation in the bone morphogenetic protein receptor type 2 gene (*BMPR2*), a member of the transforming growth factor β family, which accounts for 70% of the heritable cases. The *BMPR2* mutation has been identified in 25% of IPAH patients with no family history, raising the possibility of spontaneous mutations in some individuals or familial transmission among members without clinically evidence disease.[26,27,28] The heritable form is characterized by autosomal dominant transmission, incomplete penetrance, and genetic anticipation, in which family members in successive generations who develop PAH manifest at an earlier age with more aggressive disease course. A second, less common mutation involving activin receptor-like kinase type I, also known as endoglin, also results in a heritable form of PAH.[18]

Drug-induced PAH is primarily related to anorexigen use and accounts for up to 10% of PAH; anorexigens clearly associated with PAH include fenfluramine, amiorex, and dexfenfluramine.[29] All these agents have been removed from the market after studies demonstrated linkage between these drugs and PAH. In addition, amphetamines and methamphetamines (inhaled, smoked, oral, or IV) are very likely linked to development of IPAH.[18,30]

PAH is a potentially life-threatening complication of CTD and comprises the largest subgroup of population affected. Scleroderma is the most common CTD complicated by PAH and prevalence has been reported to be 7–12%.[31,32] Patients with PAH associated with CTD have poorer survival than IPAH patients; median survival of 12 months has been reported compared to 2.6 years in IPAH patients, and current therapies are less effective in CTD patients compared with IPAH patients.[33,34,35] Furthermore, systemic sclerosis also causes lung fibrosis and diastolic left heart disease, both conditions which increase pulmonary pressures, emphasizing the importance of a complete evaluation when PH is suspected and need for right heart catheterization (RHC) to confirm diagnosis of PH to accurately classify its etiology. The high prevalence of PAH and worse outcome in the scleroderma population, as well as the complex systemic process, mandates a practice of careful screening to ensure early detection and initiation of appropriate treatment.[35] In systemic lupus erythematosus, the prevalence is estimated at 6.2% and PAH is also seen in patients with rheumatoid arthritis and other vasculitides, though at lower frequency.[36]

HIV infection is a risk for PAH with incidence reported approximately 0.5%, or 6–12 times that of the general population.[37,38] HIV-associated PAH has clinical, hemodynamic, and histologic characteristics similar to those seen in IPAH. The occurrence of PAH is independent of the CD4 count or previous opportunistic infections, and appears to be related to the duration of the HIV infection.[39] The mechanism of development of pulmonary arteriopathy remains unclear since neither the virus nor viral DNA has been found in pulmonary endothelial cells. It is speculated that the action of the virus is indirect, through secondary messenger such as cytokines, growth factors, endothelin, or viral proteins.[18,40] Uncontrolled studies suggest that patients with severe HIV-associated PAH could benefit from PAH-directed therapy.[41]

Portopulmonary hypertension is the development of PAH in association with elevated pressure in the portal circulation. Hemodynamic studies have shown that 2–6% of patients with portal hypertension have PH.[42,43] The incidence is higher among patients undergoing liver transplant evaluation, reported to be 4–15%; the degree of PAP elevation has significant impact on perioperative morbidity and survival for patients undergoing liver transplantation.[44] RHC is essential for diagnosis since several physiologic factors may increase PAPs with liver disease, such as a high flow state due to hyperdynamic circulation or fluid overload.[18] Long-term prognosis is related to the presence and severity of cirrhosis and to cardiac function.[45]

Patients with congenital heart disease (CHD) are at increased risk of developing PAH, particularly those with increased pulmonary blood flow from systemic-to-pulmonary shunts. Over time, increased blood flow results in an elevated pulmonary vascular resistance (PVR) leading to shunt reversal (Eisenmenger syndrome) with right-to-left shunting of flow across the defect. PAH can also develop from low-pressure–high-flow shunts, such as atrial septal defect (ASD).[18] Overall, PAH arises in 1.6–12.5 per million patients with 25–50% suffering from Eisenmenger syndrome.[46] Among patients with PAH, survival is worst for patients with CTD and HIV infection.[47]

Pathophysiology

The pulmonary vasculature is a low-pressure system with normal systolic PAP ranges of 15–30 mmHg and mean PAP (mPAP) of 9–18 mmHg, essentially functioning at less than one-tenth the resistance to flow observed in the systemic vascular bed due to the large cross-sectional area of the pulmonary circulation.[48] The 5th World Symposium defined PAH as mPAP greater than 25 mmHg and pulmonary arterial wedge pressure (PAWP) 15 mmHg or less as well as PVR greater than 3 Wood units, as defined by the ACCF/AHA 2009 Expert Consensus statement.[20,40] The prior definition of PH, which also included mPAP with exercise greater than 30 mmHg, was dropped at the 4th World Symposium due to insufficient knowledge regarding PAP response to exercise across age groups and modes of exercise.[49]

PAH is a state resulting from restricted flow through the pulmonary arterial circulation, which leads to pathological increases in PAP and PVR and ultimately right heart failure and death.[15] The main abnormality is due to loss of vascular luminal cross-section from vascular remodeling as a result of excessive cell proliferation and decreased rates of apoptosis of pulmonary artery smooth muscle cells and endothelial dysfunction; excessive vasoconstriction has a significant pathological contribution in about 20% of patients.[50,51,52] Like cancer and other chronic conditions, PAH does not have a single cause; the process by which pulmonary vasculopathy is initiated results from interaction of a predisposing state and one or more inciting stimuli, a concept termed a "multiple-hit model."[52,53,54] Essentially it is thought that a genetic abnormality or substrate first renders an individual susceptible; the second "hit" may be either a systemic disorder, an environmental trigger, or an additional genetic abnormality.

Histology

The natural history and evolution of vascular lesions in PAH has been difficult to fully evaluate since biopsies are difficult to obtain. It has been shown to be characterized by a process which involves all layers of the vessel wall (panvasculopathy) including intimal hyperplasia and fibrosis, medial hypertrophy, adventitial proliferation, and in-situ thrombosis.[55] Over time, obstruction of vascular flow results in further remodeling and formation of plexiform arteriopathy, an endstage lesion in PAH. These pathologic lesions can be localized or diffuse and are present in differing degrees.

Prostacyclin and thromboxane

Prostacyclin (PGI_2) and thromboxane A_2 are the major metabolites of arachidonic acid via enzymatic action of prostacyclin synthase in the endothelium. Prostacyclin acts through the second messenger cyclic adenosine monophosphate (cAMP) to produce several effects in the vasculature: vasodilatation, antiproliferative actions of smooth muscle cells, and platelet inhibition. Conversely, thromboxane A_2 is a vasoconstrictor, and promotes cellular proliferation and platelet activation.[56] In PAH, there is an imbalance in these metabolites with decreased prostacyclin and increased thromboxane. Furthermore, prostacyclin synthase activity has shown to be decreased in small and medium-sized pulmonary arteries (Figure 22.2).[57,58]

Endothelin-1

Endothelin-1 (ET-1) is a 21-amino acid sequence belonging to a family of peptides that acts to modulate vascular tone. ET-1 is a potent vasoconstrictor and also stimulates production of pulmonary vascular smooth muscle. It exerts its effects through two receptors: ET_A receptors located on smooth muscle cells and

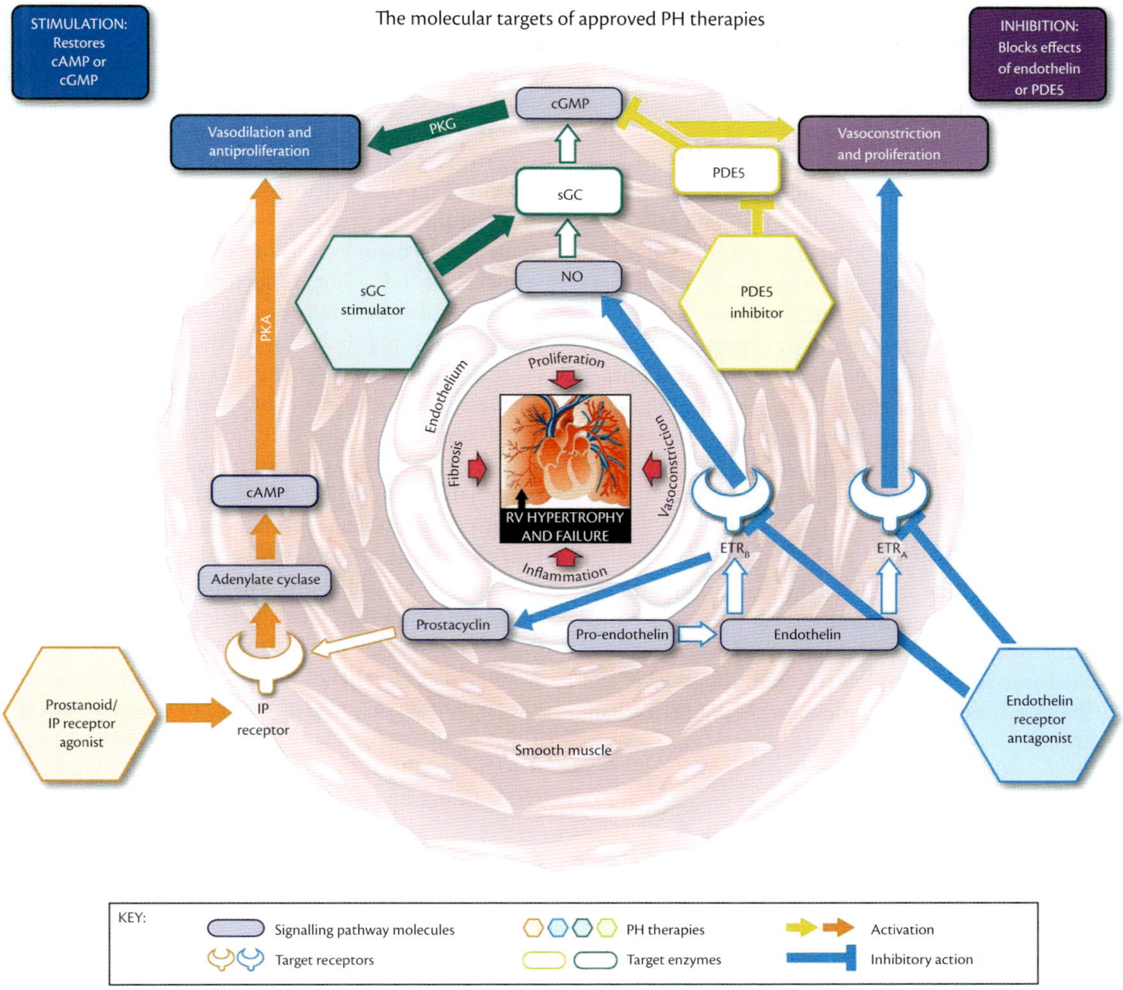

Fig. 22.2 The molecular targets, signalling pathways, and modes of action of approved pulmonary hypertension (PH) therapies. cAMP, cyclic adenosine monophosphate; cGMP, cyclic guanosine monophosphate; ETRA, endothelin receptor A; ETRB, endothelin receptor B; IP, prostacyclin; NO, nitric oxide; PDE5, phosphodiesterase type 5; PKA, phosphate kinase A; PKG, cGMP-dependent protein kinase; sGC, soluble guanylate cyclase.

Reprinted from Thorax, 2016 Jan;71(1), Humbert M, Ghofrani HA. The molecular targets of approved treatments for pulmonary arterial hypertension, 73–83.

ET_B receptors on vascular endothelial cells and smooth muscle cells.[59,60] Activation of the ET_A and ET_B receptors on smooth muscle cells induces vasoconstriction and cellular proliferation and hypertrophy, whereas stimulation of ET_B receptors on endothelial cells mediates vasodilatation via nitric oxide and prostacyclin production. Activation of the ET_A receptor results in potent vasoconstrictive response through G-protein-coupled phospholipase C activation, leading to 1,4,5-inositol triphosphate formation with resultant intracellular Ca^{2+} release. The ET_B receptor has also been shown to mediate the clearance of ET-1 from the circulatory system. The plasma level of ET-1 has been shown to be increased in PAH and correlate with disease severity and prognosis. Its level has been shown to be inversely proportional to the magnitude of the pulmonary blood flow and cardiac output (see Figure 22.2).[58,61,62]

Nitric oxide pathway

Nitric oxide (NO) is a labile gas produced from arginine by NO synthase in the vascular endothelial cells that freely diffuses across capillary membranes. Physiologically, NO stimulates dilatation of vascular smooth muscle at both the arterial and venous levels as well as exerting antiproliferative effects.[63,64] Its actions are produced through its second messenger cyclic guanosine monophosphate (cGMP), which is degraded by phosphodiesterase-5 (PDE-5). Eleven different families of PDE isoenzymes have been identified, which vary in tissue location and mechanisms of action.[65,66] PAH is associated with reduced endogenous NO production leading to decreased levels of cGMP resulting in altered calcium handling with subsequent vasoconstriction and cellular proliferation.[67] Furthermore, PDE-5 expression is upregulated in PAH, leading to increased metabolism of NO-derived cGMP. Thus PDE-5 inhibitors, by selectively blocking this enzyme, promote accumulation of intracellular cGMP and enhance NO-mediated effects (see Figure 22.2).[58,68] Since both impaired synthesis of NO and insufficient stimulation of the NO–sCG–cGMP axis is present in PAH, another mechanism to increase the effects of NO pathway is by utilizing direct soluble guanylate cyclase (sGC) stimulator, riociguat. This new therapy has a dual mode of action in that it sensitizes sGC to endogenous NO by stabilizing NO-sGC binding and also directly stimulates sGC independently of NO. Since both impaired synthesis of NO and insufficient stimulation of the NO-sCG-cGMP axis is present in PAH, another mechanism to increase the effects of NO pathway is by utilizing direct soluble guanylate cyclase (sGC) stimulator, riociguat. This new therapy has a dual mode of action in that it sensitizes sGC to endogenous NO by stabilizing NO-sGC binding and also directly stimulates sGC independently of NO.[69]

Serotonin

Serotonin (5-hydroxytryptamine) contributes to PAH through vasoconstriction and smooth muscle cell hyperplasia and hypertrophy.[70] Elevated plasma serotonin and reduced content of serotonin in platelets have been reported in idiopathic PAH (IAPH) and PAH associated with ingestion of dexfenfluramine, which increases the release of serotonin from platelets and inhibits its reuptake.[71,72] Furthermore, mutations in the serotonin transporter (5-HTT) and its receptor 5-HT2B have been described in PAH patients.[73] However, it is not certain if serotonin level alone is a determinant of PAH severity based on the observation that treatment with selective serotonin reuptake inhibitor (SSRI) does not increase incidence of PAH and may have a protective effect against hypoxia.[73]

Vasoactive intestinal peptide

Vasoactive intestinal peptide (VIP) is a member of the glucagon-growth-hormone-releasing family. It is a potent vasodilator, as well as an inhibitor of vascular smooth muscle cell proliferation. VIP levels have been found to be low in patients with PAH and treatment with VIP has been shown to decrease PAP and PVR in human subjects.[74,75]

Additional mechanisms

Inhibition of voltage-dependent potassium channels (Kv) has been linked to factors which promote PAH, such as hypoxia and fenfluamine derivatives.[76,77] Abnormalities of the coagulant cascade including increased levels of von Willebrand factor, plasminogen activator inhibitor-1, and plasma fibrinopeptide have been reported in PAH patients.[78] Furthermore, inflammatory factors such as pro-inflammatory cytokines, interleukin-6, and autoantibodies have been implicated in PAH.[79]

Genetic abnormalities

Mutations in two genes in the TGFβ receptor pathway, have been identified in patients with heritable PAH (HPAH).[80,81] BMPR2 controls the growth of smooth muscle cells in the vascular system by activation of Smad and LIM kinase. The mutations in the BMPR2 receptor protein results in aberrations of signal transduction in the pulmonary smooth muscle cell which leads to cellular proliferation and dysfunctional apoptosis. Less common mutations associated with PAH occur in activin-like kinase (Alk1), another TGFβ receptor implicated in patients with hereditary hemorrhagic telangiectasia.[82]

The right ventricle in pulmonary arterial hypertension

The critical importance of the integrity of RV function, the major determinant of functional capacity and prognosis in PAH, is well recognized. The RV is a thin walled, crescent-shaped structure, formed by the RV free wall and the interventricular septum. Designed to work optimally with the low-pressure system of the pulmonary vasculature, the compliant RV is able to pump the same stoke volume as the left ventricle (LV) with much less work.[83,84] In PAH, the RV must adapt to function in the presence of increased PVR. It is becoming apparent that even if PAH-specific treatments can improve or reverse pulmonary arterial pathology, this does not necessarily result in functional improvement or increase in survival unless it occurs in conjunction with improvement in RV function.[85]

The concept of the pulmonary arterial system and RV needing to work in concert is referred to as "PA–RV coupling". The initial adaptive response of the RV to increased afterload is usually RV hypertrophy, which has been seen within 96 hours of inducing PH in animal models.[86] RV hypertrophy can be followed by contractile dysfunction and/or RV dilatation for further compensatory maneuver to maintain cardiac output by increase in preload to offset decrease in fractional shortening. Continued remodeling of the RV soon causes alterations in RV shape from crescent to concentric, also causing flattening of the septum. Due to interventricular dependence, these changes cause LV diastolic dysfunction and decrease in LV end-diastolic volume, resulting in further decline in stroke volume and deterioration of end-organ function.[87,88] However, RV response to increased pressure and the development of RV failure in PAH is quite variable; the reasons why some RVs remain compensated, maintaining adequate cardiac output for prolonged periods of time, while others immediately dilate and fail, remain unclear. Some mechanisms have been investigated, including retention of the "fetal" genotype believed to be a contributory factor for favorable survival of PAH associated with CHD, polymorphisms in genes related to the renin–angiotensin–aldosterone system, and differences in the degree of ischemia and apoptosis.[83,89,90] There is currently intense interest in determining mechanisms of RV failure and more precise methods of imaging the RV are currently under investigation, notably using cardiac MRI (CMR).

Clinical presentation and diagnosis of pulmonary arterial hypertension

Evaluating patients with suspected PH entails the following measures: having a high index of suspicion for PAH in patients presenting with clinical symptoms and/or those who have risk factors for developing PAH; undergoing screening evaluation utilizing Doppler echocardiography, recognizing strengths and pitfalls of echocardiogram in imaging right-sided cardiac structures and estimating PAP; determining presence of any underlying cause(s) of PAH; performing RHC to confirm the diagnosis of PAH and perform acute vasodilatory challenge in appropriate patients; and assessing exercise and functional capacity to determine severity of disease and prognosis. A diagnostic approach including pivotal and contingent tests and rationale is shown in Figure 22.3.[91]

Clinical presentation: symptoms and physical examination

Diagnosing PAH can be challenging because of the nonspecific nature of the presenting symptoms, relative rarity of the disease, and the fact that routine tests are not adequate to make the diagnosis. In the NIH Registry of 187 IPAH patients, the most common presenting symptoms were dyspnea on exertion followed by fatigue, chest pain, syncope, palpitations, and lower extremity edema.[15] Patients with PAH usually do not tend to tolerate atrial arrhythmias, such as atrial fibrillation, due to loss of cardiac output contribution from the atrium kick, and this can precipitate syncope. Other causes of angina include a reduced aorta-to-RV systolic gradient and compression of the left main artery by the enlarged pulmonary artery.[40] A directed history needs to be performed to determine presence of any underlying causes and/or risk factors for PAH such as any

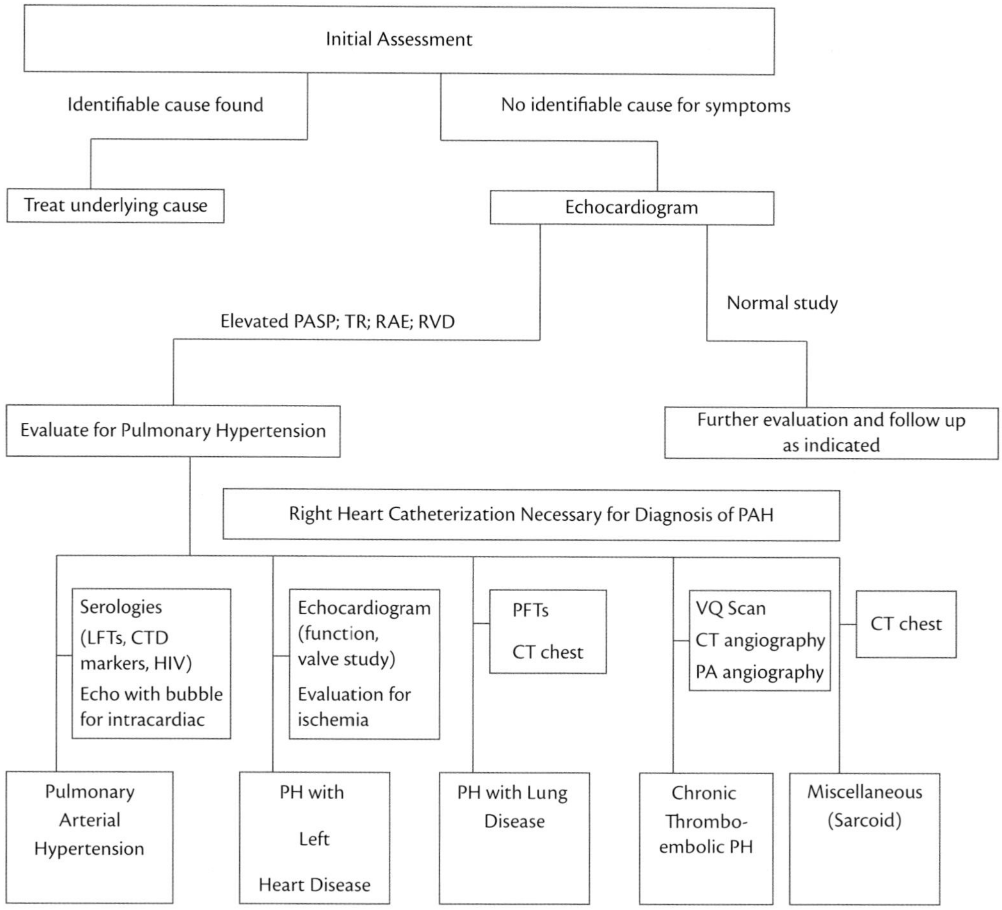

Fig. 22.3 Diagnostic algorithm for evaluation of pulmonary hypertension.
Park, MH. Pulmonary hypertension and right heart failure: Light at the end of the tunnel? In: Challenges in Heart Failure; Mehra MR, ed.

history or symptoms related to CTD, particularly systemic sclerosis; Raynaud's phenomenon has been reported in patients with IPAH in the absence of other systemic signs of CTD.[92,93] Obtaining history of other comorbidities known to be associated with PAH is important, such as HIV, portal hypertension, CHD. History of anorexigen use, especially the diet drug fenfluramine, should be elucidated since its association with development of PAH has been well documented (Table 22.1).[40,94]

Although the physical examination findings are mostly nonspecific, certain features should raise the suspicion of PAH. The classic finding is an accentuated pulmonic component of S2 which is heard best at the apex and is present in most patients with PAH due to high pulmonary pressures causing forceful closure of the pulmonic valve.[40,95] RV hypertrophy from increased pressure can cause a left parasternal lift and a right ventricular S4. An early systolic click and a midsystolic ejection murmur signify turbulent pulmonary outflow. The most common valvular dysfunction associated with PAH is tricuspid regurgitation which causes a holosystolic murmur that increases with inspiration and increased jugular v waves. Pulmonary regurgitation causes a diastolic murmur. The presence of hepatojugular reflux and pulsatile liver indicate high central venous pressure. Findings indicative of RV failure include RV S3, hepatomegaly, distended jugular veins, ascites, peripheral edema, hypotension and diminished pulse pressure, and cool extremities. Lung sounds are usually normal in patients with PAH. Some physical examination findings which can help to determine underlying cause of PAH include sclerodactyly, arthritis, Raynaud's phenomenon, rashes, and telangiectasias for CTD; obesity, large neck width, and enlarged tonsils for disordered breathing; splenomegaly, spider angiomata, palmar erythema, sclera icterus, caput medusa, and ascites for portal hypertension; central cyanosis for hypoxemia and

Table 22.1 Updated Classification for Drug- and Toxin-induced PAH

Definite	Possible
Aminorex	Cocaine
Fenfluramine	Phenylpropanolamine
Dexfenfluramine	St. John's wort
Toxic rapeseed oil	Chemotherapeutic agentsInterferon α and β
Benfluorex	Amphetamine-like drugs
SSRIs	
Likely	**Unlikely**
Amphetamines	Oral contraceptives
L-tryptophan	Estrogen
Methamphetamines	Cigarette smoking
Dasatinib	

PAH: Pulmonary arterial hypertension; SSRI: S, selective serotonin reuptake inhibitors.

Taken from Simonneau G, Gatzoulis MA, Adatia I, et al. Updated clinical classification of pulmonary hypertension. Journal of the American College of Cardiology, 2013; 62:D34–41.

Table 22.2 Patient groups with high-risk features of pulmonary arterial hypertension

Patient groups	Rationale/comments	Evaluations
Known genetic mutations predisposing to pulmonary hypertension	BMPR2 mutation identified as the main cause of inherited PAH Early detection of PAH 20% chance of developing PAH	Echocardiogram yearly RHC in echocardiogram demonstrates evidence of PAH[a]
First-degree relatives of patient with BMPR2 mutation or within pedigree of ≥2 patients with a diagnosis of PAH	Inherited as autosomal dominant trait Characterized by genetic anticipation and incomplete penetrance Phenotype may not be expressed in all generations but when expressed, it occurs at an earlier age and is associated with more severe disease	Genetic counseling as appropriate and BMPR2 genotyping Proceed as above if positive
Systemic sclerosis	Incidence of PAH about 8% by RHC and 27% by echocardiogram screening Response to approved therapy not as favorable compared with IPAH Early detection and diagnosis imperative	Echocardiogram yearly RHC if echocardiogram shows evidence of PAH[a]
Portal hypertension	Prevalence of PAH about 4% in candidates of OLT PAH associated with significant risk of perioperative morbidity and mortality in OLT	Echocardiogram for all candidates being considered for OLT RHC if echocardiogram shows evidence of PAH[a]
HIV infection	Prevalence of PAH 0.5%	Echocardiogram if symptoms or signs suggestive of PAH RHC if echocardiogram shows evidence of RHC[a]
Congenital heart disease with shunt	Overall have better prognosis compared with other subgroups High probability of PAH developing in unrepaired shunt (Eisenmenger syndrome)	Echocardiogram and RHC at time of diagnosis Consider repair of defect if shunt significant and operable
Prior appetite suppressant use	Incidence of PAH reported 0.005% if agent used >3 months	Echocardiogram if symptomatic
Recent acute PE	About 3–4% risk of CTEPH Negative V/Q scan excludes CTEPH	V/Q scan 3 months after PE if symptomatic Pulmonary angiogram if positive

CTEPH, chronic thromboembolic pulmonary hypertension; IPAH, idiopathic pulmonary arterial hypertension; OLT, orthotopic liver transplant; PE, pulmonary embolism; RHC, right heart catheterization V/Q, ventilation–perfusion.

[a] Echocardiographic evidence of PAH includes elevated right ventricular systolic pressure or right heart chamber enlargement.

shunting; digital clubbing for CHD or pulmonary venous occlusive disease (PVOD).

Screening of asymptomatic patients with risk factors

Patients with risk factors, associated conditions, or family history of PAH may need screening even if they are asymptomatic. High-risk populations for PAH include those with a *BMPR2* genetic mutation or first-degree relatives of a patient with known mutation with hereditary PAH. Other groups include patients on the scleroderma spectrum of disease, and those with HIV infection, portal hypertension, prior appetite suppressant use, recent acute pulmonary embolism, or CHD with systemic-to-pulmonary shunts (Table 22.2).[40,95]

Diagnostic evaluations for pulmonary arterial hypertension

For patients where PAH is suspected by their symptoms, physical examination, and/or presence of risk factors, an algorithm outlining pivotal and recommended tests is summarized in Figure 22.3.[91] Electrocardiography is not a particularly useful as a sole screening tool (sensitivity 55–73% and specificity 70%) but provides an essential evaluation to document baseline features.[96] There are key ECG findings that suggest presence of PAH or increase the likelihood such as right atrial (RA) enlargement, right axis deviation, and RV hypertrophy which can be present with a strain pattern; the absence of these findings does not exclude the presence of PAH or severe hemodynamic abnormalities. In the original NIH registry of IPAH patients, 87% of patients had evidence of RV hypertrophy and 79% had right axis deviation, findings consistent with an advanced stage of PAH.[15] Ventricular arrhythmias are rare in PAH but supraventricular arrhythmia may be present in advanced stages, most commonly atrial flutter but also atrial fibrillation, which usually are associated with clinical deterioration.[97] Chest radiography is useful to assess for presence of abnormalities which may suggest presence of PAH, though these are nonspecific, and to evaluate for other abnormalities such as hyperinflation (chronic obstructive pulmonary disease), kyphosis (restrictive lung disease), or pulmonary venous congestion (heart failure) which may reveal other associated conditions. Findings indicative of PAH include enlarged main and hilar pulmonary arteries, peripheral hypovascularity indicating loss of peripheral blood vessels (pruning), and RA and RV enlargement in retrosternal space as seen in lateral view (Figure 22.4a).

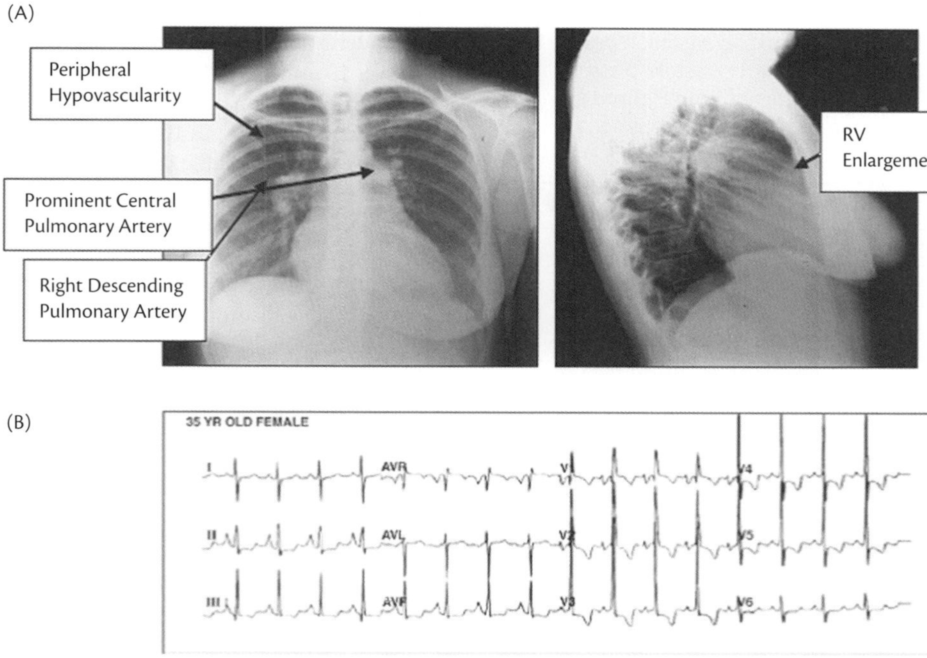

Fig. 22.4 Chest radiograph and electrocardiogram in pulmonary arterial hypertension.

Reprinted from Journal of the American College of Cardiology, 53, McLaughlin VV, Archer SL, Badesch DB, et al. ACCF/AHA 2009 expert consensus document on pulmonary hypertension: a report of the American College of Cardiology Foundation Task Force on Expert Consensus Documents, 1573–1619, (2009) with permission from Elsevier.

Echocardiography

Transthoracic Doppler echocardiography (TTE) is the most useful noninvasive screening test for patients with suspected PH by providing assessment of PAP and right-sided cardiac features, as well as identifying possible cardiac causes for PH such as LV dysfunction, valvular abnormalities, and CHD. The estimation of PAP is based on the measurement of the tricuspid regurgitation (TR) peak gradient by utilizing the modified Bernoulli equation $4v^2$, in which v is the velocity of the TR jet in meters per second. The RV systolic pressure (RVSP) is derived by adding the right atrial pressure (RAP) to the gradient: RVSP = $4v^2$ + RAP. The RAP can be estimated based on the diameter and respiratory variation of the inferior vena cava or by assigning a fixed value of 5 or 10 mmHg. A potential systolic gradient between the RV and PA should be considered in assuming equivalent estimated value between RVSP and PAP. Findings on echocardiogram that are suggestive of elevated PAP include RA and RV enlargement, RV hypertrophy, reduced RV systolic function, pulmonary artery dilatation, interatrial septal bowing to the left, and systolic flattening of the interventricular septum from chronic RV pressure overload, which results in the D-shaped appearance of the LV (Figure 22.5). Increased velocity of pulmonary valve regurgitation and a short acceleration time of RV ejection into the pulmonary artery are other echocardiographic variables that reinforce suspicion of PH. In addition to obtaining the estimation of PA systolic pressure, echocardiography also provides important prognostic information (see Assessing prognosis and response to therapy in PAH).

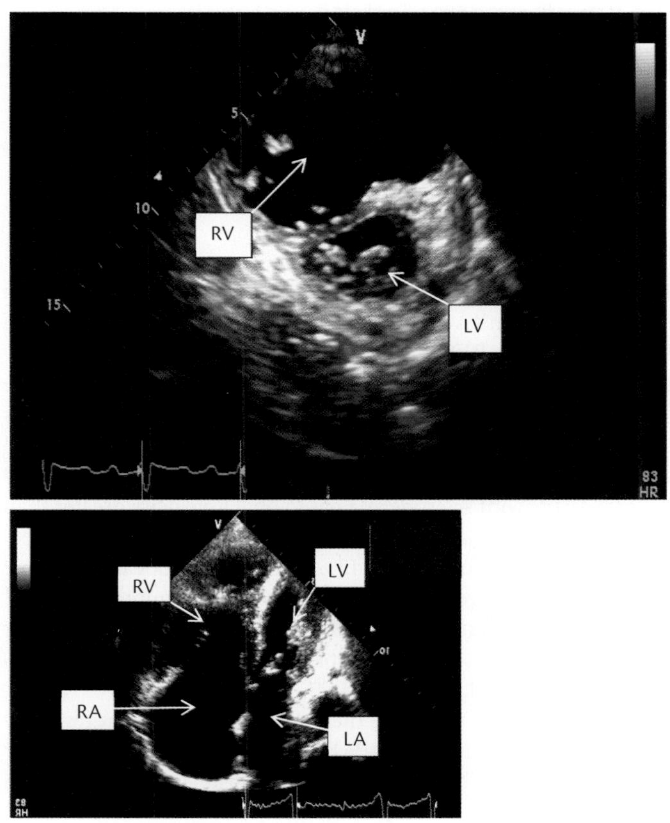

Fig. 22.5 Echocardiogram of a patient with severe pulmonary arterial hypertension.

Mild PH has been defined as a tricuspid jet velocity of 2.8–3.4 m/s or TR peak gradient of 31–46 mmHg (using RA pressure estimation of 5 mmHg) by the expert consensus at the Evian meeting in

Table 22.3 Recommended criteria for estimating the presence of pulmonary hypertension based on tricuspid regurgitation peak velocity and Doppler-calculated pulmonary artery systolic pressure at rest (assuming a normal right atrial pressure of 5 mmHg) and on additional echocardiographic variables suggestive of pulmonary hypertension

	Class[a]	Level[b]
Echocardiographic diagnosis of PH unlikely:		
◆ TR velocity ≤ 2.8 m/s ◆ PASP ≤36 mmHg ◆ No additional echocardiographic variables suggestive of PH	I	B
Echocardiographic diagnosis of PH possible:		
◆ TR velocity ≤ 2.8 m/s ◆ PASP ≤ 36 mmHg but presence of additional echocardiographic variables suggestive of PH	IIa	C
OR ◆ TR velocity 2.9–3.4 m/s ◆ PASP 37–50 mmHg with/without additional echocardiographic variables suggestive of PH	IIa	C
Echocardiographic diagnosis of PH likely:		
◆ TR velocity ≥3.4 m/s ◆ PASP >50 mmHg with/without additional echocardiographic variables suggestive of PH	I	B

[a] Class of recommendation; [b] level of evidence.

PASP, pulmonary artery systolic pressure; PH, pulmonary hypertension; TR, tricuspid regurgitation.

Galie N, Hoeper MM, Humber M, et al. Guidelines for the diagnosis and treatment of pulmonary hypertension: The task force for the diagnosis and treatment of pulmonary hypertension of the European Society of Cardiology (ESC) and the European Respiratory Society (ERS), endorsed by the International Society of Heart and Lung Transplantation (ISHLT). European Heart Journal (2009);30:2493–2537, by permission of Oxford University Press.

1998.[98] The American College of Cardiology Foundation/American Heart Association (ACC/AHA) Expert Consensus Document on PH states that an RVSP greater than 40 mmHg warrants evaluation of unexplained symptoms in the absence of left heart disease or severe lung disease.[40] Defining the TR velocity cutoff values using RHC as reference has been assessed in two large screening studies. One trial, evaluating the reliability of prospective screening of patients with scleroderma based on TR velocity greater than 2.5 m/s in symptomatic patients or greater than 3.0 m/s irrespective of symptoms, found that 45% of cases of echocardiographic diagnosis of PH were falsely positive.[32] Among symptomatic HIV patients using PH criteria based on TR velocity greater than 2.5 or greater than 2.8 m/s, this study reported false-positive rates of 72% and 29%, respectively (Table 22.3).[99]

It is imperative to recognize the limitations of echocardiography in the evaluation of PH. First, PAH is defined as mean PAP greater than 25 mmHg.[49] While it is theoretically feasible to calculate mean PAP from RVSP estimation (mean PAP = 0.61 × PASP + 2 mmHg) and thus make the diagnosis of PAH from the echocardiogram, studies evaluating correlation coefficients between RVSP derived from TR jet and PASP from RHC have been inconsistent, correlations ranging from poor to significant.[100,101,102,103] In patients with severe TR, use of the modified form of the Bernoulli equation may lead to underestimation of PA systolic pressure while overestimation by over 10 mmHg for PA systolic pressure has been reported in patients with near normal pressures.[100,104,105] Several factors attribute to the varying results: in 10–25% of patients with PH the quality of the TR Doppler profile is insufficient to reliably estimate the RVSP.[106,107] Administering a small amount of IV bolus of agitated saline contrast or encapsulated microbubble contrast agents can help to enhance the signal to improve visualization; however, these agents need to be used with caution in patients with severe PH and/or respiratory disorder. Other factors include the difficulty of obtaining reliable images in obese patients with lung disorders, and lack of accuracy of the RA pressure estimation used.[107,108,109,110]

Other limitations of echocardiography relate to the difficulty in optimal imaging of the right heart, due to its anterior position and its multiplanar morphology which make it difficult to use geometric calculations to estimate the systolic function or to use summation-type volume calculations. Furthermore, as PAH progresses and the RV fails, the tricuspid jet velocity can actually decrease, which can be misinterpreted as a sign of improvement. The TR velocity is decreasing, not because of decrease in afterload and improvement, but due to further dilatation and deterioration of RV systolic function and/or increase in RA pressure. Thus, making decisions about therapeutic changes solely based on Doppler estimates of RVSP can be misleading and it is better to consider assessing full hemodynamics via RHC.[40] Another major limitation of echocardiography is that there is no precise method to estimate the PAWP, a critical determinant in defining pulmonary arterial versus venous hypertension.

Advances in techniques have been developed to help improve the usefulness of echocardiography in the evaluation of PAH. Measurement of tricuspid annulus plane systolic excursion (TAPSE) using M-mode analysis has been shown to predict survival in PAH; TAPSE greater than 1.8 cm corresponded to an 88% 2-year survival compared to 50% survival for those with TAPSE less than 1.8 cm.[111] The Tei index, which combines information on RV systolic and diastolic time intervals independent of heart rate, RV pressure, dilatation, or TR, has also been shown to correlate with survival.[112] A recent study has proposed an echocardiographic-based prediction to differentiate between PAH and pulmonary venous hypertension, using cardiac structural indices in a stepwise scoring system which has been shown to correlate with RHC-derived PVR and PAWP[113]

Echocardiography is essential to rule out left heart disease as a cause of PH since diagnosis of PAH includes the absence of clinically significant left heart disease. Assessment of LV size, structure, and function is important to exclude LV systolic and diastolic dysfunction, enlargement, and hypertrophy. Close scrutiny for diastolic abnormalities is becoming more relevant since older patients with multiple cardiac risk factors (e.g., systemic hypertension) are being diagnosed with elevated pulmonary pressures.[24,25] Presence of LA enlargement, even in the absence of obvious LV dysfunction, should raise the suspicion of elevated left-sided pressures and a diagnosis of pulmonary venous hypertension rather than PAH (Box 22.2).[93] In these patients, it is critical to obtain a reliable PAWP during RHC; if a satisfactory PAWP wave form cannot be obtained, left heart catheterization may need to be performed to accurately measure the LV end-diastolic pressure (LVEDP) to definitively rule out pulmonary venous hypertension. PAH-specific

Box 22.2 Risk factors favoring diagnosis of diastolic heart failure

Clinical features

- Age >65 years
- Elevated systolic blood pressure
- Elevated pulse pressure
- Obesity
- Hypertension
- Coronary artery disease
- Diabetes mellitus
- Atrial fibrillation

Echocardiography

- Left atrial enlargement
- Concentric remodeling (relative wall thickness >0.45)
- Left ventricular hypertrophy
- Elevated left ventricular filling pressures (grade II–IV diastolic dysfunction)

Interim evaluation (after echocardiography)

- Symptomatic response to diuretic drugs
- Exaggerated increase in systolic blood pressure with exercise
- Re-review of chest radiograph consistent with heart failure

Data sourced from Galie N, Hoeper MM, Humber M, et al. Guidelines for the diagnosis and treatment of pulmonary hypertension: The task force for the diagnosis and treatment of pulmonary hypertension of the European Society of Cardiology (ESC) and the European Respiratory Society (ERS), endorsed by the International Society of Heart and Lung Transplantation (ISHLT). Eur Heart J 2009;30:2493–2537; Park MH, McLaughlin VV. Pulmonary hypertension: Hemodynamic assessment and response to vasodilators. In: Cardiac Catheterization, Coronary & Peripheral Angiograpy, and Interventional Procedures. London, Informa Healthcare, 2010.

therapies can worsen PH due to left-sided heart disease by precipitating pulmonary edema.[114] Echocardiography is needed to assess for valvular abnormality and CHD, which can precede or coincide with diagnosis of PH. An echocardiographic contrast ("bubble") study using agitated saline solution can screen for presence of intracardiac shunting. Transesophageal echocardiography (TEE) can add more refined structural information in diagnosing sinus venosus ASD, abnormal pulmonary venous drainage, or patent ductus arteriosus.[40,110]

Determining the etiology of pulmonary arterial hypertension

The next set of evaluations in PH is directed at determining its etiology. Routine biochemistry and hematology assessments are required in all patients. Serological testing to screen for underlying CTD, HIV, and hepatitis is mandatory. Anti-nuclear antibodies strongly predict the presence of CTD but it should be noted that up to 40% of patients with IPAH have elevated anti-nuclear antibodies, usually in low titer (<1:80).[116] Systemic sclerosis is the most important CTD to exclude since it is associated with a high prevalence of PAH. Anti-centromere antibodies are usually positive in limited scleroderma whereas U3-RNP is typically positive for the diffuse variety of scleroderma. Additional disease-specific anti-nuclear antibodies should be assessed to test for systemic lupus erythmatosus and rheumatoid arthritis. PAH is associated with HIV, and screening with a serologic test is mandatory, with positive results being confirmed by Western blot. Assessment for liver function abnormality is required since portal hypertension is associated with PAH and can be seen in the setting of cirrhosis. If liver function tests are abnormal, screening for hepatitis is recommended. Differentiating liver function abnormality as a secondary cause due to right heart failure and congestion versus portal hypertension can be difficult. Further evaluations with imaging of the liver using abdominal ultrasound and/or portal vein ultrasound, or measurement of transhepatic gradient during RHC, which is done by wedging the catheter in the hepatic vein, can help to determine the cause.[40,95] Thyroid disease is commonly seen in PAH and need to be assessed at screening and during follow-up on PAH-specific treatments, especially if there is any sudden clinical change.[117,118]

It is imperative to fully evaluate pulmonary function and physiology to rule out significant hypoxic lung disease as the primary cause of dyspnea. In patients with PAH, a pulmonary function test (PFT) usually demonstrates decreased lung diffusion capacity for carbon monoxide (LD_{CO}), typically in the range of 40–80% predicted, and mild to moderately reduced lung volumes. Any evidence of significant airway obstruction and/or restriction should prompt search for an alternative diagnosis. If PFTs suggest parenchymal lung disease, such as chronic obstructive pulmonary disease (COPD) or interstitial lung disease, high-resolution CT is needed to determine severity. Chest CT is also useful to determine the presence of interstitial and/or fibrotic changes often found in association with CTD and PAH. Pulmonary capillary hemangiomatosis can produce thickening of the septae and centrilobular ground-glass attenuations.[119] PVOD can produce local areas of congestion. Overnight oximetry or polysomnography can evaluate for obstructive sleep apnea or hypopnea.

Full evaluation for chronic thromboembolic disease in all patients with unexplained dyspnea and PH is essential since chronic thromboembolic pulmonary hypertension (CTEPH) is potentially surgically treatable. The incidence of CTEPH is estimated to be 3.8% within 2 years of surviving pulmonary embolism. Young age, a large perfusion defect, and idiopathic clinical presentation are associated with a higher probability of CTEPH.[120] Ventilation–perfusion (V/Q) scintigraphy remains the screening test of choice for CTEPH because it is more highly sensitive than a CT angiogram.[121,122] A normal or low probability V/Q scan effectively rules out CTEPH with a sensitivity of 90–100% and specificity of 94–100%. In PAH, the V/Q scan may be normal or show small peripheral unmatched and nonsegmental perfusion defects. An abnormal scan suggestive of CTEPH needs to be further studied using contrast-enhanced CT and/or pulmonary angiography with RHC for diagnosis and determination of indication for surgical thromboendarterectomy. In performing the pulmonary angiogram, a cautious approach is needed in patients with RA pressure greater than 20 mmHg; in patients with severe restriction of the pulmonary arterial bed and decreased pulmonary flow, use of nonionic or low-osmotic contrast with slowest flow rate and small volume is recommended.[123] Full evaluation for CTEPH is recommended to be done at an experienced center. Of note, patients with PVOD can present with large, asymmetrical defects which can be mistaken for CTEPH.[124]

Right heart catheterization

Complete invasive hemodynamic assessment by RHC is essential to confirm the presence of PH and to exclude elevated left-sided filling pressure to make the diagnosis of PAH. The definition of PAH requires mean PAP 25 mmHg or more and pulmonary capillary wedge pressure (PCWP) less than 15 mmHg (LVEDP or LA pressures); the ACCF/AHA Expert Consensus also includes PVR greater than 3 Wood units.[40] The essential components of RHC include RAP, PV pressure, systolic and diastolic PAP, mean PAP, PAWP (LVEDP or LA pressure), cardiac output (CO), cardiac index (CI), PVR, systemic blood pressure and heart rate, oxygen saturations (superior vena cava, inferior vena cava, RV, PA, systemic artery), and response to acute vasodilator.[40] While RHC remains the gold standard assessment of hemodynamics in PH, the utility of RHC is dependent on the accuracy and completeness of the data obtained. Furthermore, the RHC measurements are made with the patient at rest and may not reflect extent of hemodynamic burden with activity. There is currently no standardized protocol for performing or interpreting exercise RHC results but research is under way.

Components of right heart catheterization

Pulmonary artery wedge pressure

Accurate measurement of left heart filling pressure is critical for correct diagnosis of PAH, and misinterpretation of the wedge pressure is the most common error made in the invasive hemodynamic assessment of PAH. As stated, diagnosis of PAH requires both increase in mean PAP (≥25 mmHg) and normal PAWP or LVEDP (≤15 mmHg). The difference between these two measurements represents the transpulmonary gradient (TPG = mPAP − PAWP). Elevated PAWP is characteristic of PH in the setting of chronically elevated left-sided cardiac filling pressure, termed pulmonary venous hypertension, and is classified as WHO group 2 PH.[18] Pulmonary venous hypertension usually results from systolic and/or diastolic cardiac dysfunction or valvular disease. Treatments can differ significantly based on the left-sided filling pressure measurement. PAH is characterized by elevated PAP, normal PAWP, and elevated TPG whereas in pulmonary venous hypertension, PAP is elevated but TPG is normal due to elevated PAWP.[125]

The PAWP should always be measured at end-expiration of a spontaneous respiratory cycle. It is recommended that LVEDP should be obtained if there is any question about the accuracy of the wedge pressure tracing, especially if the patient has risk factors for left heart disease and diastolic dysfunction (see Box 22.2).[125] A recent study reported that as much as 50% of the patients who were presumed to have PAH based on the PAWP measurements had LVEDP greater than 15 mmHg.[126] The inaccuracy may, in large part, be due to reliance on the computer-generated mean wedge pressure, instead of assessing the value at the end-expiratory phase.[127] In patients with high suspicion of diastolic dysfunction causing PH and yet with normal PAWP, a fluid challenge of 500–1000 ml of saline may be needed to unmask the underlying physiology. Although left-sided filling pressures can be normal with diuresis, a significant increase in the wedge pressure and/or LVEDP with fluid bolus increases the likelihood that pulmonary venous hypertension (PVH) is present.[128]

The most common mistake in obtaining PAWP in PAH patients is "underwedging," which occurs when PA catheter is not advanced completely, resulting in a hybrid tracing of PAP and PAWP. This usually results in a falsely elevated PAWP reading which leads to misdiagnosing a patient as having pulmonary venous hypertension (Figure 22.6). One can measure oxygen saturation from the distal port with the catheter in the wedge position to test if the PA catheter is in the proper wedge position. If it is correctly placed, the measurement should be equal or close to the systemic arterial oxygen saturation (usually >90%) found by pulse oximetry. If it is markedly lower, the catheter is most likely underwedged. In patients with significant elevation of PAP and/or PA that is dilated, it can be challenging to obtain the correct PAWP placement. It can be helpful to allow the catheter to migrate distally with the balloon deflated and then carefully reinflate the balloon, following the pressure tracings closely; optimal placement is obtained with the balloon partially inflated. An intraluminal guide wire can also aid in advancing the catheter to a more distal position. All these maneuvers should be performed very cautiously and under direct

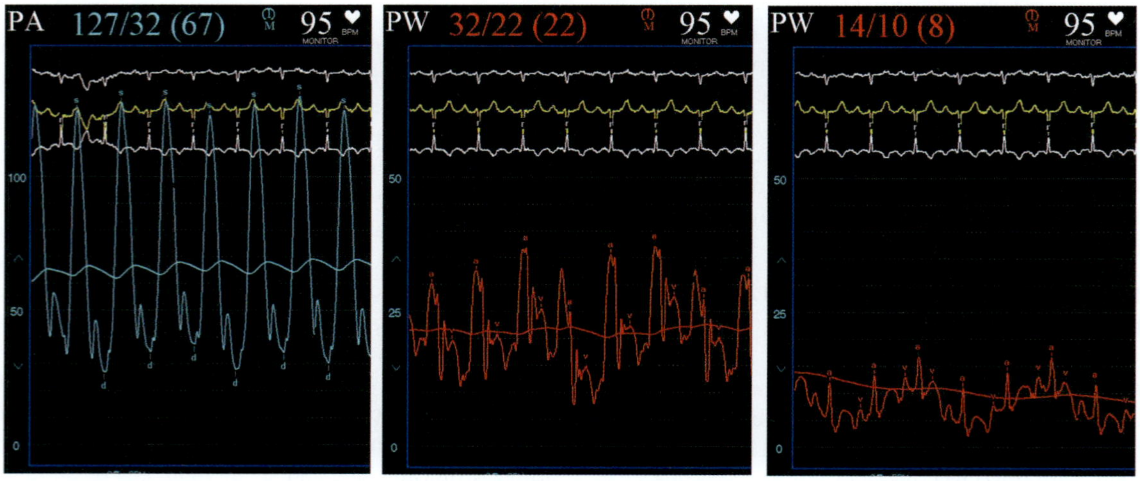

Fig. 22.6 Difference between correct pulmonary capillary wedge pressure and underwedged tracings.

Park MH, McLaughlin VV. Pulmonary hypertension: Hemodynamic assessment and response to vasodilators. In: Cardiac Catheterization, Coronary & Peripheral Angiograpy, and Interventional Procedures. London, Informa Healthcare, 2010.

fluoroscopic visualization since patients with PAH are at increased risk of PA rupture, a potentially fatal event.[125] The catheter can also be "overwedged," with excessive inflation of the balloon relative to the size of the vessel; this carries the risk of vessel rupture, which can lead to acute compromise, often fatal. The balloon should be slowly inflated at every measurement with close monitoring of the pressure tracings, with inflation stopped when a PAWP tracing is obtained. The presence of a "large" *v* wave can also lead to inaccurate reading of PAWP. The *v* wave is a normal finding on the wedge tracing and normally higher than the *a* wave, so what constitutes a "large" *v* wave is subjective. Common causes of a large *v* wave include mitral regurgitation (MR), though the height of the *v* wave is neither a sensitive nor a specific indicator of the degree of MR.[129,130] Other causes include any situations which increase volume or flow into a noncompliant LA, such as ventricular septal defect, mitral stenosis, cardiomyopathy of any etiology, or postoperative surgical conditions.

The following are characteristics of a physiologically reliable PAWP and steps that can aid in obtaining the measurement:[125,131,132,133] distinct *a* and *v* waves should be present (except in atrial fibrillation where the *a* wave will be absent); allowing a suitable length of time for steady state to occur in obtaining PAWP tracing (not immediately after the balloon is inflated) and recording at end-expiratory phase; a distinct immediate rise in pressure when balloon is deflated out of the wedge position; stable positioning of the catheter tip in PA when viewed under fluoroscopy with the balloon inflated (not moving back and forth); oxygen saturation greater than 90% measured in PCWP; multiple measurements of PCWP with similar results (Figure 22.7).

Cardiac output measurements

Accurate CO measurement is critical in calculating PVR and assessing prognosis in PAH. In the absence of an intracardiac shunt, the thermodilution method of measuring CO can be used if the results are consistent when measured in triplicate. The thermodilution method is thought to be inaccurate in the setting of severe TR and low CO, but it has been demonstrated that the thermodilution-derived CO still correlated with Fick measurements.[134] Fick determination of CO is the preferred method; however, potential errors include assumptions and inaccurate measurements of oxygen consumption.

Pulmonary artery pressure measurement

PAP varies with respiration and this needs to be considered in the interpretation of PAP measurements. During inspiration, the normal decrease in intrathoracic pressure slightly reduces the PAP relative to atmospheric pressure and increases venous return to the right heart, which results in increase in pulmonary blood flow. With normal expiration, intrathoracic pressure approaches atmospheric pressure. These hemodynamic changes can be more pronounced with large, partly artifactual swings in pressure that may occur in patients with chronic lung disease. The end-expiration phase is the recommended time for measuring PAP because the intrathoracic pressure approximates atmospheric pressure; measurements need to be averaged over 2–3 respiratory cycles.[40]

Pulmonary vascular resistance

The total pulmonary resistance (TPR) expresses the relationship between the mean PAP and CO: TPR = mean PAP × 80/CO (100–300 dyn s cm^{-5} or 10–30 MPa s m^{-3}). The PVR measures the resistance to flow imposed by pulmonary vasculature without the influence of the left-sided filling pressure: PVR = (mean PAP – PAWP) × 80/CO or PVR = TPG × 80/CO (20–130 dyn s cm^{-5} or 2–13 MPa s m^{-3}). Since PVR reflects the influence of TPG and CO and is only elevated if the vascular abnormality occurs within the precapillary pulmonary circulation, it is considered to be a more reliable diagnostic criterion for PAH. In the setting of elevated PAPs, PVR can distinguish between passive PH (elevated

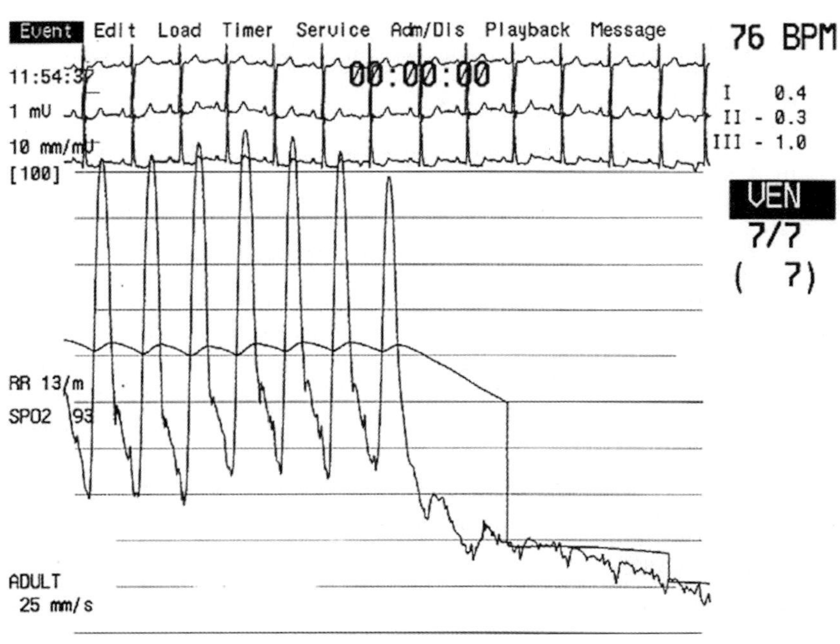

Fig. 22.7 Pulmonary artery and pulmonary arterial wedge tracing from a patient with severe pulmonary artery hypertension.
Park MH, McLaughlin VV. Pulmonary hypertension: Hemodynamic assessment and response to vasodilators. In: Cardiac Catheterization, Coronary & Peripheral Angiograpy, and Interventional Procedures. London, Informa Healthcare, 2010.

mPAP, normal PVR) from PH caused by pulmonary vascular disease (elevated mPAP, elevated PVR). By definition, in PAH both mPAP and PVR are elevated; PVR can also be elevated in patients with left-sided heart disease due to concomitant pulmonary arterial disease. However, in conditions with high flow states (sickle cell disease, portopulmonary hypertension, uncorrected CHD), PVR may be normal due to elevated CO but have elevated mPAP and pulmonary vascular disease.[40]

Safety of right heart catheterization in pulmonary arterial hypertension

Although RHC is necessary for establishing the diagnosis of PAH, concerns regarding risks in this population have been raised. A recent multicenter study which included 20 PH centers over a 5-year period with more than 7000 procedures evaluated the safety and risks of this procedure.[135] The overall incidence of serious adverse events was 1.1% (76 events). The most frequent complications were related to venous access (e.g., hematoma, pneumothorax); others included arrhythmia and hypotension due to vagal reactions or pulmonary vasoreactivity testing. Most of these complications resolved either spontaneously or after appropriate treatment. Four fatal events were reported in association with RHC and only one was directly related to performance of the procedure, which resulted in an overall procedure-related mortality of 0.05%. Thus the authors concluded that when performed in experienced centers, RHC in PAH patients is safe and associated with low morbidity rates.

Acute vasodilator testing

The use of vasodilator testing in PAH is based on the fact that acute vasodilator responsiveness identifies patients with a better prognosis and those who are more likely to have a sustained beneficial response to oral calcium channel blockers. The definition of what constitutes acute vasodilator "responder" has undergone changes over the years. The current definition is based on the retrospective study by Sitbon and colleagues who reported only 6.8% of the IPAH patients displayed long-term improvement with calcium channel blocker therapy.[136] Analysis of the data revealed the following parameters were associated with long-term success on calcium channel blocker therapy: a reduction in mean PAP to less than 37 mmHg, a fall or more than 31% in mPAP, a reduction in PVR to less than 6.7 Wood units, and a fall of over 45% in PVR. Based on this series, the European Society of Cardiology (ESC) and ACC guidelines proposed that an acute response to acute vasodilator testing be defined as a fall in mPAP of at least 10 mmHg to 40 mmHg or less, with an increased or unchanged CO.[40,136] There is a lack of data on patients with mean PAP less than 40 mmHg at baseline; if such patients demonstrate significant reduction in mean PAP in the setting of normal CO, trial of calcium channel blockers would be reasonable with close clinical follow-up.[40] For patients who meet the criteria and are placed on calcium channel blocker therapy, vigilant monitoring is essential. Those who improve to functional class I or II without the need for additional therapy are likely to do well, but this response is rare. Patients who do not meet the definition of an acute response should not be treated with calcium channel blockers.

Acute vasodilator response is even rarer in patients other than IPAH, including those with *BMPR2* genotype, anorexigen-induced PAH, or scleroderma spectrum disease.[137,138,139] Patients with advanced disease such as functional class (FC) IV symptoms, overt right heart failure, or hemodynamic markers of advanced process (high RAP and/or reduced CO, systemic hypotension) should not undergo acute vasodilator testing since these patients need prompt treatment with PAH-approved therapies and are not appropriate candidates for calcium channel blockers. The development of acute pulmonary edema during vasodilator testing should raise the suspicion of veno-occlusive disease or pulmonary capillary hemangiomatosis, in which therapy with a pulmonary vasodilator is contraindicated.[140]

Table 22.4 Agents used in acute vasodilator testing for pulmonary arterial hypertension

	Nitric oxide	Epoprostenol	Adenosine
Route of administration	Inhaled	Intravenous	Intravenous
Dose range	10–40 ppm	2–10 ng kg^{-1} min^{-1}	50–250 μg kg^{-1} min^{-1}
Dosing increments	None	1–2 ng kg^{-1} min^{-1} every 10–15 min	50 μg kg^{-1} min^{-1} every 2 min
Side effects	Increased left heart filling pressure in susceptible patients	Hypotension, headache, flushing, nausea	Chest tightness, dyspnea, atrioventricular block, hypotension

Reprinted from Journal of the American College of Cardiology, 53, McLaughlin VV, Archer SL, Badesch DB, et al. ACCF/AHA 2009 expert consensus document on pulmonary hypertension: a report of the American College of Cardiology Foundation Task Force on Expert Consensus Documents, 1573–1619, copyright (2009) with permission from Elsevier.

Intravenous epoprostenol and IV adenosine have both been studied as acute vasodilators. Both are short-acting, potent vasodilators and investigators have reported different degrees of responsiveness depending on the criteria used.[141,142,143] However, because both agents have the potential to cause systemic hypotension and side effects, using inhaled NO emerged as the vasodilator of choice due to its pulmonary selectivity, short half-life, and lack of systemic side effects (Table 22.4).[144] However, cost and the need for trained respiratory personnel for its administration have limited its availability.

Therapies for pulmonary arterial hypertension

Significant advances have been made in the treatment of PAH in the past two decades resulting in current approval by the FDA of fourteen PAH-specific therapies with different routes of administration with additional drugs under active development. Treatment of PAH with the current-era drug therapies has resulted in significant improvements in symptoms and slower clinical deterioration. A recent meta-analysis of 23 randomized clinical trials in PAH demonstrated a reduction in mortality by 43% and a 61% decrease in hospitalizations among patients treated with PAH-targeted drugs undergoing clinical trials.[145] However, PAH remains a chronic progressive disease without a cure. One of the compelling result to have emerged from these studies is that early detection and initiation of treatment is one of the most effective ways of applying therapies.[146] Treatment decisions are clinically derived based on the severity of disease, and the state of RV function is the most

Table 22.5 Assessment of risk in pulmonary arterial hypertension

Determinants of risk[a]	Lower risk (good prognosis)	Higher risk (poor prognosis)
Clinical evidence of RV failure	No	Yes
Progression of symptoms	Gradual	Rapid
WHO class	II, III[b]	IV
6MWD[c]	Longer (>400 m)	Shorter (<300 m)
Echocardiography	Normal to minimal RV dysfunction	Significant RV enlargement/ dysfunction; right atrial enlargement; pericardial effusion
Hemodynamics	Normal RAP and CI (RAP <10 mmHg; CI >2.5 L min^{-1} m^{-2})	High RAP and low CI (RAP >15 mmHg; CI <2.2 L min^{-1} m^{-2})
BNP[d]	Normal to minimally elevated	Significantly elevated

6MWD, 6 minute walk distance; BNP, brain natriuretic peptide; CI, cardiac index; IPAH, idiopathic pulmonary arterial hypertension; RAP, right atrial pressure; RV, right ventricle; WHO, World Health Organization.

[a] Most studies performed in IPAH patients. No single risk factor should be used to assess risk.

[b] Functional class III clinically encompasses a large range of disease severity. Using composite of detailed assessments of other objective characteristics is critical.

[c] 6MWD is influenced by age, gender, height, and presence of other systemic conditions.

[d] Limited data regarding utilizing BNP on risk.

Reprinted from Journal of the American College of Cardiology, 53, McLaughlin VV, Archer SL, Badesch DB, et al. ACCF/AHA 2009 expert consensus document on pulmonary hypertension: a report of the American College of Cardiology Foundation Task Force on Expert Consensus Documents, 1573–1619, copyright (2009) with permission from Elsevier.

critical determinant. Parameters which influence the prognosis of PAH are listed in Table 22.5. The use of these pharmacological therapies is a complex process and treatment algorithms have been published by the American College of Chest Physicians, the ESC/ and European Respiratory Society, the ACC/AHA, and from the 4th World Symposium meeting at Dana Point, California (Figures 22.8 and 22.9).[19,40,118,147]

General measures

Patients with PAH should be encouraged to be active with low-level graded aerobic exercise, such as walking. A study evaluating intensive exercise training in patients under treatment with PAH-specific therapies, partly done under in-patient monitoring, demonstrated significant improvements in 6 minute walk distance, quality of life, functional class, and peak oxygen consumption.[148] Heavy physical exertion and isometric exercises may induce exertional syncope and must be avoided. There is growing evidence to support the benefits of a formal rehabilitation program in PAH patients after they have achieved clinical stability with PAH-directed therapy. One study showed an improvement in exercise capacity, cardiorespiratory function, and quality of life in patients with PAH who took part in a 10-week treadmill program.[149] Maintaining oxygen saturation above 92% at rest, exertion, and with sleep is important to avoid vasoconstriction associated with hypoxia. In patients with CHD, intracardiac shunt, and right-to-left shunting/Eisenmenger physiology, the optimal oxygenation level needs to be individualized. Patient and family education about managing a sodium-restricted diet (<2400 mg/ day) is very important in the setting of RV dysfunction. Pregnancy in women with PAH is associated with high maternal mortality rates (30–50%) relating to the hemodynamic fluctuations of pregnancy, labor, and delivery.[150] Current guidelines recommend that pregnancy be avoided or terminated early in women with PAH.[147] Though there is no firm guideline relating to methods of birth control, most experts agree that dual contraception, combining a hormonal agent with a barrier method, is advisable. It needs to be noted that the endothelial receptor antagonist (ERA) bosentan may reduce the efficacy of oral contraceptive agents. Keeping up to date with routine immunizations against influenza and pneumococcal pneumonia is advised.

Background treatments

Anticoagulation has been studied in three uncontrolled studies in IPAH patients which demonstrated survival improvement among patients treated with warfarin.[151,152,153] Most guidelines

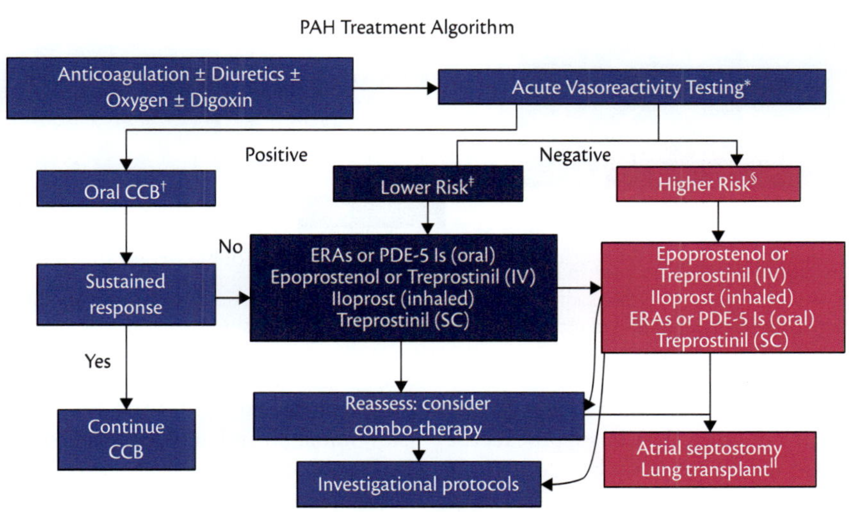

Fig. 22.8 Treatment algorithm for pulmonary arterial hypertension based on risk assessment.

Reprinted from Journal of the American College of Cardiology, 53, McLaughlin VV, Archer SL, Badesch DB, et al. ACCF/AHA 2009 expert consensus document on pulmonary hypertension: a report of the American College of Cardiology Foundation Task Force on Expert Consensus Documents, 1573–1619, copyright (2009) with permission from Elsevier.

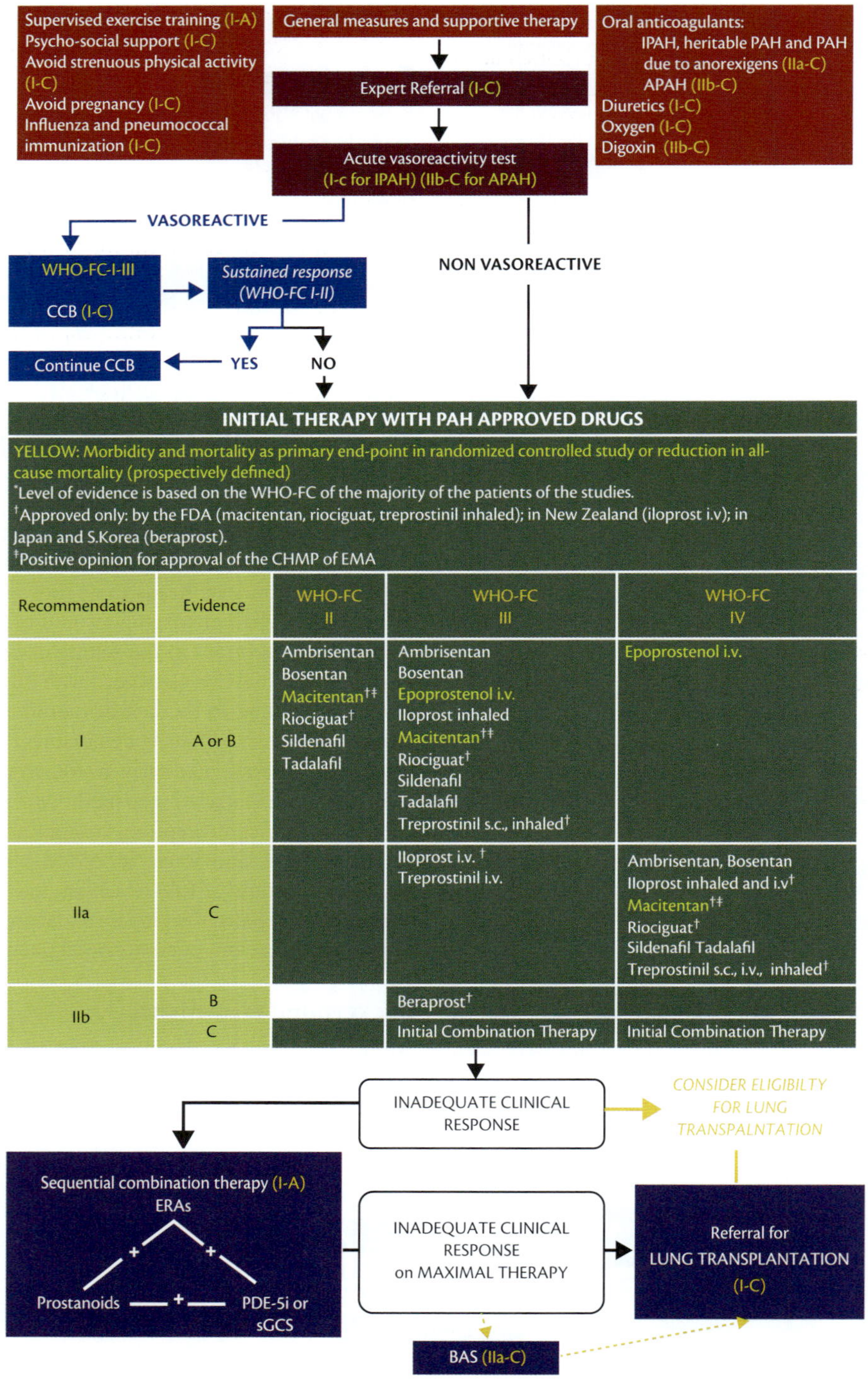

Fig. 22.9 Evidence-based treatment algorithm. APAH, associated pulmonary arterial hypertension; BAS, balloon atrial septostomy; CCB, calcium channel blockers; ERA, endothelin receptor antagonist; sGCS, soluble guanylate cyclase stimulators; IPAH, idiopathic pulmonary arterial hypertension; IV, intravenous; PDE-5i, phosphodiesterase type-5 inhibitor; PAH, pulmonary arterial hypertension; PDE-5, phosphodiesterase type 5; SC, subcutaneous; WHO, World Health Organization functional class.
Reprinted from the Journal of the American College of Cardiology, 2013 62(25) Suppl D. Galie N, Corris PA, Frost A, et al. Updated treatment algorithm of pulmonary arterial hypertension.

recommend warfarin anticoagulation targeted to an INR of 1.5–2.5 in patients with IPAH. There is not much data to support its use in patients with PAH associated with other secondary conditions. In CTD and portopulmonary patients, the risk of gastrointestinal bleeding may be increased. However, most experts recommend that warfarin anticoagulation should be considered in patients with advanced PAH being treated with IV prostanoids in the absence of contraindicating factors. Diuretics are used to treat volume overload due to right heart failure. For diuretic-naive patients, slow initiation and monitoring of renal function are recommended with goal of attaining near normal intravascular volume. In acute decompensated right heart failure and/or in the presence of diuretic resistance, IV diuretics are needed. Although digoxin has not been well studied in patients with PAH, it is used with careful monitoring in low doses in the setting of refractory right heart failure with low CO and in patients with atrial arrhythmia.

Calcium channel blockers

Calcium channel blockers are recommended for those few patients who demonstrate significant vasodilator response during an acute vasodilator testing (see Acute vasodilator testing). Patients with IPAH who meet the criteria may be considered for treatment with calcium channel blockers. Long-acting nifedipine, diltiazem, or amlodipine are the most commonly used agents. Verapamil should be avoided because of its potential negative inotropic effects. Very few patients with IPAH do well over the long term (<7%) and patients on calcium channel blockers need to be followed closely for efficacy and safety.[51] A patient who does not improve to FC I or II on calcium channel blockers should not be considered a chronic responder and PAH-directed treatment should be initiated.

PAH-targeted approved therapies

The current PAH-specific therapies exert their effects via targeting the three identified pathobiological pathways by augmenting the two deficient systems (prostacyclin and nitric oxide), and blocking the endothelin pathway. Each class and drug has its own unique side effects and challenging properties requiring thoughtful consideration in choosing the initial treatment and close follow-up to assess response and continued efficacy (Tables 22.6 and 22.7).

Prostacyclins

Epoprostenol

The advent of IV epoprostenol in 1995 as the first FDA-approved therapy for PAH transformed the field for PH. Epoprostenol is the first-line preferred agent for WHO FC IV patients, and is the therapy of choice for patients with advanced disease needing rescue treatment. The pivotal clinical trial which demonstrated its efficacy was conducted in an open-label, randomized trial of 81 FC III and IV IPAH patients comparing IV epoprostenol to conventional treatment.[154] Treatment with IV epoprostenol improved FC, exercise capacity, hemodynamics, and survival in IPAH. All eight deaths during the 12-week trial period occurred among patients who were randomized to conventional therapy, which resulted in a survival benefit ($p = 0.003$). IV epoprostenol has also been studied

Table 22.6 Summary of pivotal clinical trials in pulmonary arterial hypertension

Drug studied	Year study published	# of patients	Duration of study (wks)	FC of patients	Group of PAH patients	Background therapy	Primary endpoint 6MWD improvement	Comments
Epoprostenol[154]	1996	81	12	III/IV	IPAH	No	47 m (placebo corrected)	Only PAH trial demonstrating survival benefit
Epoprostenol[155]	2000	111	12	III/IV	PAH a/w scleroderma	No	108 m (placebo corrected)	Resulted in expansion of approved indication for epoprostenol to include CTD patients
Treprostinil SC[163]	2002	470	12	II/III/IV	IPAH, CTD, CHD	No	16 m (median; all in treatment group; unchanged in placebo)	Increase in 6MWD correlated with dose; patients underdosed due to site pain development
Bosentan[180] BREATHE-1	2002	213	16	III/IV	IPAH, CTD	No	44 m (placebo corrected)	First study to assess composite endpoint of time to clinical worsening
Iloprost[174] (AIR Study)	2002	203	12	III/IV	IPAH, CTD, appetite suppressants, CTEPH	No	36 m (placebo corrected)	Novel composite end point used as primary endpoint (see text)
Sildenafil[190] (SUPER-1)	2005	278	12	II/III	IPAH, CTD, CHD	No	45 m (placebo corrected)	Did not meet delay in time to clinical worsening
Ambrisentan[183] (ARIES 1 and 2)	2008	202 192	12	II/III	IPAH, CTD, appetite suppressants, HIV	No	31 m (5 mg) and 51 m (10 mg) for ARIES-1 32 m (2.5 mg) and 59 m (5 mg) for ARIES-2	Delayed time to clinical worsening for both ARIES trials
Tadalafil[195] (PHIRST)	2009	405	16	II/III	IPAH, CTD, CHD, appetite suppressants	~50% on bosentan	33 m (placebo corrected)	40 mg group met the pre specified level of statistical significance
Treprostinil Inhaled[173] (Triumph-1)	2010	235	12	III/IV	IPAH and all APAH	Yes	19 m (median)	

(continued)

Table 22.6 (Continued)

Drug studied	Year study published	# of patients	Duration of study (wks)	FC of patients	Group of PAH patients	Background therapy	Primary endpoint 6MWD improvement	Comments
Treprostinil Oral[171] (FREEDOM-M)	2013	228	12	II/III	IPAH and APAH	No	23 m	FREEDOM-C study (oral treprostinil on background treatment) did not show significant improvement in 6MWD
Riociguat[197]	2013	445	12	II/III	PAH	Yes	35.8 m	First therapy in soluble guanylate cyclase stimulator class to be approved for PAH Improvements in hemodynamic and clinical worsening reported
Macitentan[189] (SERAPHIN)	2013	742	Event-driven study (103.9 weeks for 10 mg arm)	II/III	PAH	Yes	Primary endpoint met (composite end points including death, lung transplant, worsening PAH)	First long-term, event-driven study in PAH
Selexipag[178] (GRIPHON)	Not published to date	1156	Event-driven study (76 ± 50 weeks for active treatment)	II/III	PAH	Yes	Primary endpoint met (composite end points including death, lung transplant, worsening PAH)	Largest PAH study to date; morbidity/mortality as primary endpoint

APAH, associated pulmonary arterial hypertension; CHD, congenital heart disease; CTD, connective tissue disease; FC, functional class; HIV, human immunodefiency virus; IPAH, idiopathic pulmonary arterial hypertension.

Park, MH. Pulmonary hypertension and right heart failure: Light at the end of the tunnel? In: Challenges in Heart Failure; Mehra MR, ed.; Park MH, McLaughlin VV. Pulmonary hypertension: Hemodynamic assessment and response to vasodilators. In: Cardiac Catheterization, Coronary & Peripheral Angiograpy, and Interventional Procedures. London, Informa Healthcare, 2010.

in PAH associated with CTD demonstrating marked improvements in 6 minute walk distance and hemodynamics but no effect on mortality in a 12-week, open-label randomized trial (see Table 22.6).[155] Observational studies have also reported beneficial effects of IV epoprostenol in patients with PAH related to HIV, CHD, and portopulmonary hypertension.[156,157,158] Two longer-term observational studies have confirmed the chronic benefits of IV epoprostenol in IPAH patients, specifically improvements in survival compared with historical controls, FC, 6 minute walk distance, and hemodynamics.[159,160]

IV epoprostenol is a challenging therapy to implement. Like endogenous prostacyclin, epoprostenol is a chemically unstable compound with a plasma half-life of less than 5 minutes which requires placement of a tunneled central venous catheter for long-term treatment. Each patient must learn the techniques of sterile preparation of the medication, operation of the ambulatory

Table 22.7 Summary of pharmacologic therapies for pulmonary arterial hypertension

Name of drug	Class of drug	Route	Dose	Common side effects	Comments
Epoprostenol (Flolan)	Prostanoid	IV	Start 1–2 ng kg^{-1} min^{-1} and titrate following side effect and PAH symptoms Dosing need to be individualized Optimal dose for chronic therapy 25–40 ng kg^{-1} min^{-1}	Prostanoid side effects[a]	Tunneled catheter needed; line infection major source of morbidity Long-term data available[157,158] Preferred drug recommended for WHO FC IV patients Complex treatment; recommend patients be referred to PH centers
Treprostinil (Remodulin)	Prostanoid	SC	Start 1.25–2.5 ng kg^{-1} min^{-1} and titrate following side effect and PAH symptoms	Prostanoid side effects[a] Injection site pain and erythema	Site pain effects majority of patients Experienced centers have reported successful outcome in managing patients with site pain Long-term survival data available

(continued)

Table 22.7 (Continued)

Name of drug	Class of drug	Route	Dose	Common side effects	Comments
Treprostinil (Remodulin)	Prostanoid	IV	Start 2 ng kg^{-1} min^{-1} and titrate following side effect and PAH symptoms	Prostanoid side effects[a] Leg pain more common than with epoporstenol	More convenient for chronic infusion than epoprostenol Revised recommendations for central tunneled catheter care (see text)
Treprostinil (Tyvaso)	Prostanoid	Inhaled	4 times a day	Prostanoid side effects[a] though generally less than SC or IV; also cough	Selective delivery of prostacyclin to lungs Rapid inhalation time Need to assess patient compliance Used in combination treatment with oral therapies
Oral Treprostinil (Orenitram)	Prostanoid	Oral	Available in 4 doses (0.125, 0.25, 1, 2.5 mg). BID or TID dosing. Maximum dose determined by tolerability	Prostanoid side effects* with GI side effects predominant	Pivotal studies used BID dosing. Clinical efficacy suggested to be enhanced by TID dosing (under study)
Iloprost (Ventavis)	Prostanoid	Inhaled	20 μg 6–9 inhalations a day; use of decreased frequency (4–5 times a day) reported with combination use of oral background therapy	Prostanoid side effects[a] though generally less than SC or IV; also cough	Selective delivery of prostacyclin to lungs Compliance can be an issue with need for frequent treatments Used in combination treatment with oral therapies
Bosentan (Tracleer)	ERA	Oral	62.5 mg BID × 4 weeks then 125 mg BID if LFT normal	Headache, dizziness, edema	Need LFTs checked monthly Shown to be effective in patients with mildly symptomatic PAH (FC II); not recommended for FC IV patients with overt right heart failure Contraindicated with ciclosporin and Glyburide Decreases effectiveness of oral hormonal contraceptives Long-term observed survival data available[173]
Ambrisentan (Letairis)	ERA	Oral	5 mg QD or 10 mg QD	Peripheral edema, nasal congestion, sinusitis	Do not need monthly LFTs checked; most clinicians follow intermittent LFTs More reported incidence of edema, especially >65 years of age Decreases effectiveness of oral hormonal contraceptives
Macitentan (Opsumit)	ERA	Oral	10 mg QD	Anemia, nasopharyngitis, headache	Do not need monthly LFT testing (LFT checked prior to initiation of treatment) H/H should be checked and monitored due to side effect of anemia
Sildenafil (Revatio)	PDE5-inhibitor	Oral	20 mg TID	Epistaxis, headache, flushing, diarrhea	Contraindicated with nitrates Some patients may need up titration of dose
Tadalafil (Adcirca)	PDE5-inhibitor	Oral	40 mg QD	Headache, myalgia, flushing	Contraindicated with nitrates
Riociguat (Adempas)	sGC stimulator	Oral	Available in 5 doses (0.5, 1, 1.5, 2, 2.5 mg). Recommended starting dose 1 mg TID (0.5 mg TID with concern for hypotension). Titrate q 2 weeks. Maximal dose 2.5 mg TID	Headache, dyspepsia, nausea, dizziness, edema, syncope	Contraindicated with PDE-5 inhibitors due to hypotension

[a] Side effects related to prostacyclin: jaw pain, diarrhea, flushing, headache, nausea.

BID, twice daily; ERA, endothelin receptor antagonist; IV, intravenous; LFT, liver function test; PDE-5, phosphodiesterase-5. QD, daily; SC, subcutaneous; TID, three times a day; sGC, soluble guanylate cyclase; WHO, World Health Organization.

Park, MH. Pulmonary hypertension and right heart failure: Light at the end of the tunnel? In: Challenges in Heart Failure; Mehra MR, ed.

infusion pump, and care of the central venous catheter. A thermostable formulation of epoprostenol (Veletri) has been approved. Incidences of sepsis and catheter-related infections are not negligible (0.1–0.6 case per patient-year) and can cause significant morbidity.[160] Any interruption of epoprostenol infusion can be potentially life threatening due to the short half-life and possible rebound PH. IV epoprostenol is commonly started in the hospital at a dose of 1–2 ng kg^{-1} min^{-1} and titrated on the basis of PAH symptoms and side effects. Most experts consider the optimal dose of chronic therapy to be between 25 and 40 ng kg^{-1} min^{-1} titrated over 6 months to 1 year, thought the dosing must be individualized. It is imperative that patients be monitored closely with periodic RHC to obtain hemodynamics on treatment because chronic overdose can lead to high CO failure and lead to recurrent symptoms.[161] Common side effects include headache, jaw pain, diarrhea, nausea, flushing, rash, and musculoskeletal pain. Thrombocytopenia has been reported with long-term treatment.[162] Most of these symptoms are common to all prostanoids, dose dependent, and generally well tolerated. Due to the complexity of administering this therapy, epoprostenol administration should be initiated by experienced physicians at designated centers (see Table 22.7).[40]

Practical management considerations for epoprostenol

- Epoprostenol is considered the most effective (gold standard) treatment as the only therapy shown to have survival benefit. It is the only drug that has received grade A recommendation for treatment of FC IV patients. Epoprostenol is the agent of choice as rescue therapy for patients presenting with severe refractory right heart failure/cardiogenic shock due to PAH.
- Initiation needs to be done in hospital under careful monitored setting. Dosing is determined by degree of symptoms, severity of disease, and amount of side effects. Usual starting dose is 1–2 ng kg^{-1} min^{-1} and discharge dose ranges 6–12 ng kg^{-1} min^{-1}.
- It is difficult therapy to administer because of its short half-life and potential for acute deterioration related to rebound PAH in the event of drug interruption. Careful assessment of patient's ability to manage the pump and mix the drug daily, as well as presence of stable support, is necessary. Identification of a "mixing partner" is mandatory—someone who can handle the intricacies involved with the therapy in the event the patient becomes unable to cope with it.
- Risks associated with tunneled catheter are major sources of morbidity, which is present for both administration of epoprostenol and IV treprostinil (see below) due to line malfunction and infection. Catheter-related infection leads to hospitalization and need for line removal and replacement. Episodes of sepsis can result in hemodynamic deterioration, shock, and death.
- Other practical aspects include the need for the drug to be kept refrigerated (the cassette needs to be kept in an ice pack), a difficult challenge for patients living in warm climates. The drug needs to be mixed daily under strict sterile procedure and the patient needs to maintain sterile care of the tunneled catheter.
- Side effects are numerous and need to be discussed with the patient and family. Acute side effects include headache, nausea, vomiting, flushing, jaw pain, and diarrhea. Supportive measures are used to manage the side effects, both acutely and chronically. Side effects are usually dose related, so decreasing the dose transiently with uptitration at a slower rate can help to decrease side effects. Thrombocytopenia is associated with chronic epoprostenol use, so platelet counts need to be followed. Thyroid dysfunction can also be seen with epoprostenol treatment and checking thyroid studies periodically is advisable.

Treprostinil

Treprostinil is a tricyclic benzene prostacyclin analog with a half-life of 4–5 hours and similar pharmacologic action to epoprostenol. Due to its longer elimination half-life, pH neutrality, and stability at room temperature, treprostinil can be delivered as a continuous subcutaneous (SC) infusion, a continuous IV infusion, or an intermittent inhaled treatment. Treprostinil was initially studied as a continuous SC infusion in a 12-week, placebo-controlled, randomized trial of 470 patients with FC II, III, or IV PAH.[163] There was a modest but statistically significant median increase of 16 m in 6 minute walk distance that was noted to be dose dependent. The major difficulty in administering SC treprostinil is pain and erythema at the infusion site, which was reported by 85% of the patients. It is now recognized that site pain is not dose related, and that some patients feel better after proper dose escalation which helps them to improve their PAH symptoms.[164]

Due to limitations of the SC delivery system, treprostnil was studied in a 12-week open-label trial of 16 patients being given by the IV route, which showed improvements in 6 minute walk distance and hemodynamics.[165] In another open-label trial, 31 FC II and III PAH patients on IV epoprostenol were transitioned to IV treprostinil;[166] 27 patients completed the transition, and 4 were transitioned back to epoprostenol. The 6-minute walk distance measurements were maintained among patients who completed the transition; however, there was a modest increase in mean PAP and decrease in CI. Noteworthy is that the dose of IV treprostinil at the end of the study period was more than twice the dose of epoprostinil at the start of the study. The FDA approval of the IV route of administration was based on the bioequivalence of subcutaneous and IV formations.[167,168] The Centers for Disease Control and Prevention (CDC) report raised concerns for increased risk of bloodstream infections, especially with Gram-negative organisms, in patients receiving IV treprostinil.[169] Significant center-dependent variability was present in reporting and no definite conclusion was made based on these reports. However, this finding has resulted in revised recommendations regarding catheter care (see Tables 22.6 and 22.7).[170]

Oral treprostinil (Orenitram®) is a novel salt form of treprostinil diethanolamine recently approved for the treatment of WHO group 1 PAH to improve exercise capacity. Oral treprostinil, available as a sustained-release tablet to be administered twice daily, was evaluated in two large clinical trials. The phase III FREEDOM-M trial was performed among 228 treatment naïve PAH patients in a randomized double-blind placebo-controlled 12-week study. It demonstrated significant improvement in primary endpoint of improving 6MWD (increase in median 6MWD of 23 m from baseline; $p = 0.0125$).[171] The FREEDOM-C(2) trial, which enrolled 310 PAH patients receiving background treatment with ERA and/or PDE-5 inhibitors, did not meet the primary end point of reaching significant improvement in 6MWD (improvement of 10 m; $p = 0.089$).[172] There is a study currently enrolling in a clinical trial assessing efficacy of oral treprostinil given three times daily.

Inhaled treprostinil was recently approved for intermittent use based on the result of a multicenter randomized placebo-controlled study of 235 PAH patients on oral bosentan or sildenafil with active symptoms. The addition of inhaled treprostinil resulted in an improvement of 6 minute walk distance, the primary endpoint.[173] The dose of inhaled treatment can be titrated and need to be administered four times daily. Common side effects reported include cough, headache, nausea, dizziness, and flushing (see Tables 22.6 and 22.7).

Practical management considerations for treprostinil

- Treprostinil is considered a "more convenient and safer" prostacyclin than epoprostenol, due to its longer half-life (4–5 hours vs. 4–5 minutes for epoprostenol). Thus in the event of drug interruption, the patient has time to arrange for care. This therapy is more frequently used for patients who live at a distance from the PH center.
- Treprostinil is room temperature stable; for the IV route the system is refilled every 2 days and for SC, every 3 days.
- There is no head-to-head study comparing the two prostacyclins. However, it takes approximately 1.5–2 times the dose of treprostinil to achieve the efficacy of epoprostenol.
- Risks related to the tunneled catheter for the IV route are the same as for epoprostenol. An increased incidence of Gram-negative bacteremia among patients receiving IV treprostinil has been reported, thought to be associated with catheter care, inadequate sterile measures during drug-mixing preparations, and different pH of the diluent used. Compulsory education of the patient and family regarding central line care is critically important. In the event of suspected infection, broad antibiotic coverage needs to be initiated until culture information is available.
- For IV treprostinil, side effects are similar to IV epoprostenol except for increased incidence of leg pain.
- For SC treprostinil, site pain is a problem experienced by most patients. It is helpful to discuss expectations with patient and the family members and point out that the pain usually decreases and dissipates with time with dose titration and improvement of PAH.

Inhaled iloprost

Iloprost is a stable prostacyclin analog that is delivered via an aerosolized device. Inhaled iloprost was the first therapy available via an inhaled delivery system; the direct dilatation of the pulmonary vasculature provided by the inhalation route provided for enhanced intrapulmonary selectivity with less systemic side effects and avoidance of right-to-left shunt blood flow. Iloprost was studied in a 12-week multicenter placebo-controlled randomized trial of 207 FC III and IV patients with either IPAH, PAH associated with CTD or appetite suppressants, or PH related to inoperable chronic thromboembolic disease.[174] Treatment with iloprost resulted in meeting a novel composite endpoint of improvement in functional class by at least one level and increase in 6 minute walk distance by at least 10% in the absence of clinical deterioration. It was generally well tolerated, with cough as the most common side effect; headache and flushing can also occur. Due to its relatively short half-life, inhaled iloprost needs to be administered 6–9 times daily (see Tables 22.6 and 22.7).

Practical management considerations for inhaled prostanoids

- Inhaled therapies allows selective delivery of prostacyclin to pulmonary systems.
- Both are generally well tolerated when used in combination with oral PAH treatments.
- Inhaled iloprost: For 20 μg/ml dose, the average treatment time reported per treatment session is approximately 5–8 minutes. Due to its short half-life, 6–9 treatments a day are needed; clinicians also prescribe 4–5 treatments a day with background oral regimen.
- Inhaled treprostinil: Inhalation duration is approximately 2–3 minutes, to be administered four times daily.
- Cough is the major side effect and is experienced by most patients for both regimens.
- Patient compliance need to be assessed when considering inhaled therapy.
- Hypoxia can worsen in patients with parenchymal lung disease and PH.

IP prostacyclin-receptor agonist

Selexipag

The second oral agent in the prostacyclin family, which has recently been approved by FDA, is selexipag (Uptravi). This is an oral selective IP prostacyclin-receptor agonist which, as a diphenylpyrazine moiety, is chemically distinct from prostacyclin and prostanoid analogues.[175] Selexipag becomes hydrolyzed via enzymatic actions to a long-acting active metabolite that has a half-life of about 8 hours. Unlike other prostanoid analogues, it has been shown to be highly selective for human prostacyclin IP receptor.[176] A phase II study demonstrated that selexipag was well tolerated at doses of less than 800 mg twice daily and treatment with the active drug resulted in decrease in PVR.[177] The results of the pivotal phase III study, GRIPHON trial, have been recently presented. This is a multicenter double-blind placebo-controlled event-driven study with the primary endpoint of time to first event.[178] This is the largest PAH study conducted to date with 1156 patients randomized to receive placebo or selexipag in 1:1 design and 80% of patients receiving background treatment with ERA and/or PDE-5 inhibitors. The study demonstrated a significant effect on the time to first event, mostly driven by decrease in morbidity. The treatment effect was seen irrespective of background therapy and it was well tolerated.

Endothelin receptor antagonists

Bosentan

Bosentan, a nonselective endothelin receptor blocker, was the first orally available therapy approved for PAH (in 2001). It was studied in two placebo-controlled randomized trials of FC III or IV patients with either PAH or PAH related to CTD.[179,180] In the pivotal BREATHE-1 trial, bosentan improved the primary endpoint of 6 minute walk distance by 36 m whereas placebo patients deteriorated by 8 m ($p = 0.0002$). Bosentan also improved the composite endpoint of time to clinical worsening, which was defined as death, initiation of IV epoprostenol, hospitalization for worsening PAH, lung transplantation, or atrial septostomy.

Long-term observational findings in survival of 169 patients treated with bosentan as first-line therapy have shown improved survival compared with expected outcome based on the NIH registry equation.[181] The Kaplan–Meier survival estimate at 2 years was 89%, compared with the predicted 2-year survival of these patients based on the NIH equation of 57%. In this study, 70% of the patients remained on bosentan monotherapy while 23% of patients received additional therapies or were transitioned to prostanoid-based therapies. Furthermore, bosentan was shown to be effective in the treatment of mildly symptomatic patients in the EARLY study, a multicenter placebo-controlled clinical trial that enrolled only FC II patients, to determine efficacy in intervening early in the course of the disease.[182] The study lasted 6 months, longer than other randomized clinical trials performed at that time, providing a longer time to determine response to treatment. The results of the 168 patients randomized demonstrated a significant decrease in PVR, which was the primary endpoint to evaluate treatment effects on vascular remodeling and RV function; furthermore, there was a significant delay in time to clinical worsening. This study showed that early diagnosis and initiation of therapy in PAH were critical factors in optimizing outcome in PAH.

The major toxicity associated with bosentan is hepatocellular injury by induction of the cytochrome P450 enzymes by the liver; the FDA requires that patients be followed with monthly liver function tests. In the BREATHE-1 trial, patients taking 125 mg and 250 mg of bosentan twice daily had a dose-dependent increase in aminotransferase elevations up to 8 times the upper limit of normal. Thus bosentan is only approved as a maximal dose of 125 mg twice daily. Patients are started on 62.5 mg twice daily with uptitration to 125 mg twice daily if no elevation of liver function enzymes is noted. Dose reduction or discontinuation of the drug usually results in resolution of liver enzyme abnormalities, although irreversible liver toxicity has been reported. Using this dosing approach, the increase in hepatic transaminases to more than three times the upper limit of normal in the BREATHE-1 trial was 10–12%.[180] Bosentan is teratogenic and may decrease the efficacy of hormonal contraception, so women of childbearing age must be counseled to use dual contraception for birth control. Other side effects include headache, flushing, lower extremity edema, and anemia. Therefore, treatment with bosentan requires monthly monitoring of liver function tests, monthly pregnancy tests on women of childbearing potential, and quarterly hemoglobin/hematocrit testing. Patients should be counseled regarding potential for lower extremity edema, especially in the initial weeks of therapy, and possible need for diuretic adjustments. Glyburide and ciclosporin A are contraindicated with bosentan due to significant drug–drug interactions.

Ambrisentan

Ambrisentan is a selective ET_A receptor antagonist studied in two placebo-controlled randomized 12-week studies of WHO group I patients (ARIES-1 and ARIES-2) which were conducted in the US and Europe/South America, respectively.[183] The treatment resulted in a significant improvement in 6 minute walk distance and delay in time to clinical worsening in all treatment groups. Ambrisentan is available in 5 mg and 10 mg oral tablets taken once a day. Long-term results showed estimates of survival and freedom from clinical worsening for the combined dose groups to be 94% and 83% respectively at 1 year and 88% and 72% respectively at 2 years.[184]

The incidence of hepatic transaminase elevation more than three times the upper limit of normal for patients receiving ambrisentan was 0.8%.[181] The lower risk of aminotransferase elevation with ambrisentan was further investigated in a study of 36 patients who, due to hepatic transaminase increases, did not tolerate bosentan or sitaxsantan (a selective endothelin receptor antagonist which is no longer available due to liver toxicity) and were placed on ambrisentan therapy.[185] Ambrisentan therapy was tolerated well in this group. Following further analysis of post-marketing use safety data, the FDA has removed the monthly liver function test monitoring requirement in patients on ambrisentan, although many experts continue to check liver function tests periodically. Peripheral edema is another side effect of endothelin receptor antagonists and was reported in mild to moderate severity in the clinical trials.[181] An increase report of incidences of peripheral edema during post-marketing use has prompted the FDA to issue a labeled warning for patients aged over 65 years.[186] The mechanism behind this observed edema is not clear. There is no drug interaction with sildenafil. Ambrisentan is teratogenic so monthly pregnancy tests for women of childbearing age are required.

Practical management considerations for oral endothelin receptor antagonists

General comments

- No direct head-to-head comparison availablefor the two agents; clinical trials demonstrate similar short-term efficacy.
- Endothelin receptor antagonists are most effective when used for treatment of patients in early stage of PAH (FC II/IIIA).
- Not recommended as first-line agent for patients with advanced PAH (e.g., clinically overt right heart failure, FC IV).
- Tolerated well when used in combination with PDE-5 inhibitors.
- Endothelin receptor antagonists shown to have anti-fibrotic effect (evidence mostly with bosentan); advocated for patients with scleroderma-related PAH.

Warnings

- Bosentan: Need monthly liver function tests; multiple drug interactions.
- Ambrisentan: No need for monthly liver function checks but most physicians follow liver function tests on a scheduled periodic basis; drug interactions not common.
- Lower extremity edema can be seen with both agents but is generally more pronounced with ambrisentan.
- Both agents known to be teratogenic; strict adherence to contraception with dual method essential for women of childbearing age.

Macitentan

Macitentan (Opsumit®) is the newest oral ERA agent approved for PAH. It is a dual (ET_A and ET_B) endothelin receptor blocker shown to have enhanced tissue penetration due to an increased proportion of the non-ionized form of the molecule related to its ability to cross the lipophilic cell membranes.[187,188,189] Initial clinical studies demonstrated that macitentan was well tolerated in healthy volunteers and had dose-dependent pharmacokinetics.[188] The pivotal phase III SERAPHIN trial is notable in that it is the first long-term event-driven outcome trial in PAH, defining morbidity and mortality as the primary endpoint. This double-blind placebo-controlled study enrolled 742 patients with 180 participating centers in over 40 countries. Two doses were studied, 3 mg and 10 mg, with the mean treatment duration of 85.3, 99.5, and 103.9 weeks. Macitentan reduced the risk of occurrence of morbidity and mortality events versus placebo by 30% in the 3mg group (97.5% CI 4–48%; $p = 0.0108$) and 45% in the 10 mg group (97.5% CI 24–61%; $p < 0.0001$), irrespective of background therapy. Treatment with macitentan also reduced the risk of the secondary endpoint, mortality due to PAH/hospitalization for PAH, by 33% for 3 mg (97.5% CI 3–54%; $p = 0.0146$) and 50% for 10 mg (97.5% CI 25–67%; $p < 0.0001$).[189] The 10 mg once-daily macitanten was approved for WHO group 1 PAH to delay disease progression. The main side effects reported are anemia, nasopharyngitis, and headache. The incidence of liver transaminase elevation in SERAPHIN study greater than 3 times the upper limits of normal range was 3.4% for macitanten and 4.5% for placebo. Liver function testing need to be performed prior to initiation of treatment and repeat during therapy as indicated; however, monthly liver function testing is not needed. For patients with anemia, macitanten use should be done with close monitoring for its known side effects of decreasing hemoglobin.

Phosphodiesterase-5 inhibitors

Sildenafil

Sildenafil was studied in a 12-week randomized placebo-controlled study (SUPER-1) of 278 symptomatic PAH patients.190 The primary endpoint of 6 minute walk distance improved by 45, 46, and 50 m in the 20, 40, and 80 mg groups, respectively ($p < 0.001$). Sildenafil treatment in all dosing groups was associated with significant improvement in functional class and reduction in mean PAP. There was no change in the time to clinical worsening at week 12. The result of 222 patients who completed 1 year of treatment demonstrated that the improvement in 6 minute walk distance was maintained; however, nearly all patients were titrated up to a dose of 80 mg 3 times a day. Analysis of 259 patients who enrolled in the long-term open-label extension study showed that about 60% of the patients who entered the SUPER-1 trial improved or maintained their functional status and 46% maintained or improved the improved 6 minute walk distance.191 Although the current FDA-approved dose is 20 mg three times daily based on the SUPER-1 study, higher off-label doses have been used safely in patients with recurrent symptoms, demonstrating effect of tolerance to treatment; however, the optimal dosing and long-term outcome regarding hemodynamics and survival is not known. Sildenafil is appropriate in FC II or III patients as a first-line treatment. However, oral therapy with either PDE5 inhibitors or endothelin receptor antagonists should not be utilized as a first-line agent for patients presenting in FC IV, for whom continuous infusion of prostanoids is recommended as first-line treatment.

Sildenafil is rapidly absorbed and has a plasma half-life of approximately 4 hours. It is metabolized through the cytochrome P450 enzymes and drug–drug interactions have been reported. The most common side effects among patients in the SUPER-1 trial included headache, flushing, dyspepsia, and epistaxis, which are dose related.[191] No significant laboratory abnormalities were reported. Because of a shared and common pathway of increased NO-mediated effects, concomitant administration with oral nitrate medications is contraindicated since the combined therapies can potentiate the effects of the drugs and produce severe hypotension and syncope.[66] Sildenafil should not be given to patients who have taken any nitrate preparations within the previous 24 hours at a minimum.

Visual disturbances have been reported with sildenafil from its use in treatment of erectile dysfunction, the most common ocular effect being dose-dependent reversible impairment of color discrimination, principally in the blue-green to blue-purple range, and increases in light sensitivity.[66,189] Sildenafil affects ocular vasculature from its concurrent crossover inhibition of phosphodiesterase type 6, which is expressed in the retinal photoreceptor layer of both rods and cones.[192] A study in PAH population receiving long-term sildenafil reported that it was well tolerated in patients receiving doses up to 80 mg three times daily.[191,192] Anecdotal reports suggesting an increased risk of nonarteritic anterior ischemic optic neuropathy (NAION) has been associated in sildenafil-treated patients. However, pooled data from clinical trials to date suggested no increased risk of NAION.[193] Patients at highest risk for development of NAION are those who have suffered NAION in one eye, and those with other risk factors for vascular disease including diabetes mellitus. It remains advisable to monitor for visual changes and for ophthalmologic examination for patients with risk factors.[194] Hearing loss has also been reported with use of sildenafil.

Tadalafil

Tadalafil, an oral longer-acting PDE-5 inhibitor, was recently studied in a 16-week double-blind placebo-controlled trial among 405 PAH patients using 2.5, 10, 20, and 40 mg tablets once a day in the PHIRST study.[195] The tadalafil-treated subjects experienced a dose-dependent increase in 6 minute walk distance, but only the 40 mg dose reached a statistically significant increase of 41 m compared with 9 m for placebo ($p < 0.001$). There was also a delay in the time to clinical worsening (defined as death, hospitalization, initiation of new PAH therapy, or worsening WHO FC). Long-term treatment during an open-label extension study found tadalafil to be well tolerated and the improvement in 6 minute walk distance to be maintained in the 52-week observation.[196] Side effects were similar to sildenafil and included headache, diarrhea, nausea, back pain, dizziness, dyspepsia, and flushing; increased report of myalgia has been noted with tadalafil use.

Practical management considerations for PDE-5 inhibitors

- Both agents are usually well tolerated.
- PDE-5 inhibitors are most often used as first-line treatment; not advised to be used as monotherapy in patients with advanced (FC IV) disease and right heart failure.
- Sildenafil has been studied in patients with PH in the setting of left heart and lung disease. Response and outcome have been shown to vary depending on the degree of underlying cardiac and pulmonary dysfunction. PDE-5 inhibitors are only approved for treatment of WHO group 1 PAH. Treating patients with "out of proportion" PAH with features of left heart or lung disease need to be considered on an individual basis.

Soluble guanylate-cyclase stimulator

Riociguat

Riociguat is a an oral soluble guanylate cyclase (sGC) stimulator that acts independently of nitric oxide (NO) and enhances the sensitivity of sGC to low levels of NO.[197,198,199] Riociguat recently completed 2 pivotal phase III clinical trials: PATENT-1, evaluating riociguat in PAH patients; CHEST-1, first clinical study to evaluate CTEPH patients. The PATENT-1 study enrolled 445 treatment-naïve patients and those receiving ERAs or inhaled/

subcutaneous prostanoids in a 12-week trial. Riociguat was given 0.5–2.5 mg three times daily and the primary outcome was the placebo-corrected change from baseline in 6MWD. The results showed an increase in 6MWD from baseline of 35.8 m with riociguat versus placebo (95% CI 20.1–51.5 m, p <0.0001) and the results were similar between treatment-naïve versus patients on background therapy. Significant improvements were also seen in PVR (p <0.0001) and clinical worsening (p = 0.0046).[197]

The CHEST-1 study enrolled 261 patients with inoperable chronic thromboembolic pulmonary hypertension (CTEPH) or recurrent PH after pulmonary thromboendareterectomy to receive either riociguat (0.5 to 2.5 mg TID) or placebo. CHEST-1 trial met its primary endpoint of showing significant improvement in 6MWD in CTEPH patients treated with riociguat, the first therapy ever to demonstrate such improvement in this population. It also demonstrated improvement in relevant secondary endpoints, including improvement in PVR and WHO functional class.[197] The most common reported side effects include headache, gastritis/reflux, dizziness, hypotension. Cases of hemoptysis have also been reported. Concomitant use of riociguat and PDE-5 inhibitors is contraindicated due to hypotension. Riociguat received dual indications in PH, namely for patients with WHO Group 1 PAH to improve exercise capacity, functional class, and delay in clinical worsening; and for WHO Group IV patients with inoperable CTEPH or recurrent PH post thromboendarterectomy. However, it must be noted that patients with surgically accessible lesions should undergo surgical evaluation and that riociguat cannot replace surgical treatment which can restore normal cardiopulmonary status.[198]

Combination therapy in pulmonary arterial hypertension

Since PAH is a progressive disease with monotherapy observed to be insufficient to maintain clinical stability for long periods of time, investigators have proposed goal-oriented strategies that utilize dual or triple therapies with the aim of optimizing hemodynamics and functional status and demonstrating improvements in outcome (see Table 22.8).[199] Combination therapy directed at the multiple PAH pathways offers the potential advantage of maximizing treatment efficacy while minimizing toxicity. Several small open-label observational studies have reported the potential benefit of combination treatment.[200,201] One of the first randomized clinical trial for combination treatment, BREATHE-2, which evaluated combining bosentan or placebo for FC III or IV patients receiving IV epoprostenol, failed to show benefit mainly because it was underpowered.[202] Two studies evaluated adding inhaled iloprost to bosentan therapy in a randomized double-blind placebo-controlled design: The STEP study enrolled 67 patients in a 12-week study which demonstrated safety as well as improvement in 6 minute walk distance (26 m, placebo corrected; p = 0.051), and the COMBI study evaluated 40 patients but failed to demonstrate benefit and was terminated.[203,204]

The PACES study investigated sildenafil as add-on therapy to IV epoprostenol.[205] This 16-week multinational double-blind placebo-controlled study enrolled 267 patients who were on stable epoprostenol therapy. Patients were randomized to receive 20 mg three times a day (TID) titrated to 40 mg and 80 mg TID, at 4-week intervals, or corresponding placebo. At the end of 16 weeks, more than 80% of patients had reached the 80 mg TID dosing level. The primary endpoint was change in 6 minute walk distance and there was a placebo-adjusted increase of 26 m for the subjects who received sildenafil. There were seven deaths in the placebo group and none among patients receiving sildenafil. Clinical worsening events, defined as death, transplant, hospitalization, or an increase in epoprostenol dose, were significantly in favor of the treated group. The TRIUMPH trial, which studied adding inhaled treprostinil to either background bosentan or sildenafil, showed improved quality of life and 6 minute walk distance favoring the combination approach.[169]

A recent multicenter, multinational, placebo controlled trial AMBITION compared first line monotherapy with tadalafil or monotherapy with ambrisentan with upfront combination therapy with tadalafil and ambrisentan in FC II and III PAH patients.[206] The primary endpoint was time-to-event analysis of the first event of clinical failure, which was defined as composite of death, hospitalization, PAH progression, and unsatisfactory long-term clinical response. The study showed 50% reduction of events in the group who received upfront combination therapy. Furthermore, improvements in exercise capacity, rate of satisfactory clinical response and decrease in NT-proBNP plasma levels were observed.

Investigational therapies

Despite the availability of multiple agents targeting the three defined pathways, long-term outcomes in PAH still remain suboptimal. There is a clear need for new treatment options that deliver via known pathways with improved safety and/or efficacy, or agents that target novel pathologic pathways not currently addressed by existing treatments.

Surgical and interventional therapies for pulmonary arterial hypertension

Despite the availability of multiple PAH-specific treatments, many patients still experience progressive functional decline which is largely due to worsening right heart failure. For these patients, interventional and surgical therapies need to be considered.

Atrial septostomy

Atrial septostomy creates a right-to-left interatrial shunt which decreases right-side filling pressure, thereby improving RV function and left-side filling. Although the created shunt decreases systemic arterial oxygen saturation, the expectation is that the improved CO will result in overall increase in systemic oxygen delivery. Reports of hemodynamic improvement with increase in CO have been noted, ranging from 15% to nearly 60%, as well as improvements in NYHA functional class and 6MWD.[207,208,209,210,211,212] However, procedural mortality is high which ranges from 5% to 50% in published case series, driven by the severity of right heart failure. Patients with advanced age, renal dysfunction, severe elevation of RA pressure, and derangements in systemic oxygenation are at greatest risk. Atrial septostomy is currently recommended for patients with severe PAH and intractable right heart failure despite maximal medical therapy, including PAH-specific agents and inotropes, and can be viewed as a possible bridge to transplantation.[40,118] This procedure should be performed only by experienced operators in centers with multidisciplinary team members to care for these critically sick patients.

Transplantation

For patients who are refractory to optimal PAH-specific therapy, lung transplantation remains the only treatment option. Identifying the high-risk subset of patients who need to be considered for transplantation is challenging; one study showed that patients who remain in NYHA class III or IV, or do not achieve a 30% drop in the PVR from baseline after 3 months following initiation of IV epoprostenol, need to be evaluated for lung transplantation.[159] Given the difficulty in predicting the course of illness in patients with PAH, it is recommended that patients be referred early to a transplant center for evaluation, and that transplantation as a potential therapeutic option be discussed with PAH patients upon diagnosis. However, only a small proportion of transplant procedures in the US, about 5%, are for the indication of PAH. Although PAH patients undergoing transplantation face an increase in operative mortality, the long-term survival outcome is comparable with patients undergoing transplantation for other indications: the International Society of Heart and Lung Transplant 2010 registry reports median survival ("half-life") for all lung transplant recipients as 5.3 years and for IPAH patients, 4.9 years.[210] The most commonly performed transplant procedure is bilateral lung, to limit the reperfusion injury that has been reported in the donor lung of PAH patients receiving a single lung transplant.[211] The decision to perform heart and lung transplantation is based on the degree and severity of right heart failure, for patients requiring inotropic support, or for patients with complex CHD.

The current prioritization scheme used by the United Network for Organ Sharing (UNOS) uses the Lung Allocation Score (LAS) which takes into account waiting list urgency and the probability of post-transplantation survival. The score ranges from 0 to 100, with a higher score reflecting a sicker patient. Since the inception of the LAS system in 2005, deaths on the waiting list have decreased for all diagnostic categories except IPAH, which remained unchanged; analysis showed that PAH patients were less likely to be transplanted than patients with idiopathic pulmonary fibrosis (IPF) and more likely to die on the waiting list than COPD patients.[212,216] Critics of the LAS system have pointed out that the equation is weighted more heavily toward PFTs and not hemodynamic factors which determine the outcome in PAH. Analysis of mortality as predicted by the REVEAL registry cohorts compared with the LAS system identified two additional variables to be independently associated with increased mortality, namely RA pressure 14 mmHg or more and 6MWD 300 m or less.[213] Modification of the current LAS system is under discussion; in the meantime, UNOS has adopted criteria for an appeal process to re-evaluate the score. A patient with IPAH can be granted LAS in the 90th percentile of all LAS if they meet all of the following criteria: deterioration despite optimal medical therapy, RAP greater than 15 mmHg, and CI less than 1.8 L min^{-1} m^{-2}.[213]

Assessing prognosis and response to therapy in pulmonary arterial hypertension

The search for prognostic predictors has been a key goal for clinicians involved in the care of PH patients for decades as the disease remains progressive despite rapid advances in the number of available treatments. The NIH registry was the first to attempt to characterize clinical factors associated with outcome, using baseline hemodynamic parameters in a formula to calculate survival.[15] However, the usefulness of these data is now limited by the fact that it was compiled 30 years ago, before approved PAH-specific treatments became available. As such, it provided a tool for assessing baseline hemodynamic markers of prognosis but did not allow a method of predicting how the patient might respond to therapy. Nevertheless it showed that markers of baseline prognosis might be relevant as treatment goals. During recent decades, with the advent of multiple clinical trials and the success of exercise tests, the focus has been toward the use of noninvasive markers as the surrogate for hemodynamic indices. The 6MWD has been utilized widely as the key treatment goal of most clinical trials as it has demonstrated correlation with hemodynamic parameters and long-term outcome. Concomitantly, other measures such as functional class and biomarkers have been shown to correlate with long-term outcome in PAH. However, it has become evident that one measure does not reflect the complexity of the disease and the possibility of using composite treatment goals is being investigated.

Prognostic factors in pulmonary arterial hypertension

Hemodynamics

Since the outcome of PAH is governed by RV function, the fact that hemodynamic parameters have been regarded as the gold standard indices of outcome is a well-accepted principle. The NIH registry demonstrated three variables to be associated with an increased mortality risk which were incorporated into a regression equation to estimate survival: increased mean PAP, increased mean RA pressure, and decreased CI.[15] In both the French and REVEAL registries, RA pressure and CO were shown to be the most important prognostic hemodynamic indicators.[21,214]

However, there are several caveats and limitations in ascertaining hemodynamic parameters to assess prognosis. First, the vasodilator response during RHC has been shown to be a strong indicator of favorable outcome since responders have up to 95% 5-year survival rate.[51] The other factor is that mPAP declines as PAH progresses and the RV dilates and fails, which is why the survival estimates utilize mean RAP and CI in the equations. This was shown by a retrospective analysis of patients on epoprostenol where lower mPAP and higher mean RAP increased mortality risk on univariate analysis and mean RAP on multivariate analysis; in a similar analysis of patients receiving epoprostenol, only mean RAP was predictive of survival.[159] However, obtaining hemodynamics requires an invasive procedure that is not widely available and associated risks, albeit small in experienced centers, limit the ability to obtain hemodynamic parameters on treatment. Hemodynamic measurements also illustrate the physiological state at a single time point at rest, in a supine position, and does not account for changes associated with activity. Although exercise-related hemodynamic effects are currently undergoing active research, there is no consensus regarding the method of performing exercise RHC or interpretation on the hemodynamic effects in PAH.[215] Furthermore, the effects of systemic processes such as anxiety, hypertension, and sedation can markedly affect the parameters.

Six-minute walk test

Exercise capacity as measured by the distance walked in 6 minutes is a major determinant of disease severity and prognosis. The advantage of the 6MWD is that it is a simple and noninvasive test that is inexpensive, reproducible, and well tolerated even among those with advanced PAH. Indeed, the 6MWD has been used as the primary objective for almost all pivotal clinical trials for PAH treatments. Barst and colleagues reported significant improvement seen in 6MWD after 12 weeks of epoprostenol infusion compared with patients receiving conventional therapy.[154] The increase in distance walked also correlated with improvement in hemodynamics, setting a precedent for future PAH clinical trials. Furthermore, baseline 6MWD was shown to be an independent predictor of survival. This initial observation was corroborated by a study performed by Miyamoto and colleagues, demonstrating correlation between baseline low and high median 6MWD groups and hemdoynamics reflective of RV function (CO, mixed venous oxygen saturation, TPR, and RAP) and long-term survival.[216] Patients who walked 332 m or more had significantly better long-term survival than those who were not able to achieve that distance baseline. Among all the noninvasive variables analyzed (distance walked, age, sex, plasma norepinephrine, heart rate, arterial oxygen saturation, presence of pericardial effusion, LV deformity index), only the distance walked was independently related to mortality. Furthermore, a well-defined correlation was observed between the severity of NYHA class and the distance walked. However, being able to assess response to treatment is the most critical measure needed in PAH and the evidence for 6MWD as a surrogate marker for long-term survival on therapy has not been consistent or robust. In one of the earlier studies of patients treated with epoprstenol, the 6MWD performed after 3 months of therapy correlated with long-term survival; specifically, patients who walked 380 m or more demonstrated a significantly better outcome than those who did not.[159] Surprisingly, analyzing outcome based on the absolute increase in the distance walked from baseline on treatment showed no correlation.

The 6MWD has many limitations, including inconsistent correlation with survival when comparing across different clinical trials. Clinical relevance of changes seen in 6MWD is often not clear, whether it is the effect of day-to-day variability or true clinical improvement or worsening; the impact of a learning effect after repeated testing must also be taken into account. Results of the 6MWD are difficult to interpret in patients with CTD or joint dysfunction. Furthermore, lack of sensitivity to detect changes in patients with early stage of PAH and those with relatively high 6MWD at baseline is a commonly encountered problem, referred to as the "ceiling effect." As well, inability to detect changes in 6MWD when utilizing combination treatment as add-on therapy is frequently encountered in clinical practice.[217,218,219]

There remain many unanswered questions in utilizing 6MWD, specifically which parameter best correlates with exercise capacity and right heart function. Is there an absolute cutoff value of 6MWD that is associated with improved survival in PAH, such as 380 m as suggested by study by Sitbon and colleauges or 440 m as shown by the REVEAL registry?[159,214] Furthermore, what improvement in distance translates to meaningful change in quality of life or survival? Or should the change be assessed by percent achieved based on individualized parameters (i.e., age, gender, height) and percent changed? There is evidence to suggest that other parameters should be incorporated in interpreting 6MWD such as heart rate recovery; one group of investigators reported among 75 PAH patients that heart rate recovery of 16 or less (measured as a difference in heart rate at the end of the 6MWD test and at 1 minute after completion of the test) correlated with clinical worsening and was a better predictor of outcome than 6MWD alone.[220]

Two recent studies evaluated the usefulness of 6MWD in determining outcome in PAH. In a meta-analysis that included 22 trials and 3112 patients, the authors conclude that pharmacological treatments resulted in significant reduction of all-cause death, hospitalization for PAH, transplantation, initiation of rescue therapy, and composite outcome, but the favorable effects on clinical events were not predicted by changes in 6MWD.[221] Another set of investigators performed a pooled analysis of 10 trials to determine whether changes in 6MWD in the 12-week treatment period correlated with clinical events to find that change in 6MWD accounted for only 22.1% of the treatment effect.[222] The average difference in 6MWD was 22.4 m and the significant threshold effect was found to be 41.8 m, therefore the change in 6MWD does not explain a large proportion of the treatment effect with only a modest validity as a surrogate endpoint for clinical events.

Functional class

The modified FC system, which is based on the NYHA functional classification, is commonly used to assess the severity of PAH (see Box 22.3).[223] It is a simple tool used by healthcare providers in assessing the tolerance and/or limitation of activities due to symptoms that a patient experiences in everyday activities. In the NIH registry, the baseline FC assessments correlated with outcome: for patients in NYHA class I or II the median survival was almost 6 years, while it was 2.5 years for patients in NYHA class III and 6 months for NYHA class IV.[15] Baseline functional assessment was also shown to be highly predictive of outcome among patients treated with long-term epoprostenol. Survival was significantly worse for patients who were FC IV at baseline compared to those who were FC III at the time of treatment initiation.[160] Furthermore, failure to achieve FC I or II after 3 months of treatment was shown to be a poor prognostic indicator.[159] The more recent French and REVEAL registries have corroborated the usefulness of FC as a tool to assess outcome at baseline and with treatment.[22,214] The FC assessment has also been shown to correlate with severity in patients with PAH associated with CHD and CTD.[224,225]

Limitations of the FC system are many, and include the subjective basis of evaluation, poor inter-observer variability, and no objective criteria for "ordinary" or "normal" activities or what defines "mild" or "moderate" limitations. Similarly, many clinicians subdivide class III into IIIA and IIIB, though there is no formal definition or data. Furthermore, as the PAH population becomes more diverse, lack of information on effects of age, gender, or PAH subtype limits its application.

Echocardiography

Although echocardiography is an essential screening test for PAH, its use as a tool to provide prognostic information is based on a relatively small amount of data. Since the integrity of the RV is the key determinant in survival, echocardiographic determinants of RV function has been shown to correlate with outcome. The Tei index, which is an index of the combined RV systolic and diastolic function obtained by dividing the sum of both isovolumetric contraction and relaxation intervals by the ejection time, has been shown to be predictive of outcome.[226] However, it is affected by loading conditions and degree of TR.

The other parameter of RV function that has been reported to correlate with survival is TAPSE.[111] Presence of a pericardial effusion to any extent has been shown to be a strong predictor of mortality; larger effusion has been shown to be directly correlated to RA dilatation and inversely correlated to exercise performance.[227] RA and RV enlargement and eccentricity index have also been shown to correlate with outcome in IPAH patients.[228] The major

Table 22.8 Combination therapy in pulmonary arterial hypertension: clinical trial results

Combination studied	6MWD improvement	Comments
IV eporpostenol ± oral treatment		
BREATHE-2 (epo + bosentan; $n = 33$)	No difference	Trend for improvement in PVR ($p = 0.08$)
PACES (epo + sildenafil; $n = 267$)	26 m ($p < 0.06$)	Improvement in hemodynamics and time to clinical worsening ($p < 0.06$)
Bosentan ± inhaled iloprost		
STEP ($n = 67$)	26 m ($p = 0.06$) at peak; no difference measured at trough	Improvement in FC, time to clinical worsening, postinhalation hemodynamics ($p < 0.06$)
COMBI ($n = 40$)	No difference	Unblinded randomized study No difference in FC or time to clinical worsening
Oral therapy ± inhaled treprostinil		
TRIUMPH-1 ($n = 236$)	19 m ($p = 0.0001$)	No improvement in FC or time to clinical worsening
Monotherapy versus upfront combination treatment		
AMBITION (n = 500) First line monotherapy of taladafil or ambrisentan with upfront combination therapy with tadalafil and ambrisentan	50% reduction with upfront combination treatment in clinical events (death, hospitalization, disease progression, unsatisfactory long-term clinical response)	Landmark study showing significant clinical benefit in utilizing upfront combination of tadalafil and ambrisentan

AMBITION – Ambrisentan and Tadalafil in patients with pulmonary arterial hypertension; BREATHE-2, Bosentan Randomized Trial of Endothelin Antagonist Therapy; COMBI, Combination Therapy of Bosentan and Aeriolized Iloprost in Idiopathic Pulmonary Arterial Hypertension; PACES, The Efficacy and Safety of Sildenafil Citrate Used in Combination With Intravenous Epoprostenol in PAH; STEPH, Iloprost Inhalation Solution Safety and Pilot Efficacy Trial in Combination with Bosentan for Evaluation in Pulmonary Arterial Hypertension; TRIUMPH-1, Clinical Investigation into Inhaled Treprostinil Sodium in Patients with Severe PAH.

6MWD, 6 minute walk distance; epo, epoprostenol; FC, functional class; IV, intravenous; PVR, pulmonary vascular resistance.

limitations of echocardiographic parameters for prognostic assessments relate to technical difficulties and reproducibility in obtaining RV measurements.

B-type natriuretic peptide

The clinical utility of natriuretic peptides in the assessment of PAH has gained much interest. Brain natriuretic peptide (BNP) and N-terminal proBNP have both been studied in this patient population as a marker of RV dysfunction and have been used interchangeably. Nagaya and colleagues, in a study of 63 patients with IPAH during a mean follow-up period of 24 months, reported that baseline BNP was an independent predictor of mortality, in that patients with BNP levels 150 pg/ml or more had a significantly lower survival rate than those with lower BNP.[229] Regarding levels obtained on treatments, the same group showed that BNP levels obtained 90 days after therapy initiation were also predictive of outcomes. Furthermore, another group of investigators found that a BNP reduction of 50% or more 3 months after initiation of epoprostenol was predictive of event-free survival up to 12 months of follow-up.[230] Furthermore, N-terminal proBNP was shown to correlate with other markers of prognosis, specifically 6MWD and hemodynamics.[231] Some of the challenges in interpreting BNP levels in PAH relate to the fact that the peptides are influenced by noncardiac factors, such as obesity and renal function.[232] Furthermore, the cutoff values which define the "normal" range are based on data from studies of patients with left heart failure and do not take gender and age into consideration.

Cardiac MRI

There is a growing interest in utilizing cardiac MRI (CMR) in PAH. CMR allows a direct assessment of RV size, morphology, and function providing reproducible measurements including stroke volume and ejection fraction, RV volume and mass, and anatomic and physiologic assessment of the pulmonary artery.[233,234] Investigators have determined a decreased stroke volume, an increased RV end-diastolic volume, and a decreased LV end-diastolic volume measured at baseline to be associated with poor prognosis. As outcome in PAH is closely associated with RV function, CMR has been shown to be a useful tool to assess for response to treatment. One study showed that increased RV end-diastolic volume may be the most relevant marker of progressive RV failure in follow-up evaluations.[235] A recent study evaluated the relationship between changes in PVR and RV ejection fraction among 76 patients with PAH on therapy with subsequent follow-up RHC and CMR after 12 months.[236] The findings showed that PVR correlated only moderately with changes in RV ejection fraction and did not correlate with survival, whereas RV ejection showed significant correlation. Furthermore, RV function could further deteriorate on PAH-targeted therapy despite reduction in PVR. Limitations in utilizing CMR in PAH include that it is an expensive test, not widely available, and difficulty to perform for patients with advanced PAH.

Prognostic variables in the era of PAH-targeted therapies

Assessments such as FC and 6MWD have served as useful tools to provide information in patients with PAH regarding disease progression, treatment response, and prognosis. However, PAH research is now evolving with new clinical trials focusing on longer-term outcomes and hard endpoints such as morbidity, mortality, and clinical worsening. In the era of multiple PAH-specific treatments, there is a need to determine which prognostic factors are most useful and relevant to reflect right heart function. Also, baseline parameters alone cannot impart long-term treatment outcomes. Nickel and colleagues reported a systemic evaluation of prognostic markers at baseline and follow-up in a series of patients with IPAH.[237] They identified four variables that were independently associated with survival at baseline as well as at follow-up: NYHA class, NT-proBNP, CI, and SvO_2. NYHA class I or II, NT-proBNP

Table 22.9 Treatment goals for pulmonary arterial hypertension

Functional class	I or II
Echocardiography/CMR	Normal/near-normal RV size and function
Hemodynamics	Normalization of RV function (RAP <8 mmHg and CI >2.5 to 3.0 l/min/m^2
6-min walk distance	>380 to 440 m; may not be aggressive enough in young individuals
Cardiopulmonary exercise testing	Peak VO_2 >15ml/min/kg and $EqCO_2$ <45 l/min/l/min
B-type natriuretic peptde level	Normal

CI, cardiac index; CMR, cardiac magnetic resonance; $EqCO_2$, ventilatory equivalent for carbon dioxide; RAP, right atrial pressure; RV, right ventricular; VO_2, peak oxygem consumption.

Reproduced from Journal of the American College of Cardiology, 2013 Dec 24;62(25 Suppl):D73–81. McLaughlin VV, Gaine SP, Howard LS, et al. Treatment goals of pulmonary hypertension.

less than 1800 ng/L, CI 2.5 L min^{-1} m^{-2} or more, and SvO_2 65% or more during follow-up were associated with a better survival. Of note, the follow-up assessments were better outcome predictors than the baseline evaluations; in fact the outcome was almost entirely determined by the variables obtained at follow-up rather than by the baseline measurements. The REVEAL risk calculator provides another method of determining outcome of patients utilizing clinical variables.[214] Furthermore, developing a heart function score that focuses on the RV has been proposed.[238] A study is under way in France for systematic assessment of a combination of variables in a cohort of newly diagnosed patients with idiopathic, heritable, or anorexigen-associated PAH. The main objective is to determine treatment goals by combining variables associated with the longest survival time.[239]

Longitudinal assessment in pulmonary arterial hypertension

Long-term management of PAH patients requires close monitoring and vigilant follow-up. However, strict guidelines with specific recommendations for longitudinal assessment are not available because most randomized controlled trials have been only short-term studies, usually 12–16 weeks in duration. There are a few long-term studies but they are mostly single-center experiences without a control cohort. Furthermore, response to treatment is very patient specific and varies widely from patient to patient which makes creating general recommendations infeasible.[95] Current treatment goal recommendations from 2013 World Symposium on PH meeting in Nice are for patients receiving PAH-specific treatments to achieve functional class I or II, 6MWD greater than 380 to 400 m, RAP less than 8 mmHg, CI greater than 2.5–3.0 L min^{-1} m^{-2}, peak VO_2 greater than 15 ml per min per kg and $EqCO_2$ less than 45L min^{-1}, /normal RV size and function on echocardiogram, and normal BNP levels (see Table 22.9).[240]

Consensus recommendations on longitudinal reassessment were formulated for the 2009 ACCF/AHA Expert Consensus Document on Pulmonary Hypertension which is based on the known clinical prognostic indicators such as FC, 6MWD, and echocardiographic and hemodynamic parameters (Box 22.3).[40] Patients who are stable, having achieved WHO FC I or II with 6MWD greater than 400 m and normal RV function on echocardiogram and normal hemodynamic parameters can be seen at 3- to 6-month intervals. High-risk patients, determined as those who remain FC III or IV with 6MWD less than 300 m and have echocardiographic evidence of RV dysfunction and abnormal parameters on RHC, merit closer follow-up with visits at 1- to 3-month intervals (Table 22.10).

Box 22.3 Functional classification of pulmonary hypertension modified after the New York Heart Association functional classification according to WHO 1998

Class I

- Patients with pulmonary hypertension but without resulting limitation of physical activity
- Ordinary physical activity does not cause undue dyspnea or fatigue, chest pain, or near syncope

Class II

- Patients with pulmonary hypertension resulting in slight limitation of physical activity
- They are comfortable at rest
- Ordinary physical activity causes undue dyspnea or fatigue, chest pain, or near syncope

Class III

- Patients with pulmonary hypertension resulting in marked limitation of physical activity
- They are comfortable at rest
- Less than ordinary activity causes undue dyspnea or fatigue, chest pain, or near syncope

Class IV

- Patients with pulmonary hypertension with inability to carry out any physical activity without symptoms
- These patients manifest signs of right heart failure
- Dyspnea and/or fatigue may even be present at rest
- Discomfort is increased by any physical activity

Reprinted from Journal of the American College of Cardiology, 43, Barst RJ, McGoon M, Torbicki A, et al. Diagnosis and differential assessment of pulmonary arterial hypertension, S40–S47. Copyright (2004) with permission from Elsevier.

Future directions

Tremendous progress has been achieved in the field of PAH with availability of disease-specific treatments resulting in improved survival and quality of life. However, much more yet remains to do. Although awareness of PAH has increased, there is still a considerable lack of recognition of the disease and significant delay in diagnosis that severely impacts prognosis. Concerted efforts are currently under way to educate the medical community, as well as patients and families, in order to optimize outcome through early detection and diagnosis. With regard to treatment, newer

Table 22.10 Longitudinal evaluation of the patient with pulmonary arterial hypertension[a] [40]

Clinical course	Stable (no increase in symptoms and/or decompensation)	Unstable (increase in symptoms and/or decompensation)
Physical examination	No evidence of right heart failure	Signs of right heart failure
Functional class	I/II	IV[b]
6MWD	>400 m	<300 m
Echocardiogram	RV size and function normal	RV enlargement/ dysfunction
Hemodynamics	RAP and CI normal	RAP high/CI low
BNP	Near normal/stable or decreasing	Elevated/increasing
Treatment	Oral therapy	IV prostacyclin and/or combination treatment
Frequency of evaluation	Q 3–6 months[c]	Q 1–3 months
Functional class assessment	Every clinic visit	Every clinic visit
6MWD	Every clinic visit	Every clinic visit
Echocardiogram[d]	Q 12 months or center dependent	Q 6–12 months or center dependent
BNP[e]	Center dependent	Center dependent
Right heart catheterization	Clinical deterioration and center dependent	Q 6–12 months or clinical deteroration

6MWD, 6 minute walk distance; BNP, brain natriuretic peptide; CI, cardiac index; FC, functional class; IV, intravenous; PAH: pulmonary arterial hypertension; Q: every; RAP: right atrial pressure; RHC: right heart catheterization; RV: right ventricle.

[a] For patients in the high-risk category, consider referral to a PH specialty center for consideration for advanced therapies, clinical trials, and/or lung transplantation.

[b] The frequency of follow-up evaluation for patients in FC III and/or 6MWD 300–400 m would depend on composite of detailed assessments on other clinical and objective characteristics listed.

[c] For patients who remain stable on established therapy, follow-up assessments can be performed by referring physician(s) or PH specialty centers.

[d] Echocardiographic measurement of pulmonary artery systolic pressure is estimation only and it is strongly advised not to rely on its evaluation as the sole parameter to make therapeutic decisions.

[e] The utility of serial BNP levels to guide management in individual patients has not beeen established.

Reprinted from Journal of the American College of Cardiology, 53, McLaughlin VV, Archer SL, Badesch DB, et al. ACCF/AHA 2009 expert consensus document on pulmonary hypertension: a report of the American College of Cardiology Foundation Task Force on Expert Consensus Documents, 1573–1619, copyright (2009) with permission from Elsevier.

therapeutic options that provide novel mechanisms of treatment and enhanced efficacy hold promise in providing improved outcome. Furthermore, intravenous prostacyclins are recognized to be the most effective therapy available but usually approached as a "last resort" for patients with advanced disease due to the complexity and complications associated with intravenous route. The availability of oral prostanoids may herald a paradigm shift in how PAH therapies are utilized. Finally, we need greater understandingof the assessment and mechanism of the target organ in PAH, namely the RV. Recent studies have shown the potential usefulness of CMR in assessing the baseline status and for follow-up evaluation of RV in PAH patients, demonstrating that RV ejection fraction may be one of the most important determinants of long-term prognosis. The need to improve understanding of the underlying mechanism of RV failure remains one of the most critical goals in the treatment of patients with pulmonary hypertension. In summary, the future of PAH includes continued efforts aimed towards early recognition and diagnosis of the disease, development of new drugs targeting novel pathways, and increasing our understanding of the mechanisms of RV failure—measures which hopefully will result in our ability to help patients live longer, better lives.

References

1. Harvey W. Exercitatio Anatomica de Motu Cordis et Sanguinis in Animabilus. Francoforti Guilemi Fitzeri, 1628 [translated by CD Leake]. Springfield, IL: Charles C. Thomas; 1928.
2. Richards DW. The J. Burns Amberson lecture: The right heart and the lung. Am Rev Respir Dis 1966;94:691–702.
3. Newman JH. Centennial review: Pulmonary hypertension. Am J Respir Crit Care Med 2005;172:1072–7.
4. Romberg E. Uebere sklerose der lungenarterien. Dtsch Arch Klin Med 1891;48:197–206.
5. Osler W. The Principles and Practices of Medicine. New York: D. Appleton; 1893.
6. Arrillaga FC. [Sclerose de l' artere pulmonaire (cardiagues noirs)]. Bull Mem Soc Med Hop Paris 1924;48:292–303.
7. Fishman AP. Primary pulmonary arterial hypertension. A look back. J Am Coll Cardiol 2004;43:2S–4S.
8. Brenner O. Pathology of the vessels of the pulmonary circulation. Arch Intern Med 1935;56:211–37.
9. Humbert M, Simonneau G, Rubin LJ. A decade of achievement in pulmonary hypertension. Eur Respir Rev 2011;20:215–17.
10. Forssman W. Die Sonderung des rechten Herzens. Klin Wockschr 1929;8:2085–7.
11. Cournand AW, Ranges HA. Catheterization of the right auricle in man. Proc Soc Exp Biol Med 1941;46:62.
12. Dresdale DT, Schultz M, Michtom RJ. Primary pulmonary hypertension: I. Clinical and hemodynamic study. Am J Med 1951;11:686–705.
13. Wood P, Besterman EM, Towers MK, et al. The effect of acetylcholine on pulmonary vascular resistance and left atrial pressure in mitral stenosis. Br Heart J 1957;19:276–86.
14. Hatano S, Strasso R, ed., Primary Pulmonary Hypertension. Geneva: World Health Organization; 1975.
15. Rich S, Dantzker DR, Ayres SM, et al. Primary pulmonary hypertension: a national prospective study. Ann Intern Med 1987,107:216–23.
16. D'Alonzo GE, Barst RJ, Ayres SM, et al: Survival in patients with primary pulmonary hypertension: results from a national prospective registry. Ann Intern Med 1991,115:343–9.
17. Simonneau G, Nazzareno G, Rubin LJ, et al. Clinical classification of pulmonary hypertension. J Am Coll Cardiol 2004;43(12,Suppl 1):S5–12.
18. Simonneau G, Robbins IM, Beghetti M, et al. Updated clinical classification of pulmonary hypertension. J Am Coll Cardiol 2009;54:S43–54.
19. Barst RJ, Gibbs SR, Hossein A, et al. Updated evidence-based treatment algorithm in pulmonary arterial hypertension. J Am Coll Cardiol 2009;54:S78–84.
20. Simonneau G, Gatzoulis MA, Adatia I, et al. Updated clinical classification of pulmonary hypertension. J Am Coll Cardiol 2013;62:D34-41.
21. Humbert M, Sibton O, Chaouat A, et al. Pulmonary arterial hypertension in France. Results from a national registry. Am J Respir Crit Care Med 2006;173:1023–30.
22. Humbert M, Sitbon O, Chaouat A, et al. Survival in patients with idiopathic, familial, and anorexigen-associated pulmonary arterial hypertension in the modern management era. Circulation 2010;122:156–63.

23. Badesch D, Raskob G, Elliott G, et al. Pulmonary arterial hypertension. Baseline characteristics from the REVEAL Registry. Chest 2010;137:376–87.
24. Frost A, Badesch D, Barst R, et al. The changing picture of patients with pulmonary arterial hypertension in the United States. How REVEAL differs from historic and non-US contemporary registries. Chest 2011;139:128–37.
25. Yigla M, Kramer MR, Bendayan D, et al. Unexplained severe pulmonary hypertension in the elderly: report on 14 patients. Isr Med Assoc J 2004;6:78–81.
26. Machado RD, James V, Southwood M, et al. Investigation of a second genetic hits at the BMPR2 locus as a modulator of disease progression in familial pulmonary arterial hypertension. Circulation 2005;111:607–13.
27. Cogan JD, Vnencak-Jones CL, Phillips JA III, et al. Gross BMPR2 gene rearrangements constitue a new cause for primary pulmonary hypertension. Genet Med 2005;7:169–74.
28. Thomson JR, Machado RD, Pauciulo MW, et al. Sporadic primary pulmonary hypertension is associated with germline mutations of the gene encoding BMPR-II, a receptor member of the TGF-B family. J Med Genet 2000;37:741–5.
29. Abenhaim L, Moride Y, Brenot F, et al. Appetite-suppressant drugs and the risk of primary pulmonary hypertension. N Engl J Med 1996;335:609–16.
30. Walker AM, Langleben D, Korelitz JJ, et al. Temporal trends and drug exposuresin pulmonary hypertension: an American experience. Am Heart J 2006;152:521–6.
31. Mukerjee D. St. George D. Coleriro B, et al. Prevalence and outcome in systemic sclerosis associated pulmonary arterial hypertension: Application of a registry approach. Ann Rheum Dis 2003;62:1088–93.
32. Hachulla E, Gressin V, Guillevin L, et al. Early detection of pulmonary arterial hypertension in systemic sclerosis: a French nationwide prospective multicenter study. Arthritis Rheum 2005;52:3792–800.
33. Koh ET, Lee P, Gladman DD, et al: Pulmonary hypertension in systemic sclerosis: An analysis of 17 patients. Br J Rheumatol 1996,35:989–93.
34. Kuhn KP, Byrne DW, Arbogast PG, et al. Outcome in 91 consecutive patients with pulmonary arterial hypertension receiving epoprostenol. Am J Respir Crit Care Med 2003,167:580–6.
35. Wigley FM, Lima JA, Mayes M, et al. The prevalence of undiagnosed pulmonary arterial hypertension in subjects with connective tissue disease at the secondary health care level of community-based rheumatologist (the UNCOVER study). Arthritis Rheum 2005;52:2125–32.
36. Tanaka E, Harigai M, Tanaka M, et al. Pulmonary hypertension in systemic lupus erythematosus: Evaluation of clinical characteristics and response to immunosuppressive treatment. J Rheumatol 2001;29:282–7.
37. Sitbon O, Lascoux-Combe C, Delfraissy JF, et al. Prevalence of HIV-related pulmonary arterial hypertension in the current antiretroviral therapy era. Am J Respir Crit Care Med 2008;177:108–13.
38. Speich R, Jenni R, Opravil M, et al. Primary pulmonary hypertension in HIV infection. Chest 1991;100:1268–71.
39. Mehta NJ, Khan IA, Metha RN, et al. HIV-related pulmonary hypertension: analytic review of 131 cases. Chest 2000;118:1133–41.
40. McLaughlin VV, Archer SL, Badesch DB, et al. ACCF/AHA 2009 expert consensus document on pulmonary hypertension: a report of the American College of Cardiology Foundation Task Force on Expert Consensus Documents. J Am Coll Cardiol 2009;53:1573–619.
41. Sitbon O, Gressin V, Speich R, et al. Bosentan for the treatment of human immunodeficiency virus-associated pulmonary arterial hypertension. Am J Repir Crit Care Med 2004;170:1212–17.
42. Kuo PC, Plotkin JS, Johnson LB, et al. Distinctive clinical features of portopulmonary hypertension. Chest 1997;112;980–6.
43. Colle IO, Moreau R, Godinho E, et al. Diagnosis of portopulmonary hypertension in candidates for liver transplantation: a prospective study. Hepatology 2003;37:401–9.
44. Krowka M, Plevak DJ, Findlay JY, et al. Pulmonary hyemodynamics and perioperative cardiopulmonary mortality in patients with portopulmonary hypertension undergoing liver transplantation. Liver Transplant 2000;6:443–50.
45. Le Pavec J, Souza R, Herve P, et al. Portopulmonary hypertension: survival and prognostic factors. Am J Respir Crit Care Med 2008;178:637–43.
46. Galie N, Manes A, Palazzini M, et al. Management of pulmonary arterial hypertension associated with congenital systemic-to-pulmonary shunts and Eisenmenger's syndrome. Drugs 2008;68:1049–66.
47. McLaughlin VV, Presberg KW, Doyle RL, et al. American College of Chest Physicians. Prognosis of pulmonary arterial hypertension: ACCP evidence-based clinical practice guidelines. Chest 2004;126:78S–92S.
48. Grossman W, Barry WH. Cardiac catheterization. In: Braunwald E, ed. Heart Disease: A Textbook of Cardiovascular Medicine. Philadelphia: WB Saunders; 1988, pp. 247–52.
49. Badesch DB, Champion HC, Sanchez MA, et al. Diagnosis and assessment of pulmonary arterial hypertension. J Am Coll Cardiol 2009;54:S55–66.
50. Rich S, Kaufmann E, Levy PS. The effect of high doses of calcium-channel blockers on survival in primary pulmonary hypertension. N Engl J Med 1992;327:76–81.
51. Sitbon O, Humber M, Jais X, et al. Long-term response to calcium channel blockers in idiopathic pulmonary arterial hypertension. Circulation 2005;111:3105–11.
52. Farber HW, Loscalzo J. Pulmonary arterial hypertension. N Engl J Med 2004;351:1655–65.
53. Yuan JXJ, Rubin LJ. Pathogenesis of pulmonary arterial hypertension: the need for multiple hits. Circulation 2005,111:534–8.
54. Machado RD, James V, Southwood M, et al. Investigation of a second genetic hits at the BMPR2 locus as a modulator of disease progression in familial pulmonary arterial hypertension. Circulation 2005;111:607–13.
55. Archer S, Rich S. Primary pulmonary hypertension: A vascular biology and translational research "Work in progress." Circulation 2000;102:2781–91.
56. Christman BW, McPherson CD, Newman JH, et al. An imbalance between the excretion of thromboxane and prostacyclin metabolites in pulmonary hypertension. N Engl J Med 1992,327:70–5.
57. Tuder RM, Cool CD, Geraci MW, et al. Prostacyclin synthase expression is decreased in lungs from patients with severe pulmonary hypertension. Am J Respir Crit Care Med 1999;159:1925–32.
58. Benza RL, Park MH, Keogh A, et al. Management of pulmonary arterial hypertension with a focus on combination therapies. J Heart Lung Transplant 2007;26:437–46.
59. Yanagisawa M, Kurihara H, Kimura S, et al.A novel potent vasoconstrictor peptide produced by vascular endothelial cells. Nature 1988;332:411–15.
60. Ogawa Y, Nakao K, Arai H, et al. Molecular cloning of a non-isopeptide-selective human endothelin receptor. Biochem Biophys Res Commun 1991,178:248–55.
61. Giad A, Yanagisawa M, Langleben D, et al. Expression of endothelin-1 in the lungs of patients with pulmonary hypertension. N Engl J Med 1993,328:1732–9.
62. Rubens C, Ewert R, Halank M, et al. Big endothelin-1 and endothelin-1 plasma levels are correlated with the severity of primary pulmonary hypertension. Chest 2001;120:1562–9.
63. Tantini B, Manes A, Fiumana E, et al. Antiproliferative effect of sildenafil on human pulmonary artery smooth muscle cells. Basic Res Cardiol 2005;100:131–8.
64. Archer SL, Machelakis ED. Phosphodiesterase type 5 inhibitors for pulmonary arterial hypertension. N Engl J Med 2009;361:1864–71.
65. Barst RJ, ed., Pulmonary Arterial Hypertension: Diagnosis and Evidence-Based Treatment. Chichester, UK: John Wiley & Sons; 2008.
66. Ramani GR, Park MH. Update on the clinical utility of sildnenafil in the treatment of pulmonary arterial hypertension. Drug Design Dev Ther 2010;4:61–70.

67. Giaid A, Saleh D. Reduced expression of endothelial nitric oxide synthase in the lungs of paients with pulmonary hypertension. N Engl J Med1995;333:214–21.
68. Corbin JD, Beaskey A, Blount MA, et al. High lung PDE5: a strong basis for treating pulmonary hypertension with PDE5 inhibitors. Biochem Biophys Res Commun 2005;334:930–8.
69. Stasch JP, Pacher P, Evgenov OV. Soluble guanylate cyclase as an emerging therapeutic target in cardiopulmonary disease. Circulation 2011 24 May;123(20):2263–73.
70. Herve P, Launay JM, Scrobohaci ML, et al. Increased plasma serotonin in primary pulmonary hypertension. Am J Med 1995;99:249–54.
71. Abenhaim L, Moride Y, Brenot F, et al. Appetite-suppressant drugs and the risk of primary pulmonary hypertension. N Engl J Med 1996;335:609–16.
72. Eddahibi S, Humbert M, Fadel E, et al. Serotonin transporter over expression is responsible for pulmonary artery smooth muscle hyperplasia in primary pulmonary hypertension. J Clin Invest 2001;108:1141–50.
73. Marcos E, Adnot S, Pham MH, et al. Serotonin transporter inhibitors protect against hypoxic pulmonary hypertension. Am J Respir Crit Care Med 2003;168:487–93.
74. Soderman C, Eriksson LS, Juhlin-Dannfelt A, et al. Effect of vasoactive intestinal popypeptide (VIP) on pulmonary ventilation-perfusion relationships and central hemodynamics in healthy subjects. Clin Physiol 1993;13:677–85.
75. Petkov V, Mosgoeller W, Ziesche R, et al. Vasoactive intestinal peptide as a new drug for treatment of primary pulmonary hypertension. J Clin Invest 2003;111:1339–46.
76. Yuan JJ, Aldinger AM, Juhaszova M, et al. Dysfunctional voltage-gated K^+ channels in pulmonary artery smooth muscle cells of patients with primary pulmonary hypertension. Circulation 1998;98:1400–6.
77. Weir EK, Reeve HL, Huang JM, et al. Anorexic agents aminorex, fenfluramine, and dexfenfluramine inhibit potassium current in rat pulmonary vascular smooth muscle and cause pulmonary vasoconstriction. Circulation 1996;94:2216–30.
78. Welsh CH, Hassell KL, Badesch DB, et al. Coagulation and fibrinolytic profiles in patients with severe pulmonary hypertension. Chest 1996;110:710–17.
79. Tuder RM, Groves BM, Badesch DB, et al. Exuberant endothelial cell growth and elements of inflammation are present in plexiform lesions in pulmonary hypertension. Am J Pathol 1994;144:275–85.
80. Lane KB, Machado RD, Pauciulo MW, et al. Heterozygous germline mutations in BMPR2, encoding a TGF-β receptor, cause familial primary pulmonary hypertension: the International PPH Consortium. Nat Genet 2000,26:81–4.
81. Deng Z, Morse JH, Slager SL, et al. Familial primary pulmonary hypertension (gene PPH1) is caused by mutations in the bone morphogenetic protein receptor-II gene. Am H Hum Genet 2000,67:737–44.
82. Trembath R, Thomson J, Machado R, et al. Clinical and molecular genetic features of pulmonary hypertension in patients with hereditary hemorrhagic telangiectasia. N Engl J Med 2001;345:325–34.
83. Voekel NF, Quaife RA, Leinwant LA, et al. Right ventricular function and failure. Report of a National Heart, Lung, and Blood Institute Working Group on Cellular and Molecular Mechanisms of Right Heart Failure. Circulation 2006;114:1883–91.
84. Dell'Italia LJ. Anatomy and physiology of the right ventricle. Cardiol Clin 2012:30;167–87.
85. Champion HC, Michelakis ED, et al. Comprehensive invasive and noninvasive approach to the right ventricle-pulmonary circulation unit: state of the art and clinical and research implications. Circulation 2009:120;992–1007.
86. Dias CA, Assad RS, Caneo LF, et al. Reversible pulmonary trunk banding, II: an experimental model for rapid pulmonary ventricular hypertrophy. J Thorac Cardiovasc Surg 2002;124:999–1006.
87. Louie EK, Lin SS, Reynertson SI, et al. Pressure and volume loading of the right ventricle have opposite effects on left ventricular ejection fraction. Circulation 1995;92:819–24.
88. Gan CT, Lankhaar J, Marcus JT, et al. Impaired left ventricular filling due to right-to-left ventricular interaction in patients with pulmonary arterial hypertension. Am J Physiol Heart Circ Physiol 2006:290;H1528–33.
89. Hopkins WE, Waggoner AD. Severe pulmonary hypertension without right ventricular failure: the unique hearts of patients with Eisenmenger syndrome. Am J Cardiol 2002;89:34–8.
90. Busjahn A, Knoblauch H, Knoblauch M, et al. Angiotensin-converting enzyme DD genotype in patients with primary pulmonary hypertension: incrased frequency and association with preserved hemodynamics. J Renin Angiotensin Aldosterone Syst 2003;4:27–30.
91. Park, MH. Pulmonary hypertension and right heart failure: Light at the end of the tunnel? In: Mehra MR, ed., Clinical Challenges in Heart Failure, Chapter 3. Dublin: Research and Markets.
92. Gaine SP, Rubin LJ. Primary pulmonary hypertension. Lancet 1998;352:719–25.
93. Rubn LJ. Primary pulmonary hypertension. N Engl J Med 1997;336:111–17.
94. Abenhaim L, Moride Y, Brenot F, et al. Appetite-suppressant drugs and the risk of primary pulmonary hypertension. International Primary Pulmonary Hypertension Study Group. N Engl J Med 1996;335:609–16.
95. McLaughlin VV, Davis M, Cornwall W. Pulmonary arterial hypertension. Curr Probl Cardiol 2011;36:461–517.
96. Ahearn GS, Tapson VG, Rebeiz A, et al. Electrocardiography to define clinical status in primary pulmonary hypertension and pulmonary arterial hypertension secondary to collagen vascular disease. Chest 2002;122:524–7.
97. Tongers J, Schwerdtfeger B, Klein G, et al. Incidence and clinical relevance of supraventricular tachyarrhythmias in pulmonary hypertension. Am Heart J 2007;153:127–32.
98. McGoon MD. The assessment of pulmonary hypertension. Clin Chest Med 2001;22:493–508.
99. Sitbon O, Lascoux-Combe C, Delfraissy JF, et al. Prevalence of HIV-related pulmonary arterial hypertension in the current antiretroviral therapy era. Am J Respir Crit Care Med 2008;177:108–13.
100. Fisher MR, Forfia PR, Chamera E, et al. Accuracy of Doppler echocardiography in the hemodynamic assessment of pulmonary hypertension. Am J Resp Crit Care Med 2009;179:615–21.
101. Bossone E, Duong-Wagner TH, Paciocco G, et al. Echocardiographic features of primary pulmonary hypertension. J Am Soc Ehocardiogr 1999;12:655–62.
102. Homma A, Anzueto A, Peters JI, et al. Pulmonary artery systolic pressures estimated by echocardiogram vs cardiac catheterization in patients awaiting lung transplantation. J Heart Lung Transplant 2001;20:833–9.
103. Yock PG, Popp RL. Noninvasive estimation of right ventricular systolic pressure by Doppler ultrasound in patients with tricuspid regurgitation. Circulation 1984;70:657–62.
104. Brecher SJ, Gibbs JS, Fox KM, et al. Comparison of Doppler derived hemodynamic variables and simultaneous high fidelity pressure measurements in severe pulmonary hypertension. Br Heart J 1994;72:384–9.
105. Arcasoy SM, Christie JD, Ferrari VA, et al. Echocardiographic assessment of pulmonary hypertension in patients with advanced lung disease. Am J Respir Crit Care Med 2003;167:735–40.
106. Hinderliter AL, Willis PW 4th, Long WA, et al. Frequency and severity of tricuspid regurgitation determined by Doppler echocardiography in primary pulmonary hypertension. Am J Cardiol 2003;91:1033–7.
107. Currie PJ, Seward JB, Chan KL, et al. Continuous wave Doppler determination of right ventricular pressure: A simultaneous Doppler-catheterization study in 127 patients. J Am Coll Cardiol 1985;6:750–6.
108. Homma A, Anzueto A, Peters JI, et al. Pulmonary artery systolic pressures estimated by echocardiogram vs cardiac catheterization in patients awaiting lung transplantation. J Heart Lung Transplant 2001;20:833–9.

109. Murata I, Kihara H, Shinohara S, et al. Echocardiographic evaluation of pulmonary arterial hypertension in patients with progressive systemic sclerosis and related syndromes. Jpn Circ J 1992;56:983–91.
110. McGoon M, Gutterman D, Steen V, et al. Screening, early detection, and diagnosis of pulmonary arterial hypertension. ACCP Evidence-based clinical practice guidelines. Chest 2004;126:14S–34S.
111. Forfia PR, Fisher MR, Mathai SC, et al. Tricuspid annular displacement predicts survival in pulmonary hypertension. Am J Respir Crit Care Med 2006;174:1034–41.
112. Yeo TC, Dujardin KS, Tei C, et al. Value of a Doppler-derived index combining systolic and diastolic time intervals in predicting outcome in primary pulmonary hypertension. Am J Cardiol 1998;81:1157–61.
113. Opotowsky AR, Ojeda J, Rogers F, et al. A simple echocardiographic prediction rule for hemodynamics in pulmonary hypertension. Circ Cardiovasc Imaging 2012;6:765–75.
114. Humbert M, Maitre S, Capron F, et al. Pulmonary edema complicating continuous intravenous prostacyclin in pulmonary capillary hemangiomatosis. Am J Respir Crit Care Med 1998;157:1681–5.
116. Rich S, Kieras K, Groves B, et al. Antinuclear antibodies in primary pulmonary hypertension. J Am Coll Cardiol 1986;8:1307–11.
117. Chu JW, Kao PN, Faul JL, et al. High prevalence of autoimmune thyroid disease in pulmonary arterial hypertension. Chest 2002;122:1668–73.
118. Galie N, Hoeper MM, Humber M, et al. Guidelines for the diagnosis and treatment of pulmonary hypertension: The task force for the diagnosis and treatment of pulmonary hypertension of the European Society of Cardiology (ESC) and the European Respiratory Society (ERS), endorsed by the International Society of Heart and Lung Transplantation (ISHLT). Eur Heart J 2009;30:2493–37.
119. Dutour B, Maitre S, Humbert M, et al. High-resolution CT of the chest in four patients with pulmonary capillary hemangiomatosis or pulmonary venoocclusive disease. Am J Radiol 1998;171:1321–4.
120. Pengo V, Lensing A, Prins MH, et al. Incidence of chronic thromboembolic pulmonary hypertension after pulmonary embolism. N Engl J Med 2004;350:2257–64.
121. Tunariu N, Gibbs SJR, Win Z, et al. Ventilation-perfusion scintigraphy is more sensitive than multidetector CTPA in detecting chronic thromboembolic pulmonary disease as a treatable cause of pulmonary hypertension. J Nucl Med 2007;48:680–4.
122. Fedulo PF, Auger WR, Kerr KM, et al. Chronic thromboembolic pulmonary hypertension. N Engl J Med 2001;345:1465–72.
123. Pitton MB, Kemmerich G, Herber S, et al. Hemodynamic effects of monomeric nonionic contrast media in pulmonary angiography in chronic thromboembolic pulmonary hypertension. Am J Roentgenol 2006;187:128–34.
124. Sol M, Garc A, Picado C, et al. Segmental contour pattern in a case of pulmonary venoocclusive disease. Clin Nucl Med 1993;18:679–81.
125. Park MH, McLaughlin VV. Pulmonary hypertension: Hemodynamic assessment and response to vasodilators. In: Cardiac Catheterization and Intervention. London, Informa Healthcare; 2010, pp. 98–117.
126. Halpern SD, Taichman DB. Misclassification of pulmonary hypertension due to reliance on pulmonary capillary wedge pressure rather than left ventricular end-diastolic pressure. Chest 2009;136:37–43.
127. Ryan JJ, Rich JD, Thiruvoipati T, et al. Current practice for determining pulmonary capillary wedge pressure predispoises to serious errors in the classification of patients with pulmonary hypertension. Am Heart J 2012;163:589–94.
128. Hoeper MM, Barberia JA, Channick RN, et al. Diagnosis, assessment, and treatment of non-pulmonary arterial hypertension pulmonary hypertension. J Am Coll Cardiol 2009;54(1 Suppl):S85–96.
129. Pichard AD, Kay R, Smith H, et al. Large V waves in the pulmonary wedge pressure tracing in the absence of mitral regurgitation. Am J Cardiol 1982;50:1044–50.
130. Fuchs RM, Henser RR, Yin FCP, et al. Limitation of pulmonary wedge V waves in diagnosing mitral regurgitation. Am J Cardiol 1982;49:849–54.
131. Pepine CJ, Hill JA, Lambert CR. Pressure measurement and determination of vascular resistance. In: Diagnostic and Therapeutic Cardiac Catheterization, 2nd edn. Philadelphia, PA: Williams & Wilkins; 1994, pp. 355–71.
132. Ragosta M. Right sided heart disorders. In: Textbook of Clinical Hemodynamics. Philadelphia, PA: Elsevier Saunders; 2008, pp. 109–22.
133. Ragosta M. Normal waveforms, artifacts, and pitfalls. In: Textbook of Clinical Hemodynamics. Philadelphia, PA: Elsevier Saunders; 2008, pp. 16–37.
134. Hoeper MM, Maier R, Tongers J, et al. Determination of cardiac output by the Fick method, thermodilution, and acetylene rebreathing in pulmonary hypertension. Am J Respir Crit Care Med 1999;160:535–41.
135. Hoeper MM, Lee SH, Voswinckel R, et al. Complications of right heart catheterization procedures in patients with pulmonary hypertension in experienced centers. J Am Coll Cardiol 2006,48:2546–52.
136. Sitbon O, Humbert M, Jais X, et al. Long-term response to calcium channel blockers in idiopathic pulmonary arterial hypertension. Circulation 2005,111:3105–11.
137. Elliott CG, Glissmeyer EW, Havlena GT, et al. Relationship of BMPR2 mutations to vasoreactivity in pulmonary arterial hypertension. Circulation 2006;113:2509–15.
138. Simonneau G, Fartoukh M, Sitbon O, et al. Primary pulmonary hypertension associated with the use of fenfluramine derivatives. Chest 1998;114:195S–9S.
139. Klings ES. Hill NS, Ieong MH, et al. Systemic sclerosis-associated pulmonary hypertension: short- and long-term effects of epoprostenol (prostacyclin). Arthritis Rheum 1999;42:2638–45.
140. Palmer SM, Robinson LJ, Wang A, et al. Massive pulmonary edema and death after prostacyclin infusion in a patient with pulmonary veno-occlusive disease. Chest 1998;113:237–40.
141. Groves BM, Badesch DB, Turkevich D, et al. Correlation of acute prostacyclin response in primary (unexplained) pulmonary hypertension with efficacy of treatemt with calcium channel blockers and survival. In:Weir K, ed. Ion Flux in Pulmonary Vascular Control. New York, NY: Plenum Press; 1993, pp. 317–30.
142. Sitbon O, Brenot F, Denjean A, et al. Inhaled nitric oxide as a screening vasodilator agent in primary pulmonary hypertension: a dose-response study and comparison with prostacyclin. Am J Respir Crit Care Med 1995;151:384–9.
143. Schrader BJ, Inbar S, Kaufmann L, et al. Comparison of the effects of adenosine and nifedipine in pulmonary hypertension. J Am Coll Cardiol 1992,19:1060–4.
144. Sitbon O, Humbert M, Jagot JL, et al: Inhaled nitric oxide as a screening agent for safely identifying responders to oral calcium-channel blockers in primary pulmonary hypertension. Eur Respir J 1998,12:265–70.
145. Galie N, Manes A, Negro L, et al. A meta-analysis of randomized controlled trials in pulmonary arterial hypertension. Eur Heart J 2009;30:394–403.
146. Galie N, Rubin LJ, Hoeper MM, et al. Treatment of patients with mildly symptomatic pulmonary arterial hypertension with bosentan (EARLY study): a duble-blind, randomized controlled trial. Lancet 2008;317:2093–100.
147. Badesch DB, Abman SH, Simonneau G, et al. Medical therapy for pulmonary arterial hypertension: Updated ACCP evidence based clinical practice guidelines. Chest 2007;131:1917–28.
148. Mereles D, Ehlken N, Kreuscher S, et al. Exercise and respiratory training improve exercise capacity and quality of life in patients with severe chronic pulmonary hypertension. Circulation 2006;114:1482–9.
149. Chan L, Chin LM, Kennedy M, et al. Benefits of intensive treadmill exercise training on cardiorespiratory function and quality of life in patients with pulmonary hypertension. Chest 2013;143:333–43.
150. Weiss BM, Zemp L, Seifert B, et al. Outcome of pulmonary vascular disease in pregnancy: A systematic overview from 1978 through 1996. J Am Coll Cardiol 1998;31:1650–7.

151. Rich S, Kaufmann E, Levy PS. The effect of high doses of calcium-channel blcokers on survival in primary pulmonary hypertension. N Engl J Med 1992;327:76–81
152. Frank H, Mlczoch J, Huber K, et al. The effect of anticoagulant therapy in primary and anorectic drug-induced pulmonary hypertension. Chest 1997;112:714–21.
153. Fuster V, Frye RL, Gersh BJ, et al. Primary pulmonary hypertension: Natural history and the importance of thrombosis. Circulation 1984;70:580–7.
154. Barst RJ, Rubin LJ, Long WA, et al. A comparison of continuous intravenous epoprostenol (prostacyclin) with conventional therapy for primary pulmonary hypertension. The Primary Pulmonary Hypertension Study Group. N Engl J Med 1996,334:296–302.
155. Badesch DB, Tapson VF, McGoon MD, et al. Continuous intravenous epoprostenol for pulmonary hypertension due to the scleroderma spectrum of disease: a randomized, controlled trial. Ann Intern Med 2000;132:425–34.
156. Aguilar RV, Farber HW. Epoprostenol (prostacyclin) therapy in HIV-associated pulmonary hypertension. Am J Respir Crit Care Med 2000;162:1846–50.
157. Rosenzweig EB, Kerstein D, Barst RJ. Long-term prostacyclin for pulmonary hypertension with associated congenital heart defects. Circulation 1999;99:1858–65.
158. Kuo PC, Johnson LB, Plotkin JS, et al. Continuous intravenous infusion of epoprostenol for the treatment of portopulmonary hypertension. Transplantation 1997;63:604–16.
159. Sitbon O, Humbert M, Nunes H, et al. Long-term intravenous epoprostenol infusion in primary pulmonary hypertension: prognostic factors and survival. J Am Coll Cardiol 2002,40:780–8.
160. McLaughlin VV, Shillington A, Rich S. Survivval in primary pulmonary hypertension: the impact of epoprostenol therapy. Circulation 2002, 106:1477–82.
161. Rich S, McLauglin VV. The effects of chronic prostacyclin therapy on cardiac output and symptoms in primary pulmonary hypertension. J Am Coll Cardiol 1999;34:1184–7.
162. Chin KM, Channick RN, de Lemos JA, et al. Hemodynamics and epoprostenol use are associated with thrombocytopenia in pulmomary arterial hypertension. Chest 2009;135:130–6.
163. Simonneau G, Barst RJ, Galie N, et al. Continuous subcutaneous infusion of treprostinil, a prostacyclin analogue, in patients with pulmonary arterial hypertension. Am J Respir Crit Care Med 2002;165:800–4.
164. Mather M, McDevitt S, Saggar R. Subcutaneous treprostinil in pulmonary arterial hypertension: practical considerations. J Heart Lung Transplant 2010;29:1210–17.
165. Tapson VF, Gomberg-Maitland M, McLaughlin V, et al. Safety and efficacy of IV treprostinil for pulmonary arterial hypertension: a prospective, multicenter, open-label, 12-week trial. Chest 2006;129:683–8.
166. Gomberg-Maitland M, Tapson VF, Benza RL, et al. Transition from intravenous epoprotenol to intravenous treprostinil in pulmonary hypertension. Am J Respir Crit Care Med 2005;172:1586–9.
167. Hiremath J, Thanikachalam S, Parikh K, et al. Exercise improvement and plasma biomarker changes with intravenous treprostinil therapy for pulmonary arterial hypertension: A placebo-controlled trial. J Heart Lung Transplant 2010;29:137–49.
168. Laliberte K, Arneson C, Jeffs R, et al. Pharmacokinetics and steady-state bioequivalence of treprostinil sodium (Remodulin) administered by the intravenous and subcutaneous route to normal volunteers. J Cardiovasc Pharmacol 2004;44:209–14.
169. Centers for Disease Control and Prevention. Bloodstream infections among patients treated with intravenous epoprostenol or intravenous treprostinil for pulmonary arterial hypertension—seven sites, United States 2003–2006. MMWR Morb Mortal Wkly Rep 2007;56:170–2.
170. Doran A, Ivy D, Barst RJ, et al. Guidelines for the prevention of central venous catheter-related bloodstream infections with prastanoid therapy for pulmonary arterial hypertension. Adv Pulm Hypertens 2008;7:245–8.
171. Jing ZC1, Parikh K, Pulido T, et al. Efficacy and safety of oral treprostinil monotherapy for the treatment of pulmonary arterial hypertension: a randomized, controlled trial. Circulation. 2013 Feb 5;127(5):624–33.
172. Tapson VF, Jing ZC, Xu KF, et al. Oral treprostinil for the treatment of pulmonary arterial hypertension in patients receiving background endothelin receptor antagonist and phosphodiesterase type 5 inhibitor therapy (the FREEDOM-C2 study): a randomized controlled trial. Chest. 2013 Sep;144(3):952–8.
173. McLaughlin VV, Benza RL, Rubin LJ, et al. Addition of inhaled treprostinil to oral therapy for pulmonary arterial hypertension: A randomized controlled clinical trial. J Am Coll Cardiol 2010;55:1915–22.
174. Olschewski H, Simonneay G, Galie N, et al. Inhaled iloprost for severe pulmonary hypertension. N Engl J Med 2002;347:322–9.
175. Mubarak KK. A review of prostaglandin analogs in the management of patients with pulmonary arterial hypertension. Respir Med 2010;104:9–21.
176. Kuwano K, Hashino A, Asaki T, et al. 2-[4-[(5,6-diphenylpyrazin-2-yl)(isopropyl)amino]butoxy]-N-(methylsulfonyl)acetamide (NS-304), an orally available and long-acting prostacyclin receptor agonist prodrug. J Pharmacol Exp Ther 2007;322:1181–8.
177. Simonneau G, Lang I, Torbicki A, et al. Efficacy, safety, and tolerability of ACT-293987, a novel oral, non-prostanoid, prostaglandin I2 (IP) receptor agonist: results from a phase IIa study in pulmonary arterial hypertension (PAH). Am J Respir Crit Care Med 2010;181:A2515.
178. McLaughlin VV, Channick R, Chin K, et al. Effect of selexipag on morbidity/mortality in pulmonary arterial hypertension: results of the GRIPHON study. JACC 2015;65(10S).
179. Channick RN, Simonneau G, Sitbon O, et al. Effects of the dual endothelin-receptor antagonist bosentan in patients with pulmonary hypertension: a randomized placebo-controlled study. Lancet 2001;358:1119–23.
180. Rubin LJ, Badesch DB, Barst RJ, et al. Bosentan therapy for pulmonary arterial hypertension. N Engl J Med 2002,346:896–903.
181. McLaughlin VV, Sitbon O, Badesch DB, et al. Survival with first-line bosentan in patients with primary pulmonary hypertension. Eur Respir J 2005,25:244–9.
182. Galie N, Rubin LJ, Hoeper MM, et al. Treatment of patients with mildly symptomatic pulmonary arterial hypertension with bosentan (EARLY study): a double-blind, randomized controlled trial. Lancet 2008;317:2093–100.
183. Galie N, Olschewski H, Oudiz R, et al. Ambrisentan for the treatment of pulmonary arterial hypertension. Results of the ambrosentan in pulmonary arterial hypertension, randomized, double-blind, placebo-controlled, multicenter, efficacy (ARIES) study 1 and 2. Circulation 2008;117:3010–19.
184. Oudiz RJ, Galie N, Olschewski H, et al. Long-term ambrisentan therapy for the treatment of pulmonary arterial hypertension. J Am Coll Cardiol 2009;54:1971–81.
185. McGoon M, Frost AE, Oudiz RJ, et al. Ambrisentan therapy in patients with pulmonary arterial hypertension who discontinued bosentan or sitaxsentan due to liver function test abnormalities. Chest 2009;135:122–9.
186. Letairis: Highlights of prescribing information <http://www.gilead.com/pdf/letairis_pi.pdf>.
187. Iglarz M, Binkert C, Morrison K, et al. Pharmacology of macitentan, an orally active tissue-targeting dual endothelin receptor antagonist. J Pharmacol Exp Ther 2008;327:736–45.
188. Raja SG. Macitentan: a tissue-targeting endthelin receptor antagonist for the potential oral treatment of pulmonary arterial hypertension and idiopathic pulmonary fibrosis. Curr Opin Invest Drugs 2010;11:1066–73.
189. Pulido T, Adzerikho I, Channick RN, et al. Macitentan and morbidity and mortality in pulmonary arterial hypertension. N Engl J Med. 2013 Aug 29;369(9):809–18.

190. Galie N, Ghofrani HA, Torbicki A, et al. Sildenafil Use in Pulmonary Arterial Hypertension (SUPER) Study Group. Sildenafil citrate therapy for pulmonary arterial hypertension. N Engl J Med 2005,353:2148–57.
191. Rubin LJ, Badesch DB, Fleming TR, et al. Long-term treatment with sildenafil citrate in pulmonary arterial hypertension: the SUPER-2 study. Chest 2011;140:1274–83.
192. Laties AM. Vision disorders and phosphodietserase type 5 inhibitors: a review of the evidence to date. Drug Saf 2009;32:1–18.
193. Gabrieli CB, Regine F, Vingolo EM, et al. Subjective visual halos after sildenafil (Viagra) administration: electroretinographic evaluation. Ophthalmology 2001;108:877–81.
194. Wirostko BM, Tressler C, Hwang LJ, et al. Ocular safety of sildenafil citrate when administered chronically for pulmonary arterial hypertension: results from phase III, randomized, double masked, placebo controlled trial and open label extension. BMJ 2012;344:1–20.
195. Galie N, Brundage BH, Ghofrani HA, et al. Tadalafil therapy for pulmonary arterial hypertension. Circulation 2009;119:2894–903.
196. Oudiz RJ, Brundate BH, Galie N, et al. Tadalafil for the treatment of pulmonary arterial hypertension: a double-blind uncontrolled extension study. J Am Coll Cardiol 2012;60:768–74.
197. Ghofrani HA, Galiè N, Grimminger F, et al. Riociguat for the treatment of pulmonary arterial hypertension. N Engl J Med. 2013 Jul 25;369(4):330–40.
198. Ghofrani HA, Hoeper MM, Halank M, et al. Riociguat for chronic thromboembolic pulmonary hypertension and pulmonary arterial hypertension: a phase II study. Eur Respir J 2010;36:792–9.
199. Hoeper MM, Markevych I, Spiekerkoetter E, et al. Goal-oriented treatment and combination therapy for pulmonary arterial hypertension. Eur Respir J 2005;26:858–63.
200. Hoeper MM, Faulenbach C, Golpon H, et al. Combination therapy with bosentan and sildenafil in idiopathic pulmonary arterial hypertension. Eur Respir J 2004;24:1007–10.
201. Ghofrani HA, Rose F, Schermuly RT, et al. Oral sildenafil as long-term adjunct therapy in severe pulmonary arterial hypertension. J Am Coll Cardiol 2003;42:158–64.
202. Humbert M, Barst RJ, Robbins IM, et al. Combination of bosentan with epoprostenol in pulmonary arterial hypertension: BREATHE-2. Eur Respir J 2004;24:353–9.
203. McLaughlin VV, Oudiz RJ, Frost AE, et al. Randomized study adding inhaled iloprost to existing bosentan in pulmonary arterial hypertension. Am J Respir Crit Care Med 2006;174:1257–63.
204. Hoeper MM, Leuchte H, Halank M, et al. Combining inhaled iloprost with bosentan in patients with idiopathic pulmonary arterial hypertension. Eur Respir J 2006;28:691–4.
205. Simonneau G, Rubin LJ, Nazzareno G, et al. Addition of sildenafil to long-term intravenous epoprostenol therapy in patients with pulmonary arterial hypertension. Ann Intern Med 2008;149:521–30.
206. Galiè N, Barberà JA, Frost AE, et al. Initial use of ambrisentan plus tadalafil in pulmonary arterial hypertension. N Engl J Med 2015;373:834.
207. Sandoval J, Gaspar J, Pulido T, et al. Graded balloon dilation atrial septostomy in severe primary pulmonary hypertension. A therapeutic alternative for patients nonresponsive to vasodilator treatment. J Am Coll Cardiol 1998;32:297–304.
208. Rothman A, Sklansky MS, Lucas VW, et al. Atrial septostomy as a bridge to lung transplantation in patients with severe pulmonary hypertension. Am J Cardiol 1999;84:682–6.
209. Reichenberger F, Pepke-Zaba J, McNeil K, et al. Atrial septostomy in the treatment of severe pulmonary arterial hypertension. Thorax 2003;58:797–800.
210. Christie JD, Edwards LB, Kucheryavaya AY, et al. The registry of the International Society for Heart and Lung Transplantation: twenty-seventh official adult lung and heart-lung transplant report-2010. J Heart Lung Transplant 2010;29:1104–8.
211. Cottini SR, Lerch N, de Perrot M, et al. Risk factors for reperfusion injury after lung transplantation. Intenxive Care Med 2006;32:557–63.
212. Orens JB, Estenne M, Arcasoy S, et al. International guidelines for the selection of lung transplant candidates: 2006 update—a consensus report from the pulmonary scientific council of the International Society for Heart and Lung Transplantation. J Heart Lung Transplant 2006;25:745–55.
213. Chen H, Shiboski SC, Goldern JA, et al. Impact of the lung allocation score on lung transplantation for pulmonary arterial hypertension. Am J Respir Crit Care Med 2009;180:468–74.
214. Benza RL, Miller DP, Gomberg-Maitland M, et al. Predicting survival in pulmonary arterial hypertension: Insights from the registry to evaluate early and long-term pulmonary arterial hypertension disease management (REVEAL). Circulation 2010;122:164–72.
215. Saagar R, Khanna D, Furst DE, et al. Exercise-induced pulmonary hypertension associated with systemic sclerosis: four distinct entities. Arthritis Rheum 2010;62:3741–50.
216. Miyamoto S, Nagaya N, Satoh T, et al. Clinical correlates and prognostic significance of six-minute walk test in patients with primary pulmonary hypertension: comparison with cardiopulmonary exercise testing. Am J Respir Crit Care Med 2000,161:487–92.
217. Macchia A, Marchioli R, Marfisi R, et al. A meta-analysis of trials of pulmonary hypertension: a clinical condition looking for drugs and research methodology. Am Heart J 2007;153:1037–47.
218. Coghlan JG, Pope J, Denton CP. Assessment of endpoints in pulmonary arterial hypertension associated with connective tissue disease. Curr Opin Pulm Med 2010:16(Suppl 1):S27–34.
219. Rubin L, Simonneau G. Perspective on the optimal endpoints for pulmonary arterial hypertension trials. Curr Opin Pulmon Med 2010:16(Suppl 1);S43–46.
220. Minai OA, Gudavalli R, Mummadi S, et al. Heart rate recovery predicts clinical worsening in patients with pulmonary arterial hypertension. Am J Respir Crit Care Med 2012;185:400–8.
221. Savarese G, Paolillo S, Costanzo P, et al. Do changes of 6-minute walk distance predict clinical events in patients with pulmonary arterial hypertension? A meta-analysis of 22 randomized clinical trials. J Am Coll Cardiol 2012:60;1192–201.
222. Gabler NB, French B, Strom BL, et al. Validation of 6-minute walk distance as a surrogate end point in pulmonary arterial hypertension trials.Circulation 2012;126:349–56.
223. Barst RJ, McGoon M, Torbicki A, et al. Diagnosis and differential assessment of pulmonary arterial hypertension. J Am Coll Cardiol 2004;43:S40–7.
224. Dimopoulos K, Inuzuka R, Goletto S, et al. Improved survival among patients with Eisenmenger syndrome receiving advanced therapy for pulmonary arterial hypertension. Circulation 2010;121:20–5.
225. Condliffe R, Kiely DG, Peacock AJ, et al. Connective tissue disease associated pulmonary arterial hypertension in the modern treatment era. Am J Respir Crit Care Med 2009;179:151–7.
226. Vonk MC, Sander MH, van den Hoogen FH, et al. Right ventricle Tei-index: a tool to increase the accuracy of non-invasive detection of pulmonary arterial hypertension in connective tissue diseases. Eur J Echocardiogr 2007;8:317–21.
227. Eysmann SB, Palevsky HI, Reichek N, et al. Two-dimensional and Doppler-echocardiographic and cardiac catheterization correlates of survival in primary pulmonary hypertension. Circulation 1989;80:353–60.
228. Raymond RL, Hinderliter AL, Willis PW, et al: Echocardiographic predictors of adverse outcomes in primary pulmonary hypertension. J Am Coll Cardiol 2002,39:1214–19.
229. Nagaya N, Nishikimi T, Uematsu M, et al. Plasma brain natriuretic peptide as a prognostic indicator in patients with primary pulmonary hypertension. Circulation 2000;102:865–70.
230. Park MH, Scott RL, Uber PA, et al. Usefulness of b-type natriuretic peptide as a predictor of treatment outcome in pulmonary arterial hypertension. Congest Heart Fail 2004;10:221–5.
231. Fijalkowska A, Kurzyna M, Torbicki A, et al. Serum N-terminal brain natriuretic peptide as a prognostic parameter in patients with pulmonary hypertension. Chest 2006;129:1313–21.

232. Cracowski JL, Leuchte HH. The potential of biomarkers in pulmonary arterial hypertension. Am J Cardiol 2012;110(6 Suppl):32S–8S.
233. Van Wolferen SA, Marcus JT, Boonstra A, et al. Prognostic value of right ventricular mass, volume, and function in idiopathic pulmonary arterial hypertension. Eur Heart J 2007;28:1250–7.
234. Bradlow WM, Gibbs JSR, Mohiaddin RH. Cardiovascular magnetic resonance in pulmonary hypertension. J Cardiovasc Magnetic Resonance 2012;14:6–12.
235. Torbicki A. Cardiac magnetic resonance in pulmonary arterial hypertension: a step in the right direction. Eur Heart J 2007;28:1187–9.
236. van de Veerdonk MC, Kind T, Marcus JT, et al. Progressive right ventricular dysfunction in patients with pulmonary arterial hypertensionresponding to therapy. J Am Coll Cardiol 2011;58:2511–19.
237. Nickel N, Golpon H, Greer M, et al. The prognostic impact of follow-up assessments in patients with idiopathic pulmonary arterial hypertension. Eur Respir J 2012;39:589–96.
238. Galie N, Rubin L, Simonneau G. Developing a heart score: next steps. Am J Cardiol 2012;110(Suppl):49S–51S.
239. <http://clinicaltrials.gov/ct2/show/NCT01600898>
240. McLaughlin VV, Gaine SP, Howard LS, et al. Treatment goals of pulmonary hypertension. JACC 2013;62:Suppl 73.

CHAPTER 23

End of life care in advanced heart failure

Jessi Khangura MD and Sarah J. Goodlin MD

Introduction

While progressive organ dysfunction or frailty are indicators that patients with heart failure (HF) are approaching death, the "end of life" is difficult to identify in many chronically ill persons with HF.

Palliative care aims to improve quality of life and support patients and their families in serious illness, often concurrently with treatment to maximize survival. Palliative care should be provided throughout the course of HF; however, patients with advanced HF and their families typically have increased needs for symptom management, support, and planning as they approach the end of life.

Many medical and device interventions in advanced HF care are palliative, in that they improve quality of life and reduce symptom severity, while also prolonging life. Other aspects of palliation, often provided by members of an interdisciplinary team, include psychological and social support, and counseling to cope with existential or spiritual distress. Optimizing end of life care involves ensuring medical care and psychosocial support for the patient and family, decreasing symptom burden, clarifying goals of care and planning care, and managing devices such as implantable cardioverter defibrillators (ICDs) and ventricular assist devices (VADs) with a view toward decreasing morbidity.

Support for patients and families

In addition to the physical limits and symptoms, patient and family distress in advanced HF results from the uncertainty of living with an unpredictable course and the stress of serious illness on finances and social relations. Psychosocial support to address spouse or family distress decreases patient distress.[1] Self-care, including sodium and fluid restriction, is more consistent among patients with advanced HF than in patients who are less ill, and it may be a way for patients and families to feel that they have control over their HF. Although not studied, providing patients and families a sense of what to expect, including decision points they may reach, gives advanced HF patients some certainty and allows them to plan their care for HF exacerbations or emergencies.

Decision-making

Goals for care should be reassessed as the patient's status changes. With chronic illness, patients often modify their appraisal of what brings quality to their life and accept more functional limitation over time; so, reasonably, a patient's preferences can change. Care goals ought to be readdressed when there is a change in health status, at the time of hospitalization and therapy decision points such as cardiac resynchronization therapy (CRT), VAD, or transplant listing.

A conversation to assess preferences and set goals of care should follow an "ask–tell–ask" framework, asking what the patient knows or believes, telling information, and then asking what questions the patient has. An initial conversation can begin by asking the patient what they believe, or what they have talked about with other clinicians regarding HF or regarding goals or end of life plans. When reviewing goals of care for a patient with previously documented goals, it is appropriate to begin by saying "I understand the goals for your care have been .... What do you think at this time about those goals?"

Clinicians worry that saying "death is possible" or that the patient "is seriously ill" may take away hope. A helpful tool is to identify what the patient hopes for, and then to also plan for what to do if things do not go as they hope. This "hope for the best but plan for the worst" conversation allows the clinician to set up a dichotomy, hoping along with the patient while simultaneously acknowledging what realistically is likely to occur, including death.[2]

The patient's preference for resuscitation should be solicited early in HF care and then again with events such as hospitalization or at changes in clinical status. Patients may change their preferences for resuscitation when their clinical status has changed. The conversation about resuscitation should simply ask whether the patient wishes to allow natural death when it comes or whether they would want an attempt at resuscitation. Those who prefer a trial of resuscitation should be asked to clarify states under which they would not want life prolonged (such as if they are unable to recognize friends and family), or specific limitations (such as length of a trial of intubation). All HF patients who indicate that they prefer a trial of resuscitation should have family and friends learn basic life support.

Advance care planning optimally will help patients and their families anticipate multiple decision points, including potential interventions, hospitalizations, and approaching the end of life. Planning for the future, as outlined in Table 23.1, is a positive endeavor. Knowing that there is a choice of several options may empower patients. Planning for possible future decisions provides patients and families time to weigh values and clarify their preferences for certain health states. It also provides a platform on which to make care plan decisions when, and if, they arise. The important points to emphasize are that doctors and nurses will assist with the decision-making, and that patients can change their minds and reset their preferences over time.

Table 23.1 Heart failure: planning for the future

Decision point	Options	Considerations
Worsened dyspnea or volume overload	Medications to manage symptoms at home Emergency care and/or hospitalization	Patients managing symptoms at home must have medications and instructions in advance Patients not improving with at-home management might then go to the ED
Worsened HF despite appropriate medications	CRT LVAD Heart transplantation Hospice care	Clinicians would not suggest advanced technologies to patients unless they would be candidates Hospice care requires the referring physician to certify death would not be surprising within 6 months
Syncope, sudden cardiac death	Try resuscitation (call 911) versus allowing natural death	Families of patients with or without ICDs should have a plan as to how to respond Sudden death may occur with an ICD
Adverse outcome from intervention or serious comorbid problem	Hospital ICU care and efforts to prolong life Hospice care	Patients can identify conditions under which they would not want to try to prolong life
End of life care	Site of care (home, hospital, nursing home) Who provides care (family, in-home paid providers, homecare or hospice staff) What medical team would manage (e.g., which physician, hospice, heart failure team)	Patients and families should identify preferred site and care providers of end of life care, and a "safety plan" alternative if the preferred is not possible
Desired symptom relief	Which symptoms and to what comfort level to manage	Medication (opioids for pain or dyspnea) and nonmedication management to achieve symptom goals

CRT, cardiac resynchronization therapy; ED, emergency department; ICD, implantable cardioverter defibrillator; ICU, intensive care unit; LVAD, left ventricular assist device.

Advance directives

Advance care planning should include completing an advance directive. Advance directives are formal documents directing decision-making when the patient loses the capacity to do so. Advance directives will help ensure that patients' goals regarding death with dignity are upheld. In the United States, advance directives are set by state law or statute. Two forms of advance directives are generally identified: the durable power of attorney for health care, and the living will.

A durable power of attorney or healthcare proxy should be appointed by all adults, and the appointee(s) should have a sense of the patient's preferences or priorities. The surrogate makes decisions for the patient if the patient loses decision-making capacity, but, should the patient retain the ability to understand and choose at a general level, the patient's preferences direct care. In that situation, the surrogate should be engaged as needed to make more complex or nuanced decisions keeping in mind the patient's general preferences.

A living will is typically governed by language requiring that the patient be "terminally ill," and thus is limited in its application. Many states have adopted a broader advance directive called "Five Wishes," which provides more guidance regarding the patient's preferences.[3] Even in states where the Five Wishes document is not a formal advance directive, the document may be completed to give guidance to the healthcare proxy.

Symptom burden

The most commonly reported symptoms in advanced HF include pain, dyspnea fatigue, anxiety, nausea or constipation, depressed mood, and sleep disturbance.[1,4] Patient self-report is the most reliable means of assessing symptoms. The Edmonton Symptom Assessment Scale, designed to follow daily symptom severity in cancer patients, has been used in a variety of formats with HF patients.[5,6]A longer, more detailed tool, the Memorial Symptom Assessment Scale—HF, has been validated for use in HF patients.[7] Two research tools, the Kansas City Cardiomyopathy Questionnaire and the Minnesota Living with Heart Failure Questionnaire, are long but can be used to identify the impact of HF on physical, emotional, social, and mental function.[8,9]

Simply asking a patient to tell you what is most bothersome or disruptive to their life is a reasonable way to target symptom evaluation and management. Symptom severity and frequency, as well as what improves and worsens the symptom, should be queried. Some symptoms (dyspnea, pain, fatigue) are so common that a query about them is warranted.

Pain

The prevalence of pain is as high as 84% of patients with advanced HF; however, some patients have infrequent or mild pain, while others have severe or disabling pain.[4,5,10,11] Patients frequently have pain at several locations. A report of pain should be followed by questions about the location and severity of the pain, as well as what makes it better or worse. Although nonsteroidal anti-inflammatory drugs (NSAIDs) are associated with worsened renal and volume status, they may be purchased over the counter, so patients need specific instructions not to use these agents, as well therapeutic alternatives. Nonacetylated salicylates (salsalate or trilisate) may be effective for some patients and do not impact renal function or platelet function. Salicylate levels should be followed. Opioid analgesics are safe and effective in alleviating dyspnea[12] and are likely safe for pain control. Local treatments such as heat or cold therapy and physical therapy should be considered in a multidisciplinary approach to pain management. Topical capsaicin, topical NSAIDs, and topical salicylates may also be considered, although limited data are available on their use or effectiveness.

Dyspnea

Sodium restriction and diuretics are essential in maintaining fluid balance to decrease dyspnea due to congestion. Dyspnea can be present in HF patients even without volume overload, and relates to the skeletal myopathy associated with the HF syndrome.[1] Thigh muscle strengthening reduces dyspnea and fatigue in patients with New York Heart Association (NYHA) class II HF, possibly by altering the skeletal myopathy.[13] Exercise therapy, including tai chi, can also assist in reducing the sensation of dyspnea in moderate HF.[14] These strategies could be employed in patients with advanced HF.

Opioid medications alter chemosensitivity to decrease the perception of dyspnea[61], reduce the responsiveness of the respiratory control center, and decrease anxiety. Opioids increase the HF patient's exercise tolerance, resulting in a decrease in respiratory effort and a decreased sensation of dyspnea.[12,15,16] Although the hemodynamic effects of opioids vary, morphine reduces preload and is appropriate for acute management of dyspnea.[13] Active morphine metabolites accumulate with renal dysfunction and cause delirium, myoclonus, and other toxicity, so morphine is not appropriate for chronic or long-term use in patients with advanced HF. Fentanyl or methadone may be safer opioids because neither relies on renal excretion, though they have not been specifically studied in HF patients. Several opioids have been documented to be safe in chronic HF.

Nitrates reduce left ventricular end-diastolic pressure and are commonly prescribed to reduce dyspnea and improve exercise tolerance in patients with and without an ischemic etiology of HF.[16]

Although the evidence behind using oxygen therapy to manage dyspnea in HF is not concrete, oxygen supplementation is indicated when the dyspnea is related to arterial hypoxemia. Oxygen supplementation is also thought to provide benefit through promoting the patient's sense of control in the management of dyspnea. There can also be a placebo effect in the use of oxygen supplementation.[17] Patients may not require constant oxygen supplementation; in some instances, using oxygen therapy while sleeping or only during exacerbations can be helpful. Nocturnal nasal oxygen supplementation has been shown to have a significant beneficial impact on exercise capacity and quality of life in HF.[18]

Noninvasive ventilation through continuous positive airway pressure (CPAP) devices can relieve dyspnea by decreasing the neuromechanical dissociation of the respiratory drive and counterbalancing the inspiratory load on respiratory muscles. CPAP can also have a beneficial response on ventricular remodeling.[19] By increasing intrathoracic pressure, CPAP decreases afterload, increases stroke volume, and reduces cardiac sympathetic activity. It also decreases preload by impeding venous return and reducing right and left ventricular end-diastolic pressures. With this redistribution of fluid in the extrathoracic cavity, lung compliance can increase. Use of CPAP has been shown to improve quality of life.[20]

Extreme temperatures, humidity, and smoking can exacerbate dyspnea. Upright positioning of a patient can improve dypsnea. Having a flow of air across the face, from a fan for example, can also relieve symptoms by activating the inhibitory fibers of the facial receptors.[21]

Exercise can also help diminish anxiety by promoting the patient's sense of control. Anxiety and dyspnea are related. The sympathetic activation of anxiety is similar to the sensation of dyspnea. Benzodiazepines can be used to relieve anxiety associated with dyspnea.

Gastrointestinal symptoms

Anorexia, weight loss, and protein malnutrition are common features of advanced HF and are related to the associated neurohormonal and cytokine abnormalities of the HF syndrome. Anorexia may also result from volume overload with right heart dysfunction, particularly when intestinal edema, ascites, and hepatic congestion are present. Optimizing volume status and treating sleep apnea and other contributors to pulmonary hypertension may decrease early satiety and stabilize right heart function. Since changes in weight may reflect changes in food intake and body size as well as fluid balance, weight targets for diuretic use may require adjustment over time. β-Blockers and angiotensin converting enzyme (ACE) inhibitors counter cachexia in HF with reduced ejection fraction (HFrEF), presumably by reducing neurohormonal and immune dysfunction.[22]

Fatigue

In patients with HF, fatigue is prevalent and is associated with worsening prognosis and increased mortality.[23,24] Fatigue may be due to decreased cardiac output, elevated neurohormones and inflammatory cytokines, deconditioning, sleep impairment, and depression and/or anxiety.[25] Thus, assessment and treatment of fatigue should be multifaceted. Effective restriction of fluid and sodium intake results in reduced fatigue, as well as reduced edema and dyspnea.[26] In HF patients with anemia, erythropoietin therapy may enhance exercise capacity.[27] Opioids, caffeine, and perhaps other stimulants can improve exertional fatigue.[15,28] Selective thigh muscle strengthening can improve fatigue in chronic HF.[13]

Frailty

In HF, pathophysiologic changes in skeletal muscle mirror those in the heart tissue, suggesting a common mechanism in heart and skeletal myopathy and perhaps a mechanism for frailty.[29] Frailty is a physiologic syndrome characterized by loss of skeletal muscle, fatigue or exhaustion, weight loss, and decreased physical reserve. Frailty commonly coexists with HF in the elderly. The clinical syndrome of frailty can be identified with one of several research indices that measure a group of functional and cognitive abilities or assign a "prefrail" or "frail" score based on the number of deficits out of the following: sedentary life, involuntary weight loss, low physical activity, exhaustion, and low grip strength.[30] Inability to stand repeatedly from a chair without using one's arms predicts a 50% 6-month mortality in hospitalized elderly HF patients, and very slow gait speed (>6 seconds to walk 5 m) is a good screen for frailty in patients with cardiovascular disease. Treatment of frailty in HF has not been specifically studied, but ACE inhibitors improve walking speed in frail elders, and other interventions to counter the neurohormonal activation in HF may help combat frailty. As thigh muscle strengthening decreases fatigue it may benefit the overall frailty syndrome.

Depression

Depression is common in HF and even more common in advanced HF. A positive response to the Patient Health Questionnaire (PHQ)-2 in HF patients is associated with an 8% increase in 1-year mortality [cite JCF PHQ-2]. Patients with HF and depressive symptoms are twice as likely to die or experience a cardiac event compared to HF patients without depressive symptoms.[31,62]

Studies of treatment for depression are limited to patients with chronic stable HF. Pharmacologic therapy for depression is not always successful, but strategies such as support groups and education may help.[32] Depression in patients with stable HF may be effectively managed with use of paroxetine.[33] Results from the Sertraline Against Depression and Heart Disease in Chronic HF (SAD-Heart-HF) trial and other recent studies suggest that non-pharmacologic interventions, such as brief cognitive therapy, may be effective for the treatment of depression in patients with HF.[34,35] SAD-Heart-HF identified that sertraline is safe in HF, though the study did not achieve therapeutic doses of sertraline in most patients and no net benefit was shown.[34] Data to support the use of other depression therapies are not available, but an "n of 1" trial, assessing depression and function before and after initiation of medication or other treatments, may well be appropriate. Selective serotonin reuptake inhibitors (SSRIs) may cause hyponatremia and can alter volume status, particularly when renal impairment is present, so serum sodium should be monitored when these medications are used.

Spiritual health

The impact of HF on quality of life for both patient and family is complex and extends beyond physical symptoms. The loss of physical and social function is significant. HF patients are frightened of dying, worried about burdening families, and experience hopelessness, isolation, disability, and uncertainty regarding their course.[36,37] Patients benefit from an active-behavioral coping style, including strategies to constructively control their HF.[38] Approaches to spiritual issues and anticipatory grief, such as used in other advanced illnesses, are appropriate in HF. At minimum, clinicians should screen for spiritual concerns and sources of support and acknowledge patients' losses and sources of grief.[39]

Goals of end of life care

At some point the clinician, patient, or both will recognize that interventions to prolong life carry more burden than benefit. At that time, the focus of care shifts to enhancing the quality of life for as long as the patient has to live. Therapies should be re-evaluated with the patient. Some treatments, such as medications that block neurohormonal alterations in HFrEF, clearly improve symptoms and should be continued as tolerated by blood pressure.[1]

A first step to maximize function and well-being in patients with advanced HF is optimized pharmacologic, device and other interventions for HF. Treatment of sleep-disordered breathing with oxygen or CPAP and thigh muscle strengthening are not yet studied, but likely improve symptoms and function in advanced HF. Patients not eligible for or not electing advanced therapies often have comorbidities or are elderly and frail, making end of life care more complex. Partnering with palliative care or geriatrics specialists can be helpful.

Provision of palliative care at the end of life for HF patients is challenged by limitations in clinician expertise. Cardiologists and HF specialists with expertise in HF management may not have training, practice, or comfort with end of life care issues; while generalists, geriatricians, and other clinicians with expertise in hospice and palliative care often lack knowledge and expertise in HF management.[40,41] Collaboration between experts in HF care and those experts in end of life care should be ensured in order to provide adequate end of life care to advanced HF patients.

Hospice care

Hospice care is an option for patients with a poor prognosis and an estimated life expectancy of approximately 6 months. The goal in hospice therapy is to provide comfort, which in HF care often means that effective HF-specific medications are continued through the end of life. Hospice utilization is lower for patients with HF than cancer, and about one-third of HF patients receive less than a week of hospice care before death,[42,43] while other HF patients are stabilized by the hospice care and exceed 6 months. Hospice care can be recertified if death within 6 months still seems likely, or patients may be discharged from hospice to be re-enrolled later. Many problems surround hospice enrollment for patients with advanced heart disease, but some hospice agencies have developed dedicated HF care programs that provide exceptional end of life care. There is a clear need for communication and comanagement by HF specialists of patients while in hospice care.[44]

Physicians may not be comfortable in assessing prognosis for HF patients. Tools that assist in prognostication for HF patients perform equivalently to HF specialist physician estimates,[63] but may add to assessment by less experienced clinicians. Both the Seattle Heart Failure Model and the EFFECT score can identify a group of HF patients unlikely to survive longer than 6 months and for whom hospice care options should therefore be considered.[45,46,47]

HF clinicians and cardiologists should work with hospice agencies to build approaches to care that continue appropriate HF treatments in hospice care. Withdrawal of evidence-based therapies may be appropriate during endstage care for certain patients with persistent advanced HF, particularly those with hypotension or left ventricular systolic dysfunction with progressive low cardiac output. When these treatments are discontinued, a plan to manage symptoms should be enacted.

Inotropic and vasoactive agents

Inotropic and vasoactive agents improve function and HF status in some patients with advanced HF due to systolic dysfunction. Patients who are inotrope dependent have a limited (in the range of 6 months) prognosis, so these patients are appropriate for hospice care. Inotropes are generally continued until the end of life, and inotrope patients are at increased risk of ventricular arrhythmias and sudden cardiac death. Not all hospice agencies have the staff or financial resources to provide intravenous inotropes, and in general these therapies are provided by agencies with average daily census of more than 200 patients.[48] Clinicians caring for inotrope-dependent patients may be able to develop collaborative relationships with hospice agencies who commit to a HF care program. Alternatively, HF specialty programs can provide palliative end of life care to inotrope-dependent patients without some of the hospice resources. Rarely a patient will choose to discontinue an intravenous inotrope. The withdrawal of inotropic and vasoactive agents can reduce cardiac output within minutes, and this may present as angina, hypotension, and pulmonary edema with increased heart rate or respiratory rate. Opioids can provide symptom relief in this setting.

Implantable cardioverter defibrillators

Many patients will approach the end of life with an ICD that was implanted at an earlier stage of illness. Few patients with ICDs engage in advanced planning specifically related to their device, or discuss deactivation.[49] As patients progress to end of life, when a patient elects to allow natural death, or when it is recognized that prognosis is bleak, discussion of the option to turn off defibrillator therapies is important.[50] This discussion can be presented to patients as deactivating the device to avoid the distress of shocks (that will not change the patient's course), and to allow a peaceful death whenever that comes. Patients and their families should understand that deactivation of a defibrillator does not lead immediately to death, and that it is an ethically sound withdrawal of a therapy to meet the goals of care. All centers that implant ICDs should have a process in place to electively deactivate the defibrillator function.

Deactivation of ICDs includes discussion of device deactivation in the context of overall goals of care,[51] and ideally such a discussion takes place at implantation as well as when the patient's condition declines near the end of life. The ease of the procedure when deactivation is conducted electively should be presented, and the uncertainties of the patient's course with advanced HF should be acknowledged.

Reprogramming the defibrillator and/or antitachycardia pacing is the preferred method of deactivating an ICD. All clinicians managing patients with advanced HF should have ready access to a donut magnet in the event a late decision is made to deactivate an ICD, for repeated distressing shock, or for rare episodes of "defibrillator storm."

Of note, after death, patients can be buried with an ICD, but they cannot be cremated with the ICD in place. Removal of the ICD is necessary if it is an investigational device or if the body is to be cremated.[52]

Cardiac resynchronization therapy and pacemakers

Although there is a general consensus that ICD therapies may become burdensome near end of life, CRT may remain of some benefit.[53] The defibrillator function of a CRT device should be addressed equivalently to an ICD. Most clinicians recommend continuing biventricular pacing as long as the patient responded to this therapy previously.

Pacemaker deactivation in pacemaker-dependent patients may be perceived as ethically questionable, especially because death may occur immediately after pacemaker deactivation.[54,55] However, an informed decision by a patient with decision-making capacity or their healthcare proxy to withdraw a pacemaker should be honored. At times, clinicians uncomfortable with withdrawing life-sustaining therapies will want to arrange for another physician to withdraw treatment.

The clinical team should be prepared to promote patient comfort during the withdrawal process of pacemakers and CRT devices, with medications if needed. Again, patients can be buried with a pacemaker in place but they cannot be cremated. Pacemakers should be removed to avoid the risk of explosion of a pacemaker battery if a patient is to be cremated.[56,57,58] A recent guideline from the Heart Rhythm Society can assist clinicians in deactivating devices thought to be burdensome.[51]

Ventricular assist devices

Until recently, patients receiving left ventricular assist devices (LVADs) as destination therapy generally were ill enough to be considered candidates for hospice care should they not elect a LVAD. A recent trend to implant the LVAD before the patient develops endstage HF means that some patients will live for several years before reaching the 6-month prognosis required by the Medicare Hospice Benefit. Patients who receive destination therapy with LVADs will eventually die with their device in place. Palliative medicine consultation should be standard prior to initiation of destination therapy care, both to present palliative and hospice care as an alternative and to present the potential benefit of palliative care following LVAD implantation. Palliative care clinicians support the patient and family when distress or adverse outcomes complicate an LVAD patient's course. Patients with adverse outcomes from LVADs, particularly disabling stroke, refractory bleeding, or sepsis, also are appropriate for hospice care.

Hospice care for LVAD patients requires partnership by the hospice with the LVAD team to provide ongoing LVAD management and troubleshooting while hospice services are provided. Some patients and families will not want to discontinue the LVAD, and this is permissible in hospice care. The timing of discontinuation of LVAD support varies depending on patient and family preferences and also on the clinical setting. Patients with sepsis and multisystem organ failure may die (cease breathing) with the LVAD still functioning. Some patients and families prefer to allow time for family to gather or other events before deactivating the LVAD, and hospice can provide anticipatory bereavement, psychosocial, and spiritual support during this time.

Discontinuation of a LVAD should be scheduled, and if it occurs outside the hospital, adequate time should be allowed to initiate care by the hospice team.

The event should be orchestrated, and the patient should identify who will be present. Alarms must be turned off, and medications to manage terminal symptoms should be in place. Anticipated symptoms include dyspnea, anxiety, agitation, pain, noisy breathing, and excessive secretions. These symptoms can be treated with combinations of opioids and benzodiazepines titrated to comfort. Noisy breathing can be reduced with anticholinergics such as scopolamine (if a patch formulation is used it must be applied many hours in advance) and repositioning, but deep suctioning is discouraged.[59]

Termination of LVAD support can result in rapid death when the device is turned off. Furthermore, because the device is in place but not functioning, there is resultant pulmonary congestion, thrombosis, and regurgitant blood flow.[60] Opioids can relieve or minimize symptoms associated with congestion; and, for an awake patient, benzodiazepines may relieve anxiety.

Summary

The need for palliative care, integrated with evidence-based HF care, has been recognized. Many interventions both improve the quality of life or diminish symptoms for patients with HF, and, so by definition, are palliative. At the end of life, palliative interventions predominate, particularly when the benefits of life-prolonging treatments are outweighed by their burdens.

Although the course of HF can be unpredictable, risk models may help with prognostication. Advanced care and end of life care planning must take place among clinicians, their patients, and their patient's families and loved ones. Communication with HF patients and their families about their preferences for care and the potential life-limiting nature of HF early in the course of illness will facilitate later conversations when the patients' disease status worsens or they approach the end of life. The majority of HF patients prefer honest communication about their illness from doctors.

Supportive and palliative care should be provided throughout the course of HF care, based upon patient and family need. Meticulous management of HF and associated symptoms is critical to palliation of symptoms in HF patients. Palliative care that is multidisciplinary is indicated to address the broad physical and psychological symptom burden in advanced HF. Hospice care can bridge the care needed for patients with complex comorbidities and a prognosis of less than 6 months of survival.

In those patients with mechanical devices such as pacemakers, ICDs, and VADs, a plan for managing the device near the end of life should be developed, ideally along with the decision to implant these devices. Deactivation of these devices needs to be discussed when a decision is made to implant the device. The end of life device plan can be integrated into advance directives.

References

1. Goodlin SJ. Palliative care in congestive heart failure. J Am Coll Cardiol 2009;54:386–96.
2. Goodlin SJ, Quill TE, Arnold RM. Communication and decision-making about prognosis in heart failure care. J Card Fail 2008;14.
3. <http://www.agingwithdignity.org/five-wishes.php>.
4. Levenson JW, McCarthy EP, Lynn J, Davis RB, Phillips RS. The last six months of life for patients with congestive heart failure. J Am Geriatr Soc 2000;48:S101–9.
5. Walke LM, Gallo WT, Tinetti ME, Fried TR. The burden of symptoms among community-dwelling older persons with advanced chronic disease. Arch Intern Med 2004;164:2321–4.
6. Ezekowitz JA, Thai V, Hodnefield TS, et al. The correlation of standard heart failure assessment and palliative care questionnaires in a multidisciplinary heart failure clinic. J Pain Symptom Manag 2011;42:379–87.
7. Zambroski CH, Moser DK, Roser LP, et al. Patients with heart failure who die in hospice. Am Heart J 2005;149:558–64.
8. Green CP, Porter CB, Bresnahan DR, Spertus JA. Development and evaluation of the kansas city cardiomyopathy questionnaire: A new health status measure for heart failure. J Am Coll Cardiol 2000;35:1245–55.
9. Naveiro-Rilo JC, Diez-Juarez DM, Romero Blanco A, et al. Validation of the minnesota living with heart failure questionnaire in primary care. Rev Esp Cardiol 2010;63:1419–27.
10. Goodlin SJ, Wingate S, Albert NM, et al. Investigating pain in heart failure patients: The pain assessment, incidence, and nature in heart failure (PAIN-HF) study. J Card Fail 2012;18:776–83.
11. Weiss SC, Emanuel LL, Fairclough DL, Emanuel EJ. Understanding the experience of pain in terminally ill patients. Lancet 2001;357:1311–15.
12. Johnson MJ, McDonagh TA, Harkness A, et al. Morphine for the relief of breathlessness in patients with chronic heart failure—a pilot study. Eur J Heart Fail 2002;4:753–6.
13. Beniaminovitz A, Lang CC, LaManca J, Mancini DM. Selective low-level leg muscle training alleviates dyspnea in patients with heart failure. J Am Coll Cardiol 2002;40:1602–8.
14. Yeh GY, Wood MJ, Lorell BH, et al.Effects of tai chi mind-body movement therapy on functional status and exercise capacity in patients with chronic heart failure: A randomized controlled trial. Am J Med 2004;117:541–8.
15. Williams SG, Wright DJ, Marshall P, et al. Safety and potential benefits of low dose diamorphine during exercise in patients with chronic heart failure. Heart 2003;89:1085–6.
16. Bitar F, Akhter MW, Khan S, et al. Survey of the use of organic nitrates for the treatment of chronic congestive heart failure in the united states. Am J Cardiol 2004;94:1465–8.
17. Booth S, Wade R, Johnson M, et al. The use of oxygen in the palliation of breathlessness. A report of the expert working group of the scientific committee of the association of palliative medicine. Respir Med 2004;98:66–77.
18. Paul B, Joseph M, De Pasquale CG. Domiciliary oxygen therapy improves sub-maximal exercise capacity and quality of life in chronic heart failure. Heart Lung Circ 2008;17:220–3.
19. Yan AT, Bradley TD, Liu PP. The role of continuous positive airway pressure in the treatment of congestive heart failure. Chest 2001;120:1675–85.
20. Bradley TD, Logan AG, Kimoff RJ, et al. Continuous positive airway pressure for central sleep apnea and heart failure. N Engl J Med 2005;353:2025–33.
21. Manning HL, Schwartzstein RM. Pathophysiology of dyspnea. N Engl J Med 1995;333:1547–53.
22. Davos CH, Doehner W, Rauchhaus M, et al. Body mass and survival in patients with chronic heart failure without cachexia: The importance of obesity. J Card Fail 2003;9:29–35.
23. Smith OR, Denollet J, Schiffer AA, et al. Patient-rated changes in fatigue over a 12-month period predict poor outcome in chronic heart failure. Eur J Heart Fail 2009;11:400–5.
24. Ekman I, Cleland JG, Swedberg K, et al. Symptoms in patients with heart failure are prognostic predictors: Insights from comet. J Card Fail 2005;11:288–92.
25. Fink AM, Gonzalez RC, Lisowski T, et al. Fatigue, inflammation, and projected mortality in heart failure. J Card Fail 2012;18:711–16.
26. Colin Ramirez E, Castillo Martinez L, Orea Tejeda A, et al. Effects of a nutritional intervention on body composition, clinical status, and quality of life in patients with heart failure. Nutrition 2004;20:890–5.
27. Mancini DM, Katz SD, Lang CC, et al. Effect of erythropoietin on exercise capacity in patients with moderate to severe chronic heart failure. Circulation 2003;107:294–9.
28. Notarius CF, Morris B, Floras JS. Caffeine prolongs exercise duration in heart failure. J Card Fail 2006;12:220–6.
29. Middlekauff HR, Vigna C, Verity MA, et al. Abnormalities of calcium handling proteins in skeletal muscle mirror those of the heart in humans with heart failure: A shared mechanism? J Card Fail 2012;18:724–33.
30. Afilalo J, Alexander KP, Mack MJ, et al. Frailty assessment in the cardiovascular care of older adults. J Am Coll Cardiol 2014;63:747–62.
31. Rutledge T, Reis VA, Linke SE, et al. Depression in heart failure a meta-analytic review of prevalence, intervention effects, and associations with clinical outcomes. J Am Coll Cardiol 2006;48:1527–37.
32. Sullivan MJ, Wood L, Terry J, et al. The support, education, and research in chronic heart failure study (SEARCH): A mindfulness-based psychoeducational intervention improves depression and clinical symptoms in patients with chronic heart failure. Am Heart J 2009;157:84–90.
33. Gottlieb SS, Kop WJ, Thomas SA, et al. A double-blind placebo-controlled pilot study of controlled-release paroxetine on depression and quality of life in chronic heart failure. Am Heart J 2007;153:868–73.
34. O'Connor CM, Jiang W, Kuchibhatla M, et al. Safety and efficacy of sertraline for depression in patients with heart failure: Results of the SADHART-CHF (sertraline against depression and heart disease in chronic heart failure) trial. J Am Coll Cardiol 2010;56:692–9.
35. Dekker RL, Moser DK, Peden AR, Lennie TA. Cognitive therapy improves three-month outcomes in hospitalized patients with heart failure. J Card Fail 2012;18:10–20.

36. Murray SA, Kendall M, Boyd K, et al. Exploring the spiritual needs of people dying of lung cancer or heart failure: A prospective qualitative interview study of patients and their carers. Palliat Med 2004;18:39–45.
37. Horne G, Payne S. Removing the boundaries: Palliative care for patients with heart failure. Palliat Med 2004;18:291–6.
38. Doering LV, Dracup K, Caldwell MA, et al. Is coping style linked to emotional states in heart failure patients? J Card Fail 2004;10:344–9.
39. Puchalski C, Romer AL. Taking a spiritual history allows clinicians to understand patients more fully. J Palliat Med 2000;3:129–37.
40. Hauptman PJ, Swindle J, Hussain Z, et al. Physician attitudes toward end-stage heart failure: A national survey. Am J Med 2008;121:127–35.
41. Goodlin SJ, Trupp R, Bernhardt P, et al. Development and evaluation of the "advanced heart failure clinical competence survey": A tool to assess knowledge of heart failure care and self-assessed competence. Patient Educ Couns 2007;67:3–10.
42. Setoguchi S, Glynn RJ, Stedman M, et al. Hospice, opiates, and acute care service use among the elderly before death from heart failure or cancer. Am Heart J 2010;160:139–44.
43. Bain KT, Maxwell TL, Strassels SA, Whellan DJ. Hospice use among patients with heart failure. Am Heart J 2009;158:118–25.
44. Goodlin SJ. Hospice care following heart failure admission: What next? J Card Fail 2012;18:478–9.
45. Lee DS, Austin PC, Rouleau JL, et al. Predicting mortality among patients hospitalized for heart failure: Derivation and validation of a clinical model. JAMA 2003;290:2581–7.
46. Levy WC, Mozaffarian D, Linker DT, et al. The seattle heart failure model: Prediction of survival in heart failure. Circulation 2006;113:1424–33.
47. Aaronson KD, Schwartz JS, Chen TM, et al. Development and prospective validation of a clinical index to predict survival in ambulatory patients referred for cardiac transplant evaluation. Circulation 1997;95:2660–7.
48. Goodlin S, Kutner J, Connor S, et al. Hospice care for heart failure patients. J Pain Symptom Manag 2005;29:525–8.
49. Epstein AE, Dimarco JP, Ellenbogen KA, et al. ACC/AHA/HRS 2008 guidelines for device-based therapy of cardiac rhythm abnormalities: Executive summary. Heart Rhythm 2008;5:934–55.
50. Jessup M, Abraham WT, Casey DE, et al. 2009 focused update: ACCF/AHA guidelines for the diagnosis and management of heart failure in adults: A report of the american college of cardiology foundation/american heart association task force on practice guidelines: Developed in collaboration with the international society for heart and lung transplantation. Circulation 2009;119:1977–2016.
51. Lampert R, Hayes DL, Annas GJ, et al. AHA/HRS expert consensus statement on the management of cardiovascular implantable electronic devices (CIEDS) in patients nearing end of life or requesting withdrawal of therapy. Heart Rhythm 2010;7:1008–26.
52. Reilly D, Morton P, Vojtko K. Implantable cardioverter-defibrillator. In: Wiegand D, Carlson K, ed. AACN Procedure Manual for Critical Care. Philadelphia, PA: Elsevier; 2005, pp. 637–42.
53. Padeletti L, Arnar DO, Boncinelli L, et al. EHRA expert consensus statement on the management of cardiovascular implantable electronic devices in patients nearing end of life or requesting withdrawal of therapy. Europace 2010;12:1480–9.
54. Mueller PS, Jenkins SM, Bramstedt KA, Hayes DL. Deactivating implanted cardiac devices in terminally ill patients: Practices and attitudes. Pacing Clin Electrophysiol 2008;31:560–8.
55. Lewis WR, Luebke DL, Johnson NJ, et al. Withdrawing implantable defibrillator shock therapy in terminally ill patients. Am J Med 2006;119:892–6.
56. Braun TC, Hagen NA, Hatfield RE, Wyse DG. Cardiac pacemakers and implantable defibrillators in terminal care. J Pain Symptom Manage 1999;18:126–31.
57. Anon. Not for burning. Lancet 1977 Jul 30;2(8031):232.
58. Anon. Hidden hazards of cremation. Br Med J 1977;ii(6103):1620–1.
59. Swetz KM, Ottenberg AL, Freeman MR, Mueller PS. Palliative care and end-of-life issues in patients treated with left ventricular assist devices as destination therapy. Curr Heart Fail Rep 2011;8:212–18.
60. Bramstedt KA, Wenger NS. When withdrawal of life-sustaining care does more than allow death to take its course: The dilemma of left ventricular assist devices. J Heart Lung Transplant 2001;20:544–8.
61. Chua TP, Harrington D, Ponikowski P, et al. Effects of dihydrocodeine on chemosensitivity and exercise tolerance in patients with chronic heart failure. J Am Coll Cardiol 1997 Jan;29(1):147–52.
62. Rollman BL, Belnap BH, Mazumdar S, et al. A positive PHQ-2 depression screen among hospitalized heart failure patients is associated with elevated 12-month mortality. J Card Fail 2012;18(3):238–45. DOI:10.1016/j.cardfail.2011.11.002.
63. Drazner MH, Hellkamp AS, Leier CV, et al. Value of clinician assessment of hemodynamics in advanced heart failure: the ESCAPE trial. Circ Heart Fail 2008 Sep;1(3):170–7. DOI: 10.1161/circheartfailure.108.769778.

CHAPTER 24

Future directions in advanced heart failure

Michael J. Domanski MD, Marc A. Pfeffer MD PhD, and Mandeep R. Mehra MD

In spite of improvements in diagnosis and treatment, heart failure (HF) remains a worldwide epidemic with the number of HF patients expected to double between now and 2030.[1] Prevalence and incidence are both increasing, the syndrome remains highly lethal, and the quality of life of those afflicted is severely impacted. About 10% of HF patients are considered to have "advanced" HF, meaning that they are severely disabled despite conventional pharmacologic therapy, cardiac resynchronization, and implantable cardioverter defibrillator (ICD) placement and are potential candidates for cardiac transplantation or placement of a mechanical circulatory support (MCS) device.[2]

In this final chapter we look to the future, not making predictions but rather setting out challenges that we believe are essential elements of a research agenda for investigation focused on significantly reducing the worldwide burden of HF. Transformative advances that reduce the burden of HF will require preventing the development of this syndrome in the first place, more effectively attenuating progression, or replacing lost function.

Prevention

A central difficulty with preventing HF is that we are dealing with a syndrome that represents the final common physiologic pathway of many different etiologic processes. As a result, a discussion of the prevention of HF becomes a discussion of preventing (or treating) the manifold diseases that produce it. Major strides seem possible in prevention of important risk factors for HF, such as coronary heart disease. Also, uncovering the genetic basis of conditions predisposing to HF may enable new approaches to early intervention. However, for the foreseeable future, the developed HF syndrome is likely to remain a common problem. So, while stipulating the importance of preventing HF, in this chapter we focus on progress to be made in treating (or curing) individuals presenting with the HF syndrome.

Transplantation

For patients with advanced HF, cardiac transplantation, with a 1-year survival of approximately 90% and a median 10-year survival of 60%, offers the best survival for patients with endstage HF.[2] The central problem with human allograft cardiac transplantation is that only about 2200 human donor hearts are available each year in the United States, about 4000 worldwide, and the number is not projected to increase.[3] Given that there are approximately 100 000 to 150 000 people in the US alone who could benefit from heart transplantation, and the fact that donor supply will not grow significantly, heart transplantation will continue to be an important therapy for a limited, carefully selected segment of the overall HF population. As yet, there is not another therapy capable of prolonging life while restoring its quality with the effectiveness and durability offered by allogeneic cardiac transplantation.

On other hand, while the number of allografts will remain tiny relative to need, advances in the science could materially improve this modality.[4] Although well-constructed randomized controlled clinical trials testing a variety of immunosuppressive therapies exist, they are limited by duration of follow-up. In this regard, most clinical trials truncate their outcomes at 1 year and, while some demonstrate the benefit of improvements in immunosuppressive efficacy on endpoints of rejection and surrogate endpoints for late complications, altering long-term outcomes with these approaches remains enigmatic.[5] In cardiac transplantation, few interventions have successfully changed the landscape of late outcomes including the adjunctive immunosuppressive agent mycophenolate mofetil and 3-hydroxy-3-methylglutaryl-coenzyme A (HMG CoA)-inhibiting statin therapy.[6]

The proper role of "high risk" or "marginal" donor hearts, potentially allocated through "alternate" lists, requires more systematic attention. An improved understanding of the long-term outcomes in patients transplanted with such hearts as a function of specific characteristics of these hearts is needed. As left ventricular assist devices (LVADs) and other mechanical circulatory assist devices evolve, trials comparing these devices to alternate list transplants will be needed. Importantly, methods to prolong the feasible ischemic time of donor hearts allowing longer safe transport distances, enhanced approaches to repairing otherwise suboptimal hearts, and techniques to reduce ischemia-reperfusion injury are central to expanding the available donor pool.

Reducing the late morbidity caused by immunosuppression requires concerted efforts. The constellation of malignancy, cardiac allograft vasculopathy (CAV), and renal failure represent the most vexing disorders in late survivors of a cardiac transplant.[2] Whether cardiovascular risk mitigation strategies, such as use of antiplatelet agents and/or renin-angiotensin-aldosterone antagonist therapy or goal-directed control of lipids, blood pressure, and obesity effectively prolong the life of cardiac allografts is unknown and large-scale trials are needed. A deeper understanding of the immune processes of rejection and their interaction with traditional risk factors may enable development of new medications and strategies for their use. For instance, a much enhanced knowledge of the fundamental biology of antibody-mediated rejection is needed, to understand its impact on CAV and late patient outcomes.[7]

Genomic, proteomic, and metabolomic biosignatures of rejection and allograft function to replace invasive techniques such as endomyocardial biopsy would be a major management improvement and should be sought by application of next-generation platforms.[8,9]

A central barrier to the randomized trials of allograft transplantation proposed is the small number of potential subjects. No single center or even small group of centers has a sufficient number of patients to do randomized trials of the size needed to answer the questions posed. As a result, the transplant community needs to come together in a coherent clinical trials enterprise that vets clinical trial proposals and performs the studies, with a collective emphasis on prolonging late outcomes. Leadership and funding would be appropriate government roles.

The heart transplantation picture would be completely different if xenografting became feasible. Were it possible to safely transplant the hearts of nonhuman species into human patients, an unlimited donor organ supply would become available. For this to be feasible, we would have to learn how to selectively suppress immunocompetent cell clones responding to the graft or, alternatively, genetically engineer animals to avoid expressing antigens that invited a human immune response. Work continues, as it should, on xenografting. However, advances in the science sufficient to permit clinical xenografting of hearts into human beings must be relegated to, at best, a distant future.[10]

Mechanical circulatory support

As discussed above, the number of patients with advanced HF refractory to conventional medical (including resynchronization) therapy may be as many as 150 000 in the US alone, a number that dwarfs the number of donor hearts that are available.[9,10] Filling the unmet need for donor hearts is the role of MCS. The indications and survival improvement that attend MCS have been extensively discussed in prior chapters.

LVADs are in widespread use. Continuous-flow LVADs have essentially replaced pulsatile devices in clinical practice.[11] In addition to providing better survival, they enable a better quality of life than the older pulsatile devices. They are, smaller, more reliable, operate silently, and so enable patients to carry on many of the usual activities of daily living.

Although used most often as a bridge to more definitive therapy, such as transplantation, or to improve end organ function and enhance transplant eligibility, they have also been used to provide lifetime support (destination therapy). Early in the use of these devices there was optimism that the hemodynamic support provided would result in recovery of myocardial function. That is, the devices would serve as a "bridge to recovery." Yet, recovery explants occur in fewer than 2% of patients.[11] We believe that appropriately constructed clinical trials to systematically address myocardial recovery using LVADs are required. Although the prospects may appear gloomy at the moment in typical advanced HF patients, we need focused investigations to predict the probability of recovery in selected subjects.

Currently available systems have external power sources requiring transcutaneous connections that are a nidus for infection. These infections are a serious limitation of current LVADs.[12] The infection may involve the driveline or pump assembly. Once the pump assembly is infected, antibiotic treatment alone is seldom effective. Thus, for device-based therapy to become commonplace, fully internal systems will need to become the norm.

Importantly, with continuous-flow pumps, a debate on the importance of pulsatility has emerged. Indeed, we now recognize that bleeding complications, especially gastrointestinal bleeding arbitrated through the generation of an acquired deficiency of von Willebrand factor, has surfaced.[13] Additionally, the continuous, rather than pulsatile, flow generated by these devices may cause or exacerbate arteriovenous malformations in the gastrointestinal tract that account for a high rate of gastrointestinal bleeding.

While the evolution of blood-compatible biomaterials has been enabling for current MCS equipment, stroke remains an important complication.[11] Also, there is a recent recognition of a significant rate of pump thrombosis, which frequently requires pump exchange to avoid devastating LVAD dysfunction.[14] The competing risks of bleeding and thrombosis make the selection of anticoagulation regimens challenging. In the future, it will be necessary to develop far more rheologically inert devices that ideally do not require anticoagulation and function as fully biocompatible devices.

Another common complication is the development of aortic insufficiency.[15] Valvular incompetence is likely related to continuing pressure on the aortic valve throughout the cardiac cycle in the presence of a closed valve. Mechanical distortion of the aortic annulus may be contributory. The aortic valve leaflets may fuse. When sufficiently severe, perfusion can be compromised and elevated left ventricular filling pressures can result in pulmonary congestion (as would occur with sufficiently severe aortic regurgitation from any cause). Progress in reducing aortic insufficiency is needed and gains may be possible based on (1) better surgical technique of outflow cannula implantation, (2) facilitation of transaortic pulsatile flow, and (3) optimizing aortic loading conditions.

A poorly functioning right ventricle preimplant may fail postimplant. Because there is no permanent right ventricular assist device (RVAD), this can be a catastrophic event. Attempts have been made to predict postimplant right ventricular dysfunction.[16] The success in predicting which right ventricles will fail is limited, with very poorly functioning right ventricles frequently providing adequate complementary flow and support. Thus, the future will require gains in understanding, predicting and avoiding post-LVAD right HF.

For some patients who require complete biventricular support, a total artificial heart is needed. One such device, the Syncardia Total Artificial Heart (Syncardia Systems, Inc., Tuscon, AZ), which is a pneumatically-driven pulsatile system, that has been implanted in well over 1000 patients.[17] It is an effective bridge to transplant and can remain in place for many months. Indeed, a driver exists that permits patients to go home. The Syncardia device can be an effective long-term bridge to transplant. However, it is large, noisy, and cumbersome and can only be implanted in individuals with a sufficiently large mediastinum. The quality of life is not comparable to the smaller continuous-flow LVADs that are also more reliable. The device has four mechanical valves and requires a higher level of anticoagulation commensurate with that required for prosthetic valves. Newer technology for biventricular support is needed.

The future of mechanical circulatory support

What should be the goals of MCS? In the near term, there will be a refinement of the indications for the use of LVAD placement. For instance, the Randomized Evaluation of VAD Intervention Before Inotrope Trial (REVIVE-IT) will assess the usefulness of LVAD (Heartmate II) placement in patients who are less ill than those who are currently candidates.[18] Specifically, patients with class IIIb symptoms and left ventricular ejection fraction (LVEF) less than 0.35 who are not inotrope dependent will be randomly assigned to optimal medical therapy or to LVAD placement (Heartmate II) in addition to optimal medical therapy. The primary endpoint is a composite outcome of survival, freedom from moderately disabling stroke (defined as Modified Rankin Scale (MRS) ≥ 3), and improvement of 6 minute walk test distance by 75 m or more from prerandomization baseline. The Risk Assessment and Comparative Effectiveness of Left Ventricular Assist Device and Medical Management in Ambulatory Heart Failure (ROADMAP) study is an observational follow-up of New York Heart Association (NYHA) IIIb/IV patients who are not inotrope dependent and who are nonrandomly assigned to optimal medical therapy or to optimal medical therapy placement of an LVAD (Heartmate II).[19] The primary endpoint is a composite of survival with improvement in 6 minute hallway walk test distance from baseline of 75 m or more over 12 months. These studies will be useful in refining the indications for use of the current generation of LVADs. However, as the LVAD systems continue to evolve, the indications are likely to evolve as well.

The major advances in the MCS field will be driven by the development of new equipment. What should we be working toward? There should come a time when a family of devices is available that allows individualization of MCS to be provided. Different patients require different forms of long-term support; some require only LVADs, others require biventricular support, and there are some patients who may require only an RVAD. Specific devices should become available for each application.

Common to all future MCS devices is a requirement to eliminate the necessity for percutaneous connections. This should dramatically lower the infection risk while immensely improving quality of life. Smaller devices would also improve tolerability. An example is the CircuLite Synergy micropump (CircuLite Inc., Teaneck, NJ).[20] This device will provide 3 L/min of flow and connect the left atrium to the descending aorta. The partial support provided will be sufficient for some patients and can be placed via minithoracotomy. These devices are plagued by the development of rheological abnormalities in the device and patient, which will need to be overcome for mainstream use.

Truly transformational would be the development of a practical, durable, fully implantable total artificial heart (TAH) that does not require any percutaneous connections. Such a device would obviate all concerns about the capacity of the right heart to perform following LVAD placement. The burden of poor right heart performance on liver and kidney function would cease to be an issue. Shock due to loss of cardiac function could be rapidly reversed. Indeed, the ability to, in effect, rapidly switch out a poorly functioning heart for a new effective one would result in a fundamental change in the practice of advanced HF.

Developing a TAH is a difficult engineering problem, but the problem is fundamentally different from bringing cell-based therapies to clinical reality. In the case of the TAH, no new science is needed. In the case of stem-cell-based therapy substantial new science is needed. In addition to new science, there are "unknown unknowns." So, with the engineering problem of developing an operational TAH, sufficient effort devoted is likely to be successful. With the cell-based therapies the probability of success is difficult to estimate.

So, why is there not a headlong charge by industry to develop a practical TAH? The answer is that the project would have a long, extremely expensive development cycle with a market that might be insufficient to justify the development cost and the money put at risk. No midcapitalization company has the resources to undertake such a project, and the opportunity cost for large engineering development firms is huge. The reality is that the development of the TAH described above would require a commitment of government resources and so the assignment of funding priority to such a project.

Even so, a device called the BiVACOR (BiVACOR, Inc., Houston, TX) is under active development and investigation. This pump is unique due to the inclusion of left and right impeller vanes positioned on a common rotating disk. Magnetic levitation technology allows this pump to operate completely by suspending and rotating this disk, which affords it the unique ability to respond to a patient's changing needs by dynamically altering its impeller position, to safely pump blood from both sides of the heart. One of the unique aspects of the BiVACOR is that it can support both sides of a failing heart (BV Assist) or may act as a TAH replacing the heart completely (BV Replace).[21]

More recently, the Carmat pump (CARMAT, 78140 Velizy Villacoublay, France) was developed with a structure similar to that of the human heart. The device has two ventricular cavities with two volume spaces separated by a flexible biomembrane: one for blood and one for the "actioning fluid." A flexible external bag contains this actioning fluid and beats at the same rate as a native heart, displacing the biomembrane and mimicking the native ventricle wall during heart contraction. The first patient implanted with this device, in 2014, was a 76-year-old who survived for 75 days. Much work needs to be done to bring these technologies into the mainstream,

Cell-based and gene therapies

At the more distal end of the spectrum from current to future management of patients with advanced HF, genetic manipulation and regenerative medicine are two tantalizingly plausible areas to reverse abnormal ventricular geometry, improve performance and hopefully prognosis. In both rapidly evolving fields, the basic investigative discoveries currently far outstrip their more modest clinical investigative programs. However, despite the current elusiveness of developing a definitive therapeutic advance utilizing either of these investigative strategies, the rate of progress in improving our basic understanding of these processes has created a great deal of positive momentum and clinical enthusiasm to encourage novel clinical developmental programs. Although lectures on the future of HF treatment would generally conclude with gene manipulation and cell therapy, on the horizon the current clinical reality would in our view position actual therapeutic products from these discoveries as more distant prospects.

Regenerative therapy

The shedding of the long-held concept that myocytes are terminally differentiated and could not be replaced opened the way for extremely productive basic investigations regarding the death and turnover of myocardium.[23] In an experimental model of myocardial infarction, the demonstration that c-kit-positive hematopoietic stem cells could be used to repair a region of damaged myocardium was one of the early major turning points in the basic investigations of cardiac regeneration.[24] This discovery resulted in the current intense investigative effort to better understand and harness the biology of the cardiac regenerative capacity in order to develop improved HF treatments. These basic discoveries have led to an explosion of potential opportunities to be explored. It is now clear that a variety of naturally occurring and derived cell populations (bone marrow mononuclear cells, more selective bone marrow progenitor cells such as mesenchymal stem cells, or mobilized endothelial precursor cells, adipose-derived mesenchymal stem cells, cardiac-derived stem cells, and others) can be used or created with the capacity to regenerate, transdifferentiate, and/or provide sufficient paracrine stimulation to improve cardiac function in experimental animal models.[25,26,27] Unfortunately, progress in basic understandings has outstripped our capacity to rigorously examine all the encouraging scientific leads. Studying potential interventions/products in rigorous clinical trials is particularly difficult because of the host of possible delivery systems including direct ventricular injections, intracoronary infusions, and pericardial approaches. The range of possible cell types and various delivery approaches, as well as the expanding list of growth promoting cofactors, combined with the difficulty of developing patentable products, make it difficult for an industrial concern to justify expenditure of the resources needed to pursue product development. Because of this, the available investigations are largely of small proof-of-concept studies representing early experiences, generally with cardiac imaging-based endpoints.[28] Due to the absence of major funding for clinical trial development programs, there are a host of small phase 1 or 2 studies, but no phase 3 studies.[29] These uncoordinated efforts have not led to randomized, placebo-controlled clinical outcome trials. This is illustrated in the recent comprehensive meta-analysis of 50 studies involving altogether only 2625 patients.[30] Since the studies were quite heterogeneous and not definitive, the overall small improvement reported in LVEF is difficult to attribute to any particular therapy.

This lack of standardization of the experimental interventions examined also applies to the patient populations which are heterogeneous, generally with reduced ejection fraction but not advanced HF.[30,31] The effect of intracoronary reperfusion of bone-marrow–derived mononuclear cells on all-cause mortality in acute myocardial infarction (BAMI) is the largest randomized trial evaluating a regenerative therapy using clinical rather than imaging outcomes. The plan is to enroll 3000 patients with acute ST-elevation myocardial infarction and LVEF of 45% or less to determine whether the intracoronary infusion of bone-marrow–derived mononuclear cells will improve survival and reduce hospitalizations (NCT01569178). At present, no regenerative therapy is being actively investigated with the objective of improving prognosis of patients with advanced HF.

This summary of the present state of affairs is meant to be realistic rather than pessimistic. We believe that cell-based therapies offer promise and need to be explored. Targeting patients with advanced HF for experimental investigations would facilitate more effective evaluation of new therapies.

Gene therapy

For a recognized single gene mutation, as in sickle cell disease, the concept of selectively altering the genetic milieu to restore cells to normal function remains the elusive holy grail. As the field progresses, there are now viral vectors that can be used to deliver a "therapeutic" DNA or RNA to the nucleus of targeted cells. Only a small minority of patients with HF have a HF etiology attributable to a specific genetic mutation. Instead, there is consistent evidence for a much more general process of altered gene expression in the failing myocardium. In both animal models of HF and human cardiac tissue, a pattern of genotypic changes occur in the failing myocardium and the general pattern of recapitulation of a more fetal gene expression, as has been described in hypertrophy and failure, is present (Chapter 2).

The activity of sarco(endo)plasmic reticulum Ca^{2+} ATPase (SERCA2a), a key regulator of myocyte calcium uptake, is consistently diminished in multiple animal models of HF as well as in myocardial tissue from patients with HF.[32,33] Although many proteins are expressed differently in the failing heart, the developmental program of using this specific gene therapy product (adeno-associated virus type 1/SERCA2a) to augment SERCA2a and improve intracellular calcium cycling in humans with HF is the most advanced. By demonstrating an apparently safe vector delivery system, the investigators have systematically addressed the important safety concerns for regulatory approval to even begin a clinical development program.[34] With a series of small and large animal models of HF, as well as in human cells, they completed sufficient preclinical proof-of-concept studies to obtain approval to conduct a phase 1 clinical exposure evaluation.[35,36,37] This initial human administration of a potential gene therapy was conducted in the Calcium Up-Regulation by Percutaneous Administration of Gene Therapy In Cardiac Disease (CUPID) trial (NCT00454818).[38] Of the 39 patients in NYHA class III/IV with LVEF 35% or less, 25 received one of three doses of the gene product by antegrade coronary artery infusion. The safety and effectiveness on a combination of surrogate outcomes compared to the 14 placebo-treated patients was sufficiently encouraging to lead to a larger, now ongoing, trial of 200 patients with a clinical event endpoint—time to all-cause death, heart transplant, or LVAD implantation (NCT01643330).[39]

Although the road ahead is long and uncertain, other gene products for HF are also in the pipeline. At present, it is fair to say that advanced HF is an appropriate target for studies of gene therapy and early studies are under way.

The establishment of a subspecialty for the care of patients with advanced HF brings with it recognition of the need for the special skills and experiences of an entire healthcare team as well as the need for a major institutional commitment of hospitals with advanced HF programs. For most fragile patients with truly advanced HF, a major concentration of resources and professional commitments are required to render optimal care and treatment to this most severely impacted HF cohort. The existence and growth of dedicated units and teams has already greatly enhanced our understanding and management of these patients. In some respects, the current status of advanced HF can be considered analogous to of the early phase of the establishment of coronary care units for the treatment of patients with acute myocardial infarction.[40,41] These units effectively concentrated clinical expertise and provided a focus for cooperation. Multi-institutional databases were created and teams to conduct quality randomized, placebo-controlled trials were established. A similar international foundation of cooperation is emerging for patients with advanced HF that will undoubtedly lead to more targeted and improved research and patient care.

References

1. Liu L, Eisen HJ. Epidemiology of heart failure and scope of the problem. Cardiol Clin 2014;32(1):1–8.
2. Lala A, Joyce E, Groarke JD, Mehra MR. Challenges in long-term mechanical circulatory support and biological replacement of the failing heart. Circ J 2014;78(2):288–99.
3. Lund LH, Edwards LB, Kucheryavaya AY, et al.; International Society for Heart and Lung Transplantation. The Registry of the International Society for Heart and Lung Transplantation: thirtieth official adult heart transplant report—2013; focus theme: age. J Heart Lung Transplant 2013;32(10):951–64.
4. Shah MR, Starling RC, Schwartz Longacre L, Mehra MR; Working Group Participants. Heart transplantation research in the next decade—a goal to achieving evidence-based outcomes: National Heart, Lung, And Blood Institute Working Group. J Am Coll Cardiol 2012;59(14):1263–9.
5. Mehra MR. Advancing immunosuppression in heart transplantation: one step forward, two steps back. Am J Transplant 2013;13(5):1119–20.
6. Garrity ER Jr, Mehra MR. An update on clinical outcomes in heart and lung transplantation. Transplantation 2004 May 15;77(9 Suppl):S68–74.
7. Nair N, Ball T, Uber PA, Mehra MR. Current and future challenges in therapy for antibody-mediated rejection. J Heart Lung Transplant 2011;30(6):612–17.
8. Kienzl-Wagner K, Pratschke J, Brandacher G. Biomarker discovery in transplantation—proteomic adventure or mission impossible? Clin Biochem 2013;46(6):497–505.
9. Mehra MR, Feller E, Rosenberg S. The promise of protein-based and gene-based clinical markers in heart transplantation: from bench to bedside. Nat Clin Pract Cardiovasc Med 2006;3(3):136–43.
10. Yang YG, Syker M. Xenotransplantation: current status and a perspective on the future. Nat Rev Immunol 2007;7:519–31.
11. Kirklin JK, Naftel DC, Kormos RL,et al. Fifth INTERMACS annual report: risk factor analysis from more than 6,000 mechanical circulatory support patients. J Heart Lung Transplant 2013;32(2):141–56.
12. Hannan MM, Husain S, Mattner F, et al.; International Society for Heart and Lung Transplantation. Working formulation for the standardization of definitions of infections in patients using ventricular assist devices. J Heart Lung Transplant 2011;30(4):375–84.
13. Uriel N, Pak SW, Jorde UP, et al. Acquired von Willebrand syndrome after continuous-flow mechanical device support contributes to a high prevalence of bleeding during long-term support and at the time of transplantation. J Am Coll Cardiol 2010;56(15):1207–13.
14. Mehra MR, Stewart GC, Uber PA. The vexing problem of thrombosis in long-term mechanical circulatory support. J Heart Lung Transplant 2014;33(1):1–11.
15. John R, Mantz K, Eckman P, et al. Aortic valve pathophysiology during left ventricular assist device support. J Heart Lung Transplant 2010;29(12):1321–9.
16. Kormos RL. The right heart failure dilemma in the era of left ventricular assist devices. J Heart Lung Transplant 2014;33(2):134–5.
17. Copeland JG, Copeland H, Gustafson M, et al. Experience with more than 100 total artificial heart implants. J Thorac Cardiovasc Surg 2012;143(3):727–34.
18. <https://clinicaltrials.gov/ct2/show/NCT01369407> (accessed May 7th 2014).
19. <https://clinicaltrials.gov/ct2/show/NCT01452802> (accessed May 7th 2014).
20. Klotz S, Meyns B, Simon A, et al. Partial mechanical long-term support with the CircuLite Synergy pump as bridge-to-transplant in congestive heart failure. Thorac Cardiovasc Surg 2010;58(Suppl 2):S173–8.
21. Greatrex NA, Timms DL, Kurita N, et al. Axial magnetic bearing development for the BiVACOR rotary BiVAD/TAH. IEEE Trans Biomed Eng 2010;57(3):714–21.
22. Jansen P, van Oeveren W, Capel A, Carpentier A. In vitro haemocompatibility of a novel bioprosthetic total artificial heart. Eur J Cardiothorac Surg 2012;41(6):e166–7.
23. Kajstura J, Leri A, Finato N, et al. Myocyte proliferation in end-stage cardiac failure in humans. Proc Natl Acad Sci U S A 1998;95(15):8801–5.
24. Orlic D, Kajstura J, Chimenti S, et al. Bone marrow cells regenerate infarcted myocardium. Nature 2001;410(6829):701–5.
25. Leri A, Anversa P. Stem cells: bone-marrow-derived cells and heart failure—the debate goes on. Nat Rev Cardiol 2013;10(7):372–3.
26. Takehara N, Matsubara H. Cardiac regeneration therapy: connections to cardiac physiology. Am J Physiol Heart Circ Physiol 2011;301(6):H2169–80.
27. Anversa P, Kajstura J, Rota M, Leri A. Regenerating new heart with stem cells. J Clin Invest 2013;123(1):62–70.
28. Sanganalmath SK, Bolli R. Cell therapy for heart failure: a comprehensive overview of experimental and clinical studies, current challenges, and future directions. Circ Res 2013;113(6):810–34.
29. Rosen MR. The math of Sisyphus: the conundrum of stem cell administration for myocardial infarction and myocardial failure. Can J Cardiol 2014;30(11):1262–4.
30. Jeevanantham V, Butler M, Saad A, et al. Adult bone marrow cell therapy improves survival and induces long-term improvement in cardiac parameters: a systematic review and meta-analysis. Circulation 2012;126(5):551–68.
31. Jakob P, Landmesser U. Current status of cell-based therapy for heart failure. Curr Heart Fail Rep 2013;10(2):165–76.
32. Kawase Y, Hajjar RJ. The cardiac sarcoplasmic/endoplasmic reticulum calcium ATPase: a potent target for cardiovascular diseases. Nat Clin Pract Cardiovasc Med 2008;5(9):554–65.
33. Braunwald E. Heart Failure. JACC Heart Fail 2013;1(1):1–20.
34. US Department of Health and Human Services, Food and Drug Administration, Center for Biologics Evaluation and Research, Center for Devices and Radiological Health Guidance for Industry. Cellular Therapy for Cardiac Disease. Washington, DC: US Dept of Health and Human Services; 2010.
35. Hajjar RJ, Kang JX, Gwathmey JK, Rosenzweig A. Physiological effects of adenoviral gene transfer of sarcoplasmic reticulum calcium ATPase in isolated rat myocytes. Circulation 1997;95(2):423–9.
36. Byrne MJ, Power JM, Preovolos A, Mariani JA, et al. Recirculating cardiac delivery of AAV2/1SERCA2a improves myocardial function in an experimental model of heart failure in large animals. Gene Ther 2008;15(23):1550–7.
37. Hadri L, Bobe R, Kawase Y, et al. SERCA2a gene transfer enhances eNOS expression and activity in endothelial cells. Mol Ther 2010;18(7):1284–92.
38. Jessup M, Greenberg B, Mancini D, et al. Calcium Upregulation by Percutaneous Administration of Gene Therapy in Cardiac Disease (CUPID): a phase 2 trial of intracoronary gene therapy of sarcoplasmic reticulum Ca^{2+}-ATPase in patients with advanced heart failure. Circulation 2011;124(3):304–13.
39. Greenberg B, Yaroshinsky A, Zsebo KM, et al. Design of a phase 2b trial of intracoronary administration of AAV1/SERCA2a in patients with advanced heart failure: the CUPID 2 Trial (Calcium Up-Regulation by Percutaneous Administration of Gene Therapy in Cardiac Disease Phase 2b). JACC Heart Fail 2014;2(1):84–92.
40. Julian DG, Valentine PA Miller GG. Disturbances of rate, rhythm and conduction in acute myocardial infarction: a prospective study of 100 consecutive unselected patients with the aid of electrocardiographic monitoring. Am J Med 1964;37:915–27.
41. Lown B, Fakhro AM, Hood WB, Jr., Thorn GW. The coronary care unit. New perspectives and directions. JAMA 1967;199(3):188–98.

Index

Tables, figures and boxes are indicated by an italic *t*, *f* and *b* following the page number.

A
abatacept 300
abdominal decompression 146
ABO matching 268
accelerometers 78
accessory pathway-mediated tachycardia 159
ACE inhibitors 142–3, 203, 209–10
α-actin 24
actin-associated LIM protein 15
actin–myosin cross-bridges 18–19
activation 57
activin-like kinase 390
actomyosin ATPase 18
acute cellular rejection 58, 97, 258, 299, 311–12, 314–17
adaptive hypertrophy 13
adenosine 167, 398, 398*t*
adherence problems 267
adhesion molecules 67–8
ADMIRE-HF 128
β-adrenergic receptors 15, 20, 22–3
adult congenital heart disease, *see* congenital heart disease
advanced heart failure
  definition 43–4
  subspecialty 7–8
advance directives 421
AF-CHF 156
affinity maturation 64*b*
AFFIRM 154, 155, 156
afterload 333–4
aging 5–6
A-HeFT 142
AHG-CDC crossmatch 270
AICAR 31
Akt 31
alcohol abuse 261, 267
aldosterone antagonists 143
alemtuzumab 287*t*, 288
ALLHAT 4–5
allograft ischemic time 257
allograft rejection 70; *see also* cardiac allograft rejection
AlloMap 309
allosensitization 268–72
alternative pathway 69–70
AMBITION 408
ambrisentan 403*t*, 406
ambulatory ECG 165
American Heart Association/American College of Cardiology (AHA/ACC) guidelines 3–7
amiloride 146*t*
amiodarone 155, 167
^{13}N-ammonia 125
AMPK 31
amplification 57
amyloid heart disease 95, 122, 161, 257, 266
anaerobic threshold 51, 52*b*
analgesics 421–2
anaphylatoxin 69
ANDROMEDA 156
anemia 244
anemnestic response 58
angiotensin II 14
angiotensin converting enzyme (ACE) inhibitors 142–3, 203, 209–10
angiotensin–neprilysin inhibitors 143–4
angiotensin receptor blockers (ARBs) 142–3
ankyrin 15
anorexigens 387
Anrep effect 20
antiarrhythmic drugs 144, 154, 155, 167
antibodies 65, 66–70
antibody-dependent cellular cytotoxicity 66
antibody-mediated rejection 97–8, 299, 307, 312, 317–18
anticoagulation
  atrial fibrillation 156–7
  chronic thromboembolic pulmonary hypertension 378
  coronary artery bypass grafting 221
  heart failure 144
  left ventricular assist device 241
  pulmonary arterial hypertension 399–400
anti-cytokine receptor antibodies 287*t*, 288
antigen 57
antigen-presenting cells 58, 70–2
antigen processing 61–2
antigen receptor genes 64*b*
anti-HLA antigens 268–9
antimicrobials
  immunosuppression with infectious comorbidity 299–300
  prophylactic 240, 319–20
antiproliferative agents 281*t*, 284–5, 315, 319
anti-thymocyte globulin 286, 287*t*, 288
aortic calcification 219
aortic regurgitation 46, 47, 208–10, 226–7, 240
aortic stenosis 202–4, 224–5, 240
  pseudo 203, 225
aortic valve area 203
aortic valve repair/replacement 202, 203–4, 209, 210, 225, 226–7
apixiban 144, 156–7
apoptosis 29–31, 342
ARC 30
arginine vasopressin 47, 237
ARIES-1/-2 406
βARK 23
β-arrestin agonists 15
arrhythmias
  atrioventricular node and above 153–62
  device-related 75–6
  see also ventricular arrhythmias
arrhythmogenic right ventricular cardiomyopathy 366–8
arterial switch 371
ASCEND-HF 147, 358
ask-tell-ask 420
asperigillus infection 320
Atgam 286, 287*t*, 288
ATLAS 143
atrial fibrillation 153–7
  antiarrhythmic drugs 154, 155
  anticoagulation 156–7
  cardiac resynchronization therapy 181–2
  catheter ablation 157, 182
  clinical features 153–4
  DC cardioversion 154
  device-related 75
  left atrial appendage closure 157
  left ventricular assist device 244, 249
  multiple wavelet theory 153
  pathophysiology 153
  pharmacological cardioversion 155
  rate control 154, 156
  reentry rotors theory 153
  rhythm control 154–6

atrial flutter 157–9
  atypical/typical 158
  catheter ablation 158–9
  left ventricular assist device 244
atrial septal defect 369
atrial septostomy 408
atrial switch 371
atrial tachycardia 159
  device-related 75
auscultation, right ventricular failure 348*b*
autocrine stimulation 67
autoimmune disease 266
autonomic nervous system 333
autophagy 31–2, 342
AVID 169, 170*t*
AV nodal reentry tachycardia 159
Ayerza's disease 385
azathioprine 281*t*, 284, 315, 319

B
B7 molecules 63–4
balance of activity hypothesis 22
balloon aortic valvotomy 204
balloon mitral valvotomy 205
BAMI 430
basiliximab 287*t*, 288
basophils 58*t*
Bax 29
B cells 58, 58*t*, 65–6
  memory B cells 66
Bcl-2 proteins 29, 30
bead assays 268–9
Beclin-1 32
belatacept 300
βARK 23
β-blockers 139–42, 154, 204, 209, 221
BH3-only proteins 29
bicuspid aortic valve 261
BIG 51
bioenergetics 341
bioimpedance systems 51, 78–82
biomarkers 5, 47, 49
biomechanical overload 15
bioptome 100
biplane Simpson method 108
BiVACOR device 429
BLOCK-HF 183
blood flow 116
blood pressure
  left ventricular assist device 244, 248
  right ventricular failure 348*b*
blood urea nitrogen 49
BMPR2 387, 390
body weight 74
bone marrow 59
bone marrow cell therapy 128
bortezomib 299
bosentan 403*t*, 405–6
bradyarrhythmias 160–1
brain natriuretic peptide (BNP) 49, 347, 349, 411
braking phenomenon 145
BREATHE-1 405–6
BREATHE-2 408
breathing reserve 51, 52*b*
bridge to transplantation 235, 257
bumetanide 146*t*, 365*t*
bundle branch reentry 175

C
C1q assay 269
C3 convertase 69
C4a 69
CABG-Patch 169, 170*t*
cachexia 219, 265–6
calcineurin inhibitors 281–2*t*, 283–4, 314–15
  avoidance 295
  monotherapy 296
  renal-sparing protocol 293–5
  toxicity 318–19
  withdrawal 295–6
calcium channel blockers 154, 204, 401
calcium cycling 17–18, 20–3
calcium-dependent signaling 15–16
calcium-induced calcium release 17, 341
calmodulin-dependent protein kinase II 15–16
cAMP response binding protein 15
cAMP response element modulator 15
cancer, *see* malignancy
candidiasis 320
cardiac allograft rejection
  acute cellular 58, 97, 258, 299, 311–12, 314–17
  antibody-mediated 97–8, 299, 307, 312, 317–18
  cardiac MRI 311
  echocardiography 310–11
  endomyocardial biopsy 97–9, 308–9, 317*t*
  frequency 307
  gene expression profiling 309–10
  hyperacute 69
  immune response 58
  outcomes 308
  surveillance 307–12
  treatment 299, 311–12, 316–17
  ventricular evoked response 311
cardiac allograft vasculopathy 129, 258, 272, 297–8, 322–5
cardiac ankyrin repeat protein 15
cardiac cachexia 219, 265–6
cardiac dyssynchrony, *see* dyssynchrony
cardiac filling pressure 74
cardiac metabolism 26–9
cardiac MRI
  cardiac allograft rejection 311
  cardiac resynchronization therapy response 119–20, 186
  coronary artery disease 216
  dilated cardiomyopathy 120–1
  displacement encoding with stimulated echoes 119
  dyssynchrony identification 119, 180–1
  heart failure 117–24
  hypertrophic cardiomyopathy 121–2
  infiltrative cardiomyopathies 122–3
  inflammatory cardiomyopathies 123–4
  ischemic cardiomyopathy 118–20
  late gadolinium enhancement 118–21, 122, 123, 124
  myocardial edema 118, 123
  myocardial tagging 119
  phase-contrast tissue velocity mapping 119
  pulmonary arterial hypertension 411
  right heart function 237
  right ventricle 353, 356*t*, 357*f*, 360*b*, 362*b*
  scar analysis 186
  techniques 117–18
  ventricular arrhythmia 165–6
cardiac myocytes
  calcium cycling 17–18, 20–3
  contractility 17–20
  death pathways 29–32
  hypertrophy 1, 12–17
  normal morphology 12–13
  passive stiffness 26
  physiologic hypertrophy 1, 13–14, 14*f*
  plasticity 33, 342
  right ventricle 330–1
  sarcomeric proteins 23–6
cardiac output
  echocardiography 102–3
  noninvasive monitors 51
  pulmonary arterial hypertension 397
cardiac resynchronization therapy 179–97
  atrial fibrillation 181–2
  atrial pacing/tracking 196
  AV interval optimization 192–7
  cardiac MRI 119–20, 186
  cardiac tamponade 189
  complications 188–90
  coronary sinus dissection/perforation 186
  device implantation 183–8
  device interrogation 188, 189*t*
  echocardiography 112, 116, 186, 193–5, 196–7
  end-of-life issues 197, 424
  follow-up 188–97
  historical background 183–4
  implantation techniques 186
  intraventricular conduction delay 182
  lead implantation troubleshooting 187
  lead problems 190
  lead technology 187–8
  loss of biventricular pacing 190–1
  mechanism of action 179
  nonresponders 181, 191–2, 193*f*, 193*b*
  patient selection 179–83, 184*t*
  premature ventricular contractions 183
  preprocedure dyssynchrony 185–6
  proarrhythmias 189
  procedural complications 186
  right bundle branch block 182
  right ventricular apical pacing 183
  scar analysis 186
  strain imaging 116
  super-responders 181
  telescoping catheter delivery systems 186
  ventricular tachycardia/fibrillation 189
cardiac tamponade
  cardiac resynchronization therapy 189
  endomyocardial biopsy 100
cardiac transplantation
  age of recipient 257, 264
  allograft ischemic time 257
  amyloidosis 257, 266
  autoimmune disease 266
  cachexia 265–6
  cardiac allograft vasculopathy 129, 258, 272, 297–8, 322–5
  cerebrovascular disease 265
  chemotherapy-induced cardiomyopathy 257
  comorbidities 257
  compliance with medical care 267
  complications 314–25
  contraindications 262–7
  coronary artery bypass grafting 325
  demographics 255, 256*t*
  desensitization protocols 271, 298–9
  diabetes 265, 321
  direct crossmatch 270
  donor evaluation 259–62
  donor management 259
  donor–recipient matching 267–72
  future directions 427–8
  gastrointestinal bleeding 266
  graft rejection, *see* cardiac allograft rejection

heparin-induced thrombocytopenia 267
hepatic disease 264–5
history of 255
hyperlipidemia 321
hypertension 266, 318, 321
immune response activation 70–2
immunosuppressive strategies, *see* immunosuppression
indications 255
infection 99, 258, 266, 299–300, 319–20
malignancy 99, 259, 266, 279, 298, 321–2
morbidity 257–9, 272
mortality 256–7, 272
muscular dystrophies 266
nuclear imaging 129
obesity 265
osteoporosis 321
outcomes 255–9
patient selection 255
peritransplant ischemic injury 99
post-transplantation care 272–3
post-transplant lymphoproliferative disorder 99, 259, 298, 321
pregnancy 319
previous sternotomy 267
pulmonary hypertension 263–4
pulmonary infarction 264
pulmonary parenchymal disease 264
Quilty lesions 98
radiation-induced heart disease 267
rejection, *see* cardiac allograft rejection
renal function 259, 264, 320–1
retransplantation 257, 325
sarcoidosis 266
subspecialty 7–8
supraventricular arrhythmias after 160
survival 255–6
tobacco abuse 266–7
vascular disease 265
ventricular tachycardia 176
virtual crossmatch 270–1
cardiogenic shock 147–8, 238
CardioMEMS 83*t*, 84, 85
cardiopulmonary exercise testing 51–3
cardiorenal syndrome 47, 50, 264, 358, 360, 365*b*
cardiovascular flow 116
cardioversion 154–5
CARE-HF 5, 189
CareLink Network 88*t*
CARGO 309
Carmat pump 429
carotid artery disease 219
carotid endarterectomy 219
CARRESS-HF 146, 358, 360, 365*b*
carvedilol 154
CASH 169, 170*t*
caspases 30, 32
catecholamines 14
catheter ablation
atrial fibrillation 157, 182
atrial flutter 158–9
supraventricular tachycardias 160
ventricular arrhythmia 172–6
Ca^{2+} transient 17
CD3 63
CD4 63
CD8 63
CD-25 65, 67, 67*t*
CD28 63–4
cell-based therapy 429–30
cell death 29–32
cellular diastole 18
cellular rejection, *see* acute cellular rejection
cellular systole 18
central venous catheter 50
central venous pressure 50
CentriMag 238
cerebrovascular disease 265
CHA2DS2-VASc 156, 158*t*
Chagas disease 161
CHARM-Added 142
chemotherapy toxicity 96, 257
CHEST-1 408
chest radiography
cardiac resynchronization therapy 188
heart failure 49
pulmonary arterial hypertension 392, 393*f*
right ventricular failure 349, 350*t*, 351*f*
CHF-STAT 156
Child–Pugh score 220, 239, 239*t*, 264
chlorothiazide 146*t*
chronic kidney disease 264
Chronicle device 50–1, 82, 83*t*, 84
chronic thromboembolic pulmonary hypertension 377–8, 395
CIBIS-II 139
ciclosporin 281*t*, 283–4, 314–15, 318–19
CIDS 169, 170*t*
CircuLite Synergy micropump 429
class II associated invariant chain peptide (CLIP) 62
classical pathway 69
clonal anergy 64
Clostridium difficile 266
coagulation, pulmonary arterial hypertension 390
cocaine 261
COMBI 408
COMPASS-HF 50–1
complement 68–70
complement-dependent cytotoxicity assay 268, 269
complete heart block 161
computed tomography (CT)
cardiac vasculature 185
right ventricle 353, 360*b*
congenital heart disease
organ donors 261
pulmonary arterial hypertension 388
right ventricle 342
right ventricular failure 368–73
congenitally corrected transposition of the great arteries 371–2
connective tissue disease 388
CONSENSUS 6, 142
CONSENSUS II 107
constant region 65
constrictive pericarditis 350–2
continuous positive airway pressure 422
contraception 399
contractile proteins 18–19, 342
proteolysis 26
contractile reserve 19, 225
COPERNICUS 139–41
coronary angiography
cardiac transplantation 129, 323
organ donors 261
ventricular arrhythmia 166–7
coronary artery bypass grafting (CABG) 216–21
anticoagulation 221
aortic calcification 219
cardiac transplantation 325
carotid artery disease 219
frailty 218–19
heparin-induced thrombocytopenia 219–20
informed consent 220
LIMA-LAD graft 217
liver function 220
lung disease 219
mitral surgery at a time of 222–3
nutritional status 219
off-pump 220, 221
on-pump beating-heart 220, 221
patient preparation 220
post-surgical care 221
preoperative issues 217–20
pulmonary hypertension 220
renal function 219
right heart failure 220
surgical technique 220–1
triage 216–17
ventricular reconstruction with 221
coronary artery disease 215–16
organ donors 261
coronary sinus
anatomy 184–5
perforation/dissection 186
corticosteroids 279–80, 281*t*, 292–3, 315–16
C-protein 20
creatinine 49
cryopreserved valves 271
CTAF 155
CT angiography 378
CTLA-4 64
CTLA-4 immunoglobulin 300
CUPID 430
cyclophilin D 32
Cylex ImmuKnow 296–7, 311
cytokines 14–15, 66–7, 340
cytomegalovirus 99, 319–20
cytoskeletal proteins 342
cytotoxic T lymphocytes 63

D
dabigatran 144, 156–7
daclizumab 287*t*, 288
DAVID 183
DC cardioversion 154
DECIDE LVAD 245
decision-making 420
decompensation
common causes 48*b*
pathophysiology 74–82
defective desmosome hypothesis 366
DEFINITE 170*t*
deformation (strain) imaging 113, 114–16
dendritic cells 58*t*, 70
DENSE imaging 119
depleting antibodies 286
depression 422–3
desensitization protocols 271, 298–9
desmosomes 366
diabetes
cardiac metabolism 27–9
cardiac transplantation 265, 321
Diamond HF 155, 156
diapedesis 68
diastole 18
differentiation 57
DIG 144
digoxin (digitalis) 144, 154, 237, 400
dilated cardiomyopathy
cardiac MRI 120–1
sarcomeric protein mutations 23–4, 24*b*

DINAMIT 169, 170*t*
direct antigen presentation 62
direct crossmatch 270
direct current cardioversion 156
direct recognition 71
displacement encoding with stimulated echoes 119
diuretics 144–5, 146*t*, 203, 204, 365*t*, 400
dobutamine 148, 148*t*, 237
dobutamine cardiac MRI 117
dobutamine stress echocardiography
  aortic stenosis 225
  cardiac allograft vasculopathy 324
  mitral regurgitation 111–12
  myocardial viability 110
dofetilide 155
donor antigen recognition 59–66
donor evaluation 259–62
donor management 259
donor–recipient matching 267–72
donor-specific antibodies 268, 270, 271
dopamine 148, 148*t*
Doppler imaging, *see* echocardiography
DOSE 145, 358
double-chambered right ventricle 369
dronedarone 155–6
drug-induced pulmonary arterial hypertension 387–8
DTPA imaging 126
d-transposition of the great arteries 370–1
durable power of attorney for health care 421
dyspnea 47, 422
dyssynchrony
  cardiac MRI 119, 180–1
  echocardiography 112, 116, 179–80, 186
  electrocardiography 179
  identification methods 179–81
  pre-CRT implantation 185–6

E
EARLY 406
Ebstein anomaly 370
echocardiography
  aortic stenosis 225
  cardiac allograft rejection 310–11
  cardiac allograft vasculopathy 324
  cardiac resynchronization therapy 112, 116, 186, 193–5, 196–7
  cardiovascular flow 116
  dyssynchrony 112, 116, 179–80, 186
  endomyocardial biopsy guidance 99–100
  heart failure 49, 102–16
  hemodynamic assessment 102–7
  left ventricular systolic function 107–9
  mitral regurgitation 110–12, 222
  myocardial viability 109–10, 115
  pulmonary arterial hypertension 393–5, 410–11
  real-time 3D 116
  right heart function 236–7
  right ventricle 352–3, 354*t*, 355–6*f*, 360*b*, 362*t*
  speckle tracking 114 115*f*, 180, 186
  strain imaging 113, 114–16
  valvular heart disease 110–12
  ventricular arrhythmia 165–6
  ventricular assist devices 112–14
ECHO-CRT 180
edema
  myocardial 118, 123
  peripheral 49

Edmonton Symptom Assessment Scale 421
edoxaban 156–7
effector cells 63
EFFECT score 423
Eisenmenger syndrome 372
elderly patients 5–6
electrical cardioversion 154
electrical storm 167
electrocardiography (ECG)
  ambulatory in ventricular arrhythmia 165
  cardiac resynchronization therapy 190
  dyssynchrony 179
  pulmonary arterial hypertension 392, 393*f*
  QRS prolongation 179
  right ventricular failure 349, 349*b*, 350*f*
  SPECT gating 125
electrophysiology study 167
ELISA 268–9
embryology 329
EMPHASIS-HF 143
end-of-life care 197, 420–5
endomyocardial biopsy 92–100
  cardiac allograft rejection 97–9, 308–9, 317*t*
  cardiomyopathy diagnosis 92–6
  chemotherapy toxicity 96
  complications 100
  echocardiography-guided 99–100
  fluoroscopy-guided 100
  guidelines 92, 93*t*
  technique 99–100
endothelin 14
endothelin-1 388–9
endothelin receptor antagonists 149, 405–7
ENDURANCE 245
engine out of fuel hypothesis 28
eosinophilic myocarditis 92, 94
eosinophils 58*t*
EPHESUS 143
epinephrine 237
epoprostenol 398, 398*t*, 401–2, 402*t*, 404
Epstein–Barr virus 99, 259, 320
equilibrium radionuclide ventriculography 126
ERK signaling 16, 33
ESCAPE 47, 48, 50, 51, 138, 147, 148
ethacrynic acid 146*t*
ethanol abuse 261
everolimus 282*t*, 285–6, 316, 319
excitation–contraction coupling 17–18, 341–2
exercise-induced hypertrophy 14
exercise stress echocardiography 111
exercise training 399
extracellular matrix 342
extracellular signal-regulated kinases (ERK) 16, 33

F
F(ab[1]) fragment 66
Fabry–Anderson disease 95, 123
F-actin 18
factor B 70
factor D 70
family support 420
fatigue 47, 422
Fc region 66
FDG-PET 125, 126, 128
fetal development 329
fetal gene program 27
fetal isoform switch 24
fetal metabolic program 27

filamentous actin 18
  filling pressure
  left heart 106–7
  right heart 104
first heart field cells 329
first-pass radionuclide ventriculography 126
Five Wishes 421
flecainide 155
fluid index 79
Fontal circulation 372–3
force–frequency response 19–20, 22
forward-mode NCX 22
fractional area change 113
frailty 218–19, 422
Framingham Heart Study 6
Frank–Staring relation 19, 20
FREEDOM 196
FREEDOM-C 404
FREEDOM-M 404
free fatty acids 27
fungal infections 320
furosemide 146*t*, 365*t*

G
gadolinium 117–18
gastrointestinal bleeding 240, 250, 266
gastrointestinal symptoms 422
gene expression profiling 309–10
gene therapy 430
genetics
  antigen receptor gene rearrangement 64*b*
  human leukocyte antigens 60
  pulmonary arterial hypertension 387, 390
  sarcomeric protein mutations 23–4, 24*b*
germinal centers 59
GESICA 155
giant cell myocarditis 92, 93–4, 161
global left ventricular systolic function 107–8
glucagon-like peptide-1 (GLP-1) 29
gout 319
G_i proteins 20, 23
graft rejection, *see* cardiac allograft rejection
GRIPHON 405
GRK2 23
growth hormone 14

H
hangout interval 332
Harefield Strategy 252
HARPS 252
Heart Failure Survival Score 137
HeartMate II 233, 240, 241, 241*f*, 242, 243*f*, 244, 250, 251, 374
HeartMate 3 245–6
HeartPOD device 51, 83*t*, 84–5
heart rate
  implantable device monitoring 76
  variability 74, 76–8
heart rhythm, implantable device monitoring 75–6
Heart Save the Nephron 295
heart-to-mediastinum ratio 128
heart transplantation, *see* cardiac transplantation
HeartWare device 244, 250
hemochromatosis 95, 161
hemodynamics
  cardiorenal syndrome 50
  echocardiography 102–7
  guide to pharmacotherapy 53, 138
  heart failure 47

implantable cardioverter defibrillators 171
implantable monitors 50–1, 82–7
invasive assessment 49–50
left ventricular assist device 236, 240
pulmonary arterial hypertension prognosis 409
right ventricular failure 349–52, 353*b*, 353*t*
hemoglobin 49
hemolysis 244
heparin-induced thrombocytopenia 219–20, 239, 267
hepatic function 220, 239, 264–5
hepatitis B 260–1, 266
hepatitis C 260–1, 266
hibernating myocardium 29
Hill coefficient 19
history-taking 47–8
HIV 260–1, 266, 388
HLA-DM 62
home monitoring 88*t*
hospice care 423
hospitalization 6
human leukocyte antigens (HLA) 58, 59–61, 62
sensitization 268–72
hybrid resistance 66
hydrochlorothiazide 146*t*
hyperacute rejection 69
hyperkalaemia 143
hyperlipidemia 321
hypersensitivity myocarditis 94
hypertension
cardiac transplantation 266, 318, 321
heart failure and 44, 46
immunosuppressive toxicity 318
left ventricular assist device 244, 248
hypertrophic cardiomyopathy
cardiac MRI 121–2
endomyocardial biopsy 94–6
genetic causes 23, 24*b*
hypertrophy 1, 12–17
hyponatremia 47, 49
hypotension 248
hypothyroidism 49
hypovolemia 244

I
ibutilide 155
ICAM 68
IgA 65, 66
IgD 65
IgE 65
IgG 65, 66
IgM 65, 66, 69
IL-2 64–5, 67, 67*t*
IL-2 receptor 65, 67, 67*t*
IL-6 67, 67*t*
IL-17 67, 67*t*
iloprost 403*t*, 405
IMAGE 310
ImmuKnow 296–7, 311
immune response 57–8
cardiac transplantation 70–2
immune system 58–9
donor–recipient matching 268–72
immunoglobulins 65, 66
immunoglobulin superfamily adhesion molecules 68
immunosuppression
adverse events 283*t*
cardiac allograft vasculopathy 297–8
clinical trials of 289–92
conventional agents 279–86
high circulating antibodies/ sensitization 298–9
induction therapy 272, 286–9, 316
infectious comorbidity 299–300
maintenance therapy 314–16
malignancy management 298
minimization 292–7
monitoring 296–7, 311
novel agents 300
strategies and regimen 286–92
tapering 272, 320
toxicity 318–19
impedance cardiography 78
implantable cardioverter defibrillators (ICDs)
arrhythmogenic cardiomyopathy 367–8
deactivation 424
end-of-life 424
indications and contraindications 166*b*
left ventricular assist device and 241, 249
tetralogy of Fallot 370
tricuspid regurgitation associated with 373
ventricular arrhythmia 165, 167–72
implantable monitoring devices 74–89
financial aspects 88–9
hemodynamics 50–1, 82–7
medicolegal aspects 88–9
pathophysiological insights 74–82
remote monitoring systems 86, 88*t*, 89
strategies for use 86–7
indirect antigen presentation 62
indirect recognition 71
inducibility 57
infection
cardiac transplantation 99, 258, 266, 299–300, 319–20
ICD-related 171
left ventricular assist device 239–40, 249–50
organ donor screening 260*t*, 260–1
inferior vena cava 104
infiltrative cardiomyopathies
bradyarrhythmias 161
cardiac MRI 122–3
endomyocardial biopsy 94–6
inflammation 14–15, 390
inflammatory cardiomyopathies
bradyarrhythmias 161
cardiac MRI 123–4
infrahisian block 161
innate immunity 72
inotropes 148, 148*t*, 423
inpatient care 6
insulin 14
insulin-like growth factor (IGF1) 14
insulin resistance 27
inteferon-γ 67, 67*t*
integrins 15, 68
interdigitating dendritic cells 70
interleukins 14–15, 67, 67*t*
IL-2 64–5, 67, 67*t*
IL-6 67, 67*t*
IL-17 67, 67*t*
INTERMAC classification 7, 137, 138*t*, 231, 232*t*
International Society for Heart and Lung Transplantation (ISHLT)
antibody-mediated rejection 307*t*, 317, 318*t*
cardiac allograft vasculopathy nomenclature 323*b*
endomyocardial biopsy grading system 308*t*, 317*t*
interventricular septum 330, 335
intra-abdominal pressure 146
intra-aortic balloon counterpulsation pump 175, 206, 220
intracardiac pressures 104–6
intrathoracic bioimpedance 51, 78–82
intravascular ultrasound 323–4
intravenous immunoglobulin 271, 298
intraventricular conduction defects 112, 182
INTrEPID 233
IRIS 169, 170*t*
iron overload 95, 122, 161
ischemia–reperfusion injury 30–1, 32
ischemic cardiomyopathy
bradyarrhythmias 161
cardiac MRI 118–20
catheter ablation 175
ventricular reconstruction with CABG 221
ischemic preconditioning 29
isoform switches 24–5
isoproterenol 237
isotypes 65
isotype switching 66
ivabradine 144

J
Jatene operation 371
jugular venous pressure 48, 348*b*
jugular venous pulsation 48
c-Jun N-terminal kinases (JNK) 16

K
Kansas City Cardiomyopathy Questionnaire 421
kidneys, *see* renal function
killer immunoglobulin-like receptors 66
Kussmaul's sign 48, 348*b*

L
LAMP2 31
Lariat atrial occluder 157
late gadolinium enhancement 118–21, 122, 123, 124
late preconditioning 31
Latitude Patient Management System 88*t*
LCZ696 143–4
LEA29Y 300
lean body mass 53
lectin-like receptors 66
left atrial appendage closure 157
left heart filling pressure 106–7
left ventricle
compared to right ventricle 336, 337*b*
remodeling 337–8
systolic function 107–9
volumes 107–8
left ventricular assist device (LVAD)
adult cardiac life support 251–2
anemia 244
anticoagulation 241
antimicrobial prophylaxis 240
associated drug and device therapy 241
atrial fibrillation/flutter 244, 249
blood pressure 244, 248
bridge to transplantation 235, 257
cardiogenic shock 238
cardiopulmonary resuscitation 252
critical care situations 251–2
data display 242, 243*f*

left ventricular assist device (LVAD) (*Contd.*)
decompensated heart failure 238
destination therapy 7
echocardiography 112–14
end-of-life 424
explantation 252
follow-up frequency 248
future directions 428–9
gastrointestinal bleeding 240, 250
hemodynamics 236, 240
hemolysis 244
heparin-induced thrombocytopenia 239
hepatic function 239
HLA sensitization 270, 271
hypertension 244, 248
hypotension 248
hypovolemia 244
ICDs and 241, 249
inadequate preload 244
indications 231–5
infection 239–40, 249–50
lung disease 239
magnetically levitated pumps 245–6
myocardial recovery 33–4, 252–3
nontransplant candidates 231–5
nutritional status 239
optimal device function 248, 249*t*
outflow or inflow obstruction 243
outpatient management 248–53
patient selection and optimization 235–40
postimplant considerations 240–1
pulsatility index 243
pump thrombosis 250–1
renal function 238–9
reverse remodeling 33–4
right heart function 235–8, 249
right ventricular failure 237–8, 363–4, 374–7
rotor clots 244
sepsis 243
shunting 114
speed optimization 240–1
stroke risk 245–6, 250
suction events 244, 249
termination 424
tricuspid regurgitation associated with 373, 374*t*
trouble shooting 242–4
valvular disease 113, 240
ventricular arrhythmias 176, 244, 249
left ventricular ejection fraction 2, 107, 108, 114
left ventricular end-diastolic volume 44
left ventricular hypertrophy 44
organ donors 261
left ventricular outflow tract 102–3
length-dependent force production 20
levosimendan 148, 148*t*
LFA-2 68
lipotoxicity hypothesis 27–8
liraglutide 29
liver function 220, 239, 264–5
living will 421
loop diuretics 144–5, 365*t*
l-transposition of the great arteries 371–2
L-type Ca^{2+} channels 17, 20–1, 341
Luminex 268–9
lung allocation score 409
lung disease 219, 239
lung transplantation 408–9
Lyme disease 161
lymph nodes 59
lymphocytic myocarditis 92, 94
lymphoid organs 59

M

macitentan 403*t*, 406–7
macrophages 58*t*
MADIT I 170*t*
MADIT II 169, 170*t*
MADIT-CRT 182, 183, 189, 190, 191
Mahan's equation 105
major histocompatibility complex (MHC) 60
malignancy
cardiac transplant recipients 99, 259, 266, 279, 298, 321–2
organ donors 260
MAPK signaling 16
mast cells 58*t*
matrix metalloproteinases 128
maximal voluntary ventilation 51
mean fluorescent index 269
mean heart rate 76
mean pulmonary artery pressure 105–6
mechanical circulatory support
cardiac transplantation outcomes 257
future directions 428–9
HLA sensitization 270, 271
myocardial recovery 252–3
see also left ventricular assist device; total artificial heart
mechanical ventilation 104, 357
mechanosensing systems 15
Medawar, Peter 57–8
MELD Score 220, 239, 239*t*, 264–5
membrane attack complex 70
Memorial Symptom Assessment Scale–HF 421
memory 57, 58
memory B cells 66
MERIT-HF 139
Merlin.net Patient Care Network 88*t*
metabolic derangement 26–9
metabolic syndrome 27
metformin 31
methylprednisolone 281*t*
metolazone 146*t*
^{123}I-MIBG imaging 128
β_2- microglobulin 60
microRNA 24, 338
milrinone 148, 148*t*, 237
Minnesota Living with Heart Failure Questionnaire 421
minute ventilation 51, 78
MIRACLE-ICD 189, 191
mitochondria 13
remodeling 341
mitochondrial permeability transitions 32
mitogen-activated protein kinase 16
MitraClip 208
mitral annular calcification 205–6
mitral leaflet tenting 110
mitral regurgitation 46–7, 206–8, 221–4
echocardiography 110–12, 222
functional (secondary) 110–12, 206, 208
ischemic 222–4
left ventricular assist device 240
nonischemic 224
primary 206–7
mitral stenosis 204–6, 240
mitral valve repair/replacement 205, 207–8, 223–4
with CABG 222–3
minimally invasive 224
Mobitz I/II block 161
Model for End-Stage Liver Disease (MELD) score 220, 239, 239*t*, 264–5
MOMENTUM 3 246
monoclonal antibodies 287*t*, 288
morphine 422
mTOR inhibitors 282*t*, 284–5, 316, 319
multigated acquisition (MUGA) scan 126
multiple wavelet theory 153
muromonab-CD3 287*t*, 288
muscle LIM protein 15
muscular dystrophies 266
Mustard procedure 371
mycophenolate mofetil 281*t*, 284–5, 315, 319
myocardial dyssynchrony, *see* dyssynchrony
myocardial edema 118, 123
myocardial hibernation 29
myocardial infarction
biomechanical overload 15
heart failure and 5, 44
right ventricular failure and 364–6
myocardial performance index 339
myocardial plasticity 33, 342
myocardial stunning 26
myocardial tagging 119
myocardial viability
echocardiography 109–10, 115
nuclear imaging 126–8
myocarditis, endomyocardial biopsy 92–4
myocytes, *see* cardiac myocytes
myofibrils 13
myopalladin 15
myosin 18
myosin essential light chain 24
myosin heavy chain isoform switch 24

N

^{13}N-ammonia 125
natural killer (NK) cell 58*t*, 66
nebulette 15
necrosis 32, 342
necrostatin-1 32
necrotizing eosinophilic myocarditis 92, 94
nesiritide 146–7, 147*t*, 148, 237
neurohormones 47, 49, 340
neurohumoral mediators 14–15
neutrophils 58*t*
New York Heart Association (NYHA) classification system 2–3
NICO device 51
NICOM device 51
nighttime heart rate 76
nitrates 422
nitric oxide 237, 340–1, 389–90, 398, 398*t*
nitroglycerine 147*t*, 148
nitroprusside 147–8, 147*t*
NK-κB 32
nominal antigen presentation 62
nonadherence 267
nonarteritic anterior ischemic optic neuropathy 407
nondepleting antibodies 286
noninvasive programmed stimulation 167
noninvasive ventilation 422
norepinephrine 237
Norwood procedure 372
novel anticoagulants 144, 156–7
N-terminal proBNP 49, 411
nuclear factor of activated transcription 15

nuclear imaging 124–9, 353, 360*b*
nutritional status 219, 239

O
obesity
cardiac metabolism 27–9
cardiac transplantation 265
obscurin 15
OKT3 287*t*, 288
^{15}O-labeled water 125
opioids 421, 422
opsonization 69
OPTIME-CHF 148
OPTIMIZE-HF 141
OptiVol Fluid Status Monitoring System 51
O_2 pulse 52*b*
organ donors
donor–recipient matching 267–72
evaluation 259–62
management 259
orthopnea 47–8
osteoporosis 321
oxygen saturation 52*b*
oxygen therapy 422

P
p38 MAP kinases 16
PABA-CHF 157
PACE 183
pacemakers/pacing
end-of-life 424
tricuspid regurgitation associated with 373
PACE-RBBB 182
PACES 408
pain 421–2
palladin 15
pAMR 98
panel reactive antibody level 268, 269
papillary muscles 110, 121
PARADIGM-HF 143
paroxetine 423
paroxysmal nocturnal dyspnea 48
PARTNER 225
PA–RV coupling 390
PATENT-1 407–8
patent ductus arteriosus 329
patient assessment 47–51
Pcr:ATP ratio 28–9
peak endocardial acceleration 86
peak oxygen uptake 51, 52*b*
peak VO_2 lean 52*b*
PECAM 68
peptide-binding groove 60
percutaneous coronary intervention 325
perfusion pressure 147–8
peripheral edema 49
peripheral neuropathy 318
peritransplant ischemic injury 99
PET scan 124, 125, 126, 128, 129, 353
phase-contrast tissue velocity mapping 119
PHIRST 407
phosphodiesterase-5 inhibitors 149, 340–1, 407
phospholamban 22, 341
photochemotherapy 299
photopheresis 299
physical examination 48–9, 347, 348*b*, 391–2
physiologic hypertrophy 1, 13–14, 14*f*
planning for the future 420, 421*t*
plasma cells 58*t*, 65
plasmapheresis 271, 298
plasticity 33, 342
polyclonal antibodies 286, 287*t*, 288
polymorphic ventricular tachycardia 175
portopulmonary hypertension 388
positron emission tomography (PET) 124, 125, 126, 128, 129, 353
posterior reversible encephalopathy syndrome 318
post-transplant lymphoproliferative disorder 99, 259, 298, 321
potassium, serum 49
prednisolone 281*t*
prednisone 281*t*
pregnancy
cardiac transplantation 319
HLA sensitization 269–70
pulmonary arterial hypertension 399
premature ventricular contractions 165
cardiac resynchronization therapy 183
catheter ablation 175
PREVENT-HF 183
proarrhythmia 189
procainamide 167
prognosis
cardiac MRI 121
cardiopulmonary exercise testing 52–3
myocardial strain imaging 115
pulmonary arterial hypertension 409–12
proliferation 57
proliferative signal inhibitors 282*t*, 285–6, 316, 319
propafenone 155
properdin 70
PROSPECT 112, 180
prostacyclins 388, 401–2, 404–5
proteasome 61
protein kinase A (PKA) 25
protein kinase C (PKC) 16–17, 25–6
proteolysis 26
pseudo aortic stenosis 203, 225
psychiatric factors 267
psychological issues 172
psychosocial factors 267, 420
pulmonary arterial hypertension 385–413
anticoagulation 399–400
atrial septostomy 408
calcium channel blockers 401
classification 386–7
clinical presentation 390–2
combination therapy 408
congenital heart disease 388
connective tissue disease 388
contraception 399
definition 388
diagnosis 391*f*, 392–5
digoxin 400
diuretics 400
drug-induced 387–8
endothelin receptor antagonists 405–7
epidemiology 386–8
etiology 395
exercise training 399
functional classification 410, 412*b*
heritable 387, 390
historical background 385
idiopathic 387
investigational therapies 408
longitudinal assessment 412, 413*t*
lung transplantation 408–9
pathophysiology 388–90
phosphodiesterase-5 inhibitors 407
physical examination 391–2
pregnancy 399
prognosis 409–12
prostacyclin therapy 401–2, 404–5
right heart catheterization 396–8
right ventricle 390
right ventricular failure 358
risk assessment 399*t*
screening 392
soluble guanylate-cyclase stimulator therapy 389–90, 407–8
symptoms 390–1
therapy 398–409
vasodilator testing 398
pulmonary artery catheterization 49–50, 147, 147*b*, 349, 362*b*
pulmonary artery end-diastolic pressure 105
pulmonary artery mean pressure 105–6
pulmonary artery pressures 104–6, 397
pulmonary artery systolic pressure 104–5
pulmonary artery wedge pressure 396–7
pulmonary capillary wedge pressure 106
pulmonary function 239, 263–4
pulmonary function tests 219, 395
pulmonary hypertension
cardiac transplantation 263–4
coronary artery bypass grafting 220
pharmacological management 148–9
pulmonary rales 49
pulmonary stenosis 368–9
pulmonary thromboembolism 377–8
pulmonary thromboendarterectomy 378
pulmonary vascular impedance 333
pulmonary vascular resistance 107, 236, 263–4, 397–8
pulmonary vasodilators 204–5
pulmonary vein isolation 157, 182
pulmonic insufficiency 211
pulsatility index 243
pulse contour analysis 51
pulsus paradoxus 348*b*

Q
QuickOpt™ 196
Quilty lesions 98

R
RAB7 31
RACE-2 154
radiation-induced heart disease 267
radionuclide ventriculography 125–6, 353, 360*b*
RALES 143
rales, pulmonary 49
rapamycin (sirolimus) 282*t*, 285, 316, 319
Rastelli procedure 371
rate control 154, 156, 204
real-time 3D echocardiography 116
receptor-interacting protein (RIP) 32
red blood cells 269
reentry rotors theory 153
reference impedance 79
refractory heart failure 6–7, 137–8
regenerative therapy 429–30
regional left ventricular systolic function 108–9
regulatory T cells 65
rejection, *see* cardiac allograft rejection
RELAX-AHF 147, 149
RELY 156–7
REMATCH 138, 231–3
RemonCHF 83*t*
remote monitoring systems 86, 88*t*, 89

renal function
- cardiac transplantation 259, 264, 320–1
- coronary artery bypass grafting 219
- heart failure 47, 50
- immunosuppressive toxicity 318, 319
- left ventricular assist device 238–9

renal vein compression 146
renin–angiotensin–aldosterone system 47, 142
respiratory exchange ratio 51, 52*b*
RESPOND 181
resting heart rate 76
restrictive cardiomyopathy
- constrictive pericarditis and 350–2
- endomyocardial biopsy 94–6

ReThinQ 180
REVERSE 189
reverse modeling 32–4, 342
reverse-mode NCX 22
REVIVE-1 148
REVIVE-2 148
REVIVE-IT 429
rheumatic heart disease 204, 205–6
rheumatoid arthritis 388
rhythm control 154–6
right bundle branch block 182
right heart
- coronary artery bypass grafting 220
- left ventricular assist device 235–8, 249

right heart catheterization
- chronic thromboembolic pulmonary hypertension 378
- heart failure 49–50
- pulmonary arterial hypertension 396–8

right heart filling pressure 104
right ventricle
- anatomy 329–31
- apical pacing 183
- cardiac contraction cycle 331–3
- cardiodynamics 331–5
- cardiomyocytes 330–1
- compared to left ventricle 336, 337*b*
- congenital heart disease 342
- coronary demand and supply 336
- diastolic filling and function 334–5, 335*t*, 354
- double-chambered 369
- imaging 352–4, 358*t*, 359*t*, 360*b*
- mechanical ventilation and 357
- myocardial infarction 364–6
- plasticity 342
- pre-LVAD insertion 237–8
- pulmonary arterial hypertension 390
- pulmonary vascular impedance and 333
- regulation of function 333
- remodeling 338–42
- reverse modeling 342
- structure and function 329–36
- systolic function 332–3, 334*t*

right ventricular assist devices 238
right ventricular end-systolic pressure–volume relation 332
right ventricular failure 346–78
- acute 347*t*, 354–5, 357–8, 360–6
- adult congenital heart disease 368–73
- arrhythmogenic cardiomyopathy 366–8
- cardiorenal syndrome 358, 360, 365*b*
- chest radiography 349, 350*t*, 351*f*
- chronic 347*t*, 361*f*, 363*b*
- chronic pulmonary thromboembolism 377–8
- definition 346
- differential diagnosis 346
- ECG 349, 349*b*, 350*f*
- etiologies 346, 347*b*
- hemodynamics 349–52, 353*b*, 353*t*
- imaging 352–4, 358*t*, 359*t*, 360*b*
- laboratory assessment 347, 349
- left ventricular assist device 237–8, 363–4, 374–7
- pharmacological therapy 148–9
- physical examination 347, 348*b*
- pseudo-restriction and 350
- pulmonary arterial hypertension 358
- pulmonary artery catheterization 349, 362*b*
- remodeling and 338–42
- right ventricular myocardial infarction 364–6
- symptoms and signs 346–7, 347*t*
- tricuspid regurgitation 352, 373

right ventricular filling pressure difference 334–5
right ventricular outflow tract acceleration time 105
right ventricular stroke work index 236
riociguat 389–90, 403*t*, 407–8
rituximab 299, 320
rivaroxaban 144, 156–7
ROADMAP 245, 429
ROSE 147
rubidium 125
ryanodine receptor 17, 21

S

S100A1 23
SAD-Heart-HF 423
SAFE-T 155
sarcoidosis 94, 124, 161, 266
sarcomeres 13
- thick and thin filaments 18

sarcomeric proteins 23–6
sarcoplasmic reticulum 13
sarcoplasmic reticulum Ca-ATPase (SERCA) 18, 22
- SERCA2 341
- SERCA2a 430

SAVE 4
SCD-HeFT 167, 169
scleroderma 388
SDI index 112
Seattle Heart Failure Model 137, 423
second heart field cells 329
segmental wall motion analysis 108–9
seizures 318
selectins 68
selective serotonin reuptake inhibitors 423
selexipag 405
Senning procedure 371
sepsis 243
septal-posterior wall mechanical delay 112
SERAPHIN 406–7
SERCA 18, 22
SERCA2 341
SERCA2a 430
serelaxin 147
serotonin 390
sertraline 423
serum potassium 49
SHIFT 144
shunting 114
signal 57, 63
sildenafil 149, 205, 237, 340–1, 403*t*, 407
Simpson biplane method 108
sinoatrial node inhibition 144
sirolimus (rapamycin) 282*t*, 285, 316, 319
six-minute walk test 409–10
skin cancer 259
slow force response 20
SMART-AV 195
smoking 266–7
social support 267
sodium–calcium exchanger 18, 22
sodium intake 145
sodium levels 47, 49
sodium nitroprusside 147–8, 147*t*
solid-phase immunoassays 268–9
soluble guanylate-cyclase stimulator 389–90, 407–8
SOLVD 4, 44, 142
SOLVD-T 6
sotalol 167
specificity 57–8
speckle tracking echocardiography 114, 115*f*, 180, 186
SPECT imaging 124, 126, 128, 129, 353
spiritual health 423
spironolactone 146*t*
spleen 59
stage A heart failure 3
stage B heart failure 3–4
stage C heart failure 5–6, 7
stage D heart failure 6–7, 8*b*
standard deviation of the 5-minute median atrial sensed A-A intervals (SDAAM) 76–8
STAR 116
STARTER 186
statins 286, 321
stem cell therapy 430
STEP 408
steroids 279–80, 281*t*, 292–3, 315–16
STICH 216–17, 221, 222
strain imaging 113, 114–16
stroke risk, left ventricular assist device 245–6, 250
stroke volume 102–3
stunned myocardium 26
substance abuse 261–2, 267
suction events 244, 249
sudden death
- arrhythmogenic cardiomyopathy 366
- tetralogy of Fallot 370

SUPER-1 407
support services 420
supraventricular tachycardias 159–60
switch recombination 66
sympathetic nervous system 47, 128
symptom burden 421–3
SynCardia total artificial heart 238, 244–5, 252, 428
syndromic approach 1, 43
systemic lupus erythematosus 388
systemic sclerosis 388
systemic vascular resistance 107
systole 18
systolic area index 351–2
systolic dyssynchrony index 112
systolic heart failure 27

T
T1-mapping 121, 122
tachycardia 47
tachycardia-mediated cardiomyopathy 159–60
tacrolimus 282*t*, 283, 284, 314–15, 318–19
tadalafil 403*t*, 407
TAP protein 61
TAPSE 113, 237, 394, 410
TARGET 186
target of rapamycin 285
T cell activation 63–5
T cell receptor 58, 62–5
T cells 58–9, 58*t*, 62–5
technetium-99m imaging 124–5, 126
Tei index 339
telethonin 15
tetralogy of Fallot 369–70
TH1 subset 65
TH2 subset 65
Th17 65, 67
thallium-201 imaging 124–5, 126
thiazide diuretics 145
thick filaments 18
thin filaments 18
third heart sound 49
Thoratec HeartMate II 233, 240, 241, 241*f*, 242, 243*f*, 244, 250, 251, 374
threshold-crossing event 79–82
thromboxane 388
thymoglobulin 286, 287*t*, 288
thymus 59
thyroid hormone 14
TICTAC 289, 296
time to peak systolic velocity 112
titin 15, 20, 24–5, 26
tobacco abuse 266–7
torsemide 146*t*, 365*t*
total artificial heart 238, 244–5, 252, 428, 429
total blood volume 47
total pulmonary resistance 397
transcatheter aortic valve replacement 225
transfusion, HLA sensitization 269
transient receptor potential ion channels 15
transplant immunology 57–72
  antibody responses 66–70
  donor antigen recognition 59–66
  immune response 57–8, 70–2
  immune system 58–9
transposition of the great arteries 370–2
Treg cells 65
treprostinil 402–3*t*, 404–5
trials
  ADMIRE-HF 128
  AF-CHF 156
  AFFIRM 154, 155, 156
  A-HeFT 142
  ALLHAT 4–5
  AMBITION 408
  ANDROMEDA 156
  ARIES-1/-2 406
  ASCEND-HF 147, 358
  ATLAS 143
  AVID 169, 170*t*
  BAMI 430
  BIG 51
  BLOCK-HF 183
  BREATHE-1 405–6
  BREATHE-2 408
  CABG-Patch 169, 170*t*
  CARE-HF 5, 189
  CARGO 309
  CARRESS-HF 146, 358, 360, 365*b*
  CASH 169, 170*t*
  CHARM-Added 142
  CHEST-1 408
  CHF-STAT 156
  CIBIS-II 139
  CIDS 169, 170*t*
  COMBI 408
  COMPASS-HF 50–1
  CONSENSUS 6, 142
  CONSENSUS II 107
  COPERNICUS 139–41
  CTAF 155
  CUPID 430
  DAVID 183
  DECIDE LVAD 245
  DEFINITE 170*t*
  Diamond HF 155, 156
  DIG 144
  DINAMIT 169, 170*t*
  DOSE 145, 358
  EARLY 406
  ECHO-CRT 180
  EMPHASIS-HF 143
  ENDURANCE 245
  EPHESUS 143
  ESCAPE 47, 48, 50, 51, 138, 147, 148
  FREEDOM 196
  FREEDOM-C 404
  FREEDOM-M 404
  GESICA 155
  GRIPHON 405
  HARPS 252
  Heart Save the Nephron 295
  IMAGE 310
  INTrEPID 233
  IRIS 169, 170*t*
  MADIT I 170*t*
  MADIT II 169, 170*t*
  MADIT-CRT 182, 183, 189, 190, 191
  MERIT-HF 139
  MIRACLE-ICD 189, 191
  MOMENTUM 3 246
  OPTIME-CHF 148
  OPTIMIZE-HF 141
  PABA-CHF 157
  PACE 183
  PACE-RBBB 182
  PACES 408
  PARADIGM-HF 143
  PARTNER 225
  PATENT-1 407–8
  PHIRST 407
  PREVENT-HF 183
  PROSPECT 112, 180
  RACE-2 154
  RALES 143
  RELAX-AHF 147, 149
  RELY 156–7
  REMATCH 138, 231–3
  RESPOND 181
  ReThinQ 180
  REVERSE 189
  REVIVE-1 148
  REVIVE-2 148
  REVIVE-IT 429
  ROADMAP 245, 429
  ROSE 147
  SAD-Heart-HF 423
  SAFE-T 155
  SAVE 4
  SCD-HeFT 167, 169
  SERAPHIN 406–7
  SHIFT 144
  SMART-AV 195
  SOLVD 4, 44, 142
  SOLVD-T 6
  STAR 116
  STARTER 186
  STEP 408
  STICH 216–17, 221, 222
  SUPER-1 407
  TARGET 186
  TICTAC 289, 296
  TRIUMPH 408
  V-HeFT 52
  VHeFT-1 142
  VHeFT II 142
  WARCEF 144
tricuspid annular plane systolic excursion (TAPSE) 113, 237, 394, 410
tricuspid annular systolic velocity 113
tricuspid regurgitation 210–11, 236, 352, 373
tricuspid regurgitation jet 104
tricuspid valve repair/replacement 373
TRIUMPH 408
tropomyosin 18
troponin complex 18, 19, 20
troponins 347, 349
TRPC1/6 15
T-tubules 13
tumor necrosis factor alpha (TNFα) 14–15, 32, 67, 67*t*

U
UCF-101 31
ultrafiltration 146
urinary cotinine 267

V
valvular heart disease 202–11
  echocardiography 110–12
  heart failure and 46–7
  left ventricular assist device 113, 240
  organ donors 261
variable region 65
vascular disease 265
vascular resistance 107
vasoactive intestinal peptide 390
vasodilators 142–3, 147–8, 204–5
vasodilator testing 398
vasopressin 47, 237
VCAM 68
velocity-time integral 102, 103, 193–5
venovenous ultrafiltration 146
ventilation/carbon dioxide production ratio 52*b*
ventricular arrhythmias 165–76
  cardiac resynchronization therapy 189
  cardiac transplantation 176
  catheter ablation 172–6
  diagnosis 165–7
  implantable cardioverter defibrillators 165, 167–72
  left ventricular assist device 176, 244, 249
  nonsustained ventricular tachycardia 167
  physical signs 165
  sustained ventricular tachycardia 167
  symptoms 165

ventricular evoked response 311
ventricular fibrillation 175, 189
ventricular interdependence 335, 336*f*
ventricular remodeling 1–2, 336–42
  reverse 32–4, 342
ventricular septal defect 369
V-HeFT 52
VHeFT-1 142
VHeFT II 142
virtual crossmatch 270–1
voltage-dependent potassium channels 390
volume assessment 48–9
volume overload, refractory 144–7

W

wall motion analysis 108–9
WARCEF 144
warfarin 144, 156
Watchman device 157
water retention 47
Weibel–Palade bodies 68
weight gain 49
Wenckebach block 161

X

XIAP 30

Y

Yu index 112